The 5-Minute Sports Medicine Consult Premium

3rd EDITION

EDITORS

Suraj A. Achar, MD, FAAFP, CAQSM
Clinical Professor of Family Medicine
University of California, San Diego, School of Medicine
Associate Director
University of California San Diego Primary Care Sports Medicine Fellowship
Head Team Physician
San Diego Sockers
San Diego, California
Team Physician
UCSD Tritons
U.S. Olympic Training Center

Kenneth S. Taylor, MD, FAAFP, CAQSM
Clinical Professor of Family Medicine/ Sports Medicine
University of California, San Diego, School of Medicine
Chief, Primary Care Sports Medicine
Director, UCSD Primary Care Sports Medicine Fellowship
Head Primary Care Sports Physician, San Diego Padres
Head Team Physician UCSD Tritons, San Diego Sockers
Team Physician US Olympic Training Center; San Diego Seals Professional Lacrosse
San Diego, California

ASSISTANT EDITOR

Andrea L. Pana, MD, MPH
Direct Orthopedic Care
Austin, Texas

SECTION EDITORS

Kenneth P. Barnes, MD, MSc, CAQSM, FACSM
Sports Medicine Physician
Greensboro Orthopaedics
Adjunct Professor, Kinesiology
University of North Carolina Greensboro
Greensboro, North Carolina
Internal Medicine, Pediatrics, and Sports Medicine
Adjunct Faculty
Cone Sports Medicine Fellowship Program
Adjunct Professor, Exercise Science
Elon University
Elon, North Carolina
Team Physician, Alamance-Burlington School System
Burlington, North Carolina

Holly J. Benjamin, MD, FAAP, FACSM
Professor
Orthopaedic Surgery, Rehabilitation Medicine, and Pediatrics
Director, Primary Care Sports Medicine
University of Chicago
Chicago, Illinois

Kevin E. Burroughs, MD, CAQSM
Professor
Department of Family Medicine
Carolinas HealthCare System
Associate Professor, Department of Family Medicine
University of North Carolina
Director, Cabarrus Sports Medicine Fellowship
Team Physician, Catawba College; AL Brown High School
Concord, North Carolina

Jeffrey R. Bytomski, DO, FAOASM
Professor
Department of Community and Family Medicine
Head Medical Team Physician
Duke University
Durham, North Carolina

James M. Daniels, MD, MPH, RMSK, FAAFP, FACOEM, FACPM
Southern Illinois University School of Medicine
Professor, Departments of Family and Community Medicine and Orthopedic Surgery
Director, Primary Care Sports Medicine Fellowship—Quincy
Quincy, Illinois

George D. Harris, MD, MS, FAAFP, CAQSM
Chair and Professor
Department of Family Medicine
West Virginia University School of Medicine—Eastern Campus
University Healthcare Physicians Medical Director—Primary Care
Martinsburg, West Virginia

Marc I. Harwood, MD
Associate Professor
Department of Family and Community Medicine
Department of Orthopaedic Surgery
Sidney Kimmel Medical College
Thomas Jefferson University
Rothman Orthopaedic Institute
Philadelphia, Pennsylvania

Suzanne Hecht, MD
Associate Professor
Department of Family Medicine and Community Health
Director, Sports Medicine Fellowship
University of Minnesota
Minneapolis, Minnesota

Chris Koutures, MD, FAAP
Pediatric and Sports Medicine Specialist
ActiveKidMD
Anaheim Hills, California
Clinical Instructor, Department of Pediatrics
University of California, Irvine
Children's Hospital of Orange County
Team Physician, USA Volleyball National Teams; Cal State Fullerton Athletics
Department of Dance, Chapman University
Orange, California

Amy Leu, DO, FAAFP, CAQSM
Assistant Clinical Professor, Family Medicine
University of California, San Diego, School of Medicine
Assistant Director, UCSD Primary Care Sports Medicine Fellowship
Team Physician, UCSD Tritons
Consulting Physician, San Diego Padres
San Diego, California
Consulting Physician, U.S. Olympic Training Center
Chula Vista, California

James L. Moeller, MD, FACSM, CAQSM
Director
Primary Care Sports Medicine Fellowship
Henry Ford Health System
Detroit, Michigan
Head Team Physician
Oakland University
Rochester, Michigan

Dusty Marie Narducci, MD, Board Certified Family Medicine, CAQSM
Assistant Director
The University of South Florida-Morton Plant Mease Primary Care Sports Medicine Fellowship
Assistant Professor, Morsani College of Medicine
Team Physician, Department of Athletics at the University of South Florida
Team Physician, Saint Leo University
St. Leo, Florida

Rathna R. Nuti, MD, CAQSM
Assistant Team Physician
Dallas Stars NHL Hockey Club
Frisco, Texas

Deepak S. Patel, MD, FAAFP, FACSM
Assistant Professor
Rush Medical College
Chicago, Illinois
Director, Sports Medicine
Rush Copley Family Medicine Residency
Medical Director, Sports Medicine
Rush Copley Medical Center
Aurora, Illinois
Family Medicine and Sports Medicine
Yorkville Primary Care and Sports Medicine
Aurora and Yorkville, Illinois

Stephen R. Paul, MD, CAQSM
Associate Professor, Family and Community Medicine
Assistant Team Physician, Intercollegiate Athletics
Head Team Physician, Club Sports
University of Arizona
Tucson, Arizona

George G.A. Pujalte, MD, FACSM
Senior Associate Consultant, Family Medicine and Sports Medicine
Assistant Professor, Mayo Clinic College of Medicine
Vice-Chair for Academics, Department of Family Medicine
Associate Program Director, Sports Medicine Fellowship Program
Vice-Chair for Communications, American Medical Society for Sports Medicine
Team Physician, USA Taekwondo
Mayo Clinic
Jacksonville, Florida

Margot Putukian, MD, FACSM
Director, Athletic Medicine
Head Team Physician
Assistant Director Medical Services
Princeton University
Princeton, New Jersey
Associate Clinical Professor
Rutgers-Robert Wood Johnson Medical School
New Brunswick, New Jersey
Team Physician, U.S. Lacrosse Men's National Team; U.S. Soccer
Chief Medical Officer, Major League Soccer

Alan Shahtaji, DO, CAQSM
Associate Clinical Professor
University of California at San Diego Health Sciences
Department of Family Medicine and Public Health
Assistant Director, Primary Care Sports Medicine Fellowship
Director, UCSD Sports Medicine Concussion Clinic
Team Physician, U.S. Soccer Federation; UCSD Tritons
San Diego, California
Team Physician, Hoover High School
Birmingham, Alabama

Kevin Waninger, MD, MS, FAAFP, FACEP, FACSM, CAQSM
Coordinated Health Sports Medicine
Allentown, Pennsylvania

David Webner, MD
Board Certified, Sports Medicine
Board Certified, Brain Injury Medicine
Board Certified, Family Medicine and Community Health
Team Physician, Philadelphia Union
Director, Sports Medicine Fellowship
Director, Running Medicine
Crozer-Keystone Health System
Suburban Philadelphia
Healthplex Sports Medicine Institute
Springfield, Pennsylvania

The 5-Minute Sports Medicine Consult Premium

3rd EDITION

1-Year Enhanced Online Access + Print

Editors

Suraj A. Achar, MD, FAAFP, CAQSM
Clinical Professor of Family Medicine
University of California, San Diego, School of Medicine
Associate Director
University of California San Diego Primary Care Sports Medicine Fellowship
Head Team Physician
San Diego Sockers
San Diego, California
Team Physician
UCSD Tritons
U.S. Olympic Training Center

Kenneth S. Taylor, MD, FAAFP, CAQSM
Clinical Professor of Family Medicine/Sports Medicine
University of California, San Diego, School of Medicine
Chief, Primary Care Sports Medicine
Director, UCSD Primary Care Sports Medicine Fellowship
Head Primary Care Sports Physician, San Diego Padres
Head Team Physician UCSD Tritons, San Diego Sockers
Team Physician US Olympic Training Center; San Diego Seals Professional Lacrosse
San Diego, California

Assistant Editor

Andrea L. Pana, MD, MPH
Direct Orthopedic Care
Austin, Texas

Wolters Kluwer

Philadelphia • Baltimore • New York • London
Buenos Aires • Hong Kong • Sydney • Tokyo

5MinuteConsult™

Director, Medical Practice: Rebecca Gaertner
Digital Product Development Editor: Leanne Vandetty
Editorial Assistant: Brian Convery
Production Project Manager: Bridgett Dougherty
Design Coordinator: Holly McLaughlin
Manufacturing Coordinator: Beth Welsh
Marketing Manager: Rachel Mante Leung
Prepress Vendor: Absolute Service, Inc.

3rd edition

9 8 7 6 5 4 3 2 1

Printed in China

Library of Congress Cataloging-in-Publication Data

Names: Achar, Suraj A., editor. | Taylor, Kenneth S., editor.
Title: The 5-minute sports medicine consult / editors, Suraj A. Achar, Kenneth S. Taylor ; assistant editor, Andrea L. Pana ; section editors, Kenneth P. Barnes [and 18 others].
Other titles: Five minute sports medicine consult
Description: 3rd edition. | Philadelphia : Wolters Kluwer, [2020] | Includes bibliographical references and index.
Identifiers: LCCN 2018061449 | ISBN 9781496396938
Subjects: | MESH: Sports Medicine | Athletic Injuries | Handbook
Classification: LCC RC1211 | NLM QT 29 | DDC 617.1/027--dc23 LC record available at https://lccn.loc.gov/2018061449

shop.lww.com

CCS0219

This book is dedicated to the entire team of health care professionals who work with athletes of all ages and abilities, often in time-sensitive environments where accurate diagnoses and treatment plans are critical. *The 5-Minute Sports Medicine Consult* in both printed and web-based format is ideal for this setting.

It is our hope that the information contained in this body of work will help guide you and your patients along the path to recovery and peak performance.

PREFACE

Since the publication of the second edition of *The 5-Minute Sports Medicine Consult* (5MSMC), technology has changed our lives. As the computer and mobile devices permeate our professional and personal lives, health care professionals have increasingly turned to web-based formats as a source of medical information in our busy practices. Building on our success with the first two editions of the 5MSMC, progress with the third edition was streamlined by utilizing the expertise of sports medicine authors and editors from around the country and world. Users of the first two editions will be pleased to note that the format has remained by and large the same with new focused chapters and updated evidence-based information. In addition, a new web-based format will integrate the tools of the entire 5MinuteConsult series with a mobile platform to make searches and cross-referencing information easier.

The basic concept for this book parallels teaching techniques at our collaborative sports medicine fellowship at the University of California, San Diego (UCSD). As part of our regular weekly Sports Medicine didactic program, fellows and faculty from four separate Accreditation Council for Graduate Medical Education (ACGME)-approved sports fellowships are asked to present lectures on topics in sports medicine clinical practice covering the essential elements in the diagnosis and management of problems as seen through the eyes of a primary care sports physician. The audience consists of experienced clinicians, including orthopedic surgeons, radiologists, physical therapists, athletic trainers, and other members of the "Sports Medicine Team." The organization and presentation of these didactics follow those found in this book with an emphasis on evidence-based medicine and clinical relevance.

We would like to express our sincerest gratitude to Mark Bracker, MD, who started the UCSD sports medicine fellowship and who led the efforts to create the first edition in 2001. We also want to thank all our section editors and authors who used their expertise to provide organized and useful reviews on each topic in the book. Our more fervent gratitude goes toward our assistant editor Andrea L. Pana, MD, MPH, and administrative assistant and international research fellow Ibraheem Algarni, MD. Dr. Pana worked diligently reviewing chapters and communicating with the team of section editors and Dr. Algarni worked closely with the publisher and authors to keep this project moving forward and completed on time.

SURAJ A. ACHAR, MD, FAAFP, CAQSM
KENNETH S. TAYLOR, MD, FAAFP, CAQSM

CONTRIBUTORS

Suraj A. Achar, MD, FAAFP, CAQSM
Clinical Professor of Family Medicine
University of California, San Diego, School of Medicine
Associate Director
University of California San Diego Primary Care Sports Medicine Fellowship
Head Team Physician
San Diego Sockers
San Diego, California
Team Physician
UCSD Tritons
U.S. Olympic Training Center

Jessalynn Adam, MD
Attending Physiatrist, Sports Medicine
Department of Orthopedics
Mercy Orthopedic Specialty Hospital
Baltimore, Maryland

Ayo Adu, MD, CAQSM
Team Physician
University of Houston—Victoria
Victoria, Texas

Giselle Aerni, MD
Assistant Director, York Hospital Sports Medicine Fellowship
Associate Director, York Hospital Family Medicine Residency
Head Team Physician, Spring Grove Area High School
Team Physician, Gettysburg College
Team Physician, Skipjacks Hockey
York, Pennsylvania

Arturo J. Aguilar, MD, CAQSM†
Primary Care Sports Medicine
MemorialCare Medical Group
Huntington Beach, California

Sonya S. Ahmed, MD
Co-Director, Nilssen Orthopedics Ankle and Foot Center
Andrews Institute Foot and Ankle Physician Provider
Consulting Physician to United States Olympic Committee
Pensacola, Florida

Muath Alammar, MD, SBFM
Assistant Consultant of Family Medicine
Assistant Professor at College of Medicine
Shaqra University
Shaqra, Saudi Arabia

Ibraheem Algarni, MD
Sports Medicine Research Fellow
University of California, San Diego
San Diego, California
Family Medicine Teaching Assistant
King Abdulaziz University
Jeddah, Saudi Arabia

Joseph E. Allen, MD, MS, FAAFP, CAQSM†
Commander, Medical Corps (Flight Surgeon), United States Navy
Squadron Flight Surgeon, VFC-13 Fighting Saints
Naval Air Station Fallon, Nevada
Federal Aviation Administration Senior Aviation Medical Examiner
San Diego, California

Fahad Anwer, FCPS, MRCGP (Int.)
Assistant Professor of Family Medicine
Department of Family and Community Medicine
Faculty of Medicine in Rabigh
King Abdulaziz University
Jeddah, Makkah Province, Saudi Arabia

Cesar Arguelles, MD, CAQSM
Assistant Professor of Family Medicine
Southern Illinois University School of Medicine
Associate Director, SIU Quincy Primary Care Sports Medicine Fellowship
Head Team Physician, Culver Stockton College Wildcats, Culver, Missouri
Team Physician, Quincy University Hawks, Quincy, Illinois
Quincy, Illinois

Kamel Azhar, MD, MAS
Family Medicine Resident
Assistant Curriculum Director
Texas Tech University Health Sciences Center
Lubbock, Texas
Family Medicine Teaching Assistant
University of Jeddah
Jeddah, Saudi Arabia

Amanda Babcock, MD, CAQSM
Family and Sports Medicine
Clinical Faculty
Family Health Centers of San Diego
Team Physician, Grossmont College
San Diego, California

Rebecca Bacharach, DO
Primary Care Sports Medicine Fellow
San Diego Sports Medicine and Family Health Center
San Diego, California

Aaron L. Baggish, MD, FACC, FACSM†
Associate Professor of Medicine
Harvard Medical School
Director, Cardiovascular Performance Program
Massachusetts General Hospital
Boston, Massachusetts

Marwan A. Bakarman, MBBS, FFCM
Associate Professor and Consultant, Family Medicine
King Abdulaziz University, Jeddah, Rabigh Faculty of Medicine
Chairman Department of Family and Community Medicine
Jeddah, Saudi Arabia

Robert J. Baker, MD, PhD, FAAFP, FACSM
Professor of Family and Community Medicine and Orthopedics
Homer Stryker MD School of Medicine
Western Michigan University
Program Director
Primary Care Sports Medicine Fellowship
Team Physician
Western Michigan University
Kalamazoo, Michigan

Aleem Bakhtiar, MS, MD†
Sports Medicine Fellow
Texas A&M University
College Station, Texas

Larry Balle II, MD, MPH
Primary Care Sports Medicine Fellow
Department of Family and Preventative Medicine
University of Arkansas for Medical Sciences, Northwest
Fayetteville, Arkansas

Ilona Barash, MD, PhD, CAQSM
Physician
Scripps Clinic Torrey Pines Urgent Care
Volunteer Clinical Professor of Emergency Medicine
University of Colorado, San Diego
Physician
University of California, San Diego Student Health Sports Medicine
San Diego, California

Erin S. Barnes, MD
Department of Physical Medicine and Rehabilitation
Temple University Hospital/Moss Rehab
Philadelphia, Pennsylvania

Kenneth P. Barnes, MD, MSc, CAQSM, FACSM
Sports Medicine Physician
Greensboro Orthopaedics
Adjunct Professor, Kinesiology
University of North Carolina, Greensboro
Greensboro, North Carolina
Internal Medicine/Pediatrics/Sports Medicine
Adjunct Faculty
Cone Sports Medicine Fellowship Program
Adjunct Professor, Exercise Science
Elon University
Elon, North Carolina
Team Physician
Alamance-Burlington School System
Burlington, North Carolina

Evan S. Bass, MD, FAAFP, CAQSM
Associate Professor of Family Medicine
University of California, Los Angeles, School of Medicine
Associate Director, Harbor-UCLA/Team to Win Primary Care Sports Medicine Fellowship
Director of Primary Care Sports Medicine
Department of Family Medicine
Kaiser Permanente
Harbor City, California

David E.J. Bazzo, MD, FAAFP, CAQSM
Clinical Professor of Family Medicine
University of California, San Diego School of Medicine
Assistant Director
UCSD Primary Care Sports Medicine Fellowship
Team Physician UCSD Tritons, U.S. Olympic Training Center, Mira Mesa High School
San Diego, California

Briana Beach, DO
Resident
Carilion Clinic
Virginia Tech Carilion Family Medicine Residency Program
Roanoke, Virginia

Holly Beach, MD, CAQSM†
Associate Professor of Family and Community Medicine
Fellowship Director Primary Care Sports Medicine
University of Arizona
Tucson, Arizona

Holly J. Benjamin, MD, FAAP, FACSM†
Professor of Orthopaedic Surgery, Rehabilitation Medicine and Pediatrics
Director of Primary Care Sports Medicine
University of Chicago
Chicago, Illinois

Kenneth Bielak, MD, FACSM, FAAFP, CAQSM
Professor
Department of Family Medicine
University of Tennessee Health Science Center
Graduate School of Medicine, Knoxville Campus
Associate Director
University of Tennessee Primary Care Sports Medicine Fellowship
Knoxville, Tennessee

W. Scott Black, MD
Associate Professor
Department of Clinical Sciences
Program Director
Physician Assistant Studies Program
College of Health Sciences
University of Kentucky
Medical Director
Sports Medicine Research Institute
Team Physician
University of Kentucky
Lexington, Kentucky

Brandon M. Bockewitz, MD, CAQSM
Associate Professor
University of Illinois College of Medicine at Peoria
Team Physician
Peoria Rivermen Hockey
Head Team Physician
Robert Morris University Peoria
Peoria, Illinois

Delmas Bolin, MD, PhD, FACSM†
Professor, Sports and Family Medicine
Virginia College of Osteopathic Medicine
Blacksburg, Virginia
Head Team Physician, Radford University
Radford Virginia
Medical Director and Team Physician, Roanoke College
Salem, Virginia
Director, Performance Medicine of Southwest Virginia
Roanoke, Virginia

James R. Borchers, MD, MPH†
Professor, Department of Family Medicine
Director, Division of Sports Medicine, Department of Family Medicine
Head Team Physician, Athletic Department
Associate Director, Primary Care Sports Medicine Fellowship
The Ohio State University Wexner Medical Center Jameson Crane Sports Medicine Institute
Columbus, Ohio

Christopher Bossart, MD
Emergency Medicine Resident Physician
University of New Mexico
Albuquerque, New Mexico

Benjamin Boswell, DO†
Division of Sports Medicine
Primary Care Sports Medicine
Department of Orthopaedic Surgery
Department of Emergency Medicine
Case Western Reserve University School of Medicine
University Hospitals Cleveland
Assistant Medical Physician, Cleveland Browns
Cleveland, Ohio

Anne S. Boyd, MD, FAAFP, FACSM
LifeWellness Institute
San Diego, California

William W. Briner Jr., MD, FACSM, FAAFP, CAQSM
Team Physician, USA Volleyball National Teams
Hospital for Special Surgery
Uniondale, New York

David L. Brown, MD, MBA
Director, Sports Medicine
Providence Medical Group
Southwest Washington Service Area
Olympia, Washington

Steven T. Brown, MD
Sports Medicine Fellow
University of Louisville Primary Care Sports Medicine Fellowship
Louisville, Kentucky

Benjamin D. Brusch, MD
Team Physician, UNC-Charlotte 49ers, JCSU Golden Bulls
Charlotte, North Carolina

Sean T. Bryan, MD, FAAFP, CAQSM
Sidney Kimmel Medical College of Thomas Jefferson University
Philadelphia, Pennsylvania
Sports Medicine Physician, Rothman Institute
Willow Grove, Pennsylvania
Team Physician, Perkiomen Valley High School
Collegeville, Pennsylvania

Chau Bui, DO
Sports Medicine Fellow
University of California, San Diego
Team Physician, SDSU Aztecs, San Diego Legion
San Diego, California

Randall Burgett, DO
Sports Medicine Fellow
Riverside Methodist Hospital
Ohio Health
Columbus, Ohio

Kevin E. Burroughs, MD, CAQSM
Professor
Department of Family Medicine
Carolinas HealthCare System
Associate Professor
Department of Family Medicine
University of North Carolina
Director
Cabarrus Sports Medicine Fellowship
Team Physician, Catawba College, AL Brown High School
Concord, North Carolina

Jeffrey R. Bytomski, DO, FAOASM[†]
Professor
Department of Community and Family Medicine
Head Medical Team Physician
Duke University
Durham, North Carolina

Greg Canty, MD
Medical Director, Sports Medicine Center
Fellowship Director, Pediatric Sports Medicine
Children's Mercy Kansas City
Assistant Professor of Orthopedics and Pediatrics
University of Missouri–Kansas City School of Medicine
Kansas City, Missouri

Nicholas M. Cardinale, MD
Family Practice CAQSM
Vancouver, British Columbia, Canada

Nathan Cardoos, MD, CAQSM
Instructor of Family Medicine
Boston University School of Medicine
Team Physician, Boston University
Team Physician, Boston College
Boston, Massachusetts

Stephen Carek, MD
Primary Care Sports Medicine Fellow
Department of Community Health and Family Medicine
University of Florida College of Medicine
Gainesville, Florida

David Carfagno, DO, CAQSM[†]
Scottsdale Sports Medicine
Assistant National Medical Director, Rock and Roll Marathon
Physician, Arizona State Boxing and MMA Commission
Physician, USA Boxing
Scottsdale, Arizona

Rebecca L. Carl, MD, MSCI
Institute for Sports Medicine
Ann & Robert H. Lurie Children's Hospital of Chicago
Director
Northwestern McGaw Primary Care Sports Medicine Fellowship
Assistant Professor of Pediatrics
Northwestern Feinberg School of Medicine
Chicago, Illinois

Corey Carson, MD, CAQSM
Sports Medicine Physician
Family Medicine Residency Clinical Faculty
Family Health Centers of San Diego
Team Physician, Grossmont College Griffins
San Diego, California

Alejandro Centurion, MD
Primary Care Sports Medicine Fellow
University of Florida at Orlando Health Primary Care Sports Medicine Fellowship
Orlando, Florida

Scott Chandler, DO
Family Medicine/Sports Medicine Fellow
PeaceHealth Southwest Medical Center
Vancouver, Washington

Amanda Chaney, DO, FAAFP, CAQSM
TriHealth Event Medicine Physician
Team Physician, Xavier University, Mount Saint Joseph University, Walnut Hills High School
Cincinnati, Ohio

Andrew Cheung, DO
Resident Physician
John Muir Health Family Medicine Residency Program
Member, USA Weightlifting Sports Medicine Society
Colorado Springs, Colorado

Alicia Chitanand, DO
Cone Health Sports Medicine Fellow
Guilford College Team Physician
Greensboro, North Carolina

Jin Choi, DO
Primary Care Sports Medicine Fellow
University of California, San Diego, School of Medicine
Former Chief Resident
Dignity Health Northridge Family Medicine Residency
San Diego, California

Joseph Chorley, MD, FAAP, FACSM, CAQSM
Associate Professor of Pediatrics
Section of Adolescent Medicine and Sports Medicine
Baylor College of Medicine/Texas Children's Hospital
Fellowship Director
Primary Care Sports Medicine
Associate Medical Director
Houston Marathon
Team Physician, Texas Southern University, Chavez, Sterling, Austin High Schools
Houston, Texas

Dwaipayan Choudhury, MD
Sports Medicine Fellow
Southern Illinois University Sports Medicine Fellowship
Team Physician, Quincy Hawks, Culver-Stockton Wildcats
Quincy, Illinois

Adam T. Chrusch, MD, CAQSM[†]
Assistant Professor of Community and Family Medicine
Sidney Kimmel Medical College of Thomas Jefferson University
Philadelphia, Pennsylvania

Julie Chuan, MD, FAAFP, CAQSM
Overlake Hospital
Bellevue, Washington

Matthew Chung, DO
VCOM Primary Care Sports Medicine Fellow (2018–2019)
Associate Professor of Family Medicine
Division of Sports Medicine, VCOM
Assistant Team Physician, Virginia Tech
Team Physician, Auburn High School
Blacksburg, Virginia

Rachel A. Coel, MD, PhD, FAAP, CAQSM
Medical Director
Center for Sports Medicine
The Queen's Medical Center
Clinical Assistant Professor
Department of Family Medicine
University of Hawai'i John A. Burns School of Medicine
Team Physician
Hawai'i Pacific University
Chaminade University
Honolulu, Hawaii

Philip H. Cohen, MD, CSQSM
Diplomate of the American Board of Internal Medicine
Clinical Associate Professor of Medicine
University of California, Los Angeles David Geffen School of Medicine
Los Angeles, California

David Cole, MD
Primary Care Sports Medicine Fellow (2018–2019)
WellSpan Health York Hospital
York, Pennsylvania

Ryan P. Cole, MD, CAQSM
Instructor of Medicine
Northwestern University Feinberg School of Medicine
Team Physician
Northwestern University Athletics
Chicago, Illinois

William M. Collins, DO
Primary Care Sports Medicine Fellow
University of California, San Diego
San Diego, California

Douglas Comeau, DO, CAQSM, FAAFP
Medical Director, Sports Medicine
Director, Boston University Sports Medicine Fellowship
Ryan Center for Sports Medicine
Boston Medical Center
Assistant Professor, Family Medicine
Boston University School of Medicine
Head Team Physician, Boston University
Team Physician, Boston College
Boston, Massachusetts

Michael Connolly, MD
Associate Professor of Family Medicine
Southern Illinois University Center for Family and Community Medicine
Quincy, Illinois

Steven Cuff, MD, FAAP, CAQSM
Division of Sports Medicine
Nationwide Children's Hospital
Associate Professor of Pediatrics
The Ohio State University College of Medicine
Columbus, Ohio

Adam Culver, MD
Family Medicine Resident
Atrium Health
Charlotte, North Carolina

Claudia Dal Molin, DO
Assistant Professor in Primary Care Sports Medicine, MSK Ultrasound, and Osteopathy
University of Maryland School of Medicine
Team Physician, University of Maryland Terrapins
Baltimore, Maryland

Kayla Daniel, MD[†]
Department of Pediatrics
Nationwide Children's Hospital
Columbus, Ohio

James M. Daniels, MD, MPH, RMSK, FAAFP, FACOEM, FACPM
Professor
Southern Illinois University School of Medicine
Departments of Family and Community Medicine and Orthopedic Surgery
Director
Primary Care Sports Medicine Fellowship—Quincy
Quincy, Illinois

Alexei DeCastro, MD, FAAFP, CAQSM[†]
Assistant Professor
Department of Family Medicine
Medical University of South Carolina
Program Director
Trident/MUSC FMRP
Chief of Primary Care Sports Medicine
Team Physician, Charleston Battery, Charleston RiverDogs
Tournament Physician, Volvo Car Open
Charleston, South Carolina

Timothy Dekker, MD
Resident in Family Medicine
Mayo Clinic Florida
Jacksonville, Florida

Marjorie Delo, MD, CAQSM, RMSK
Director of Sports Medicine
Lakeshore Orthopaedics
Assistant Clinical Professor
Medical College of Wisconsin
Manitowoc, Wisconsin

Rania L. Dempsey, MD, MS
Director, Center for Whole Health
Delafield, Wisconsin

Kevin deWeber, MD, FAAFP, FACSM, RMSK
Program Director
Southwest Washington Sports Medicine Fellowship
Affiliate Associate Professor of Family Medicine
Oregon Health and Science University
Team USA Olympic Physician 2012, 2016
Team Physician, Clark College
Vancouver, Washington

William W. Dexter, MD, FACSM
Professor, Family Medicine
Tufts University School of Medicine
Faculty, MMC Sports Medicine Fellowship
Medical Director of Athletic Training and Team Physician
University of Southern Maine
Maine Medical Partners Orthopedics and Sports Medicine
South Portland, Maine

Mark A. Diamond, MD
Physical Medicine and Rehabilitation and Physiatry
Avera Health Medical Group
Sioux Falls, South Dakota

Joshua Dilley, MD
Family Medicine Resident
Department of Family and Community Medicine
Wake Forest University
Winston-Salem, North Carolina

Douglas J. DiOrio, MD
Assistant Program Director
Riverside Sports Medicine Fellowship
Chairman OhioHealth Sports Medicine
Team Physician Columbus Crew
Columbus, Ohio

Laura M. Distel, MD, CAQSM
Community Health Care Sports Medicine and Family Practice
Team Physician, Norton High School
Wadsworth, Ohio

William H. Dixon, MD
Assistant Professor of Family and Community Medicine
Residency Program Director
Southern Illinois University—Quincy Family Medicine Residency
Quincy, Illinois

Timothy Ryan Draper, DO, ABFM, CAQSM
Assistant Clinical Professor of Family Medicine
University of North Carolina, Chapel Hill School of Medicine
Associate Program Director
Cone Health Primary Care Sports Medicine Fellowship
Team Physician, Guilford College
Greensboro, North Carolina

Brandon Eck, DO†
Sports, Osteopathic and Regenerative Medicine Physician
Sports and Spine Division
Premier Orthopaedics
Philadelphia, Pennsylvania

Angelina R. Edwards, MD
Assistant Professor of Medicine
Division of Renal Diseases and Hypertension and Division of Immunology and Organ Transplantation
McGovern Medical School
University of Texas Health Science Center
Transplant Nephrologist
Memorial Hermann Transplant Center
Texas Medical Center
Houston, Texas

David S. Edwards, MD, CAQSM
Associate Professor
Associate Director, Primary Care Sports Medicine Fellowship
Department of Family and Community Medicine
Texas Tech University Health Sciences Center, Lubbock
Lubbock, Texas

Angelene M. Elliott, DO†
Primary Care Sports Medicine
Boston University/Boston Medical Center
Boston, Massachusetts

Dina Elnaggar, MD, MS†
Indiana University Sports Medicine Fellow
Indianapolis, Indiana

Johnnie Faircloth, MD, CAQSM
Associate Professor
Pediatrics and Sports Medicine
Texas Tech University Health Sciences Center
Amarillo, Texas
Associate Program Director
Assistant Team Physician PRCA with Justin Sports Medicine
Ringside Physician, USA Boxing

Lisa Falotico, DO, CAQSM
Family Practice Physician
Parkview Physician Group
Fort Wayne, Indiana

Melissa Faubert, DO
Primary Care Sports Medicine Fellow
University of Chicago/NorthShore University HealthSystem
Chicago, Illinois

Marcia Faustin, MD, CAQSM
Associate Physician
Primary Care Network (Family Medicine) and Department of Sports Medicine
University of California, Davis
Sacramento, California

Jeffrey P. Feden, MD, FACEP, CAQSM
Associate Professor (Clinical) of Emergency Medicine
Alpert Medical School of Brown University
Providence, Rhode Island

Karl B. Fields, MD, CAQ
Professor of Family Medicine and Sports Medicine
University of North Carolina School of Medicine
Cone Health Sports Medicine Fellowship
Greensboro, North Carolina

Diana Filtz, MD
Pediatric Sports Medicine Fellow
Cincinnati Children's Hospital Medical Center
Cincinnati, Ohio

Anastasia Fischer, MD, FAAFP, FACSM
Associate Professor of Pediatrics
Department of Sports Medicine
Nationwide Children's Hospital
The Ohio State University College of Medicine
Columbus, Ohio

Ryan C. Fowler, MD, CAQSM
Director of Sports Medicine
Coryell Memorial Healthcare System
Gatesville, Texas

Cody Franzen, MD, CAQSM
Providence West Olympia Sports Medicine
Primary Care Sports Medicine
Immediate Care
Team Physician for Black Hills High School
Adjunct Faculty for Providence St. Peter Family Medicine Residency
Olympia, Washington

Samuel J. Galloway, MD
Sports Medicine Fellow
University of California, San Diego
Team Physician, UCSD Tritons
San Diego, California

Shaun P. Garff, DO
Sports Medicine Fellow
Intermountain Healthcare
Utah Valley Sports Medicine
Provo, Utah

Anne M. Garrison, DO, CAQSM
Humble, Texas

Kevin B. Gebke, MD
Chair
Department of Family Medicine
Indiana University School of Medicine
Director
Indiana University Center for Sports Medicine
Indianapolis, Indiana

Christopher A. Gee, MD, MPH, FACEP, CAQSM
Clinical Associate Professor
Department of Orthopaedics
University of Utah School of Medicine
Associate Director
University of Utah Primary Care Sports Medicine Fellowship
Head Team Physician, Salt Lake City Stars
Team Physician, US Speedskating
Medical Director, United States Olympic Committee High Performance Center
Kearns, Utah

Alecia Gende, DO
Primary Care Sports Medicine Fellow
UI Sports Medicine
University of Iowa Hospitals and Clinics
Iowa City, Iowa

Jordan F. Geroski, DO
Saint Joseph Regional Medical Center—Family Medicine Center
Mishawaka, Indiana

Chad J. Giles, DO
Sports Medicine Fellow
Summa Health System
Summa Health Sports Medicine
Akron, Ohio

Kory Gill, DO, FAAFP, CAQSM
Clinical Professor
Texas A&M Health Science Center
Program Director
Texas A&M Primary Care Sports Medicine Fellowship Program
Texas A&M Team Physician
College Station, Texas

Rodney S. Gonzalez, MD, FAAFP[†]
Deputy Commanding Officer
Blanchfield Army Community Hospital
Fort Campbell, Kentucky

Miranda Gordon-Zigel, MD[†]
Resident Physician
Department of Community and Family Medicine
Hospital of the University of Pennsylvania
Philadelphia, Pennsylvania

Aaron Gray, MD, CAQSM
Associate Professor in Orthopedics
Associate Professor in Family Medicine
University of Missouri, School of Medicine
Medical Director, MU Human Performance Institute
Columbia, Missouri

Steven A. Greer, MD, CAQ, FAAFP
Medical Director, TRIA St. Paul
HealthPartners Orthopaedics and Sports Medicine
Team Physician, Mounds View High School
St. Paul, Minnesota

Andrew J.M. Gregory, MD, FAAP, FACSM[†]
Associate Professor of Orthopedics, Neurosurgery and Pediatrics
Vanderbilt University School of Medicine
Assistant Director
Pediatric Sports Medicine Fellowship
Team Physician, Nashville Christian School, Vanderbilt University, Nashville Sounds, USA Volleyball National Teams
Nashville, Tennessee

Claire Gross, MD
Primary Care Sports Medicine Fellow
MacNeal Hospital
Berwyn, Illinois

Sunny Gupta, DO
Clinical Assistant Professor of Family and Community Medicine
Sidney Kimmel Medical College, Thomas Jefferson University
Sports Medicine
Rothman Institute
Marlton, New Jersey

Mario Gutierrez, MD
Sports Medicine Fellow
Texas Tech University Health Science Center El Paso
El Paso, Texas

Tarek S. Hadla, MD, CAQSM
President, Founder and Owner
Sports Medicine
Interventional Spine
Michigan Sports Medicine
Dearborn Heights, Michigan

Mark Halstead, MD, FAAP
Associate Professor of Pediatrics and Orthopedics
Washington University in St. Louis
Medical Director, Young Athlete Center
Medical Director, Sports Concussions Clinic
Team Physician, St. Louis Blues, Washington University Bears
St. Louis, Missouri

John W. Hariadi, MD, FAAFP[†]
Chief Medical Officer, Safe Use Initiatives
Professional Affairs and Stakeholder Engagement
Office of the Center Director
Center for Drug Evaluations and Research
U.S. Food and Drug Administration
Silver Spring, Maryland

Kimberly G. Harmon, MD[†]
Professor Departments of Family Medicine and Orthopaedics and Sports Medicine
University of Washington School of Medicine
Head Football Physician, University of Washington
Seattle, Washington

Mark D. Harris, MD, MPH, MBA, MDiv, FAAFP, CAQSM[†]
Chief of Staff
Family, Sports, and Preventive Medicine
Veterans Administration Medical Center
Beckley, West Virginia

Abdullah Hasan-Pratt, MD
Emergency Medicine Resident
University of Chicago Medicine
Chicago, Illinois

Daniel C. Herman, MD, PhD, FAAPMR, FACSM, CAQSM
Assistant Professor
Divisions of PM&R, Sports Medicine, and Research
Department of Orthopaedics and Rehabilitation
University of Florida College of Medicine
Faculty
University of Florida Primary Care Sports Medicine Fellowship
Gainesville, Florida

Fernando Enrique Hernandez, MD
Sports Medicine Fellow
Department of Sports Medicine/ Department of Family Medicine
Texas Tech University Health Sciences Center
Lubbock, Texas

Marc P. Hilgers, MD, PhD, FAAFP
Associate Medical Director
Sports Medicine
Aurora, Illinois

Vihangi Hindagolla, DO
Family Medicine Residency of Southwest Washington
PeaceHealth Southwest Medical Center
Vancouver, Washington

David Milo Hirschi III, MD
Team Physician
University of Southern Indiana
Evansville, Indiana

Quynh Hoang, MD, FAAP, CAQSM
Pediatric Primary Care Sports Medicine
The Adolescent & Children's Orthopedic Surgeons, Inc.
Encino, California

Brandon Hockenberry, MD
Primary Care Sports Medicine Fellow
University of New Mexico School of Medicine
Albuquerque, New Mexico

Matthew Horn, MD
Department of Family and Community Medicine
Wake Forest University
Winston-Salem, North Carolina

Michal Kalli Hose, MD[†]
Clinical Professor of Internal Medicine
University of California, San Diego
Staff Physician
VA San Diego Healthcare System
Medical Director
National Veterans Summer Sports Clinic
Co-Director
VA Musculoskeletal Clinic
San Diego, California

Robert Hosey, MD, FACSM, CAQSM
Professor
Departments of Orthopaedic and Sports Medicine, Family Medicine
Director
University of Kentucky Primary Care Sports Medicine Fellowship
Director of Athletic Medicine
University of Kentucky
Lexington, Kentucky

Antonio Howard, MBBS, MSc, FAAPMR, CAQSM[†]
Assistant Professor, Physical Medicine and Rehabilitation
Clerkship Director, College of Medicine
University of Arkansas for Medical Sciences
Little Rock, Arkansas

Robert L. Howard, MA, ATC
Assistant Director of Athletics—Head Athletic Trainer
Department of Sports Medicine
University of Connecticut Division of Athletics
Storrs, Connecticut

Shane Hudnall, MD, CAQSM
Cone Health Sports Medicine
High Point, North Carolina

Tudor Hughes, FRCR
Professor of Clinical Radiology
Radiology Resident Program Director
Vice Chair of Education
Department of Radiology
University of California, San Diego Medical Center
San Diego, California

Yaffa Ilyaguyeva
Brooklyn, New York

Krishna Israni, MD, MS, BS[†]
Mayo Clinic Family Medicine Residency
Jacksonville, Florida
Saba University School of Medicine
The Bottom, Saba, Dutch Caribbean
University of Arizona
Tucson, Arizona

Dominic Jacobelli, MD
Primary Care Sports Medicine Fellow
University of Tennessee, Knoxville
Knoxville, Tennessee

Bjorn Allan Jacobson, MD
Primary Care Sports Medicine Fellow
TriHealth Bethesda Family Practice
Cincinnati, Ohio

Carrie A. Jaworski, MD, FAAFP, FACSM
Director, University of Chicago/NorthShore Primary Care Sports Medicine Fellowship
Division Head, Primary Care Sports Medicine, NorthShore University HealthSystem
Clinical Assistant Professor of Family Medicine, Pritzker School of Medicine
University of Chicago
Chicago, Illinois

Patrick Jenkins III, MD
Fellow, University of South Carolina Sports Medicine Fellowship
Palmetto Health
Columbia, South Carolina

Matthew J. Jepson, MD, MS
Primary Care Sports Medicine Fellow
Palmetto Health USC Sports Medicine Fellowship
Columbia, South Carolina

David Johnson, MD
Resident Physician in Family Medicine
Philadelphia, Pennsylvania

Robert L. Jones, MD, CAQSM
Head Team Physician
Medical Director, Student Health Center
University of North Carolina at Charlotte
Charlotte, North Carolina

Christopher Jordan, MD, ATC, CAQSM
Associate Director Sports Medicine
South Bend-Notre Dame Sports Medicine Fellowship
Mishawaka, Indiana

Vijay Jotwani, MD
Assistant Professor of Family Medicine
Weill Cornell Medical College
Texas A&M College of Medicine
Head Team Physician, Houston Dash
Primary Care Sports Medicine Physician, Houston Astros
Team Physician, Rice University Athletics
Team Physician, Houston Ballet
Houston, Texas

Kimberly Kaiser, MD, CAQSM[†]
Assistant Professor of Orthopaedic Surgery and Sports Medicine
Assistant Professor of Family and Community Medicine
University of Kentucky College of Medicine
Team Physician, University of Kentucky
Head Team Physician, Eastern Kentucky University
Lexington, Kentucky

Amy Kakimoto, MD, DAAFP, CAQSM
North Coast Family Medical Group
Encinitas, CA

Rahul Kapur, MD, CAQSM
Associate Professor, Family Medicine and Sports Medicine
Director, Penn Primary Care Sports Medicine Fellowship
Chief Medical Physician, Penn Athletics
University of Pennsylvania
Philadelphia, Pennsylvania

Julie M. Kerr, MD, CAQSM[†]
Clinical Associate Professor of Pediatrics
Northeast Ohio Medical University
Program Director
Akron Children's Hospital Primary Care Sports Medicine Fellowship
Team Physician, University of Akron, St. Vincent-St. Mary High School
Akron, Ohio

Misha Khalighi, MD
Chief Resident at the University of California, Irvine—Children's Hospital of Orange County General Pediatrics Residency, AY 2017–2018
Jefferson Medical College
Philadelphia, Pennsylvania

Razib Khaund, MD
Clinical Assistant Professor in Internal Medicine
Warren Alpert Medical School
Brown University
Director of Sports Medicine
Care New England Health Care System
Providence, Rhode Island

John Kiel, DO, MPH[†]
Primary Care Sports Medicine Fellow
University of Kentucky School of Medicine
Department of Family and Community Medicine
Lexington, Kentucky

Brian Young Kim, MD, MS, CAQSM
Assistant Professor of Family Medicine
Director of Medical Student Education
Department of Family Medicine
University of California, Irvine School of Medicine
Associate Team Physician, UC Irvine Athletics
Irvine, California

Spencer Kirk, MD, MS
Primary Care Sports Medicine Fellow
Presence Resurrection Medical Center
Chicago, Illinois

Jennifer Scott Koontz, MD, MPH, FAAFP, CAQSM
Newton Orthopaedics and Sports Medicine
Assistant Professor of Family and Community Medicine
University of Kansas School of Medicine—Wichita
Wichita, Kansas
Head Team Physician, Bethel College
North Newton, Kansas
Head Team Physician, Hesston College
Hesston, Kansas
Head Team Physician, Newton High School
Newton, Kansas

Chris Koutures, MD, FAAP
Pediatric and Sports Medicine Specialist
ActiveKidMD
Anaheim Hills, California
Clinical Instructor
University of California Irvine/CHOC Children's Department of Pediatrics
Team Physician, USA Volleyball National Teams, CS Fullerton Athletics, Chapman University Department of Dance
Orange, California

David W. Kruse, MD
Orthopaedic Specialty Institute
Athlete Care Coordinator, USA Gymnastics
Team Physician, USA Gymnastics Men
Team Physician, UC Irvine Associate
Team Physician, Biola University, Orange County Soccer Club
Associate Faculty
Long Beach Memorial Primary Care Sports Medicine Fellowship
Orange, California

Jason A. Krystofiak, MD
Sports Medicine Fellow
Primary Care Sports Medicine Fellowship
Rutgers Robert Wood Johnson Medical School
New Brunswick, New Jersey

Geoffrey S. Kuhlman, MD, FAAFP, CAQSM
Director of Sports Medicine
Hinsdale Family Medicine Residency
Private Practice
Hinsdale, Illinois

Daniel Kuo, DO, MA[†]
Resident Physician
Department of Physical Medicine and Rehabilitation
Tufts Medical Center
Boston, Massachusetts

Bittu Kuruvilla, MD, FAAPMR, CAQSM
Assistant Professor of Physical Medicine and Rehabilitation
Montefiore Medical Center
University Hospital for Albert Einstein College of Medicine
Faculty, Montefiore PM&R Sports Medicine Fellowship
Bronx, New York

Andrea Kussman, MD, CAQSM
Clinical Assistant Professor
Primary Care Sports Medicine
Stanford University Department of Orthopaedics
Team Physician
Stanford University
Palo Alto, California

Anthony Kwon, MS
John A. Burns School of Medicine
Honolulu, Hawaii

Michael Ladewski, DO
Associate Director
Family Medicine Residency Program
Assistant Director
Primary Care Sports Medicine Fellowship
Chicago, Illinois

Lindsay A. Lafferty, MD
Primary Care Sports Medicine Fellow
Penn State Medical Center
Hershey, Pennsylvania

Mike LaGrange, MD, FAAFP, CAQSM
Volunteer Professor of Family Medicine
Indiana University School of Medicine
Team Physician
Indiana University Athletics
Bloomington, Indiana

Christopher P. Lake, MD
Sports Medicine Fellow
Cone Health Sports Medicine Fellowship
Greensboro, North Carolina

Mark E. Lavallee, MD, CSCS, FACSM
Director
York Hospital Sports Medicine Fellowship Program
York, Pennsylvania
Assistant Clinical Professor
Pennsylvania State University College of Medicine
Hershey, Pennsylvania
Adjunct Clinical Professor
Drexel University School of Medicine
Philadelphia, Pennsylvania
Head Team Physician
Gettysburg College
Gettysburg, Pennsylvania
Chairman, USA Weightlifting Sports Medicine Society
Colorado Springs, Colorado
Medical Director
International Weightlifting Federation—Masters World Championships
Budapest, Hungary

Se Won Lee, MD
Associate Professor of Physical Medicine and Rehabilitation
Albert Einstein College of Medicine
Program Director
Montefiore Medical Center Primary Care Sports Medicine Fellowship
Bronx, New York

Jeffrey C. Leggit, MD, CAQSM[†]
Director of Healthcare Operations
Family and Primary Care Sports Medicine
Associate Professor
Department of Family Medicine
Uniformed Services University of the Health Sciences
Bethesda, Maryland

Amy Leu, DO, FAAFP, CAQSM
Assistant Clinical Professor of Family Medicine
University of California, San Diego, School of Medicine
Assistant Director
UCSD Primary Care Sports Medicine Fellowship
Team Physician
UCSD Tritons
Consulting Physician
San Diego Padres and the U.S. Olympic Training Center
Chula Vista, California

Emily Levy, MD, CAQSM
Clinical Professor of Family Medicine, Drexel COM
Assistant Program Director of Sports Medicine, Drexel Sports Medicine Fellowship
Philadelphia, Pennsylvania

Michael M. Linder, MD, CAQSM
Professor of Family Medicine
University of South Alabama, School of Medicine
Mobile, Alabama

Ryan J. Lingor, MD, AT-C, RD, CSCS
Associate Attending Physician
Hospital for Special Surgery
Medical Director, HSS Same Day Sports
Team Physician, New York Rangers Hockey Club
Faculty, Weill Cornell Medical College
New York, New York

Laura Lintner, DO, CAQSM
Assistant Professor of Family Medicine
Wake Forest University School of Medicine
Assistant Director
Wake Forest University Primary Care Sports Medicine Fellowship
Winston-Salem, North Carolina

Fernando Liquido, MD
University of California San Diego Family Medicine Residency
San Diego, California

Jayson Loeffert, DO
Assistant Professor of Family and Community Medicine and Orthopedics and Rehabilitation
Penn State Health Milton S. Hershey Medical Center
Faculty Member
PSU Hershey Primary Care Sports Medicine Fellowship
Team Physician, Harrisburg Senators, Lebanon Valley College
Hershey, Pennsylvania

Kelsey Logan, MD, MPH, FAAP, FACP
Director
Division of Sports Medicine
Cincinnati Children's Hospital Medical Center
Associate Professor of Pediatrics and Internal Medicine
University of Cincinnati College of Medicine
Cincinnati, Ohio

Frank E. Lorch, MD, FAAPMR
Director, Nonsurgical Sports Medicine
AAPMR Board Certified Sports Medicine
Institute for Western Surgery
Shanghai, China

Brian Lowell, MD, CAQSM
Teacher Clinician of PeaceHealth Medical Group
Southwest Family Medicine and Sports Medicine
Vancouver, Washington

James H. Lynch, MD, MS, FACSM†
U.S. Army Special Operations Command
Fort Bragg, North Carolina

Adam Lyons, MD
Primary Care Sports Medicine Fellow
Department of Family Medicine and Community Health
Perelman School of Medicine at the University of Pennsylvania
Philadelphia, Pennsylvania

Navid Mahooti, MD, MPH, CAQSM
Sports Medicine and Nonsurgical Orthopedics Specialist
North Shore Physicians Group
Mass General/North Shore Center for Outpatient Care
Clinical Instructor of Sports Medicine
North Shore Medical Center Internal Medicine Residency
Head Team Physician, Gordon College
Danvers, Massachusetts

Britt Marcussen, MD, FAAFP, CAQSM
Clinical Associate Professor of Family Medicine
University of Iowa College of Medicine
Director, University of Iowa Primary Care Sports Medicine Fellowship
Team Physician, University of Iowa
Iowa City, Iowa
Team Physician, U.S. Ski Team

Anthony Martin, MD, CAQSM
Assistant Professor of Family Medicine
Associate Director, Atrium Health Primary Care Sports Medicine Fellowship
Head Team Physician, East Mecklenburg High School
Team Physician, Charlotte 49ers
Ringside Physician, Golden Gloves Tournament
Charlotte, North Carolina

Robert D. Martin, MD
Assistant Professor of Orthopaedic Surgery
University of Arkansas for Medical Sciences
Foot and Ankle Division
Little Rock, Arkansas

Julio A. Martinez-Silvestrini, MD, FAAPMR, CAQSM
Clinical Associate Professor in Physical Medicine and Rehabilitation
Department of Neurology
University of Massachusetts—Baystate
Worcester, Massachusetts
Adjunct Clinical Associate Professor
Department of Physical Medicine and Rehabilitation
Tufts University School of Medicine
Boston, Massachusetts
Medical Director, Baystate Rehabilitation Care
East Longmeadow, Massachusetts

David McClaskey, MD, ATC
Primary Care Sports Medicine
Kaiser Permanente
San Diego, California

Christopher McGrew, MD, FACSM, CAQSM†
Professor
Department of Family and Community Medicine
Department of Orthopedics and Rehabilitation
University of New Mexico Health Sciences Center
Director
Primary Care Sports Medicine Fellowship
Assistant Team Physician, University of New Mexico Athletics
Albuquerque, New Mexico

Ian D. McKeag, MD, MS
Cone Health Sports Medicine
Greensboro, North Carolina

Sean McKeown, MS, PT, Cred MDT
Center Director/Owner
PRN Physical Therapy
Mission Valley
San Diego, California

Gary Means, MD†
LTC, MC
United States Army Special Operations Command
Fort Bragg, North Carolina

Joseph Medellin, MD, MPH, MBA†
Sports Medicine Fellow (2018–2019)
Wellspan York Hospital
York, Pennsylvania

Paul Meirick, MD†
Clinical Instructor, Orthopaedics and Rehabilitation
Clinical Instructor, Internal Medicine
Vanderbilt University Medical Center
Team Physician, Vanderbilt Commodores, Nashville Sounds, Nashville Soccer Club
Nashville, Tennessee

Sarah Merrill, MD, CAQSM
Assistant Clinical Professor of Family Medicine, Step III
Loyola University Chicago Stritch School of Medicine
Chicago, Illinois
Assistant Program Director
University of California San Diego Family Medicine Residency
Medical Director
UCSD Scripps Ranch Family Medicine Clinic
Team Physician, UCSD Tritons
San Diego, California

Brent H. Messick, MD, MS, FAAFP, CAQSM
Associate Professor, Atrium Health
Assistant Professor
University of North Carolina at Chapel Hill
Chapel Hill, North Carolina
Sports Medicine and Injury Care
Concord, North Carolina
Assistant Director, Cabarrus Sports Medicine Fellowship
Team Physician, Catawba College, Carolina Energy Arena Football

Kyle Meyer, DO
Sports Medicine Fellow
University of Pennsylvania
Philadelphia, Pennsylvania

Christopher Miles, MD, CAQSM
Associate Director
Primary Care Sports Medicine Fellowship
Assistant Professor
Department of Family and Community Medicine
Wake Forest School of Medicine
Medical Director of Athletics
Wake Forest University
Winston-Salem, North Carolina

Jennifer J. Mitchell, MD, FAAFP, CAQSM
Professor
Sports Medicine Fellowship Director
Department of Family and Community Medicine
Texas Tech University Health Sciences Center School of Medicine
Team Physician Texas Tech University
Lubbock, Texas

Kelly T. Mitchell, MD
Associate Professor
Co-Director Retina Service
Residency Program Director
Department of Ophthalmology
Adjunct Faculty, Department of Pediatrics
Texas Tech University Health Sciences Center
Ophthalmology Consultant, Athletic Department Texas Tech University
Lubbock, Texas

Jeffrey M. Mjaanes, MD, CAQSM, FAAP, FACSM
Assistant Professor
Director of Sports Medicine/Head Team Physician
Northwestern University
Evanston, Illinois

Caitlyn C. Mooney, MD, FAAP, CAQSM†
Staff Physician
University Medical Associates/University Health System
Adjunct Professor
University of Texas Health—San Antonio
San Antonio, Texas

Kinshasa Morton, MD, CAQSM
Assistant Professor of Family Medicine
Rutgers Robert Wood Johnson Medical School
Team Physician, Rutgers University
New Brunswick, New Jersey

John Munyak, MD
Sports Medicine/Nonoperative Orthopedic Surgery
Maimonides Bone and Joint Center
Medical Director, National Basketball Association
Team Physician, St. Francis College, Brooklyn
Team Physician, New York Islanders
Former Team Physician, Brooklyn Nets
Brooklyn, New York

Daniel Murphy, MD, FAAFP
Assistant Professor
Department of Family and Community Medicine
Paul L. Foster School of Medicine
Texas Tech University Health Science Center El Paso
El Paso, Texas

Laura J. Murphy, DO†
Family Medicine Resident
University of California, San Diego
San Diego, California

Tenley Murphy, MD, FAAFP, CAQSM
Assistant Professor
Department of Family and Preventive Medicine
Program Director
Palmetto Health—University of South Carolina Primary Care Sports Medicine Fellowship
Team Physician
University of South Carolina
Columbia, South Carolina

Priya Nagarajan, DO†
Family Medicine Resident
University of Minnesota North Memorial Family Medicine Residency
Minneapolis, Minnesota

Dhiren J. Naidu, MD, FRCPC, Dip. Sport Med.
Associate Professor, Division of Physical Medicine and Rehabilitation
Faculty of Medicine and Dentistry, University of Alberta
President, HealthPointe Medical
Head Team Physician, Edmonton Oilers Hockey Club
Head Team Physician, Edmonton Eskimos Football Club
Varsity Physician, University of Alberta Athletics
Edmonton, Alberta, Canada

Greg Nakamoto, MD, FACP
Department of Orthopedics and Sports Medicine
Virginia Mason Medical Center
Clinical Assistant Professor of Medicine
University of Washington School of Medicine
Seattle, Washington

Dusty Marie Narducci, MD, Board Certified Family Medicine, CAQSM
Assistant Director, University of South Florida—Morton Plant Mease Primary Care Sports Medicine Fellowship
Assistant Professor, Morsani College of Medicine
Team Physician, Department of Athletics at the University of South Florida
Team Physician, Saint Leo's University
Tampa, Florida

Melissa Nayak, MD, CAQSM
Assistant Program Director
Primary Care Sports Medicine Fellowship
Henry Ford Health System
Clinical Assistant Professor
Wayne State University School of Medicine
Detroit, Michigan

Sara Neal, MD, MA, CAQSM†
Associate Professor of Family Medicine
University of North Carolina, Chapel Hill, School of Medicine
Associate Program Director, Cone Health Family Medicine Residency
Assistant Director, Cone Health Primary Care Sports Medicine Fellowship
Greensboro, North Carolina

Giorgio A. Negron, MD†
Department of Physical Medicine and Rehabilitation
Emory University
Atlanta, Georgia

Mark L. Nelson, MD†
Family Medicine Resident Physician
University of Minnesota, Twin Cities School of Medicine
Minneapolis, Minnesota

Vicki R. Nelson, MD, PhD
Clinical Assistant Professor of Family Medicine
Steadman Hawkins Clinic of the Carolinas
University of South Carolina School of Medicine—Greenville
Greenville, South Carolina

Mark W. Niedfeldt, MD
Associate Clinical Professor
Departments of Family and Community Medicine, Cell Biology, Neurobiology, and Anatomy
Medical College of Wisconsin
Private Practice
Mequon, Wisconsin

Rochelle M. Nolte, MD, FAAFP, CAQSM†
Assistant Professor of Family Medicine
Uniformed Services University of the Health Sciences
Staff Physician
Metropolitan Correctional Center
San Diego, California

Rathna R. Nuti, MD, CAQSM
Assistant Team Physician
Dallas Stars NHL Hockey Club
Frisco, Texas

Richard Okragly, MD
Fellowship Director
TriHealth Primary Care Sports Medicine Fellowship
Head Team Physician, Mount St. Joseph University, Cincinnati Rollergirls
Team Physician, Athletics Health Care Administrator, Xavier University
Cincinnati, Ohio

David E. Olson, MD, CAQSM, FACSM†
Assistant Professor Family Medicine and Community Health
University of Minnesota
Associate Director, University of Minnesota Primary Care Sports Medicine Fellowship
Team Physician, University of Minnesota Athletics, Minnesota Vikings, Bethel University, University of St. Thomas, U.S. Soccer and Roseville Area High School
Minneapolis, Minnesota

Ross Osborn, MD, FAAFP, CAQSM
Medical Director
The Center for Health and Sports Medicine
Nova Southeastern Physician Assistant Program Jacksonville
Associate Clinical Professor
Philadelphia College of Osteopathic Medicine
Medical Director
University of North Florida Athletic Training Program
Jacksonville, Florida

Sona Patel, MD, FAAP
Urgent Care Physician
Montefiore Medical Center
Bronx, New York

Stephen R. Paul, MD, CAQSM†
Associate Professor of Family and Community Medicine
University of Arizona
Assistant Team Physician, Intercollegiate Athletics
Head Team Physician, Club Sports University of Arizona
Tucson, Arizona

Bernadette Pendergraph, MD
Associate Professor of Family Medicine
David Geffen School of Medicine
Program Director, Harbor-UCLA/Team to Win Sports Medicine Fellowship
Los Angeles, California

Timothy Perdue, DO†
Fort Bragg, North Carolina

Evan D. Perez, MD
Primary Care Sports Medicine Fellow
Texas Tech University Health Sciences Center El Paso
El Paso, Texas

Shawn Phillips, MD, MSPT
Assistant Professor of Family and Community Medicine and Orthopedics and Rehabilitation
Penn State College of Medicine/ Milton S. Hershey Medical Center
Department of Family and Community Medicine
Hershey, Pennsylvania
Medical Director
Penn State Health Mount Joy
Mount Joy, Pennsylvania

Brent Pickett, DO†
Memorial Hospital of South Bend Family Medicine Residency
South Bend, Indiana

David J. Pohl, DO
Primary Care Sports Medicine Fellow
Advocate Lutheran General Hospital
Park Ridge, Illinois

Katherine M. Pohlgeers, MD, MS, CAQSM
Team Physician, University of Louisville
Assistant Professor, University of Louisville School of Medicine
Medical Director, Newburg Clinic
Louisville, Kentucky

Thomas L. Pommering, DO, FAAFP
Division Chief for Sports Medicine
Nationwide Children's Hospital
Associate Director, Nationwide Children's Hospital Sports Medicine Fellowship Program
Associate Professor of Pediatrics and Family Medicine
The Ohio State University College of Medicine
Head Team Physician, Ohio Dominican University
Columbus, Ohio

Steven K. Poon, MD, CAQSM
Team Physician, Sun Devil Athletics
Arizona State University
Sports Medicine Section, Student Health Services
Tempe, Arizona

Emily B. Porter, MD, ATC
Sports Medicine Physician
SSM Health Dean Medical Group
Madison, Wisconsin

Shannon Powers, DO
Primary Care Sports Medicine Fellow
Rush University Medical Center
Chicago, Illinois

David E. Price, MD, FAAFP, CAQSM
Clinical Professor of Family Medicine
Atrium Health
Director, Primary Care Sports Medicine Fellowship
Head Team Physician, Johnson C. Smith University Golden Bulls
Team Physician, Charlotte Knights
Charlotte, North Carolina

Aaron J. Provance, MD, FAAP, CAQSM†
Associate Professor
Department of Orthopedics
University of Colorado, School of Medicine
Medical Director, Sports Medicine Center
Children's Hospital Colorado
Aurora, Colorado

James C. Puffer, MD
President and Chief Executive Officer
American Board of Family Medicine
Professor of Family and Community Medicine
College of Medicine
University of Kentucky
Lexington, Kentucky

George G.A. Pujalte, MD, FACSM†
Senior Associate Consultant, Family Medicine and Sports Medicine
Assistant Professor, Mayo Clinic College of Medicine
Vice Chair for Academics, Department of Family Medicine
Associate Program Director, Sports Medicine Fellowship Program
Vice Chair for Communications, American Medical Society for Sports Medicine
Team Physician, USA Taekwondo
Mayo Clinic
Jacksonville, Florida

Margaret Pusateri, MD
Emergency Medicine Sports Medicine Fellow
University of New Mexico
Albuquerque, New Mexico

Anna P. Quan, MD†
Clinical Professor of Medicine
University of California, San Diego School of Medicine
General Internal Medicine Section
Chief, San Diego VAMC Sorrento Valley CBOC
Co-Director San Diego VAMC Musculoskeletal Clinic
San Diego, California

Kristina Quirolgico, MD
Sports Medicine Fellow
Primary Care Sports Medicine Fellowship
Rutgers Robert Wood Johnson Medical School
New Brunswick, New Jersey

Matthew Rachwalski, DO
Primary Care Sports Medicine Fellow
Indiana University-Purdue University Indianapolis
Indianapolis, Indiana

Sara N. Raiser, MD
Primary Care Sports Fellow
Stanford University
Stanford, California

Z. Victor Ratajczak, MD
Sports Medicine Physician
OrthoVirginia
Lynchburg, Virginia

Reno Ravindran, MD, CAQSM†
Assistant Clinical Professor of Pediatrics and Family Medicine
Nationwide Children's Hospital Sports Medicine
The Ohio State University College of Medicine
Columbus, Ohio

Tracy Ray, MD, FACSM, CAQSM
Associate Professor of Community and Family Medicine and Orthopaedic Surgery
Duke University
Director, Sports Medicine/Primary Care
Director, Primary Care Sports Medicine Fellowship Program
Durham, North Carolina

Ziad Fahad Rayes, MBBS, MBA, Ccfp(Sem), Dip Sport Med(Casem)†
Lecturer, Department of Family Medicine
University of Toronto, Canada
Toronto, Ontario, Canada
Clinical Adjunct Faculty, Family Medicine
Alfaisal University
Deputy Director Business Development
Program Delivery Director, Corporate Transformation Office
King Faisal Specialist Hospital and Research Center
Member of the Hearing Committee
Saudi Anti-Doping Agency
Managing Director, MSK Sport Medicine Clinic
Riyadh, Saudi Arabia

Ryan Reese, DO†
Family Medicine Resident
WellSpan York Hospital
York, Pennsylvania

Brent S.E. Rich, MD, ATC†
Fellowship Director, Utah Valley Sports Medicine
Intermountain Health Care
Team Physician, Brigham Young University
Provo, Utah

Brittney M. Richardson, MD, CAQSM†
Assistant Professor of Family Medicine
Department of Family and Geriatric Medicine
University of Louisville School of Medicine
Team Physician, University of Louisville
Rotation Coordinator, University of Louisville Primary Care Sports Medicine Fellowship
Assistant Clerkship Director, Family Medicine
Louisville, Kentucky

James C. Ritchey, MD, MS, FAAFP
Family Medicine Physician and Sports Medicine Fellow
Eisenhower Health
Rancho Mirage, California

Tara Robbins, MD
SIMCA
Team Physician, Southern Illinois Miners
Marion, Illinois

Richard E. Rodenberg, MD, FAAP, CAQSM
Program Director, NCH Sports Medicine Fellowship Program
Nationwide Children's Hospital Division of Sports Medicine
Associate Professor, Departments of Pediatrics
The Ohio State University College of Medicine
Columbus, Ohio
Team Physician, Ohio Dominican University and Big Walnut High School

Stephen Rohrer, DO, FAOASM
San Diego Sports Medicine & Family Health Center
Team Physician, San Diego State University
Assistant Clinical Professor, UCSD, nonsalaried
Assistant Clinical Professor, SDSU, nonsalaried
San Diego, California

Gregory Rubin, DO
Sports Medicine Fellow
University of Kentucky College of Medicine
Lexington, Kentucky

Alana Ryan, DO
Family Medicine Physician
Primary Care Sports Medicine Fellow
Wake Forest University
Winston-Salem, North Carolina

Anthony J. Saglimbeni, MD, Board Certified Internal Medicine, CAQSM
President, South Bay Sports and Preventive Medicine Associates, Inc
Head Team Physician, San Francisco Giants
Team Physician, San Francisco 49ers
Team Physician, Santa Clara University Broncos
San Jose, California

Glenn H. Sapp II, MD†
Department of Physical Medicine and Rehabilitation
University of Virginia
Charlottesville, Virginia

Uziel Sauceda, MD, ABFM certified
Sports Medicine Fellow
University of California, San Diego Primary Care Sports Medicine
Team Physician, UCSD Tritons
USA Boxing Volunteer Ringside Physician
San Diego, California

Fouad Sayde, MD, ABIM, FACP
Sports Medicine Fellow
Henry Ford Health System
Detroit, Michigan

Daniel Schlegel, MD, MHA
Assistant Professor of Family and Community Medicine
Penn State Health Milton S. Hershey Medical Center
Penn State College of Medicine
Program Director, Family Medicine Residency Program
Hershey, Pennsylvania

Andrew Schleihauf, DO, CAQSM
Primary Care Sports Medicine Fellow
University of Kentucky
Lexington, Kentucky

Jeremy Schmitz, MD, ABFM
Cone Health Primary Care Sports Medicine Fellow
Greensboro, North Carolina

W. Franklin Sease Jr., MD, FAAFP, FACSM[†]
Associate Professor of Clinical Sports Medicine
University of South Carolina
School of Medicine Greenville
Greenville, South Carolina

Michael K. Seifert, MD, CAQSM
Assistant Professor of Sports and Internal Medicine
University of Central Florida College of Medicine
Orlando, Florida

Nicholas Sgrignoli, MD
Primary Care Sports Medicine Fellow, 2018
University of California, San Diego School of Medicine
San Diego, California

Nilesh Shah, MD, FAAFP, CAQSM
Medical Director, Summa Health Sports Medicine
Fellowship Director, Summa Health Sports Medicine Fellowship
Associate Professor of Family and Community Medicine
Northeast Ohio Medical University
Clinical Assistant Professor of Family Medicine and Sports Medicine
Ohio University College of Osteopathic Medicine
Head Team Physician, Akron RubberDucks
Medical Director, Akron Marathon Race Series
Akron, Ohio

Stephen Shaheen, MD, CAQSM
Assistant Professor, Emergency Medicine and Primary Care Sports Medicine (Orthopedic Surgery)
Associate Director, Primary Care Sports Medicine Fellowship
Assistant Team Physician, Duke University Athletics
Durham, North Carolina

Alan Shahtaji, DO, CAQSM
Associate Clinical Professor
University of California at San Diego Health Sciences
Department of Family Medicine and Public Health
Assistant Director, Primary Care Sports Medicine Fellowship
Director, UCSD Sports Medicine Concussion Clinic
Team Physician, U.S. Soccer Federation, UCSD Tritons, Hoover High School
San Diego, California

David C. Shin, MD
Sports Medicine Fellow
Long Beach Memorial Primary Care Sports Medicine
Long Beach, California

Matthew L. Silvis, MD[†]
Professor, Departments of Family and Community Medicine and Orthopedics and Rehabilitation
Vice Chair Clinical Operations, Department of Family and Community Medicine
Program Director, Penn State Primary Care Sports Medicine Fellowship, Hershey
Penn State Milton S. Hershey Medical Center
Head Team Physician, Hershey Bears Hockey Club
Head Team Physician, Hershey High School
Team Physician, Lebanon Valley College
Hershey, Pennsylvania

Stephen M. Simons, MD, FACSM
Director of Sports Medicine
Saint Joseph Health System
Mishawaka, Indiana
Co-Director, South Bend-Notre Dame Sports Medicine Fellowship
Team Physician, University of Notre Dame Cross Country and Track and Field
Bethel College, St. Mary's College
Volunteer Physician, United States Olympic Committee
Assistant Clinical Professor, Indiana University School of Medicine
Indianapolis, Indiana

Shawn Skarpnes, MD, CAQSM[†]
Family and Sports Medicine Physician
Elevation Physicians and V5 Medical Campus
Folsom, California
Team Physician, Folsom and Vista Del Lago High Schools
2016–2017 Graduate at UCSD Primary Care
Sports Medicine Fellowship
San Diego, California

Andrew Smith, MD, FAAP[†]
Lieutenant, Medical Corps, United States Navy
Assistant Professor of Pediatrics
Uniformed Services University of the Health Services
Fellow, Naval Hospital Camp Pendleton Primary Care Sports Medicine Fellowship
San Diego, California

Kristy Smith, MD
Clinical Assistant Professor
Department of Community Health and Family Medicine
University of Florida
Gainesville, Florida

Michael Seth Smith, MD, CAQSM, PharmD
Assistant Clinical Professor
Department of Orthopedics and Rehabilitation
University of Florida
Gainesville, Florida

M. Kyle Smoot, MD[†]
Associate Professor
Associate Program Director
Associate Head Team Physician, UK Athletics
University of Kentucky
Lexington, Kentucky

Ryan Sorell, MD
Family Medicine Resident
St. Joseph Regional Medical Center
Mishawaka, Indiana

Jason J. Stacy, MD[†]
Director of Sports Medicine & Physical Therapy
Associate Medical Director
Student Health Services
University of South Carolina
Columbia, South Carolina

Mark Stovak, MD
Professor
Reno School of Medicine Department of Family and Community Medicine
University of Nevada
Team Physician
University of Nevada, Reno
Reno, Nevada

Keith A. Stuessi, MD, CAQSM†
Subject Matter Expert, Traumatic Brain Injury
Defense and Veterans Brain Injury Center (DVBIC)
Marine Corps Base Camp Pendleton
Camp Pendleton, California
Contractor, General Dynamics Health Solutions
Fairfax, Virginia

Jessica Stumbo, MD, CAQSM
Associate Professor of Medicine
University of Louisville, Department of Family and Geriatric Medicine
Program Director, University of Louisville Primary Care Sports Medicine Fellowship
Team Physician, University of Louisville
Louisville, Kentucky

James Suchy, MD
Primary Care Sports Medicine Fellow
Department of Family Medicine
Oregon Health & Science University
Portland, Oregon

Yaqoob Syed, DO
Sports Medicine Fellow
Presence Resurrection Sports Medicine Fellowship
Chicago, Illinois

Isaac P. Syrop, MD
Assistant Professor, Department of Rehabilitation and Regenerative Medicine
Columbia University School of Medicine
New York, New York

Adrian Tabares, MD, CAQSM
Family Medicine, Sports Medicine
Crossover Health
Menlo Park, California

Kenneth S. Taylor, MD, FAAFP, CAQSM
Clinical Professor of Family Medicine/Sports Medicine
University of California, San Diego, School of Medicine
Chief, Primary Care Sports Medicine
Director, UCSD Primary Care Sports Medicine Fellowship
Head Primary Care Sports Physician, San Diego Padres
Head Team Physician UCSD Tritons, San Diego Sockers
Team Physician U.S. Olympic Training Center; San Diego Seals Professional Lacrosse
San Diego, California

Johnny Tenegra, MD, MS
Assistant Professor, Family and Community Medicine
Southern Illinois University School of Medicine
Decatur Family Medicine Residency
Decatur, Illinois

Timothy Tiu, MD, FAAPMR, CAQSM
Assistant Professor
Sports Medicine
Department of Rehabilitation Medicine
Montefiore Medical Center
Albert Einstein College of Medicine
Bronx, New York

Christopher C. Trigger, MD, FACEP, CAQSM
Clinical Assistant Professor of Emergency Medicine
Michigan State University College of Osteopathic Medicine
Core Faculty and Research Director
Lakeland Health Emergency Medicine Residency, an Affiliate of MSUCOM
Co-Founder and Medical Director
Great Lakes Sports Medicine and Concussion Clinic
Saint Joseph, Michigan

Thomas Trojian, MD†
Director
Sports Medicine Fellowship
Chief
Division of Sports Medicine
Professor
Department of Family, Community and Preventative Medicine
Chief Medical Officer
Drexel Athletics
Drexel University College of Medicine
Philadelphia, Pennsylvania

Priscilla Tu, DO, FAAFP, FAOASM, DABMA
Director of Osteopathic Education
Carilion Clinic—Virginia Tech Carilion Family Medicine Residency Program
Assistant Professor of Family Medicine
Virginia Tech Carilion School of Medicine
Assistant Professor of Family Medicine
Edward Via College of Osteopathic Medicine—Virginia
Director of Student Medical Education
Edward Via College of Osteopathic Medicine—Roanoke
Head Team Physician, Northside Vikings
Team Physician, USA Volleyball
Roanoke, Virginia

Amity Tung, MD
BS in Physiological Science
San Diego, California

Philipp J. Underwood, MD, FAAEM, FACEP, FAAFP, CAQSM, RDMS
Assistant Professor of Emergency Medicine
Hofstra—Northwell School of Medicine
Program Director, Sports Medicine Fellowship
North Shore University Hospital
Manhasset, New York

Saif Usman, MD, FAAFP, CAQSM
Primary Care Sports Medicine
Facey Medical Group
Valencia, California

Jean Pierre Valette, MD
Family Medicine Resident Physician
University of California, San Diego School of Medicine
San Diego, California

Gerardo Vazquez, MD, CAQSM
Assistant Program Director
Texas Tech University Health Sciences Center El Paso Sports Medicine Fellowship
El Paso, Texas

Kenneth Vitale, MD, FAAPMR
Associate Professor, Department of Orthopaedic Surgery
Physical Medicine and Rehabilitation
Subspecialty Certification in Sports Medicine
University of California San Diego School of Medicine
San Diego, California

Natalie Voskanian, MD
Associate Clinical Professor
Department of Orthopaedic Surgery
University of California, San Diego Sports Medicine
San Diego, California

Bryant Walrod, MD, CAQSM
Assistant Professor, Clinical
Department of Family Medicine
Team Physician, Ohio State Buckeyes
Columbus, Ohio

David A. Wang, MD
Assistant Attending Physician
Primary Care Sports Medicine Service
Hospital for Special Surgery
Assistant Professor of Clinical Medicine
Weil Cornell Medical College
New York, New York

Kevin Waninger, MD, MS, FAAFP, FACEP, FACSM, CAQSM
Coordinated Health Sports Medicine
Allentown, Pennsylvania

Andrew M. Warner, MD
Clinical Staff, USA Family Medicine
Resident Physician
University of South Alabama
Mobile, Alabama

Anna L. Waterbrook, MD, FACEP, CAQSM†
Associate Professor
Department of Emergency Medicine
Associate Program Director, South Campus Residency Program
Associate Program Director, Sports Medicine Fellowship
Assistant Team Physician, Intercollegiate Athletics
The University of Arizona
Tucson, Arizona

Charles W. Webb, DO, FAAFP, CAQSM
Sports Medicine Physician
Legacy Medical Group
Portland, Oregon

Kathleen Weber, MD, MS†
Assistant Professor
Rush University Medical Center
Midwest Orthopaedics at Rush
Director, Primary Care Sports Medicine
Director, Primary Care Sports Medicine Fellowship
Team Physician, Chicago Bulls, Chicago White Sox, DePaul University, Malcolm X College
Company Physician, Hubbard Street Dance and Chicago Luvabulls
Chicago, Illinois

William H. West, MD†
Graduate, School of Medicine
University of Tennessee Health Science Center
Knoxville Campus
Knoxville, Tennessee

Nancy White, MD†
Program Director
Henry Ford Health System
Departments of Orthopedics and Family Medicine
Primary Care Sports Medicine Fellowship
Detroit, Michigan
Team Physician, Lawrence Tech University, Cranbrook-Kingswood Schools, U.S. Figure Skating

Elizabeth A. Williams, DO
Team Physician, San Diego State University, University of San Diego
San Diego, California

Kristina Wilson, MD, MPH, FAAP, CAQSM
Medical Director, Pediatric and Adolescent Sports Medicine
Phoenix Children's Hospital
Co-Medical Director, Brain Injury and Concussion Program
Barrow Neurologic Institute at Phoenix Children's Hospital
Clinical Assistant Professor, Department of Child Health
The University of Arizona School of Medicine—Phoenix
Phoenix, Arizona

Jason P. Womack, MD†
Assistant Professor
Director, Sports Medicine Fellowship
Assistant Team Physician, Rutgers Athletics
Department of Family Medicine and Community Health
Rutgers Robert Wood Johnson Medical School
New Brunswick, New Jersey

Justin M. Wright, MD, CAQSM
Associate Professor
Program Director, Family Medicine Residency Program
Program Director, Sports Medicine Fellowship Program
Department of Family and Community Medicine
Texas Tech University Health Sciences Center El Paso
Team Physician, UTEP Miners
El Paso, Texas

Jarrod Yamanaka, MD
Fairview Sports and Orthopedic Care
Orthopedics and Sports Medicine
Fairview Health Services
Minneapolis, Minnesota

Michael Y. Yang, MD
Sports Medicine Physician
Department of Orthopedics
Mercy Philadelphia Hospital
Philadelphia, Pennsylvania

Ramon Ylanan, MD, CAQSM†
Head Team Physician, University of Arkansas Razorbacks
Assistant Professor, Family and Preventative Medicine
Program Director, Primary Care Sports Medicine Fellowship
University of Arkansas for Medical Science Northwest Campus
Fayetteville, Arkansas

Craig C. Young, MD
Professor of Orthopaedic Surgery and Community & Family Medicine
Medical College of Wisconsin
Team Physician, Milwaukee Brewers, Milwaukee Bucks, U.S. Ski & Snowboard
Company Physician, Milwaukee Ballet, Skylight Opera
Milwaukee, Wisconsin

Warren Young, MD, FAAP
Assistant Attending Physician
Primary Care Sports Medicine
Hospital for Special Surgery
New York, New York

Eric Yuan, MD
Resident Physician of Family Medicine
University of California, School of Medicine
San Diego, California

Jason L. Zaremski, MD, CAQSM, FAAPMR, FACSM
Assistant Professor, Divisions of PM&R, Sports Medicine, and Research
Department of Orthopaedics and Rehabilitation
Co-Medical Director Adolescent and High School Sports Medicine Outreach Program
University of Florida College of Medicine
Gainesville, Florida

Carrie Zaslow, MD[†]
Ophthalmologist
Draga Eye Care
Bayside, New York
Assistant Clinical Professor
Hofstra University School of Medicine
Long Island, New York

Tracy Zaslow, MD, FAAP, CAQSM
Children's Orthopaedic Center (COC) at Children's Hospital Los Angeles
Medical Director, CHLA Sports Medicine Program
Director, CHLA Sports Concussion Program
Assistant Professor, University of Southern California
Team Physician, LA Galaxy
Los Angeles, California

Roman Zolotoy, DO
Pain Medicine Fellow
Baystate Health
Springfield, Massachusetts

[†] *The views expressed are those of the authors and do not reflect the official policy of the Department of the Army, Department of the Navy, Department of the Air Force, the Department of Defense, or the United States Government.*

SECOND EDITION AUTHOR ACKNOWLEDGMENTS

The editors and authors of the third edition gratefully acknowledge the past contributions of the following previous edition authors:

Adam Abdulally
Safdar Akbar
Keith A. Anderson
Chad A. Asplund
Elizabeth Austin
James Bales
Karrn Bales
Tricia Beatty
Clint Beaver
Brent R. Becker
Jonathan A. Becker
David T. Bernhardt
Krystian Bigosinski
Warren Bodine
Blake Boggess
Matthew P. Boyd
Robert Bramante
James E. Bray
Stacey L. Brown Brocklehurst
Steve Burdine
Michelle Burke
Seth M. Burkey
Matthew D. Capuano
Nick Carter
Kyle J. Cassas
Yvonne Chow
Christopher Cieurzo
Kristen Samuhel Clarey
Justin A. Classie
Kara D. Cox
Rafael daFonseca
Jeffrey W. R. Dassel
Matt DesJardins
Rajwinder Deu
Alex B. Diamond
Masha Diede
Martha A. Dodson
Jonathan Drezner
Anna Dumont
Kevin Eerkes
Kevin E. Elder
Benjamin D. England
Robyn Fean
David Z. Frankel
R. Michael Galbraith
Coley Gatlin
Nicole Y. Gesik
Andrew Getzin
Gordon Givan
Jason Glowney
Orlando V. Gonzalez
Alysia L. Green
Tanya J. Hagen
Andrew Harcourt
Natasha Harrison
Benjamin A. Hasan
Eugene Hong
Stephen Huang
Andrew Hunt
Nadim Ilbawi
Arthur Islas
Sandeep Johar
Matthew John
Christopher Johnson
Rob Johnson
Scott Fister Johnson
Pankaj Kaw
Roberta Kern
Thomas Kern
Jacklyn Kiefer
Jane Kim
Jeff Kindred
Kari Kindschi
Robert B. Kiningham
K. Michele Kirk
Michael A. Krafczyk
Jeffrey B. Kreher
Steve Kroll
Sebastian Ksionski
Michele LaBotz
Shanyn Lancaster
Adrian Lavina
Aaron Lee
Jason Lee
Jason M. Leinen
Aaron P. Leininger
Daniel Lewis
Brian Lindenmayer
Emily Lott
Brian Macy
Christopher C. Madden
Danielle L. Mahaffey
Navid Mahooti
Aaron V. Mares
Peter D. Marshall
Catharine Mayer

Jeffrey McDaniel
Emily C. McDevitt
Paul B. McKee
Dominic McKinley
Robert D. Menzies
Tara Merrit
Christopher D. Meyering
Mark H. Mirabelli
Jason Mogonye
Anna G. Monroe
Carter W. Muench
Vikram Narula
Rodolfo R. Navarro
Lisa Palazollo
Susan Park
Eric D. Parks
Matthew Pecci
K. Brooke Pengel
Jayson Pereira
Andrew R. Peterson
Deena C. Petrocelli
Thomas A. Phipps
Sourav K. Poddar
Mitchell Pratte
Catherine Rainbow
Neha P. Raukar
Steven G. Reece
Paul Reehal
L. Shay Richardson
Allen Richburg
Leland S. Rickman
James Robinson
Jorge O. Rodriguez
Daryl A. Rosenbaum
Jeffrey Rosenberg
Matt Roth
Mark Rowand
Cherise Russo
Tomoya Sakai
Bradley Sandella
Thomas Sargent
Michael Schettino
David A. Scott
Ramsey Shehab
John Shelton
Matthew D. Shores
Ian Shrier
Robby S. Sikka
David V. Smith
Dan Somogyi
Luke M. Spellman
Jason E. Spring
Harry Stafford
David A. Stone
Paul Stricker
Payal Sud
Tod Sweeney
Michael Devin Taylor
Todd Toriscelli
Verle Valentine
Jake Veigel
Nadya Volsky
Jason Wander
C. Thayer White
Russell D. White
John J. Wilson
Lauren Wood
Shannon Woods
Ronald Yee
Alan Zakaria

CONTENTS

ABDOMINAL MUSCLE STRAINS

Brittney M. Richardson, MD, CAQSM

BASICS

DESCRIPTION

Injury to the abdominal wall musculature, including the rectus abdominis, internal/external obliques, and transverse abdominis muscles:

- Typically a noncontact injury but may be caused by trauma
- Can be acute or subacute.
- Acute injury typically is the result of an abrupt movement of the trunk.
- Subacute injury caused by repetitive activity
- A specific variant known as a side strain most commonly involves the internal oblique at or near the inferior rib attachments.

EPIDEMIOLOGY

Somewhat uncommon injuries, but specific sports have a higher prevalence:

- Account for <2% of athletic injuries (1)
- Sports with repetitive trunk rotation have higher rates:
  - Soccer, tennis, baseball, ice hockey, gymnastics, pole vault, cricket, bowling (2)
- Seen in runners, because the abdominal muscles are used for pelvic stabilization
- Attributed to weight training and abdominal workouts as well

ETIOLOGY AND PATHOPHYSIOLOGY

Acute or chronic muscle-tendon injury of the abdominal wall musculature from a sudden intrinsic eccentric contraction of the abdominal musculature (3)

RISK FACTORS

- Poorly conditioned abdominal musculature or deficits in core strength
- Previous abdominal wall muscle strain/tear
- Poor weight training or conditioning techniques
- Participation in activities that require abrupt and/or repetitive movements of the torso early in the sport season

GENERAL PREVENTION

Appropriate weight training and conditioning techniques with attention to core strength

DIAGNOSIS

HISTORY

- Acute abdominal wall pain associated with stretching or twisting mechanism
- Chronic pain due to repetitive activity of the trunk or torso
- Direct trauma associated with a minority of these injuries
- Pain usually focal and exacerbated by specific movements or positions
- Pain with active contraction of affected muscle during sneezing or coughing
- Symptoms generally subside in the absence of activity.
- In throwing or overhead athletes typically on the side contralateral to the throwing arm, in baseball batters contralateral to the dominant batting side (4)

PHYSICAL EXAM

- Appearance is typically normal with swelling and evidence of contusion rare in the absence of preceding trauma.
- Splinting may be noted if pain is severe.
- Tenderness of the abdominal wall is usually focal and discrete but may be more diffuse in overuse injuries.
- Muscle defect may be notable if an associated tear or herniation is present.
- Peritoneal signs are absent.
- Symptoms are reproduced by contraction of the affected muscle.

DIFFERENTIAL DIAGNOSIS

- Abdominal wall contusion
- Abdominal wall hematoma:
  - Swelling, periumbilical contusion, and a mass with rigidity and/or guarding are signs of a rectus sheath hematoma.
- Abdominal wall hernia (umbilical, spigelian)
- Intra-abdominal injury (contusion, laceration, perforation)
- Intra-abdominal process (e.g., infection, mass)
- Iliac apophysitis
- Osteitis pubis

DIAGNOSTIC TESTS & INTERPRETATION

- Typically not indicated (5)[C]
- Plain films, computed tomographic (CT) scan indicated if there is concern for rib fracture or intra-abdominal process
- Magnetic resonance imaging (MRI) can be used to assess for muscle tear or to assess the extent of injury:
  - Reserved for more severe injuries
- Musculoskeletal ultrasound (US) can help confirm the diagnosis of muscle tear or hematoma and aid in clinical follow-up (3)[C].

TREATMENT

Acute treatment:

- Remove the athlete from the offending activity.
- Ice
- Compressive wrap
- Nonsteroidal anti-inflammatory drugs (NSAIDs) or acetaminophen PRN only
- Once pain subsides, a rehabilitation program may be initiated (1,6)[C].

MEDICATION

First Line

NSAIDs or acetaminophen:

- Avoid NSAIDs if there is concern for bleeding or hematoma.

Second Line

Low-dose opioids or muscle relaxants may be used for more severe injuries but are rarely needed. Use should be limited to 3 days.

ADDITIONAL THERAPIES

- Rehabilitation:
  - Assess abdominal muscle strength and core strength/stability.
  - Initiate a rehab program once pain has subsided:
    - Start with passive stretching.
    - Advance to strengthening activities as tolerated with isometrics starting 5 to 7 days; concentrics at day 12; and advancement to eccentrics, core strength, and plyometrics (4)[C].
    - Progress to sport-specific activities (1,6)[C].
- Modalities such as US or muscle stimulation may help alleviate symptoms.
- Thoracic spine mobilization may help restore unrestricted motion.
- Platelet-rich plasma injection at the site of injury may help improve pain relief and introduce growth factors to the injured muscle group (3)[C].
- Corticosteroid injection at the site of muscle tear/strain may be considered for acute pain relief or refractory cases.

SURGERY/OTHER PROCEDURES

Surgery may be necessary in cases of rectus sheath hematoma, hernia, or intra-abdominal process.

ONGOING CARE

FOLLOW-UP RECOMMENDATIONS

- The athlete may return to activity once pain subsides and he or she can engage in sport-specific activity.
- Side strain–type injury has been reported to take up to 30 days in some athletes.

PROGNOSIS

Overall prognosis for recovery is excellent:

- Duration of symptoms is variable and may persist for months.
- Recurrence rates are high (>20%).

REFERENCES

1. Johnson R. Abdominal wall injuries: rectus abdominis strains, oblique strains, rectus sheath hematoma. *Curr Sports Med Rep*. 2006;5(2):99–103.
2. Nealon AR, Cook JL. Trunk side strain has a high incidence in first-class cricket fast bowlers in Australia and England. *Clin J Sport Med*. 2018;28(3):284–288.
3. Dauty M, Menu P, Dubois C. Uncommon external abdominal oblique muscle strain in a professional soccer player: a case report. *BMC Research Notes*. 2017;7:684.
4. Nealon AR, Kountouris A, Cook JL. Side strain in sport: a narrative review of pathomechanics, diagnosis, imaging and management for the clinician. *J Sci Med Sport*. 2017;20(3):261–266.
5. Cartwright SL, Knudson MP. Diagnostic imaging of acute abdominal pain in adults. *Am Fam Physician*. 2015;91(7):452–459.
6. Maquirriain J, Ghisi JP, Kokalj AM. Rectus abdominis muscle strains in tennis players. *Br J Sports Med*. 2007;41(11):842–848.

CLINICAL PEARLS

- Athletes can return to play when there is minimal-to-no tenderness, normal muscle strength and stamina, and can perform sport-specific tasks.
- Usual duration of symptoms varies from weeks to months.

ACHILLES TENDINOPATHY

Craig C. Young, MD • Mark W. Niedfeldt, MD

BASICS

DESCRIPTION

- Achilles tendinitis is an overuse injury of the Achilles tendon that causes pain in the posterior calf and heel.
- Synonym(s): Achilles tendinosis; Achilles tendinopathy

EPIDEMIOLOGY

- Accounts for 6.5–18% of injuries in runners
- Accounts for up to 4% of patients in sports medicine clinics
- Most common site is midportion (80–90%); pure insertional is rare (5%).

Incidence

- Lifetime incidence in competitive athletes is estimated to be 24%.
- Athletes in running and jumping sports are especially at risk:
  - Lifetime incidence in competitive runners may be as high as 50%.

ETIOLOGY AND PATHOPHYSIOLOGY

- Higher risk areas:
  - Musculotendinous junction
  - The region of distal Achilles tendon that is 2 to 6 cm proximal to insertion. This is a region with a relative lack of mesotenon and intratendinous vessels.
- Tendinosis: Chronic degenerative condition is more common than tendinitis, which is an inflammatory condition.
- Disruption of normal tendon architecture:
  - Chronic intratendinous degeneration, collagen disorientation, and increases in mucoid ground substance
  - Neovascularization and increase in sympathetic nerve ingrowth around the ventral surface of the Achilles tendon

RISK FACTORS

- Training errors: recent increase in distance, intensity, or length of activity
- Worn and/or old shoes
- Inflexibility, especially tight heel cords
- Higher body mass index (BMI)
- Hypertension
- Diabetes
- Hypothyroidism
- Older patients: decreased tensile strength and increased stiffness of tendon
- Malalignment of the leg (excessive genu valgum, external tibial torsion) or ankle/foot (pes planus)
- Medications:
  - Fluoroquinolones: Recent use of these antibiotics has been associated with increased risk for Achilles tendinopathy and rupture.
  - Glucocorticoids
  - Aromatase inhibitors
  - Statins have been theorized to cause tendinopathy and have been shown in some animal models.

COMMONLY ASSOCIATED CONDITIONS

- Retrocalcaneal bursitis
- Posterior ankle impingement syndrome
- Superficial Achilles bursitis ("pump bump" or Haglund deformity)
- Achilles tendon rupture: Chronic changes in tendon may predispose to rupture.

DIAGNOSIS

HISTORY

- Pain that initially subsides with use but returns with continued use or after use suggests an overuse injury.
- Morning stiffness is a hallmark of Achilles tendinitis.
- Training errors are a factor in a large percentage of cases.
- Worn or old shoes: Shoes need to be changed every 250 to 500 miles because of shoe padding breakdown:
  - Older shoes, even new, unused shoes, may have decreased shock absorption from age-related breakdown of the shock-absorbing materials.
- Patients may report weakness and intermittent swelling.

PHYSICAL EXAM

- Pain and stiffness 2 to 6 cm above Achilles tendon insertion
- Pain with running, especially sprinting
- Tenderness over the distal Achilles tendon (2 to 6 cm above the insertion):
  - Tenderness near insertion suggests insertional Achilles tendinopathy (enthesopathy) or bursitis.
- Thickening of distal Achilles tendon in chronic cases
- Tenderness with resisted plantar flexion
- Weakness with repetitive single leg heel raises
- Crepitus with ankle motion
- Negative Simmonds-Thompson test: Compression of the calf will cause normal passive plantar flexion of the foot:
  - A positive test (absence of plantar flexion with calf compression) suggests complete Achilles tendon rupture.
- Decreased ankle dorsiflexion (from tight heel cord)

DIFFERENTIAL DIAGNOSIS

- Retrocalcaneal bursitis
- Superficial Achilles bursitis
- Calcaneal apophysitis (Sever condition) in adolescents
- Haglund deformity: prominent superior tuberosity of calcaneus
- Achilles tendon rupture
- Gastrocsoleus tear
- Plantaris tendinopathy
- Overuse myositis
- Chronic exertional compartment syndrome
- Os trigonum irritation or posterior ankle impingement syndrome
- Vascular/neurogenic claudication
- Deep venous thrombosis
- Hematoma
- Infection

DIAGNOSTIC TESTS & INTERPRETATION

- Not usually needed for initial evaluation. X-rays should be obtained if other potential injuries are suspected (e.g., fracture or tumor) or if injury is not responding to appropriate treatment.
- Standard ankle series (anteroposterior, lateral, and mortise) may show calcification of tendon; however, presence of calcification does not affect initial treatment.
- Ultrasound:
  - Hypoechoic regions, intratendinous calcifications, disorganization of fibers, fusiform expansion, intrasubstance/partial-thickness tears, and neovascularization may be seen with Achilles tendinopathy:
    - Degenerative changes may be seen in ~60% of healthy uninjured persons:
      - Higher activity individuals are more likely to have changes.
      - Studies have shown that these abnormalities are related to an increased risk of future tendinopathy (1)[A], but that resolution of these changes is not necessarily related to resolution of symptoms (2)[B].
    - Neovascularization at baseline does not predict clinical outcome of nonoperative treatment.
- MRI shows thickening of the tendon with intratendinous changes.

TREATMENT

GENERAL MEASURES

- Relative rest: Especially eliminate sprinting, speed work, and running hills or stairs. Overall decrease in running intensity, duration, and/or frequency.
- Ice after activity; proper warm-up prior to activity
- Use properly fitted, activity-appropriate shoes.
- Stretching: Ensure athlete is on appropriate conditioning program, preactivity warm-up, and postactivity cool-down programs.
- Strengthening: Include a gastrocnemius and soleus strengthening program with emphasis on eccentric exercises.

MEDICATION

- Nonsteroidal anti-inflammatory drugs (NSAIDs): may be useful as an adjunct for pain control particularly in cases of acute injury
- Nitric oxide via topical nitroglycerin particularly for noninsertional chronic Achilles tendinopathy
- Injections:
  - Autologous blood or platelet-rich plasma: theoretically makes the environment of fibroblasts more conducive to healing (3)[B]
  - Injection of sclerosing agents to destroy the sensory nerves that travel with the blood vessels of neovascularization
  - Avoid injection of cortisone into the Achilles tendon because of risk of rupture.

ISSUES FOR REFERRAL

Consider referral for surgical débridement for individuals whose symptoms have not responded to 3 to 6 or more months of nonoperative treatment.

- Minimally invasive techniques result in clinical outcomes equivalent to traditional open techniques but with lower complications (4)[A].

ADDITIONAL THERAPIES

- Short-term immobilization (7 to 10 days) with walking boot for severe acute symptoms or recalcitrant symptoms:
  - Alternatively, a heel lift (or high-heeled shoes):
    - Use of heel lifts or high heels often can acutely decrease symptoms. However, chronic use of these devices may increase risk of developing symptoms in the future.
- Night splints may also be useful in patients with recalcitrant symptoms; physical therapy with emphasis on lower extremity flexibility and gastrocsoleus strengthening:
  - Progression to eccentric exercise programs has been shown to shorten time to return to full activity.
  - Aggressive or instrument-assisted soft tissue mobilization: techniques thought to break up scar tissue and stimulate healing (5)[B]
- Gait retraining: Consider converting forefoot strikers to rearfoot strikers.
- Modalities: Although some studies have shown that these modalities are useful in returning an athlete to activity sooner, they also show no long-term benefit:
  - Ultrasound
  - Low-level laser therapy: thought to modulate inflammation and regeneration of collagen
- Orthotics or arch supports may be useful in patients with pes planus and those who overpronate.
- Extracorporeal shock wave therapy: thought to induce neovascularization and a new inflammatory process that leads to tissue healing (6)[B]

ONGOING CARE

- Gradual return to activity: gradual increase in running intensity, duration, and/or frequency. General rule of thumb is no >10% increase per week.
- New shoes: Avoid shoes with high heel counters or other structures that place pressure over irritated area. Running shoes should be changed every 250 to 500 miles.

REFERENCES

1. McAuliffe S, McCreesh K, Culloty F, et al. Can ultrasound imaging predict the development of Achilles and patellar tendinopathy? A systematic review and meta-analysis. *Br J Sports Med*. 2016;50(24):1516–1523.
2. de Jonge S, Tol JL, Weir A, et al. The tendon structure returns to asymptomatic values in nonoperatively treated Achilles tendinopathy but is not associated with symptoms: a prospective study. *Am J Sports Med*. 2015;43(12):2950–2958.
3. Guelfi M, Pantalone A, Vanni D, et al. Long-term beneficial effects of platelet-rich plasma for non-insertional Achilles tendinopathy. *J Foot Ankle Surg*. 2015;21(3):178–181.
4. Baltes TPA, Zwiers R, Wiegerinck JI, et al. Surgical treatment for midportion Achilles tendinopathy: a systematic review. *Knee Surg Sports Traumatol Arthrosc*. 2017;25(6):1817–1838.
5. McCormack JR, Underwood FB, Slaven EJ, et al. Eccentric exercise versus eccentric exercise and soft tissue treatment (Astym) in the management of insertional Achilles tendinopathy. *Sports Health*. 2016;8(3):230–237.
6. Taylor J, Dunkerley S, Silver D, et al. Extracorporeal shockwave therapy (ESWT) for refractory Achilles tendinopathy: a prospective audit with 2-year follow up. *Foot (Edinb)*. 2016;26:23–29.

ADDITIONAL READING

- Gerdesmeyer L, Mittermayr R, Fuerst M, et al. Current evidence of extracorporeal shock wave therapy in chronic Achilles tendinopathy. *Int J Surg*. 2015;24(Pt B):154–159.
- Habets B, van Cingel RE. Eccentric exercise training in chronic mid-portion Achilles tendinopathy: a systematic review on different protocols. *Scand J Med Sci Sports*. 2015;25(1):3–15.
- Holmes GB, Lin J. Etiologic factors associated with symptomatic Achilles tendinopathy. *Foot Ankle Int*. 2006;27(11):952–959.
- Kirchgesner T, Larbi A, Omoumi P, et al. Drug-induced tendinopathy: from physiology to clinical applications. *Joint Bone Spine*. 2014;81(6):485–492.
- Krogh TP, Ellingsen T, Christensen R, et al. Ultrasound-guided injection therapy of Achilles tendinopathy with platelet-rich plasma or saline: a randomized, blinded, placebo-controlled trial. *Am J Sports Med*. 2016;44(8):1990–1997.
- Lohrer H, David S, Nauck T. Surgical treatment for Achilles tendinopathy—a systematic review. *BMC Musculoskelet Disord*. 2016;17:207.
- McClinton S, Luedke L, Clewley D. Nonsurgical management of midsubstance Achilles tendinopathy. *Clin Podiatr Med Surg*. 2017;34(2):137–160.
- Nicol AM, McCurdie I, Etherington J. Use of ultrasound to identify chronic Achilles tendinosis in an active asymptomatic population. *J R Army Med Corps*. 2006;152(4):212–216.
- Paoloni JA, Murrell GA. Three-year follow-up study of topical glyceryl trinitrate treatment of chronic noninsertional Achilles tendinopathy. *Foot Ankle Int*. 2007;28(10):1064–1068.
- Sadoghi P, Rosso C, Valderrabano V, et al. The role of platelets in the treatment of Achilles tendon injuries. *J Orthop Res*. 2013;31(1):111–118.
- Scott LA, Munteanu SE, Menz HB. Effectiveness of orthotic devices in the treatment of Achilles tendinopathy: a systematic review. *Sports Med*. 2015;45(1):95–110.
- Smith WB, Melton W, Davies J. Midsubstance tendinopathy, percutaneous techniques (platelet-rich plasma, extracorporeal shock wave therapy, prolotherapy, radiofrequency ablation). *Clin Podiatr Med Surg*. 2017;34(2):161–174.
- Sode J, Obel N, Hallas J, et al. Use of fluroquinolone and risk of Achilles tendon rupture: a population-based cohort study. *Eur J Clin Pharmacol*. 2007;63(5):499–503.
- Stergioulas A, Stergioula M, Aarskog R, et al. Effects of low-level laser therapy and eccentric exercises in the treatment of recreational athletes with chronic Achilles tendinopathy. *Am J Sports Med*. 2008;36(5):881–887.
- Zwiers R, Wiegerinck JI, van Dijk CN. Treatment of midportion Achilles tendinopathy: an evidence-based overview. *Knee Surg Sports Traumatol Arthrosc*. 2016;24(7):2003–2011.

CLINICAL PEARLS

- Because of the high stresses placed on the Achilles tendon with weight-bearing activities and the risk of rupture, corticosteroid injection into the Achilles tendon should be avoided.
- Categorization of the problem into paratendinopathy, insertional tendinopathy, or midportion tendinopathy may be helpful in guiding treatment decisions.
- A walking boot, night splint, or heel lift may be useful for pain relief especially in cases of acute injury.

ACHILLES TENDON RUPTURE

Carrie A. Jaworski, MD, FAAFP, FACSM • Melissa Faubert, DO

BASICS

- Achilles tendon ruptures are caused by laceration or by indirect forces applied to the tendon.
- Three types of indirect forces have been described:
  - Pushing off with the weight-bearing forefoot while extending the knee, such as with sprint starts and the push off in basketball
  - Sudden, unexpected dorsiflexion of the ankle, as when the foot slips in a hole
  - Violent dorsiflexion of a plantarflexed foot, as with a fall from a height

DESCRIPTION

- Achilles tendon rupture is a complete disruption of the Achilles tendon, usually occurring 2 to 6 cm proximal to its calcaneal insertion, where blood supply is the poorest.
- It can be associated with preexisting tendon degeneration and microtrauma.
- It most commonly occurs in 30- to 40-yr-old men.
- Synonym(s): heel-cord rupture; Achilles tear

EPIDEMIOLOGY

- >75% of Achilles tendon ruptures occur in patients 30 to 40 yr old while they partake in sports activities.
- Males > females: Ratio ranges from 1.7:1 to 19:1.
- Left Achilles > right Achilles: thought to be due to higher prevalence of right-side dominant individuals using left lower limb to push off during activity
- Yearly incidence is around 2 in 10,000.

ETIOLOGY AND PATHOPHYSIOLOGY

- Is the largest tendon in the human body and is designed to endure stresses up to 10 times the body's weight
- Is formed by the confluence of the tendons of the gastrocnemius and soleus muscles. The gastrocnemius medial and lateral heads originate from the medial and lateral femoral condyles, respectively. The soleus originates from a large attachment on the posterior tibia and fibula. Together, these tendons insert onto the calcaneus and form the Achilles tendon.
- Receives its blood supply intrinsically from both the musculotendinous junction and the osteotendinous insertion site
- Additional vascular supply comes from an external source known as the paratenon. The paratenon is a thin layer of areolar tissue that encases the Achilles tendon. The further the tendon is from its musculotendinous origin and calcaneal insertion, the more it relies on the paratenon for vascular support.
- The area with the poorest vascular supply is ~2 to 6 cm proximal to the calcaneal insertion site.
- Prior to inserting into the calcaneus, the Achilles tendon internally rotates, which imparts a structural torque stress in the tendon. This is thought to contribute to decreased vascularity in the tendon and ensuing tendon failure.

RISK FACTORS

- Disease processes: connective tissue disorders, seronegative spondylopathies, rheumatoid arthritis, collagen vascular disease, diabetes mellitus, gout, hyperparathyroidism, renal insufficiency, hypothyroidism

ALERT

Medications: Anabolic steroids or prolonged oral corticosteroid as well as fluoroquinolone antimicrobial usage leads to degradation of collagen fibrils and decreased Achilles tendon strength. Corticosteroid injections weaken tendon structure.

- Disuse atrophy and sedentary lifestyle
- Prolonged immobilization
- Advanced age
- History of Achilles tendonitis/tendinosis, regardless of history of injection therapy
- Mechanical imbalances (i.e., decreased flexibility of gastrocnemius-soleus complex)
- Body weight/obesity
- Possibility of genetic predisposition (possibility of association with human leukocyte antigen [HLA]-B27, blood group 0)

DIAGNOSIS

HISTORY

- Patients commonly report feeling as if they have been kicked or struck in the back of the heel, only to find no one is nearby.
- May feel or hear a "pop" or snap
- Pain with weight-bearing
- Weakness or stiffness of posterior ankle
- May give history of chronic Achilles tendinitis with or without history of injection therapy

PHYSICAL EXAM

- Acute complete rupture of the Achilles tendon involves a sudden, sharp pain behind the ankle, usually associated with a painful, palpable defect in the tendon.
- Swelling and/or ecchymosis
- "Hatchet strike" defect: palpable, tender defect, usually 2 to 6 cm from the tendon insertion site
- Positive Thompson test is diagnostic. Have patient lie prone or kneel with ankles clear of the table. Perform on uninvolved side first for comparison. Squeeze bulk of calf muscle and observe for plantar flexion. Absence of plantar flexion is consistent with complete tendon rupture (sensitivity 0.96, specificity 0.93) (1).

ALERT

Note that for the Achilles to function normally, only 25% of the fibers are needed; therefore, partial tears may be missed on manual examination.

- Plantar flexion strength and ability to toe rise may be decreased compared to unaffected side.
- Passive dorsiflexion may be increased compared to unaffected side.
- These signs may be absent because of recruitment of other intact muscles, such as tibialis posterior, plantaris, peroneus longus and brevis, and flexor digitorum and hallucis longus.

DIAGNOSTIC TESTS & INTERPRETATION

- Routine plain films should be obtained to avoid missing a calcaneal avulsion rupture, which would require surgical treatment. This finding usually can be appreciated on the lateral ankle radiograph.
- Ultrasound (US) and magnetic resonance imaging (MRI) should be reserved for when the diagnosis of a complete rupture is questionable or if one is considering a partial tear.

DIFFERENTIAL DIAGNOSIS

- Achilles tendinitis
- Ankle sprain
- Peritendinitis
- Retrocalcaneal bursitis
- Superficial Achilles bursitis
- Periostitis
- Plantar tendon rupture
- Calcaneal avulsion

TREATMENT

- Analgesia should be based on the patient's degree of pain.
- Rest, ice, compression, and elevation (RICE) should be used in the initial treatment of complete and partial tears.

- Controversy in the literature exists as to the best treatment approach for Achilles tendon rupture.
- Careful patient selection is based on the patient's activity level and goals.
- Nonoperative treatment:
  - Fewer complications than surgery (infection, risk of deep vein thrombosis [DVT]) (2,3,4)[A]
  - Nonoperative treatment is targeted to ruptures with <1 cm of gapping on US examination.
  - Partial tears, or a tear in continuity diagnosed by MRI, also treated conservatively
  - Traditionally, nonoperative treatment was almost exclusively used by older, more sedentary patients, or those with medical contraindications to surgery. Now more young, active people are undergoing nonoperative treatment with comparable results.
  - Older studies show risk of rerupture greater than with surgical repair: 10–12% for nonsurgical versus 1–3% for surgical repair (5)[A].

ALERT
Early weight-bearing and range of motion have improved outcomes and decreased risk of rerupture in randomized control trials, equivalent to that of operative repair (2,3,4,5)[A].

ALERT
When early functional rehabilitation was not used, surgical repair reduced the absolute rerupture rate by 8.8% (number needed to treat [NNT] = 12) (2)[A].

  - The option exists to use a functional dorsal block splint that restricts dorsiflexion and gradually increases the amount of plantar flexion. Functional splints have been shown to help prevent gastrocnemius atrophy, quicker return to full dorsiflexion, and better tolerance by patients.

ADDITIONAL THERAPIES

ALERT
Both treatment approaches should be followed by a well-outlined rehabilitation program.

- Advances in therapy should be supervised by the treating physician.
- Cardiovascular fitness during treatment can be sustained through arm ergometer use, then recumbent cycling once no longer using crutches.
- Once the cast is removed (nonoperative treatment), active movement is initiated with the knee bent to 90 degrees; wound care and edema reduction is administered if patient underwent surgical treatment.
- Progress to passive movement, but focus on limiting maximum stretch on the tendon as to not let ankle progress past neutral for at least 12 to 16 wk (1)[A].
- Slowly start strength exercises with isometrics, then progress to resisted range of motion exercises.
- To restore functional activity, progress to closed kinetic chain exercises focusing on eccentric gastrocnemius strength.

SURGERY/OTHER PROCEDURES

Open repair or closed, percutaneous technique:
- Associated with a lower incidence of rerupture compared to nonoperative with no early functional training
- Increased restoration of calf strength/less loss of push-off power (4,6)[A]
- Surgical complications can include infection, DVT, pulmonary embolism, and death (3,5)[A].
- Other postoperative risks include delayed healing, scar adhesions, infection, persistent equinus, overlengthening, and fistulas and sural nerve injury in percutaneous techniques.
- Usually recommended for high-level athletes, those returning to high-risk activities (basketball, tennis, soccer, and sprinting), and for treatment of rerupture

ONGOING CARE

FOLLOW-UP RECOMMENDATIONS

Return to activity guidelines in nonoperative treatment with functional rehabilitation available (1)[A]:
- 0 to 2 wk: equinus cast in 15 to 20 degrees plantar flexion and non–weight-bearing with crutches
- 2 to 6 wk: removable controlled ankle motion (CAM) boot with 1- to 2-inch heel lift. Partial weight-bearing with crutches progressing to full weight-bearing as tolerated (WBAT) by week 4. Boot should be removed for active unrestricted plantar flexion and dorsiflexion to neutral.
- 6 to 8 wk: full weight-bearing in the boot. Decrease heel lift by 25% each week. Start resisted plantar flexion exercises with resistance bands, gentle dorsiflexion stretching with belt.
- 8 to 12 wk: Discontinue boot 1 wk after ambulation with no heel lift; physical therapist to guide patient through strengthening, range of motion, and proprioception
- 16 wk: Start run–walk program, and continue strengthening.
- 6 mo: Return to full activity.

REFERENCES

1. Cooper MT. Acute Achilles tendon ruptures: does surgery offer superior results (and other confusing issues)? *Clin Sports Med*. 2015;34(4):595–606.
2. Soroceanu A, Sidhwa F, Aarabi S, et al. Surgical versus nonsurgical treatment of acute Achilles tendon rupture: a meta-analysis of randomized trials. *J Bone Joint Surg Am*. 2012;94(23):2136–2143.
3. Zhang H, Tang H, He Q, et al. Surgical versus conservative intervention for acute Achilles tendon rupture: a PRISMA-compliant systematic review of overlapping meta-analyses. *Medicine (Baltimore)*. 2015;94(45):e1951.
4. Jiang N, Wang B, Chen A, et al. Operative versus nonoperative treatment for acute Achilles tendon rupture: a meta-analysis based on current evidence. *Int Orthop*. 2012;36(4):765–773.
5. Willits K, Amendola A, Bryant D, et al. Operative versus nonoperative treatment of acute Achilles tendon ruptures: a multicenter randomized trial using accelerated functional rehabilitation. *J Bone Joint Surg Am*. 2010;92(17):2767–2775.
6. Nilsson-Helander K, Silbernagel KG, Thomeé R, et al. Acute Achilles tendon rupture: a randomized, controlled study comparing surgical and nonsurgical treatments using validated outcome measures. *Am J Sports Med*. 2010;38(11):2186–2193.

ADDITIONAL READING

Pedowitz D, Kirwan G. Achilles tendon ruptures. *Curr Rev Musculoskelet Med*. 2013;6(4):285–293.

CLINICAL PEARLS

- New literature is emerging suggesting nonoperative treatment with early functional rehabilitation has similar rerupture rates to surgical treatment; however, overall power is reduced by about 10% with nonoperative treatment.
- Nonoperative treatment has less complication overall compared to surgery.
- Early weight-bearing and range of motion are preferred for ruptures <1 cm, but it is best to discuss surgical treatment approaches with your local sports medicine or orthopedic group to determine their philosophy.

ACL INJURIES

Suraj A. Achar, MD, FAAFP, CAQSM • Kenneth S. Taylor, MD, FAAFP, CAQSM

BASICS

DESCRIPTION

- The anterior cruciate ligament (ACL) is a critical stabilizer of the knee.
- The ACL provides stability against anterior translation of the knee and is a secondary stabilizer of tibial rotation.
- The ACL has two important bundles: The posterolateral bundle is tight in extension, whereas the anteromedial bundle is tight in flexion.
- ACL tears can occur with trauma but occur more often with noncontact hyperextension or twisting injuries (1)[B],(2,3).

EPIDEMIOLOGY

- The ACL is the most commonly injured knee ligament accounting for almost half of knee injuries in sport.
- An estimated 200,000 ACL injuries occur annually in the United States with ~100,000 ACL reconstructions.
- The incidence of ACL injury is greater in active adults and children participating in cutting sports such as basketball, football, skiing, soccer, and gymnastics.
- Female gender confers higher risk. A meta-analysis in 2007 noted a roughly 3 to 4 times greater incidence of ACL tears in female gymnastics, soccer and basketball players versus male athletes. Year-round female athletes who play soccer and basketball have an ACL tear rate approaching 5% (2)[A].

RISK FACTORS

- High-risk sports and female gender are the primary risk factors for ACL injuries (1)[B]:
  - ~70% of ACL injuries occur in the high-risk sports, such as football (i.e., soccer), American football, basketball, volleyball, gymnastics, and downhill skiing.
  - Female risk factors being evaluated include differences in quadriceps-dominant deceleration, > valgus knee angulation with pivoting, decelerating or landing, different strength-to-weight ratios, joint laxity, and muscle recruitment patterns. The role of the notch index or Q angle is controversial.
  - Kinematics and electromyography studies suggest that females prepare for landing with decreased hip and knee flexion, increased quadriceps activation, and decreased hamstring activation, which may result in increased ACL loading and injury. An exception of the relative muscle weakness is female dancers who sustain relatively fewer ACL tears than their field counterparts.
- Factors that increase traction have been associated with a higher incidence of ACL tears:
  - Early studies of artificial turf ("Astroturf") in the National Football League noted an increased risk.
  - Cleats that have a predominant grip on the periphery may also increase the risk, especially when used with artificial turf.

GENERAL PREVENTION

- Neuromuscular training programs:
  - A recent analysis of ACL prevention programs demonstrated a significant effect of neuromuscular training programs on ACL incidence in athletes ($p < .0001$). Authors note risk of publication bias. The reviewers noted the following (3)[B]:
    - Studies that incorporated high-intensity plyometrics reduced ACL risk, whereas the studies that failed to use this regimen did not reduce ACL injuries.
    - Training sessions need to be performed at least 3 times a week and should last 15 to 20 min or longer.
    - Duration: minimum of 6 wk
    - Plyometrics, feedback on landing, balance, static stretching and strengthening exercises all need to be incorporated into a comprehensive training protocol.
- Bracing:
  - Bracing has been used to reduce knee injuries in American football for many years.
  - Randomized and observational studies suggest that prophylactic bracing does not prevent ACL tears or reduce re-tears in ACL reconstructed knees.

COMMONLY ASSOCIATED CONDITIONS

- Injuries to the medial and lateral meniscus are commonly associated with an ACL tear.
- ~50% of ACL injuries are associated with meniscal tears (most often lateral initially and medial when the ACL injury is chronic).
- Chondral and subchondral injuries are often noted.

DIAGNOSIS

HISTORY

- Many patients with an ACL tear feel a "pop" in their knee, followed by an acute swelling of the knee within hours.
- In the absence of bony trauma, an immediate effusion is believed to have a strong correlation with an ACL injury of some degree.
- Symptoms of an ACL-deficient knee include feeling of "giving out" and instability aggravated by squatting, pivoting, and stepping laterally or bearing the entire body weight when walking down stairs.

PHYSICAL EXAM

- If evaluated within 12 hr of an acute injury, the athlete will have difficulty bearing weight and will have an effusion.
- Loss of full knee extension can occur when an ACL stump gets caught in the intercondylar notch, an associated bucket meniscal tear is present, or a loose body fragment gets stuck.
- Examination should begin with inspection to look for an effusion and examination of the uninjured knee.
- Palpation of bony structures is important to evaluate for associated tibial plateau fractures or growth plate injuries in the case of growing adolescents.
- Palpation of the joint line is critical to evaluate for meniscal tears or medial collateral ligament (MCL) injuries.
- Valgus stress testing can be of further help in evaluating the MCL.
- Specific tests to determine an ACL tear include the Lachman test, the pivot shift, the anterior drawer test, and the flexion-rotation drawer examination:

ALERT

The anterior drawer test was found to be only 50% positive, especially if the posterior horn of the medial meniscus is intact. It is important to first examine for posterior translation, which can occur with a PCL injury.

  - The flexion-rotation drawer/pivot shift examination is performed by cradling the calf and flexing the knee. A posteriorly directed force on the tibia will cause reduction of the tibia as the femur rotates from an externally rotated position.
  - The pivot shift test, although useful, is often painful and leads to guarding.
  - The Lachman test is an accurate predictor of anterior cruciate injury. The sensitivity of this test decreases with hemarthrosis, guarding, and experience of the performer but is still reported to have a pooled sensitivity of 85%. One key to using the Lachman test is to first examine the uninjured side for comparison. Patients may have increased laxity that is not pathologic (4)[A].
  - The Lachman test should be the first special test performed for evaluation of a possible ACL-injured athlete. Performance of the test is described below:
    - Allow the hip to rotate externally, and support the knee in slight flexion to facilitate relaxation.
    - One hand should firmly grasp the femur, while the other is positioned below the joint, grasping the tibia to allow anterior translation.
    - The knee should be flexed around 20 to 30 degrees.
    - A quick, firm motion pulling the tibia anteriorly while stabilizing the femur should be performed.
    - The examiner will appreciate the degree of translation and quality of endpoint.
    - A soft endpoint has a greater specificity for a positive ACL tear. Asymmetry in side to side laxity >3mm is also helpful.
    - It is more important to interpret the Lachman test as positive or negative rather than to quantify the degree of laxity.

Imaging

- Standard radiography:
  - Plain radiography should be performed on all patients suspected of acute ACL tears because of the risk of fractures.
  - X-ray studies have a pivotal role in the evaluation of adolescents and children because of the risk of growth plate fractures and tibial spine fractures.
  - In children, plain x-rays should be performed before aggressive maneuvers are performed, especially in the case of decreased active range of motion (ROM) or tenderness at the distal femoral physis.
  - X-rays should include anteroposterior (AP); lateral; and sometimes, oblique views to better visualize fractures. In some cases, an avulsion fracture of the anterolateral tibial plateau at the attachment of the lateral capsular ligament (segond fracture) is noted.
- Advanced imaging:
  - Magnetic resonance imaging (MRI) should be used to evaluate for other concomitant injuries and, in some cases, either to confirm the diagnosis or help to plan surgery.
  - The surgical consent and plan will depend on associated injuries, such as meniscal or MCL injuries.
  - MRI, if used for evaluation of a presumed ACL tear, should be non-contrast-enhanced.
  - The accuracy and sensitivity of MRI are excellent when compared with arthroscopic findings.
  - Sonography is another modality that can be used to assess the ACL; has limited use in the United States owing to the widespread use of MRI

TREATMENT

- Most patients who sustain an ACL injury are active in some type of sports. Expectations after injury vary based on age and activity. Reconstruction is an elective procedure for most individuals. Many can maintain an active lifestyle with an ACL-deficient knee. High-level athletes and the young do the worst without surgery and have frequent episodes of instability.

- The adolescent with open growth plates poses a significant challenge. There is some concern about damaging the growth plates in adolescents with tunnels. However, the risk of growth disturbance is very low.
- To date, there is a lack of evidence to support a protective role of reconstructive surgery of the ACL against osteoarthritis development. At 10 to 20 yr, 50% of those diagnosed with an ACL tear have osteoarthritis and functional impairment—"the young patient with an old knee" (5).
- No studies have shown that bracing an ACL-deficient knee will prevent episodes of instability when an athlete returns to cutting and pivoting sports. The data on bracing do show a decrease in anterior tibial translation at low levels of force. Activity modification provides the best method outside of surgery to prevent "giving way" episodes. If an athlete attains and maintains full ROM and at least 90% strength of the contralateral lower extremity, low-risk sports such as running, bicycling, and swimming can be performed.
- An athlete's inability to return to sports determines whether that athlete elects surgery. A positive pivot-shift test at 3 mo after injury in an awake patient is a strong predictor of the future need for reconstruction. Dynamic functional testing (a series of hopping tests) may be a useful adjunct to predict who may be a "coper" and can continue nonoperative treatment.
- In most cases, incomplete or partial tears of the ACL can be managed nonoperatively. A hinged knee brace can be worn during the early stages of rehab.

SURGERY/OTHER PROCEDURES

- Operative treatment: The procedure selected for ACL reconstruction must restore normal stability and full ROM. Primary ACL suturing does not restore stability and has been abandoned. One exception to primary repair is a bony avulsion, seen mostly in adolescents.
- Graft selection:
  - Autogenous tissue:
    - Patellar tendon (with bone attached both proximally and distally)
    - Hamstring tendons
  - Allograft tissue: Most allografts are taken from the patellar tendon, or Achilles from cadaver donors. However, hamstring and quadriceps tendons can also be used. The use of synthetic materials such as Dacron and Gore-Tex has been abandoned because of long-term failure.
- Patellar tendon autograft: The patellar tendon autograft is an example of bone-to-bone ACL reconstruction and has been used more for high-demand athletes. Of all the procedures, it appears to have the least laxity on KT-1000 testing on follow-up. The potential bone-to-bone fixation promotes earlier graft fixation. Long-term follow-up shows no difference in return to full participation for either autograft procedure.
- Hamstring tendon autograft: The hamstring graft has several advantages. Use of the hamstring tendon avoids patellar tendon morbidity. Studies have shown a decrease in anterior knee pain among those who undergo a hamstring autograft compared with those undergoing bone-to-bone fixation (relative risk 0.49, 95% confidence interval 0.32–0.76, $p = .001$, $I^2 = 0\%$). Hamstring donor-site pain heals within 3 mo while hamstring strength returns within 12 mo (6)[A].
- Allografts: Allografts are used commonly for ACL reconstruction. These are often employed as 2nd-option surgeries in those who have already had a hamstring or bone-to-bone patellar graft:
  - The risks of infection are extremely low but can be dangerous. The benefits of decreased surgical morbidity and easier rehabilitation must be weighed against the potential for greater failure of biologic incorporation, infection, and possibly slower return to activities.
  - The overall risk of infection is extremely low because donors are tested and the grafts are irradiated.
  - Significant bacterial infections occur in fewer than 1%, and no reports of HIV or hepatitis transmission have occurred after 2002.
  - New data now suggest increased failure rates with allografts compared with hamstring tendon or patellar tendon autografts.
- Timing of surgery:
  - The timing of surgery is controversial because some surgeons perform surgery at the site where patients are injured (i.e., the ski area).
  - Negative outcomes, especially arthrofibrosis, are not directly associated with surgical timing but rather with signs of inflammation marked by periarticular swelling, effusion, and hyperthermia.
  - Other factors that predict arthrofibrosis include decreased ROM and perioperative pain.
  - Surgery should be delayed until these factors are improved (often $>$ 3 wk).
  - Early surgery is absolutely indicated only in bony avulsions.

ONGOING CARE

- Patients are now returning to activity sooner after reconstruction. Return to sport depends more on strength and proprioception than on time from surgery. Usual return to sport may fall between 6 and 12 mo or longer after surgery. Early return prior to full proprioception and strength may lead to prolonged instability and possible reinjury (8)[A],(9).
- Therapy protocols may be divided into four categories:
  - Phase 1: preoperative; maintain ROM.
  - Phase 2 (0 to 2 wk): Achieve full extension; maintain quadriceps strength, reduce swelling, and achieve flexion to 90 degrees.
  - Phase 3 (3 to 5 wk): Maintain full extension and increase flexion up to full ROM; stair climbers and stationary cycle may be used.
  - Phase 4 (6 wk to 9 mo): Increase strength and agility; progressive return to sports
- Prior to return to sport, athletes should meet discharge criteria including isokinetic strength, running T-test, single hop, triple hop, and crossover tests.
- The use of custom ACL bracing has also been controversial. A systemic review of several randomized, controlled trials (level I evidence, 12 trials) found no evidence that pain, ROM, graft stability, or protection from subsequent injury was affected by postoperative bracing (7)[A].

FOLLOW-UP RECOMMENDATIONS

- If arthrofibrosis is evident after surgery, early surgical intervention ($<$1 yr) improves the outcome.
- Full ROM should be achieved to prevent degenerative joint disease.

PROGNOSIS

- Most patients with ACL injuries do well with activities of daily living even after follow-up in the range of 5 to 15 yr. Most can participate in some sports activity if they are inclined to do so, but most will have some limitations in vigorous sports, and only a few will be entirely asymptomatic.
- The presence of clinically significant chondral and meniscal injuries that occur at the time of injury or after injury determines long-term prognosis more than the ACL injury itself. Over time, the prevalence of meniscal injuries increases, leading to increasing disability, surgery, and arthrosis in high-risk patients.
- Ligament reconstruction has not been shown to prevent arthrosis, but in prospective studies, it appears to reduce the risk of subsequent meniscal injury and to facilitate return to high-level sporting activities (8).

REFERENCES

1. Chappell JD, Creighton RA, Giuliani C, et al. Kinematics and electromyography of landing preparation in vertical stop-jump: risks for noncontact anterior cruciate ligament injury. *Am J Sports Med*. 2007;35(2):235–241.
2. Prodromos CC, Han Y, Rogowski J, et al. A meta-analysis of the incidence of anterior cruciate ligament tears as a function of gender, sport, and a knee injury-reduction regimen. *Arthroscopy*. 2007;23(12):1320.e6–1325.e6.
3. Sugimoto D, Myer GD, McKeon JM, et al. Evaluation of the effectiveness of neuromuscular training to reduce anterior cruciate ligament injury in female athletes: a critical review of relative risk reduction and numbers-needed-to-treat analyses. *Br J Sports Med*. 2012;46(14):979–988.
4. Benjaminse A, Gokeler A, van der Schans CP. Clinical diagnosis of an anterior cruciate ligament rupture: a meta-analysis. *J Orthop Sports Phys Ther*. 2006;36(5):267–288.
5. van Meer BL, Meuffels DE, van Eijsden WA, et al. Which determinants predict tibiofemoral and patellofemoral osteoarthritis after anterior cruciate ligament injury? A systematic review. *Br J Sports Med*. 2015;49(15):975–983.
6. Poolman RW, Farrokhyar F, Bhandari M. Hamstring tendon autograft better than bone patellar-tendon bone autograft in ACL reconstruction: a cumulative meta-analysis and clinically relevant sensitivity analysis applied to a previously published analysis. *Acta Orthop*. 2007;78(3):350–354.
7. Wright RW, Fetzer GB. Bracing after ACL reconstruction: a systematic review. *Clin Orthop Relat Res*. 2007;455:162–168.
8. Czuppon S, Racette BA, Klein SE, et al. Variables associated with return to sport following anterior cruciate ligament reconstruction: a systematic review. *Br J Sports Med*. 2014;48(5):356–364.
9. Kyritsis P, Bahr R, Landreau P, et al. Likelihood of ACL graft rupture: not meeting six clinical discharge criteria before return to sport is associated with a four times greater risk of rupture. *Br J Sports Med*. 2016;50(15):946–951.

CLINICAL PEARLS

- Nearly all patients with an acute ACL tear have an effusion.
- Noncontact injuries account for the majority of ACL tears.
- ACL reconstruction does not protect against the development of osteoarthritis.

ACL TEAR: MANAGEMENT IN SKELETALLY IMMATURE ATHLETES

Holly J. Benjamin, MD, FAAP, FACSM • Michael Ladewski, DO

BASICS

DESCRIPTION

- Acute injury sustained by known mechanism that leads to knee instability with significant effect on the athlete's ability to perform at the highest levels of sport
- Considerable variation exists regarding specific treatment in the skeletally immature population with operative treatment becoming more favorable when compared to non- or delayed operative treatment (1,2,3)[B].

EPIDEMIOLOGY

- Higher risk in female athletes than in male athletes participating in similar sports (4)
- The higher incidence in females is thought to be due to differences in biomechanics, joint laxity, hormonal influences, intercondylar notch dimensions, and ligament size (4).
- Sporting activity associated with anterior cruciate ligament (ACL) injury involves cutting, pivoting, and sudden deceleration (4).

Incidence

- 0.11/ (virgule)10,000 at 8 yr of age (4)
- 2.42/ (virgule)10,000 by 14 yr of age (4)
- 19% increase in patients 10 to 14 yr of age from 2007 to 2011 (4)

ETIOLOGY AND PATHOPHYSIOLOGY

- Midsubstance tear most common
- Tibial spine avulsion fracture more frequent in the skeletally immature athletes
- Femoral ACL avulsion fractures are rare causes of ACL injury.
- Mechanisms of injury:
  - Hyperextension, sudden deceleration, or a valgus and rotator force with a planted foot
  - External rotation of the femur on a fixed tibia combined with a valgus load often the result of a noncontact pivoting injury

GENERAL PREVENTION

Neuromuscular balance training and core strengthening have been shown to decrease the incidence in athletes of various ages (1)[C].

COMMONLY ASSOCIATED CONDITIONS

- Bone bruise: lateral compartment more than medial compartment
- Meniscus tears: lateral more commonly in acute knee injury; medial more common in athlete with chronic ACL deficiency
- Associated medial meniscus tears and medial collateral ligament (MCL) injury in patient with valgus stress mechanism

DIAGNOSIS

HISTORY

- May be a "pop" sensation at the time of injury
- Effusion usually develops acutely.
- Athlete unable to continue play
- Instability of knee after injury

PHYSICAL EXAM

- It can be difficult to perform an accurate physical exam after significant hemarthrosis develops.
- Loss of normal knee contour secondary to effusion is often present.
- The Lachman test is the most sensitive physical examination test and is the "gold standard" for diagnosis (4)[A].
- Anterior drawer and pivot-shift tests are positive but are less sensitive tests (4)[A].
- Evaluation of the uninjured knee can help establish a baseline when compared to the injured knee.
- Testing for other ligamentous, tendon, and meniscal injury is indicated.
- Palpate the distal femur and proximal tibia physes for tenderness that might indicate the presence of a physeal fracture.
- Tenderness at the ends of long bones is a fracture until proven otherwise in skeletally immature patients.
- Perform a complete neurologic and vascular exam of the lower extremity.

DIFFERENTIAL DIAGNOSIS

- Tibial spine avulsion fractures
- Physeal fractures of the distal femur or proximal tibia
- Meniscal injury
- Articular cartilage injury
- Patellar subluxation
- Other ligamentous injury of the knee

DIAGNOSTIC TESTS & INTERPRETATION

Initial Tests (lab, imaging)

- Knee radiographs to rule out tibial spine avulsion fracture, physeal fractures, Segond fracture, and osteochondral fractures
- Magnetic resonance imaging (MRI) to evaluate ACL and concomitant meniscal, posterior cruciate ligament, collateral ligament, and chondral injuries:
  - 3-Tesla images are 97–100% sensitive when correlated with arthroscopic findings (5)[B].
  - Tear imaging shows increased signal intensity with a disrupted pattern.
  - May have a higher false-positive rate in adolescents (5)[B]
- Consider wrist x-rays to assess bone age, which may influence surgical technique.

Diagnostic Procedures/Other

- Diagnostic arthroscopy is sometimes required when physical exam and imaging studies are equivocal.
- KT-1000 device may be helpful in quantifying relative ACL laxity.

TREATMENT

GENERAL MEASURES

- Compression
- Ice
- Pain management
- Weight-bearing as tolerated unless physeal fracture is suspected
- Therapeutic aspiration can be performed on the hemarthrosis.
- If fat is noted in the hemarthrosis, then a fracture is present.

ISSUES FOR REFERRAL

- Patients with suspected ACL injuries should be referred to an orthopedic or sports medicine specialist.
- Preference for specialist with experience in surgical techniques in the skeletally immature athlete

ADDITIONAL THERAPIES

Nonoperative therapy may be considered depending on physical demands and age of athlete:

- Restoration of range of motion (ROM)
- Strengthening quadriceps and hamstrings
- Activity modification
- May be recommended if ACL reconstruction delayed owing to skeletal immaturity or for partial ACL tears
- Specific physical therapies and bracing can significantly improve functional status of injured knee (1)[B].
- Increased risk of recurrent instability and further meniscal and articular cartilage damage with nonoperative treatment (2)[A]
- Bracing with derotational ACL-stabilizing brace does not restore stability when athlete returns to high-demand sport.

SURGERY/OTHER PROCEDURES

Variation related to approach and risk for early physeal closure:

- Degree of knee instability is primary driving force to pursue early surgical treatment (1,2,3)[B].
- Options include physeal sparing, partial transphyseal, and complete transphyseal ACL reconstruction (2,3,4,6,7)[A].
- Degree of skeletal maturity is a factor in decision making for treatment (2,3,4,6,7)[C].
- Undertaken only after restoration of ROM and resolution of joint effusion
- Early surgical treatment most common treatment compared to non- or delayed operative treatment in a survey of pediatric orthopedists (3)[C]

ONGOING CARE

FOLLOW-UP RECOMMENDATIONS

- Patients will require substantial physical therapy to regain ROM and strength as well as to address functional and sports-specific mechanics to address prevention of recurrence.
- Use of postsurgical ACL bracing may be more effective in pediatric compared to adult patients possibly due to compliance with activity restriction guidelines and therapy protocols (1,2,3,4,6,7)[C].
- Consistent clinical follow-up post-ACL reconstruction until skeletal maturity for complication surveillance

PROGNOSIS

- Typical postoperative recovery and rehabilitation period is usually 9 to 12 mo, prolonged period of rehab of possible benefit for skeletally immature.
- Return to previous level of sport can be as high as 90% after operative treatment (2,3,4,6,7)[C].
- Natural history of the ACL-deficient knee is chronic instability, chondral injury, subsequent meniscal pathology, pain, and joint arthrosis.

COMPLICATIONS

- Associated MCL and meniscal injuries
- Surgical complications:
  - Graft failure
  - Premature physeal closure
  - Leg-length discrepancy
  - Limb malalignment
  - Slow recovery in ROM
  - Usual risks of infection and anesthesia

REFERENCES

1. Moksnes H, Engebretsen L, Eitzen I, et al. Functional outcomes following a non-operative treatment algorithm for anterior cruciate ligament injuries in skeletally immature children 12 years and younger. A prospective cohort with 2 years follow-up. *Br J Sports Med*. 2013;47(8):488–494.
2. Ramski DE, Kanj WW, Franklin CC, et al. Anterior cruciate ligament tears in children and adolescents: a meta-analysis of nonoperative versus operative treatment. *Am J Sports Med*. 2014;42(11):2769–2776.
3. Popkin CA, Wright ML, Pennock AT, et al. Trends in management and complications of anterior cruciate ligament injuries in pediatric patients: a survey of the PRiSM Society. *J Pediatr Orthop*. 2018;38(2):e61–e65.
4. Frank JS, Gambacorta PL. Anterior cruciate ligament injuries in the skeletally immature athlete: diagnosis and management. *J Am Acad Orthop Surg*. 2013;21(2):78–87.
5. Schub DL, Altahawi F, F Meisel A, et al. Accuracy of 3-Tesla magnetic resonance imaging for the diagnosis of intra-articular knee injuries in children and teenagers. *J Pediatr Orthop*. 2012;32(8):765–769.
6. Anderson CN, Anderson AF. Management of the anterior cruciate ligament-injured knee in the skeletally immature athlete. *Clin Sports Med*. 2017;36(1):35–52.
7. Ludwig M, Atanda A Jr. Management of anterior cruciate ligament tears in skeletally immature athletes. *Phys Sportsmed*. 2015;43(4):440–447.

ADDITIONAL READING

- Pennock A, Murphy MM, Wu M. Anterior cruciate ligament reconstruction in skeletally immature patients. *Curr Rev Musculoskelet Med*. 2016;9(4):445–453.
- Siow HM, Cameron DB, Ganley TJ. Acute knee injuries in skeletally immature athletes. *Phys Med Rehabil Clin N Am*. 2008;19(2):319–345, ix.

CLINICAL PEARLS

- Injury that is increasing in incidence in the skeletally immature population
- Early surgical therapies are becoming more favorable when compared to non- or delayed surgical treatment.
- Type of ACL reconstruction and timing of surgery in the skeletally immature athlete vary widely, and cases should be decided on an individual basis.
- Primary and secondary prevention programs have been shown to be effective.

ACROMIOCLAVICULAR SEPARATIONS (TYPES 1–6)

Anne S. Boyd, MD, FAAFP, FACSM

BASICS

- Separation of the clavicle and acromion due to injury of the acromioclavicular (AC) and coracoclavicular (CC) ligaments
- Classified based on radiographic findings, indicating severity of injury to the capsular and extracapsular ligaments and supporting structures (types I to VI) (1)
- AC and CC ligaments are responsible for maintaining the joint in physiologic position (2).
- AC ligament is the main static stabilizing force for the AC joint in the anterior-posterior direction (3):
  - This ligament blends with the trapezius and deltoid fascia to form the AC capsule.
- CC ligament is an indirect stabilizing force for the AC joint in the inferior direction:
  - The two CC ligaments can be divided into two parts: the trapezoid and conoid ligaments.
- Synonym(s): shoulder separation; shoulder sprain; AC sprain; AC dislocation
- Note: The term *shoulder dislocation* primarily refers to glenohumeral dislocation, not disruption of the AC joint.

DESCRIPTION

- Type I:
  - Sprain of the AC ligament, some fiber disruption
  - Intact CC ligament and AC joint capsule
- Type II:
  - Complete tear of the AC ligament
  - Sprained but intact CC ligament
  - Disrupted, widened AC joint
- Type III:
  - Complete tear of AC and CC ligaments
  - Dislocated AC joint
  - Superior displacement of distal clavicle (<100%)
  - Probable disruption of deltoid and trapezius attachments
- Type IV:
  - Complete tear of AC ligament
  - Partial or complete disruption of CC ligament
  - Dislocation of AC joint
  - Posterior displacement of distal clavicle into trapezius muscle
  - High probability of detachment of deltoid and trapezius muscle from distal clavicle

ALERT

Axillary view on radiographs demonstrates posterior displacement of distal clavicle in relation to the acromion. Type IV injury may be missed without this view (3,4).

- Type V:
  - Complete tear of AC and CC ligaments
  - Dislocated AC joint
  - >100% superior displacement of distal clavicle
  - Position of clavicle: also thought of as a large type III; there is 100–300% widening of CC interval.
  - High probability of detachment of deltoid and trapezius muscle from distal clavicle
- Type VI: rare
  - Complete tear of AC
  - CC ligaments intact or torn
  - Dislocated AC joint
  - Inferior displacement of the distal clavicle relative to the acromion or coracoid
  - Position of clavicle: 100% inferior AC joint displacement, usually with distal clavicle wedged underneath coracoid process. There is potential damage to the underlying brachial plexus and subclavian vessels.

EPIDEMIOLOGY

- Commonly occurs during sports involving direct contact (2,3,4)
- Severity of injury is directly related to the force of impact (2).
- Mechanism of injury is primarily by direct impact over the superolateral shoulder forcing the AC joint inferiorly (2,4).
- Primary injury is depression of the scapular complex (not elevation of the clavicle) causing disruption of the AC and CC ligaments (3).
- Direct trauma commonly due to tackling with the shoulder or falling directly on the "point" of shoulder
- Indirect trauma: fall on outstretched hand, causing the humeral head to be driven upward into the inferior aspect of the AC joint (2,5)
- Downward indirect force, sudden change in load through upper extremity, usually heavier weight

Incidence

- Common, representing 9% of all shoulder injuries (1,2)
- Nearly 50% of all AC dislocations occur to individuals in their 20s (1,2,3).
- Males are 5 times more likely to suffer injuries than females (1,2).
- Types I and II injuries account for most AC separations.

COMMONLY ASSOCIATED CONDITIONS

- Fracture injuries are associated with types III to V AC separations in 5% of patients.
- Intra-articular injuries are associated with types III to V AC dislocations in 18% of patients (3):
  - Shoulder labrum/superior labrum anterior and posterior (SLAP) tears reported in 5–14%
  - Rotator cuff tears reported in ~4%

DIAGNOSIS

HISTORY

- Present following a fall on the shoulder or collision and pain at the AC joint
- Exact mechanism of injury helpful to indicate severity of the injury and potential associated injuries
- Assess for neurologic symptoms or vascular symptoms (which indicate a more severe injury and may require immediate surgical intervention).

PHYSICAL EXAM

- Inspection should be done bilaterally for comparison to the uninjured side.
- Inspection may show asymmetry of the shoulders or swelling at the AC joint.
- Deformity (step-off) of AC joint with type III injuries and higher
- Palpation (point tenderness of the affected AC joint)
- Types III and V may show instability of the lateral clavicle when depressed manually ("piano key" phenomenon) (3).
- Range of motion is usually reduced due to pain acutely.
- Pain with adduction of the shoulder and possibly with shoulder abduction and flexion
- Cross body adduction test (77% sensitivity); forward flexion of shoulder to 90 degrees, then assisted adduction across chest, reproduces pain over the AC joint (3).
- Careful neurovascular examination should always be performed with any significant musculoskeletal injury.

DIFFERENTIAL DIAGNOSIS

- Fractures of the coracoid, acromion, or clavicle
- Rotator cuff injuries
- SLAP/shoulder labrum lesion
- Glenohumeral dislocation
- Burner/stinger (neurogenic)
- Cervical spine injuries
- Pneumothorax (rare)
- Gorham massive osteolysis
- Gout
- Neoplasm (multiple myeloma)

DIAGNOSTIC TESTS & INTERPRETATION

Initial Tests (lab, imaging)

- Radiographs: True anteroposterior (AP), scapular Y lateral, and an axillary view are the initial images of choice for this injury (1)[B],(3,4)[C]:
  - Vertical displacement of the distal clavicle may be seen on the AP view, whereas AP displacement may be evident on the axillary view.

- If suspecting a posterior dislocation, consider adding lateral view of the acromion.
- Axillary lateral view is essential to help distinguish a type III from a type IV injury. A type IV will show the scapula anterior to the clavicle.
- Axillary view may be uncomfortable and takes some time to obtain.

- Zanca view: an AP of the shoulder with the central beam directed 10 to 15 degrees cephalad toward the clavicle and with reduced beam penetration (because the AC joint is superficial and will be over-penetrated with regular beam strength) (3,4):
  - Zanca views of both shoulders provide superior AC joint evaluation while avoiding the superimposition of the acromion on the distal clavicle.
  - Helps identify fractures of the clavicle, acromion, or coracoid, and to preliminarily evaluate AC joint separation and CC ligament disruption
- A wide plate should be used with AP and Zanca views to incorporate bilateral shoulders for direct comparison views on a single cassette (4).
- Stress views (weighted views) can be used to differentiate types I to III, but are not recommended, because the results do not affect treatment, and disruption of the CC ligament (larger space between coracoid and clavicle on the affected side) can be seen on the standard AP (4).
- The average distance between the inferior aspect of the clavicle and the coracoid is 1.1 to 1.3 cm. This value can vary, so it is important to compare to the unaffected side.
- Stryker notch views to assess for coracoid fracture when indicated

Diagnostic Procedures/Other

- Computed tomography (CT) scan has not been shown to improve diagnostic reliability (1)[B].
- Magnetic resonance imaging (MRI) in coronal oblique plane parallel to the CC ligament may be used to identify higher grade or additional injuries if surgery intervention is being considered (1)[B].

TREATMENT

GENERAL MEASURES

- Types I and II:
  - Types I and II injuries involve minimal disruption of the joint and are stable. Treatment is conservative (nonoperative) (2)[A].
  - Conservative treatment includes a sling and activity modification for comfort, ice, and analgesics until symptoms subside and range of motion is comfortable.
  - Shoulder sling for several days (average of 3 to 7 days) alleviates stress at the affected ligaments and allows for healing.
  - Ice and analgesics for pain and swelling:
    - Generally, <1 to 2 wk of analgesia are needed.
  - Type II injuries receive similar treatment as those with type I injuries but generally require addition of an early rehabilitation program with passive and active shoulder range of motion exercises.
  - Rotator cuff, scapular stabilization, and trunk strengthening exercises as pain resolves
  - Heavy lifting and contact activities to resume only once the extremity is pain free and symmetric range of motion is achieved
- Type III:
  - The most controversial regarding management
  - Most studies show comparably high satisfaction and long-term functional outcomes with operative and nonoperative treatment, yet higher incidence of complications in those treated surgically (2)[A],(6)[B].
  - Generally, consensus is to advocate for initial nonoperative management. However, this injury likely requires initial and continued individualization of treatment based on patient activity level, impairment, and occupation (3,4).
- Types IV to VI (3,4)[A]:
  - Surgical referral

ADDITIONAL THERAPIES

- Types I and II: Shoulder range of motion exercises should be started as pain eases, followed by a strengthening program for the rotator cuff and scapular stabilizers. Return to contact when full, painless range of motion and normal strength resumes.
- Type III: Shoulder strengthening exercises are introduced when range of motion and pain are improved. Return to contact sports usually is anticipated in 6 wk to 6 mo, depending on resumption of full painless range of motion and normal strength.

SURGERY/OTHER PROCEDURES

Types IV to VI usually require operative treatment.

ONGOING CARE

- If types IV to VI, refer to orthopedics.
- Refer type III AC separations for discussion of surgical options for high-level athletes, patients refusing conservative therapy, heavy manual laborers, patients unable to tolerate the deformity, and patients who have failed nonoperative treatment after 6 mo (3).

PROGNOSIS

- In most, pain resolves, and an athlete may return to sports within several weeks. Recovery generally takes 6 wk for type II and 12 wk for type III injuries.
- Reports suggest that up to 40% of individuals with type I or II injures will go on to develop osteoarthritis at the AC joint.

COMPLICATIONS

- Persistent instability or residual pain with activity
- Cosmetic deformity and AC joint arthritis are common complications.
- Some patients note intermittent pain and/or clicking, often referred to as nuisance symptoms. These symptoms may require an injection or further physical therapy.
- Although uncommon, severe, persistent symptoms may require surgical intervention.
- Rarely, distal clavicle osteolysis may occur.

REFERENCES

1. Gorbaty JD, Hsu JE, Gee AO. Classifications in brief: rockwood classification of acromioclavicular joint separations. *Clin Orthop Relat Res*. 2017;475(1):283–287.
2. Chillemi C, Franceschini V, Dei Giudici L, et al. Epidemiology of isolated acromioclavicular joint dislocation. *Emerg Med Int*. 2013;2013:171609.
3. Van Bergen CJA, Van Bemmel AF, Alta TDW, et al. New insights in the treatment of acromioclavicular separation. *World J Orthop*. 2017;8(12):861–873.
4. Lee S, Bedi A. Shoulder acromioclavicular joint reconstruction options and outcomes. *Curr Rev Musculoskelet Med*. 2016;9(4);368–377.
5. Johansen JA, Grutter PW, McFarland EG, et al. Acromioclavicular joint injuries: indications for treatment and treatment options. *J Shoulder Elbow Surg*. 2011;20(Suppl 2):S70–S82.
6. Joukainen A, Kröger H, Niemitukia L, et al. Results of operative and nonoperative treatment of Rockwood types III and V acromioclavicular joint dislocation: a prospective, randomized trial with an 18- to 20-year follow-up. *Orthop J Sports Med*. 2014;2(12):2325967114560130.

CLINICAL PEARLS

- Types I and II AC separations generally do well with conservative treatment.
- Management of type III injuries should be made on a case-by-case basis.
- In general, full return to contact sports is possible when painless range of motion and normal, symmetrical strength are achieved.
- Cosmetic deformity and AC joint arthritis are common complications.

ADDUCTOR TENDON INJURY

Sara N. Raiser, MD • Daniel C. Herman, MD, PhD, FAAPMR, FACSM, CAQSM

BASICS

DESCRIPTION

- Medial thigh/groin pain and weakness resulting from injury to muscle
- May be acute or chronic
- The hip adductors include adductor longus, magnus, and brevis; gracilis; obturator externus; and pectineus.
- Adductor longus is the most commonly injured adductor muscle; other muscles involved in groin injuries may include gracilis, iliopsoas, rectus femoris, sartorius, and/or abdominal muscles.
- 3-tier grading system: (i) mild partial tear with pain but minimal loss of strength or range of motion; (ii) moderate partial tear with pain, +/− swelling, and noticeable decrease in strength and range of motion without complete loss of function; (iii) complete tear with severe limitation or complete loss of function
- Synonym(s): groin strain; pulled groin

EPIDEMIOLOGY

Most common cause of groin pain in athletes, but symptoms overlap with a wide differential

ETIOLOGY AND PATHOPHYSIOLOGY

- Eccentric loading of adductor muscle (muscle is passively being stretched while it is contracting) is usual mechanism of injury.
- Sudden acceleration/deceleration, change of direction, kicking, jumping, and/or overstretching are commonly involved mechanisms.

RISK FACTORS

- Increasing age
- Previous adductor injury (1)[A]
- Weak, inactive, or fatigued adductor muscles have less ability to absorb energy and are more likely to undergo acute strain.
- Core muscle weakness

DIAGNOSIS

HISTORY

- Acutely, often a stretch injury with an abrupt cutting motion as in soccer or a straddling injury as in gymnastics, cheerleading, or horseback riding
- Usually an acute episode is reported, but symptoms may become chronic after initial injury if undertreated and repeatedly strained.
- Chronic injury may also result from overuse through repetitive activity such as skating, kicking, or rollerblading.
- Typically unilateral but may become bilateral
- May have only minor discomfort with walking, but pain and weakness are noticeable with cutting or running
- An unusual presentation, nocturnal pain, or lack of response to appropriate treatment may be concerning for a nonmusculoskeletal etiology.

PHYSICAL EXAM

- Classic triad of tenderness to palpation of the muscle and its bony attachments (proximal third of medial thigh and tendinous origin in pubic region), pain with passive stretching (hip abduction), and pain with resisted contraction (hip adduction)
- Swelling, ecchymosis, and significant weakness increase suspicion for tear.
- With complete rupture, palpable depression and retraction of torn muscle may be present.

DIFFERENTIAL DIAGNOSIS

- Osteitis pubis
- Stress fracture of femoral neck or pubic ramus
- Iliopsoas or rectus femoris tendonitis, iliopsoas bursitis
- Avascular necrosis of femoral head
- Groin disruption (sports hernia, Gilmore groin, athletic pubalgia)
- Femoro-acetabular impingement, labral tear, osteochondral lesion, hip osteoarthritis
- Myositis ossificans
- Avulsion fracture, apophysitis in adolescents
- Slipped capital femoral epiphysis (usually seen in early teens)
- Inguinal hernia
- Nerve entrapment, specifically obturator nerve
- Referred pain from spine
- Conjoined tendon lesions
- Nonmusculoskeletal considerations include urologic, gynecologic, and gastrointestinal disorders as well as malignancies.

DIAGNOSTIC TESTS & INTERPRETATION

ALERT

- Straightforward cases may not require imaging.
- Hip and pelvis films should be obtained for the following concerns: pubic ramus tenderness; persistent pain despite conservative treatment; or suspicion of hip involvement, myositis ossificans following direct trauma, or avulsion fracture in an adolescent.
- Bone scan or magnetic resonance imaging (MRI) if stress fracture is suspected
- MRI may also be used for definitive diagnosis (2,3)[C].
- Musculoskeletal ultrasound (US) may be used to evaluate for tendon fiber discontinuity or hematoma if there is a palpable mass or retraction (2,3)[C] and to periodically monitor during the recovery phase.

TREATMENT

GENERAL MEASURES

- Protection, rest, ice, compression, and elevation (PRICE) is beneficial.
- Ice for 20 min every 2 to 3 hr for the first 2 to 3 days
- Heat may be added after 2 to 3 days.

- Gentle compression with compression shorts (4)[C], neoprene sleeve, or elastic wrap
- Strict immobilization generally is not recommended, and rehabilitation should be initiated early within the first few days.
- Limited activity as tolerated for 1 to 2 wk; longer for more protracted cases
- For severe, incomplete tears, crutches for walking while symptomatic with ambulation. Pain is usually controlled with over-the-counter (OTC) analgesics, but topical anesthetics and/or muscle relaxants may be occasionally used.

ISSUES FOR REFERRAL

- Grade 3 tears or skeletally mature pelvic avulsion fractures should be referred to an orthopedic surgeon to consider surgical repair.
- If suspicion for nonmusculoskeletal etiology exists, refer to the appropriate specialist for further workup and treatment.

ADDITIONAL THERAPIES

- Isometric strengthening (5)[A] should be instituted as symptoms subside.
- Avoid excessive passive stretching.
- Progress to dynamic, eccentric strengthening, balance training, and proprioceptive exercises of hip and groin musculature (5,6)[A].
- When active range of motion reaches at least 50% of the noninjured side with good muscle activation and pain free with exercises, may increase to full loading for conditioning (5)[A]
- Strength and range of motion should be nearly 100% and pain free prior to return to sport (5)[A].
- Stretching and physical therapy modalities, such as US or electrical stimulation, may benefit more chronic cases.

SURGERY/OTHER PROCEDURES

- Peritendinous adductor corticosteroid injections are not recommended given no evidence of long-term benefit.
- Regenerative therapies may potentially play a role in adductor injury treatment, although there is currently no evidence specifically regarding use with adductor injuries.
- Surgical repair may be indicated for complete avulsion from the femur or complete muscle/tendon tears.
- Early repair is generally recommended if surgery is deemed appropriate.

ONGOING CARE

PATIENT EDUCATION

- Correction of predisposing factors, such as muscle tightness, weakness, or imbalance, should be addressed (6)[B].
- Adequate stretching and warm-up may help prevent reinjury (6)[B].
- Decision on return to play is dependent on extent of injury and underlying predisposing factors. Pain is usually a fair measure, so unrestricted play is generally permitted if pain free.

PROGNOSIS

- Prognosis is generally favorable.
- Healing of an adductor strain may take from 1 to 3 wk for a grade 1 injury and up to 4 to 8 wk for grade 3 injuries and longer for chronic injuries.

REFERENCES

1. Nicholas SJ, Tyler TF. Adductor muscle strains in sport. *Sports Med*. 2002;32(5):339–344.
2. Lee SC, Endo Y, Potter HG. Imaging of groin pain: magnetic resonance and ultrasound imaging features. *Sports Health*. 2017;9(5):428–435.
3. Branci S, Thorborg K, Nielsen MB, et al. Radiological findings in symphyseal and adductor-related groin pain in athletes: a critical review of the literature. *Br J Sports Med*. 2013;47(10):611–619.
4. Chaudhari AM, Jamison ST, McNally MP, et al. Hip adductor activations during run-to-cut manoeuvres in compression shorts: implications for return to sport after groin injury. *J Sports Sci*. 2014;32(14):1333–1340.
5. Hölmich P, Uhrskou P, Ulnits L, et al. Effectiveness of active physical training as treatment for long-standing adductor-related groin pain in athletes: randomised trial. *Lancet*. 1999;353(9151):439–443.
6. Tyler TF, Silvers HJ, Gerhardt MB, et al. Groin injuries in sports medicine. *Sports Health*. 2010;2(3):231–236.

ADDITIONAL READING

- Anderson M, Hall S, Martin M. *Foundations of Athletic Training: Prevention, Assessment, and Management*. Philadelphia, PA: Lippincott Williams & Wilkins; 2005:475–477.
- Bahr R, Machlum S. *Clin Guide Sports Injur*. 2004:266–268.
- Dahan R. Rehabilitation of muscle-tendon injuries to the hip, pelvis and groin areas. *Sports Med Arthrosc Rev*. 1997;5:326–333.
- Gilmore J. Groin pain in the soccer athlete: fact, fiction, and treatment. *Clin Sports Med*. 1998;17(4):787–793, vii.
- Lacroix VJ. A complete approach to groin pain. *Phys Sports Med*. 2000;28(1):66–86.
- Macleod DA, Gibbon WW. The sportsman's groin. *Br J Surg*. 1999;86(7):849–850.
- Weir A, Homlich P, Thorborg K. Groin pain. In: Hutchinson M, Brukner P, Khan K, et al, eds. *Brukner & Khan's Clinical Sports Medicine*. Vol 1. 5th ed. North Ryde NSW, Australia: McGraw-Hill; 2017:629–658.

CLINICAL PEARLS

- Although initial symptoms may not be debilitating enough to impair performance, pain is a marker for injury.
- Left untreated, adductor strains can become chronic and ultimately take longer to rehabilitate or fail to fully recover.
- A history of prior groin injury is the greatest risk factor for subsequent injury (1,5,6)[A].
- The clinical examination is neither sensitive nor specific for identifying the exact etiology of athletic groin pain in the majority of cases (6).
- Return to full competitive play should not occur until the athlete is pain free due to the high risk of chronic pain or complications.

ADHESIVE CAPSULITIS

Adam Lyons, MD • Rahul Kapur, MD, CAQSM

BASICS

DESCRIPTION

- Commonly known as "frozen shoulder"
- Painful restriction of glenohumeral joint range of motion (ROM)
- Caused by thickening, fibrosis, and contraction of glenohumeral joint capsule with adherence to the humeral head
- Classified into two categories:
  - Primary, which has an insidious idiopathic onset with no precipitating event
  - Secondary, which follows trauma, immobilization, or underlying systemic illness

EPIDEMIOLOGY

- Slight predominance in females, 1.4:1
- Mean age of onset is ~55 yr of age; rare before 40 yr
- 15% experience bilateral disease
- No known racial or ethnic predilection

Prevalence

3% of the general population; prevalence is 10–20% in patients with diabetes mellitus.

ETIOLOGY AND PATHOPHYSIOLOGY

- Exact pathophysiology of condition is unclear.
- Increasing evidence suggests the process involves synovial inflammation with subsequent reactive fibrosis.
- Pain is due to synovial inflammation.
- Resultant capsular fibrosis restricts ROM.
- Generally idiopathic
- Can result from period of shoulder immobilization
- Rarely, also arises from clinically significant trauma to shoulder, cervical radiculopathy, brachial plexus pathology, or rotator cuff tendonitis
- Autoimmune theory of disease: Microvascular disease causes abnormal collagen repair, leading to capsular fibrosis.

RISK FACTORS

- Shoulder immobilization increases risk by 5 to 9 times over the general population (1).
- Diabetes mellitus: 10–20% prevalence (1,2)
- Thyroid disease
- Stroke
- Female gender
- Age 40 to 70 yr

GENERAL PREVENTION

Avoidance of prolonged shoulder immobilization or severe restriction of movement

COMMONLY ASSOCIATED CONDITIONS

- Diabetes
- Thyroid disorders
- Hypertriglyceridemia
- Cervical spondylosis

DIAGNOSIS

HISTORY

- Progressive shoulder pain over weeks to months
- Pain worse with any shoulder movement, both active and passive. Pain is worse at night and may interfere with sleep. Pain usually is not only present in the region of the deltoid but also may radiate into the upper arm and neck regions.
- Common functional impairments include difficulty dressing, combing one's hair, and reaching into one's back pocket for a wallet.
- A careful medical history to exclude associated conditions should be conducted.
- Three clinical phases (1,2):
  - Phase 1: painful phase, insidious onset of nocturnal pain, progresses to pain at rest, no restriction of ROM, may last 2 to 9 mo
  - Phase 2: frozen or adhesive phase, progressive limitation of ROM in all directions, lasts 4 to 12 mo or longer
  - Phase 3: thawing or regressive phase; symptoms gradually improve over 5 to 24 mo.

PHYSICAL EXAM

- The hallmark of adhesive capsulitis is a decreased glenohumeral ROM associated with pain.
- Observation usually reveals limited use of the limb and lack of arm swing in walking.
- Often occurs in nondominant arm first
- Pain at extremes of ROM may be the only finding in the early phase. The greatest limitation is usually seen in external rotation initially. In later stages, all ranges of motion usually are limited. The loss of motion commonly occurs in the following order: external rotation → abduction → internal rotation → forward flexion.
- There is a limitation of both active and passive ROM.
- Active ROM may show inverted scapulothoracic motion to compensate.
- Impingement (Neer, Hawkins) and biceps tendinopathy (Speed) maneuvers may be positive.
- The scapula usually is elevated, laterally placed, and protracted. Wasting of the shoulder girdle muscles may be present due to disuse atrophy.

DIFFERENTIAL DIAGNOSIS

- Rotator cuff disease
- Impingement syndrome
- Biceps tendinopathy
- Posterior shoulder dislocation
- Arthritis/degenerative arthrosis of the glenohumeral joint
- Cervical radiculopathy
- Polymyalgia rheumatica
- Fracture of the humerus or glenoid
- Referred pain from the cervical spine, thorax, or abdomen
- Nonmusculoskeletal etiology

DIAGNOSTIC TESTS & INTERPRETATION

- Radiographs are useful to assess the presence of degenerative joint disease (DJD), calcific tendonitis, or other diagnosis(es) but are often normal in appearance.
- Periarticular osteopenia may be present as a result of disuse.
- Dynamic ultrasound may show limitations in the movement of the supraspinatus tendon below the acromion during abduction.
- MRI may reveal slight thickening in the joint capsule and the coracohumeral ligament.

TREATMENT

- A high rate of spontaneous recovery within 18 to 30 mo for this condition should be kept in mind when choosing treatment options. Treatment should be focused on relief of symptoms and optimization of ROM (1)[A].
- Topical and potentially a short course of oral nonsteroidal anti-inflammatory drugs (NSAIDs) can be used, if tolerated, to aid with pain control in the initial painful phase (2)[B].
- Distention with saline and steroid can reduce pain and improve ROM and function in the short term. At 2 yr of follow-up, distention was as effective as manipulation under anesthesia (MUA) without the risks associated with MUA.
- Oral steroids also can provide short-term benefit in pain relief and improved ROM and function. However, oral steroids have side effects that limit the patient population for which they can be used (3)[B].
- Intra-articular corticosteroid injections have been shown to decrease pain, improve function, and increase ROM. Multiple injections have been shown to be beneficial, specifically up to three injections within a 16-wk period. However, there is a theoretical risk of weakening ligaments, tendons, and/or other capsular structures with repetitive cortisone injections (3)[B].
- A program of therapeutic exercise comprising gentle ROM exercises, stretching, and graded resistance training has been associated with increased ROM and decreased pain. The program should be guided by the patient within the limits of his or her pain, and vigorous programs that increase symptoms should be avoided (2)[B],(4)[C].
- Suprascapular nerve blocks may decrease pain.
- MUA is recommended if conservative measures fail.
- Surgical capsular release also may be used for refractory cases.

REFERENCES

1. Wong CK, Levine WN, Deo K, et al. Natural history of frozen shoulder: fact or fiction? A systematic review. *Physiotherapy*. 2017;103(1):40–47.
2. Ewald A. Adhesive capsulitis: a review. *Am Fam Physician*. 2011;83(4):417–422.
3. Sun Y, Zhang P, Liu S, et al. Intra-articular steroid injection for frozen shoulder: a systematic review and meta-analysis of randomized controlled trials with trial sequential analysis. *Am J Sports Med*. 2017;45(9):2171–2179.
4. Chan HBY, Pua PY, How CH. Physical therapy in the management of frozen shoulder. *Singapore Med J*. 2017;58(12):685–689.

ADDITIONAL READING

- Buchbinder R, Green S, Youd JM, et al. Arthrographic distension for adhesive capsulitis (frozen shoulder). *Cochrane Database Syst Rev*. 2008;(1):CD007005.
- Juel NG, Brox JI, Brunborg C, et al. Very high prevalence of frozen shoulder in patients with type 1 diabetes of ≥45 years' duration: the Dialong Shoulder Study. *Arch Phys Med Rehabil*. 2017;98(8):1551–1559.

CLINICAL PEARLS

- Frozen shoulder typically presents with insidious shoulder stiffness, and near-complete loss of both active and passive motion of the shoulder most prevalent, often with limitations of external rotation
- Shoulder immobilization, thyroid disease, and diabetes are risk factors for developing adhesive capsulitis.
- The three clinical phases include the painful phase with maintained ROM and lasts 2 to 9 mo, the frozen phase with decreased ROM and lasts 4 to 12 mo, and the thawing phase with gradually resolving symptoms and lasts 12 to 24 mo.
- There are high rates of spontaneous recovery after 18 to 30 mo.
- Conservative treatment options include a home exercise program and physical therapy but may also include NSAIDs and intra-articular corticosteroids.

ANAPHYLAXIS

Kristina Wilson, MD, MPH, FAAP, CAQSM

BASICS

- The causative agent in anaphylaxis remains unknown in up to 1/3 of cases.
- Food is the most common causative agent (about 1/3 of known cases) in children.
- Pharmacotherapeutic agents are the most common cause in adults.
- Other common causes include *Hymenoptera* stings and latex.
- Key to management and treatment is early recognition and immediate initiation of appropriate medical therapy.
- Epinephrine is the undisputed initial therapy for anaphylaxis, and its administration should never be delayed.
- Failure to inject epinephrine promptly has been identified as the most important factor contributing to death in patients experiencing anaphylaxis.

DESCRIPTION

- Severe, potentially life-threatening systemic hypersensitivity reaction
- Allergic type mediated by immunoglobulin E (IgE):
  - Involves the respiratory and/or cardiovascular systems
  - Patients may have a history of less severe reaction previously on exposure to relevant allergen.
- Exercise-induced anaphylaxis (EIAn):
  - Occurs in response to physical exertion
  - Subset of patients must have associated food trigger—food-dependent exercise-induced anaphylaxis (FDEIAn).
- Cold urticaria:
  - Reproducible, rapid onset of erythema, pruritus, and edema after exposure to cold
  - Most idiopathic
  - Occasionally involves abnormal circulating proteins (i.e., cryoglobulins or cryofibrinogens); agglutinates or precipitates at lower temperatures

EPIDEMIOLOGY

Death rates from the most common causes of anaphylaxis have varied:

- Food induced has increased.
- Insect sting has declined.
- Drug induced has increased.

Incidence

- 8 to 50/100,000 person-years in Western countries
- Incidence rates vary widely owing to differences in sample populations, data-collection methods, and varying definitions of anaphylaxis.

Prevalence

Lifetime prevalence of 0.05–2.0% in Western countries (1), rising especially in children

ETIOLOGY AND PATHOPHYSIOLOGY

- Allergic: IgE-mediated:
  - Drugs
  - Venom
  - Latex
  - Vaccines
  - Food
- Nonallergic: direct basophil/mast cell–mediated:
  - Radiocontrast dye
  - Opioid drugs

RISK FACTORS

- Prior anaphylaxis event can predict subsequent anaphylaxis:
  - As the only risk factor, prior anaphylaxis has a poor ability to identify patients who might develop anaphylaxis.
  - 14% of anaphylaxis admissions for peanut sensitivity have a prior history of anaphylaxis.
- Often occurs following a previous mild allergic reaction to the same allergen
- Most proposed risk factors have limited value owing to a low specificity:
  - Coexisting atopic disease; especially poorly controlled asthma
  - Older age at first reaction to food allergy
- Clinical risk factors for fatality in anaphylactic reactions (2):
  - Severe or uncontrolled asthma
  - Cardiovascular disease
  - Mastocytosis

GENERAL PREVENTION

- Avoidance of known allergen
- No available tests exist to predict the likelihood of a person developing anaphylaxis.
- Neither size of skin prick test wheal nor the level of serum-specific IgE correlate with reaction severity.
- Immunotherapy:
  - *Hymenoptera* venom and penicillin: currently available
  - Oral immunotherapy (OIT) mg doses or sublingual immunotherapy (SLIT) microgram doses over months
  - Milk, egg, and peanut
  - 20% drop out due to serious side effects such as anaphylaxis
  - Temporary tolerance maintained with regular ingestion
  - Permanent immunologic tolerance difficult to demonstrate
  - Only available in controlled trials
- Cold-induced anaphylaxis:
  - Avoidance of:
    - Cold water and air
    - Cold food and beverages
- Promising outlooks: characterization of β-cell epitope responses:
  - Specific allergenic epitopes may correlate with severity of reaction.
  - Individuals have a unique fingerprint of IgE-specific allergenic epitopes, and characterization of this profile may help to determine risk of anaphylaxis.

DIAGNOSIS

- Diagnosis is made based on clinical symptoms:
  - Do not underestimate the potential severity of an allergic reaction in its early stages.
  - Symptoms may progress rapidly.
- Suspicion of anaphylaxis requires immediate medical intervention and should not be delayed by diagnostic tests.
- Biphasic reactions reported in up to 20% of reactions (3)
- Clinical criteria for diagnosing anaphylaxis (3)[C]:
  - Acute onset of an illness (minutes to several hours) with involvement of the skin, mucosal tissue, or both (e.g., generalized hives; pruritus or flushing; swollen lips, tongue, and/or uvula) and *at least one* of the following:
    - Respiratory compromise (e.g., dyspnea, wheeze/bronchospasm, stridor, reduced peak expiratory flow [PEF], hypoxemia)
    - Reduced blood pressure (BP) or associated symptoms of end-organ dysfunction (e.g., hypotonia/collapse, syncope, incontinence)
  - Two or more of the following that occur rapidly after exposure to a likely allergen for that patient:
    - Involvement of the skin–mucosal tissue (e.g., generalized hives; itch or flush; swollen lips, tongue, and/or uvula)
    - Respiratory compromise (e.g., dyspnea, wheeze/bronchospasm, stridor, reduce PEF, hypoxemia)
    - Reduced BP or associated symptoms (e.g., hypotonia/collapse, syncope, incontinence)
    - Persistent gastrointestinal (GI) symptoms (e.g., crampy abdominal pain, vomiting)
  - Reduced BP after exposure to known allergen for that patient:
    - Infants and children: low systolic BP (age specific) or >30% decrease in systolic BP
    - Adults: systolic BP of <90 mm Hg or >30% decrease from that person's baseline

HISTORY

- Previous history of anaphylaxis
- Symptoms:
  - Fatigue
  - Pruritus
  - Urticaria
  - Angioedema
  - Wheezing
  - Rhinitis
  - GI distress
  - Cardiovascular collapse
- Time between exposure or suspected exposure and event may happen within seconds.
- Recent changes in baseline health
- Contributing environmental factors:
  - Extremes of temperature
  - Elevated humidity
  - Increased pollen count
- Contributing personal factors:
  - Physical exertion
  - Ethanol consumption
  - Insect sting
  - Food consumption
  - Stress
  - Menses
  - Fever
- Medications:
  - Nonsteroidal anti-inflammatory drugs (NSAIDs)
  - Aspirin
  - Antibiotics
  - Angiotensin-converting enzyme (ACE) inhibitors
- Comorbid medical conditions:
  - Asthma
  - Chronic obstructive pulmonary disease (COPD)
  - Cardiovascular disease
  - Mastocytosis
- If patient has a history of anaphylaxis: previous treatments and their effects

PHYSICAL EXAM

- Respiratory: bronchospasm, laryngeal edema
- Cardiovascular: hypotension, dysrhythmias, myocardial ischemia
- GI: nausea, vomiting, diarrhea
- Cutaneous: urticaria, angioedema
- Hematologic: activation of intrinsic coagulation pathway sometimes leading to disseminated intravascular coagulation (DIC), thrombocytopenia
- Neurologic: seizures
- Death can occur from airway obstruction or circulatory collapse.

DIFFERENTIAL DIAGNOSIS

- Pulmonary embolism
- Acute myocardial infarction
- Airway obstruction
- Asthma
- Tension pneumothorax
- NSAID reaction
- Vasovagal collapse
- Septic shock
- Hereditary angioedema
- Serum sickness
- Systemic mastocytosis
- Pheochromocytoma
- Carcinoid syndrome

DIAGNOSTIC TESTS & INTERPRETATION

Initial Tests (lab, imaging)

- There are no specific tests to make the diagnosis of anaphylaxis, and evaluation should not delay diagnosis and treatment.
- For respiratory distress after administration of epinephrine, an arterial blood gas analysis may be helpful in evaluating ventilatory status.
- These changes can be noted during anaphylaxis:
  - Elevation of plasma histamine level
  - Increase in hematocrit secondary to fluid extravasation
- May obtain tryptase levels:
  - Must be drawn within 3 hr of symptom onset
  - Must be placed on ice
  - Rarely elevated in food-induced anaphylaxis

Diagnostic Procedures/Other

Electrocardiogram (ECG): abnormalities including dysrhythmias, ischemic changes, infarction

TREATMENT

- Prehospital:
  - Airway, breathing, and circulation (ABCs)
  - Remove trigger (i.e., stinger from insect).
  - Early administration of epinephrine intramuscular (IM) in the anterolateral thigh positively affects outcome (3)[B]:
    - If preloaded epinephrine is available, it is prudent to administer prior to emergency personnel arriving if anaphylaxis is suspected.
    - May be administered every 5 to 15 min as needed based on patient's condition
    - Call 911 for emergent transfer to hospital.
  - Recumbent position with legs elevated (3)[B]: maintenance of central vascular compartment volume
  - Albuterol: metered-dose inhaler (MDI) or nebulized solution if bronchospasm not relieved by administration of epinephrine: every 20 min or continuously
  - Diphenhydramine: Cochrane Review 2007 of H_1 antihistamines in anaphylaxis revealed no studies that provided evidence for the use of H_1 antihistamines in anaphylaxis (4)[B]:
    - Onset of action takes 1 to 2 hr.
    - Relieves pruritus, urticaria, and angioedema
    - Works synergistically with epinephrine
    - Does not relieve upper or lower respiratory tract obstruction or circulatory collapse
    - Does not prevent fatality
- Emergency department (ED) treatment:
  - Continuous cardiac and vital sign monitoring until stable
  - Persistent bronchospasm can be treated with β-agonist bronchodilators.
  - Hypotension should be treated with isotonic volume. Vasopressors and Trendelenburg positioning are useful adjuncts.
  - Antihistamines (both H_1 and H_2 blockers) have been shown to be helpful in preventing histamine interactions with target tissues:
    - *Not* a first-line treatment
    - Does not treat life-threatening symptoms of anaphylaxis (4)[B]
    - Most helpful treating cutaneous symptoms
  - Corticosteroids have never been shown in placebo-controlled trials to affect the course of anaphylaxis but are used to treat associated conditions (e.g., asthma, allergic rhinitis):
    - Onset 4 to 6 hr
    - May decrease the chance of having a biphasic reaction:
      - Second episode of anaphylaxis after treatment for first episode
      - Occurs 2 to 72 hr after onset of first episode
      - 80% occur within the first 4 hr of initial episode.
  - Glucagon is useful in epinephrine-resistant anaphylaxis from β-adrenergic blocking agents.

MEDICATION

First Line

Epinephrine (EpiPen):

- Adult: 0.3 to 0.5 mg (Use 1:1,000 dilution for subcutaneous [SC] route.)
- Children: 0.01 mg/kg SC (maximum dose 0.3 mg)
- Preloaded syringe: 0.15 mg per injector (EpiPen Jr) and 0.30 mg per injector (EpiPen)
- Refractory hypotension:
  - Epinephrine drip 0.1 to 1.0 μg/kg/min (maximum 10 μg/min)
  - Titrated based on clinical effect; must be on cardiac monitor owing to risk of lethal cardiac arrhythmias

Second Line

- β-agonist: albuterol:
  - MDI
  - Continuous nebulizer treatment
- H_1 antagonist: diphenhydramine:
  - Adult: 50 mg intravenous (IV)
  - Children: 1 to 2 mg/kg slow IV pump (IVP)
- Steroids:
  - Methylprednisolone: severe reactions:
    - Adult: 125 mg IV
    - Children: 1 to 2 mg/kg IV (maximum single dose 60 to 80 mg)
  - Prednisone: mild reactions:
    - Adult: 60 mg PO
    - Children: 1 to 2 mg/kg PO (maximum single dose 60 to 80 mg)
  - Hydrocortisone:
    - Adults: 500 mg IV
    - Children: 4 to 8 mg/kg per dose IV
- Oxygen: respiratory distress/hypoxia
- H_2 antagonist:
  - Ranitidine: adult: 50 mg IV *or*
  - Cimetidine: 300 mg IV; children: 1 to 2 mg/kg (maximum dose 75 to 150 mg)

- Glucagon: for refractory hypotension, especially if patient is on a β-blocker:
  - Adult: 1 mg IV
  - Children: 20 to 30 μg/kg (maximum dose 1 mg) given over 5 min; followed by an infusion of 5 to 15 μg/min titrated to effect

ADMISSION, INPATIENT, AND NURSING CONSIDERATIONS

- Initial stabilization:
  - ABCs:
    - Ensure adequate ventilation.
    - Endotracheal intubation may be required but is difficult because of laryngeal edema or spasm.
    - Transtracheal jet insufflation or cricothyrotomy may be necessary to control the airway.
  - Epinephrine IM
  - Aggressive volume resuscitation with crystalloids to maintain BP; transfer of as much as 50% of the intravascular fluid into the extravascular space may occur within 10 min.
  - In volume-refractory hypotension, may need continuous IV epinephrine or other vasopressors (e.g., vasopressin or dopamine)
  - Monitor for biphasic reaction.
- Admission criteria:
  - Intubated patients, patients in respiratory distress, and patients with refractory hypotension should be admitted to an intensive care unit (ICU) setting.
  - A monitored bed may be necessary for the patient who has not had substantial response to initial therapy.
  - Patients with significant generalized reactions and persistent symptoms should be admitted for observation for 24 hr.
- Discharge criteria:
  - Individualized based on the following criteria (5)[C]:
    - Initial presentation
    - Response to therapy
    - Availability of close observation at home
    - Accessibility of a medical facility from home
  - Patients with complete resolution of symptoms may be discharged after 4 to 6 hr of ED observation:
    - Epinephrine duration—1 hr
    - Majority of biphasic reactions occur within the first 4 hr of initial episode.
  - Continuation of H_1 antagonist, H_2 antagonist, and corticosteroids for minimum 48 hr after discharge
  - Patients with allergic reactions should have follow-up within 48 hr of discharge to evaluate effectiveness of outpatient therapy.
  - Severity of the reaction should be emphasized to each patient and family.
  - Anaphylaxis action plans:
    - Education about prevention and prehospital management
    - Prescription for self-administered epinephrine and instructions on its use
    - Patients with a known trigger should be counseled on strict avoidance of that trigger.
    - Limited evidence on their impact on recurrence of anaphylaxis or reduction in fatal events (5)[B]
  - A follow-up visit with an allergist is also recommended for consideration of allergy testing exercise ± food provocation test.

REFERENCES

1. Lieberman P, Camargo CA Jr, Bohlke K, et al. Epidemiology of anaphylaxis: findings of the American College of Allergy, Asthma and Immunology Epidemiology of Anaphylaxis Working Group. *Ann Allergy Asthma Immunol*. 2006;97(5):596–602.
2. Simons FE, Ardusso LR, Dimov V, et al. World Allergy Organization Anaphylaxis guidelines: 2013 update of the evidence base. *Int Arch Allergy Immunol*. 2013;162(3):193–204.
3. Muraro A, Roberts G, Worm M, et al. Anaphylaxis: guidelines from the European Academy of Allergy and Clinical Immunology. *Allergy*. 2014;69(8):1026–1045.
4. Sheikh A, ten Broek VM, Brown SGA, et al. H1-antihistamines for the treatment of anaphylaxis with and without shock. *Cochrane Database Syst Rev*. 2007;(1):CD006160.
5. Nurmatov U, Worth A, Sheikh A. Anaphylaxis management plans for the acute and long-term management of anaphylaxis: a systematic review. *J Allergy Clin Immunol*. 2008;122(2):353–361, 361.e1–361.e3.

ADDITIONAL READING

- Liberman DB, Teach SJ. Management of anaphylaxis in children. *Pediatr Emerg Care*. 2008;24(12):861–866.
- Lieberman P. Epidemiology of anaphylaxis. *Curr Opin Allergy Clin Immunol*. 2008;8(4):316–320.
- Oswalt ML, Kemp SF. Anaphylaxis: office management and prevention. *Immunol Allergy Clin North Am*. 2007;27(2):177–191.
- Pumphrey RSH. When should self-injectible epinephrine be prescribed for food allergy and when should it be used? *Curr Opin Allergy Clin Immunol*. 2008;8(3):254–260.
- Sheikh A, Shehata YA, Brown SG, et al. Adrenaline for the treatment of anaphylaxis: Cochrane systematic review. *Allergy*. 2009;64(2):204–212.
- Soar J; for Guideline Development Group. Emergency treatment of anaphylaxis in adults: concise guidance. *Clin Med (Lond)*. 2009;9(2):181–185.
- Soar J, Pumphrey R, Cant A, et al; for Working Group of the Resuscitation Council. Emergency treatment of anaphylactic reactions—guidelines for healthcare providers. *Resuscitation*. 2008;77(2):157–169.
- Tang ML, Osborne N, Allen K. Epidemiology of anaphylaxis. *Curr Opin Allergy Clin Immunol*. 2009;9(4):351–356.

SEE ALSO

Exercise-Induced Anaphylaxis; Exercise-Induced Urticaria

CLINICAL PEARLS

- Epinephrine is the undisputed initial therapy for anaphylaxis, and its administration should never be delayed.
- There are no specific tests to make the diagnosis of anaphylaxis, and evaluation should not delay diagnosis and treatment.
- Failure to inject epinephrine promptly has been identified as the most important factor contributing to death in patients experiencing anaphylaxis.

ANKLE IMPINGEMENT

Marcia Faustin, MD, CAQSM

BASICS

DESCRIPTION

- Impingement is a clinical syndrome of end-range joint pain or restricted motion caused by direct abutment and/or compression of bone or soft tissues.
- Classifications: based on types of impingement:
  - Posttraumatic synovitis
  - Bony spur
  - Intra-articular fibrous band/scar
  - Capsular scarring
- Ankle impingement syndromes are classified based on location:
  - Anterior
  - Anterolateral
  - Anteromedial (less common)
  - Posterior
  - Posteromedial (less common)

EPIDEMIOLOGY

- 1–2% of ankle inversion injuries lead to chronic disability requiring surgical intervention.
- Common in athletes who play on grass or turf (1)
- 10–25% of population have os trigonum.

ETIOLOGY AND PATHOPHYSIOLOGY

- Arises from either traumatic or repetitive hyperdorsiflexion (anterior impingement) or hyperplantar flexion (posterior impingement)
- Microtrauma from repetitive movements such as kicking soccer ball can lead to spur formation.
- Initial ankle injuries in the subacute or chronic phase can lead to the development of abnormal osseous or soft tissue thickening.
- Pain generators are typically the soft tissue caught between traction spurs and osteophytes, not the actual osteophytes/bone spurs.
- Anterior impingement is typically easier to diagnose than posterior impingement, due to superficial location:
  - Anterior impingement:
    - Anterior lateral gutter—damage to lateral collateral ligament complex and joint capsule, resulting in synovitis, irregular thickening, and/or scarring of ligaments after inversion ankle sprain
    - Anterior:
      - Repeated capsuloligamentous traction or microtrauma in plantar flexion may induce spur formation (kicking a ball).
      - Tibial or talar osteophytes impinge soft tissue.
  - Anteromedial—unclear mechanism; possibly secondary to eversion ankle injury or inversion injury with rotational component that leads to soft tissue impingement
  - Posterior impingement: Spectrum of disorders characterized by posterior ankle pain after acute fracture or recurrent plantar flexion or hyperplantar flexion. Symptoms can arise due to impingement and mechanical irritation of the soft tissues between these posterior structures:
    - Os trigonum (accessory ossicle connected by a fibrous band to the posterolateral tubercle of the talus) (2)[C]
    - Talar compression syndrome
    - Prominent posterolateral process of talus (Stieda process)
    - Prominent medial malleoli process
    - Prominent posterior process of calcaneus

RISK FACTORS

- Anterior impingement:
  - Risk factors include sports requiring recurrent forceful dorsiflexion of the ankle, recurrent ankle sprains (supination and plantar flexion) and/or chronic ankle instability, and acute ankle sprains/fractures.
  - Athletes: soccer players, gymnasts, basketball players, football players, high jumpers, running uphill
- Posterior impingement:
  - Risk factors include acute or recurrent hyperplantar flexion (ballet on pointe), recurrent ankle sprains, or ankle instability.
  - Athletes: ballet dancers ("en pointe" and "demi pointe"), cheerleaders, running downhill (forced plantar flexion)
  - Poor shoe wear without appropriate support
  - Overuse injury is more common than traumatic injury (3)[C].

GENERAL PREVENTION

- Preventing recurrent ankle sprains
- Early exercise protocol for acute ankle sprain
- Proper rehabilitation, including ankle strengthening, range of motion, and proprioception
- Proper footwear/orthotics
- Recognizing the condition early in order to allow early rest and rehabilitation

DIAGNOSIS

HISTORY

- Typically, a clinical diagnosis of exclusion
- Prior history of single or multiple episodes of traumatic ankle injuries (typically inversion injuries)
- Mild swelling or effusion after activity (2,3,4,5)[C]
- Anterior impingement:
  - Pain with activities requiring ankle in dorsiflexion (uphill running/walking)
  - Pain with kicking a soccer ball, especially a dead ball
  - Popping or snapping sensation of isolated soft tissue lesions
  - Subjective feeling of limited range of motion or blocking on dorsiflexion
- Exacerbating factors: climbing stairs, ascending ladders, and deep squat (1,2,3,4,6)[C]
- Posterior impingement:
  - Pain is difficult to localize, typically anterior to the Achilles tendon.
  - Pain described as consistent, sharp, dull and/or radiating
  - Prior history of inversion (supination) and plantar flexion injury
  - Posterior ankle pain exacerbated by either plantar flexion (compression of soft tissues or bony prominence) or dorsiflexion (stretching of the posterior capsule and ligaments)
- History of repetitive push off or plantar flexion maneuvers (i.e., downhill running/walking, descending stairs, and high-heeled shoe wear) (1,2,3,5,6)[C]

PHYSICAL EXAM

- Complete neurovascular exam, strength, and range of motion
- Possible soft tissue swelling or effusion
- Anterior impingement:
  - Tenderness to palpation over the anterior, anterolateral, or anteromedial ankle (most important clinical finding)
  - Pain in the anterior aspect of the ankle with either forced plantar flexion or dorsiflexion
  - Possible palpable mass with tenderness to palpation (1,2,3,6)[C]
- Posterior impingement:
  - Tenderness to palpation in the posterior aspect of ankle, typically anterior to and not involving the Achilles tendon
  - Possible palpable soft tissue thickening with tenderness to palpation
  - Positive plantar flexion test: pain in posterior ankle with plantar flexion (pathognomonic)
  - Reproducible pain with pressure over posteromedial aspect of the ankle during passive inversion and plantar flexion
- Pain with dorsiflexion (stretching of the capsule and ligament) (1,2,3,5)[C]

DIFFERENTIAL DIAGNOSIS

- Anterior impingement:
  - Lateral ankle ligament sprain
  - Synovial thickening/synovitis
  - Loose/intra-articular bodies, avulsion fragments
  - Chondral or osteochondral lesions of anterior tibial plafond or talar dome
  - Osteoid osteoma of the talus
  - Ganglion cyst
  - Osteoarthritis (1,2,3,4,6)[A]

- Posterior impingement:
  - Deltoid ligament sprain
  - Posterior tibial tendonitis/tenosynovitis
  - Flexor hallucis tendonitis/tenosynovitis
  - Achilles tendonitis/tenosynovitis
  - Peroneal tendonitis/tenosynovitis
  - Retrocalcaneal bursitis
  - Haglund deformity
  - Tarsal coalition
  - Thickening of posteromedial ankle capsule
  - Tarsal tunnel syndrome
  - Osteochondral lesions of talar dome (medial)
  - Shepherd fracture (acute fracture of the posterolateral process of the talus)
  - Ganglion cyst
  - Osteoarthritis (1,2,3,5,6)[C]

DIAGNOSTIC TESTS & INTERPRETATION

Initial Tests (lab, imaging)

- Weight-bearing ankle x-rays:
  - Anteroposterior (AP), lateral, oblique
- Anterior impingement:
  - Oblique anterior impingement view: beam tilted in 45-degree craniocaudal direction with leg in 30-degree external rotation and foot in plantar flexion) (2,4,6)[C]
- Posterior impingement:
  - Posterior impingement view: lateral, 25-degree external rotation, oblique view (os trigonum) (2,5,6)[C]

Follow-Up Tests & Special Considerations

- Magnetic resonance imaging (MRI) (evaluates osseous and soft tissue) (1,2,5,6)[C]
- Ultrasound (evaluates soft tissue and tendons) (6)[C]
- Computed tomography (CT) (evaluates osseous pathologies and for surgical planning) (1,2,5,6)[C]
- MR arthrogram (1,4)[C]

Diagnostic Procedures/Others

Ultrasound-guided injection of local anesthetic and/or corticosteroid into:

- Anterolateral gutter
- Area of synovitis or focal capsular thickening (anterior or posterior impingement)
- Os trigonum synchondrosis (1,2,4,6)[C]

Test Interpretation

MRI:

- Most useful to diagnose soft tissue pathology and excluding other pathology (such as an osteochondral lesion)
- Bone marrow edema, fracture line, fluid in synchondrosis (in case of os trigonum fracture), posterior capsular or ligament thickening with intermediate to low intensity on T2-weighted images (3)[C]

TREATMENT

GENERAL MEASURES

- Rest, avoid provocative activities, ice
- Cast immobilization (severe cases)
- Shoe modifications, heel lifts, orthotics
- Physical therapy with emphasis on:
  - Range of motion exercises, proprioceptive (balance) training, and strengthening exercises to improve ankle stability
  - Address core/gluteal weakness.
  - Modalities: electrotherapy, transcutaneous electrical nerve stimulation (TENS) unit, deloading taping, soft tissue massage (1,2,3,4,5,6)[C]

MEDICATION

First Line

Nonsteroidal anti-inflammatory drugs (NSAIDs)

Second Line

Ultrasound-guided local anesthetic and/or corticosteroid injection (diagnostic and therapeutic)

ISSUES FOR REFERRAL

- 3 to 6 mo of failed conservative treatment affected normal daily activities or athletic performance and correlated physical exam and imaging findings (1,2,3)[C]
- Posteromedial impingement typically fails conservative treatment, which leads to surgical débridement (3)[C].

SURGERY/OTHER PROCEDURES

- Surgical goals are to improve function and pain by removing offending pathologic bony and/or soft tissue lesions.
- Arthroscopic (more common) or open procedures (3,5,6)[C]
- Prognosis decreases with higher degree of tibiotalar osteoarthritis (2,4)[A].

COMPLEMENTARY & ALTERNATIVE MEDICINE

Limited data suggest the use of biologics such as platelet-rich plasma (PRP) and concentrated bone marrow aspirate (CBMA) at the time of surgery. They are injected into degenerative tendon or the bed of the lesion (5)[C].

ONGOING CARE

FOLLOW-UP RECOMMENDATIONS

Postsurgical treatment:

- Weight-bearing as tolerated immediately postoperative with early range of motion
- Physical therapy focuses on increasing available joint space for more mobility and less pain during activity.
- Ankle immobilization is recommended if there is intraoperative evidence of extensive osseous injury (5)[A].
- Return to play average ~9 to 16 wk (1,2,5)[C]

PROGNOSIS

- Majority of patients have resolution of symptoms with conservative/nonoperative care (3,5)[C].
- Posterior impingement secondary to overuse has better prognosis than traumatic injury (2,3)[C].

Pediatric Considerations

Pediatric patients will present with similar symptoms and exam findings as adults. They are typically treated conservatively; if they fail nonoperative management, surgical treatment may be indicated.

REFERENCES

1. Lavery KP, McHale KJ, Rossy WH, et al. Ankle impingement. *J Orthop Surg Res*. 2016;11(1):97.
2. Niek van Dijk C. Anterior and posterior ankle impingement. *Foot Ankle Clin*. 2006;11(3):663–683.
3. Russo A, Zappia M, Reginelli A, et al. Ankle impingement: a review of multimodality imaging approach. *Musculoskelet Surg*. 2013;97(Suppl 2):S161–S168.
4. Vaseenon T, Amendola A. Update on anterior ankle impingement. *Curr Rev Musculoskelet Med*. 2012;5(2):145–150.
5. Yasui Y, Hannon CP, Hurley E, et al. Posterior ankle impingement syndrome: a systematic four-stage approach. *World J Orthop*. 2016;7(10):657–663.
6. Dimmick S, Linklater J. Ankle impingement syndromes. *Radiol Clin North Am*. 2013;51(3):479–510.

ADDITIONAL READING

- John S, Mendicino R, Catanzariti A. Mastering ankle impingement syndromes. *Podiatry Today*. 2007;(20)8:52–60.
- McMurray TP. Footballer's ankle. *J Bone Joint Surg Br*. 1950;32(1):68–69. (first article to discuss ankle impingement in the literature)
- Vasukutty NV, Akrawi H, Theruvil B, et al. Ankle arthroscopy in children. *Ann R Coll Surg Engl*. 2011;93(3):232–235.
- Witjes S, Gresnigt F, van den Bekerom MP, et al. The ANKLE TRIAL (ankle treatment after injuries of the ankle ligaments): what is the benefit of external support devices in the functional treatment of acute ankle sprain? A randomised controlled trial. *BMC Musculoskelet Disord*. 2012;13:21.

CLINICAL PEARLS

- Ankle impingement is classified according to type of impingement and location of impingement.
- Largely a clinical diagnosis of exclusion
- Typically, conservative treatment will resolve majority of cases.

ANKLE SPRAINS, LATERAL

Christopher A. Gee, MD, MPH, FACEP, CAQSM

BASICS

DESCRIPTION

- Lateral ankle sprains are the most common injury sustained by athletes (1) and comprise approximately 14% of all sports-related injuries (2).
- Over 80% of sprains are due to an inversion type of mechanism that injures the lateral ankle ligaments.
- Whereas the medial side of the ankle has the broad, strong deltoid ligament as a restraint, the lateral side of the ankle has three smaller ligaments that act as the static restraint system.
- Primary static restraints to ankle inversion:
  - Anterior talofibular ligament (ATFL): passes from the tip of the fibula to the lateral talar neck; taut in plantar flexion; injured most commonly
  - Calcaneofibular ligament (CFL): passes inferior and posterior from the tip of the fibula to the lateral calcaneus; usually injured with the ATFL
  - Posterior talofibular ligament (PTFL): passes posteriorly from the fibula to the talus; injured less often
- These ligaments are injured in a sequential pattern as extreme inversion and plantarflexion forces are placed on the ankle. The ATFL is injured first (isolated ATFL injuries occur in approximately 2/3 of injuries). After the small ATFL is injured, the CFL then is stressed and injured, followed by the PTFL. The ankle joint capsule is also sprained during an inversion injury. Given this pattern, isolated CFL injuries are uncommon.
- Increasing inversion force leads to more damage to lateral ligaments and capsule.
- Bony support of the distal fibula assists the deltoid ligament in restricting eversion stress to the ankle.
- The smaller medial malleolus provides less protection and allows inversion stress to injure the lateral ankle ligaments more easily.
- Ankle sprain grading:
  - Grade 1: stretch or partial tearing of ligaments but no gross laxity
  - Grade 2: partial tear of ligaments with increased laxity of ankle but still firm end point
  - Grade 3: complete rupture of ligaments; gross laxity of ankle with no end point

EPIDEMIOLOGY

Incidence

Very common injury in athletes and the general population, with around 23,000 cases every day (3)

ETIOLOGY AND PATHOPHYSIOLOGY

Lateral ankle sprains occur when the ankle is stressed with extreme inversion and plantarflexion forces that overcome the static restraints (ligaments, capsule). Spraining and tearing of the ligaments leads to pain, swelling, and varying degrees of disability.

RISK FACTORS

- Athletes (especially those involved in sports with jumping near other players and quick "cutting" motions, i.e., basketball, soccer, football) (4)
- Dancers
- Congenital tarsal coalition (allows less "give" in the foot and results in more stress to ankle)
- Prior ankle injury (Previously injured or stretched ligaments provide less overall stability.) (5)

DIAGNOSIS

HISTORY

Patients report history of inversion-type injury often with an audible pop. This is followed by rapid swelling, pain, and an inability to walk.

PHYSICAL EXAM

- Physical examination reveals ecchymosis and diffuse swelling about the ankle joint.
- Tenderness to palpation is noted along the course of injured ligaments and can be diagnostic of which ligaments are injured.
- Palpation of the anterior ankle joint and the talar dome with the foot in full plantarflexion can help to diagnose other forms of pathology (i.e., osteochondral defects).
- It is important to palpate both the medial and lateral malleoli and the base of the 5th metatarsal to examine for possible fracture (i.e., Ottawa Ankle Rules) (6).
- Occasionally, the ankle ligaments can be disrupted, and the stress passed up the tibiofibular syndesmosis. This leads to syndesmotic injuries or the so-called high ankle sprain.
- Assess neurovascular status by feeling distal pulses and manually testing appropriate muscle groups.
- Grading of ankle injury can be accomplished by testing the integrity of various ligaments. Examiner also should take into account the fact that prior ankle sprains may have left residual laxity on either side.
- Anterior drawer:
  - Tests stability of ATFL; performed by holding the distal tibia and pulling the heel forward. Increased laxity relative to the opposite side indicates a tear of the ATFL. The anterior drawer test in the ankle has poor sensitivity and specificity.
  - Inversion tilt: tests stability of CFL; performed by holding the distal tibia and moving the foot from a neutral position to an inversion position. Increased laxity compared with opposite side indicates a tear of the CFL.

DIFFERENTIAL DIAGNOSIS

- Tibia fracture (shaft, malleolus, etc.)
- Pilon fracture
- Fibula fracture (malleolus, Maisonneuve)
- Avulsion fracture
- Osteochondral defect in talar dome/tibial plafond
- Anterior ankle impingement
- Os trigonum syndrome
- Talus fracture
- Calcaneal fracture
- Peroneal subluxation
- Bimalleolar/trimalleolar fracture

DIAGNOSTIC TESTS & INTERPRETATION

- Plain radiographs of affected ankle (including anteroposterior, lateral, and mortise views) to rule out fracture (weight-bearing if able)
- May not need to perform x-rays if patient doesn't have tenderness along posterior 6-cm edge of lateral and medial malleoli and can bear weight initially after injury (Ottawa Ankle Rules) (6)
- Computed tomography (CT) scans may be performed to evaluate for occult fracture.
- Magnetic resonance imaging (MRI) is rarely useful in ankle sprains but may be useful in assessing integrity of various ligaments in patients with chronic ankle instability or in evaluation of osteochondral defects that are not apparent on radiographs.

TREATMENT

GENERAL MEASURES

- Initial therapy focuses on PRICE (protection [bracing], rest, ice, compression, elevation) protocol to decrease pain and swelling.
- Crutches can be used until patient is able to bear weight as tolerated.
- Various kinds of braces, compression devices, stirrup splints, and walking boots can be used to provide protection and support and to encourage walking.
- Should advise patients to begin gentle range of motion as soon as pain allows and to keep limb elevated to decrease swelling
- Severe sprains may be best treated with more motion restriction in devices such as casts or walking boots (7).
- Progressive therapy through a three-phase approach may best promote rapid recovery:
  - Phase 1 consists of RICE protocols to improve pain and swelling (often weeks 1 to 2).
  - Phase 2 consists of progressive range of motion exercises to improve motion and decrease swelling. Patients should continue to use a protective brace when walking to prevent further injury. Patients should be working toward full weight-bearing during this stage (weeks 2 to 4).
  - Phase 3 begins more aggressive strengthening and rehabilitation exercises. Specifically, patients should work on proprioception and endurance. This can be a formalized physical therapy program as needed (weeks 4 to 6).

MEDICATION

Acetaminophen or nonsteroidal anti-inflammatory drugs (NSAIDs) can be used after initial injury for pain. NSAIDs should be avoided in patients at risk for gastrointestinal (GI) bleeding.

ADDITIONAL THERAPIES

- Physical therapy can be used to assist patients in strengthening and generally rehabilitating the injured ankle.
- Electrical stimulation and iontophoresis may have a role in pain and swelling control.

SURGERY/OTHER PROCEDURES

- In general, most patients recover spontaneously and are able to go back to activities as pain allows. More unstable joints, recurrent injuries, and higher level athletes may need formal physical therapy.
- Often, general rehabilitation principles and conservative therapy are adequate to return athletes to their sport without more aggressive interventions. Patients rarely need primary repair of ligaments after an acute lateral ankle sprain.
- Occasionally, severe laxity of lateral ankle restraints may lead to recurrent ankle injuries and chronic ankle instability. These patients may benefit from ligament repair or ankle reconstruction to improve stability.

ONGOING CARE

FOLLOW-UP RECOMMENDATIONS

Patient Monitoring

- Patients may return to play once they have achieved a full range of motion and strength as well as being able to perform their sport-specific activities without limitations. Some may be able to return to play with a supportive device to protect from further injury depending on the sport and the patient's position.
- Depending on the sport, certain patients may need to go through a progression of sport-specific activities to return to play.

PROGNOSIS

- Prognosis depends on the extent of injury and any concurrent injuries, but for most patients, prognosis is excellent. More severe injuries may require more extensive rehabilitation for a patient to return to full function and prevent recurrence.
- Patients with recurrent instability and those in high-risk sports (e.g., volleyball, basketball) may benefit from functional bracing or taping.
- Patients who fail to undergo proper rehabilitation are often left with chronic instability and recurrent ankle injuries.

COMPLICATIONS

- Stiffness from prolonged immobilization
- Recurrent instability
- Osteochondral defects
- Chronic regional pain syndromes

REFERENCES

1. Roos KG, Kerr ZY, Mauntel TC, et al. The epidemiology of lateral ligament complex ankle sprains in National Collegiate Athletic Association sports. *Am J Sports Med*. 2017;45(1):201–209.
2. Fong DT, Chan YY, Mok KM, et al. Understanding acute ankle ligamentous sprain injury in sports. *Sports Med Arthrosc Rehabil Ther Technol*. 2009;1:14.
3. Kannus P, Renström P. Treatment for acute tears of the lateral ligaments of the ankle. Operation, cast, or early controlled mobilization. *J Bone Joint Surg Am*. 1991;73(2):305–312.
4. Nelson AJ, Collins CL, Yard EE, et al. Ankle injuries among United States high school sports athletes, 2005–2006. *J Athl Train*. 2007;42(3):381–387.
5. Malliaropoulos N, Ntessalen M, Papacostas E, et al. Reinjury after acute lateral ankle sprains in elite track and field athletes. *Am J Sports Med*. 2009;37(9):1755–1761.
6. Stiell IG, Greenberg GH, McKnight RD, et al. A study to develop clinical decision rules for the use of radiography in acute ankle injuries. *Ann Emerg Med*. 1992;21(4):384–390.
7. Lamb SE, Marsh JL, Hutton JL, et al. Mechanical supports for acute, severe ankle sprain: a pragmatic, multicentre, randomised controlled trial. *Lancet*. 2009;373(9663):575–581.

CLINICAL PEARLS

- Extremely common injury that can present with swelling, ecchymosis, and inability to walk
- Thorough exam and proper imaging (when indicated) can help to avoid missing associated fractures.
- Treatment involves progression from RICE protocol to progressive weight-bearing and range of motion and finally to strengthening and proprioceptive exercises.

ANKLE SPRAINS, MEDIAL

Daniel C. Herman, MD, PhD, FAAPMR, FACSM, CAQSM • Giorgio A. Negron, MD

BASICS

DESCRIPTION

- Injury to the deltoid ligament complex of the medial ankle occurs when the foot is forced into eversion and external rotation.
- Medial ankle sprains are less common than their lateral counterpart due to the vast strength of the deltoid ligament:
  - Deltoid ligament complex is composed of four superficial and two deep components (1).
- Grade I sprain results from mild stretching of the deltoid ligament with microscopic tears (1). Patients have mild swelling and tenderness. There is no joint instability on exam, and the patient is able to bear weight and ambulate with minimal pain. Owing to their benign nature, these injuries are not seen frequently in the office.
- Grade II sprain is a more severe injury involving an incomplete tear of the deltoid ligament. Patients have moderate pain, swelling, tenderness, and ecchymosis. There is mild to moderate joint instability on exam with some restriction in the range of motion and loss of function. Weight-bearing and ambulation are painful.
- Grade III sprain involves a complete tear of the deltoid ligament. Patients have severe pain, swelling, tenderness, and ecchymosis. There is significant mechanical instability on exam and significant loss of function and motion. Patients are unable to bear weight or ambulate.
- May progress to chronic ankle instability (constant sensation of ankle "giving away") if lingering symptoms persist a year after initial ankle sprain (2)
- Synonym(s): medial ankle sprain, deltoid ligament sprain

EPIDEMIOLOGY

- Although the majority of ankle injuries are lateral etiology (>90%), the incidence of medial ankle sprains is ~6% (2).
- Deltoid ligament sprains are often accompanied by a lateral malleolar fracture and/or syndesmotic injury (1).

RISK FACTORS

- Previous ankle sprain
- High-risk sports, including football, basketball, and long jumping
- Valgus-flat foot deformity (3)
- Low arch of the foot (i.e., pes planus)
- Dysfunction of the spring ligament
- Dysfunction of the posterior tibialis
- Extreme fatigue of peroneus (fibularis) longus muscle

GENERAL PREVENTION

- Exercise therapy and taping/bracing are effective in the management of primary and recurrent ankle sprains (4).
- Proprioceptive training appears to be effective in secondary prevention of ankle injuries (4).

COMMONLY ASSOCIATED CONDITIONS

- Syndesmosis disruption (3)
- Fracture of the fibula and/or tibia
- Avulsion fracture of the medial malleolus
- Bimalleolar and trimalleolar fracture
- Severe lateral ligament injury
- Spring ligament injury
- Posterior tibial tendon injury
- Flexor hallucis longus injury
- Posterior tibial and/or saphenous nerve traction injury

DIAGNOSIS

HISTORY

- Mechanism of injury: Athletes typically report an off-balanced, pronated foot landing, which leads to forced external rotation, abduction, and eversion.
- Alternate mechanism includes supination and excessive external rotation of the ankle (3).
- Should inquire about previous ankle injury and history of "giving way." This would suggest that there is an acute injury superimposed on chronic ankle instability.

PHYSICAL EXAM

- Signs and symptoms include:
  - Medial ankle pain.
  - Swelling on the medial aspect of the ankle.
  - Ecchymosis around the medial aspect of the ankle.
  - Sensation of a "pop."
  - Inability to walk.
- Physical examination includes:
  - Evaluation of the ability to bear weight.
  - Careful palpation to identify tender structures.
  - Determination of tenderness over the deltoid ligament.
  - A check for tenderness over the anterior syndesmosis ligament, Achilles tendon, lateral ankle, and fibula (distal and proximal).
  - A check of posterior tibial tendon function with resisted inversion.
  - A check of extensor hallucis longus tendon function with resisted extension of the great toe.
  - A check of range of motion of the ankle joint.
  - A check of flexor hallucis longus tendon function with resisted flexion of the great toe.
  - An eversion stress test determines the stability of the deltoid ligament; this is done with passive eversion of the ankle (1)[C].
  - A squeeze test and external rotation test are highly specific tests to rule out syndesmotic injury (1)[C].
  - An anterior drawer test may evaluate anterior and medial subluxation with deltoid ligament injury (1)[C].
  - Examine the patient's gait and while standing for valgus-flat foot deformity.

DIFFERENTIAL DIAGNOSIS

- Syndesmosis tear or sprain
- Posterior tibial tendon tear or subluxation
- Flexor hallucis longus tendon tear or sprain
- Distal tibia fracture
- Osteochondral fracture of the talar dome
- Fracture of the calcaneus
- Fracture of the lateral process of the talus
- Medial ankle sprain with associated proximal fibular fracture (Maisonneuve fracture)

DIAGNOSTIC TESTS & INTERPRETATION

- In the setting of acute injury, follow the Ottawa Ankle Rules to determine if radiographs are indicated (inability to bear weight, tenderness over posterior edge or tip of lateral/medial malleolus, the base of the 5th metatarsal, or navicular bone).
- Anteroposterior, lateral, and mortise views of the injured ankle are essential to rule out fracture when indicated (5)[B].
- >3 mm of medial clear space between the lateral border of the medial malleolus and the medial border of the talus at the level of talar dome is abnormal and suggestive of a deltoid ligament disruption (3)[C].
- Consider a valgus talar tilt stress radiograph to assess for significant instability and possible surgical treatment: >10 degrees difference in abduction tilt of the talus compared with opposite ankle is abnormal (perform this test *only* if there are no associated fractures) (3)[C].
- Magnetic resonance imaging (MRI) has high sensitivity and high specificity for injury to superficial/deep deltoid ligaments. Consider MRI if deltoid ligament rupture is unclear (partial vs. complete) and surgical treatment is being considered (5)[C].
- Ultrasonography may be an alternative when MRI is not readily available (high sensitivity and high specificity) (5)[C].

TREATMENT

GENERAL MEASURES

Prehospital:

- PRICE protocol: protection from further injury, rest, ice, compression, and elevation (1)[C]
- Protection can be achieved through an Aircast or a boot with a bladder to restrict inversion/eversion stress while also maintaining sagittal plane motion.
- Rest is achieved by limiting weight-bearing by having patients use crutches or other assistive devices until they are able to walk with a normal gait.
- Ice or cold-water immersion is recommended for 15 to 20 min q2–3h for the first 48 hr or until swelling improves, whichever comes first.
- Compression to control and decrease swelling should be applied early, usually with an Ace wrap or stirrup brace. Compression should be supportive but not constrictive.
- The injured ankle should be kept elevated above the level of the heart to further alleviate swelling.

ISSUES FOR REFERRAL

- >4 mm of medial clear space on the mortise view (bilateral and preferably weight-bearing if able)
- Significant instability on reverse talar tilt stress radiograph or weight-bearing views (5)[C]
- Grade III injury may need operative repair to prevent long-term complications (5)[C].
- Medial malleolus fracture
- Displaced lateral malleolus fracture
- Wound penetrating into the joint
- Conservative treatment has failed and the injury has progressed to chronic ankle instability.
- Patients with neurovascular compromise
- Uncertain diagnosis

ADDITIONAL THERAPIES

- Grade I sprain: functional rehabilitation and possibly a splint or a brace, with the recognition that return to sports generally is more delayed (3 to 6 wk) than with a lateral sprain (1 to 3 wk) (3)[C]
- Grade II sprain: same as grade 1, but in addition, may need a short period prior of immobilization in posterior splint or walking boot (3 to 4 wk)
- Grade III sprain: Treatment is controversial; requires immobilization (6 to 8 wk) or may need operative repair (see "Issues for Referral")
- Nonsteroidal anti-inflammatory drugs (NSAIDs) are the first-line medication for pain control (4)[A].
- Functional rehabilitation is of great importance in aiding return to activity and preventing chronic instability. The exercises should begin as soon as the initial pain and swelling have subsided sufficiently to allow the patient to perform simple exercises and should continue until the patient has returned to pain-free activity (4,5)[A].
- Achilles tendon stretch
- Foot circles
- Alphabet exercises: Although leg is stable, patient should use the great toe and foot to "write" the letters of the alphabet in the air.
- Isometric and isotonic plantar flexion, dorsiflexion, inversion, eversion, and toe curls
- Marble pickups (using toes)
- Heel walks
- Toe walks
- Circular wobble board
- Walking on different surfaces
- Walk–jog, jog–run
- During functional rehabilitation, it may be of benefit to use splints, braces, and taping to try to reduce instability, protect the ankle from further injury, and limit swelling.

COMPLEMENTARY & ALTERNATIVE MEDICINE

Neither ultrasound therapy, low-level laser therapy, nor hyperbaric therapy appears to be effective in the treatment of medial ankle sprains (4)[B].

ONGOING CARE

PROGNOSIS

- Pain decreases rapidly during the first 2 wk following injury:
  - Up to 70% of patients report residual symptoms or recurrence (4).
- Healing rates vary widely among studies, with 36–85% of patients reporting full recovery over the first 3 yr (6).
- Lack of proper rehabilitation contributes to recurrent and/or chronic ankle symptoms, complaints, and problems.

COMPLICATIONS

Deltoid ligament injury generally is a more serious injury than lateral ankle sprain and frequently is associated with concomitant injury to the lateral ligaments or fibula.

REFERENCES

1. Czajka CM, Tran E, Cai AN, et al. Ankle sprains and instability. *Med Clin North Am*. 2014;98(2):313–329.
2. Doherty C, Delahunt E, Caulfield B, et al. The incidence and prevalence of ankle sprain injury: a systematic review and meta-analysis of prospective epidemiological studies. *Sports Med*. 2014;44(1):123–140.
3. Savage-Elliott I, Murawski CD, Smyth NA, et al. The deltoid ligament: an in-depth review of anatomy, function, and treatment strategies. *Knee Surg Sports Traumatol Arthrosc*. 2013;21(6):1316–1327.
4. Doherty C, Bleakley C, Delahunt E, et al. Treatment and prevention of acute and recurrent ankle sprain: an overview of systematic reviews with meta-analysis. *Br J Sports Med*. 2017;51(2):113–125.
5. McCollum GA, van den Bekerom MP, Kerkhoffs GM, et al. Syndesmosis and deltoid ligament injuries in the athlete. *Knee Surg Sports Traumatol Arthrosc*. 2013;21(6):1328–1337.
6. van Rijn RM, van Os AG, Bernsen RM, et al. What is the clinical course of acute ankle sprains? A systematic literature review. *Am J Med*. 2008;121(4):324.e6–331.e6.

ADDITIONAL READING

- Birrer RB, Fani-Salek MH, Totten VY, et al. Managing ankle injuries in the emergency department. *J Emerg Med*. 1999;17(4):651–660.
- Mei-Dan O, Kahn G, Zeev A, et al. The medial longitudinal arch as a possible risk factor for ankle sprains: a prospective study in 83 female infantry recruits. *Foot Ankle Int*. 2005;26(2):180–183.

CLINICAL PEARLS

- An athlete may return to full activity once he or she is able to do a progressive rehabilitation program without pain and instability. Return to sports may be prolonged over several months depending on the degree of injury.
- To prevent future injuries, athlete should wear an ankle brace for sporting activities and complete rehabilitation.
- Untreated, severe sprain may result in chronic pain, instability, and the possibility of ankle arthritis.
- Effect of external ankle support on performance:
  - Dependent on the specific brace or method (such as taping) used
  - Decrease in performance ≤5%

ANKYLOSING SPONDYLITIS

Scott Chandler, DO • Kevin deWeber, MD, FAAFP, FACSM, RMSK

BASICS

DESCRIPTION

- Ankylosing spondylitis (AS) is a chronic inflammatory, autoimmune arthritis characterized by inflammatory back pain (IBP).
- It is the most common and potentially severe subtype of spondyloarthritis (SpA), which includes:
  - Reactive (Reiter) arthritis.
  - Arthritis/spondylitis with inflammatory bowel disease (IBD).
  - Arthritis/spondylitis with psoriasis.
  - Unspecified spondylitis.
  - AS without confirmed radiographic findings is classified as nonradiographic axial spondyloarthropathy (nr-axSpA) and has similar outcomes and response to treatment.
- AS causes inflammation of the sacroiliac (SI) joints, peripheral joints, and entheses (sites where ligaments or tendons attach to bone).
- Common sites for enthesopathy include:
  - Calcaneus (Achilles and plantar fascia insertions).
  - Patella.
  - Tibial tubercle.
  - Vertebral bodies.
- The involvement of vertebral body entheses leads to the characteristic findings of syndesmophytes (vertical bony growths) and eventual fusion, which are responsible for the classic radiographic "bamboo" appearance of the spine in advanced disease.
- Synonym(s): axial spondyloarthritis; inflammatory spine disease

EPIDEMIOLOGY

Incidence

- Overall incidence: 0.5 to 8.2/100,000/yr
- Incidence rate varies directly with prevalence of human leukocyte antigen (HLA)-B27 in given population.
- Commonly presents in young adulthood
- Predominant age:
  - 80% of patients with AS develop symptoms before age 30 yr.
  - <5% of patients with AS present after age 45 yr.
- Predominant gender: male > female (~3:1)

Prevalence

- Prevalence of AS is 9 to 30/10,000 depending on HLA-B27 prevalence in the population (1).
- Higher in Alaskan Eskimos and some Native American populations owing to higher than average HLA-B27 rate
- Lower in African Americans secondary to a lower HLA-B27 rate
- Up to 5% of patients evaluated for chronic low back pain are ultimately diagnosed with AS.

ETIOLOGY AND PATHOPHYSIOLOGY

- A clear etiologic pathway has not been established.
- Speculated that an environmental/infectious trigger in a genetically susceptible individual leads to an inflammatory (T cell and macrophage) immune response that specifically targets SI, peripheral joint, and enthesis inflammation, eventually causing bony proliferation, erosions, sclerosis, and joint destruction.

Genetics

- Expression of HLA-B27 antigen is clearly linked to the development of AS, but the exact mechanism is unknown.
- Prevalence of HLA-B27 in African Americans is 2–4% and in Caucasians is 8%.

RISK FACTORS

- Positive family history of SpA or HLA-B27
- 90% or more of individuals with AS are HLA-B27 positive, although an individual who is HLA-B27 positive has a 5% chance of having AS.
- Reactive arthritis triggered by *Chlamydia trachomatis* and certain enteric infections (e.g., *Shigella*, *Salmonella*, *Yersinia*, and *Campylobacter* spp.) predisposes to development of AS.

GENERAL PREVENTION

- Currently no preventive therapies or screening tests
- Early recognition and initiation of treatment can prevent disease progression and complications; unfortunately, it is common for there to be 5 to 6 yr delay in diagnosis.

COMMONLY ASSOCIATED CONDITIONS

- Enthesitis—29% (2)
- Uveitis/iritis—23%
- Psoriasis—10%
- Dactylitis—6%
- IBD—4%
- Rarely, cardiac valve/aortic root involvement

DIAGNOSIS

- Diagnosis is primarily based on history of IBP (see "History") and exam findings with imaging used to confirm diagnosis.
- The modified New York criteria have historically been used for research inclusion but have never been validated for clinical use. Their limitation is requirement of radiographic evidence of disease, which may take years to develop; need at least one radiographic criteria and one clinical criteria for definitive diagnosis:
  - Radiologic criteria:
    - Bilateral sacroiliitis grades 2 to 4 *or*
    - Unilateral sacroiliitis grade 3 or 4
  - Clinical criteria:
    - Low back pain and stiffness of at least 3 mo duration that improves with exercise but is not relieved by rest
    - Limited lumbar spinal motion in sagittal (sideways) and frontal (forward and backward) planes
    - Chest expansion decreased relative to normal values corrected for age and sex
- New criteria to diagnose all causes of IBP, not just AS, have been developed by the Assessment for SpondyloArthritis International Society (ASAS); intended to detect early disease without dependence on radiographic evidence of disease
- ASAS-endorsed criteria for IBP (validated clinical rule) (3)[A]:
  - Age of onset <45 yr
  - >3 mo of back pain of insidious onset
  - Sacroiliitis on imaging + one SpA feature *or* positive HLA-B27 + two SpA features
    - SpA features: IBP, arthritis, enthesitis, uveitis, dactylitis, psoriasis, IBD, responds to nonsteroidal anti-inflammatory drugs (NSAIDs), family history of SpA, HLA-B27 positive, elevated C-reactive protein (CRP)
  - 82.9% sensitive, 84.4% specific for SpA

HISTORY

- 3 mo of back pain with insidious onset
- IBP: morning stiffness >30 min, improves with exercise but not with rest, alternating buttock pain, back pain at night

PHYSICAL EXAM

Physical exam should include assessment of:

- Entire spine: Range of motion, tenderness (although clinical spinal mobility measurements do not correlate with degree of inflammation or radiographic measure of spinal mobility):
  - Decreased cervical motion can be tested with occiput to wall test (distance between occiput to the wall when standing erect against a wall) and brow to chin angle (the degree of forward vertical angulation using a line drawn from the eyebrow to the chin compared to a vertical line perpendicular to the ground).
  - Increased thoracic kyphosis and decreased chest expansion (usually <2 cm)
  - Decreased lumbar motion can be determined by Schober test: Mark area on patient's back at L5 and 10 cm above that point. Once patient bends forward, remeasure that distance. In normal persons, it should be >5 cm greater in flexion; <5 cm suggests loss of motion in lumbar spine.
- Peripheral joints, especially in the lower extremity: limited range of motion, inflammatory signs such as effusion, warmth, tenderness
- Major entheses: calcaneus for Achilles and plantar fascia attachments, patella, tibial tubercle
- Eyes: inflammatory findings, may require slit-lamp exam
- Skin: rash characteristic of psoriasis

DIFFERENTIAL DIAGNOSIS

- Mechanical low back pain
- Myofascial low back pain
- SI joint dysfunction
- Herniated nucleus pulposus
- Degenerative disk disease
- Degenerative joint disease
- Spondylolysis
- Discitis
- Other causes of IBP

DIAGNOSTIC TESTS & INTERPRETATION

Initial Tests (lab, imaging)

- No definitive serologic markers, although rheumatologic labs will be negative (antinuclear antibody [ANA], rheumatoid factor [RF], cyclic citrullinated peptide [CCP], etc.)
- HLA-B27 with erythrocyte sedimentation rate (ESR) or CRP:
  - CRP and ESR can be elevated in 50–70% of patients with AS, but normal values do not negate presence of disease. Furthermore, normal or elevated levels in patients with established disease do not correlate with disease activity.
- Plain radiograph of SI joints and lumbar spine:
  - Sacroiliitis is a hallmark of disease: graded 1 (suspicious), grade 2 (minimal), grade 3 (moderate), or grade 4 (ankylosis).
  - 20–30% of patients with the first 2 yr of developing IBP will have structural changes detectable by radiographs, confirming diagnosis.
  - In established AS, 95% of patients have detectable structural changes; however, structural changes may take several years or longer to become apparent radiographically.
  - Absence of radiographic findings in patients with IBP does not imply a lack of inflammation, nor does it negate the possibility of AS.

Follow-Up Tests & Special Considerations

- Magnetic resonance imaging (MRI) (T_2 and short-tau inversion recovery [STIR]):
  - Becoming more widely used due to the ability to identify early inflammatory changes before structural changes are apparent on plain radiographs
  - Not as sensitive as plain radiographs to assess degree of structural changes
- Computed tomography (CT) scan:
  - Can detect chronic changes in SI joints, although role is limited due to high radiation exposure and the high sensitivity of the other imaging modalities

TREATMENT

GENERAL MEASURES

- A multidisciplinary approach of drug therapy along with exercises/physiotherapy helps decrease disease activity and progression while improving function.
- Treatment is generally lifelong and divided into active versus stable disease.
- Recent literature review performed by American College of Rheumatology, Spondylitis Association of America, and Spondyloarthritis Research and Treatment Network have provided the latest guidelines for treatment and are reviewed here.
- Treatment same for AS and nr-axSpA

MEDICATION

Depending on location and severity of disease, the following treatment modalities may be indicated:

- NSAIDs
- Tumor necrosis factor inhibitors (TNFi)
- Disease-modifying antirheumatic drugs (DMARDs) have limited recommendations.
- Interleukin inhibitors showing success in early trials
- Corticosteroid injections
- No role for systemic glucocorticoids

First Line

NSAIDs (4)[A]:

- No one NSAID recommended over another diclofenac, naproxen, celecoxib, and others
- Use full dose and regular scheduling to maximize symptom relief for active disease but can use as needed for stable disease.
- Beneficial for both axial (spine) and peripheral (joint, enthesis) involvement
- Data suggest that long-term therapy may have disease-controlling properties evidenced by suppression of radiographic progression.
- Trial of two separate NSAIDs for 1 to 2 mo each prior to moving onto second-line therapy
- Must monitor for gastrointestinal (GI), cardiovascular, renal, and hepatic side effects with ongoing NSAID use.

Second Line

- TNFi (4)[A]:
  - Infliximab, adalimumab, and etanercept
  - No clear recommendation for one TNFi versus another; infliximab and adalimumab considered for recurrent iritis or concomitant IBD
  - Try two separate TNFi before moving onto DMARD if no clinical response.
  - With extended therapy, up to 1/3 of patients may develop remission.
  - TNFi increases risk for infection; should screen for tuberculosis, HIV, and hepatitis before initiating. Ensure vaccinations are up to date; do not give live vaccines while on therapy.
- DMARDs (4)[A]:
  - Considered if failure to NSAID and TNFi contraindicated; use over non-TNFi biologics.
  - Limited role for sulfasalazine; some benefit with peripheral disease only.
  - High-dose pamidronate may be beneficial but needs further studies.
  - No role for methotrexate
- Interleukin-17A inhibitor (5)[B]:
  - Secukinumab has shown significant reduction in signs/symptoms of disease.
  - Considered if contraindications or failure of NSAIDs and/or TNFi

ISSUES FOR REFERRAL

- Early rheumatology referral for patients with IBP may help prevent a delay in diagnosis and can help with initiating biologics.
- Refer to ophthalmology if signs/symptoms of iritis, which may consider prescription of topical steroids to use PRN for flares.

ADDITIONAL THERAPIES

- Physiotherapy/physical therapy helps improve spinal mobility and overall function (6)[A].
- Supervised training and home exercises improve long-term functional outcomes when compared to no intervention or educational/behavioral intervention.

SURGERY/OTHER PROCEDURES

- Local corticosteroid injections: for isolated sacroiliitis or peripheral joint disease if more than three joints involved
- Hip arthroplasty as indicated for progressive arthropathy
- Thoracolumbar osteotomy can be considered for severe kyphotic disease, or cervicothoracic osteotomy for chin to chest deformity to restore horizontal gaze, but should be performed at specialized spine centers.

ONGOING CARE

FOLLOW-UP RECOMMENDATIONS

Patient Monitoring

- Can continue to monitor response to treatment using validated AS disease activity measures (Bath Ankylosing Spondylitis Disease Activity Index [BASDAI], Bath Ankylosing Spondylitis Functional Index [BASFI], or Ankylosing Spondylitis Disease Activity Score [ASDAS]) and regular interval CRP (5)[A]
- The BASDAI is a valid and appropriate composite to defining disease activity during treatment:
  - Five major symptoms (fatigue, spinal pain, joint pain/swelling, areas of tenderness, and duration/severity of morning stiffness) are individually rated on 0 to 10 scale and the sum of each score is divided by 5 to obtain final score.
  - A score >4 suggest suboptimal disease control and is a candidate for change in therapy.
- The BASFI is a set of 10 questions used to assess and follow functional limitations.

PROGNOSIS

- The key to good outcomes and prevention of disease progression and severe complications is early recognition and initiation of treatment.
- AS has an unpredictable clinical course independent of age of onset or sex.
- Most patients have a fluctuating course with flares and periods of relative remission.

COMPLICATIONS

- Fusion of vertebrae leading to loss of function or restrictive lung disease
- Aortitis or aortic insufficiency, rare
- Hip arthritis with refractory pain or disability requiring arthroplasty

REFERENCES

1. Wang R, Ward M. Epidemiology of axial spondyloarthritis: an update. *Curr Opin Rheumatol*. 2018;30(2):137–143.
2. De Winter JJ, van Mens LJ, van der Heijde D, et al. Prevalence of peripheral and extra-articular disease in ankylosing spondylitis versus non-radiographic axial spondyloarthritis: a meta-analysis. *Arthritis Res Ther*. 2016;18(1):196.
3. Sieper J, van der Heijde DM, Landewé RB, et al. New criteria for inflammatory back pain in patients with chronic back pain: a real patient exercise of the Assessment in SpondyloArthritis International Society (ASAS). *Ann Rheum Dis*. 2009;68(6):784–788.
4. Ward MM, Deodhar A, Akl EA, et al. American College of Rheumatology/Spondylitis Association of America/Spondyloarthritis Research and Treatment Network 2015 recommendations for the treatment of ankylosing spondylitis and nonradiographic axial spondyloarthritis. *Arthritis Rheumatol*. 2016;68(2):282–298.
5. Braun J, Baraliakos X, Deodhar A, et al. Effect of secukinumab on clinical radiographic outcomes in ankylosing spondylitis: 2-year results from the randomised phase III MEASURE 1 study. *Ann Rheumatic Dis*. 2017;76(6):1070–1077.
6. Dagfinrud H, Kvien TK, Hagen KB. Physiotherapy interventions for ankylosing spondylitis. *Cochrane Database Syst Rev*. 2008;(1):CD002822.

ADDITIONAL READING

- Braun J, Sieper J. Ankylosing spondylitis. *Lancet*. 2007;369(9570):1379–1390.
- Sieper J, Rudwaleit M, Khan MA, et al. Concepts and epidemiology of spondyloarthritis. *Best Pract Res Clin Rheumatol*. 2006;20(3):401–417.

CLINICAL PEARLS

- Diagnosing AS can be difficult because there is no clear diagnostic criteria, yet a delay in diagnosis can lead to unnecessary disease progression and irreversible changes.
- Identifying the features of IBP is key to the diagnosis of AS.
- Plain radiographs are typically diagnostic, but MRI can show early evidence of disease/inflammation when radiographs are normal.
- Treatment is multimodal and typically includes both drug therapy with NSAIDs ± TNFi along with physical therapy/physiotherapy.

ANTERIOR INTEROSSEOUS SYNDROME

Jarrod Yamanaka, MD

BASICS

- The anterior interosseous nerve (AIN) is a motor branch of the median nerve that innervates the pronator quadratus, flexor pollicis longus, and flexor digitorum profundus serving the index finger.
- *Anterior interosseous syndrome* (AIS) is a "catch-all" term for neuropathies that result in paralysis of these muscles secondary to several causes.
- Overall AIS is a rare condition with a paucity of research (1).

ETIOLOGY AND PATHOPHYSIOLOGY

The most frequent causes of AIS are direct traumatic nerve damage and external compression. Insidious onset of the condition thought to be a transient neuritis (1):

- Traumatic causes:
  - Penetrating trauma
  - Blunt injury
  - Traction injury
  - Chronic vibration (cyclists)
  - Fracture
  - Surgery
  - Venipuncture
  - Injection
  - Cast pressure
- External compression:
  - Bulky, tendinous origin of the deep head of the pronator teres
  - Soft tissue mass such as lipoma, ganglion, or tumor
  - Accessory muscle
  - Fibrous band originating from the superficial flexor
  - Vascular abnormality

DIAGNOSIS

HISTORY

- Pain in the forearm
- Sensory loss not noted
- Weakness noted as difficulty with writing or with fine-pinch activities

PHYSICAL EXAM

- The signature finding is weakness of the flexor pollicis longus, flexor digitorum profundus indicis, and partial innervation of the 3rd digit as well as pronator quadratus.
- Weakness of the flexor pollicis longus and flexor digitorum profundus to the index finger is indicated by an inability to make the "OK sign." Rather, the distal interphalangeal (DIP) joint of the index finger and interphalangeal (IP) joint of the thumb are hyperextended during attempted tip-to-tip pinch.
- The pronator quadratus is difficult to isolate clinically. Weakness may be detected by asking the patient to forcibly pronate the forearm against resistance (resist supination) with the elbow flexed at 90 degrees (1)[C].
- The AIN provides no sensory fibers to the skin; therefore, abnormal sensation testing suggests another etiology (1)[C].
- Electrodiagnostic testing (2)[C]:
  - Should include electromyography (EMG) of the flexor pollicis longus, pronator quadratus, and flexor digitorum profundus indicis.
  - The latency and amplitude of compound muscle action potential are compared with those of the unaffected side.
  - Sensory nerve action potentials are normal.
- Imaging modalities:
  - Both magnetic resonance imaging (MRI) and ultrasound (US) may be helpful in confirming the clinical diagnosis of AIS.
  - MRI findings of edema in the muscles innervated by the AIN on T2-weighted fat-suppressed images
  - The AIN may appear swollen on US when compared with the normal contralateral nerve.
  - US of the AIN-innervated muscles may show a loss of bulk, increased reflectivity, reduced perfusion on Doppler sonography, and lack of active contraction of the affected muscles.

DIFFERENTIAL DIAGNOSIS

- Tendon rupture
- Brachial plexus neuritis (Parsonage-Turner syndrome)
- Congenital absence of the flexor digitorum longus and flexor pollicis longus
- Partial lesion of the median nerve

TREATMENT

- Once an accurate diagnosis of AIS is made, treatment must be guided by the underlying etiology (1)[C].
- Penetrating trauma suggests nerve disruption or compression and is best treated with surgical exploration and nerve decompression or repair.
- With blunt trauma, an EMG suggestive of a complete lesion may mandate early surgical exploration. Partial injuries may be given an opportunity to recover spontaneously. If no improvement is noted after 6 to 12 wk of conservative management, surgical exploration is necessary (2)[C].
- The typical nonsurgical treatment regimen includes rest, splinting, and observation.
- Spontaneous paralysis of the AIN may be treated nonsurgically for 12 wk with surgical exploration if no clinical or EMG improvement is evident (2)[C].
- Spontaneous recovery after 12 mo is documented, and some advocate nonsurgical management for at least this long before proceeding with surgical exploration.
- Tendon transfers allow functional reconstruction of the thumb and index finger should the AIN fail to recover, be unreconstructable, or irreversible muscle atrophy is present after prolonged muscle denervation.

REFERENCES

1. Rodner CM, Tinsley BA, O'Malley MP. Pronator syndrome and anterior interosseous nerve syndrome. *J Am Acad Orthop Surg*. 2013;21(5):268–275.
2. Pham M, Bäumer P, Meinck H, et al. Anterior interosseous nerve syndrome: fascicular motor lesions of median nerve trunk. *Neurology*. 2014;82(7):598–606.

ADDITIONAL READING

- Chin DH, Meals RA. Anterior interosseous nerve syndrome. *J Am Soc Surg Hand*. 2001;1:249–257.
- Dang AC, Rodner CM. Unusual compression neuropathies of the forearm, part II: median nerve. *J Hand Surg Am*. 2009;34(10):1915–1920.
- Dunn AJ, Salonen DC, Anastakis DJ. MR imaging findings of anterior interosseous nerve lesions. *Skeletal Radiol*. 2007;36(12):1155–1162.
- Singh V, Ericson WB. Median nerve entrapments. In: Trescot AM, ed. *Peripheral Nerve Entrapments: Clinical Diagnosis and Management*. Basel, Switzerland: Springer; 2016:369–382.

CLINICAL PEARLS

- Dysfunction of the AIN is characterized by weakness of the pronator quadratus, flexor pollicis longus, and flexor digitorum profundus serving the index finger.
- On examination, the patient cannot make the "OK sign" with the thumb and index finger.
- The AIN does not provide sensory nerves to the skin; therefore, abnormal sensation suggests an alternative diagnosis.
- Penetrating trauma or blunt trauma with an EMG suggestive of a complete AIN lesion mandates surgical exploration.
- Insidious onset of condition can signify transient neuritis; usually resolves in 12 mo. Intense rehabilitation is first-line treatment.

ANTERIOR METATARSALGIA

Dominic Jacobelli, MD • Kenneth Bielak, MD, FACSM, FAAFP, CAQSM

BASICS

DESCRIPTION

- Pain in the plantar aspect of the metatarsal (MT) heads
- Metatarsalgia can be thought of as a symptom rather than a specific disease.
- Primary metatarsalgia develops from intrinsic factors, such as a long first ray, hallux valgus, or other congenital deformities.
- Secondary metatarsalgia may result from trauma, overuse, or poor footwear.

EPIDEMIOLOGY

Athletes in high-impact sports involving the lower extremities (dancing, running, jumping)

ETIOLOGY AND PATHOPHYSIOLOGY

- Repetitive/excessive stress combined with intrinsic and extrinsic factors
- The 1st MT head usually carries 30% of the load in weight-bearing. A normal MT arch ensures this balance by providing adequate padding around the 1st MT head. A pronated or splayfoot can disturb this balance, resulting in an abnormally high pressure over the 2nd through 5th MT heads. Over time, reactive tissue can form a callus around the MT heads, which further compounds pain.

RISK FACTORS

- Foot deformities: overpronation, pes planus, pes cavus, hallux valgus, prominent MT heads, hammertoe deformity, Morton foot (short 1st MT and a relatively long 2nd MT)
- Muscle imbalance or soft tissue dysfunction: tight Achilles tendon or toe extensors, weak toe flexors, laxity in the Lisfranc ligament
- Extrinsic factors: obesity, high heels, poorly fitted or worn-down shoes
- Dermatologic issues: calluses and warts
- Fat pad atrophy or displacement
- Iatrogenic changes from surgeries resulting in unequal force distribution

GENERAL PREVENTION

- Wear properly fitted shoes with adequate padding.
- Gradual progression of weight-bearing exercise programs

COMMONLY ASSOCIATED CONDITIONS

- Intrinsic foot muscle weakness
- Calluses and warts
- Hallux valgus or rigidus
- Hammertoe or claw toe
- Morton syndrome (long 2nd MT)
- Freiberg infraction (aseptic necrosis of a MT head, most commonly the 2nd, as seen in adolescent sprinters)

DIAGNOSIS

HISTORY

- Pain over the plantar surface of the MT heads, typically described as walking with a "pebble in the shoe"
- Pain is typically gradual and chronic in onset rather than acute.
- Pain is worse in midstance and propulsion phases of walking and running.

PHYSICAL EXAM

- Inspect for the presence of callus, edema, erythema, deformity, and skin breaks.
- Palpate for tenderness, which is typically located over the distal half of the MT shaft and head.
- Pain in the interdigital space or positive MT squeeze test suggests interdigital neuroma.
- Range of motion of the phalanges, metatarsophalangeal (MTP) joint, and ankle, especially to dorsiflexion, to evaluate tight gastrocsoleus complex
- Gait analysis should be performed.

DIFFERENTIAL DIAGNOSIS

- Neuroma (plantar or Morton neuroma)
- Idiopathic MTP joint synovitis
- Freiberg disease: ischemic epiphyseal necrosis of the 2nd MT
- Inflammatory arthritis of MT joint (rheumatoid arthritis, seronegative spondyloarthropathy, crystalline-induced arthritis, osteoarthritis, septic arthritis)
- Stress fracture
- Salter I fracture (pediatric population)
- Sesamoiditis or sesamoid fracture
- Lisfranc injury
- Traumatic arthritis
- Foreign body
- Cellulitis or infection (diabetic foot, Lyme disease)
- Ganglion cyst
- Vasculitis (diabetes)
- Tumor (rare)

DIAGNOSTIC TESTS & INTERPRETATION

Initial Tests (lab, imaging)

- Lab usually not required but may be considered based on differential diagnosis
- White blood cell (WBC) count and erythrocyte sedimentation rate (ESR) may be elevated in infection or inflammatory arthritis.
- Consider testing for:
  - Gout—uric acid level.
  - Pseudogout—synovial fluid.
  - Systemic disease—rheumatoid factor.
- Imaging usually not required but may be considered based on differential diagnosis
- Weight-bearing anteroposterior (AP), lateral, and oblique films often normal but may demonstrate foot deformities that may predispose to metatarsalgia
- Bone scan or magnetic resonance imaging (MRI) may be considered based on suspicion for stress fracture.
- Ultrasonography can be used to evaluate for neuromas, bursitis, and joint effusions.

Diagnostic Procedures/Other

- Diagnostic injection (MTP joint) with local anesthetic can help differentiate intra-articular pathology (synovitis/capsulitis) from extra-articular pathology (neuroma).
- Plantar pressure distribution analysis may help to distinguish patterns of pressure distribution due to malalignment.

TREATMENT

- Acute:
  - Ice and rest with activity modification
  - Well-cushioned, correctly fitted athletic shoes (1)[C]
  - Analgesics such as acetaminophen or nonsteroidal anti-inflammatory drugs (NSAIDs)
  - Calluses should be pared down, preferably after soaking the foot in warm water and using a stone or emery board.
  - An MT pad may be placed just proximal to the MT heads to relieve pressure (avoid the pad directly beneath MT heads).
  - Stretching a tight Achilles tendon
- Long-term treatment:
  - Prescriptive orthotics are beneficial:
    - Pes cavus (2)[C]
    - Hallux valgus (2)[C]
  - Arch support and a well-fitted, low-heel shoe for daily wear
  - Energy-absorbing running shoes, which are replaced every 350 miles or when showing early wear
  - Maintenance of gastrocsoleus flexibility
  - Physical therapy for the correction of postural or gait imbalance
  - Avoid hard surfaces and prolonged standing.

MEDICATION

Analgesics, NSAIDs, or acetaminophen for symptom control

ISSUES FOR REFERRAL

- Athletes may warrant early podiatric or orthopedic evaluation.
- If no improvement with conservative therapy for 3 to 6 mo, consider referral to foot/ankle orthopedist or surgical podiatrist.
- Multiple types of osteotomies with varying success rates have been described as surgical interventions for metatarsalgia.
- The Weil osteotomy, which is a shortening osteotomy performed to decrease pressure on a prominent MT head and performed by shifting the MT head back toward the heel, appears to be a safe and effective surgical procedure for the treatment for metatarsalgia of the second and 3rd MT (3)[B].
- More recently, percutaneous surgical techniques have been developed, which in retrospective analysis, show significantly better long-term outcomes and lower rates of late metatarsalgia compared to open procedures (4)[B].

ADDITIONAL THERAPIES

Corticosteroid injection should be avoided because it may cause fat pad atrophy.

ONGOING CARE

PATIENT EDUCATION

- Instruct patient about wearing proper shoes and gradual return to activity.
- Cross training until symptoms subside

COMPLICATIONS

- Back, knee, and hip pain owing to compensatory gait change
- Transfer metatarsalgia following surgical intervention as stress transfers to other areas

REFERENCES

1. Espinosa N, Maceira E, Myerson MS. Current concept review: metatarsalgia. *Foot Ankle Int*. 2008;29(8):871–879.
2. Hockenbury RT. Forefoot problems in athletes. *Med Sci Sports Exerc*. 1999;31(Suppl 7):S448–S458.
3. Pérez-Muñoz I, Escobar-Antón D, Sanz-Gómez TA. The role of Weil and triple Weil osteotomies in the treatment of propulsive metatarsalgia. *Foot Ankle Int*. 2012;33(6):501–506.
4. Bauer T, Gaumetou E, Klouche S, et al. Metatarsalgia and Morton's disease: comparison of outcomes between open procedure and neurectomy versus percutaneous metatarsal osteotomies and ligament release with a minimum of 2 years of follow-up. *J Foot Ankle Surg*. 2015;54(3):373–377.

ADDITIONAL READING

- Baker CL, Flandry F, Henderson JM, eds. Reactive synovitis of the foot—metatarsalgia. In: *The Hughston Clinic Sports Medicine Field Manual*. Baltimore, MD: Williams & Wilkins; 1996:270.
- Besse JL. Metatarsalgia. *Orthop Traumatol Surg Res*. 2017;103(1S):S29–S39.
- DiPreta JA. Metatarsalgia, lesser toe deformities, and associated disorders of the forefoot. *Med Clin North Am*. 2014;98(2):233–251.
- Gregg J, Marks P. Metatarsalgia: an ultrasound perspective. *Australas Radiol*. 2007;51(6):493–499.
- Gregg JM, Schneider T, Marks P. MR imaging and ultrasound of metatarsalgia—the lesser metatarsals. *Radiol Clin North Am*. 2008;46(6):1061–1078.
- Maceira E, Monteagudo M. Transfer metatarsalgia post hallux valgus surgery. *Foot Ankle Clin*. 2014;19(2):285–307.
- Tóth K, Huszanyik I, Kellermann P, et al. The effect of first ray shortening in the development of metatarsalgia in the second through fourth rays after metatarsal osteotomy. *Foot Ankle Int*. 2007;28(1):61–63.
- Weber PC. Resolution of metatarsalgia following oblique osteotomy. *Clin Orthop Relat Res*. 2007;458:248.

CLINICAL PEARLS

- Pain of the plantar surface of the forefoot, usually over the MT heads
- May be caused by abnormal pressure distribution over the plantar surface of the MT heads
- Common in athletes involved in high-impact sports (running, jumping, dancing)
- Athletes may warrant early referral to podiatry or orthopedic surgery.

ATHLETIC HEART SYNDROME

Evan D. Perez, MD • Daniel Murphy, MD, FAAFP • Justin M. Wright, MD, CAQSM

BASICS

DESCRIPTION

- A benign condition consisting of physiologic adaptations to increased cardiac workload. Primary features include biventricular hypertrophy and bradycardia.
- Associated with normal systolic and diastolic function
- Characteristics may overlap with pathologic conditions.
- Synonym(s): athlete's heart; physiologic cardiac hypertrophy; exercise-induced cardiac remodeling; exercise-related cardiac remodeling

EPIDEMIOLOGY

- These adaptations are common in highly trained athletes.
- Cardiac remodeling has been observed in moderately active adults who exercise 3 to 5 hr per week (1).
- Mistaken for pathologic conditions

ETIOLOGY AND PATHOPHYSIOLOGY

- Changes in cardiac structure vary based on type of exercise (2).
- Cardiac dimensions rarely exceed upper limits of normal.
- Dynamic exercise (e.g., distance running) (2):
  - Increased heart rate, augmented stroke volume, and decreased systemic vascular resistance
  - Adaptive responses due to volume overload and increased systolic blood pressure (BP)
  - Increase left ventricular (LV) end-diastolic diameter with proportional increases in septal and free-wall thickness
- Static exercise (e.g., weight lifting, bodybuilding) (2):
  - Increased peripheral resistance with smaller increases in heart rate and cardiac output
  - Increased septal and free-wall thickness without an increase in LV end-diastolic diameter
- Combined exercise (e.g., cycling, rowing) (2):
  - Extreme volume and pressure load
  - Largest increase in LV end-diastolic diameter, septal wall, and free-wall thickness

RISK FACTORS

- Chronic endurance exercise
- Genetic predisposition

DIAGNOSIS

HISTORY

- Differentiate benign physiologic change from pathologic conditions.
- History of chest pain, dizziness, impaired exercise capacity, or syncope with exercise may be suggestive of pathology.
- Inquire about heart disease risk factors, including hypertension (HTN), hyperlipidemia, tobacco use, and family history of sudden cardiac death.
- History of cardiac murmur should be investigated.

PHYSICAL EXAM

- Decreased body fat and increased muscle mass
- Bradycardia (sinus bradycardia or bradycardia with 1st- and 2nd-degree blocks)
- Grade 1 or 2 midsystolic murmurs (benign functional ejection murmur, which resolves with Valsalva maneuver)
- Third and fourth heart sounds are common (benign filling).
- BP remains normal.
- Point of maximal ventricular impulse displaced lateral to the midclavicular line.

DIFFERENTIAL DIAGNOSIS

- Hypertensive cardiac hypertrophy
- Hypertrophic cardiomyopathy (HCM)
- Dilated cardiomyopathy
- Arrhythmogenic right ventricular cardiomyopathy (ARVC)
- Aortic stenosis

DIAGNOSTIC TESTS & INTERPRETATION

Initial Tests (lab, imaging)

- Electrocardiography (ECG) normal findings (3)[C]:
  - Increased vagal tone:
    - Sinus bradycardia:
      - 40 to 60 beats/min at rest is common; 30 to 40 beats/min in highly trained athletes
      - Sinus pauses <3 sec
    - Early repolarization:
      - J-point elevation, ST elevation, J waves, or terminal QRS slurring in the inferior and/or lateral leads
      - Normal when present in isolation
    - "Black athlete heart":
      - J-point elevation, convex ST segment elevation followed by T-wave inversion in leads V_1 to V_4
    - Juvenile T-wave pattern (<16 yr old):
      - T-wave inversion in leads V_1 to V_3
    - Sinus arrhythmia:
      - Physiologic heart rate variation associated with respirations (increased with inspiration; decreased with expiration)
      - Resolves with onset of exercise
    - Junctional escape rhythm:
      - QRS rate faster than resting P wave
      - Regular R-R interval
      - Sinus rhythm should resume with activity.
    - Ectopic atrial rhythm:
      - Morphologically different ectopic P waves from the sinus P wave
      - "Wandering pacemaker" (dynamic athletes)
      - Sinus rhythm should resume with exercise.
    - Atrioventricular (AV) blocks:
      - 1st-degree AV block present only at rest; P-R interval normalizes with exercise.
      - Mobitz type I (Wenckebach) 2nd-degree AV block: present only at rest; common in marathon runners
      - Higher grade AV blocks (Mobitz II, 3rd degree) rare in athletes; workup indicated

- Increased chamber size:
  - Voltage criteria for the following:
    - LV hypertrophy
    - Right ventricular hypertrophy, common in dynamic athletes
    - Incomplete right bundle branch block (RBBB)
- ECG borderline findings (3)[C]:
  - Isolated borderline ECG findings do not warrant further investigation (if asymptomatic and negative cardiac family history).
  - Two or more of the following borderline ECG findings need further investigation:
    - Left axis deviation
    - Left atrial enlargement
    - Right axis deviation
    - Right atrial enlargement
    - Complete RBBB
- Chest radiography (4)[C]:
  - Heart is globular in appearance, particularly in endurance athletes.
  - Cardiomegaly (cardiothoracic ratio >0.50)
  - Pulmonary vascular marking may be increased.
- Echocardiography (2)[C]:
  - Biventricular hypertrophy
  - LV wall hypertrophy with LV wall thickness 11 to 13 mm is common in athletes.
  - LV wall thickness measuring 13 to 15 mm considered a "gray zone"
  - LV wall thickness >15 mm suggestive of HCM; requires a multimodality evaluation
  - Diastolic dysfunction is suspicious for pathology.
  - High-dynamic athletes:
    - Eccentric hypertrophy with increased left and right ventricular wall thickness
    - Left and right ventricular chamber dilation
    - Normal to mildly enlarged left and right atria
    - Supranormal LV diastolic indices
    - Normal to low normal systolic function
  - High-static athletes:
    - Mild symmetric LV concentric hypertrophy with normal to subnormal chamber size
    - Normal right ventricle dimensions
    - Normal to mildly enlarged left atrium
    - May be more pronounced in high-static athletes with HTN
  - Combined static/dynamic athletes:
    - Eccentric LV hypertrophy with a balanced increase in wall thickness and chamber size
- Cardiac magnetic resonance imaging (MRI) (5)[C]:
  - Precise assessment of chamber size, myocardial mass, and systolic function
  - Not influenced by body habitus
  - Capable of measuring both ventricles
  - Useful in identifying athlete's heart, HCM, or early and subtle ARVC

Diagnostic Procedures/Other

- Cardio pulmonary exercise testing (6)[C]:
  - VO_2 max >50 mL/kg/min or >120% predicted is consistent with an athlete's heart.
- Prescribed detraining (6)[C]:
  - Leads to a decrease in wall thickness and a reversal of ECG and echocardiographic abnormalities
  - 8 to 12 wk is sufficient for changes.
  - Can be used to differentiate from HCM if other methods are unrevealing

TREATMENT

GENERAL MEASURES

- Unwarranted discontinuation of exercise may have unintended psychological ramifications to the athlete.
- Reassure the athlete that the observed changes are normal physiologic adaptations to exercise and encourage the athlete to continue exercising.

ISSUES FOR REFERRAL

Patients with overlapping features of athletic heart and pathologic features (i.e., exertional symptoms, family history, LV wall thickness "gray zone") should be evaluated by a cardiologist prior to returning to physical activity.

ONGOING CARE

FOLLOW-UP RECOMMENDATIONS

- Many of the physiologic adaptations observed in athletic heart syndrome resolve when exercise is stopped.
- The adaptations that occur in resistant or static athletes are similar to those caused by chronic HTN.
- These individuals are encouraged to incorporate dynamic exercise to their weight-lifting routine.
- Routine follow-up is recommended.

REFERENCES

1. Dawes TJ, Corden B, Cotter S, et al. Moderate physical activity in healthy adults is associated with cardiac remodeling. *Circ Cardiovasc Imaging*. 2016;9(8):e004712.
2. Baggish AL, Battle RW, Beckerman JG, et al. Sports cardiology: core curriculum for providing cardiovascular care to competitive athletes and highly active people. *J Am Coll Cardiol*. 2017;70(15):1902–1918.
3. Drezner JA, Sharma S, Baggish A, et al. International criteria for electrocardiographic interpretation in athletes: consensus statement. *Br J Sports Med*. 2017;51(9):704–731.
4. Rich BS, Havens SA. The athletic heart syndrome. *Curr Sports Med Rep*. 2004;3(2):84–88.
5. Paterick TE, Gordon T, Spiegel D. Echocardiography: profiling of the athlete's heart. *J Am Soc Echocardiogr*. 2014;27(9):940–948.
6. D'Silva A, Sharma S. Exercise, the athlete's heart, and sudden cardiac death. *Phys Sportsmed*. 2014;42(2):100–113.

ADDITIONAL READING

- Baggish AL. Exercise-induced cardiac remodeling: competitive athletes are just the tip of the iceberg. *Circ Cardiovasc Imaging*. 2016;9(8):e005321.
- Drezner JA, O'Connor FG, Harmon KG, et al. AMSSM position statement on cardiovascular preparticipation screening in athletes: current evidence, knowledge gaps, recommendations, and future directions. *Clin J Sport Med*. 2016;26(5):347–361.

CLINICAL PEARLS

- Physiologic response to exercise; no increased risk with participation
- Important to differentiate from pathologic conditions that place athlete at risk for sudden cardiac death
- ECG, echocardiography, and cardiac MRI may help distinguish physiologic from pathologic changes.
- Detraining can aid in differentiation.

ATLANTOAXIAL INSTABILITY

Rebecca L. Carl, MD, MSCI

BASICS

DESCRIPTION

- Atlantoaxial instability (AAI) is the term for increased motion at the joint between the 1st and 2nd cervical vertebrae (the atlas and the axis).
- Congenital, inflammatory, traumatic, or infectious conditions may weaken the structures supporting the C1–C2 joint leading to AAI.
- Many patients who meet the radiographic definition of AAI are asymptomatic and at low risk for neurologic sequelae.
- Synonym(s): atlantoaxial subluxation

EPIDEMIOLOGY

- The incidence of radiographic/asymptomatic AAI in individuals with Down syndrome is estimated between 10% and 20%.
- The incidence of *symptomatic* AAI is much lower at ~2.6%.
- Incidence of AAI increases with age, and progression may occur during growth spurts.
- For individuals with Down syndrome, males age >10 yr are most likely to have progression of AAI.

RISK FACTORS

- Down syndrome
- Rheumatoid arthritis
- Juvenile idiopathic arthritis
- Many forms of dwarfism/skeletal dysplasias
- Marfan syndrome: increased incidence of C1–C2 hypermobility, but symptoms are rare

DIAGNOSIS

Lateral cervical radiographs with flexion and extension views are used for screening. AAI is defined radiographically as an increased distance between the odontoid process and the anterior arch of the axis.

- Obtaining screening x-rays for AAI in asymptomatic patients with Down syndrome is controversial:
  - Because of poor radiographic reproducibility and because many radiographic signs of AAI often resolve over time in asymptomatic patients, the American Academy of Pediatrics does not endorse routine screening (1)[A],(2)[C].
  - The Special Olympics requires a history and physical evaluation that includes screening for AAI. Individuals with symptoms that could represent AAI must have a comprehensive workup (3)[C].

HISTORY

- Most individuals with AAI are asymptomatic.
- AAI can be acute or chronic. However, acute AAI without a history of preceding symptoms is rare:
  - Patients with acute AAI often present after injury. Injury can be due to direct or indirect trauma. Mechanisms of injury include hyperextension, hyperflexion, and direct loading.
  - In patients who have an acute worsening of AAI, participation in organized sports is an uncommon triggering event.
  - Patients with chronic AAI often present with gait changes, progressive weakness, and fatigue. Neck pain, bowel and bladder incontinence, ataxia, spasticity, and quadriplegia can be present with longstanding, severe chronic AAI (4)[B].

PHYSICAL EXAM

- Hyperreflexia
- Sensory changes
- Weakness
- Gait changes
- Cervical spine range of motion is often normal.

DIAGNOSTIC TESTS & INTERPRETATION

- Lateral neck radiographs with flexion/extension views:
  - AAI is defined as a space of 5 mm or more between the odontoid process of the axis and the anterior arch of the atlas.
- Further evaluation with computed tomography (CT) or magnetic resonance imaging (MRI) in cervical flexion and extension is often needed to assess for spinal cord compression in patients with AAI on plain radiographs.

DIFFERENTIAL DIAGNOSIS

- Neck sprain/strain
- Cervical disc herniation
- Torticollis
- Vertebral fracture
- Ligamentous laxity
- Spinal contusion
- Epidural hemorrhage

TREATMENT

GENERAL MEASURES

- Management of athletes with acute worsening of AAI symptoms
- If worsening occurs with trauma, assume a potentially unstable injury is present until proven otherwise.
- The cervical spine must be stabilized in the field.
- Protect the airway if respiratory difficulties arise.

ADDITIONAL THERAPIES

Anesthesia administration:

- Blind endotracheal intubation of a patient with AAI should be avoided.
- Tracheal intubation with a flexible bronchoscope under topical anesthesia avoids neck flexion and maintains cervical spine stability.
- For elective procedures, consider regional anesthesia with minimal sedation (5)[C].

SURGERY/OTHER PROCEDURES

- Atlantoaxial fusion should be considered for patients with progressive, symptomatic AAI and/or cervical myelopathy (4)[B].
- Because atlantoaxial fusion is a very high-risk procedure, nonoperative management is recommended for patients without neurologic symptoms.

ONGOING CARE

Long-term management:

- Individuals who exhibit signs and symptoms should be restricted from contact sports and other activities that place stress on the neck (4)[B].
- Restriction of asymptomatic patients with only radiographic evidence of AAI is somewhat controversial, particularly for noncontact activities:
  - Special Olympics requires that patients with radiographic evidence of AAI be *temporarily* restricted from the following:
    - Butterfly stroke
    - Diving (including diving starts in swimming)
    - Pentathlon
    - High jump
    - Squat lifts
    - Equestrian sports
    - Artistic gymnastics
    - Soccer
    - Skiing
  - These restrictions can be removed if an asymptomatic athlete (or the athlete's parents in the case of a minor) signs a waiver after having the risks of AAI explained by two physicians.

FOLLOW-UP RECOMMENDATIONS

- Primary care physicians should counsel families of patients with Down syndrome, rheumatoid arthritis, juvenile inflammatory arthritis, and skeletal dysplasias about possible signs and symptoms of AAI (2,6)[C].
- Physicians should counsel parents of children with Down syndrome about the increased risk of AAI and potential spinal cord injury with contact sports and activities with a high risk of collision or fall (e.g., trampoline) (2)[C].

REFERENCES

1. Cremers MJ, Bol E, de Roos F, et al. Risk of sports activities in children with Down's syndrome and atlantoaxial instability. *Lancet*. 1993;342(8870):511–514.
2. Bull MJ; and Committee on Genetics. Health supervision for children with Down syndrome. *Pediatrics*. 2011;128(2):393–406.
3. Special Olympics General Rules. http://www.specialolympicswisconsin.org/wp-content/uploads/2015/04/Athletes-with-Down-Syndrome-Special-Examination-Form.pdf. Accessed June 18, 2018.
4. Atlantoaxial instability in Down syndrome: subject review. American Academy of Pediatrics Committee on Sports Medicine and Fitness. *Pediatrics*. 1995;96(1, Pt 1):151–154.
5. Lewanda AF, Matisoff A, Revenis M, et al. Preoperative evaluation and comprehensive risk assessment for children with Down syndrome. *Paediatr Anaesth*. 2016;26(4):356–362.
6. Laiho K, Savolainen A, Kautiainen H, et al. The cervical spine in juvenile chronic arthritis. *Spine J*. 2002;2(2):89–94.

ADDITIONAL READING

- Torg JS, Ramsey-Emrhein JA. Suggested management guidelines for participation in collision activities with congenital, developmental, or postinjury lesions involving the cervical spine. *Med Sci Sports Exerc*. 1997;29(Suppl 7):S256–S272.
- Wills BP, Dormans JP. Nontraumatic upper cervical spine instability in children. *J Am Acad Orthop Surg*. 2006;14(4):233–245.
- Winell J, Burke SW. Sports participation of children with Down syndrome. *Orthop Clin North Am*. 2003;34(3):439–443.

CLINICAL PEARLS

Athletes with radiographic evidence of AAI who are asymptomatic appear to be at low risk for experiencing acute worsening during participation in organized sports (particularly noncontact activities) (1)[B]. Each individual athlete should discuss sports participation guidelines with his or her physician(s) (2)[C].

AURICULAR HEMATOMAS

Steven K. Poon, MD, CAQSM • Kimberly G. Harmon, MD

BASICS

ALERT
Failure to diagnose and promptly treat this condition with evacuation of the hematoma may lead to permanent deformation of the ear.

DESCRIPTION

- Auricular hematoma is an injury caused by trauma or friction of the ear that often occurs in contact sports such as wrestling, rugby, boxing, and judo.
- Trauma or continuous friction to the auricle leads to bleeding into the soft tissues of the ear.
- Bleeding often occurs anteriorly at the junction of the perichondrium and elastic cartilage of the ear.
- Recognition of this condition as a result of trauma led to the development of treatments during the latter half of the 20th century.

EPIDEMIOLOGY

Incidence

Most injuries occur while engaged in combat sports such as wrestling while not wearing protective headgear.

Prevalence

Studies estimate ear injuries account for up to 23.4% of all reported wrestling related injuries.

ETIOLOGY AND PATHOPHYSIOLOGY

- The condition is caused by trauma owing to a direct blow or frictional forces to the auricle.
- Bleeding into the auricle, specifically between the skin and auricular cartilage, results in a hematoma in this space.
- Untreated, the hematoma can cause pressure, necrosis, and scarring of the auricular cartilage leading to a "cauliflower ear," which is the name given to the characteristic deformity to the ear:
  - Neocartilage formation at the site of the clot also plays a role in the associated deformity.
  - This deformity is disfiguring and permanent.

RISK FACTORS

Failure to wear headgear while participating in sports such as wresting, rugby, or martial arts disciplines such as judo may increase the risk of ear trauma.

GENERAL PREVENTION

- General prevention is based on proper use of headgear during participation.
- Ill-fitting headgear may provide inadequate protection to the auricle.
- Awareness of the importance and use of proper fitting headgear by athletes, coaches, and athletic training staff may prevent this injury.

COMMONLY ASSOCIATED CONDITIONS

- Auricle laceration
- Rupture of tympanic membrane owing to associated trauma
- Concussions related to head trauma
- Cellulitis and perichondritis may mimic or be associated with this disorder.

DIAGNOSIS

- Diagnosis is made based on clinical exam and history of trauma/excessive friction to the ear (1)[C].
- The absence of associated factors that may lead to cellulitis of the ear may aid in the correct diagnosis.

HISTORY

- History of direct and recent trauma to the auricle with resulting hematoma
- Lack of protective headgear while participating in high-risk sports for this injury should raise level of suspicion.
- The athlete complains of a painful ear and may have associated hearing loss.

PHYSICAL EXAM

- Examination of the auricle reveals a soft hematoma with tenderness of the auricle presenting within a few hours after the inciting injury.
- Loss of the normal architecture of the auricle compared with the contralateral side
- Exam should include an assessment of the athlete's hearing.
- Associated ear drainage should prompt consideration for rupture of the tympanic membrane.
- Assessment to rule out signs and symptoms of concussion should be performed.

DIFFERENTIAL DIAGNOSIS

- Ear laceration
- Cellulitis of ear
- Perichondritis

DIAGNOSTIC TESTS & INTERPRETATION

Diagnosis of this condition is based on history and clinical exam:

- No specific lab tests confirm diagnosis.
- Complete blood count (CBC) or erythrocyte sedimentation rate (ESR) may aid in the diagnosis of associated infection.

TREATMENT

GENERAL MEASURES

- Once frictional and/or direct pressures have resulted in a hematoma between the skin and auricular cartilage, the initial goal in treatment is to aspirate this area to prevent further complications.
- Following anesthesia with lidocaine without epinephrine, aspiration can be attempted with a 18- to 22-gauge needle and syringe (2)[C]:
  - This aspiration must be done in the acute phase when the hematoma is palpable.
- If left untreated, the hematoma can lead to neocartilage formation, scarring, and necrosis, all of which can lead to permanent deformity.
- Antibiotics are sometimes given as a preventive measure because infection of the auricle will result in further poor outcomes. Antibiotics should cover common gram-positive skin bacteria. Cephalexin is used commonly.

MEDICATION

- Consider antibiotics for prophylactic coverage (e.g., cephalexin × 7 days). If suturing or incision and drainage are done, antibiotics definitely should be used (3)[B].
- Nonsteroidal anti-inflammatory drugs (NSAIDs) and aspirin should be avoided to minimize hematoma recurrence risk.

ADDITIONAL THERAPIES

- The importance of acute aspiration of hematoma has been described as well as the possible need for attempted hematoma evacuation with a larger bore needle.
- On occasion, a pressure dressing may not be needed if the hematoma does not recur within 1 hr of successful aspiration.
- To prevent reaccumulation of the hematoma and the need for additional aspirations, a compression dressing commonly is placed over the area:
  - Compression must stay over the ear until it is fully healed.
  - Compression dressing may be needed for 3 days or more.
- Multiple reports have described using through-and-through mattress sutures for better cosmetic outcomes and lower risk of hematoma reaccumulation (3,4)[B]:
  - Anesthesia was achieved by using an auricular block and lidocaine 1% without epinephrine.
  - Incision and drainage performed with a number 15 blade scalpel over the area of fluid accumulation and allowing for full evacuation of hematoma. Hemostats may be needed to break up loculations.
  - After copious irrigation, horizontal mattress sutures are placed through and through the ear cartilage with 4-0 or 5-0 absorbable sutures.
  - Cover the suture and incision site with topical antimicrobial ointment and start oral antibiotics as described above.
  - Sutures remain in place for 7 to 10 days.
  - This can be done in a training room setting but may require referral to ear, nose, and throat (ENT) if provider is not comfortable with this procedure.

SURGERY/OTHER PROCEDURES

The possibility of surgery may be entertained, as mentioned earlier, in consultation with ENT or plastic surgery.

ONGOING CARE

FOLLOW-UP RECOMMENDATIONS

Daily follow-up is needed to observe for signs of hematoma redevelopment, pressure necrosis, allergic reaction to materials, and infection.

Patient Monitoring

Follow-up with ENT or plastic surgery after acute treatment is recommended because of the risk of poor cosmetic result even with proper treatment of the condition.

PATIENT EDUCATION

- Return to play too early, prior to fully healing of the injury, will increase the risk of a poor outcome:
  - No definitive return-to-play protocol exists.
  - Some authors recommend no competition while wearing ear compression dressing, whereas others allow full activity with ear protection being worn.
  - Bolsterless mattress suture repair often allows for immediate return to activity.
  - The decision should be made in consultation with the athlete, recognizing the potential for poor cosmesis with recurrence of the injury.
- Ear protectors and headgear always should be worn in high-risk sports.
- Ice and pressure applied at the end of practices and matches may help to prevent recurrence of injury.

PROGNOSIS

- Best prognosis is achieved by prompt aspiration and compression if needed.
- Poorer outcomes are associated with repeated need for aspiration and earlier return to contact sports/reinjury.

COMPLICATIONS

- Permanent scarring and cosmetic deformity
- Chondritis and perichondritis
- Prompt treatment, including aseptic technique, may prevent these consequences.

REFERENCES

1. Cassaday K, Vazquez G, Wright JM. Ear problems and injuries in athletes. *Curr Sports Med Rep*. 2014;13(1):22–26.
2. Kiningham R, Monseau A. Caring for wrestlers. *Curr Sports Med Rep*. 2015;14(5):404–412.
3. Kakarala K, Kieff DA. Bolsterless management for recurrent auricular hematomata. *Laryngoscope*. 2012;122(6):1235–1237.
4. Giles WC, Iverson KC, King JD, et al. Incision and drainage followed by mattress suture repair of auricular hematoma. *Laryngoscope*. 2007;117(2):2097–2099.

ADDITIONAL READING

- Hewett TE, Pasque C, Heyl R, et al. Wrestling injuries. *Med Sport Sci*. 2005;48:152–178.
- Skidmore K, Gossman WG. *Ear, Cauliflower Ear*. Treasure Island, FL: StatPearls Publishing; 2018.

CLINICAL PEARLS

- Diagnosis of this condition is based on history and clinical exam.
- Early recognition and treatment of this condition with hematoma aspiration may prevent long-term sequelae and disfigurement.
- Return to contact sports without sufficient time for injury to fully heal/allow adequate retreatment increases the risk for a poor cosmetic result.
- Compression treatment options include bolsters and horizontal mattress suture repair.
- ENT/plastic surgery consultation may be required.
- Use of ear protection/headgear is effective in prevention of this condition.

AXILLARY NERVE INJURY

Laura M. Distel, MD, CAQSM • James R. Borchers, MD, MPH

BASICS

DESCRIPTION

- Originates from the C5–C6 rami (and occasionally C4) and is a branch of the posterior cord of the brachial plexus (1)
- Courses from the brachial plexus and below the coracoid process along the anterior surface of the subscapularis and then heads posteriorly and through the quadrilateral space (1)
- The quadrilateral space is an anatomic entity created by the teres minor muscle inferiorly, the long head of the triceps medially, the neck of the humerus laterally, and the subscapularis and teres major muscles superiorly. The axillary nerve and posterior humeral circumflex artery travel within the space (1).
- Once through the space, the nerve travels further posteriorly and branches into an anterior and posterior trunk.
- The anterior trunk courses around the posterolateral (surgical) neck of the humerus and innervates the anterior and middle deltoid.
- The posterior trunk bifurcates into a motor branch, the teres minor and posterior deltoid muscles, and a sensory branch innervating the superolateral brachial cutaneous nerve, which innervates the lateral upper extremity.

EPIDEMIOLOGY

Has been reported to encompass <1% of all nerve injuries (2)

Incidence

True incidence unknown owing to underrecognition of the diagnosis

ETIOLOGY AND PATHOPHYSIOLOGY

- Traction injury to the nerve during an anterior dislocation or fracture (2)
- Presumed compression injury of the nerve as a result of a direct blow to the anterolateral deltoid (2)
- Quadrilateral space syndrome: Proposed mechanisms include compression of the nerve by fibrous bands, hypertrophied muscles that border the space, any space-occupying lesion (e.g., aneurysm or cyst), or shear between the teres minor and major (2).
- Iatrogenic damage to the nerve during shoulder surgery (2)

RISK FACTORS

- Anterior shoulder (glenohumeral) dislocation
- Humeral neck fracture
- Direct blunt trauma to the anterior lateral deltoid, which is common in contact sports such as hockey, football, or rugby
- Repetitive overhead sports (e.g., volleyball, tennis, or baseball): This can lead to quadrilateral space syndrome.
- Iatrogenic damage (e.g., shoulder instability surgery, rotator cuff surgery, and rarely, shoulder arthroscopy)

COMMONLY ASSOCIATED CONDITIONS

- Anterior glenohumeral dislocation
- Humeral neck fracture

DIAGNOSIS

Nerve injury should be suspected in any athlete with anterior shoulder dislocation or humeral neck fracture.

HISTORY

- Easy fatigability with overhead activities or heavy lifting (3)
- Decreased strength with shoulder abduction (3)
- Paresthesias or loss of sensation in the lateral upper arm (Sensation is spared after anterior shoulder dislocation.)
- Quadrilateral space syndrome: vague, nonspecific aching or burning of the posterolateral shoulder and/or generalized weakness with overhead activities (1)

PHYSICAL EXAM

- Assess for deltoid or teres minor atrophy compared with the unaffected side (more common in chronic cases).
- Active and passive range of motion (ROM) about the shoulder, including abduction, forward elevation, and external rotation
- Strength testing of abduction and forward elevation (deltoid function) and external rotation (teres minor function)
- Neurovascular exam, especially assessing for sensation over the lateral deltoid area known as the "sergeant's patch"
- Perform the Spurling maneuver (rotate the patient's head to the affected side and hyperextend the neck) to assess for cervical radiculopathy.
- Tenderness to palpation of the posterior shoulder at the quadrilateral space (often the only positive finding in quadrilateral space syndrome)

DIFFERENTIAL DIAGNOSIS

- Brachial plexus syndromes:
  - Thoracic outlet syndrome
  - Neuralgic amyotrophy (Parsonage-Turner syndrome)
- Quadrilateral space syndrome
- Cervical spine lesions
- Aneurysm, neoplasm, or cystic mass near the axillary nerve

DIAGNOSTIC TESTS & INTERPRETATION

Initial Tests (lab, imaging)

- Plain x-rays of the shoulder to evaluate glenohumeral dislocation or evidence of fracture (3)
- Consider cervical spine x-rays to rule out cervical spine causes of deltoid paresthesias, weakness, or atrophy (1).
- Magnetic resonance imaging (MRI) can be helpful in chronic cases to identify a combined nerve injury, to determine prognosis of functional recovery by evaluating fatty replacement of the muscle, or to evaluate other soft tissue causes of shoulder weakness but is often not needed (3).

Diagnostic Procedures/Other

- Electromyography (EMG) and nerve conduction velocity (NCV) should be obtained no sooner than 3 wk after injury to establish baseline dysfunction (3,4)[A].
- Repeat EMG and NCV after 3 mo to assess for nerve recovery if no clinical improvement in deltoid function (2,4)[A].
- Arteriogram of the posterior circumflex humeral artery to evaluate for quadrilateral space syndrome but there are conflicting recommendations regarding the use of this test (1)[B]

TREATMENT

GENERAL MEASURES

- Nonoperative treatment is preferred initially (2,4)[A].
- Emphasize active and passive ROM of the shoulder.
- Relative rest
- Strengthening exercises of the shoulder
- Avoidance of exacerbating triggers or activities
- Emergency department (ED) treatment:
  - Reduction of glenohumeral dislocation or treatment of fracture

ADDITIONAL THERAPIES

Electrical stimulation of the deltoid is an option to prevent atrophy while the nerve is recovering (3)[C].

SURGERY/OTHER PROCEDURES

- Appropriate interval for surgical intervention is unclear, but there is some evidence to suggest that surgery within 6 mo of injury yields superior return of function and strength (3)[B].
- Generally indicated if no improvement using nonoperative treatments or if EMG/NCV shows no interval nerve recovery in 3 to 12 mo postinjury (2)[A]
- Operative procedures include (2,5,6)[A]:
  - Neurolysis.
  - Sural nerve grafting.
  - Neurorrhaphy.
  - Nerve transfer.
  - Neurotization.
- Surgical decompression can be performed for quadrilateral space syndrome to release fibrous bands (3)[B].

ONGOING CARE

FOLLOW-UP RECOMMENDATIONS

- Routine clinical follow-up every 4 to 8 wk while patient is undergoing therapy to assess for return of strength and sensation
- Repeat EMG/NCV if no improvement in 3 mo.
- Return to contact sports once full ROM and adequate strength of the shoulder are achieved

PROGNOSIS

- Depends on mechanism and severity of nerve damage
- Functional shoulder recovery is usually excellent (2).
- 85–100% of axillary nerve injury owing to fracture or dislocation will recover fully by 6 to 12 mo with nonoperative treatment (1).
- Poorer prognosis for functional recovery in symptomatic patients who undergo surgical intervention >12 mo after date of injury (3)

REFERENCES

1. Safran MR. Nerve injury about the shoulder in athletes, part 1: suprascapular nerve and axillary nerve. *Am J Sports Med*. 2004;32(3):803–819.
2. Perlmutter GS, Apruzzese W. Axillary nerve injuries in contact sports: recommendations for treatment and rehabilitation. *Sports Med*. 1998;26(5):351–361.
3. Steinmann SP, Moran EA. Axillary nerve injury: diagnosis and treatment. *J Am Acad Orthop Surg*. 2001;9(5):328–335.
4. Galvin JW, Eichinger JK. Outcomes following closed axillary nerve injury: a case report and review of the literature. *Mil Med*. 2016;181(3):e291–e297.
5. Yang X, Xu B, Tong JS, et al. Triceps motor branch transfer for isolated axillary nerve injury: outcomes in 9 patients. *Orthop Traumatol Surg Res*. 2017;103(8):1283–1286.
6. Baltzer HL, Kircher MF, Spinner RJ, et al. A comparison of outcomes of triceps motor branch-to-axillary nerve transfer or sural nerve interpositional grafting for isolated axillary nerve injury. *Plast Reconstr Surg*. 2016;138(2):256e–264e.

CLINICAL PEARLS

- Axillary nerve injury should be suspected in individuals with a glenohumeral dislocation or humeral neck fracture.

ALERT

Normal sensation of the lateral upper arm does *not* rule out axillary nerve injury.

- EMG/NCV tests should be performed in a suspected axillary nerve injury but no sooner than 3 wk postinjury.
- Despite variable recovery rates of the axillary nerve and deltoid muscle, functional recovery of the shoulder is excellent.

BAROTRAUMA

Dusty Marie Narducci, MD, Board Certified Family Medicine, CAQSM

BASICS

- Barotrauma is defined as physical damage to the body from the mechanical effects of pressure.
- Can occur due to overpressurization (during ascent) or more commonly underpressurization (during descent)
- Boyle law states that at a constant temperature, pressure (*P*) is inversely related to volume (*V*):
  - $PV = K$ (constant) or $P_1V_1 = P_2V_2$
  - Increase in pressure mandates a reduction in volume by same factor.
  - Example: If an average breath-hold diver (lungs contain ~5 L of gas) takes a full breath at the surface and descends to 10 m, the volume of air in his lungs may be reduced from 5 ℓ to 2.5 ℓ.
- Gas-filled cavities in the body are subject to expansion/contraction:
  - Lung
  - Middle ear
  - Sinus
  - Teeth
  - Gastrointestinal (GI) system
- Barotrauma is the most common form of diving-related injury (1).
- Following drowning, pulmonary barotrauma (PBT) is the second leading cause of death in scuba divers (1).
- Volume changes experienced during diving are greatest in the few feet nearest the surface.

ALERT

- For barotrauma of descent, unless an air-filled cavity has ruptured, no progression of the disease on return to normal atmospheric pressure expected
- If patient transport requires air evacuation, maintain air cabin pressure at 1 atm or fly below 1,000 feet to avoid aggravating barotrauma.

ETIOLOGY AND PATHOPHYSIOLOGY

- During descent: Increase in pressure with subsequent decrease air volume in a space that also contains tissue can lead to vascular engorgement, mucosal edema, and hemorrhage.
- During ascent: Decrease in pressure with subsequent increase in gas volume in a confined space can result in disruption or rupture of tissue.
- There are several different causes of ear barotrauma; most common etiology is flying.
- Blast injuries have become a more prevalent cause of barotrauma (war and terrorist attacks):
  - Barotrauma results from a rapid air pressure wave generated by an explosion without time to equalize the pressure.
  - Injuries include bruising of the eardrum, bleeding into the drum and middle ear, eardrum rupture, ossicular disruption, and inner ear injury.
- Middle ear:
  - Barotrauma of descent
  - Most common type of barotrauma
  - Seen in 30% of inexperienced divers and 10% of experienced divers
  - Results from inadequate equalization of pressure between the middle ear and the external ear canal
  - Eustachian tube provides the sole route of pressure equalization for the middle ear.
  - Upper respiratory infections may cause blockage or dysfunction of the eustachian tube.
  - The resulting tissue damages include congestion, hemorrhage, outward or inward bulging, and possible rupture of tympanic membrane (TM).
- External ear:
  - Barotrauma of descent or ascent
  - Due to the presence of a tight-fitting hood, ear plugs, a cerumen plug, or bony growths (exostoses)
  - Pressure cannot equalize throughout the canal, and a relative intracanal vacuum is created as the pressure differential across the obstruction increases.
- Inner ear:
  - Barotrauma of descent
  - Infrequent
  - Results from forceful attempts at equalizing middle ear pressure
  - Increased middle ear pressure can raise intracranial pressure and cause rupture of the round or labyrinth windows, allowing perilymph to enter the middle ear.
- Paranasal sinus (2):
  - Barotrauma of descent
  - Relatively common diving injury usually resulting from sinus outflow compromise, such as inflammatory mucosal thickening, polyps, and structural deviations
  - Nasal ostia act as a valve to regulate sinus pressure.
  - If the ostia fail to allow pressure equalization, congestion, edema, and hemorrhage can occur.
  - Frontal sinus most commonly affected
- Teeth (barodontalgia):
  - Barotrauma of ascent
  - Rapid volume change in the air spaces of adjacent fillings or at the roots of infected teeth
  - Common in novice and experienced divers
- GI (aerogastralgia):
  - Barotrauma of ascent
  - Swallowed air in the GI tract expands as external pressure decreases.
  - Risk of stomach rupture, resulting in pneumoperitoneum
- PBT or pulmonary overpressurization syndrome (POPS):
  - Occurs with ascent
  - Lungs expand against a closed glottis.
  - Ascending diver due to inadequate exhalation and overexpansion of the lungs; can occur from depths as shallow as 4 feet
  - Can result in pneumomediastinum, pneumothorax; interstitial gas dissecting the esophagus can result in pneumoperitoneum.
  - Most serious complication is arterial gas embolism.
  - Divers with decrease lung compliance/increased lung volumes at increased risk (chronic obstructive pulmonary disease [COPD], asthma)

GENERAL PREVENTION

- Avoid diving with upper respiratory infection, which may not allow for equalization of pressures across the TM because of eustachian tube blockage.
- Predive medical examination can help to identify individuals at increased risk for barotrauma.
- Taking pseudoephedrine 30 min prior to diving was shown to decrease the incidence and severity of middle ear barotrauma (3)[C].
- Oxymetazoline is somewhat less effective.
- Ongoing studies are considering inhaled surfactant and decompression in near zero-gravity environments to reduce the incidence of barotrauma.
- Attempt to equilibrate pressure in the middle ear to the outside by swallowing to open the eustachian tube or Valsalva maneuver.

DIAGNOSIS

Essential workup:

- Head, eyes, ears, nose, and throat (HEENT) exam with particular attention paid to the TM to determine if rupture has occurred
- Pulmonary exam looking for signs of subcutaneous (SC) emphysema and pneumothorax
- Neurologic exam looking for signs of inner ear pathology or arterial gas embolism

PHYSICAL EXAM

Signs and symptoms:

- Middle ear (barotitis media):
  - Begins as a clogged sensation
  - Increasingly painful as the pressure differential across the TM increases
  - Associated symptoms include nausea, vertigo, tinnitus, conductive hearing loss, and, occasionally, facial nerve palsy.
  - Progresses to rupture of the TM: appearance: TM congestion → TM edema → gross hemorrhage → TM rupture

- External ear: Canal mucosa becomes edematous, then hemorrhagic, and ultimately may tear.
- Inner ear:
  - Sudden, severe vertigo
  - Tinnitus
  - Sensorineural hearing loss in the affected ear
  - Symptoms begin or are associated with forceful attempt to equalize pressures of middle ear during descent.
  - Normal external canal and TM exam with isolated inner ear barotrauma
- Paranasal sinuses (2):
  - Sinus congestion
  - Headache
  - Pain
  - Epistaxis
- External objects:
  - Mask: conjunctival hemorrhage, facial edema, diplopia, and swelling
  - Tight-fitting dive suit: edema and erythema of the skin
- Barodontalgia:
  - Severe tooth pain
  - Possible tooth breakdown
- Aerogastralgia:
  - Excessive belching
  - Flatulence
  - Abdominal distension
  - In divers, abdominal pain during ascent increases in severity as depth becomes shallower.
- Pulmonary:
  - Dyspnea
  - Chest pain
  - Cough with a frothy red sputum
  - SC emphysema of the neck and chest
  - Delayed symptoms, including a bull neck appearance, dysphagia, and changes in voice character
  - Hamman sign: crackling sound heard over the heart during systole (crepitation in the neck associated with SC emphysema)
- Sinus imaging:
  - Computed tomography (CT) scan
  - Plain films
- Chest and neck radiographs for pneumothorax, pneumomediastinum
- Abdominal series (upright, decubitus) for free air from a ruptured viscus

DIFFERENTIAL DIAGNOSIS

- Decompression sickness (DCS)
- Otitis media/externa
- Sinusitis
- Arterial gas embolism
- Substance abuse/intoxication
- Asthma exacerbation
- Head injury
- Pneumothorax

DIAGNOSTIC TESTS & INTERPRETATION

Arterial blood gas determinations for pulmonary symptoms

TREATMENT

- Hospital admission criterion: PBT, arterial gas embolism, unstable patients
- Emergency department (ED) treatment:
  - Establish intravenous (IV) access for unstable patients.
  - Intubation in patients with massive SC emphysema of the neck
  - Immediate needle thoracostomy for evidence of tension pneumothorax
  - Control bleeding from the ear or nose.
  - Antibiotics with TM or sinus rupture
  - Analgesics
  - Consult Divers Alert Network (DAN): 1–919–684–4DAN (4326).
- Outpatient considerations:
  - Middle ear barotrauma:
    - Most TM ruptures heal spontaneously (4 to 6 wk) if infection is controlled and normal eustachian tube function is restored; large or marginal perforations may require surgery.
    - Spontaneous healing less likely with blast injury
    - Avoid all Cortisporin products in TM rupture (3)[C].
    - Antibiotics only with TM rupture; ofloxacin otic, ciprofloxacin eye drops (Ciloxan), Ciprodex (4)[C]
    - Decongestants, glucocorticoids, and antihistamines are not proven to expedite recovery.
    - Analgesics as needed
  - Inner ear barotrauma:
    - Complete bed rest with head elevation (avoids increase in cerebrospinal fluid [CSF] pressure, which can lead to perilymph leakage)
    - May require tympanotomy and patching of the round or oval window
    - Permanent inner ear damage possible → persistent vestibular deficits
  - Myringotomy may be considered to prevent and treat barotrauma related to flying.
  - Sinus barotrauma:
    - Consider prophylactic antibiotics for meningitis; coverage should be directed at nasopharyngeal flora (penicillin or cephalosporin classes) (2)[C].

ONGOING CARE

- Good prognosis, with most cases being self-limited
- No diving until TM has healed and other symptoms have resolved.
- Predive medical clearance is recommended for anyone with prior PBT or decompression illness.
- Absolute contraindications to diving: acute asthma, spontaneous pneumothorax, cystic/cavitary/obstructive/restrictive lung disease, seizures, atrial septal defect (ASD), symptomatic coronary artery disease (CAD), chronic perforated TM, inability to equalize sinus or middle ear pressure, or intraorbital gas
- Educate proper scuba technique; divers who hold their breath as they ascend are at increased risk of barotrauma.
- Ear, nose, and throat (ENT) referral for severe TM, inner ear, or sinus pathology
- Modern commercial aircrafts (lowered barometric pressure, ambient oxygen partial pressure, and low humidity) are safe for most healthy individuals; could be potentially dangerous following neurosurgical, plastic, and otolaryngologic procedures (craniotomy, skull base surgery)

REFERENCES

1. Glazer TA, Telian SA. Otologic hazards related to scuba diving. *Sports Health*. 2016;8(2):140–144.
2. Vaezeafshar R, Psaltis AJ, Rao VK, et al. Barosinusitis: comprehensive review and proposed new classification system. *Allergy Rhinol (Providence)*. 2017;8(3):109–117.
3. Livingstone DM, Smith KA, Lange B. Scuba diving and otology: a systematic review with recommendations on diagnosis, treatment and post-operative care. *Diving Hyperb Med*. 2017;47(2):97–109.
4. Becker GD, Parell GJ. Barotrauma of the ears and sinuses after scuba diving. *Eur Arch Otorhinolaryngol*. 2001;258(4):159–163.

ADDITIONAL READING

- Bove A. Diving medicine. *Am J Respir Crit Care Med*. 2014;189(12):1479–1486.
- Divers Alert Network: http://www.diversalertnetwork.org
- Lee YI, Ye BJ. Underwater and hyperbaric medicine as a branch of occupational and environmental medicine. *Ann Occup Environ Med*. 2013;25(1):39.
- Schipke JD, Cleveland S, Drees M. Sphenoid sinus barotrauma in diving: case series and review of the literature. *Res Sports Med*. 2018;26(1):124–137.
- van Rijswijk JB, Dubach P. Binaural tympanic-membrane perforations after blast injury. *N Engl J Med*. 2017;11;376(19):e41.

CLINICAL PEARLS

- Barotrauma is the most common form of diving-related injury; most common is middle ear barotrauma.
- Most serious complication of barotrauma is arterial gas embolism.
- Divers with lung disease are at high risk for PBT.
- Most TM ruptures heal spontaneously within 4 to 6 wk; antibiotics *only* when the TM is ruptured
- Decongestants, glucocorticoids, and antihistamines are not the standard of care for ear barotrauma.
- Consider prophylactic antibiotics for meningitis for sinus barotrauma.
- Modern commercial aircrafts can be dangerous following neurosurgical, plastic, and otolaryngologic procedures.

BICEPS TENDINOPATHY

Daniel C. Herman, MD, PhD, FAAPMR, FACSM, CAQSM • Giorgio A. Negron, MD

BASICS

DESCRIPTION

- Overuse injury of the long head of the biceps muscle
- Initially begins as inflammation in the tendon sheath known as *tenosynovitis* and then progresses to tendon degeneration and disordered arrangement of collagen fibers, otherwise known as *tendinosis* or *biceps tendinopathy*
- Primary biceps tendinitis (inflammation of the tendon) is estimated to represent only 5% of cases (1).

EPIDEMIOLOGY

80% of bicep tendinopathy cases are seen in males with peak incidence in the 5th and 6th decade of life (2).

ETIOLOGY AND PATHOPHYSIOLOGY

- Anatomy:
  - The long head of the biceps muscle arises from the superior glenoid labrum and the supraglenoid tubercle of the scapula.
  - It is an intra-articular but extrasynovial structure.
  - Primary blood supply proximally is the anterior humeral circumflex artery.
- Biomechanics:
  - Primary function of the biceps at the elbow is a flexor and supinator.
  - In the shoulder, the biceps tendon may act as a humeral head depressor and a secondary stabilizer of the glenohumeral joint.
  - During throwing, it assists in deceleration of the humerus.

RISK FACTORS

Repetitive use of upper extremities (especially overhead), such as throwing/hitting, swimming, racquet sports, and gymnastics

COMMONLY ASSOCIATED CONDITIONS

- Rotator cuff pathology (tendinopathy, impingement, tears)
- Glenoid labral tears (superior labrum anterior and posterior [SLAP] lesions)
- Subluxation/dislocation of the long head of the biceps
- Biceps tendon rupture

DIAGNOSIS

HISTORY

- Anterior shoulder pain localized over the bicipital groove, which may radiate distally toward the biceps
- Pain is aggravated by overhead activities or lifting objects.

PHYSICAL EXAM

- Point tenderness over the bicipital groove with the arm in 10 degrees internal rotation (sensitivity: 54%; specificity: 72%) (3)
- An audible or palpable snap during arc of motion while throwing may indicate instability or subluxation of the biceps tendon.
- A large mass ("Popeye deformity") in the upper arm, ecchymosis, and swelling following a painful audible pop with quick resolution of pain could indicate biceps tendon rupture.
- Any positive testing for biceps tendon pathology may also signify a glenoid labral tear (SLAP lesion).
- Special tests:
  - Uppercut test: With the patient's shoulder in neutral position and forearm supinated, elbow is flexed 90 degrees with hand in a fist. Patient then rapidly brings fist toward chin against resistance. Pain in the shoulder is considered a positive test (sensitivity: 73%; specificity: 78%) (3).
  - Speed test: With the patient's shoulder elevated to 90 degrees of forward flexion, elbow extended and forearm supinated, the patient flexes the shoulder against resistance. Pain in or about the bicipital groove is considered a positive test (sensitivity: 54%; specificity: 81%) (3).
  - Yergason test: With the patient's elbow flexed to 90 degrees, the patient supinates against resistance. Pain over the biceps tendon in the bicipital groove is considered a positive test (sensitivity: 41%; specificity: 79%) (3).
  - Performing the uppercut test and biceps groove tenderness together has the highest sensitivity and specificity to clinically diagnose long head biceps pathology (3)[A].

DIFFERENTIAL DIAGNOSIS

- Rotator cuff tendinopathy
- Impingement syndrome
- Glenoid labral tears
- Biceps tendon subluxation/dislocation
- Subacromial bursitis
- Acromioclavicular joint separation or arthritis
- Pectoralis minor strain
- Glenohumeral joint arthritis
- Thoracic outlet syndrome
- Cervical disk disease
- Brachial plexus injuries
- Rheumatoid arthritis
- Pancoast tumor

DIAGNOSTIC TESTS & INTERPRETATION

- Plain-film radiographs are not helpful in the diagnosis of biceps tendon pathology. Magnetic resonance imaging (MRI) may show increased signal on T2-weighted images in the area of the biceps tendon and is beneficial for detecting complete tears (sensitivity: ~60%; specificity: ~100%) (4)[B]. Also useful in detecting pathology of the superior labrum and rotator cuff. Magnetic resonance (MR) arthrography may be superior to conventional MRI in diagnosing biceps tendon lesions and SLAP lesions but is invasive (sensitivity: ~90%; specificity: ~50%) (1,4)[B].
- Dynamic musculoskeletal ultrasound (US) is becoming more popular in diagnosing biceps tendon rupture, subluxation, and dislocation (sensitivity: 49%; specificity: 97%) (1). It is not reliable in evaluating intra-articular tears or the glenoid labrum. US is very operator- and facility-dependent. Advantages include low cost and lack of radiation exposure.

TREATMENT

Acute treatment:

- Rest, ice, nonsteroidal anti-inflammatory drugs (NSAIDs), and/or acetaminophen
- Rest should not include prolonged immobilization because this may lead to adhesive capsulitis (frozen shoulder).
- Gentle stretching and range of motion (ROM) exercises should be initiated early once symptoms begin to improve.
- Consider physical therapy for persistent symptoms.
- Surgery is reserved for refractory cases.

ADDITIONAL THERAPIES

- Physical therapy:
  - Gentle ROM exercises are begun first.
  - Scapulothoracic stabilization exercises
  - Rotator cuff strengthening
  - Biceps strengthening
- Include:
  - US: uses sound waves to heat up the affected tissues
  - Phonophoresis: uses US waves to drive topical corticosteroid medication into the affected tissue
  - Iontophoresis: uses electric current to drive a corticosteroid into the affected tissue (5)[C]

SURGERY/OTHER PROCEDURES

- Injections:
  - Corticosteroid injection into the biceps tendon sheath may be considered providing short-term pain control up to 6 wk, but controversy exists regarding the accuracy of such injections (5):
    - US may increase the accuracy and analgesic effect (1).
  - Injection into the tendon itself has been associated with tendon rupture and should be avoided.
- Surgical options may be considered for patients who fail conservative treatment after 3 mo or have refractory pain (1):
  - Tenotomy: surgical release of the long head of the biceps tendon at or near its superior glenoid labral origin:
    - Recommended in older patients with low activity requirements
    - Disadvantage includes a cosmetic "Popeye deformity" and possible loss of some strength with supination.
    - Minimal rehabilitation is required.
  - Tenodesis: fixation of the long head of the biceps tendon in the bicipital groove:
    - Minimal loss of function compared with tenotomy
    - No cosmetic defect
    - Recommended in younger, more active individuals
    - Disadvantages include a more complex operation, a period of immobilization, and longer postoperative rehabilitation.
- Proximal rupture of the long head of the biceps typically relieves symptoms of pain without significant loss of function. Surgery may be considered if there is significant loss of strength or function.

REFERENCES

1. Churgay CA. Diagnosis and treatment of biceps tendinitis and tendinosis. *Am Fam Physician*. 2009;80(5):470–476.
2. Donaldson O, Vannet N, Gosens T, et al. Tendinopathies around the elbow part 2: medial elbow, distal biceps and triceps tendinopathies. *Shoulder Elbow*. 2014;6(1):47–56.
3. Rosas S, Krill MK, Amoo-Achampong K, et al. A practical, evidence-based, comprehensive (PEC) physical examination for diagnosing pathology of the long head of the biceps. *J Shoulder Elbow Surg*. 2017;26(8):1484–1492.
4. Dubrow SA, Streit JJ, Shishani Y, et al. Diagnostic accuracy in detecting tears in the proximal biceps tendon using standard nonenhancing shoulder MRI. *Open Access J Sports Med*. 2014;5:81–87.
5. Andres BM, Murrell GA. Treatment of tendinopathy: what works, what does not, and what is on the horizon. *Clin Orthop Relat Res*. 2008;466(7):1539–1554.

ADDITIONAL READING

- Ahrens PM, Boileau P. The long head of biceps and associated tendinopathy. *J Bone Joint Surg Br*. 2007;89(8):1001–1009.
- Friedman DJ, Dunn JC, Higgins LD, et al. Proximal biceps tendon: injuries and management. *Sports Med Arthrosc Rev*. 2008;16(3):162–169.
- Longo UG, Franceschi F, Ruzzini L, et al. Characteristics at haematoxylin and eosin staining of ruptures of the long head of the biceps tendon. *Br J Sports Med*. 2009;43(8):603–607.
- Patton WC, McCluskey GM III. Biceps tendinitis and subluxation. *Clin Sports Med*. 2001;20(3):505–529.

CLINICAL PEARLS

- Primary biceps tendinitis is very rare and thought to be ~5% of cases.
- Performing the uppercut test and biceps groove tenderness together has the highest sensitivity and specificity to clinically diagnose long head biceps pathology.
- Imaging should be considered with shoulder radiography to rule out primary causes of impingement followed by advanced imaging with either US and/or MRI.
- Nonsurgical measures include rest, NSAIDs, acetaminophen, and physical therapy. Corticosteroid injection in bicipital tendon sheath may provide short-term alleviation of pain.

BICEPS TENDON RUPTURE

Saif Usman, MD, FAAFP, CAQSM

BASICS

DESCRIPTION

- Biceps brachii muscle is composed of a long head originating from the apex of the glenoid and a short head originating from the tip of coracoid process.
- Distally both heads insert onto the distal radial tuberosity.
- Complete or partial tear of the long bicipital tendon can occur at a proximal or distal location from repetitive microtrauma or acute traumatic injury.

EPIDEMIOLOGY

- Occurs most commonly in males 30 to 60 yr of age
- Occurs most commonly concomitantly with supraspinatus and subscapularis tears (1)
- 90–97% of biceps tendon ruptures are proximal, at the intertubercular sulcus.
- 3–10% occur distally at the elbow.

RISK FACTORS

- Male
- Age >30 yr
- Smokers have 7.5 times increased risk of distal biceps rupture.
- Preexisting bicipital tendinopathy
- Rotator cuff tendinopathy or tear (biceps tendon pathologically loaded)
- Overhead athlete (contributes to anterior shoulder stability with repeated abduction/external rotation)
- Prior corticosteroid injection into biceps tendon sheath
- Anabolic steroid use

COMMONLY ASSOCIATED CONDITIONS

- Rotator cuff impingement: Subacromial impingement in combination with repetitive overhead motion, such as with throwing, can lead to proximal biceps tendon degeneration.
- Superior labrum anterior-to-posterior (SLAP) lesions: may involve the biceps anchor (2)
- Supraspinatus rupture/partial rupture
- Subscapularis rupture/partial rupture: Following subscapularis tears, the biceps tendon can sublux medially out of the bicipital groove, causing a painful clicking sensation.
- Rotator interval lesions: The biceps tendon can sublux medially over the lesser tuberosity after tears to the rotator interval, but there usually is an associated subscapularis injury (2).

DIAGNOSIS

HISTORY

- Mechanism is usually forceful eccentric biceps contraction applied to a flexed elbow.
- Pain is usually located more proximal than distal.
- Prior symptoms are indicative of prior rotator cuff or bicipital tendinopathy.
- An injury with minimal symptoms in elderly patients showing acceptable strength may be managed nonsurgically.

PHYSICAL EXAM

- Proximal rupture:
  - Patient may report a sudden tearing or "pop" in the shoulder.
  - Acute pain and later ecchymosis and swelling about the anterior shoulder
  - Visible lump type of deformity in the midupper arm anteriorly, secondary to muscle belly retracting distally ("Popeye sign")
  - In some cases of chronic shoulder pain, there may be notable improvement after inflammation subsides.
  - Patients with accompanying rotator cuff pathology may complain of overhead pain and weakness and night pain.
  - Inspect for "Popeye sign" deformity in anterior brachium.
  - Ecchymosis may involve entire anterior biceps.
  - Elbow function generally is preserved. Patient may have mild weakness of elbow flexion and supination.
  - Shoulder function may be diminished, and careful evaluation of rotator cuff integrity is advised.
  - Specialized tests for biceps pathology include the Speed, Yergason, and Ludington tests.
- Distal rupture:
  - History is usually of a sudden eccentric load with elbow at 90 degrees of flexion.
  - Acute tearing sensation with sudden loss of elbow flexion and supination strength
  - Pain, ecchymosis, and swelling localized over the antecubital fossa
  - Variable degree of proximal retraction of muscle belly ("reverse Popeye sign") (3)
  - May visualize absence of distal biceps tendon as it crosses the elbow flexion crease
  - Hook test is useful in differentiating between complete avulsion and sprain or partial tear.
  - Hook test is 100% sensitive and specific in detecting complete distal ruptures (4).
  - Biceps squeeze test is 96% sensitive in detecting distal biceps ruptures.
  - Usually significant losses in strength on resisted elbow flexion and supination
  - A partial rupture may have many of the same features as a complete rupture, but generally, the tendon still can be palpated in continuity.

DIFFERENTIAL DIAGNOSIS

- Proximal rupture:
  - Superior labral lesion (i.e., SLAP tear)
  - Subscapularis injury
  - Rotator cuff/rotator interval injury
  - Biceps tendon subluxation (rupture of transverse ligament)
  - Long head of biceps tendinitis or tendinosis; onset usually insidious
  - Greater or lesser tuberosity fractures may occur following shoulder dislocation.

- Distal rupture:
  - Distal biceps tendinitis or tendinosis; onset usually insidious
  - Partial distal biceps tendon rupture
  - Anterior capsule strain; occurs with hyperextension injuries, and tenderness is more diffuse anteriorly
  - Coronoid process fractures directly tender over coronoid process; no palpable biceps defect
  - Lateral antebrachial cutaneous nerve entrapment syndrome

DIAGNOSTIC TESTS & INTERPRETATION

Initial Tests (lab, imaging)

- Plain films of shoulder are often negative with isolated tendon rupture.
- Shoulder magnetic resonance imaging (MRI) confirms diagnosis if clinical exam not straightforward and if rotator cuff pathology is suspected.
- MRI findings may include absence of the tendon within the intertubercular groove as a result of tendon retraction.
- Shoulder ultrasound is reliable for diagnosing complete rupture, subluxation, or dislocation of biceps tendon (5)[C].
- Standard elbow x-ray series for distal injuries:
  - Check for avulsion fragment of radial tuberosity.
  - Degenerative changes or lipping at the radial tuberosity can be associated with biceps tendinopathy.
- Elbow ultrasound is reliable for detecting complete versus partial distal biceps tendon tears (6)[C].

TREATMENT

GENERAL MEASURES

- Proximal rupture:
  - Acute immobilization in posterior elbow splint with the elbow at 90 degrees for comfort and forearm in full supination; add sling for comfort.
  - Younger patients should begin immediate shoulder and elbow passive range of motion (ROM) exercises.
  - Strengthening can begin in 4 to 5 wk or when there is resolution of pain.
  - Return to unrestricted activities after 2 to 3 mo.
  - Patients >50 yr of age may require longer period of immobilization prior to strengthening rehab.
  - Younger patients may prefer surgical treatment (tenodesis vs. tenotomy) for cosmetic reasons or to return to their previous level of functioning, especially if overhead athletes (2).
  - Most patients are older and will have little to no change in elbow flexion/supination strength; they may opt for surgery, however, if there is additional rotator cuff pathology.
- Distal rupture:
  - Acute management is the same as for proximal injuries.
  - Nonoperative treatment is reserved for older, lower demand patients or those with unacceptably high risk for surgery.
  - Nonoperative management is associated with significant loss of elbow supination endurance and strength as well as elbow flexion weakness (2)[C].
  - Majority of patients require surgical repair as soon as possible after injury.

ADDITIONAL THERAPIES

- The main complaint after conservative management of biceps tendon ruptures, especially distal ruptures, is loss of elbow flexion and forearm supination strength, especially endurance.
- Most young people and athletes require surgical repair of complete biceps tendon injuries. Many advocate surgical repair of partial ruptures in this population, especially if the ruptures are distal.

REFERENCES

1. Kowalczuk M, Kohut K, Sabzevari S, et al. Proximal long head biceps rupture: a predictor of rotator cuff pathology. *Arthroscopy*. 2018;34(4):1166–1170.
2. Burns JP, Bahk M, Snyder SJ. Superior labral tears: repair versus biceps tenodesis. *J Shoulder Elbow Surg*. 2011;20(Suppl 2):S2–S8.
3. Schmidt CC, Savoie FH III, Steinmann SP, et al. Distal biceps tendon history, updates, and controversies: from the closed American Shoulder and Elbow Surgeons meeting—2015. *J Shoulder Elbow Surg*. 2016;25(10):1717–1730.
4. O'Driscoll SW, Goncalves LB, Dietz P. The hook test for distal biceps tendon avulsion. *Am J Sports Med*. 2007;35(11):1865–1869.
5. Armstrong A, Teefey SA, Wu T, et al. The efficacy of ultrasound in the diagnosis of long head of the biceps tendon pathology. *J Shoulder Elbow Surg*. 2006;15(1):7–11.
6. Lobo Lda G, Fessell DP, Miller BS, et al. The role of sonography in differentiating full versus partial distal biceps tendon tears: correlation with surgical findings. *AJR Am J Roentgenol*. 2013;200(1):158–162.

ADDITIONAL READING

- Beall DP, Williamson EE, Ly JQ, et al. Association of biceps tendon tears with rotator cuff abnormalities: degree of correlation with tears of the anterior and superior portions of the rotator cuff. *AJR Am J Roentgenol*. 2003;180(3):633–639.
- Ward J, Shreve M, Youm T, et al. Ruptures of the distal biceps tendon. *Bull Hosp Jt Dis (2013)*. 2014;72(1):110–119.
- Zappia M, Reginelli A, Russo A, et al. Long head of the biceps tendon and rotator interval. *Musculoskelet Surg*. 2013;97(Suppl 2):S99–S108.

CLINICAL PEARLS

- Biceps tendon ruptures occur most commonly concomitantly with supraspinatus and subscapularis tears.
- Popeye sign is highly indicative of proximal biceps tendon rupture.
- Hook test is 100% sensitive and specific for distal biceps rupture.
- Musculoskeletal ultrasound can reliably diagnose proximal and distal biceps tendon ruptures, both partial and complete.
- Most cases of distal biceps tendon rupture will require surgical repair as soon as possible after injury.

BITES AND STINGS

Steven A. Greer, MD, CAQ, FAAFP

BASICS

Arthropods inoculate poison or invading tissue and transmit diseases. Inoculation of poison may occur as either a bite or a sting. This discussion is limited to the irritative, poisonous, allergic effects of these pests.

DESCRIPTION

- Harmful arthropods of the United States include (1):
  - Ants: fire ants, harvester ants
  - Bees: bumblebees, sweat bees, honeybees, Africanized (killer) bees
  - Bugs: kissing, bed, wheel
  - Caterpillars: puss, browntail, buck, moth saddleback
  - Centipedes
  - Fleas: human, cat, dog
  - Flies: deer, horse, black, stable, and biting midges
  - Lice: body, head, pubic
  - Mites: itch mite (scabies), red bugs (chiggers)
  - Mosquitoes
  - Scorpions
  - Spiders: brown recluse, black widow, hobo
  - Ticks: deer, lone star
  - Wasps: hornets, wasps
- Characteristic reactions include:
  - Local tissue irritation, inflammation, and destruction.
  - Systemic effects related to inoculated poisons.
  - Allergic reactions: immediate or delayed.
- System(s) affected: skin/exocrine

EPIDEMIOLOGY

- Affects all ages with 0- to 4-yr-olds and 20- to 24-yr-olds at highest risk for nonfatal bites/stings (2)
- Males = females

Incidence

- Common, with ~1 million nonfatal and 50 fatal cases per year (3,4)
- Anaphylaxis is estimated at 3% in adults and 0.4–0.8% in children.
- Individual stings from Africanized (killer) bees are no more potent than other bees; the danger lies in their predilection to swarm, causing death by multiple stings.

Prevalence

Ubiquitous, varies by region and season (2)

ETIOLOGY AND PATHOPHYSIOLOGY

- Local tissue inflammation and destruction from poison (5)
- Allergic reaction from previous sensitization (0.4–3%)
- Toxic reaction from large inoculation of poison

Genetics

No genetic predilection

RISK FACTORS

- Living environment (3,5)
- Climate
- Season
- Clothing
- Lack of protective measures
- Perfumes, colognes
- Previous sensitization
- Young or elderly at more risk for morbidity/mortality

GENERAL PREVENTION

Prevention/avoidance (3,4,5):

- Avoid reexposure in known hypersensitive individuals.
- Prescribe anaphylactic (ANA kit) or self-administered epinephrine (EpiPen), if indicated.
- Educate on risks of increasing anamnestic responses in the future.
- Consider desensitization with immunotherapy in severe cases.
- Cover as much skin as possible.
- Use repellants on uncovered areas.
- Apply sunscreen first, then repellant.
- N-Diethyl-meta-toluamide (DEET), picaridin, or other proven insect repellants
- Oil of lemon eucalyptus, p-menthane-3,8-diol (PMD), and IR3535 are considered biopesticides by the Environmental Protection Agency (EPA), but be sure to use EPA-approved products because many versions have not been tested.
- Permethrin applied to clothes is effective through multiple washings.
- Permethrin-infused clothing is commercially available and effective.
- Consider immunization/prophylaxis for travel to endemic areas.

DIAGNOSIS

PHYSICAL EXAM

- Signs and symptoms (1,3,4,5):
  - Erythema
  - Pain
  - Heat
  - Swelling
  - Itching
  - Blisters
  - Secondary infection: cellulitis, abscess
  - Necrosis
  - Ulceration
  - Drainage
- Toxic reactions (nonantigenic):
  - Nausea
  - Vomiting
  - Headache
  - Fever
  - Diarrhea
  - Light-headedness
  - Syncope
  - Drowsiness
  - Muscles spasms
  - Edema
  - Convulsions
- Systemic reactions (allergic):
  - Itching eyes
  - Facial flushing
  - Generalized urticaria
  - Dry cough
  - Chest/throat constriction
  - Wheezing
  - Dyspnea
  - Cyanosis
  - Abdominal cramps
  - Diarrhea
  - Nausea
  - Vomiting
  - Vertigo
  - Chills/fever
  - Stridor
  - Shock
  - Loss of consciousness
  - Involuntary bowel/bladder action
  - Frothy sputum
  - Respiratory failure
  - Cardiovascular collapse
  - Death
- Delayed reaction:
  - Serum-sickness–like reactions
  - Fever
  - Malaise
  - Headache
  - Urticaria
  - Lymphadenopathy
  - Polyarthritis
- Unusual reactions:
  - Encephalopathy
  - Neuritis
  - Vasculitis
  - Nephrosis
  - Extreme fear/anxiety

DIFFERENTIAL DIAGNOSIS

- Local reaction: infection, cellulitis, dermatoses, punctures, foreign bodies
- Toxic reaction: chemical exposure/ingestion, medications, intravenous (IV) drug abuse, environmental, plants
- Allergic reaction: medications, illicit drugs, foods, topical products, environmental, plants, chemicals

DIAGNOSTIC TESTS & INTERPRETATION

- Lab: Leukocytosis, thrombocytopenia, hypofibrinogenemia, abnormal coagulation, disseminated intravascular coagulation, proteinuria, hemoglobinemia, hemoglobinuria, myoglobinemia, myoglobinuria, and azotemia are uncommon but possible manifestations in severe reactions.
- Pathologic findings: inflammation, ulceration, vesiculation, pustulation, rupture, eschar, swelling (1,5)

TREATMENT

- Long-term treatment (5):
  - Recommended for those with hypersensitivity reaction but may be considered for individuals with large local reactions
  - Self-administered epinephrine device
  - Hypersensitivity identification
  - Venom immunotherapy for 3 to 5 yr is 80–90% effective even after cessation of treatment.
- Acute treatment (1,5,6):
  - Outpatient or inpatient, depending on individual response to injury
  - Hospitalize for severe systemic reactions with threatened airway obstruction, bronchospasm, hypotension, severe angiodermatitis, or pain.

GENERAL MEASURES

- First aid measures, local treatment, activate emergency services in severe reactions. If history of allergy or large envenomations, don't wait to seek emergency care (1,3,5).
- Use ANA kit and over-the-counter antihistamines, if available and required.
- Local (depending on severity):
  - Remove stinger (scrape it out—don't squeeze with tweezer).
  - Cleanse wound.
  - Ice packs to bite or sting site (alternate 10 min on or 10 min off)
  - Elevation of affected part
  - Débride ulcers.
  - Drain abscesses.
- Systemic (depending on severity and type of reaction): home use—EpiPen:
  - Adequate airway (intubation, tracheostomy): if needed to bypass obstruction
  - Oxygen (4 to 6 L/min): if needed for respiratory distress
  - Hospitalize and observe 24 to 48 hr.

MEDICATION

First Line

- Local (depending on severity):
  - Analgesics
  - Antihistamines: diphenhydramine (Benadryl) 25 to 50 mg QID.
  - Steroids topical or oral: Prednisone 20 to 40 mg/day is unproven but may be helpful for large local reactions.
  - Antibiotics only if there is a secondary infection
- Systemic (depending on severity and reaction type):
  - Epinephrine (1:1,000) subcutaneous (SC): to combat urticaria, wheezing, angioedema—child: 0.01 mL/kg; adult 0.3 to 0.5 mL/kg
  - Diphenhydramine: 25 to 50 mg IV or intramuscular (IM) to combat urticaria, wheezing, angioedema
  - Albuterol 5 mg Inhalation and ipratropium bromide 0.5 mg Inhalation: bronchospasm
  - IV fluids (Ringer lactate): if needed for hypotension, hypovolemia
  - Dopamine: 200 mg in 250 mL at 5 μg/kg/min to correct vascular collapse
- Titrate to maintain systemic blood pressure (BP) over 90 mm Hg:
  - Hydrocortisone: 100 to 250 mg IV, if needed, for severe urticaria or spider bite
  - Tetanus prophylaxis and antibiotics: only if secondary infection, rarely indicated
  - Diazepam (Valium): 5 to 10 mg, if needed, for severe muscle spasms
  - Morphine or meperidine (Demerol): if needed for pain
- Antivenins may be appropriate based on availability, identification of organism, and previous sensitivity.
- Topical insecticides:
  - Lice: 1% permethrin (Nix, Elimite) is still considered first line despite up to 50% resistance. 0.5% malathion (Ovide) may be used as initial choice or for permethrin failure. 1% lindane (Kwell) or pyrethrin (Rid) is also effective.
  - Scabies: 5% permethrin is drug of choice, but 10% crotamiton (Eurax) and lindane are effective.
- Contraindications: Refer to manufacturer's literature.
- Precautions:
  - Dosing appropriate to age
  - If severe reaction, don't delay treatment.
  - Severe vascular collapse may require central pressure monitor.
- Significant possible interactions: Refer to manufacturer's literature.

Second Line

Alternative drugs (6):

- Other H_1 antihistamines (e.g., loratadine [Claritin], fexofenadine [Allegra])
- H_2 blockers (e.g., ranitidine [Zantac], cimetidine [Tagamet], famotidine [Pepcid])
- Oral ivermectin (Mectizan) appears effective for lice and scabies but is not FDA approved for this purpose.

SURGERY/OTHER PROCEDURES

Optimal treatment of necrotic spider bites is not well defined. Surgical repair may be required for severe ulcerative lesions but not until primary necrotizing process is complete (1,3).

COMPLEMENTARY & ALTERNATIVE MEDICINE

- Oil of lemon eucalyptus, PMD, and IR3535 are considered biopesticides by the EPA, but be sure to use EPA-approved products because essential oils have not been tested (3,7).
- Turmeric may help inflammation. Animal studies show promise but no proof in humans and no dose data.

ONGOING CARE

FOLLOW-UP RECOMMENDATIONS

No activity restrictions

Patient Monitoring

Follow-up wound care

DIET

No special diet; nothing by mouth if severe systemic reaction

PATIENT EDUCATION

- Protective measures, ANA kit/EpiPen use, risks (3,5)
- Individuals with known sensitivity should wear medical identification (bracelet, tag) or carry a card.

PROGNOSIS

Expected course (5):

- Minor reactions—excellent
- Severe reactions—excellent with early, appropriate treatment

COMPLICATIONS

- Infection (5,6):
  - Bacterial
  - Arthropod-associated diseases with tick, fly, bug, and mosquito bites (e.g., Lyme borreliosis, rickettsial disease [Rocky Mountain spotted fever], arboviral encephalitis, malaria, leishmaniasis, trypanosomiasis, dengue)
- Scarring
- Drug reactions
- Multisystem failure
- Death

Pediatric Considerations

Not a contraindication to appropriate management

REFERENCES

1. Centers for Disease Control and Prevention. Necrotic arachnidism—Pacific Northwest, 1988-1996. *MMWR Morb Mortal Wkly Rep*. 1996;45(21):433–436.
2. Centers for Disease Control and Prevention. Injury prevention & control. http://www.cdc.gov/injury/wisqars/index.html.
3. Centers for Disease Control and Prevention. *CDC Health Information for International Travel 2016*. New York, NY. Oxford University Press; 2015.
4. Fradin MS. Mosquitoes and mosquito repellants: a clinician's guide. *Ann Intern Med*. 1998;128(11):931–940.
5. Moffitt JE, Golden DB, Reisman RE, et al. Stinging insect hypersensitivity: a practice parameter update. *J Allergy Clin Immunol*. 2004;114(4):869–886.
6. Pickering L, ed. *Red Book: 2009 Report of the Committee on Infectious Diseases*. 28th ed. Itasca, IL: American Academy of Pediatrics; 2009.
7. Jurenka JS. Anti-inflammatory properties of curcumin, a major constituent of Curcuma longa: a review of preclinical and clinical research. *Altern Med Rev*. 2009;14(2):141–153.

CLINICAL PEARLS

- Prevention is often more effective than treatment.
- Vigilant observation for systemic reaction allows for early treatment and better recovery.
- Allergic reactions worsen with each successive exposure.

BRACHIAL PLEXUS INJURIES (BURNERS AND STINGERS)

Geoffrey S. Kuhlman, MD, FAAFP, CAQSM

BASICS

DESCRIPTION

- Acute trauma to the neck and shoulder area injuring the brachial plexus
- Typically causes burning or stinging pain in the upper shoulder radiating down the entire upper extremity, hence, the names "burner" and "stinger"
- Most commonly involves the upper trunk of the plexus or cervical nerve roots C5 and C6
- Mechanism of injury:
  - Traction to the plexus when the shoulder is depressed and the head is forced away from the injured side
  - Compression of cervical nerve roots when the head is forced toward the side of injury
  - Direct blow to the brachial plexus at the supraclavicular fossa

EPIDEMIOLOGY

Incidence

- Exact incidence unknown due to underreporting by athletes
- Common in contact sports (football, wrestling, hockey); football career incidence reported between 49% and 65%
- Frequent recurrence, reported as high as 87% (1)

ETIOLOGY AND PATHOPHYSIOLOGY

- Most are limited to neurapraxia, nerve dysfunction with demyelination.
- Minority involve axonotmesis with subsequent wallerian degeneration and eventual regeneration of axons.

RISK FACTORS

- Previous burner
- Limited range of motion of the neck or shoulder
- Cervical canal and foraminal stenosis

GENERAL PREVENTION

Neck roll, shoulder pad lifter, or rigid collar (e.g., cowboy collar) in football might reduce injury risk.

DIAGNOSIS

HISTORY

- Mechanism of injury (Falling on an outstretched arm suggests alternative injury.) (2)
- Details of symptom quality, severity, and location (Bilateral or lower extremity symptoms indicate cervical fracture or cord injury until proven otherwise; symptoms not typical of burners mandate search for an alternative diagnosis.)
- Modifying factors (Limitation or pain with shoulder motion suggests alternative shoulder diagnosis.)
- Initial versus recurrent injury (Recurrence typically requires more aggressive rehabilitation.)

PHYSICAL EXAM

- Signs and symptoms (1):
  - Burning or stinging pain radiating down one arm circumferentially (i.e., nondermatomal pattern)
  - Sometimes numbness, paresthesias, and weakness in the extremity
  - Athlete often immediately holds the arm close to the body or even shakes the upper extremity.
  - Symptoms often last a few minutes but can persist for weeks, particularly in recurrent episodes.
- Physical examination:
  - Inspection (asymmetry or postural abnormality to address in therapy)
  - Palpation (Tenderness suggests alternative diagnosis; spasm is common but nonspecific.)
  - Neurologic examination (strength, sensation, reflexes to localize injury, rule out cord injury)
  - Weakness most common in deltoid, biceps, and rotator cuff (1)
  - Spurling test may be positive.
  - Tinel sign at the supraclavicular fossa (Positive result indicates plexus injury.)
  - After serious cervical injury is ruled out, Spurling neuroforaminal compression test (disk herniation, burner from cervical foraminal stenosis)

DIFFERENTIAL DIAGNOSIS

- Cervical injury (fracture, dislocation, spinal cord injury, disc herniation):
  - Bilateral symptoms, cervical vertebral tenderness, or lower extremity findings indicate cervical fracture or spinal cord injury until proven otherwise.
- Glenohumeral dislocation
- Acromioclavicular separation
- Clavicle fracture
- Thoracic outlet syndrome (when chronic, recurrent):
  - Repetitive athletic movements with pitching or swimming

DIAGNOSTIC TESTS & INTERPRETATION

Initial Tests (lab, imaging)

- Not routine
- Cervical spine x-rays if recurrent injury, findings localizing to one cervical level, or symptoms in more than one extremity (2)

- X-ray cervical spine if fracture, dislocation, or cervical instability suspected:
  - Required if severe nerve pain, focal cervical spine tenderness, limited range of motion, weakness or recurrence
  - Anteroposterior (AP), lateral, oblique, flexion, extension
- Magnetic resonance imaging (MRI) or computed tomography (CT) cervical spine if x-rays are unrevealing to identify neuroforaminal stenosis, disk herniation, or mass as possible causes of nerve root impingement (3); often not needed and some risk of false positive:
  - Indications:
    - Neurologic symptoms and signs that are not improving daily
    - Bilateral symptoms (burning hands syndrome)
    - Recurrence within 1 yr

Diagnostic Procedures/Other

Electromyography/nerve conduction velocity (EMG/NCV) if symptoms last at least 3 wk for confirmation, localization, and prognosis (EMG normalization lags far behind clinical and neurologic recovery, so follow-up EMG generally not indicated.) (2)

TREATMENT

GENERAL MEASURES

- Stretch tight muscles at neck and shoulder.
- Strengthen neck, shoulder, and muscles weakened by injury.
- These strategies apply, regardless of injury mechanism.
- Schedule follow-up until symptoms and examination normalize.
- Enhancing protective equipment
- Return to play only when asymptomatic and normal neurologic examination (2).

COMPLEMENTARY & ALTERNATIVE MEDICINE

Football players can consider neck roll, shoulder pad lifter, or rigid collar when returning to play.

ONGOING CARE

Prevention:

- Chest-out posture
- Ensure correct playing technique.
- Maintain strength and flexibility of neck and shoulder.

REFERENCES

1. Kuhlman GS, McKeag DB. The "burner": a common nerve injury in contact sports. *Am Fam Physician*. 1999;60(7):2035–2040, 2042.
2. Standaert CJ, Herring SA. Expert opinion and controversies in musculoskeletal and sports medicine: stingers. *Arch Phys Med Rehabil*. 2009;90(3):402–406.
3. Safran MR. Nerve injury about the shoulder in athletes, part 2: long thoracic nerve, spinal accessory nerve, burners/stingers, thoracic outlet syndrome. *Am J Sports Med*. 2004;32(4):1063–1076.

ADDITIONAL READING

- Aval SM, Durand P Jr, Shankwiler JA. Neurovascular injuries to the athlete's shoulder: part I. *J Am Acad Orthop Surg*. 2007;15(4):249–256.
- Aval SM, Durand P Jr, Shankwiler JA. Neurovascular injuries to the athlete's shoulder: part II. *J Am Acad Orthop Surg*. 2007;15(5):281–289.
- Charbonneau RME, McVeigh SA, Thompson K. Brachial neurapraxia in Canadian Atlantic University sport football players: what is the incidence of "stingers"? *Clin J Sport Med*. 2012;22(6):472–477.
- Dimberg EL, Burns TM. Management of common neurologic conditions in sports. *Clin Sports Med*. 2005;24(3):637–662.
- Rihn JA, Anderson DT, Lamb K, et al. Cervical spine injuries in American football. *Sports Med*. 2009;39(9):697–708.

CLINICAL PEARLS

- Nerve damage is generally not permanent, but a few patients have symptoms lasting months to years (2).
- Conditioning and rehabilitation should begin immediately. You can return to contact activity when the symptoms are gone and your strength and sensation are back to normal (1).
- Continue stretching and strengthening at least the rest of the season. Continuance of exercises throughout your career will lower the chance of having another burner (1).

BRUGADA SYNDROME

Chau Bui, DO • Paul Meirick, MD

BASICS

DESCRIPTION

- Channelopathies refer to a group of inherited arrhythmogenic diseases caused by mutations in genes encoding for ion channel proteins in cardiomyocytes that disrupt the balance of currents in the cardiac action potential. These disruptions may lead to ventricular arrhythmias and sudden cardiac death (SCD).
- The channelopathies include Brugada syndrome, long QT syndrome (LQTS) (see chapter on QT syndromes), short QT syndrome (SQTS) (see chapter on QT syndromes), and catecholaminergic polymorphic ventricular tachycardia (CPVT) (see supplemental materials for CPVT).
- Brugada syndrome: mostly commonly affects the cardiac sodium channel and is characterized by electrocardiogram (ECG) findings of a pseudo–right bundle branch block (RBBB), ST-segment elevation in leads V_1 to V_3, and an increased risk of SCD

EPIDEMIOLOGY

- Most commonly presents in the 3rd or 4th decades of life. Average age at diagnosis is 41 yr (1).
- Majority of affected individuals are Asian.

Prevalence

- Approximately 1:2,000
- Prevalence higher in South Asia than in Western countries

ETIOLOGY AND PATHOPHYSIOLOGY

- Autosomal dominant inheritance of a mutation affecting the cardiac sodium channel gene
- >12 genes associated with Brugada syndrome

Genetics

The most common cause is the autosomal dominant inheritance of an SCN gene mutation that affects the cardiac sodium channel with variable penetrance (2); clinical penetrance 8-fold higher in men than women (3)

RISK FACTORS

The primary risk factor for channelopathies is genetic:

- Risk factors for precipitating a fatal arrhythmia in Brugada syndrome are swimming, fever or any cause of hyperthermia, intake of abundant meals and imbibing excessive alcohol, cocaine use, and overdose of psychotropic drugs (neuroleptics, tricyclic antidepressants).
- Arrhythmic events with Brugada syndrome occur most commonly at rest or during sleep when vagal tone predominates.

GENERAL PREVENTION

- SCD resulting from a Brugada syndrome may be prevented by carefully screening and identifying athletes with the condition. The preparticipation evaluation is the most important tool for identifying athletes with symptoms that may represent an inherited channelopathy. Any athlete with symptoms of palpitations, syncope, presyncope, any collapse, or with a family history of SCD or "accidental" death should be further evaluated with the tools reviewed below.
- Automatic external defibrillators (AEDs) are another important tool in preventing SCD from undiagnosed Brugada syndrome.

DIAGNOSIS

- Brugada pattern is used to describe those with typical ECG features but no other clinical criteria.
- Brugada type 1 is diagnosed on the basis of (4):
  - Type 1 ST-segment elevation (coved type) in >1 right precordial lead (V_1 to V_3) in the presence or absence of a sodium channel blocker plus at least one of the following:
    - Documented ventricular fibrillation (VF)
    - Self-terminating polymorphic ventricular tachycardia (VT)
    - Family history of SCD at <45 yr
    - Type 1 ST-segment elevation in family members
    - Electrophysiologic inducibility of VT
    - Unexplained syncope suggestive of a tachyarrhythmia
    - Nocturnal agonal respiration
- Brugada type 2 or 3 is diagnosed on the basis of (4):
  - Type 2 or 3 ST-segment elevation (saddleback type) in >1 right precordial lead under baseline conditions with conversion to type 1 ST-segment elevation following challenge with a sodium channel blocker plus at least one of the following:
    - Documented VF
    - Self-terminating polymorphic VT
    - Family history of SCD at <45 yr
    - Type 1 ST-segment elevation in family members
    - Electrophysiologic inducibility of VT
    - Unexplained syncope suggestive of a tachyarrhythmia
    - Nocturnal agonal respiration
- Prehospital:
  - In the case that any patient with a Brugada syndrome converts into a life-threatening arrhythmia in the field, the most useful immediate tool and treatment is an AED.

HISTORY

- Pertinent history in screening athletes: Gathering a detailed and careful history during the preparticipation physical or during the evaluation of an athlete who comes to your attention is critical. The following questions should be included when interviewing an athlete:
  - Have you ever passed out, become dizzy, or had chest pain during or after exercise?
  - Do you get tired more quickly than others during exercise?
  - Has anyone in the family died suddenly and unexpectedly before the age of 50 yr? (Remember to ask about family members who died of accidental causes such as sudden infant death syndrome, drownings, and motor vehicle accidents because they may be clues to an undiagnosed family history of channelopathy.)
  - Have you ever had a heart abnormality or murmur diagnosed by a doctor?
  - Have you ever had an abnormal heart rate, palpitations, or irregular heartbeats?
  - Have you had high blood pressure (BP) or high cholesterol?
  - Has a physician ever denied or restricted your participation in sports for heart problems?
  - Have any of your relatives ever had cardiomyopathy, Marfan syndrome, LQTS, SQTS, or significant heart arrhythmias?
- Pertinent history in potentially affected athletes:
  - Most common clinical presentation in Brugada syndrome is life-threatening arrhythmia.
  - More common at night and while sleeping
  - Not usually related to exercise
  - Inquire about a history of syncope, presyncope, past history of sudden cardiac arrest, or a family history of SCD.

PHYSICAL EXAM

- The most important elements of the exam are general (including level of consciousness), cardiac, and pulmonary examinations and, in the case of a patient who has sustained a life-threatening arrhythmia, complete trauma examination.
- Because patients with Brugada syndrome typically have structurally normal hearts, it is not uncommon to observe a completely normal examination when a life-threatening arrhythmia is not present.
- When arrhythmias are present, the examination may be notable for bradycardia or tachycardia, either regular or irregular, depending on the patient's rhythm.

DIFFERENTIAL DIAGNOSIS

QT syndromes, CPVT, acquired LQTS with its many reversible metabolic and drug-induced causes, acute coronary syndrome, true RBBB, pericarditis, drug-induced VT or VF

DIAGNOSTIC TESTS & INTERPRETATION

Initial Tests (lab, imaging)

In the setting of a life-threatening arrhythmia, it may be indicated to rule out ischemic or metabolic causes with a basic or comprehensive metabolic panel and cardiac enzymes.

Diagnostic Procedures/Other

ECG is the most important initial diagnostic tool. Holter monitors and echocardiograms may be of use as well:

- Brugada syndrome:
  - Classic Brugada type 1: Elevated ST segment (≥2 mm) descends with an upward convexity to an inverted T wave—"coved type" Brugada pattern.
  - Brugada types 2 and 3:
    - "Saddle back" ST-T wave: Elevated ST segment descends toward the baseline and then rises again to the upright or biphasic T wave.
    - ST segment elevated ≥1 mm in type 2 and <1 mm in type 3
    - Moving the right precordial chest leads up to the 2nd or 3rd intercostal space may increase the sensitivity.
    - The ECG findings may be transient and not present each time an ECG is performed.
    - Electrophysiology testing may be used in evaluating Brugada syndrome but is not heavily relied on.

TREATMENT

The mainstay of treatment in Brugada syndrome is implantable cardioverter defibrillator (ICD), although quinidine has shown promising data as a preventative pharmacotherapy.

MEDICATION

- Adjunctive pharmacotherapy for patients with frequent ICD discharges includes amiodarone and quinidine.
- Electrical storm in Brugada syndrome is treated with isoproterenol or quinidine.

SURGERY/OTHER PROCEDURES

- ICD implantation can prevent SCD in Brugada syndrome (3)[B].
- Selection of patients for ICD is not entirely clear, but ICD may be used in higher risk patients such as those with syncope or with VT without cardiac arrest (3)[C].

ADMISSION, INPATIENT, AND NURSING CONSIDERATIONS

As always, all patients who present with a life-threatening arrhythmia should be treated emergently with cardioversion and/or pharmacotherapy as dictated by standard advanced cardiac life support (ACLS).

ONGOING CARE

All patients with channelopathies should be followed regularly by a cardiologist. Education and restrictions regarding exercise are crucial to survival.

FOLLOW-UP RECOMMENDATIONS

Return-to-play decisions:

- SCD in Brugada syndrome usually is not related to exercise.
- New American Heart Association/American College of Cardiology (AHA/ACC) 2015 participation guidelines: In a symptomatic athlete, competitive sports participation may be considered following expert consultation from electrophysiologist and cardiologist, initiation of treatment, appropriate precautionary measures, and the athlete has been asymptomatic for at least 3 mo (5)[C].
- Asymptomatic athlete with genotype-positive/phenotype-negative (concealed channelopathy) may participate in all competitive sports with appropriate precautionary measures (avoidance of Brugada exacerbating drugs, appropriate electrolyte/hydration replenishment, avoidance of hyperthermic conditions, acquire personal AED, and establish appropriate emergency action plan) (5)[C].
- Competitive sports participation may be considered for an athlete with either previously symptomatic or electrocardiographically evident Brugada syndrome, assuming appropriate precautionary measures and disease specific treatments are in place, and that the athlete has been asymptomatic on treatment for at least 3 mo (5)[C].
- Caution should be used to avoid sports where impaired consciousness would be dangerous or lethal, such as with SCUBA diving, swimming, weight lifting with free weights, and horseback riding.
- Avoidance of medications or substances (alcohol overdose, cannabis, and cocaine) that can exacerbate Brugada syndrome (6).

REFERENCES

1. Brugada J, Brugada R, Brugada P. Determinants of sudden cardiac death in individuals with the electrocardiographic pattern of Brugada syndrome and no previous cardiac arrest. *Circulation*. 2003;108(25):3092–3096.
2. Drezner JA, Ackerman MJ, Cannon BC, et al. Abnormal electrocardiographic findings in athletes: recognising changes suggestive of primary electrical disease. *Br J Sports Med*. 2013;47(3):153–167.
3. Mazzanti A, O'Rourke S, Ng K, et al. The usual suspects in sudden cardiac death of the young: a focus on inherited arrhythmogenic diseases. *Expert Rev Cardiovasc Ther*. 2014;12(4):499–519.
4. Wilde AA, Antzelevitch C, Borggrefe M, et al; for Study Group on the Molecular Basis of Arrhythmias of the European Society of Cardiology. Proposed diagnostic criteria for the Brugada syndrome: consensus report. *Circulation*. 2002;106(19):2514–2519.
5. Ackerman MJ, Zipes DP, Kovacs RJ, et al. Eligibility and disqualification recommendations for competitive athletes with cardiovascular abnormalities: task force 10: the cardiac channelopathies: a scientific statement from the American Heart Association and American College of Cardiology. *Circulation*. 2015;132(22):e326–e329.
6. Postema PG, Wolpert C, Amin AS, et al. Drugs and Brugada syndrome patients: review of the literature, recommendations, and an up-to-date website (www.brugadadrugs.org). *Heart Rhythm*. 2009;6(9):1335–1341.

ADDITIONAL READING

Priori SG, Wilde AA, Horie M, et al. HRS/EHRA/APHRS expert consensus statement on the diagnosis and management of patients with inherited primary arrhythmia syndromes: document endorsed by HRS, EHRA, and APHRS in May 2013 and by ACCF, AHA, PACES, and AEPC in June 2013. *Heart Rhythm*. 2013;10(12):1932–1963.

CLINICAL PEARLS

- Brugada syndrome most often affects the cardiac sodium channel and is characterized by ECG findings of a pseudo–RBBB, ST-segment elevation in leads V_1 to V_3, and an increased risk of SCD.
- Risk factors for precipitating a fatal arrhythmia in Brugada syndrome are swimming, fever or any cause of hyperthermia, intake of abundant meals and imbibing excessive alcohol, cocaine use, and overdose of psychotropic drugs (neuroleptics, tricyclic antidepressants), although most events occur during sleep or rest.
- Diagnosis of Brugada syndrome is made by ECG.
- The first-line treatment of Brugada syndrome is an ICD.
- Return to play after diagnosis of Brugada syndrome should be a careful conversation between physician and athlete and follow the AHA/ACC 2015 participation guidelines.

BURSITIS

Ziad Fahad Rayes, MBBS, MBA, Ccfp(Sem), Dip Sport Med(Casem) • Muath Alammar, MD, SBFM

BASICS

- May be difficult to distinguish from fractures. Suspicious joints should be immobilized, particularly in the setting of trauma. Also, septic joint is a possibility that needs to be excluded.
- Inflammation or irritation of the bursa (fluid-filled sacs located between mobile structures that decrease friction and provide a cushion between bones, tendons, muscles, and skin)
- Two types of bursa and potentially any of them may be affected:
  - Superficial bursa:
    - Olecranon bursa: lies between the olecranon process and the overlying skin (usually secondary to trauma)
    - Prepatellar bursa: lies between the patella and the skin (usually secondary to trauma or frequent forward kneeling)
    - Pes anserine bursa: lies between the tibia and the insertions of the sartorius, gracilis, and semitendinosus muscles
  - Deep bursa:
    - Subacromial (subdeltoid) bursa: lies between the acromion and the rotator cuff
    - Scapulothoracic bursa: lies between superior-medial angle of the scapula and the adjacent ribs
    - Iliopsoas bursa: lies between the iliopsoas tendon and the lesser trochanter (largest bursa in the body):
      - Trochanteric bursa: has superficial and deep components. The superficial bursa lies between the tensor fascia lata and skin; the deep bursa is located between the greater trochanter and the tensor fascia lata.
      - Calcaneal bursitis: two bursae at the level of insertion of the Achilles tendon. The superficial one is located between the skin and the tendon, and the deep one is located between the calcaneus and the tendon.

DESCRIPTION

- Bursae are flattened sacs that serve as a protective buffer between bones and overlapping muscles (deep bursae) or between bones and tendons/skin (superficial bursae). In the normal state, they contain minimal amounts of fluid to reduce friction and facilitate pain-free movement during muscle contraction.
- Bursitis can be acute or chronic. Acute bursitis is result of an injury, infection, or inflammation. Chronic bursitis follows a long period of repetitive use or motion. Chronic bursal swelling is often due to tendinopathy of the underlying tendons.
- Humans have >160 bursae.

ETIOLOGY AND PATHOPHYSIOLOGY

- Trauma (acute and chronic): most common cause
- Prolonged pressure: prolonged kneeling or leaning on an elbow
- Overuse
- Infection (septic bursitis): direct introduction of microorganisms through traumatic injury or hematogenous
- For septic bursitis: *Staphylococcus aureus* causes 80%, followed by *Streptococcus*.
- Crystal deposition: gout or pseudogout
- Inflammatory arthritis: rheumatoid arthritis or spondyloarthritis

RISK FACTORS

- If you work in a profession or have a hobby that requires repetitive motion or pressure on particular bursae (e.g., carpet laying, tile setting, gardening, bicycling, baseball, ice skating)
- Rheumatoid arthritis
- Osteoarthritis
- Gout
- Thyroid disease
- Diabetes

DIAGNOSIS

- Full assessment of regional musculoskeletal function
- Any suspicion of infection warrants aspiration of bursae (especially superficial bursa).
- Aspiration of hip and other deep bursae should be deferred to orthopedics or rheumatology, or may be guided in emergency department (ED) by ultrasound (US).

PHYSICAL EXAM

- Localized tenderness (1)[A]
- Swelling (1)[A]
- Decreased range of motion or pain with movement
- Erythema or edema (seen in superficial bursitis) (1)[A]
- Traumatic bursitis often follows traumatic event or overuse of related joints.
- Muscle atrophy (seen in chronic bursitis related to immobility)

DIFFERENTIAL DIAGNOSIS

- Arthritis: rheumatoid, septic, osteoarthritis
- Cellulitis
- Gout and pseudogout
- Fracture, tendon/ligament tear, contusion, sprain
- Tendonitis

DIAGNOSTIC TESTS & INTERPRETATION

- Complete blood count (CBC) with differential, erythrocyte sedimentation rate, serum protein electrophoresis, rheumatoid factor, serum uric acid (1)[A]
- Aspiration and analysis of bursa fluid: cell count with differential, glucose and total protein, crystal determination, Gram stain, and culture (1)[A]
- Normal fluid: Fluid is clear yellow with 0 to 200 white blood cells (WBCs), 0 red blood cells (RBCs), low protein, and glucose is same as serum (1)[A].
- Traumatic bursitis: Fluid is bloody/xanthochromic with <2,000 WBCs, many RBCs, high protein, and normal glucose.

- Infective bursitis: Fluid is cloudy yellow with >50,000 WBCs, few RBCs, slightly increased protein, and decreased glucose; bacteria on Gram stain (1)[A]
- Rheumatoid and microcrystalline inflammation: Fluid is yellow, can be cloudy, has >2,000 WBCs, few RBCs, slightly increased protein, and variable glucose; use polarizing microscope to identify crystals.
- Chronic or recurrent bursitis should be sent for acid-fast staining and cultured on special media for mycobacteria, *Brucella*, and algae.
- Monosodium urate crystals seen in gout; calcium pyrophosphate crystals seen in pseudogout
- X-rays to exclude other suspected pathologies (i.e., fractures, dislocations, or foreign body) (1)[A]
- X-rays may demonstrate chronic arthritic changes or calcium deposits or rheumatologic features.
- US for diagnostic aspiration or treatment injections (1)[A]
- Magnetic resonance imaging (MRI) helps depict bursa/prebursal fluid, associated abscesses, and adjacent soft tissue structures.

TREATMENT

ED treatment:

- Shoulders should not be immobilized for >2 to 3 days due to the risk of adhesive capsulitis.
- Aseptic bursitis: Rest, ice (application of an ice pack for 20 min for superficially bursa), compression, elevation, nonsteroidal anti-inflammatory drugs (NSAIDs), physical therapy (stretching, strengthening, and maintaining range of motion), bursa aspiration, and intrabursal steroid injections (1,2)[A]
- Septic bursitis: If suspected, treat with antibiotics while awaiting culture results and drain bursae; may require repeat aspiration
- Superficial septic bursitis can be treated with oral therapy (1)[A].
- Septic bursitis with fulminant onset, systemic symptoms, or those who are immunocompromised require hospitalization and/or intravenous (IV) antibiotics.

MEDICATION

- NSAIDs: Ibuprofen: adult: 600 to 800 mg PO q8h; pediatric: 10 mg/kg PO q8h. Naproxen: adult: 375 to 500 mg PO BID. Ketorolac: adult: 30 mg IV/intramuscular (IM) q6h or 10 mg PO q4–6h
- Most patients may be treated as an outpatient.

SURGERY/OTHER PROCEDURES

In general, bursitis is not treated surgically. However, surgical release may be indicated when adhesive bursitis develops, recurrent refractory bursitis, and severely limiting joint motion. During surgery, the adhered bursa is removed, and the contiguous tissues are released (1)[A].

ADMISSION, INPATIENT, AND NURSING CONSIDERATIONS

- Immobilize joint if pain is severe.
- Admission criteria: septic bursitis with high fevers, surrounding cellulitis, unable to take oral antibiotics, failed outpatient therapy, or immunocompromised

ONGOING CARE

FOLLOW-UP RECOMMENDATIONS

- Most patients respond to therapy within 1 wk.
- Rheumatology or orthopedic referral is recommended for patients with repetitive acute bouts, necessitating repeated joint/bursa aspirations or, eventually, surgical excision of involved bursa.

REFERENCES

1. Baumbach SF, Lobo CM, Badyine I, et al. Prepatellar and olecranon bursitis: literature review and development of a treatment algorithm. *Arch Orthop Trauma Surg*. 2014;134(3):359–370.
2. Lustenberger DP, Ng VY, Best TM, et al. Efficacy of treatment of trochanteric bursitis: a systematic review. *Clin J Sport Med*. 2011;21(5):447–453.

ADDITIONAL READING

- Kim JY, Chung SW, Kim JH, et al. A randomized trial among compression plus nonsteroidal antiinflammatory drugs, aspiration, and aspiration with steroid injection for nonseptic olecranon bursitis. *Clin Orthop Relat Res*. 2016;474(3):776–783.
- Lieber SB, Fowler ML, Zhu C, et al. Clinical characteristics and outcomes of septic bursitis. *Infection*. 2017;45(6):781–786.
- Sayegh ET, Strauch RJ. Treatment of olecranon bursitis: a systematic review. *Arch Orthop Trauma Surg*. 2014;134(11):1517–1536.

CLINICAL PEARLS

- Bursitis could happen in any tendon mobilizing over skin or bone.
- Conservative treatment with ice, NSAIDs, and modifying activity is the treatment in most cases.
- Any suspicion of infection warrants aspiration of bursae (especially superficial bursa).

CALCIFIC TENDONITIS

Shawn Skarpnes, MD, CAQSM

BASICS

DESCRIPTION

- A condition that causes the formation of calcium deposition within a tendon
- Pain and dysfunction is related to impingement, inflammation, and increased intratendinous pressure from the calcific deposit.
- Calcific tendonitis (CT) can occur anywhere but predominately involves the rotator cuff of the shoulder.
- Symptoms often resolve spontaneously within 3 to 6 mo (1).
- Synonym(s): calcific tendinopathy, calcific tendinitis, calcific periarthritis

EPIDEMIOLOGY

- Occurs in 3–10% of the general population
- 50% of calcific deposits are asymptomatic.
- Bilateral occurrence in 10–20% cases
- Most common in females 30 to 60 yr of age (2,3,4).

ETIOLOGY AND PATHOPHYSIOLOGY

- No clear etiology established
- Unlikely related to trauma or overuse
- CT progresses through three stages:
  - Precalcific stage: Tendon undergoes fibrocartilaginous transformation, in which calcifications proliferate in the transformed tissue.
  - Calcific stage:
    - Resting phase: Calcific deposits are stable. Deposits may or may not be painful. If large enough, calcifications may cause mechanical symptoms.
    - Resorptive phase: An inflammatory reaction arises by an unknown trigger (5)[B]. Vascular invasion occurs around the deposit with migration of macrophages and giant cells that absorb the calcification; most painful phase
  - Postcalcific stage: The deposit is resorbed, and fibroblasts reconstitute the normal collagen pattern of tendon.

Genetics

Possible genetic predisposition given the high frequency of bilateral occurrences but no clear evidence identified

RISK FACTORS

CT is rarely part of a systemic disease but has been associated with diabetes mellitus, nephrolithiasis, and thyroid and estrogen disorders.

DIAGNOSIS

HISTORY

- Localized pain is the cardinal symptom.
- Clinical presentation varies depending on stage.
- Typically gradual pain unassociated with trauma
- Severe acute pain often presents during the resorptive phase due to spontaneous leakage of calcium crystals from the deposit into the overlying bursa. Pain improves within 1 to 2 wk (6).
- Increased pain at night and inability to sleep on affected area
- Individuals involved with strenuous manual labor or athletic activities are not at increased risk.

PHYSICAL EXAM

- Acute pain phase: guarding of affected joint with limited motion causing marked tenderness
- Chronic or subacute phase: Pain increases considerably with active range of motion (ROM) versus minimal symptoms with passive ROM.
- Shoulder impingement tests (Hawkins and Neer) are often positive.

DIFFERENTIAL DIAGNOSIS

- Rotator cuff tear
- Osteoarthritis of glenohumeral or acromioclavicular joint
- Adhesive capsulitis
- Biceps tendonitis
- Cervical radiculopathy
- Gout

DIAGNOSTIC TESTS & INTERPRETATION

Initial Tests (lab, imaging)

- Plain radiographs or ultrasound (US) reveals characteristic calcific deposits.
- X-ray: Obtain multiple views to adequately assess location, size, and morphology: Shoulder views should include anteroposterior (AP) with internal and external rotation, axillary, and outlet views.
- Appearance on x-ray (7)[A]:
  - Resting phase: dense and homogenous calcification with well-defined borders
  - Resorptive phase: fluffy with poorly defined limits and may have increased density at its center
- US: highly sensitive modality with diagnostic and therapeutic capacity
- Appearance on US (7)[A]:
  - Resting phase: appears as hyperechoic lesions with acoustic shadowing
  - Resorptive phase: fluffy and appearing fragmented, cystic, or nodular in shape. Power Doppler shows increased vascularity around deposit.
- Tenderness with sonopalpation of deposit is confirmatory (7)[A].
- Magnetic resonance imaging (MRI) or computed tomography (CT) scan: not indicated for routine evaluation

Follow-Up Tests & Special Considerations

Repeat radiographs or US helpful to assess interval change

TREATMENT

GENERAL MEASURES

- Often a self-limited benign course
- First-line therapy is conservative and focused on symptom relief.
- Initial treatment options include oral anti-inflammatories, analgesics, glucocorticoid injection, and physical therapy.
- Low evidence to suggest one treatment is preferred over others.
- A subacromial bursa (SAB) glucocorticoid injection (e.g., 20 to 40 mg of triamcinolone, methylprednisolone) indicated if acute inflammation evident clinically and with US. US will reveal a thickened and enlarged adjacent bursa and/or increased vascularity surrounding the deposit with power Doppler.
- If initial treatment fails, consider US-guided needling and lavage, also known as barbotage versus extracorporeal shock wave therapy (ESWT).
- ESWT is a modality that uses high-frequency sound waves to break up a targeted calcification.
- Improved outcomes with barbotage when compared to SAB glucocorticoid injection alone or ESWT (8)[A]
- Superior clinical and radiographic outcomes are reported when comparing barbotage to ESWT at 6 wk, but no difference at 1 yr (8)[A].
- Superior clinical and radiographic outcomes are reported when barbotage is combined with a SAB glucocorticoid injection and then an isolated glucocorticoid injection at 1 yr but no difference at 5 yr (8)[A].
- US-guided aspiration of calcium possible in most cases but occasionally is too firm to aspirate. A decrease in size of deposit over time is seen regardless of how much calcium is initially aspirated.
- Aspiration is most easily obtained during the acutely painful resorptive phase in which the calcium has a toothpaste-like consistency.

ADDITIONAL THERAPIES

Dry needling studied in small trials but further research needed

SURGERY/OTHER PROCEDURES

- 10% of patients do not respond to conservative treatment, ESWT, or barbotage; may benefit from surgery (9)
- Surgery reserved for patients not responding to conservative therapy >6 mo (7)[A]
- Surgery is arthroscopic and involves calcification removal with or without acromioplasty of the shoulder. Acromioplasty has not resulted in improved outcomes for this condition and will delay return to unrestricted activity without pain (10)[B].

COMPLEMENTARY & ALTERNATIVE MEDICINE

- Iontophoresis: introducing acetic acid as an ionized compound on the skin and applying a low electric current to make the hydroxyapatite crystals soluble and susceptible to resorption
- Radial shock wave therapy: Acoustic waves are generated by a shock wave trigger with focal point at the tip of the applicator versus ESWT which has its focal point on the target zone.
- Therapeutic/heat US: increases blood flow and metabolism of tissue, thus facilitating disintegration of calcium deposition
- Microwave diathermy: produces hyperthermia of tissue, which favors resorption of calcium deposits

ONGOING CARE

FOLLOW-UP RECOMMENDATIONS

- Conservative management follow-up:
  - Follow-up at 4 mo or after completion of physical therapy. Evaluate mobility and strength; repeat imaging by sonography or radiographs reserved for patients with persistent symptoms to guide treatment plan
  - If still symptomatic and calcific deposit visualized on imaging, then consider barbotage or ESWT > surgery.
- Barbotage or ESWT follow-up:
  - Should complete a 4-mo posttreatment physical therapy program aimed at restoring shoulder mobility and function with follow-up exam and reimaging
  - If still symptomatic and calcific deposit visualized on imaging, then consider second barbotage treatment of calcific deposit >5 mm or surgery if <5 mm. This is because small, ill-defined deposits are challenging to locate and treat with US-guided barbotage.
- Acute painful episode follow-up:
  - Early follow-up evaluation within 1 to 2 wk
  - If SAB glucocorticoid injection effective (pain reduced or absent) at previous visit, then proceed with gentle physiotherapy exercise program
  - If patient symptoms only mildly improve, with unchanged calcification on imaging, then barbotage treatment recommended
  - If significant pain persists, proceed with a second glucocorticoid injection supplemented with oral pain medication.

PROGNOSIS

- 50% are asymptomatic within 3 mo spontaneously or with conservative treatment (1).
- 70% are asymptomatic within 1 yr of onset (11).
- 30% have persistent symptoms for several years. Of these, 66% improve with barbotage or ESWT (12).
- 10% remaining symptomatic patients are referred to surgery (9).
- Negative prognostic indicators: female, bilateral limbs, dominant limb involvement, and large or multiple calcifications. In these selected patients, more aggressive treatments earlier in the disease course can improve long-term outcomes (5)[B].

COMPLICATIONS

- Adhesive capsulitis
- Rotator cuff tears
- Greater tuberosity osteolysis: very rare
- Ossifying tendonitis: very rare and associated with arthroscopic surgical intervention
- Osteonecrosis: extremely rare and related to ESWT

REFERENCES

1. Noël E. Treatment of calcific tendinitis and adhesive capsulitis of the shoulder. *Rev Rhum Engl Ed*. 1997;64(11):619–628.
2. Bosworth BM. Calcium deposits in the shoulder and subacromial bursitis: a survey of 12,122 shoulders. *JAMA*. 1941;116(22):2477–2482.
3. Luime JJ, Koes BW, Hendriksen IJ, et al. Prevalence and incidence of shoulder pain in the general population; a systematic review. *Scand J Rheumatol*. 2004;33(2):73–81.
4. Uhthoff HK, Loehr JW. Calcific tendinopathy of the rotator cuff: pathogenesis, diagnosis, and management. *J Am Acad Orthop Surg*. 1997;5(4):183–191.
5. de Witte PB, van Adrichem RA, Selten JW, et al. Radiological and clinical predictors of long-term outcome in rotator cuff calcific tendinitis. *Eur Radiol*. 2016;26(10):3401–3411.
6. Kachewar SG, Kulkarni DS. Calcific tendinitis of the rotator cuff: a review. *J Clin Diagn Res*. 2013;7(7):1482–1485.
7. Merolla G, Singh S, Paladini P, et al. Calcific tendinitis of the rotator cuff: state of the art in diagnosis and treatment. *J Orthop Traumatol*. 2016;17(1):7–14.
8. de Witte PB, Kolk A, Overes F, et al. Rotator cuff calcific tendinitis: ultrasound-guided needling and lavage versus subacromial corticosteroids: five-year outcomes of a randomized controlled trial. *Am J Sports Med*. 2017;45(14):3305–3314.
9. Rochwerger A, Franceschi JP, Viton JM, et al. Surgical management of calcific tendinitis of the shoulder: an analysis of 26 cases. *Clin Rheumatol*. 1999;18(4):313–316.
10. Balke M, Bielefeld R, Schmidt C, et al. Calcifying tendinitis of the shoulder: midterm results after arthroscopic treatment. *Am J Sports Med*. 2012;40(3):657–661.
11. Wölk T, Wittenberg RH. Calcifying subacromial syndrome—clinical and ultrasound outcome of non-surgical therapy. *Z Orthop Ihre Grenzgeb*. 1997;135(5):451–457.
12. Lee SY, Cheng B, Grimmer-Somers K. The midterm effectiveness of extracorporeal shockwave therapy in the management of chronic calcific shoulder tendinitis. *J Shoulder Elbow Surg*. 2011;20(5):845–854.

ADDITIONAL READING

- Lam F, Bhatia D, van Rooyen K, et al. Modern management of calcifying tendonitis of the shoulder. *Current Orthopaedics*. 2006;20(6):446–452.
- Sansone VC, Meroni R, Boria P, et al. Are occupational repetitive movements of the upper arm associated with rotator cuff calcific tendinopathies? *Rheumatol Int*. 2015;35(2):273–280.

CLINICAL PEARLS

- Calcium deposition from CT usually disappears spontaneously with time.
- CT is not precipitated by strenuous manual labor or athletic activities and occurs equally among sedentary individuals.
- Growing evidence supports the use of US-guided barbotage as a safe and effective treatment for patients that don't respond to conservative measures.
- Acute severe pain from CT is caused by leakage of calcium crystals from the deposit into the overlying bursa and improves <2 wk.

C

CALCIUM PYROPHOSPHATE DEPOSITION DISEASE (CPPD) (PSEUDOGOUT)

Kenneth Bielak, MD, FACSM, FAAFP, CAQSM

BASICS

DESCRIPTION

- Calcium pyrophosphate deposition disease (CPPD) is a crystal arthropathy characterized by deposition of calcium pyrophosphate (CaPPi) dihydrate crystals in joints.
- Synonym(s):
  - Pseudogout: describes an acute attack of CPPD crystal-induced synovitis (similar to gout) but less intense symptoms
  - Chondrocalcinosis: radiographic calcification but is not absolutely specific for CPPD because it can be caused by other calcific deposits on hyaline cartilage
  - Pyrophosphate arthropathy: specifically associated with inorganic pyrophosphate metabolism as the etiology for CPPD
  - CaPPi dihydrate crystal deposition disease

EPIDEMIOLOGY

- Prevalence of chondrocalcinosis is 5–8% in the general population but 15% by the 9th decade.
- Due to asymptomatic depositions and need for confirmatory aspiration for diagnosis, incidence has not been reliably recorded.
- Female-to-male ratio: 2 to 7:1
- Peak age: 65 to 75 yr

ETIOLOGY AND PATHOPHYSIOLOGY

CPPD crystal formation is initiated in cartilage located near the surface of chondrocytes. The CPPD crystal formation may be a combination of elevated levels of either calcium or pyrophosphate and/or matrix changes that enhance local CaPPi supersaturation. Many cases of CPPD deposition are idiopathically sporadic but more commonly are precipitated by trauma or various metabolic disorders.

Genetics

<1% of cases may show an autosomal dominant inheritance pattern.

RISK FACTORS

- Gout (20% may be hyperuricemic)
- Hemochromatosis
- Hypothyroidism
- Trauma
- Osteoarthritis
- Hyperparathyroidism
- Hemosiderosis
- Hypophosphatasia
- Hypomagnesemia
- Aging
- Amyloidosis

GENERAL PREVENTION

- There are no absolute prevention measures, but mainstays include adequate hydration (to prevent crystal precipitation) and decreasing purine-rich foods, such as organ meats, mushrooms, legumes, asparagus, and coffee.
- For three or more attacks per 1 yr, colchicine has been found to reduce the recurrence rate (1)[B],(2)[A].

COMMONLY ASSOCIATED CONDITIONS

- Pseudorheumatoid arthritis: a nonerosive, inflammatory arthritis with demonstrable CPPD crystals in the joint fluid. Both are clinically similar with morning stiffness, fatigue, synovial thickening, edema, and loss of motion. Both conditions may coexist but must be differentiated because the treatment options vary.
- Pseudoarthritis: progressive joint degeneration involving multiple joints. CPPD differs by radiographic evidence of calcifications in the absence of a preceding trauma.
- Case reports of CPPD associated with Charcot joints
- Several case reports involving bisphosphonates and CPPD deposition have been reported (3)[C].
- CPPD, especially familial patterns, can be found along the spine and resemble ankylosing spondylitis.

DIAGNOSIS

HISTORY

- Acute joint swelling in one or more joints with previous episodes involving the same joint (characteristic of crystal arthropathies)
- The most common joint is the knee, followed by the wrist, shoulder, and hip.
- May be severe and associated with malaise and fever
- Period of previous episodes (typically several days to weeks)
- Patients often are symptom-free between attacks.

PHYSICAL EXAM

- Involved joint:
  - Warmth
  - Edema/effusion
  - Tender
  - Limited range of motion
- Uncommon presentations include tendinopathy, tenosynovitis, and bursitis.
- Chronic CPPD: symmetrical polyarthritis affecting knees, metacarpophalangeal joints, wrists, ankles, and shoulders:
  - May involve the spine
  - Affected joints show signs of osteoarthritis with varying degrees of synovitis.
  - Predominantly affects women

DIFFERENTIAL DIAGNOSIS

- Gout (can coexist)
- Septic arthritis (can coexist)
- Rheumatoid arthritis
- Osteoarthritis
- Trauma (hemarthrosis)
- Human leukocyte antigen B27–related peripheral arthritis (psoriatic arthritis, ankylosing spondylitis, reactive arthritis)
- Hypertrophic osteoarthropathy
- Pseudorheumatoid arthritis: severe synovitis in rheumatoid pattern

DIAGNOSTIC TESTS & INTERPRETATION

- Initial diagnosis of CPPD should be followed with calcium, magnesium, thyroid-stimulating hormone, ferritin, transferrin, iron, phosphorus, and alkaline phosphatase levels.
- Synovial fluid microscopy with compensated polarized light microscopy showing weakly positive birefringent rhomboidal-shaped crystals is diagnostic; Gram stain and culture should be considered to rule out differential diagnoses. In addition, crystal analysis up to 3 days postaspiration does not adversely affect crystal identification (4)[B].
- Erythrocyte sedimentation rate, C-reactive protein, rheumatoid factor, uric acid, white blood cell count (leukocytosis), and blood cultures may be considered to rule out differential diagnoses.
- Leukocyte concentration typically in the range of 15,000 to 30,000/mm^3 with 90% neutrophils
- Plain radiography to evaluate for calcium crystal deposition (5)[C]

- X-ray: calcification of articular fibrocartilage (chondrocalcinosis) in menisci of the knee, triangular fibrocartilage complex in the wrist. Other sites include glenoid and acetabular labra and symphysis pubis.
- High-resolution ultrasound (US) may improve noninvasive diagnosis of the crystal-induced arthropathies and allow monitoring of intra-articular tophi if radiation is a concern.
- Features may show a homogeneously punctate pattern or sharply defined hyperechoic bands within the articular cartilage (5,6)[C].
- Optimal imaging is best with computed tomography (CT) for further definition of tophi and bone erosion, and 3D CT assessment of tophus volume is a promising outcome measure in gout.
- Magnetic resonance imaging (MRI) is also a reliable method for assessment of tophus size in gout and has an important role in detection of complications of disease in clinical practice.
- Emerging imaging techniques include 3D US and dual-energy CT. Advanced imaging modalities also offer new insights into the mechanisms of cartilage and bone damage in the crystal-induced arthropathies.
- Pathologic findings:
  - Tissue sections are best examined with alizarin red looking for crystals because the hematoxylin and eosin stains may cause dissolution of the crystalline CPPD due to their acidity.

TREATMENT

- Acute treatment:
  - Joint aspiration often significantly reduces pain (7)[C].
  - Intra-articular corticosteroid injection can be effective (8)[C].
  - Joint rest and splinting if needed
  - Nonsteroidal anti-inflammatory drugs (NSAIDs) and oral analgesia
  - Colchicine and systemic corticosteroids can be used if other treatments are contraindicated.
- Long-term treatment:
  - For patients suffering recurrent attacks of pseudogout, oral daily colchicine may be effective as a prophylactic agent at a usual dosage of 0.6 mg BID (1)[B].
  - Repeat joint aspiration may be required.
  - Once acute attacks have settled, the aims of treatment are to relieve symptoms and regain function.
  - No specific treatment exists for chronic CPPD, and no treatments are available that reverse joint damage.

MEDICATION

NSAIDs are first-line treatment.

ADDITIONAL THERAPIES

Antibiotics if septic arthritis is suspected until joint and blood cultures return negative

SURGERY/OTHER PROCEDURES

Joint arthroplasty may be required for severely damaged joints.

COMPLEMENTARY & ALTERNATIVE MEDICINE

There have been anecdotal reports of cured acute attacks by the consumption of dark cherries or cherry juice or herbs that contain xanthene oxidase inhibitors to decrease urate formation, but none have been well studied.

ONGOING CARE

- Primary metabolic disorders or familial predisposition is uncommon but should be considered if CPPD occurs before 55 yr of age or if there is florid polyarticular CPPD.
- After the age of 55 yr, hyperparathyroidism should be considered in all patients.

COMPLICATIONS

Although acute pseudogout usually responds well to therapy, chronic CPPD often is progressive and may cause considerable disability.

REFERENCES

1. Alvarellos A, Spilberg I. Colchicine prophylaxis in pseudogout. *J Rheumatol*. 1986;13(4):804–805.
2. Rainer TH, Cheng CH, Janssens HJ, et al. Oral prednisolone in the treatment of acute gout: a pragmatic, multicenter, double-blind, randomized trial. *Ann Intern Med*. 2016;164(7):464–471.
3. Couture G, Delzor F, Bagheri H, et al. First cases of calcium pyrophosphate deposition disease after zoledronic acid therapy. *Joint Bone Spine*. 2017;84(2):213–215.
4. Tausche AK, Gehrisch S, Panzner I, et al. A 3-day delay in synovial fluid crystal identification did not hinder the reliable detection of monosodium urate and calcium pyrophosphate crystals. *J Clin Rheumatol*. 2013;19(5):241–245.
5. Ciapetti A, Filippucci F, Gutierrez M, et al. Calcium pyrophosphate dihydrate crystal deposition disease: sonographic findings. *Clin Rheumatol*. 2009;28(3):271–276.
6. Grassi W, Meenagh G, Pascual E, et al. "Crystal clear"-sonographic assessment of gout and calcium pyrophosphate deposition disease. *Semin Arthritis Rheum*. 2006;36(3):197–202.
7. Dalbeth N, McQueen FM. Use of imaging to evaluate gout and other crystal deposition disorders. *Curr Opin Rheumatol*. 2009;21(2):124–131.
8. Announ N, Guerne PA. Treating difficult crystal pyrophosphate dihydrate deposition disease. *Curr Rheumatol Rep*. 2008;10(3):228–234.

ADDITIONAL READING

- Courtney P, Doherty M. Joint aspiration and injection and synovial fluid analysis. *Best Pract Res Clin Rheumatol*. 2013;27(2):137–169.
- Couto AR, Brown MA. Genetic factors in the pathogenesis of CPPD crystal deposition disease. *Curr Rheumatol Rep*. 2007;9(3):231–236.
- Doherty M. Crystal arthropathies: calcium pyrophosphate dihydrate. In: Klippel JH, Dieppe PA, eds. *Rheumatology*. London, United Kingdom: Mosby-Year Book Europe Limited; 1994:7.13.1–7.13.12.
- Ea HK, Lioté F. Advances in understanding calcium-containing crystal disease. *Curr Opin Rheumatol*. 2009;21(2):150–157.
- Fodor D, Albu A, Gherman C. Crystal-associated synovitis—ultrasonographic feature and clinical correlation. *Ortop Traumatol Rehabil*. 2008;10(2):90–110.
- Richette P, Bardin T, Doherty M. An update on the epidemiology of calcium pyrophosphate dihydrate crystal deposition disease. *Rheumatology (Oxford)*. 2009;48(7):711–715.
- Ryan LM, McCarty DO. Calcium pyrophosphate crystal deposition disease, pseudogout and articular chondrocalcinosis. In: Koopman WJ, ed. *Arthritis and Allied Conditions: A Textbook of Rheumatology*. 13th ed. Baltimore, MD: Williams & Wilkins; 1997:2103–2125.
- Shah K, Spear J, Nathanson LA, et al. Does the presence of crystal arthritis rule out septic arthritis? *J Emerg Med*. 2007;32(1):23–26.

CLINICAL PEARLS

- The cause of CPPD is unknown (unlike gout, in which hyperuricemia leads to precipitation of uric acid crystals into joints).
- Aspiration of joint fluid is key to diagnosis.
- There is no preventive treatment for recurrent attacks, although colchicine may be useful as prophylaxis in those with frequent recurrences (2)[A].

CALLUSES AND CORNS

Kathleen Weber, MD, MS • Shannon Powers, DO

BASICS

- Calluses and corns are common skin conditions.
- They result from increased pressure or friction; typically located on the hands and feet
- A callus is an adaptive response to repetitive friction.
- Calluses and corns may lead to considerable discomfort and pain.

DESCRIPTION

- A callus is a plaque of hyperkeratosis of relatively even thickness caused by repetitive friction, pressure, or trauma, and commonly occurs over bony prominences (1).
- A corn is a localized, tender, sharply defined area of hyperkeratosis found usually on the foot (1).
- A corn has a central core that penetrates into the dermis.

EPIDEMIOLOGY

Calluses and corns are common skin conditions.

ETIOLOGY AND PATHOPHYSIOLOGY

- Calluses and corns develop as a result of hyperkeratosis and thickening of the stratum corneum, a normal physiologic response of the skin to chronic friction, pressure, or trauma and commonly occur over bony prominences (1,2).
- Calluses commonly develop overlying bony prominences as a normal adaptation of the body to protect the skin when chronic pressure or friction is encountered (3).
- Abnormal stresses may be either extrinsic (e.g., tight toe box) or intrinsic (e.g., hammer toe) or a combination of both (3).

RISK FACTORS

- Activity: occupational (e.g., manual workers); musicians (e.g., guitarists); athletic activities that apply increased stress to the skin (i.e., racquet sports—hands, runners—feet, rowers—hands, sacrum) (4)
- Ill-fitting footwear: tight, loose irregularities in shoe, or not wearing shoes (3)
- Bony prominences
- Faulty foot mechanics or foot structure (3)
- Toe deformities

GENERAL PREVENTION

- Proper footwear (low-heeled, a soft upper portion, and wide toe box) (1,2)
- Orthotics
- Toe separators (3)
- Place felt pads over bony prominences or areas of increased friction to the skin (2,3).
- Wear gloves to protect the hands (4).
- Keep the hands and feet skin soft by applying a moisturizer.

DIAGNOSIS

- The diagnosis of calluses and corns is based on their clinical appearance.
- Radiographs may be obtained if your physician suspects an underlying bony prominence is a contributing factor.

HISTORY

- Corns and calluses are typically located at sites of friction, pressure, repetitive trauma, or at bony prominences (2,3).
- Factors that typically provoke the formation of corns and calluses are:
  - Sports that require cutting, turning, racquets, weight lifting, and sudden stops; callus formation is sometimes desired to allow pain-free play (2).
  - Occupations that are categorized as manual labor requiring the repetitive use of the hands or kneeling, such as a carpenter or landscaper (3).
  - Leisure activity that involves activities that cause repeated friction or pressure.
  - Poorly fitting footwear.
  - Coexisting illnesses (e.g., diabetes, rheumatoid arthritis) (5).
  - Inherited disposition (autosomal-dominant inheritance).

PHYSICAL EXAM

- The most common site for calluses is under the metatarsal heads and over bony prominences; may occur anywhere on the skin as a result of friction
- A callus may be asymptomatic or painful, often appearing as a thick yellowish plaque that retains the natural skin lines (helps distinguish from warts) (4).
- A hard corn is a dry horny mass found commonly over the interphalangeal joints (dorsally) or the 5th toe (dorsolaterally) (1).
- Soft corns are extremely painful; occur interdigitally; skin appears white and macerated; commonly located between the 4th interdigital space (often mistaken for tinea) (1)
- Observe gait and the alignment of the feet for any faulty mechanics (3).
- Note the location and appearance of the hyperkeratotic lesions:
  - Common sites for corns and calluses: plantar surface (over the metatarsal heads, sides of the arch, and the heel) and dorsum of the foot (over the interphalangeal joints) (3)
  - Common sites for calluses on hands: palmar surface and over metacarpophalangeal joints
- Palpate for any abnormal bony prominences (3).
- Assess for pain or tenderness.
- Physical examination of the area is typically all that is necessary to make the diagnosis.

DIFFERENTIAL DIAGNOSIS

- Verruca vulgaris or plantaris (differentiated by paring the skin; the corn becomes more normal in appearance, and the wart displays the characteristic tiny red dots when pared)
- Tinea pedis (interdigital)
- Psoriatic plaque: hyperkeratosis with red base

DIAGNOSTIC TESTS & INTERPRETATION

- Imaging usually not necessary
- Radiographs: hands and weight-bearing views of the feet used to identify bony prominences or abnormalities, especially in lesions that are refractory to treatment (3)[C]

TREATMENT

GENERAL MEASURES

Treatment is aimed at providing symptomatic relief and avoiding the underlying mechanical forces that caused the development of the callus or corn (1,2,3,4)[C]:

- Careful and regular paring
- Use an emery board or a pumice stone daily, if necessary, to remove excess thickened skin.
- The pumice stone works best after bathing when the thickened skin has softened.
- Soft corn: toe separator or lamb's wool
- Doughnut-shaped corn pads
- Proper footwear with soft upper and a roomy toe box
- Orthotics can reduce pressure by redistributing forces.
- Use a skin-softening cream to prevent cracking of the callus or corn.

MEDICATION

First Line

- Salicylic acid pad (40%): careful application of pads containing keratolytic agents (4)[C]. Repeat as needed every 48 hr for up to 2 wk. Avoid pads in patients with peripheral neuropathy.
- Can also use salicylic acid gel (10–20%) when pad is too small for lesion

ISSUES FOR REFERRAL

Consider referral to dermatology, podiatry, or orthopedic surgery (foot and ankle) if failed conservative measures or need for surgical intervention.

ADDITIONAL THERAPIES

Antibiotics are only indicated when there is evidence of an infected corn or callus.

SURGERY/OTHER PROCEDURES

- Shaving or sharp débridement can be therapeutic (2)[C].
- Surgery may be required to correct the bony abnormalities or deformities (claw toe, hammer toe, etc.) and is indicated only if all conservative measures have failed (1,2)[C].
- There is limited data on intralesional bleomycin as additional therapy (6)[C].

ONGOING CARE

FOLLOW-UP RECOMMENDATIONS

Follow-up is needed for ongoing corns and calluses despite conservative management, signs of infection, or severe pain.

Patient Monitoring

- Diabetics, the elderly, and individuals with peripheral arterial disease or peripheral neuropathy should consult with their health care providers before initiating treatment for calluses or corns.
- These individuals should be monitored closely for signs of nonhealing or infection.

COMPLICATIONS

- Recurrence
- Pain from procedure
- Although unlikely, there is potential for nonhealing and/or infection.

REFERENCES

1. Freeman DB. Corns and calluses resulting from mechanical hyperkeratosis. *Am Fam Physician*. 2002;65(11):2277–2280.
2. Phillips S, Seiverling E, Silvis M. Pressure and friction injuries in primary care. *Prim Care*. 2015;42(4):631–644.
3. Singh D, Bentley G, Trevino SG. Callosities, corns, and calluses. *BMJ*. 1996;312(7043):1403–1406.
4. Cordoro KM, Ganz JE. Training room management of medical conditions: sports dermatology. *Clin Sports Med*. 2005;24(3):565–598.
5. Siddle HJ, Redmond AC, Waxman R, et al. Debridement of painful forefoot plantar callosities in rheumatoid arthritis: the CARROT randomised controlled trial. *Clin Rheumatol*. 2013;32(5):567–574.
6. Lee WJ, Lee SM, Won CH, et al. Efficacy of intralesional bleomycin for the treatment of plantar hard corns. *Int J Dermatol*. 2014;53(12):e572–e577.

ADDITIONAL READING

- Robbins JM. Recognizing, treating, and preventing common foot problems. *Cleve Clin J Med*. 2000;67(1):45–47, 51–52, 55–56.
- Spink MJ, Menz HB, Lord SR. Distribution and correlates of plantar hyperkeratotic lesions in older people. *J Foot Ankle Res*. 2009;2:8.

CLINICAL PEARLS

- Calluses and corns are common skin conditions resulting from repetitive friction or pressure.
- Diagnosis is often clinical, but imaging may be needed to evaluate an underlying bony prominence.
- Treatment is often aimed toward alleviating symptoms and removing contributing mechanical forces.
- First-line medical therapy is use of a salicylic acid pad.
- In some sports, calluses are desired by athletes to allow for pain-free participation.

CARDIAC ARRHYTHMIAS: ATRIAL FIBRILLATION, SVT

Charles W. Webb, DO, FAAFP, CAQSM • David L. Brown, MD, MBA

BASICS

Any deviation from normal (sinus) heart rhythm broadly classified as bradyarrhythmias (slow) or tachyarrhythmias (fast) (1)

EPIDEMIOLOGY

Incidence

- Bradyarrhythmias (2,3):
  - Common in aerobically trained athletes secondary to elevated resting vagal tone
  - Sinus bradycardia (50–65% of athletes vs. 23% in general population)
  - Sinus arrhythmias (13.5–69% of athletes vs. 2.4–20% in general population)
  - Sinus pause of >2 sec (37.1% of athletes vs. 5.7% in general population)
  - First-degree atrioventricular (AV) block (6–33% of athletes vs. 0.65% in general population)
  - Second-degree AV block, Mobitz I (2.4–10% of athletes vs. 0.003% in general population)
  - Third-degree AV block (0.017% in athletes vs. 0.00002% in general population)
  - Junctional rhythms (0.031–7% of athletes vs. 0.06% in general population)
  - These changes are readily reversed in athlete's heart as increased sympathetic drive overcomes resting vagal tone; if presents with symptoms (impaired consciousness or fatigue) or not readily reversed, often associated with underlying cardiac disease
- Tachyarrhythmias (2,3):
  - Atrial fibrillation more common in competitive athletes (0.063%) than general population (0.004%)
  - Other supraventricular atrial or AV nodal tachyarrhythmias are not more common in athletes in comparison to the general population.
  - Wolff-Parkinson-White syndrome (electrocardiogram [ECG] showing short PR interval with wide QRS and slurred upstroke or delta wave) equal in athletes and general population (0.15%)
  - Premature ventricular contractions occur at similar rates in athletes versus general population.
  - Complex ventricular arrhythmias are always pathologic and should seek prompt cardiology examination.

ETIOLOGY AND PATHOPHYSIOLOGY

Special considerations (3,4):

- Systematic training may cause physiologic adaptations, including a variety of abnormal ECG findings, in about 40% of elite athletes, termed the "athlete's heart."
- Increased QRS voltage, incomplete right bundle branch block, early repolarization, and peaked T waves related to increase in overall cardiac mass
- Endurance athletes develop cardiac alterations that are associated with atrial fibrillation in nonathletes including increased vagal tone, bradyarrhythmias, increased atrial pressures during exercise, left atrial enlargement, elevated inflammatory markers, and myocardial remodeling with fibrosis.
- Increased vagal tone in trained athletes favors a reduced refractoriness and enhanced myocardial excitability.

RISK FACTORS

- Structural heart disease (hypertrophic cardiomyopathy, anomalous coronary syndrome, arrhythmogenic right ventricular dysplasia, Marfan syndrome, aortic stenosis, dilated cardiomyopathy) (3,4)
- Myocarditis
- Atherosclerotic coronary artery disease (especially if >35 yr old)
- Drugs (amphetamines, cocaine, ephedrine)
- Long QT syndrome with QTc >0.46 sec (congenital vs. iatrogenic, including medications such as class IA antiarrhythmics, antifungals, nonsedating antihistamines, antibiotics, promotility agents)
- Commotio cordis (direct nonpenetrating trauma to chest wall)
- Metabolic abnormalities (electrolyte disturbances, hyperthyroidism)

DIAGNOSIS

- Wide range of clinical presentations, from occasional palpitations to sudden cardiac death (3)
- Bradyarrhythmias can present with impaired consciousness or fatigue.
- Tachyarrhythmias can cause palpitations, chest pain, and exertional dyspnea.
- Unstable ventricular tachyarrhythmias may cause lightheadedness or syncope.
- Supraventricular tachycardia (SVT):
  - Evaluation:
    - 12-lead ECG (4)[B]
    - Echocardiogram (4)[B]
    - Ambulatory cardiac/ECG monitoring
    - Identify rate response of SVT during activity or exercise.
    - If unable to induce SVT with exercise, can induce with either atrial/esophageal pacing, then monitor with exercise stress test
- Atrial fibrillation:
  - May be present intermittently or chronically
  - More common with diseases such as coronary artery disease and hypertension
  - Evaluation:
    - 12-lead ECG (4)[B]
    - Echocardiogram (4)[B]
    - Ambulatory cardiac/ECG monitoring
    - Determination of ventricular response with athletic activity

HISTORY

Based on American Heart Association (AHA) consensus panel recommendations for preparticipation athletic screening (3):

- Family history:
  - Premature sudden cardiac death
  - Heart disease in relatives <50 yr old
- Personal history:
  - Heart murmur, fatigue, systemic hypertension, exertional chest pain, syncope/near syncope during or after exercise, unexplained or disproportionate exertional dyspnea
  - Presence of palpitations, chest pain, lightheadedness, syncope, and relation of symptoms to activity or rest
  - Note prescription and over-the-counter (OTC) medications, especially cold or diet remedies (especially those containing ephedra), nutritional supplements, alcohol use, and recreational drugs (especially cocaine).

PHYSICAL EXAM

- Vital signs (pulse, temperature, blood pressure [BP], respiration rate)
- Dynamic heart evaluation looking for heart murmur documented in at least two positions (usually supine and standing) to discern murmurs with outflow obstruction
- Hypertrophic obstructive cardiomyopathy murmur *increases* with maneuvers that decrease venous return (such as Valsalva or moving from squat or stand).
- Aortic stenosis murmur decreases with the same maneuvers.
- Pathologic murmur identified as any systolic murmur graded 3/6 or greater, any diastolic murmur, or any holosystolic murmur
- Palpation of radial and femoral pulses to exclude coarctation of the aorta (3,4)

DIFFERENTIAL DIAGNOSIS

- Anxiety disorder, panic attacks
- Angina
- Costochondritis
- Neurocardiogenic syncope
- Heat stroke
- Seizure
- Thyroid dysfunction

DIAGNOSTIC TESTS & INTERPRETATION

Workup for athletes with significant arrhythmia includes (3,4):

- 12-lead ECG (4)[B].
- Echocardiogram (evaluate for hypertrophic cardiomyopathy, dilated cardiomyopathy, and valvular abnormalities) (4)[B].

- Exercise stress test to identify exertional arrhythmias or induced ischemia; may need to be adapted specifically for athlete (i.e., at peak energy for sprinter) as well as sport (maximal ergometer stress test for rower reproducing training conditions that produce symptoms):
  - Nonpathologic bradycardias in athlete usually resolve with exercise testing.
  - Nonpathologic premature ventricular complexes usually resolve with exercise testing.
- Ambulatory cardiac monitoring, if possible during specific type of participation exercise
- Electrophysiologic studies (when ablation is being considered)
- Implanted loop recorder, cardiac magnetic resonance imaging (MRI) rarely required

TREATMENT

- Acute treatment (1,4,5,6):
  - Symptomatic athletes should initially have airway, breathing, and circulation (ABCs) assessed and stabilized.
  - If athlete is unstable, may require advanced cardiac life support, immediate direct current (DC) cardioversion, and emergent transport to a medical facility.
  - Suspected SVT may respond to efforts to increase parasympathetic tone (e.g., Valsalva maneuver, carotid massage, and ice applied to face/neck).
- Long-term treatment atrial fibrillation:
  - Treatment of underlying cardiac disease, rate control medications, antiarrhythmic medications
  - β-Adrenergic blocking agents banned in some competitive sports
  - Catheter ablation may eliminate the need for antiarrhythmics and should be considered (4)[B].
  - Should be reevaluated every 6 to 12 mo after trained to determine if conditioning affects arrhythmia
- Long-term treatment SVT:
  - Catheter ablation is the treatment of choice for athletes with symptomatic SVT (4)[C].
  - If athlete has a short refractory period bypass tract capable of anterograde conduction and a history of atrial fibrillation, they should have ablation of the bypass tract due to risk of life-threatening arrhythmias (4)[B].

ONGOING CARE

- Return to play guidelines (2)[C]:
  - Important for thorough cardiac examination because underlying structural heart disease may place athlete at increased risk for sudden cardiac death with exertion
  - Athletes with syncope or near syncope should not participate in sports where the likelihood of loss of consciousness could be hazardous until the cause has been determined and treated.
  - Athletes with symptoms such as impaired consciousness and fatigue attributed to arrhythmias should be treated, and, if asymptomatic for 2 to 3 mo during treatment, may participate in all sports.
  - Athletes with symptomatic tachycardia/bradycardia arrhythmias should be treated, if no structural heart disease, for 2 to 3 mo and then they can return to sports.
- Atrial flutter:
  - Athletes with atrial flutter in the absence of structural heart disease may participate in all sports if without flutter for 2 to 3 mo.
  - Athletes with atrial flutter and structural heart disease can participate in sports such as billiards, bowling, cricket, curling, golf, and rifle (Bethesda Guidelines class 1A sports).
  - Athletes without structural heart disease who have had ablation or surgery can participate in all sports after 2 to 4 wk without recurrence.
  - Athletes who require anticoagulation cannot participate in competitive sports where the chance of collision is present.
- Atrial fibrillation:
  - Athletes with asymptomatic atrial fibrillation without structural heart disease who maintain a ventricular rate that appropriately increases and slows, with or without treatment, can participate in all sports. (Use caution because β-blockers are banned in some sports.)
  - Athletes with atrial fibrillation and structural heart disease who have rate control can participate to the limits and recommendations of the structural disease.
  - Athletes without structural heart disease who have had ablation or surgery can participate in all sports after 4 to 6 wk without recurrence.
  - Athletes who require anticoagulation cannot participate in competitive sports where the chance of collision is present.
- SVT:
  - Athletes without structural heart disease who have controlled SVT may participate in all sports.
  - Athletes with syncope, near syncope, or significant symptoms due to arrhythmia, or who have structural heart disease may participate in class 1A sports once treated and have no recurrence for 2 to 4 wk.
  - Athletes without structural heart disease who have had ablation or surgery can participate in all sports after 2 to 4 wk without recurrence.
  - Asymptomatic athletes with SVT ranging 5 to 10 sec without increased duration with exercise can play in all sports.

REFERENCES

1. Page RL, Joglar JA, Caldwell MA, et al. 2015 ACC/AHA/HRS guideline for the management of adult patients with supraventricular tachycardia: a report of the American College of Cardiology/American Heart Association Task Force on Clinical Practice Guidelines and the Heart Rhythm Society. *J Am Coll Cardiol*. 2016;67(13):e27–e115.
2. Pelliccia A, Zipes DP, Maron BJ. Bethesda Conference #36 and the European Society of Cardiology Consensus Recommendations revisited a comparison of U.S. and European criteria for eligibility and disqualification of competitive athletes with cardiovascular abnormalities. *J Am Coll Cardiol*. 2008;52(24):1990–1996.
3. Goldberger JJ, Cain ME, Hohnloser SH, et al. American Heart Association/American College of Cardiology Foundation/Heart Rhythm Society scientific statement on noninvasive risk stratification techniques for identifying patients at risk for sudden cardiac death: a scientific statement from the American Heart Association Council on Clinical Cardiology Committee on Electrocardiography and Arrhythmias and Council on Epidemiology and Prevention. *Circulation*. 2008;118(14):1497–1518.
4. Zipes DP, Link MS, Ackerman MJ, et al. Eligibility and disqualification recommendations for competitive athletes with cardiovascular abnormalities: task force 9: arrhythmias and conduction defects: a scientific statement from the American Heart Association and American College of Cardiology. *J Am Coll Cardiol*. 2015;66(21):2412–2423.
5. Elliott AD, Mahajan R, Lau DH, et al. Atrial fibrillation in endurance athletes: from mechanism to management. *Cardiol Clin*. 2016;34(4):567–578.
6. Flannery MD, Kalman JM, Sanders P, et al. State of the art review: atrial fibrillation in athletes. *Heart Lung Circ*. 2017;26(9):983–989.

CLINICAL PEARLS

- Document pertinent negatives in history (1,5).
- Document a dynamic heart exam during physicals and evaluations of symptomatic individuals.
- Consider ECG as first step in evaluation of arrhythmias.

C

CARPAL TUNNEL SYNDROME

Stephen Shaheen, MD, CAQSM

BASICS

DESCRIPTION

- Clinical condition caused by entrapment of the median nerve in the carpal tunnel at the wrist
- Classically presents as pain, weakness, and paresthesias on the palmar surface on the first 3½ digits
- Can be acute or chronic (idiopathic)

EPIDEMIOLOGY

- Carpal tunnel syndrome (CTS) accounts for ~90% of all entrapment neuropathies (1).
- Predominant gender: female > male (from 3:1 to as high as 10:1)
- Predominant age: Peak prevalence is among women aged 55 yr and older; prevalence increases with age.
- Higher prevalence in the dominant extremity; bilateral up to 50% of the time

Incidence

- Lifetime incidence is ~10%.
- Estimated that 1 million adults annually in the United States require medical treatment (1)

Prevalence

Prevalence is 1–16% of the population depending on the criteria for diagnosis.

ETIOLOGY AND PATHOPHYSIOLOGY

Exact pathogenesis of CTS is unclear. Most accepted theories are mechanical compression, microvascular insufficiency, and vibration:

- Acute:
  - Acute cases are less common but can be caused by a sudden rise in pressure in the carpal tunnel.
  - Most commonly seen with radial fracture; also associated with burns, coagulopathy, local infection, and injections
- Chronic:
  - Idiopathic: Only 50% of cases have an identifiable cause, which can be local, regional, or systemic in origin.
  - Local: inflammation, trauma, tumors, and anatomic anomalies
  - Regional: osteoarthritis, rheumatoid arthritis, amyloidosis, and gout
  - Systemic: diabetes, obesity, hypothyroidism, pregnancy, menopause, systemic lupus erythematosus (SLE), scleroderma, dermatomyositis, renal failure, long-term hemodialysis, acromegaly, multiple myeloma, sarcoidosis, leukemia, alcoholism, and hemophilia (1)

RISK FACTORS

- Repetitive wrist motion is the most widely recognized risk factor for occupational CTS.
- Narrow bony measurements of the wrist, elevated body mass index, increased age, female gender, and pregnancy are other common risk factors.

Pregnancy Considerations

- Common during pregnancy
- Usually in the 3rd trimester and often bilateral
- Usually symptoms will resolve spontaneously after delivery or with conservative treatment during pregnancy.

COMMONLY ASSOCIATED CONDITIONS

- Activities involving repetitive wrist motion, vibration, and excessive forces through the wrist
- Diabetes, thyroid disease, advancing age, and rheumatoid arthritis all have been associated with the development of CTS.
- Traumatic carpal bone dislocation or wrist fracture can disrupt the median nerve through the carpal tunnel through direct trauma to the nerve or mechanical entrapment secondary to cortical disruption and subsequent compression.
- Lipomas, ganglion cysts, and other anatomic anomalies can grow and directly compress the median nerve.
- Proximal upper extremity nerve entrapment or nerve root compression—the "double crush" syndrome

DIAGNOSIS

HISTORY

- Complaints of pain, weakness, and paresthesias on the palmar surface on the first 3½ digits
- Exacerbated by specific wrist motion in sport, occupational task, sleeping, driving, and so forth
- Nighttime symptoms
- Improved with "shaking of the hands" (a.k.a. flick sign)
- Consider cervical root pathology or radiculopathy if complaint of "shooting pain" down arm; consider generalized peripheral polyneuropathy if complaint of "sock and glove" distribution of pain in upper and lower extremities.

PHYSICAL EXAM

- Classically presents as pain, weakness, and paresthesias on the palmar surface on the first 3½ digits; however, there can be variations.
- Nocturnal acroparesthesia (i.e., extremity numbness, tingling, or other abnormal sensation) is the symptom most characteristic of CTS (2).
- Flick sign, in which a patient may demonstrate vigorous shaking of the hand and wrist in order to relieve symptoms, may be present.
- Pain or paresthesia evoked by hand grip
- Observe and palpate the region of the thenar muscle mass for atrophy (late finding).
- Usually normal hand and wrist range of motion
- Strength testing of the abductor pollicis brevis muscle
- Sensory testing, especially in the median nerve distribution
- Provocative tests:
  - Tinel sign: Percuss over the region of the carpal tunnel at wrist to elicit paresthesias in the distribution of the nerve; 38–100% sensitive and 80% specific (2)[A]
  - Phalen test: Position wrists adjacent to each other in complete flexion for at least 60 sec to elicit paresthesias; 42–85% sensitive and 80% specific (2)[A]
  - Carpal compression test: Press with thumbs over the carpal tunnel for 30 sec to elicit symptoms; reported 87% sensitivity and 90% specificity for CTS (2)[A]
  - Square wrist sign: Increased wrist ratio (thickness: width) has an increased odds ratio for CTS (3)[A].
  - Tourniquet test: Temporary increase in carpal tunnel pressure and symptoms can be elicited by blood pressure cuff application to arm or forearm.
  - Diagnosis usually can be made on history and physical examination alone.

DIFFERENTIAL DIAGNOSIS

- de Quervain tenosynovitis
- Cervical radiculopathy, C6–C7
- Proximal median nerve entrapment, pronator teres syndrome, or anterior interosseous syndrome
- Ulnar neuropathy at the elbow or wrist
- Brachial plexus neuropathy
- Wrist arthritis or other lesions in the wrist
- Colles fracture, lunate dislocation
- Generalized peripheral polyneuropathy
- Angina pectoris
- Upper motor neuron pathology
- Syringomyelia
- Mononeuritis multiplex
- Multiple sclerosis

DIAGNOSTIC TESTS & INTERPRETATION

Initial Tests (lab, imaging)

- Indicated when the classic defining features of CTS are not present:
  - Plain films generally are normal. Occasionally, carpal tunnel views may be helpful to rule out anatomic variants, fractures with trauma, and narrowing or calcification in the carpal tunnel.
  - Ultrasound (US) of the wrist may show structural abnormalities with nerve swelling. Cross-sectional area of the median nerve is significantly greater in patients with CTS than healthy controls (4).
  - Sensitivity of diagnosis with US of median nerve enlargement can be up to 97.9% (4).
- Magnetic resonance imaging (MRI) has been used to visualize structural abnormalities in and around the nerve:
  - There are limited studies examining the sensitivity and specificity of MRI for this purpose.
  - One small study showed no difference in diagnostic accuracy between MRI and US.
  - MRI is costly and cumbersome and cannot assess the physiologic integrity of the median nerve across the carpal tunnel segment.

Diagnostic Procedures/Other

- Electrodiagnostic examinations can confirm and/or support the diagnosis of CTS.
- Nerve conduction studies provide a highly sensitive (>85%) and specific (>95%) means for assessing the physiologic integrity of the median nerve across the carpal tunnel segment (2)[A].
- Can be used to classify severity of CTS and to monitor progression of median nerve entrapment
- Needle electromyography is useful for documenting the presence of axonal loss to intrinsic hand muscles innervated by the median nerve distal to the carpal tunnel segment and if the study includes structures proximal to the carpal tunnel, identifying other or coexisting neuromuscular pathology (e.g., cervical radiculopathy).

TREATMENT

- Conservative treatment:
  - ~80% of patients with CTS respond initially to conservative treatment; however, symptoms recur in 80% after 1 yr (5).
  - Restriction of precipitating activities may relieve symptoms.
  - Splinting:
    - Splinting the wrist at a neutral angle helps to decrease repetitive flexion and rotation, thus relieving mild soft tissue swelling or flexor tenosynovitis.
    - Compared with nighttime-only splint use, full-time use has been shown to provide greater improvement of symptoms and electrophysiologic measures; however, compliance with full-time use is more difficult (5)[B].
  - Corticosteroids:
    - With regard to symptoms management, oral corticosteroids have shown efficacy for up to 8 wk. Nonsteroidal anti-inflammatory drugs (NSAIDs) or diuretics are not effective in short-term treatment (5),(6)[A].
    - Corticosteroid injection into or proximal to the carpal tunnel provides greater clinical improvement at 10 wk than placebo (5).
    - Surgery should be considered if patient needs more than two injections.
  - Other conservative treatments and their evidence:
    - Level 1 (strong evidence of efficacy): local and oral steroids
    - Level 2 (moderate evidence of efficacy): Splints and therapeutic US are effective; NSAIDs, diuretics, and vitamin B_6 are ineffective (5,6).
    - Level 3 (limited/conflicting evidence of efficacy): Yoga, laser, and nerve glide exercises are effective short-term (5).
- Surgical treatment:
  - Patients who fail conservative therapy or who have severe symptoms (e.g., nerve entrapment on nerve conduction studies, thenar atrophy, or motor weakness)
  - Surgical decompression of the carpal tunnel segment by sectioning of the transverse carpal ligament has been reported to result in good symptomatic improvement in 70–90% of patients and may prevent further median nerve axon loss.
  - Slightly quicker return to work noted in endoscopic repair versus open repair (5)
  - Complications of surgery include injury to median nerve, scar tenderness, hypotrophic scarring, loss of grip strength, pillar pain (i.e., tenderness on the base of the palm), reflex sympathetic dystrophy, and bow stringing of flexor tendons.

Geriatric Considerations

Surgery has been found to provide better symptom relief, functional status, and general satisfaction than nonoperative therapy.

ONGOING CARE

PATIENT EDUCATION

- Use of wrist wraps and taping may minimize forces through the carpal tunnel by limiting excessive motion through the wrist in upper extremity weight-bearing sports such as gymnastics and weight lifting.
- Improvements in wrist pain and paresthesias may be noted within a few weeks after CTS surgery, but maximal improvements in thenar strength and numbness may take as long as 9 mo.
- Diagnosis often can be made based on history and physical examination findings alone.
- Corticosteroids (oral and injection), splinting, and surgery have the best evidence for treatment.

REFERENCES

1. Aroori S, Spence RA. Carpal tunnel syndrome. *Ulster Med J*. 2008;77(1):6–17.
2. Wilder-Smith EP, Seet RC, Lim EC. Diagnosing carpal tunnel syndrome—clinical criteria and ancillary tests. *Nat Clin Pract Neurol*. 2006;2(7):366–374.
3. Shiri R. A square-shaped wrist as a predictor of carpal tunnel syndrome: a meta-analysis. *Muscle Nerve*. 2015;52(5):709–713.
4. McDonagh C, Alexander M, Kane D. The role of ultrasound in the diagnosis and management of carpal tunnel syndrome: a new paradigm. *Rheumatology (Oxford)*. 2015;54(1):9–19.
5. Wipperman J, Goerl K. Carpal tunnel syndrome: diagnosis and management. *Am Fam Physician*. 2016;94(12):993–999.
6. Graham B, Peljovich AE, Afra R, et al. The American Academy of Orthopaedic Surgeons evidence-based clinical practice guideline on: management of carpal tunnel syndrome. *J Bone Joint Surg Am*. 2016;98(20):1750–1754.

ADDITIONAL READING

- Gerritsen AA, de Vet HC, Scholten RJ, et al. Splinting vs surgery in the treatment of carpal tunnel syndrome: a randomized controlled trial. *JAMA*. 2002;288(10):1245–1251.
- Wainner RS, Fritz JM, Irrgang JJ, et al. Development of a clinical prediction rule for the diagnosis of carpal tunnel syndrome. *Arch Phys Med Rehabil*. 2005;86(4):609–618.

CLINICAL PEARLS

- CTS is a very common compressive neuropathy of the upper extremity.
- It classically presents as pain, weakness, and paresthesias on the palmar surface on the first 3½ digits.
- Patients also complain of nighttime symptoms and needing to shake their hands to help the pain.

CATECHOLAMINERGIC POLYMORPHIC VENTRICULAR TACHYCARDIA (CPVT)

Chau Bui, DO • Paul Meirick, MD

BASICS

DESCRIPTION

- Channelopathies refer to a group of inherited arrhythmogenic diseases caused by mutations in genes encoding for ion channel proteins in cardiomyocytes that disrupt the balance of currents in the cardiac action potential. These disruptions may lead to ventricular arrhythmias and sudden cardiac death (SCD).
- The channelopathies include catecholaminergic polymorphic ventricular tachycardia (CPVT), long QT syndrome (LQTS) (see chapter on "Congenital QT Syndromes"), short QT syndrome (SQTS) (see chapter on "Congenital QT Syndromes"), and Brugada syndrome (see chapter on "Brugada Syndrome").
- CPVT: characterized by exercise or catecholamine-induced biventricular tachycardia, polymorphic ventricular premature beats, or ventricular tachycardia (VT) in young individuals with a structurally normal heart

EPIDEMIOLOGY

CPVT often presents with symptoms in 1st decade of life, but cases have been reported to present in the 4th decade (1,2).

Prevalence

Prevalence is generally unknown but estimated at ~1/10,000.

ETIOLOGY AND PATHOPHYSIOLOGY

- Sporadic or inherited mutations in the cardiac ryanodine receptor or calsequestrin (2)
- Genetic defects in *RyR2* and *CASQ2* genes alter calcium homeostasis in cardiac myocytes and lead to delayed after repolarizations that may precipitate supraventricular and ventricular arrhythmias (2).

Genetics

Two genetic variants known: autosomal dominant related to mutations in the *RyR2* gene encoding for the cardiac ryanodine receptor and an autosomal recessive form, resulting from mutations in *CASQ2* gene encoding for cardiac calsequestrin (2)

RISK FACTORS

The primary risk factor for most channelopathies is genetic:

- Physical effort (including swimming) and emotional stress are the most common precipitants of VT or ventricular fibrillation (VF).
- Strong association between arrhythmic events and exercise or catecholamine stimulation

GENERAL PREVENTION

- SCD resulting from channelopathies may be prevented by carefully screening and identifying athletes with the condition, although CPVT generally first presents with life-threatening arrhythmia. The preparticipation evaluation is the most important tool for identifying athletes with symptoms that may represent an inherited channelopathy. Any athlete with symptoms of palpitations, syncope, presyncope, any collapse, or with a family history of SCD or "accidental" death should be further evaluated with the tools reviewed below.
- Automatic external defibrillators (AEDs) are another important tool in preventing SCD from undiagnosed CPVT.

DIAGNOSIS

- Most patients present only after experiencing life-threatening VT or VF.
- Prehospital:
  - In the case that any patient with a CPVT converts into a life-threatening arrhythmia in the field, the most useful immediate tool and treatment is an AED.

HISTORY

- Pertinent history in screening athletes: Gathering a detailed and careful history during the preparticipation physical or during the evaluation of an athlete who comes to your attention is critical. The following questions should be included when interviewing an athlete:
  - Have you ever passed out, become dizzy, or had chest pain during or after exercise?
  - Do you get tired more quickly than others during exercise?
  - Has anyone in the family died suddenly and unexpectedly before the age of 50 yr? (Remember to ask about family members who died of accidental causes such as sudden infant death syndrome, drownings, and motor vehicle accidents because they may be clues to an undiagnosed family history of channelopathy.)
  - Have you ever had a heart abnormality or murmur diagnosed by a doctor?
  - Have you ever had an abnormal heart rate, palpitations, or irregular heartbeats?
  - Have you had high blood pressure (BP) or high cholesterol?
  - Has a physician ever denied or restricted your participation in sports for heart problems?
  - Have any of your relatives ever had cardiomyopathy, Marfan syndrome, LQTS, SQTS, or significant heart arrhythmias?
- Pertinent history in potentially affected athletes:
  - CPVT is most commonly asymptomatic until initial presentation with syncope or life-threatening VT or VF.
  - May have a family history of sudden cardiac arrest or SCD

PHYSICAL EXAM

- The most important elements of the exam are general (including level of consciousness), cardiac, and pulmonary examinations and, in the case of a patient who has sustained a life-threatening arrhythmia, complete trauma examination.
- Because patients with CPVT typically have structurally normal hearts, it is not uncommon to observe a completely normal examination when a life-threatening arrhythmia is not present.
- When arrhythmias are present, the examination may be notable for bradycardia or tachycardia, either regular or irregular, depending on the patient's rhythm.

DIFFERENTIAL DIAGNOSIS

QT syndromes, acquired LQTS with its many reversible metabolic and drug-induced causes, Brugada syndrome, acute coronary syndrome, true right bundle branch block (RBBB), pericarditis, drug-induced VT or VF

DIAGNOSTIC TESTS & INTERPRETATION

Initial Tests (lab, imaging)

In the setting of a life-threatening arrhythmia, it may be indicated to rule out ischemic or metabolic causes with a basic or comprehensive metabolic panel and cardiac enzymes.

Diagnostic Procedures/Other

Electrocardiogram (ECG) is the most important initial diagnostic tool. Holter monitors and echocardiograms may be of use as well:

- No distinguishing ECG diagnostic markers. Resting ECG usually normal until a life-threatening ECG pattern of VT or VF develops.
- Reported findings include sinus bradycardia, U waves, or a short PR interval.
- Exercise stress testing or strong emotions can elicit a pathognomonic bidirectional or polymorphic VT. Exercise-induced supraventricular tachyarrhythmias are common.

TREATMENT

The primary treatment is implantable cardioverter defibrillator (ICD) placement with careful programming and β-blockers.

MEDICATION

- β-Blockers are the cornerstone of CPVT therapy.
- Flecainide also has been shown to be effective.

SURGERY/OTHER PROCEDURES

- ICD is recommended for patients who continue to experience syncope and/or documented VT despite treatment with β-blockers (3)[C].
- ICD should be programmed with long delays before shock delivery and high cutoff rates due to inappropriate shocks that may lead to proarrhythmic effect (3).
- Left cardiac sympathetic denervation considered when β-blockers are ineffective (3)[C]

ADMISSION, INPATIENT, AND NURSING CONSIDERATIONS

As always, all patients who present with a life-threatening arrhythmia should be treated emergently with cardioversion and/or pharmacotherapy as dictated by standard advanced cardiovascular life support (ACLS).

ONGOING CARE

All patients with CPVT should be followed regularly by a cardiologist. Education and restrictions regarding exercise are crucial to survival.

FOLLOW-UP RECOMMENDATIONS

Return-to-play decisions:

- Participation in all competitive sports except those of very low intensity is not advised for symptomatic athletes or asymptomatic athletes with exercise-induced premature ventricular contractions in bigeminy, couplets, or nonsustained VT (4)[C].
- Exceptions should only be made after consultation with a CPVT specialist.

REFERENCES

1. Cheung C, Laksman Z, Mellor G, et al. Exercise and inherited arrhythmias. *Can J Cardiol*. 2016;32(4):452–458.
2. Priori SG, Napolitano C, Memmi M, et al. Clinical and molecular characterization of patients with catecholaminergic polymorphic ventricular tachycardia. *Circulation*. 2002;106(1):69–74.
3. Mazzanti A, O'Rourke S, Ng K, et al. The usual suspects in sudden cardiac death of the young: a focus on inherited arrhythmogenic diseases. *Expert Rev Cardiovasc Ther*. 2014;12(4):499–519.
4. Ackerman MJ, Zipes DP, Kovacs RJ, et al. Eligibility and disqualification recommendations for competitive athletes with cardiovascular abnormalities: Task Force 10: the cardiac channelopathies: a scientific statement from the American Heart Association and American College of Cardiology. *Circulation*. 2015;132(22):e326–e329.

CLINICAL PEARLS

- CPVT is a channelopathy that can be induced by physical or emotional stress in a structurally normal heart.
- CPVT generally first presents with life-threatening arrhythmia, therefore the preparticipation evaluation is the most important tool for identifying athletes with symptoms that may represent an inherited channelopathy.
- Resting ECG is usually normal until a life-threatening ECG pattern of VT or VF develops.
- The primary treatment is placement of an ICD with careful programming and β-blockers.
- Return to play in all competitive sports except those of very low intensity is not advised for symptomatic athletes or asymptomatic athletes with exercise-induced premature ventricular contractions in bigeminy, couplets, or nonsustained VT.

CAUDA EQUINA SYNDROME

Frank E. Lorch, MD, FAAPMR • Ibraheem Algarni, MD

BASICS

- Cauda equina syndrome (CES) is a rare condition associated with mechanical compression and/or dysfunction of the components of the cauda equina within the lumbosacral spinal canal.
- It is characterized by a variable combination of symptoms and signs that can include back pain, bowel and bladder dysfunction, saddle anesthesia, and varying degrees of loss of lower extremity sensory and motor function.
- When diagnosed, the treatment is urgent surgical decompression.

DESCRIPTION

- CES can have an acute or chronic presentation with "saddle anesthesia" (sensory changes in the groin and perineal area); bladder, rectal, and/or sexual dysfunction with back pain; and often with radicular symptoms and signs.
- Bladder dysfunction is a required element for diagnosis.
- CES can be classified into:
  - Incomplete syndrome (CES-I): Patients present with motor and sensory changes, including saddle anesthesia, but have yet to develop full retention or incontinence of either bowel or bladder. Instead, symptoms include altered urinary sensation, loss of urgency, poor urinary stream, and straining to urinate. Saddle and genital area sensory deficits are usually unilateral or partial.
  - Complete syndrome with true retention (CES-R): characterized by painless urinary retention and overflow incontinence. Similarly, either retention or incontinence of the bowel may be experienced. This is usually concurrent with extensive or complete saddle and genital sensory deficit along with deficient trigone sensation.

EPIDEMIOLOGY

Incidence

- CES is a relatively uncommon condition with an estimated incidence in the population ranging between 1 in 33,000 and 1 in 100,000 (1).
- CES is reported in approximately 0.04% of all patients presenting with low back pain (LBP).
- Peak incidence is in the 4th and 5th decades.
- It is estimated that CES occurs in approximately 0.12–2% of cases of lumbar herniated discs (1,2).
- 50–70% of patients with CES have urinary retention (CES-R) on presentation and 30–50% have CES-I (1).
- Men and women are affected equally.

ETIOLOGY AND PATHOPHYSIOLOGY

- The most common cause of CES is mechanical compression arising from a large central lumbar disc herniation.
- Other etiologies include:
  - Tumors; trauma; vertebral fractures; epidural hematoma; epidural abscess; lumbar stenosis; inflammatory conditions such as ankylosing spondylitis, spinal arachnoiditis, chronic inflammatory demyelinating polyneuropathy, sarcoidosis; and infections such as tuberculosis, Lyme disease, and herpes zoster.
- Nerve root injury may be due to compression, ischemia, venous congestion, or inflammation.
- Interruption of the sympathetic and parasympathetic bladder reflex arcs by the lower motor neuron lesion of CES results in loss of sensory and motor innervation to the bladder with subsequent urinary retention and overflow incontinence.

RISK FACTORS

- A congenitally stenotic spinal canal or acquired spinal narrowing can predispose to the development of CES.
- History of trauma, including falls, motor vehicle accident (MVA), weight lifting, and chiropractic manipulation
- Previous spine surgery
- Anticoagulation
- Spine infections

ALERT
High index of suspicion with trauma and anticoagulation

COMMONLY ASSOCIATED CONDITIONS

- Bladder dysfunction
- Lumbar spondylolisthesis and stenosis
- Motor weakness

DIAGNOSIS

ALERT

- Early identification of the patient's neurologic deficits and prompt surgical intervention reduces the likelihood of permanent neurologic sequelae.
- The widely varying clinical presentation of CES is a major cause of delayed recognition.
- CES must be considered in the presence of:
  - Severe LBP.
  - Sciatica: often bilateral, sometimes absent.
  - Saddle and/or genital sensory disturbance.
  - Bladder, bowel, and sexual dysfunction.

HISTORY

- Most cases are of sudden onset and progress rapidly within hours or days.
- Less frequently, CES can evolve slowly.
- Pain often described as progressively worsening
- Acute severe or sudden increase in LBP with or without radicular symptoms
- Patients do not always complain of pain or can have chronic, intermittent LBP with gradually worsening sciatica over weeks to months with incomplete deficits of bowel/bladder function.
- Inquire about changes in bowel and bladder habits and sexual function.
- Bowel disturbance may include fecal incontinence or constipation.
- Inquire about saddle and perianal area sensory changes.
- Unilateral or bilateral sensory changes or numb sensation in the lower limbs

PHYSICAL EXAM

- Motor exam:
  - Most patients have 4/5 or less strength in one or more spinal nerve distributions often manifesting as:
    - Gait difficulties.
    - Difficulty with heel/toe walking.
    - Difficulty with sit-to-stand test.
    - Foot drop.
- Sensory exam must include comparison of pin prick to light touch testing:
  - Most patients present with an objective sensory deficit in the lower extremities.
  - 76% of patients have decreased perianal, perineum, buttock sensation, and posterior thigh sensation to pin prick (2).
- Rectal exam to evaluate for decreased tone, often an early sign of CES
- Reflexes: absent or diminished bulbocavernosus, anal, and lower limb reflexes

DIFFERENTIAL DIAGNOSIS

- Conus medullaris syndrome
- Herniated nucleus pulposus
- Spine injuries
- Guillain-Barré syndrome
- Multiple sclerosis
- Peripheral neuropathy
- Lumbosacral plexopathy
- Polyradiculopathy
- Spinal tumor

DIAGNOSTIC TESTS & INTERPRETATION

Initial Tests (lab, imaging)

- Urgent magnetic resonance imaging (MRI) of the lumbosacral spine is essential in the setting of neurologic compromise to confirm the diagnosis (3)[B].
- If MRI contraindicated, computed tomography (CT) scan and myelography indicated
- Spine radiographs useful to evaluate spine trauma, listhesis, and disc degeneration in suspected cases
- Urodynamic studies useful in bladder function assessment subacutely

Follow-Up Tests & Special Considerations

Clinical diagnosis of CES is difficult and has a 43% false-positive rate, so accurate confirmatory imaging is important (3)[B].

TREATMENT

GENERAL MEASURES

- Immediate surgical consultation
- Although not always reversible, surgical decompression may be the only chance to reverse the neurologic deficits.
- Surgical decompression is necessary within 48 hr after the onset of symptoms and preferably performed within 6 hr of injury (4,5)[B].

ISSUES FOR REFERRAL

- Recent bowel or bladder changes
- Sexual dysfunction
- Saddle anesthesia
- Lower extremity weakness or paralysis
- Sensory loss in a nerve root distribution
- Muscle atrophy
- Absent bulbocavernosus, anal, patellar, Achilles, and plantar reflexes
- Gait disturbance
- Upper motor neuron (UMN) signs such as clonus, spasticity, hyperreflexia, or Babinski sign

SURGERY/OTHER PROCEDURES

- The timing of surgical intervention is controversial, with immediate, early, and late surgical decompression showing varying results (1)[C].
- It is well established that the outcome for patients with CES-I at the time of surgery is generally favorable, whereas those who have deteriorated to CES-R when the compression is relieved have a poorer outcome (4,5)[B],(6)[C].
- Surgical technique is often wide laminectomy and extensive decompression with foraminotomies if needed for stenosis (2)[C].
- Surgical treatment might also include instrumentation/fusion for stabilization or discectomy.

ADMISSION, INPATIENT, AND NURSING CONSIDERATIONS

- Malignant disease that is considered inoperable may be treated with radiation therapy and chemotherapy.
- Glucocorticoids indicated in CES cases associated with spinal cord compression or other conditions amenable to steroids
- Pain management as needed
- Antibiotic treatment if infection is suspected
- Establishment of a bowel and bladder program

ONGOING CARE

FOLLOW-UP RECOMMENDATIONS

- Early involvement of rehabilitation team, including a spinal cord injury rehabilitation physician, physical therapist, and occupational therapist to identify and monitor community and home integration issues and other issues associated with deficits in toileting, strength, coordination, transfers, activities of daily living, and ambulation
- Primary care physician follow-up to monitor post-hospital medications and other laboratory tests
- Regular follow-up for patients with renal or bladder complications and impotence due to the increased tendency for recurrent urinary tract infection and calculi
- Regular follow-up urodynamic studies, renal ultrasound, and general cancer screening should be performed.

PROGNOSIS

- Time since symptom onset inversely correlates with chances of return of function (2)[C].
- Patients have a significantly better chance of improvement in retention than in incontinence.
- Onset of erectile dysfunction is an uncommon but prognostically poor symptom.
- Although most presenting symptoms improve significantly after surgery, urinary and bowel incontinence and sexual dysfunction might persist with sexual dysfunction being the most prevalent (5)[B].

REFERENCES

1. Gardner A, Gardner E, Morley T. Cauda equina syndrome: a review of the current clinical and medicolegal position. *Eur Spine J*. 2011;20(5):690–697.
2. Gitelman A, Hishmeh S, Morelli BN, et al. Cauda equina syndrome: a comprehensive review. *Am J Orthop (Belle Mead NJ)*. 2008;37(11):556–562.
3. Bell D, Collie D, Statham P. Cauda equina syndrome: what is the correlation between clinical assessment and MRI scanning? *Br J Neurosurg*. 2007;21(2):201–203.
4. Srikandarajah N, Boissaud-Cooke M, Clark S, et al. Does early surgical decompression in cauda equina syndrome improve bladder outcome? *Spine (Phila Pa 1976)*. 2015;40(8):580–583.
5. Venkatesan M, Nasto L, Haddad S, et al. Cauda equina syndrome: a single centre review of 147 operated cases. *Spine J*. 2017;17(3):S6.
6. Todd N, Dickson R. Standards of care in cauda equina syndrome. *Br J Neurosurg*. 2016;30(5):518–522.

ADDITIONAL READING

- Cauda Equina Syndrome Resource Group: www.caudaequina.org
- Haswell K, Gilmour J, Moore B. Clinical decision rules for identification of low back pain patients with neurologic involvement in primary care. *Spine (Phila Pa 1976)*. 2008;33(1):68–73.
- Kim J, Seong J. Endoscope-assisted oblique lumbar interbody fusion for the treatment of cauda equina syndrome: a technical note. *Eur Spine J*. 2017;26(2):397–403.
- Lavy C, James A, Wilson-MacDonald J, et al. Cauda equina syndrome. *BMJ*. 2009;338:b936.
- Maynard FM Jr, Bracken MB, Creasey G, et al. International standards for neurological and functional classification of spinal cord injury. American Spinal Injury Association. *Spinal Cord*. 1997;35(5):266–274.
- Small SA, Perron AD, Brady WJ. Orthopedic pitfalls: cauda equina syndrome. *Am J Emerg Med*. 2005;23(2):159–163.
- Spector LR, Madigan L, Rhyne A, et al. Cauda equina syndrome. *J Am Acad Orthop Surg*. 2008;16(8):471–479.
- Tan K, Sewell M, Markmann Y, et al. Anterior lumbar discectomy and fusion for acute cauda equina syndrome caused by recurrent disc prolapse: report of 3 cases. *J Neurosurg Spine*. 2017;27(4):352–356.

CLINICAL PEARLS

- CES should be considered in all patients with severe LBP from any cause.
- It is a rare disorder that is usually a surgical emergency.
- It is important to try to prevent CES-I, with its more favorable prognosis, from progressing to CES-R.

CELLULITIS IN SPORTS

Kenneth P. Barnes, MD, MSc, CAQSM, FACSM • Shane Hudnall, MD, CAQSM

BASICS

An inflammation of the skin and underlying subcutaneous tissues (specifically the dermal and subcutaneous fat layers) caused by a spreading infiltration of bacteria through the skin surface

DESCRIPTION

- Typically results from entry of bacteria through a break in the skin, from contiguous foci (abscess), or from metastatic dissemination via bacteremia
- Most commonly involves the lower extremities
- Can occur anywhere on the body, including periorbital area, upper extremities, and abdominal wall
- Gram positives (*Streptococcus pyogenes* and *Staphylococcus aureus*) comprise >80% of the organisms responsible.
- Methicillin-resistant *S. aureus* (MRSA) is a concern due to increasing prevalence in the community setting.

EPIDEMIOLOGY

Incidence

1 case per 500 patient-years

RISK FACTORS

- Previous cellulitis
- Wounds (including human and animal bites)
- Edema (related to venous insufficiency)
- Disruption of skin from trauma or scratching
- Eczema or other inflammation
- Underlying skin infections (i.e., tinea pedis)
- Obesity
- Elderly
- Intravenous (IV) drug use
- Surgeries
- MRSA risk factors:
  - Recent antibiotics
  - Recent hospitalization
  - Residence in long-term care facility
  - Homelessness
  - Previous MRSA infection
  - IV drug abuse
  - Immunocompromised
  - Prisoners
  - Military recruits
  - Contact sports

COMMONLY ASSOCIATED CONDITIONS

Consider treating for the specific organisms identified in these populations:

- Diabetes: anaerobes and gram negatives
- Neutropenia: *Pseudomonas*
- Human bite: *Eikenella corrodens*, *Fusobacterium* species
- Cat bite: *Pasteurella multocida*
- Dog bite: *Pasteurella multocida*, *Capnocytophaga canimorsus*
- Hot tub: *Pseudomonas*
- Fresh water: *Aeromonas hydrophila*
- Salt water: *Vibrio* species
- IV drug abuse: MRSA, *Pseudomonas*
- Immunocompromised: *Cryptococcus neoformans*

DIAGNOSIS

HISTORY

- Breakdown in normal skin barriers almost always precedes this infection.
- Preexisting venous stasis alone may predispose to cellulitis.

PHYSICAL EXAM

- Area of involvement denoted by spreading erythema, warmth, and swelling with ill-defined margins
- Associated pain and tenderness
- Streaks of erythema and tenderness indicative of lymphatic spread
- Bullae may develop but, generally, rash is not raised.
- Fever, sweats, shaking chills common but bacteremia infrequent
- Regional lymphadenopathy
- Look for evidence of predisposing factors: lower extremity venous stasis, tinea infection, IV drug abuse track marks, eczema, radiation (irritation and thinning of skin).
- Use of pen/marker to demarcate the leading edge of cellulitis is helpful in monitoring during follow-up.

DIFFERENTIAL DIAGNOSIS

- Erysipelas (infection of the superficial layers of the skin, usually caused by group A streptococci)
- Fasciitis/necrotizing fasciitis
- Myonecrosis/gas gangrene
- Toxic epidermal necrolysis
- Osteomyelitis
- Cutaneous candidal infection
- Septic arthritis
- Gout
- Zoster
- Erythema migrans
- Contact dermatitis
- Eczema
- Deep venous thrombosis
- Ruptured Baker cyst
- Drug rash
- Insect bite

DIAGNOSTIC TESTS & INTERPRETATION

- Blood testing nonspecific and typically not helpful (may include increased white blood cell [WBC] count, erythrocyte sedimentation rate [ESR], C-reactive protein [CRP])
- Wound culture for bacterial identification and antimicrobial sensitivity in abscesses unless <2 cm and uncomplicated
- Blood cultures rarely helpful (<10% positive) (1)
- Needle aspiration of abscess or bullae most likely to be helpful if present
- Culture of overlying intact skin is not helpful and recommended against.
- Imaging not recommended unless concerned about osteomyelitis (magnetic resonance imaging [MRI]), underlying abscess (ultrasound), or other conditions in differential (i.e., deep vein thrombosis)

TREATMENT

If staph is isolated, consider treating for MRSA if patient has MRSA risk factors and/or if local prevalence of MRSA is high.

GENERAL MEASURES

- If abscess present, incision and drainage required
- If bullae noted, typically do not rupture as part of treatment
- If underlying venous stasis noted, elevation of affected limb and, if possible, compression stockings (not over area of skin involvement) recommended

MEDICATION

- Treat presumptively with close follow-up.
- Duration of therapy 5 to 14 days total
- Improvement anticipated in 1 to 2 days
- If no improvement or clinical deterioration, admit for parenteral antibiotics and broaden differential diagnosis to include possibility of potentially fatal infections such as necrotizing fasciitis.
- Should admit for parenteral antibiotics and monitoring if two or more of the following are also present: temp >38°C or <36°C, heart rate (HR) >90/min, respiratory rate (RR) >20/min, WBC count >12,000 or <4,000/mm^3 (2)[C]
- In uncomplicated cellulitis without MRSA risk factors, addition of antibiotics targeting MRSA does not improve outcomes (3)[A].
- Treatment recommendations (1)[A]:
  - Outpatient for non-MRSA infections: dicloxacillin 500 mg PO QID, cephalexin 500 mg PO QID; may use clindamycin 300 to 450 mg PO q6–8h or fluoroquinolones if allergic to penicillins
  - Inpatient for non-MRSA infections: nafcillin or oxacillin 1 to 2 g IV q4h, ceftriaxone 1 to 2 g/day IV
  - Outpatient for MRSA infections: Bactrim DS 2 tabs PO BID or doxycycline 100 mg PO BID (not recommended for children <8 yr old) or clindamycin 300 to 450 mg PO q6–8h (Check local resistance patterns.)
  - Inpatient for MRSA infections: vancomycin (15 mg/kg/dose IV q12h), linezolid 600 mg PO or IV BID (expensive and need to monitor for thrombocytopenia)

ISSUES FOR REFERRAL

- If patient not responding to antibiotic treatment in timely manner
- If development of crepitance suggesting a gas-forming organism
- If the cellulitis is on the face, there is a low threshold for referral.
- If a high-risk patient or immunocompromised for any reason, have a low threshold for involvement of an infectious disease specialist if not readily responding to treatment.

ADDITIONAL THERAPIES

- Human bites: Augmentin (outpatient), ampicillin/sulbactam (inpatient); penicillin allergy: moxifloxacin + clindamycin or Bactrim + Flagyl
- Animal bites: Augmentin (outpatient), ampicillin/sulbactam (inpatient); penicillin allergy: (doxycycline or moxifloxacin or Bactrim) + (clindamycin or Flagyl) (1)
- Use of cell-wall active antibiotics (i.e., β-lactams) causes an initial worsening prior to improvement due to rapid release of a bolus of exotoxins (4)[B].
- Patients with recurrent cellulitis may benefit from antibiotic prophylaxis with a risk ratio of 0.46 in the treatment group (5)[A].

ONGOING CARE

PATIENT EDUCATION

- Early identification is important.
- If infection considered contagious, must not participate in contact or collision sports
- MRSA becoming more prevalent in locker rooms as well as in the community
- Do not share towels, razors, and/or other products.
- Frequent skin inspections
- Cover all wounds.
- Disinfect all shared athletic equipment and whirlpools.
- Education and posters recommended in all training rooms and locker rooms
- Liberal use of antibacterial soap or alcohol-based hand sanitizer
- Return to play:
  - 72 hr after initiation of therapy, with clinical improvement and no new lesions for 48 hr
  - No participation with exudative, moist, or draining lesions
  - Active lesions should not be covered to allow participation (6).

REFERENCES

1. Stevens DL, Bisno AL, Chambers HF, et al; for Infectious Diseases Society of America. Practice guidelines for the diagnosis and management of skin and soft-tissue infections. *Clin Infect Dis*. 2005;41(10):1373–1406.
2. Raff AB, Kroshinsky D. Cellulitis: a review. *JAMA*. 2016;316(3):325–337.
3. Pallin DJ, Binder WD, Allen MB, et al. Clinical trial: comparative effectiveness of cephalexin plus trimethoprim-sulfamethoxazole versus cephalexin alone for treatment of uncomplicated cellulitis: a randomized controlled trial. *Clin Infect Dis*. 2013;56(12):1754–1762.
4. Melzer M, Eykyn SJ, Gransden WR, et al. Is methicillin-resistant *Staphylococcus aureus* more virulent than methicillin-susceptible *S. aureus*? A comparative cohort study of British patients with nosocomial infection and bacteremia. *Clin Infect Dis*. 2003;37(11):1453–1460.
5. Oh CC, Ko HCH, Lee HY, et al. Antibiotic prophylaxis for preventing recurrent cellulitis: a systematic review and meta-analysis. *J Infect*. 2014;69(1):26–34.
6. Zinder SM, Basler RSW, Foley J, et al. National Athletic Trainers' Association position statement: skin diseases. *J Athl Training*. 2010;45(4):411–428.

ADDITIONAL READING

- Benjamin HJ, Nikore V, Takagishi J. Practical management: community-associated methicillin-resistant *Staphylococcus aureus* (CA-MRSA): the latest sports epidemic. *Clin J Sport Med*. 2007;17(5):393–397.
- Eron LJ, Laine C, Goldmann DR, et al. Cellulitis and soft-tissue infections. *Ann Intern Med*. 2009;150:ITC1-1.
- Gilbert DN, Chambers HF, Eliopoulos GM, et al, eds. *The Sanford Guide to Antimicrobial Therapy 2018*. 48th ed. Sperryville, VT: The Sandford Guide; 2018.
- McNamara DR, Tleyjeh IM, Berbari EF, et al. Incidence of lower-extremity cellulitis: a population-based study in Olmsted county, Minnesota. *Mayo Clin Proc*. 2007;82(7):817–821.
- Moran GJ, Krishnadasan A, Mower WR, et al. Effect of cephalexin plus trimethoprim-sulfamethoxazole vs cephalexin alone on clinical cure of uncomplicated cellulitis: a randomized clinical trial. *JAMA*. 2017;317(20):2088–2096.
- Quirke M, Ayoub F, McCabe A, et al. Risk factors for nonpurulent leg cellulitis: a systematic review and meta-analysis. *Br J Dermatol*. 2017;177(2):382–394.

CLINICAL PEARLS

- Admit patients for parenteral antibiotics if they have severe cellulitis or worsen despite oral antibiotics.
- If patient has uncomplicated cellulitis without MRSA risk factors, addition of antibiotics targeting MRSA does not improve outcomes.
- Incision and drainage if abscess is present
- Consider prophylaxis for patients with recurrent cellulitis.

CENTRAL SLIP AVULSION AND PSEUDOBOUTONNIÈRE DEFORMITIES

Jeffrey P. Feden, MD, FACEP, CAQSM • Razib Khaund, MD

BASICS

DESCRIPTION

- Boutonnière deformity describes a characteristic flexion deformity of the proximal interphalangeal (PIP) joint and hyperextension deformity of the distal interphalangeal (DIP) joint resulting from disruption of the central slip at or near its insertion onto the dorsal aspect of the base of the middle phalanx.
- Mechanism of injury is often forced flexion of an extended PIP joint or volar dislocation of the middle phalanx, causing avulsion of the central slip.
- Deformity of the finger may develop several weeks after an untreated injury.
- Pseudoboutonnière deformity results from hyperextension of the PIP joint; the volar plate is ruptured, whereas the central slip remains intact.

EPIDEMIOLOGY

Unknown incidence but relatively uncommon

ETIOLOGY AND PATHOPHYSIOLOGY

- Boutonnière deformity:
  - Following avulsion of the central slip, the intact lateral bands slowly migrate in a volar direction as the central slip retracts.
  - The head of the proximal phalanx "buttonholes" through the injured extensor mechanism.
  - The lateral bands become flexors of the PIP joint and extenders of the DIP joint.
- Pseudoboutonnière deformity: Contracture and fibrosis of the volar plate following injury lead to a flexion deformity of the PIP joint.

RISK FACTORS

Ball-handling sports

DIAGNOSIS

HISTORY

- Always consider injury to the central slip when an athlete "jams" a finger or has a PIP joint dislocation reduced.
- Knowledge of the mechanism of injury and/or direction of a PIP joint dislocation also may localize the injury and guide treatment:
  - Forced flexion of an extended PIP joint or *volar* dislocation of the middle phalanx may cause *central slip* injury.
  - Hyperextension of the PIP joint or *dorsal* dislocation of the middle phalanx may cause *volar plate* injury.

PHYSICAL EXAM

- Early: swollen PIP joint with dorsal tenderness, weak active extension, full passive extension; classic deformity is rarely seen in the acute setting.
- Late: flexion deformity of the PIP joint with hyperextension of the DIP joint
- Positive Elson test: With a flexed PIP joint at 90 degrees at edge of table, the patient attempts to extend middle phalanx against resistance; if central slip is disrupted, there is weak PIP extension with a rigidly extended DIP (normal: DIP remains lax) (1,2)[C].
- Unlike a true boutonnière deformity, pseudoboutonnière deformity is characterized by a *fixed* flexion contracture of the PIP joint, inability to achieve passive extension, and mild or absent DIP joint hyperextension.

DIFFERENTIAL DIAGNOSIS

- Fracture
- PIP joint dislocation
- Volar plate disruption
- Collateral ligament tears

DIAGNOSTIC TESTS & INTERPRETATION

Plain radiographs (especially a true lateral view) to evaluate for fracture and/or dislocation

TREATMENT

GENERAL MEASURES

- Boutonnière deformity:
  - Strict immobilization of the PIP joint in continuous extension for 4 to 6 wk; nighttime splinting for another 2 to 3 wk (3,4,5)[C]
  - Allow active and passive flexion of the DIP joint without immobilization (3,4,5)[C].
  - Gentle active and passive range of motion after splinting is completed (3,4,5)[C]
  - Splinting is appropriate initial treatment even for chronic deformity (5)[C].
- Pseudoboutonnière deformity:
  - May be treated with progressive extension splinting if the flexion contracture is <45 degrees; otherwise, surgical release should be considered (6)[C].
  - Acute volar plate injuries should be treated initially with an extension block splint and active flexion for 3 wk, followed by gradual extension (6)[C].

ISSUES FOR REFERRAL

Referral is recommended for:

- Inability to reduce a PIP joint dislocation or a large, displaced intra-articular PIP joint fracture
- Failure of nonoperative treatment with splinting
- Chronic flexion contractures of >45 degrees

SURGERY/OTHER PROCEDURES

Consider surgical management for:

- Interposed soft tissue preventing congruent reduction of a volar PIP dislocation.
- Large, displaced intra-articular PIP fracture at the base of the middle phalanx.
- Flexion contractures of >45 degrees.
- Symptomatic, chronic deformities.

ONGOING CARE

The athlete's sport and position will dictate his or her ability to participate with the injured finger immobilized.

REFERENCES

1. Carruthers KH, Skie M, Jain M. Jam injuries of the finger: diagnosis and management of injuries to the interphalangeal joints across multiple sports and levels of experience. *Sports Health*. 2016;8(5):469–478.
2. Chauhan A, Jacobs B, Andoga A, et al. Extensor tendon injuries in athletes. *Sports Med Arthrosc Rev*. 2014;22(1):45–55.
3. Hong E. Hand injuries in sports medicine. *Prim Care*. 2005;32(1):91–103.
4. Peterson JJ, Bancroft LW. Injuries of the fingers and thumb in the athlete. *Clin Sports Med*. 2006;25(3):527–542.
5. Lee SJ, Montgomery K. Athletic hand injuries. *Orthop Clin North Am*. 2002;33(3):547–554.
6. Rettig AC. Athletic injuries of the wrist and hand: part II: overuse injuries of the wrist and traumatic injuries to the hand. *Am J Sports Med*. 2004;32(1):262–273.

ADDITIONAL READING

- Aronowitz ER, Leddy JP. Closed tendon injuries of the hand and wrist in athletes. *Clin Sports Med*. 1998;17(3):449–467.
- Hogan CJ, Nunley JA. Posttraumatic proximal interphalangeal joint flexion contractures. *J Am Acad Orthop Surg*. 2006;14(9):524–533.

CLINICAL PEARLS

- Central slip injury may not be immediately recognized; careful history, examination, and suspicion are essential in addition to close follow-up.
- An acutely injured PIP joint with dorsal tenderness and weak active extension should be treated empirically even in the absence of a classic boutonnière deformity.
- Accidental flexion of the PIP joint during the treatment period must be avoided to prevent disruption of the healing process.
- The majority of central slip injuries can be treated nonoperatively with satisfactory results.
- The mechanism and direction of injury at the PIP joint may help to differentiate boutonnière from pseudoboutonnière deformities.

CERVICAL DISC DISEASE

Sara Neal, MD, MA, CAQSM

BASICS

DESCRIPTION

- Cervical radiculopathy is a syndrome of pain and/or sensorimotor deficits resulting from compression and inflammation of a cervical nerve root at or near the neural foramen.
- The most common causes of nerve root compression and irritation are herniated cervical discs and spondylosis.
- Spondylosis describes the degenerative aging process of the intervertebral discs, ligaments, facet joints, and vertebral bodies.
- Mechanical compression can be a result of facet and uncovertebral joint hypertrophy, vertebral body osteophytes, disc protrusion, or some combination of all three.

EPIDEMIOLOGY

- Peak age for cervical radiculopathy is 50 to 54 yr.
- Male > female with ratio 1.7:1

Incidence

Annual incidence rates of cervical radiculopathy:

- 107.3 cases/100,000 men
- 63.5 cases/100,000 women (1)

ETIOLOGY AND PATHOPHYSIOLOGY

- Cervical radiculopathy occurs when the nerve root becomes dysfunctional from compression, stretch, and/or irritation.
- Radiculopathy can also be a result of infection (herpes zoster, Lyme disease), granulomatous infiltration (sarcoid), vasculitis, or tumor.
- Causes of nerve root dysfunction: spondylosis > disc herniation > infection > granulomatous > tumor
- Pathophysiology of spondylosis:
  - As discs age, they undergo desiccation, loss of compressibility, and bulging with result of loss in disc height.
  - As the bony spine ages, osteophytes form at the uncovertebral and facet joints.
  - The ligamentum flavum undergoes hypertrophy.
  - These changes can cause narrowing of the neural foramen, impinging the nerve as it exits the cord.
- Pathophysiology of disc herniation:
  - Disc herniation is more common in the older age group. It can occur in adults <45 yr, but more force generally is needed to cause herniation because the discs are more resilient in the younger population.
  - With progressive age, the annular fibers surrounding the nucleus pulposus degenerate.
  - Under certain conditions such as mechanical force, the nucleus pulposus can herniate through the annular fibers.
  - Herniated disc material impacts and compresses the nerve root.
  - Herniation also incites inflammatory cytokines causing irritation of the nerve.
- Pathoanatomy:
  - Cervical nerve roots exit above their correspondingly numbered pedicles.
  - C6 nerve root exits between C5 and C6.
  - C7 nerve root exits between C6 and C7.
  - C8 nerve root exits between C7 and T1.
  - Most common level for the disc herniation is C6–C7 (70%), affecting the seventh cervical nerve.
  - C5–C6 is the next most common level (20%). Herniation here affects the sixth cervical nerve.
  - Disc herniations usually prolapse laterally into the neural foramen.
  - Occasionally, herniation disc material protrudes directed posteriorly, impacting the spinal cord; can cause myelopathy (cord compression); may have bilateral symptoms

DIAGNOSIS

HISTORY

- If the radiculopathy is from a herniated disc, symptoms are usually acute; symptoms from spondylosis are typically more insidious.
- Acute symptoms from herniation may be coincident with trauma such as axial loading and/or hyperflexion.
- Symptoms are typically unilateral and can include neck, shoulder, or arm pain; paresthesias; numbness; muscle weakness; and/or diminished deep tendon reflexes.
- Classically, pain in the limb is in the distribution of the cervical nerve myotome.
- If present, numbness and paresthesia occur in a dermatomal distribution; however, due to overlap of dermatomes, this may not be clinically evident or follow the classic dermatomal pattern.
- The patient may report relief of symptoms by abducting the upper limb because this maneuver decreases the amount of stretch on the nerve root.
- Weakness can develop in the muscles supplied by the nerve.
- Red flags:
  - Symptoms indicating a myelopathy (cord compression) rather than a radiculopathy include gait disturbance, bowel/bladder dysfunction, hand clumsiness or loss of manual dexterity, hyperreflexia, and/or clonus.
  - Fever, chills, unexplained weight loss
  - Constant and progressive symptoms
  - Bilateral symptoms
  - Unremitting night pain
  - Immunosuppression
  - History of cancer
  - Intravenous (IV) drug abuse

PHYSICAL EXAM

- Evaluate neck range of motion (ROM) with attention to any movement that worsens or alleviates symptoms.
- Motor testing of shoulders, arms, forearm/wrist, hand, and finger; evaluating for weakness/asymmetry
- Deep tendon reflexes should be symmetrical.
- Test sensation of dermatomes evaluating for asymmetry or abnormality.
- Spurling maneuver may be positive:
  - This position increases foraminal narrowing/compression and may reproduce symptoms.
  - To perform, extend the neck, rotate the head toward the side of symptoms, and apply downward pressure to the head. It is positive if symptoms are reproduced or increased.
  - Specificity of this test is moderate to high, whereas the sensitivity is moderate (2).
- Red flags: physical exam findings that may suggest myelopathy rather than radiculopathy:
  - Hyperreflexia
  - Note that a classic pattern of myelopathy at the C5–C6 interspace is suggested by hyperreflexia at the tricep reflex (C7) with diminished bicep and supinator reflexes (C5 and C6).
  - Babinski sign
  - Ankle clonus
  - Lhermitte sign: shock-like sensation radiating down the spine with neck flexion
  - Lower extremity weakness
  - Muscle atrophy in bilateral hands
  - Gait disturbance

DIFFERENTIAL DIAGNOSIS

- Peripheral nerve entrapment
- Myelopathy (from central disc herniation)
- Brachial plexus lesion, inflammation, or injury
- Thoracic outlet syndrome
- Spinal tumor
- Spinal infection/discitis
- Complex regional pain syndrome
- Herpes zoster
- Rotator cuff disorders
- Pancoast tumor

DIAGNOSTIC TESTS & INTERPRETATION

Initial Tests (lab, imaging)

- X-rays:
  - Obtain on initial visit if red flags; otherwise, optional
  - Anteroposterior, lateral, and oblique views
  - Spondylosis is a common finding, not diagnostic of radiculopathy.
- Magnetic resonance imaging (MRI; noncontrast): reveals good soft tissue detail of discs and nerves:
  - Indications:
    - Symptoms or signs of myelopathy
    - Red flags suggestive of tumor or infection (Get contrast MRI.)
    - Progressive or disabling neurologic deficit
    - Consider MRI if no improvement after 6 to 8 wk of conservative treatment.
  - Disc herniation seen best on T2 images
  - Caution should be used when interpreting MRIs because findings *must* correspond with symptoms to be clinically significant.
- Computed tomography (CT) myelogram:
  - Useful if patient has metallic surgical hardware in the neck because there can be distortion of MRI images
  - May offer better analysis of bony impingement on foramina
  - Disadvantages: It is invasive and uses radiation.

Diagnostic Procedures/Other

Electrodiagnostic studies (nerve conduction study with electromyogram):

- Obtain only if diagnosis is unclear.
- Can help differentiate from peripheral nerve entrapment
- False-negative results common if test performed too early in workup (must wait at least 3 wk minimum)

TREATMENT

- Optimal treatment is controversial. Most recognize conservative therapy as the initial treatment choice.
- Subsequent options include physical therapy, epidural steroid injections, and surgical procedures. The data for each of these treatment options is limited to relatively small studies. No large well-controlled studies have shown clear evidence of improved outcome for any specific treatment versus conservative treatment alone (3)[C].
- Because of a relatively high rate of spontaneous resolution, initial treatment is usually nonoperative. Exceptions that may require further workup and subspecialty consultation include:
  - Progressive neurologic deficit.
  - Disabling weakness.
  - Infection or tumor.
  - Vertebral fracture or subluxation from trauma (3)[C].
- Traditionally, conservative therapy has included some combination of the following modalities: oral analgesics, avoidance of provocative activities, short-term neck immobilization with soft collar, cervical traction, a short course of oral steroids, and physical therapy. Recent guidelines call into question the appropriateness of oral glucocorticoids and benzodiazepines given their unfavorable risk/benefit ratio (4)[A].
- Patients should be reevaluated at regular intervals during the treatment process so that worsening symptoms can be identified promptly.

MEDICATION

First Line

- Nonsteroidal anti-inflammatory drugs (NSAIDs):
  - Use at anti-inflammatory doses (e.g., ibuprofen 600 mg QID).
  - Block formation of inflammatory mediators at the site of the disc herniation.
  - Use cautiously if:
    - Risk factors for gastrointestinal (GI) bleeding
    - Risk factors for renal disease
    - In older patients (>65 yr)
- Oral steroids:
  - More potent anti-inflammatory agents than NSAIDs, although greater potential side effects
  - May consider using if:
    - Not responding to NSAIDs
    - Severe pain
    - Weakness
    - Renal insufficiency
  - Avoid using with NSAIDs.
  - Dose:
    - Typical regimen: Start with 50 to 70 mg/day of prednisone; taper over next 10 days (3)[C].
  - Side effects: have not been shown to alter the natural history of cervical radiculopathy, and risk/benefit ratio is unfavorable (4)[A]

Second Line

- Narcotics:
  - May be considered for short-term use if pain is severe and not controlled by other medications and modalities (5)[A].
  - Have additive effect with NSAIDs on pain relief.
  - Typical prescription: hydrocodone/acetaminophen—5/325 mg q4–6h PRN for pain
  - Potential side effects: drowsiness, vomiting, constipation, dependency
- Antispasmodic agents (muscle relaxants):
  - Consider using if muscle spasm is prominent.
  - Additive effect on pain relief when used with a NSAID or narcotic; drowsiness when combined with a narcotic may be intolerable.
  - Typical prescription: cyclobenzaprine—10 mg TID
  - Avoid using for >2 to 3 wk.
  - Potential side effects: sedation, dependency

ADDITIONAL THERAPIES

- Rest and avoidance of provocative activities:
  - "Relative rest" is typically recommended. Patient is encouraged to be as active as the pain allows.
- Cervical collar to limit motion:
  - Limited data on efficacy
  - May consider initially if severe pain when moving head
  - Limit use to <1 to 2 wk (to avoid weakness and stiffness).
  - Come out of the collar several times per day for ROM exercises within limits of pain.
- Formal physical therapy or home exercise program:
  - Start ROM exercises as early as possible within limits of pain.
  - Heat/cold, active ROM, isometric strengthening as tolerated
  - Add resistive exercises as tolerated.
  - May add nonimpact aerobic exercise; gear toward an activity that allows the neck to remain in neutral position (e.g., walking, stationary bike)
  - Postural education
  - Ergonomic adjustments
- Traction:
  - Limited reliable data
- Spinal manipulation (chiropractic treatment):
  - No consistent data showing benefit. Possible complications include spinal cord and vertebral artery injury if done improperly.
- Fluoroscopically guided epidural steroid injections:
  - May be effective in reducing pain and reducing need for surgery, but evidence of effectiveness is of low quality and serious complications are possible (6)[A]
  - Specific risks of procedure:
    - Dural puncture
    - Nerve damage
    - Spinal cord and brain stem infarction

SURGERY/OTHER PROCEDURES

- Consider referring to spine surgeon if:
  - Progressive or severe neurologic deficit
  - Recalcitrant radicular pain or numbness despite nonoperative treatment for 6 to 12 wk; no data on the optimal timing
  - Instability of the spine with radicular symptoms
  - Moderate to severe myelopathy
  - Muscle atrophy
- Surgical outcomes for relief of arm pain range from 80% to 90% (2)[C].
- Typical procedure for cervical radiculopathy:
  - Anterior cervical discectomy and fusion (ACDF): allows removal of the disc and uncovertebral spur without neural retraction. Bone graft or plate is placed anteriorly to vertebral body.
  - Addition of physical therapy postoperatively may improve outcome (7)[A].
- Total disc arthroplasty (experimental):
  - Diseased disc is removed, and an artificial disc is placed.
  - Allows preservation of motion, thereby theoretically decreasing the incidence of adjacent segment disease (5)[B].
  - Preliminary results have been equivocal compared with ACDF surgical procedures (8)[B].

ONGOING CARE

PATIENT EDUCATION

In attempts to decrease recurrence of symptoms:

- Keep the neck and shoulder girdle muscles strong.
- Use correct posture when sitting (head centered over shoulders).
- Set up workstations ergonomically.
- Avoid forcing the neck into extremes of motion.
- Regular aerobic exercise

PROGNOSIS

- Resolution of all or most symptoms occurs within 6 to 12 wk in most patients.
- Acute cervical radiculopathy has up to a 75% rate of spontaneous improvement (3).

COMPLICATIONS

Waiting too long to treat: If weakness is present for too long, patient may never regain full strength and function.

REFERENCES

1. Radhakrishnan K, Litchy WJ, O'Fallon WM, et al. Epidemiology of cervical radiculopathy. A population-based study from Rochester, Minnesota, 1976 through 1990. *Brain*. 1994;117(Pt 2):325–335.
2. Thoomes EJ, van Geest S, van der Windt D, et al. Value of physical tests in diagnosing cervical radiculopathy: a systematic review. *Spine J*. 2018;18(1):179–189.
3. Rhee JM, Yoon T, Riew KD. Cervical radiculopathy. *J Am Acad Orthop Surg*. 2007;15(8):486–494.
4. Chou R, Cote P, Randhawa K, et al. The Global Spine Care Initiative: applying evidence-based guidelines on the non-invasive management of back and neck pain to low- and middle-income communities [published online ahead of print February 19, 2018]. *Eur Spine J*. doi:10.1007/s00586-017-5433-8.
5. Eisenberg E, McNicol E, Carr DB. Opioids for neuropathic pain. *Cochrane Database Syst Rev*. 2006;(3):CD006146.
6. Engel A, King W, MacVicar J. The effectiveness and risks of fluoroscopically guided cervical transforaminal injections of steroids: a systematic review with comprehensive analysis of the published data. *Pain Med*. 2014;15(3):386–402.
7. Engquist M, Löfgren H, Öberg B. A 5- to 8-year randomized study on the treatment of cervical radiculopathy: anterior cervical decompression and fusion plus physiotherapy versus physiotherapy alone. *J Neurosurg Spine*. 2017;26(1):19–27.
8. Skeppholm M, Lindgren L, Henriques T, et al. The Discover artificial disc replacement versus fusion in cervical radiculopathy—a randomized controlled outcome trial with 2-year follow-up. *Spine J*. 2015;15(6):1284–1294.

ADDITIONAL READING

- Brown S, Guthmann R, Hitchcock K, et al. Clinical inquiries. Which treatments are effective for cervical radiculopathy? *J Fam Pract*. 2009;58(2):97–99.
- Caridi JM, Pumberger M, Hughes AP. Cervical radiculopathy: a review. *HSS J*. 2011;7(3):265–272.
- Childs JD, Cleland JA, Elliott JM, et al. Neck pain: clinical practice guidelines linked to the International Classification of Functioning, Disability, and Health from the orthopedic section of the American Physical Therapy Association. *J Orthop Sports Phys Ther*. 2008;38(9):A1–A34.
- Ellis JL, Gottlieb JE. Return-to-play decisions after cervical spine injuries. *Curr Sports Med Rep*. 2007;6(1):56–61.
- Kelly JC, Groarke PJ, Butler JS, et al. The natural history and clinical syndromes of degenerative cervical spondylosis. *Adv Orthop*. 2012;2012:393642.
- Nikolaidis I, Fouyas IP, Sandercock PA, et al. Surgery for cervical radiculopathy or myelopathy. *Cochrane Database Syst Rev*. 2010;(1):CD001466.
- Nordin M, Carragee EJ, Hogg-Johnson S, et al; for Bone and Joint Decade 2000-2010 Task Force on Neck Pain and Its Associated Disorders. Assessment of neck pain and its associated disorders: results of the Bone and Joint Decade 2000-2010 Task Force on Neck Pain and Its Associated Disorders. *Spine (Phila Pa 1976)*. 2008;33(Suppl 4):S101–S122.
- Young IA, Michener LA, Cleland JA, et al. Manual therapy, exercise, and traction for patients with cervical radiculopathy: a randomized clinical trial. *Phys Ther*. 2009;89(7):632–642.

CLINICAL PEARLS

- Distinguish radiculopathy from myelopathy.
- Weakness is the most serious complication of cervical radiculopathy and should be followed closely.
- MRI is the test of choice for imaging the discs and nerves.
- Treatment in most patients is nonoperative.
- The timing of surgical intervention for cervical radiculopathy has not been established, but surgery should be considered if there is significant weakness or symptoms that are refractory to nonoperative treatment.
- Don't miss the red flags: cervical myelopathy, tumor, and infection.

CERVICAL STENOSIS/MYELOPATHY

Julio A. Martinez-Silvestrini, MD, FAAPMR, CAQSM • Roman Zolotoy, DO

BASICS

DESCRIPTION

- Defined by the National Center for Catastrophic Sports Injury Research (NCCSIR) as a congenital or acquired process, which causes narrowing of the cervical spinal canal
- Functional spinal stenosis manifests by loss of the cerebrospinal fluid (CSF) around the spinal cord or a clear deformation of the cord demonstrated by computed tomography (CT) scan, magnetic resonance imaging (MRI), or myelography.
- Degenerative disk disease, spondylosis, and/or other degenerative pathology can progressively narrow the cervical spinal canal and can result in neurologic impairment due to compression of the cervical spinal cord.
- Compression of the cervical spinal cord can produce a syndrome of spinal cord dysfunction known as cervical spondylotic myelopathy (CSM).
- CSM is the most common cause of spinal cord dysfunction/impairment and the most common cause of myelopathy in adults >55 yr (1,2).
- Other potential sequelae include functional decline, progressive disability, reduction of quality of life, compromise of independence, and ability to perform activities of daily living (1).
- Synonym(s): cervical cord neurapraxia; cervical spondylotic myelopathy; degenerative cervical myelopathy (DCM)

EPIDEMIOLOGY

Incidence

- The incidence of cervical stenosis is unknown; the incidence of DCM in North America is approximately 41 per million (2).
- However, Torg reported that in a single football season, 6 of 10,000 exposures resulted in transient paresthesia in all four extremities, and 1.3 of 10,000 exposures resulted in transient quadriplegia (3):
  – This describes cervical cord neurapraxia, which is thought to be a sequela of stenosis.
- Male to female ratio of cervical spondylosis is 3:2.
- No evidence of gender predisposition to increased risk of deterioration or neurologic compromise (2)

Prevalence

- In a cadaveric data estimate the prevalence of cervical spinal stenosis to be 4.9% of the adult population: 6.8% of population 50 yr and older, and 9% of population 70 yr and older.
- Cervical stenosis also was found to increase with age.
- Prevalence of DCM in North America is about 605 per million (2).
- CSM occurs in 5–10% of patients with symptomatic cervical spondylosis (4).

ETIOLOGY AND PATHOPHYSIOLOGY

- Narrowing of the cervical spinal canal is often incited by degeneration of intervertebral disks resulting in disk herniation. This alters cervical spine biomechanics and leads to hypertrophy of the ligamentum flavum as well as laxity of facet joints. In addition, there is also uncovertebral degeneration, vertebral body osteophyte formation, and ossification of the posterior longitudinal ligament.
- Combination of mechanical compression of neural elements, spinal cord ischemia due to compression of the arterial, and/or venous blood supply to the cord can cause dysfunction of the adjacent spinal cord.
- Flexion and extension of the neck may exacerbate compression and cause further neurologic deficits.
- Most common affected levels are C5–C7 (2).
- Given that microvascular dysfunction plays a significant role in diabetic pathophysiology, diabetes could theoretically compound the symptomatology of CSM, but further studies into this potential sequelae are needed (1).
- Chronic compression of the spinal cord can also result in spinal cord vascular disruption, loss of blood-spinal cord barrier integrity, glutamate excitotoxicity, microglia activation, apoptosis, demyelination, astrogliosis, and axonal degeneration all contribute to deterioration (1).

RISK FACTORS

- Congenital or acquired defects, which include bulging disk, hypertrophied or unstable ligaments, and degenerative changes
- Congenital spinal stenosis or instability secondary to Down syndrome, Klippel-Feil syndrome, Ehlers-Danlos syndrome, odontoid abnormality, atlantooccipital fusion
- Progressive cervical kyphosis has been linked with CSM (5).
- Involvement in sports that engage in potential axial loading, such as football, ice hockey, diving, headfirst sliding in baseball, wrestling, soccer, gymnastics, and rugby
- Potential hereditary component of ossification of the posterior longitudinal ligament, ossification of ligamentum flavum, and degenerative disk disease
- Athletes who participate in sports with excessive forces to cervical spine such as football and rugby
- High-performance athletes such as cyclists and triathletes have also been found to higher incidence of cervical spine degenerative conditions.

DIAGNOSIS

HISTORY

- During preparticipation physical examination, determination of any prior history of neurologic events, such as burners/stingers or transient neurologic events, is critical.
- If the athlete gives a positive response, all data from previous evaluations must be reviewed. If no workup has been done, then consider imaging before allowing the athlete to begin contact/collision sports.
- Some athletes experience a slow and stepwise deterioration, whereas others experience prolonged periods of stability. Abrupt worsening can occur, often following minor neck injuries (2).
- If the athlete has risk factors, as delineated above, that may predispose him or her to cervical stenosis, the athlete must be further evaluated.

PHYSICAL EXAM

- Cervical stenosis is asymptomatic until forced hyperflexion or hyperextension occurs with an axial load, which causes neurapraxia.
- The athlete develops acute transient sensory paresthesia and/or motor paresis.
- Subtle gait dysfunction is the most common presentation of CSM.
- Other CSM symptoms can include upper and/or lower extremity weakness, neck pain and/or stiffness, numbness and/or paresthesias in the upper extremities, urinary and/or rectal sphincter dysfunction, and Lhermitte phenomenon.
- Upper motor neuron characteristics (hyperreflexia, increased tone, and Hoffman and/or Babinski signs)
- Lower motor neuron findings (weakness, atrophy, and suppressed reflexes)
- Findings are usually bilateral.
- Paresthesia is described as burning pain, numbness, or tingling of the affected region.
- Motor changes can range from weakness to complete paralysis.
- Neurapraxia commonly lasts 10 to 15 min but can take up to 48 hr to resolve (6).
- During the preparticipation physical examination, the Spurling foraminal compression test can be done. If symptoms are elicited, further workup can be started. The yield is very low unless the patient already has stenosis. It should be done on any athlete who gives a history of neurologic events.
- If the initial event occurs on the field, start with assessment of the athlete's level of consciousness. If unconscious, immobilize and transport. If conscious, proceed to assess neck pain:
  – If neck pain is present, or if there is no neck pain and the athlete has neurologic symptoms, immobilize and transport for further workup.

DIFFERENTIAL DIAGNOSIS
- Stable spinal fracture
- Any cause of permanent spinal cord injury
- Spear tackler's spine
- Unstable fracture
- Spinal fracture with dislocation
- Ligamentous injury
- Herniated cervical disk
- Amyotrophic lateral sclerosis
- Guillain-Barré syndrome
- Normal pressure hydrocephalus

DIAGNOSTIC TESTS & INTERPRETATION
- The initial radiographic examination should start with cervical spine x-rays, which can be used to evaluate for gross fracture or dislocation. In addition, some measurements of the spinal canal can be done. The normal canal measures >15 mm; <13 mm is considered spinal stenosis (4).
- CSM is considered unlikely if canal measures >16 mm and probable if <10 mm (2).
- On the lateral x-ray, the Torg ratio can be calculated. Measure (in millimeters) the distance from the posterior aspect of the vertebral body to the spinolaminar line (*a*) and the width of the vertebral body (*b*) and then calculate the ratio *a*/*b*. A value <0.8 is abnormal and needs further evaluation (4).
- A large vertebral body can result in a false-positive result; the false-positive rate has been reported as high as 88%. If the patient has spinal stenosis, the ratio almost always is abnormal.
- Cervical x-ray limitations include the failure of roentgenography to appraise the width of the cord and an inability to appreciate stenosis resulting from ligamentous hypertrophy, ligamentous laxity, or disk protrusion.
- Therefore, the next step is to use MRI or CT myelography.
- MRI can evaluate spinal stenosis caused by most abnormalities and is superior in providing intramedullary detail of spinal cord pathology. It is not as effective as CT myelography in evaluating bone and calcified tissues (2). Overall, MRI is sufficient in most cases (4,6).
- MRI is done in a neutral position. With hyperextension, spinal canal diameter decreases by 30% owing to infolding of the interlaminar ligaments.
- "Functional" spinal stenosis, defined as loss of CSF around the cord or, in more extreme cases, deformation of the spinal cord, whether documented by CT myelography, MRI, or standard myelography, is a more accurate measure of stenosis (4).

TREATMENT

Conservative treatment:
- Cervical immobilization
- Restriction of high-risk activities, including avoidance of collision sports and sports with high potential for cervical load
- Physical therapy for gait training
- Pain management with analgesics, muscle relaxants, antidepressants, or anticonvulsants

ADDITIONAL THERAPIES
- After the first episode of neurapraxia, if the initial workup is negative for stenosis, a generalized neck strengthening program should be started.
- Athletes involved in collision sports should be able to support their body weight with the cervical spine in neutral and in all directions when positioned at a 45-degree angle.

SURGERY/OTHER PROCEDURES
- Surgical interventions involve anterior cervical discectomy and corpectomy with fixation. Posterior approaches include laminectomy and laminoplasty (2).
- If an acquired cause for spinal stenosis is detected, consultation with a neurosurgeon or orthopedic spine surgeon for consideration of surgery can be undertaken.
- Surgery should also be considered in athletes with progressive deterioration and/or myelopathy causing neurologic deficits.
- 20–60% of patients with CSM will deteriorate neurologically over time without surgical intervention (1).
- However, after surgery, the athlete probably cannot participate in contact/collision sports.

ONGOING CARE

FOLLOW-UP RECOMMENDATIONS
- Team physicians should be concerned with functional spinal stenosis. If present, and the athlete incurs spinal cord symptoms, the athlete should not continue in contact/collision sports because such activities predispose athletes to a worse neurologic outcome in the context of cervical spine injuries (4).
- Data collected by the NCCSIR from 1987 to 1996 showed that no athlete with functional spinal stenosis and cervical spinal fracture recovered from quadriplegia:
  - This finding needs to be compared with nearly 20% of athletes with cervical spinal fracture and normal canal sizes who had initial quadriplegia and recovered fully.
  - During the same period, in all cases of quadriplegia without cervical spinal fracture dislocation, severe spinal stenosis was present.
- If the athlete redevelops neurapraxia, the workup should proceed again, from plain radiographs to MRI or CT myelography.
- According to a review performed by Torg et al., 56% of National Football League players with one episode of neurapraxia went on to develop a repeat episode after return to play (3).
- Given the excellent sensitivity of the Torg ratio, any athlete with an abnormal ratio along with spinal cord symptomatology should undergo MRI, myelography, or CT myelography (4).
- If surgery is deferred, close neurologic follow-up is recommended.

REFERENCES

1. Karadimas SK, Erwin WM, Ely CG, et al. Pathophysiology and natural history of cervical spondylotic myelopathy. *Spine (Phila Pa 1976)*. 2013;38(22 Suppl 1):S21–S36.
2. Nouri A, Tetreault L, Singh A, et al. Degenerative cervical myelopathy: epidemiology, genetics, and pathogenesis. *Spine (Phila Pa 1976)*. 2015;40(12):E675–E693.
3. Torg JS, Pavlov H, Genuario SE, et al. Neurapraxia of the cervical spinal cord with transient quadriplegia. *J Bone Joint Surg Am*. 1986;64(9):1354–1370.
4. Cantu RC. Cervical spine injuries in the athlete. *Semin Neurol*. 2000;20(2):173–178.
5. Scheer JK, Tang JA, Smith JS, et al. Cervical spine alignment, sagittal deformity, and clinical impressions. *J Neurosurg*. 2013;19(2):141–159.
6. Eddy D, Congeni J, Loud K. A review of spine injuries and return to play. *Clin J Sport Med*. 2005;15(6):453–458.

CLINICAL PEARLS

- During preparticipation physical examination, it is critical to determine of any prior history of spinal cord–related neurologic events, and consider imaging before allowing the athlete to begin contact/collision sports.
- Although subtle gait dysfunction is the most common presentation of CSM, bilateral upper and lower motor neuron findings are common.
- Cervical spine x-rays are the initial radiographic modality, which can be used to evaluate for gross fracture or dislocation, whereas MRI/CT myelography provide a more accurate measure of spinal cord pathology.
- Cervical immobilization, restriction of high-risk activities, physical therapy, and pain management are the initial treatment steps.
- Surgical intervention is considered for acquired causes of spinal stenosis, failure to respond to conservative care, or progressive deterioration and/or myelopathy.

CERVICAL STRAINS

Jeffrey M. Mjaanes, MD, CAQSM, FAAP, FACSM • Ryan P. Cole, MD, CAQSM

BASICS

DESCRIPTION

- Cervical strain refers to a stretch-type injury within the muscle substance or at the myotendinous junction of the cervical and upper back muscles. In addition to the muscle and tendons, injury may involve the ligamentous structures of the cervical spine.
- Synonym(s): cervical sprain; whiplash (whiplash-associated disorders)

EPIDEMIOLOGY

- Most frequently caused by whiplash injury, that is, hyperextension of the cervical spine from a rear-end motor vehicle collision
- >1 million cases per year are reported in the United States; more common in urban areas with a greater number of motor vehicles
- Higher incidence seen in females
- More common in adults than children (especially persons ages 30 to 50 yr)
- Incidence associated with sports is unknown.
- In general, collision sports are responsible for a high number of injuries to the head and neck.

ETIOLOGY AND PATHOPHYSIOLOGY

- In sports, cervical strain often occurs as the result of a blow to the head or neck during muscular contraction. In motor vehicle accidents, the causative force is usually a rear-end collision leading to a hyperextension then hyperflexion of the neck. The applied force often creates an eccentric contraction causing microscopic or gross tensile failure, most often at the myotendinous junction and in ligamentous structures.
- Muscles with high ratios of type II or fast-twitch muscle fibers demonstrate a higher risk for strains or shearing-type injuries.
- Cervical strains can also be chronic in nature and related to repetitive stress or abnormal postural biomechanics.

RISK FACTORS

Speculated: age, level of conditioning, prior history of neck injury, cervical degenerative disc disease, head position at time of impact, mechanism of injury, personality traits, and psychosocial factors

DIAGNOSIS

HISTORY

- When taking the history, it is essential to determine the mechanism of injury. For example, if the injury is the result of a motor vehicle accident, important information includes the approximate speed of the vehicles, the location of the patient within the vehicle (driver, front seat passenger, etc.), and whether the patient was restrained.
- Onset, time course, and location of symptoms (Anatomical pain drawings may be helpful in providing an overview of the pain pattern.)
- Presence of any neurologic symptoms and course: upper or lower extremity sensory changes, pain radiating into the arms past the elbows, or weakness in upper extremities
- Activities and head positions that aggravate or alleviate symptoms
- Prior episodes of similar symptoms, previous neck injury or surgery
- Previous treatment, including modalities, medications, physical therapy, traction, manipulation, injection, and surgical treatments
- Social history, including level of physical activity, occupation, job satisfaction, ongoing litigation, and use of nicotine, alcohol, and/or other substances
- Pain is the most common presenting complaint in cervical strains. Frequently, patients may have minimal pain immediately after the injury but have increasing pain severity several hours to days later. Pain may be referred to the shoulder, upper limb, and occipital or temporal regions of the head.
- Soft tissue swelling may be present.
- Muscle spasm or tightness
- Limitation in range of motion at the neck
- Neck fatigue, stiffness, pain at rest and/or with movement
- Other symptoms may include unusual skin sensations at head/face, dizziness, lightheadedness, concentration and memory deficits, tinnitus, blurred vision, hearing difficulties, and other cranial nerve deficit complaints.

PHYSICAL EXAM

- Observation: head and neck posture, movement during normal conversation, weak or stiff movement
- Range of motion: active range of motion, usually reduced, particularly in directions stretching the injured muscles
- Palpation: tenderness, usually noted along the cervical paraspinal muscles; may be present along muscles where symptoms are referred, muscles with associated hypertonicity, or "spasm"
- Generally normal neurologic examination, although subjective sensory deficits may be present
- Careful manual muscle testing for evidence of deficits in myotomal distribution
- Sensory examination for dermatomal deficits in sensation, hyperesthesia, inconsistent or "nonanatomical" pattern
- Deep tendon reflexes/muscle stretch reflexes and Hoffman or Babinski signs helpful in identifying myelopathy, radiculopathy, and brachial plexopathy
- By definition, all provocative tests are negative in an isolated soft-tissue strain.
- Spurling test is performed by extending the neck and rotating the head, and then applying downward pressure on the head. Considered positive if pain radiates into the limb ipsilateral to the side the head is rotated; specific but not sensitive in diagnosing acute radiculopathy
- Lhermitte sign is performed by passively flexing the neck. Considered positive if "electric-like" sensation radiates down the spine; positive with cervical stenosis, myelopathy, spinal cord injury due to tumor, multiple sclerosis, and other conditions
- Axial compression test is performed by gently applying an axially directed pressure on top of the seated patient's head. The patient's neck is in neutral. Pain radiating distal to the elbow is considered positive for likely radicular origin. Manual distraction often greatly reduces neck and limb symptoms in patients with radiculopathy.

DIFFERENTIAL DIAGNOSIS

- In evaluation of the patient with acute and subacute neck pain, it is essential to rule out more serious conditions, such as fractures, dislocations, instability, and spinal cord injury. In chronic neck pain, other diagnoses, such as neoplasia, must be considered.
- Differential diagnosis includes:
  - Cervical fracture.
  - Cervical instability, subluxation, or dislocation.
  - Disc annulus fibrosis injury.
  - Facet joint injury.
  - Myofascial pain.
  - Cervical radiculopathy.
  - Myelopathy.
  - Brachial plexus injury.
  - Thoracic outlet syndrome.
  - Peripheral nerve entrapment (e.g., suprascapular nerve).

DIAGNOSTIC TESTS & INTERPRETATION

Initial Tests (lab, imaging)

- In the management of cervical strain, radiographs are usually not necessary. In trauma patients, however, plain radiographs are used to rule out other potentially serious conditions, such as fractures or dislocations.
- Minimum views include anteroposterior, lateral, and oblique cervical spine views for evidence of acute fracture or subluxation with trauma.
- Open mouth view for evidence of atlantoaxial instability and odontoid fractures. Flexion and extension lateral views are helpful to look for evidence of spinal instability.
- According to the National Emergency X-Radiography Utilization Study (NEXUS) low-risk criteria, cervical spine radiography is indicated for patients with trauma unless they meet all of the following five criteria:
  - No posterior midline cervical spine tenderness
  - No evidence of intoxication
  - A normal level of alertness
  - No focal neurologic deficit
  - No painful distracting injuries
- Computed tomography (CT) offers superior sensitivity for detection of acute fractures than plain radiographs. When combined with myelography, CT has significant sensitivity and specificity for radiculopathy and stenosis.
- Magnetic resonance imaging (MRI) is the study of choice to detect soft tissue pathology including disc or ligament disruption, nerve root or spinal cord compression/injury.
- MRI is also indicated for patients with deterioration in neurologic findings in order to detect spinal cord changes.

Diagnostic Procedures/Other

- Electrodiagnostic studies used to diagnose nerve root dysfunction when the diagnosis is uncertain or to distinguish a cervical radiculopathy from other lesions that are unclear on physical examination
- Ideally performed 3 or more weeks after injury because diagnostic abnormalities will first be seen 18 to 21 days after the onset of radiculopathy

TREATMENT

- Early discussion involving reassurance, treatment, recovery, and maintaining daily activity as tolerated are important in the initial management.
- A multimodal treatment approach (medications, soft tissue treatment, stretching, exercises as tolerated) has been shown to be superior to a minimal intervention approach (advice and medications only) (1)[A].
- Acute treatment directed at reducing pain and inflammation. Therapies include local icing, nonsteroidal anti-inflammatory drugs (NSAIDs), and avoidance of positions that increase symptoms. Patient should be encouraged to be as active as pain allows; bed rest is discouraged.

- In addition to NSAIDs, other pharmacologic therapies include muscle relaxants to decrease spasm and tonicity and other analgesics such as acetaminophen. Narcotic analgesics are often used for pain relief, but in general, their use should be limited due to the potential of opioid-associated side effects.
- Consider myofascial trigger point injections or modalities such as electrical stimulation if pain not controlled by initial therapies in the acute phase.
- Gentle stretching; first passive mobilization and then active to begin to reestablish nonpainful range of motion
- Gentle strengthening: isometric cervical strengthening in a single plane (flexion, extension, lateral flexion, rotation), scapular stabilization, and cervicothoracic stabilization programs. All exercises should be performed without pain.
- If unable to engage cervicothoracic region due to persistent pain, consider isometric strengthening of uninvolved musculature (i.e., quadriceps). This has been shown to help decrease pain in chronic whiplash-associated disorders (2)[C].
- Low-level aerobic cross-training (e.g., stationary bike, stair stepper, treadmill, aquatic running, etc.) begun as soon as tolerated to avoid deconditioning.
- Use of soft and rigid collars for cervical strain management is controversial and has not been proven effective. Several randomized studies, including one by Kongsted et al. in 2007, showed no significant difference in outcomes (headache and neck pain intensity, disability, and work capability) between those treated with immobilization and those treated with an "act-as-usual" approach (3)[A].
- Recover phase directed toward normalizing active range of motion, neuromuscular control, strength, and posture
- Progressive passive and active stretching, mobilization, and manipulation as appropriate
- Progressive strengthening (isometric to isotonic) with independent single-plane and complex multiple-plane coordinated motions to include cervicothoracic, scapulothoracic, and scapulohumeral stabilization activities
- Maintenance phase directed toward sport/activity-specific training
- Guidelines for returning to competition: no pain at rest, full pain-free range of motion, normal posture, normal strength, and normal physical examination; athletes should not return to competition until they can perform at the level of their preinjury abilities.
- Prehospital:
  - Any victim of blunt cervical trauma who is unconscious, *or* conscious and complaining of neck pain or extremity paresthesias/paralysis should be assumed to have a cervical spine injury. The cervical spine must be stabilized and the patient transported to the emergency department (ED) on a backboard and with a semirigid cervical collar in place (4)[B].
- ED treatment:
  - All posttrauma patients with cervical pain should be "clinically cleared" using NEXUS low-risk criteria or the Canadian C-spine rule to guide the use of cervical spine radiography.
  - Initial treatments for cervical strain include:
    - Ice, analgesics or NSAIDs, muscle relaxants.

MEDICATION

- Analgesics, such as acetaminophen, can be used in the acute phase for pain relief.
- NSAIDs have anti-inflammatory as well as analgesic effects and are often used successfully in the management of cervicalgia. Examples include ibuprofen and naproxen.
- Muscle relaxants are often prescribed acutely as adjunct therapy to decrease the spasm and hypertonicity experienced in acute muscle strain.

ADDITIONAL THERAPIES

- Follow-up is recommended to ensure there has been no deterioration in symptoms or exam findings. Ideally, patients should follow up with their primary care physician within 1 wk.
- Often, referral to physical therapy may be necessary, especially in patients who have significant spasm and decreased cervical motion.
- For chronic pain, consider adding supervised exercise programs such as tai chi, qigong, or yoga (5)[A].
- Therapy focusing on progressive motion, stretching, and finally strengthening is often beneficial. Vassiliou et al. demonstrated in a randomized controlled trial involving 200 patients with whiplash injury that those who participated in a consistent physical therapy regimen had decreased pain intensity scores after 6 wk and 6 mo compared to controls (4,6)[A].
- Osteopathic manipulation may be helpful in treating cervical strains. Avoid manipulation in the following scenarios: focal neurologic deficits, severe cervical spasm or pain, advanced age, rheumatoid arthritis, point tenderness over bone, cervical fusion or fracture, osteoporosis, and cervical laxity.
- Acupuncture
- Ultrasound
- Topical analgesic creams

ONGOING CARE

COMPLICATIONS

Neck strain can result in stiffening in the cervical region with resultant decreased motion. The prolonged muscle spasm itself can become a source of long-term pain and disability. Morbidity from cervical strains comes from disuse, weakness, and spasm. Cervical strain can lead to chronic pain syndromes in certain patients.

REFERENCES

1. Sutton DA, Côté P, Wong JJ, et al. Is multimodal care effective for the management of patients with whiplash-associated disorders or neck pain and associated disorders? A systematic review by the Ontario Protocol for Traffic Injury Management (OPTIMa) Collaboration. *Spine J*. 2016;16(12):1541–1565.
2. Smith A, Ritchie C, Pedler A, et al. Exercise induced hypoalgesia is elicited by isometric, but not aerobic exercise in individuals with chronic whiplash associated disorders. *Scand J Pain*. 2017;15:14–21.
3. Kongsted A, Qerama E, Kasch H, et al. Neck collar, "act-as-usual" or active mobilization for whiplash injury? A randomized parallel-group trial. *Spine (Phila Pa 1976)*. 2007;32(6):618–626.
4. Vassiliou T, Kaluza G, Putzke C, et al. Physical therapy and active exercises—an adequate treatment for prevention of late whiplash syndrome? Randomized controlled trial in 200 patients. *Pain*. 2006;124(1–2):69–76.
5. Southerst D, Nordin MC, Côté P, et al. Is exercise effective for the management of neck pain and associated disorders or whiplash-associated disorders? A systematic review by the Ontario Protocol for Traffic Injury Management (OPTIMa) Collaboration. *Spine J*. 2016;16(12):1503–1523.
6. Dorshimer GW, Kelly M. Cervical pain in the athlete: common conditions and treatment. *Prim Care*. 2005;32(1):231–243.

ADDITIONAL READING

- Bogduk N, Teasell R. Whiplash: the evidence for an organic etiology. *Arch Neurol*. 2000;57(4):590–591.
- Cantu R, Bailes J, Wilberger JE Jr. Guidelines for return to contact or collision sport after a cervical spine injury. *Clin Sports Med*. 1998;17(1):137–146.
- Cole AJ, Farrell FP, Stratton SA, et al. Cervical spine athletic injuries: a pain in the neck. *Phys Med Rehabil Clin N Am*. 1994;5(1):37–68.
- Eyre A. Overview and comparison of NEXUS and Canadian C-spine rules. *Am J Med*. 2006;3(4):12–15.
- Johnson G. Hyperextension soft tissue injuries of the cervical spine—a review. *J Accid Emerg Med*. 1996;13(1):3–8.
- Jónsson H Jr, Cesarini K, Sahlstedt B, et al. Findings and outcome in whiplash-type neck distortions. *Spine (Phila Pa 1976)*. 1994;19(24):2733–2743.
- Lagattuta FP, Falco FJE. Assessment and treatment of cervical spine disorders. In: Braddom RL, ed. *Physical Medicine Rehabilitation*. 1st ed. Philadelphia, PA: WB Saunders; 1996:747–748.
- Malanga GA. The diagnosis and treatment of cervical radiculopathy. *Med Sci Sports Exerc*. 1997;29(Suppl 7):S236–S245.
- Maujean A, Sterling J, Sterling M. What information do patients need to know following a whiplash injury? The perspectives of patients and physiotherapists. *Disabil Rehabil*. 2018;40(10):1135–1141.
- Panjabi M, Vasavada A, White AA III, et al. Cervical spine biomechanics. *Semin Spine Surg*. 1993;5:10–16.
- Pettersson K, Hildingsson C, Toolanen G, et al. Disc pathology after whiplash injury. A prospective magnetic resonance imaging and clinical investigation. *Spine (Phila Pa 1976)*. 1997;22(3):283–288.
- Ronnen HR, de Korte PJ, Brink PR, et al. Acute whiplash injury: is there a role for MR imaging?—a prospective study of 100 patients. *Radiology*. 1996;201(1):93–96.
- Squires B, Gargan MF, Bannister GC. Soft-tissue injuries of the cervical spine. 15-year follow-up. *J Bone Joint Surg Br*. 1996;78(6):955–957.
- Sturzenegger M, DiStefano G, Radanov BP, et al. Presenting symptoms and signs after whiplash injury: the influence of accident mechanisms. *Neurology*. 1994;44(4):688–693.
- Torg JS, Glasgow SG. Criteria for return to contact activities following cervical spine injury. *Clin J Sports Med*. 1991;1:12–26.
- Zmurko M, Tannoury T, Tannoury C, et al. Cervical sprains, disc herniations, minor fractures, and other cervical injuries in the athlete. *Clin Sports Med*. 2003;22(3):513–521.

CLINICAL PEARLS

- Cervical strain is common and is usually a benign, self-limited condition.
- Management should be multimodal including analgesics, muscle relaxers, soft tissue massage/mobilization, and various exercises.
- Care must be taken not to miss more serious conditions such as fractures or dislocations, especially in patients with acute neck pain.
- Victims of trauma with neck pain or tenderness and unconscious victims need to be treated with cervical stabilization until the spine can be fully evaluated with imaging.
- At 1 to 10 yr after whiplash injury associated with motor vehicle trauma, 60–80% of patients are asymptomatic and only 5–15% are severely symptomatic. Prognosis associated with sports activities is believed to be excellent, although no data are available.

CLIMBING INJURIES

Ilona Barash, MD, PhD, CAQSM

BASICS

DESCRIPTION

- Rock climbing is becoming more mainstream with the range of climbing styles, including competitive indoor climbing and outdoor pursuits such as bouldering, sport climbing, and traditional climbing to big wall and alpine climbing seeing increased popularity.
- Climbing-related injuries are categorized as:
  - Impact injury from either the climber falling or something falling onto the climber, nonimpact acute injury, chronic overuse injuries.
- Focus will be on finger injuries because these are fairly climbing specific.

EPIDEMIOLOGY

Incidence

- Estimates vary but approximately 4.2 injuries per 1,000 participation hours (1).
- Career incidence 1.5 to 4.2 injuries per subject
- Overuse injuries are most common (2).

Prevalence

Estimates vary, approximately:

- 10–81% irrespective of cause.
- 10–50% impact injuries.
- 28–81% nonimpact acute injury.
- 33–44% chronic overuse injury.

ETIOLOGY AND PATHOPHYSIOLOGY

Finger injuries represent 33–52% of all injuries:

- Most commonly middle and ring fingers
- Annular pulleys most commonly injured:
  - Five pulleys per finger: A1, A2, A3, A4, A5
  - A2 (proximal phalanges) and A4 (distal phalanges) directly attached to underlying bone
- Grip: method by which climber holds the rock
- Crimp: proximal interphalangeal joint (PIPJ) flexed to 100 degrees, distal interphalangeal (DIP) hyper-extended to 120 degrees. Thumb over index finger; highest force and also highest likelihood of injury to A2 pulley
- Open handed: thumb not in contact with index finger, PIPJ not as flexed, DIP somewhat flexed; less force on A2, more on A4

RISK FACTORS

Inconsistent data, but the following factors may affect risk of injury:

- Intrinsic: sex, age, skill level, experience, body mass index (BMI), grip strength
- Extrinsic: type of climbing (indoor vs. outdoor, lead climbing vs. top roping vs. bouldering), climbing volume, climbing intensity, drugs/alcohol

GENERAL PREVENTION

- No consistent reduction in injury with warm-up or stretching
- Taping fingers/wrists and weight training may help.
- Avoid sudden increases in load or training intensity.

COMMONLY ASSOCIATED CONDITIONS

- Impact: fractures (usually lower extremity), abrasions/lacerations, head injuries, ankle sprains, knee ligament injuries, spinal fractures
- Nonimpact: finger pulley injury, strain finger flexor tendon or joint capsule, capsulitis, superior labrum anterior and posterior (SLAP) tear
- Overuse: tenosynovitis, epicondylitis, shoulder impingement, Dupuytren disease, ganglion cyst

Pregnancy Considerations

- Data are very limited on the safety of climbing while pregnant.
- One study showed no difference in preterm birth in women who climbed (3).
- Generally recommended to limit lead climbing and fall potential (even while bouldering) during pregnancy, but no evidence that top roping in itself is harmful (3)[B]

DIAGNOSIS

HISTORY

- Sudden versus gradual onset
- May report hearing or feeling a "pop" if finger pulley rupture with sudden pain and reduced grip strength

PHYSICAL EXAM

- Pain and tenderness palmar aspect of pulley site
- Often accompanied by swelling +/− bruising
- Pain with grip testing, reduced grip strength
- Sometimes reduced range of motion of fingers or chronic PIPJ flexion contracture
- Grade 4: may have palpable or visible bowstringing

DIFFERENTIAL DIAGNOSIS

- Other relatively climbing-specific upper extremity injuries include:
  - Hamate fractures.
  - Epiphyseal overuse fractures in fingers.
  - Third or fourth lumbrical tear.
- Common upper extremity/hand injuries in climbers, not climbing specific:
  - Flexor tendinopathies
  - Capsular inflammation
  - Extensor hood rupture
  - Collateral ligament damage
  - Osteoarthritis
  - Medial > lateral epicondylitis
  - De'Quervain tenosynovitis
  - Intersection syndrome
  - Rotator cuff injuries
  - Shoulder impingement syndrome
  - SLAP tears
  - Biceps tendinopathy

DIAGNOSTIC TESTS & INTERPRETATION

Initial Tests (lab, imaging)

- X-ray
- Ultrasound:
  - A2 pulley rupture will show >2 mm of dehiscence between tendon and bone, also known as bowstringing.
  - Pulley strain if <2 mm dehiscence
  - Can have chronic dehiscence without acute rupture
- Magnetic resonance imaging (MRI):
  - Sagittal MRI with fingers flexed may show the 2 mm dehiscence.
- Grading:
  - Grade 1: pulley strain
  - Grade 2: rupture of A4 or partial rupture of A2 or A3
  - Grade 3: complete rupture of A2 or A3
  - Grade 4: multiple pulley ruptures (A2/A3, A2/A3/A4) or A2 or A3 plus collateral ligament or lumbrical rupture

Pediatric Considerations
- Epiphyseal fractures of the PIPJ in adolescent sport climbers have been reported.
- Increased risk with dynamic finger training such as use of a campus board
- Pain and/or tenderness of dorsal aspect of the PIPJ, usually middle or ring finger
- Must be recognized and treated to avoid premature growth plate closure

TREATMENT

GENERAL MEASURES
- Conservative measures usually work.
- Relative rest
- Taping (see below)
- Progressive resistance training
- Climber's media (magazines and Web sites) and fellow climbers are full of rehabilitation advice.

MEDICATION

First Line
Nonsteroidal anti-inflammatory drugs (NSAIDs), topical or systemic

Second Line
Corticosteroids (4)[C]:
- Only for chronic tendinitis or tenosynovitis who have failed conservative treatment
- Great caution needed to avoid causing rupture
- Generally not indicated

COMPLEMENTARY & ALTERNATIVE MEDICINE
- Conservative treatment for grade 1 to 2 injuries (4,5)[C]:
  - Immobilization 10 to 14 days in palmar splint with metacarpophalangeal joint in flexion, interphalangeal joints in extension or slight flexion
  - Functional rehabilitation
  - Consider pulley protection splint with taping or soft ring splint.
- Grade 3 injuries (4,5)[C]:
  - Resume easy sport-specific activity in 6 to 8 wk.
  - Consider pulley protection with tape or ring for 6 mo after injury.
- Taping (4,5)[C]:
  - Consider for prophylactic and therapeutic uses after injury.
  - H-tape figure-of-8 technique resulting in slight PIPJ flexion may help.

ISSUES FOR REFERRAL
- Grade 4 injury: high-grade pulley injury associated with ligamentous or lumbrical injury
- Surgical intervention may be needed with return to full climbing in 6 mo (4,5)[C].
- Failure of conservative therapy

ADDITIONAL THERAPIES
Time for full return to climbing:
- Pulley strain: 6 wk
- Pulley rupture: 6 to 12 wk
- High-grade injury: 6 mo
- A4 generally heals faster than A2.

SURGERY/OTHER PROCEDURES
- Palmaris longus tendon graft or extensor retinaculum in a loop:
  - Allows early active motion
  - Multiple methods reconstruct the pulley.
- Most climbers can return to previous level of climbing after surgery.

ADMISSION, INPATIENT, AND NURSING CONSIDERATIONS
Not routine

ONGOING CARE

FOLLOW-UP RECOMMENDATIONS
- Consider taping for prolonged period after injury.
- Physical therapy and strengthening exercises can continue indefinitely:
  - Finger tendon glides (gradual flexion of all finger joints from distal to proximal and then reverse this)
  - Strengthening: rubber bands, putty, grip balls, fingers moving in rice

Patient Monitoring
Worsening pain/symptoms should prompt further assessment.

PATIENT EDUCATION
- Appropriate rest and rehab is key.
- Consider H taping—the climbing literature has good resources for how to do this effectively.

PROGNOSIS
Most climbers will recover from pulley injury with minimal complications, if they follow sufficient rehabilitation.

COMPLICATIONS
- Chronic stiffness
- Further injury

REFERENCES

1. Woollings KY, McKay CD, Emery CA. Risk factors for injury in sport climbing and bouldering: a systematic review of the literature. *Br J Sports Med*. 2015;49(17):1094–1099.
2. Schöffl V, Popp D, Küpper T, et al. Injury trends in rock climbers: evaluation of a case series of 911 injuries between 2009 and 2012. *Wilderness Environ Med*. 2015;26(1):62–67.
3. Drastig J, Hillebrandt D, Rath W, et al. Pregnant women in sport climbing—is there a higher risk for preterm birth? *Z Geburtshilfe Neonatol*. 2017;221(1):25–29.
4. King E, Lien J. Flexor tendon pulley injuries in rock climbers. *Hand Clin*. 2017;33(1):141–148.
5. Jones G, Johnson MI. A critical review of the incidence and risk factors for finger injuries in rock climbing. *Curr Sports Med Rep*. 2016;15(6):400–409.

ADDITIONAL READING
Gnecchi S, Moutet F. *Hand and Finger Injuries in Rock Climbers*. New York, NY: Springer; 2015.

CLINICAL PEARLS
- Finger pulley injuries are a relatively common, climbing-specific injury.
- Most will respond well to conservative therapy.
- Refer the high-grade/grade 4 injuries to a hand surgeon for evaluation.
- The high forces and unique stresses imposed by climbing result in some unique injuries, either from acute trauma or overuse.

COMPARTMENT SYNDROME, ANTERIOR

Brian Lowell, MD, CAQSM

BASICS

DESCRIPTION

- Chronic exertional compartment syndrome (CECS) is a rare condition that can cause significant pain to the lower extremity.
- Cases have been reported in the forearm, thigh, and foot, but the majority are reported in the lower leg.
- CECS is caused by an increase in interstitial pressure in a closed fascial compartment, which leads to ischemic pain that may be associated with paresthesias and muscular dysfunction.
- CECS can be easily misdiagnosed due to the vague nature of symptoms experienced by the patient. Delayed diagnosis can increase severity of condition.
- It is seen in a variety of sports, but most often those associated with lower extremity stresses:
  - Runners.
  - Soccer players.
  - Speed skaters.
  - Military populations (marching).
- The anterior compartment is most commonly affected and consists of the tibialis anterior, extensor hallucis longus, extensor digitorum longus, peroneus tertius, and deep peroneal nerve. The other compartments of the lower extremity include the lateral (peroneal longus, peroneus brevis, and superficial peroneal nerve), the superficial posterior (gastrocnemius, soleus, plantaris, and tibial nerve), and the deep posterior (tibialis posterior, flexor hallucis longus, flexor digitorum longus, popliteus, and the tibial nerve).

EPIDEMIOLOGY

Incidence

- CECS has an incidence reported at up to 27–33% in competitive athletes with pain related to exercise.
- Described in athletic populations at a rate of approximately 0.49 cases per 1,000 person-years
- Younger patients more likely to develop CECS. Mean age of presentation is in the late 20s.

Prevalence

- The prevalence of CECS decreases with age.
- Male > female (1)

ETIOLOGY AND PATHOPHYSIOLOGY

The etiology of CECS is unknown. The most described theory involves transient ischemia during exercise caused by an increase in intramuscular pressure which compromises blood supply to the affected compartment.

RISK FACTORS

- Rapid increase in repetitive activity
- Participation in high-risk sport activities
- Significant musculature of the lower extremity
- Diabetes mellitus

DIAGNOSIS

HISTORY

- Typically, no associated trauma or injury
- Pain is described as fullness, cramp-like, or tightness.
- Pain reoccurs consistently with specific amounts of exertion (time, distance, or intensity).
- Pain is typically bilateral in nature.
- Pain generally associated with neurologic abnormalities that include paresthesia or weakness (e.g., foot drop).
- Symptoms generally resolve <30 min after cessation of inciting activity.

PHYSICAL EXAM

- Exam is usually normal at rest. A physical exam without abnormal findings largely assists in narrowing the differential.
- Postexertional examination can greatly assist with diagnosis of CECS. Following exertion, pain may become present, muscle/facial tightness may be palpable, and neurovascular abnormalities may become present. Passive stretching of the muscles in the affected compartment may also cause pain.

DIFFERENTIAL DIAGNOSIS

- Acute compartment syndrome
- Stress fracture
- Medial tibial stress syndrome
- Fascial hernia
- Tendonitis
- Popliteal artery entrapment syndrome
- Peripheral nerve entrapment
- Thrombosis
- Peripheral vascular disease

DIAGNOSTIC TESTS & INTERPRETATION

Initial Tests (lab, imaging)

- Radiographs, magnetic resonance imaging (MRI), and computed tomography (CT) are not useful in diagnosis of CECS but are instead used to evaluate for other causes of lower extremity pain, such as stress reactions or tumors.
- MRI/magnetic resonance angiography (MRA) is useful in identifying popliteal artery entrapment.

Diagnostic Procedures/Other

- Needle manometry is currently the gold standard test of choice.
- Intracompartmental pressure measurements before and after exercise are useful in validating the clinical diagnosis of CECS. Although scrutinized, most clinicians use the modified Pedowitz criteria to indicate a positive test (2)[C]:
  - Preexercise pressure ≥15 mm Hg
  - 1-min postexercise pressure ≥30 mm Hg
  - 5-min postexercise pressure ≥20 mm Hg (2)

TREATMENT

GENERAL MEASURES

- Conservative measures have largely been lacking evidence and include stretching, prolonged rest, decreasing activity levels, avoiding activities that exacerbate symptoms, and orthoses (2)[C].
- Physical therapy to address any biomechanical predisposition

C

MEDICATION

No evidence for benefit with pharmacologic intervention; specifically nonsteroidal anti-inflammatory drugs (NSAIDs) or acetaminophen

ADDITIONAL THERAPIES

Nonsurgical therapeutic modalities have recently been studied in small number, some with promising results. These conservative therapies include the following:

- Massage: no change in postexercise compartment pressure, but decrease in postexercise pain (3)[C]
- Gait changes: Forefoot training led to a significant change in compartment pressure postintervention (3)[C].
- Chemodenervation: treatment via botulinum toxin A assisted with pain relief; however, there were concerns with lower extremity weakness associated with such therapies (3)[C].
- Ultrasound-guided fascial fenestration: no significant surgical risks. Full return to sport without reoccurring pain. Case report; further research needed (3)[C]

SURGERY/OTHER PROCEDURES

- Surgery is the definitive treatment. The gold standard is decompressive fasciotomy (4)[C].
- Surgery consists of a fasciotomy of the affected compartment or compartments; open or endoscopic. Endoscopic release is hypothesized to decrease surgical healing time and minimize risk for dehiscence. There is no evidence for improvement in postsurgical fibrosis formation.
- Studies report satisfactory results in 60–80% of patients. Greater successes were seen with anterior compartment intervention, whereas less favorable outcomes were seen with intervention to the other three compartments.
- Common surgical complications include infection, wound dehiscence, bleeding, hematoma, nerve injury (peroneal neuritis), venous injury (saphenous), and inadequate release of fascia during initial surgical intervention and postsurgical fibrosis.
- Reoccurring symptoms are seen in approximately 20–30% of postsurgical patients and typically occur from localized muscle constrictions secondary to fibrosis (4).
- Special considerations:
  - Acute compartment syndrome and acute exertional compartment syndrome are different from CECS:
    - Acute compartment syndrome: typically associated with fracture or crush injury
    - Acute exertional compartment syndrome: commonly associated with significant increase in activity
  - Remember pain out of proportion to physical exam along with neurovascular abnormalities on physical exam at rest.
  - The acute compartment syndromes are surgical emergencies that must be treated with emergent fasciotomy to avoid muscle necrosis (5).

ONGOING CARE

- Very little literature on rehabilitation after fasciotomy
- Small study rehabilitation protocol includes:
  - Crutches for ambulation immediately postfasciotomy.
  - Remove crutches when one can bear weight without significant limp.
  - Control swelling with ice, elevation, and compression.
  - Gait training and progression to full weight-bearing.
  - Progressive strengthening of the lower extremity with goal of sport-specific training between 6 and 8 wk (6).
- >80% of elite athletes return to previous sports participation in 8 to 12 wk.

REFERENCES

1. de Bruijn JA, van Zantvoort APM, van Klaveren D, et al. Factors predicting lower leg chronic exertional compartment syndrome in a large population. *Int J Sports Med*. 2018;39(1):58–66.
2. Vajapey S, Miller T. Evaluation, diagnosis, and treatment of chronic exertional compartment syndrome: a review of current literature. *Phys Sportsmed*. 2017;45(4):391–398.
3. Rajasekaran S, Hall MM. Nonoperative management of chronic exertional compartment syndrome: a systematic review. *Curr Sports Med Rep*. 2016;15(3): 191–198.
4. Campano D, Robaina JA, Kusnezov N, et al. Surgical management for chronic exertional compartment syndrome of the leg: a systematic review of the literature. *Arthroscopy*. 2016;32(7):1478–1486.
5. Livingston KS, Meehan WP III, Hresko MT, et al. Acute exertional compartment syndrome in young athletes: a descriptive case series and review of the literature. *Pediatr Emerg Care*. 2018;34(2):76–80.
6. Irion V, Magnussen RA, Miller TL, et al. Return to activity following fasciotomy for chronic exertional compartment syndrome. *Eur J Orthop Surg Traumatol*. 2014;24(7):1223–1228.

ADDITIONAL READING

Roscoe D, Roberts AJ, Hulse D. Intramuscular compartment pressure measurement in chronic exertional compartment syndrome: new and improved diagnostic criteria. *Am J Sports Med*. 2015;43(2):392–398.

CLINICAL PEARLS

- Typical presentation is a young athlete who has recurrent lower extremity pain that is aggravated with repetitive activity and alleviated with rest.
- A high index of suspicion if athletes endorse symptoms, but physical exam findings on exam are benign
- The diagnosis of CECS is clinical. Needle manometry assists with diagnosis.
- Surgical treatment via fasciotomy is the gold standard, but successful treatment of pain may be achieved with nonsurgical interventions.
- Surgical treatment success rates are high, but complications and postsurgical reoccurrences are seen.

COMPLEX REGIONAL PAIN SYNDROME

Julio A. Martinez-Silvestrini, MD, FAAPMR, CAQSM • Daniel Kuo, DO, MA

BASICS

DESCRIPTION

- Severe, continuing pain, disproportionate to any inciting event
- Manifested by four clinical characteristics: based on Budapest criteria:
  - Intense pain
  - Vasomotor disturbances
  - Sudomotor (sweat glands) disturbances, as increased sweating or clammy skin
  - Various associated motor or trophic changes
- Functional recovery delay may be observed if the patient is not treated properly.
- A consensus statement grouped several previously identified syndromes as "complex regional pain syndrome" (CRPS):
  - CRPS type I
  - Not related to a nerve injury
  - 90% of CRPS cases
  - CRPS type II ("causalgia")
  - Directly related to a nerve injury
  - The clinical syndrome is diffuse and not following the usual nerve injury distribution of pain and muscle dysfunction.
- Also known as:
  - Reflex sympathetic dystrophy
  - Shoulder-hand syndrome
  - Sudeck atrophy

EPIDEMIOLOGY

- Adult:
  - Female: male = 4:1
  - Median age at onset: 46 yr (1)[C]; incidence may vary (40 to 70 yr). This large variability has been attributed to differences in ethnic and socioeconomic background of the cohorts as well as the application of the diagnostic criteria (2)[C].
  - Upper limb twice as common as lower limb
  - Most report a triggering event
  - Most common trigger: fracture (46%)
  - Most common triggering fracture: distal radius:
    - Only 1% of radius fractures develop CRPS.
  - Incidence following peripheral nerve injury: 2–14%
- Children:
  - Majority are female (67–86%).
  - Symptoms typically start just prior to puberty.
  - Lower limb more likely to be involved than upper limb (5:1)
  - Often less clear inciting event
  - Higher recurrence rate
  - More responsive to treatment than adults

Incidence

5.46 per 100,000 person-years at risk (1,2)[C]

Prevalence

20.57 per 100,000 person-years

ETIOLOGY AND PATHOPHYSIOLOGY

Pathogenesis is unclear, but several theories exist:

- Reflex arc following inciting event
- Sympathetic nerve reflex arc causes central sympathetic dysfunction, causing peripheral vascular dysfunction.
- Increased sensitivity of injured nerves to endocrine and paracrine substances
- Inappropriate inflammatory mediator control (especially interleukin [IL]-6, IL-1β, tumor necrosis factor [TNF]-α, substance P, neuropeptide, and calcitonin gene-related peptide)
- Several studies have demonstrated central nervous system (CNS) modulation as cause of CRPS.
- A model of "neurogenic inflammation" attempts to tie the above theories together into a unifying theory of pathogenesis.

Genetics

Human leukocyte antigen (HLA) type:

- Increased incidence in those with HLA-A3, B7, and DR2 (15)
- HLA-DR2 (15) may predict poor treatment outcome.
- HLA testing has no role in clinical management of CRPS.
- No specific single-gene polymorphisms have been clearly linked to CRPS.

RISK FACTORS

- Precipitating event (adults):
  - Fracture
  - Surgery (especially arthroscopic procedures)
  - Sprain
  - Myocardial infarction
  - Hemiplegia
  - Immobilization (bracing, casting, stroke)
  - Placement of arteriovenous graft for hemodialysis
  - Peripheral nerve injury
  - May be observed in the absence of a precipitating event
- Precipitating event (children):
  - 50% have a vague, minor, or no precipitating event:
    - Sprains
    - Strains
    - Minor contusions
  - Surgery (especially arthroscopic procedures of the knee)
  - Henoch-Schönlein purpura
  - Emotional stress
  - Injections or vaccination
- Constitutional or psychiatric predisposition:
  - Suspected by many clinicians but no evidence to support
  - Clearly not present in most patients with CRPS
  - "Sympathetic hyperreactors" described as those with a history of increased sweating in the palms, poor cold tolerance, and emotional lability

GENERAL PREVENTION

- Stroke:
  - Early mobilization following stroke decreases risk of CRPS.
  - Limited evidence supports early mobilization following injury and myocardial infarction.
- Fracture:
  - Recent studies suggest that vitamin C supplementation is not effective in preventing CRPS (3)[A].
- Regional anesthesia:
  - Intravenous regional anesthesia (IVRA) is commonly used to provide anesthesia during extremity surgery.
  - IVRA with or without clonidine may decrease the chance of developing postsurgical CRPS (1)[C].

COMMONLY ASSOCIATED CONDITIONS

- Precipitating injury or event
- Possible psychiatric or personality disorders
- Other pain syndromes have been reported as associated conditions:
  - May represent heterogeneity of a single disease or susceptible phenotype

DIAGNOSIS

- Clinical diagnosis
- Positive response to sympathetic block confirms the presence of sympathetically mediated pain.
- Laboratory and imaging studies are only indicated if diagnosis is uncertain.

HISTORY

- Stage 1: early disease following inciting event or spontaneous initiation:
  - Nondermatomal progressive limb pain
  - Burning pain
  - Occasional throbbing
  - Diffuse aching
  - Sensitivity to cold and/or touch
  - Localized edema
- Stage 2: progressive physical changes (see "Physical Exam"):
  - Progressive functional limitation
- Stage 3: severe disease:
  - Worsening pain
  - Permanent functional limitation
  - Increasingly dramatic physical findings (see "Physical Exam")
- Other symptoms (not stage specific): urinary urgency, frequency, and/or incontinence

PHYSICAL EXAM

- Stage 1:
  - Allodynia
  - Localized edema
  - Vasomotor disturbances:
    - Color changes
    - Temperature changes (usually cool but can be warm)
- Stage 2:
  - Progressively worsening soft tissue edema
  - Thickening of the skin
  - Muscle wasting
  - Dystonia
- Stage 3:
  - Joint contractures
  - Waxy appearance to skin
  - Brittle nails
- Other findings (not stage specific):
  - Hyperhidrosis
  - Abnormal hair growth (patchy, sparse, or excessive hair)
  - Urinary retention
- Budapest criteria (3)[A]:
  - Must report at least one symptom in three of the four following categories:
    - Sensory: hyperalgesia and/or allodynia
    - Vasomotor: temperature asymmetry and/or skin color changes
    - Sudomotor/edema: edema and/or sweating changes and/or sweating asymmetry
    - Motor/trophic: decreased range of motion and/or motor dysfunction (weakness, tremor, dystonia) and/or trophic changes (hair, nails, skin)
  - Must display at least one sign at time of evaluation in two or more of the following categories:
    - Sensory: hyperalgesia (to pinprick) and/or allodynia (severe pain with light skin stroking, touch, local temperature changes, or joint movement):
      - Vasomotor: temperature asymmetry and/or skin color changes
      - Sudomotor/edema: edema and/or sweating changes
      - Motor/trophic: decreased range of motion and/or motor dysfunction
  - There is no other diagnosis that better explains the signs and symptoms.

DIFFERENTIAL DIAGNOSIS

- Fracture/stress fracture
- Infection
- Tumor (especially Pancoast syndrome)
- Nerve root impingement
- Vasculitis
- Rheumatoid arthritis
- Peripheral neuropathy
- Deep vein thrombosis
- Angioedema
- Other pain syndromes

DIAGNOSTIC TESTS & INTERPRETATION

Initial Tests (lab, imaging)

- Tests to exclude other systemic causes of pain:
  - Complete blood count (CBC)
  - Erythrocyte sedimentation rate (ESR)
  - Fasting blood glucose
  - Serum ionized calcium level
  - Thyroid-stimulating hormone and free thyroxine (T_4) levels

C

- Bone scan (triple-phase technetium-99m bone scintigraphy):
  - Increased uptake in 2/3 of adult patients with reflex sympathetic dystrophy
  - Findings vary by phase:
    - 30 sec: increased flow but decreased tracer uptake in affected limb
    - 3 min: capillary leak around affected joint
    - 3 hr: increased uptake of tracer at periarticular bone of affected joint
  - Findings less reliable in pediatric patients:
    - 1/3 exhibit increased uptake (usually in late stages of disease).
    - 1/3 exhibit normal findings.
    - 1/3 exhibit decreased uptake (usually in early stages).
  - Can also be used to help rule out other diagnoses, such as stress fracture or tumor
- Plain radiography:
  - Initially normal
  - After 3 mo, may show patchy subchondral osteopenia
  - Late stages show profound bone demineralization.
  - Radiographic findings are less common in children.
- Magnetic resonance imaging (MRI):
  - Multiple nonspecific changes (edema, skin thickening)
  - Useful to rule out constant stimulants (such as meniscal tear or loose body)
- Thermography:
  - Significant skin temperature asymmetry
  - Cold challenge may increase sensitivity and specificity.
- Computed tomography (CT) scan:
  - Focal areas of osteoporosis
  - "Swiss cheese" appearance of bone in stage 3 CRPS can be dramatic.
  - Costs, radiation dose, and poor sensitivity and specificity limit use.

Diagnostic Procedures/Other

- Autonomic testing:
  - Resting sweat output (RSO)
  - Resting skin temperature (RST)
  - Quantitative sudomotor axon reflex test (QSART)
  - Abnormal RSO and QSART are highly sensitive for CRPS.
  - Use of these tests should be limited to patients with uncertain diagnosis.
- Sympathetic blockade:
  - Typically causes abrupt improvement in symptoms
  - Those with cool affected limbs typically have increase of 1–3°C in skin temperature.
  - Lack of response has high negative predictive value.
  - Relief is typically transient.
  - Stellate or lumbar sympathetic blocks are more diagnostically useful than regional blocks (e.g., Bier block, although both may provide relief of symptoms).
  - This procedure can be done with fluoroscopic or ultrasound guidance.

TREATMENT

- Usually more effective early in disease (4)[B]
- Follow a stepwise approach, starting with least risky/invasive and progressing to more invasive as needed (1)[C].
- An interdisciplinary program seems to be the most effective approach to CRPS (1)[C]:
  - Physical therapy
  - Occupational therapy
  - Psychotherapy
  - Medications
  - Interventional procedures

MEDICATION

First Line

- Bisphosphonates and short course of steroids are recommended early in the disease (1)[B],(5)[A]:
  - Pamidronate, alendronate, and clodronate have been the most studied.
- Tricyclic antidepressants have been shown to decrease pain in multiple studies and should be considered (1)[C].

Second Line

- Antiepileptic drugs:
  - Thoroughly tested for other pain syndromes but cannot extrapolate results to CRPS
  - Gabapentin most widely used, but studies have demonstrated variable efficacy
  - Pregabalin is also widely used but has not been studied for treatment of CRPS.
- Selective serotonin and norepinephrine reuptake inhibitors have not been studied for treatment of CRPS.
- Topical capsaicin cream is effective in other types of neuropathic pain. It is generally safe and may be a useful adjuvant treatment for CRPS (1)[C].
- Ketamine may decrease pain immediately with effects lasting up to 3 mo (3)[A].
- Opioid use should be limited (4)[C].
- Several other medications have been reported to be effective in small trials but are rarely used:
  - Free radical scavengers (dimethyl sulfoxide and *N*-acetylcysteine)
  - Topical and epidural clonidine
  - Intrathecal agents
  - Memantine
  - Botulism toxin
  - Plasma exchange
  - Chemotherapeutic agents

ADDITIONAL THERAPIES

- Physical therapy is the mainstay of CRPS treatment.
- Tactile desensitization is most effective if used early.
- Joint mobilization, progressive weight-bearing, strengthening, and return to daily activities are important aspects of care directed by physical therapy.
- Transcutaneous electrical nerve stimulation can be beneficial.
- Behavioral management
- Relaxation techniques
- Stress management
- Mirror therapy
- Aerobic exercise
- Somatosensory rehabilitation (6)[B]

SURGERY/OTHER PROCEDURES

- Nerve blockade:
  - Sympathetic nerve blockade can be both therapeutic and diagnostic:
    - Lumbar sympathetic block for lower extremity
    - Stellate ganglion block for upper extremity
  - Unclear which patients are good candidates for sympathetic blocks
  - Unpredictable response to repeated sympathetic blocks
- Spinal cord stimulation:
  - Improves pain and quality of life (3)[A]
- Other interventional procedures:
  - Peripheral nerve stimulation
  - Chemical and surgical sympathectomy
  - Implanted spinal infusion pumps and/or intrathecal injections:
    - Baclofen may be useful if significant dystonia.
  - Deep brain stimulation

COMPLEMENTARY & ALTERNATIVE MEDICINE

Acupuncture:

- Popular complementary therapy
- High patient satisfaction
- Well-designed studies have shown no difference when compared to placebo (4)[C].
- May have a role as part of an interdisciplinary approach to CRPS

ONGOING CARE

FOLLOW-UP RECOMMENDATIONS

A strong partnership with the patient and all participating caregivers is essential, including pain management specialists, physiatrists, psychiatrists and other behavioral health specialists, and physical and occupational therapists.

Patient Monitoring

- Weekly or biweekly follow-up is appropriate.
- Have a flexible treatment plan:
  - Stepwise approach to care
  - Therapeutic trials of only 1 to 2 wk before moving on to the next treatment modality

PROGNOSIS

- Early diagnosis and treatment can lead to resolution by 6 to 12 mo.
- Late diagnosis is associated with permanent residual symptoms.
- Children are more likely to relapse than adults.
- Three distinct phases (described above):
  - Patients in stage 1 and 2 respond better to therapy.
  - Stage 3 disease is often more refractory to treatment.

REFERENCES

1. Hsu ES. Practical management of complex regional pain syndrome. *Am J Ther*. 2009;16(2):147–154.
2. Goh EL, Chidambaram S, Ma D. Complex regional pain syndrome: a recent update. *Burns Trauma*. 2017;5:2.
3. Urits I, Shen AH, Jones MR, et al. Complex regional pain syndrome, current concepts and treatment options. *Curr Pain Headache Rep*. 2018;22(2):10.
4. Dowd GS, Hussein R, Khanduja V, et al. Complex regional pain syndrome with special emphasis on the knee. *J Bone Joint Surg Br*. 2007;89(3):285–290.
5. Duong S, Bravo D, Todd KJ, et al. Treatment of complex regional pain syndrome: an updated systematic review and narrative synthesis. *Can J Anaesth*. 2018;65(6):658–684.
6. Packham TL, Spicher CJ, MacDermid JC, et al. Somatosensory rehabilitation for allodynia in complex regional pain syndrome of the upper limb: a retrospective cohort study. *J Hand Ther*. 2018;31(1):10–19.

ADDITIONAL READING

- American Academy of Orthopaedic Surgeons. Complex regional pain syndrome. In: Armstrong AD, Hubbard MC, eds. *Essentials of Musculoskeletal Care*. 5th ed. Rosemont, IL: American Academy of Orthopaedic Surgeons; 2016:65–71.
- Tran J, Ramachandran VS, Altschuler EL. Complex regional pain syndrome. In: Frontera WR, Silver JK, Rizzo TD, eds. *Essentials of Physical Medicine and Rehabilitation*. 3rd ed. Philadelphia, PA: Elsevier; 2015:495–499.

C

CLINICAL PEARLS

- Clinical diagnosis of an exaggerated response to injury of a limb with intense prolonged pain, vasomotor disturbances, delayed functional recovery, and trophic changes
- Pathology is unclear, but there is central sympathetic dysregulation that causes or modulates peripheral symptoms.
- Diagnostic tests should be reserved for unclear cases and to rule out other diagnoses.
- Treatment should be initiated immediately at diagnosis and follow a rapid stepwise approach from least to most invasive.
- In patients with an unclear but high level of suspicion of CRPS, an oral steroids taper and gabapentin can be used safely with minimal adverse effects, if not contraindicated. In some instances, early intervention may prevent the development of the syndrome.

CONCUSSION

Marc P. Hilgers, MD, PhD, FAAFP

BASICS

DESCRIPTION

- Sport-related concussion (SRC) is a traumatic brain injury (TBI) induced by biomechanical forces.
- The clinical signs and symptoms cannot be explained by drug, alcohol, or medication use; other injuries (e.g., cervical injuries, peripheral vestibular dysfunction); or other comorbidities (e.g. psychological factors or coexisting medical conditions).
- Several common features that may be used in clinically defining the nature of a concussive head injury include:
  - SRC may be caused either by a direct blow to the head, face, neck, or elsewhere on the body with an impulsive force transmitted to the head.
  - SRC typically results in the rapid onset of short-lived impairment of neurologic function that resolves spontaneously. However, in some cases, signs and symptoms evolve over a number of minutes to hours.
  - SRC may result in neuropathologic changes, but the acute clinical signs and symptoms largely reflect a functional disturbance rather than a structural injury and, as such, no abnormality is seen on standard structural neuroimaging studies.
  - SRC results in a range of clinical signs and symptoms that may or may not involve loss of consciousness (LOC). Resolution of the clinical and cognitive features typically follows a sequential course. However, in some cases symptoms may be prolonged (1).
  - Synonym(s): mild TBI; minor head trauma; commotio cerebri; MTBI; mild TBI, SRC

EPIDEMIOLOGY

- 207,830 emergency department (ED) visits for nonfatal sports-related TBIs per year between 2001 and 2005 (2)
- In 2012, an estimated 329,290 children (age 19 yr or younger) were treated in U.S. EDs for sports and recreation-related injuries that included a diagnosis of concussion or TBI (3).
- 1.6 to 3.8 million concussions per year in the United States; falls, motor vehicle accidents, and assaults being the most common etiologies
- 20% are sports related, but percentage is higher in adolescents.
- Adolescents (aged >11 yr) percentage of concussions related to sports activity is much greater (41%) than for younger children (8%) (4,5,6,7).
- Before age 10 yr, children tend to sustain concussions primarily from non–sports-related falls and then transition to sports-related injuries after age 10 yr (4,5,6,7).
- Limitations in that data only evaluate certain organized sports and do not include all sports or recreational activities.
- There might also be some overreporting of concussions because many athletes, parents, health care providers do not know what exactly a concussion is, and therefore might make that diagnosis when something else is more likely.
- The incidence may be higher because athletes, coaches, or medical providers may fail to recognize the signs and symptoms of a concussion or athletes try to minimize the symptoms in order to continue to play (8,9).
- Self-reported concussion rates have not changed significantly, but the rate at which athletes report suspected concussions has increased significantly (78.6% in 2013 vs. 47.3% in 1999 to 2002) (10).
- In a study of high school and collegiate athletes, almost 3/4 withheld information about a concussion because they did not think their symptoms needed medical care. Almost 2/3 wanted to avoid being withheld from play, and a little >1/3 simply lacked understanding of concussion (10).
- Possible underreporting of concussion especially in children because many do not seek medical care (9)
- Some evidence of a higher reported incidence of concussion in female high school and college athletes even when comparing the same sports; the reason is unclear but could be due to more honest reporting of concussion in females (9,11).
- 572 concussions per year for college athletes between 1988 and 2004 (12)
- 54.8% of the total concussions during that period of time occurred in American football (12).
- Women's soccer, men's ice hockey, men's soccer, and women's basketball each represented between 5% and 7% of total college concussions for the same time period (12).
- Given the limitations in epidemiology, more research is necessary addressing SRC in all populations.

ETIOLOGY AND PATHOPHYSIOLOGY

- Complicated pathophysiology that is incompletely understood (9,13,14)
- Impact and resulting forces create shear injury to vessels and neurons (9,14).
- Biochemical chain reactions are set in place, some of which may involve the release of excitatory amino acids (9,14,15).
- Resulting decrease in cerebral metabolism occurs (9,14,15).
- Temporarily decreased cerebral blood flow
- Alternatively, the blow may create immediate neuronal depolarization followed by a refractory period where neural transmission does not happen (14).

RISK FACTORS

- The most consistent risk predictor of slower recovery is the severity of the acute and subacute symptoms. Subacute headaches (HAs) or depression is likely a risk factor for persistent symptoms lasting a month or more. Preexisting mental illnesses also appear to have a greater risk for persistent symptoms. Contrary to prior belief, a learning disability or ADHD does not appear to carry a substantially greater risk. Teenage years, in particular high school, might be the most vulnerable time period for having persistent symptoms, with greater risk for girls than for boys (16); participation in contact and collision sports (2,8,9,12)
- An athlete with more than one previous concussion may be more likely to have a repeat concussion or any other injury than an athlete without a history of a concussion (8).
- Improper technique (e.g., leading with the head, or "spearing," in football) (12), heat exposure (17)
- Investigations ongoing as to the significance of apolipoprotein (Apo) E4, ApoE promoter gene, tau polymerase, and others in concussion (13,14)

GENERAL PREVENTION

- Helmets are not designed to prevent concussions but instead to prevent skull fractures.
- Mouth guards do not prevent concussion but do decrease dental and orofacial injuries (9,13,18).
- Rules that promote safe and proper techniques (e.g., outlawing "spearing" in football, leading with the head, and head-to-head contact) should be coached and enforced to limit concussion (12,13,15).
- Encourage fair competition but discourage violent behavior in sports, especially among young athletes (13).

DIAGNOSIS

- SRC is a TBI induced by biomechanical forces.
- The diagnosis of a concussion is a clinical assessment.

HISTORY

- Direct blow to the head, sudden rotational or acceleration–deceleration force to the head in the absence of direct trauma, or transmitted force to head from blow to other body parts (19)
- Athletes often fail to recognize or report their symptoms. Concussion should be considered in anyone demonstrating signs of a concussion (1,9).
- Standardized symptom checklists such as the one found in the Sport Concussion Assessment Tool 5 (SCAT5 or Child SCAT5) that allow the athlete to score his or her complaints on a scale of 0 to 6 may be useful when evaluating the concussed athlete (1,13)[C].

- Athletes may complain of any of the following: HA or neck pain; feeling off-balance or dizzy; nausea or vomiting; problems with vision or hearing including ringing in the ears; confusion; slowness, fatigue, or sleepiness; irritability or other emotional problems; concentration difficulty; memory problems; "dinged"; "dazed"; or "don't feel right" (8)[B].
- Prospectively validated symptoms include HA, dizziness, blurred vision, attention deficit, memory problems, and nausea (8)[A].
- On-field:
  - Use of SCAT5, providing standardized on-field and off-field assessment of SRC
  - Address airway, breathing, and circulation (ABCs) (9)[C].
  - Consider cervical spine (C-spine) immobilization (all unconscious athletes should have C-spine immobilization) (9)[C].
  - In general, do not remove the helmet in football or ice hockey players if C-spine injury is suspected (19)[C].
  - Prehospital helmet removal might be indicated if (20):
    - The helmet and chin strap fail to hold the head securely.
    - The helmet and chin strap design prevent adequate airway control, even after facemask removal.
    - The facemask cannot be removed.
    - The helmet prevents adequate proper immobilization for transport.
  - Assess level of consciousness with the Glasgow Coma Scale (GCS) as part of the SCAT5 (19)[C].
  - Evaluate for other trauma such as skull fractures (including basilar skull fractures) or lacerations (19)[C].
  - Perform a neurologic exam, including cognitive evaluation and balance assessment (19)[C].
  - Conscious athletes in whom C-spine trauma is not suspected may exit the field and undergo a more thorough exam (19)[C].
  - Immediately transfer athletes with prolonged LOC, focal neurologic deficits, including asymmetric pupils and declining GCS or worsening symptoms, athletes with comorbidities (e.g., hemophiliacs), and those with persistent vomiting (8)[C].

PHYSICAL EXAM

- The suspected diagnosis of SRC can include one or more of the following clinical domains:
  - Symptoms: somatic (e.g., HA), cognitive (e.g., feeling like in a fog), and/or emotional symptoms (e.g., lability)
  - Physical signs (e.g., LOC, amnesia, neurologic deficit)
  - Balance impairment (e.g., gait unsteadiness)
  - Behavioral changes (e.g., irritability)
  - Cognitive impairment (e.g., slowed reaction times)
  - Sleep/wake disturbance (e.g., somnolence, drowsiness)
- Remove a player who shows any signs or symptoms of an SRC:
  - The player should be evaluated by a physician or other licensed health care provider on site using standard emergency management principles, and particular attention should be given to excluding a C-spine injury:
    - The appropriate disposition of the player must be determined by the treating health care provider in a timely manner. If no health care provider is available, the player should be safely removed from practice or play and urgent referral to a physician arranged.
    - Once the first aid issues are addressed, an assessment of the concussive injury should be made using the SCAT5 or other sideline assessment tools.
    - The player should not be left alone after the injury, and serial monitoring for deterioration is essential over the initial few hours after injury.
    - A player with diagnosed SRC should not be allowed to return to play (RTP) on the day of injury (1).
- The SCAT5 was developed by the 5th International Conference on Concussion in Sport and incorporates two prospectively validated tests, the Maddocks score and the Standardized Assessment of Concussion (SAC), into a comprehensive tool (8,13,21).
- The on-field includes a C-spine assessment, GCS, Maddocks, and observable signs.
- The off-field includes history, GCS, SAC with now 5 to 10 words, the Modified Balance Error Scoring System (m-BESS) and a new neurologic screening exam, as well as disposition recommendations, RTP, and Return to learn sections (1).
- The SCAT5 should not be used as the only tool to diagnose concussions, to determine whether recovery has occurred, or to decide when to allow an athlete to RTP (13,21)[C].

DIFFERENTIAL DIAGNOSIS

- Subdural hematoma, which may be acute or subacute (22)
- Epidural hematoma, which can result in rapid deterioration after a "lucid interval" (22)
- Intraparenchymal hemorrhage (22)
- Diffuse axonal injury (DAI) or shear injury to white matter that leads to prolonged LOC and often causes residual deficits (22)
- Second impact syndrome (SIS) is a rare yet often fatal process that occurs when an athlete who has not recovered completely from one concussion sustains a second blow to the head. Cerebral edema and increased intracranial pressure result. The patient can decline rapidly as cerebral herniation occurs (9).
- Other medical conditions, including trauma-induced migraine, peripheral vestibular dysfunction, C-spine injury, medical or psychological comorbidities

DIAGNOSTIC TESTS & INTERPRETATION

Initial Tests (lab, imaging)

- Research conducted on more severe head injury suggests that many genetic and cytokine factors are induced (23).
- As yet, the significance of these factors in concussion is not fully known, and no routine laboratory testing is recommended (23).
- Cranial computed tomography (CT) scan: useful in acute imaging to rule out intracranial bleed. Consider if prolonged LOC or if symptoms are worsening or failing to resolve in a timely manner (1,8,13)[C].
- The Centers for Disease Control and Prevention (CDC) recommends against routine CT scans (in pediatric patients) (24).
- Imaging usually contributes little to routine concussion management (1,8,13).
- Magnetic resonance imaging (MRI) modalities such as gradient echo and perfusion and diffusion imaging may diagnose structural lesions better than CT scan, but routine use of MRI does not add to concussion evaluation (1,13)[C].
- Functional MRI (fMRI) may illustrate degree of symptoms and their resolution but is not yet part of standard concussion management (1,13).
- Experimental imaging technology includes positron emission tomography (PET), diffusion tensor imaging, MRI spectroscopy, magnetoencephalography (MEG), and functional connectivity (1,13).

Diagnostic Procedures/Other

- Neuropsychological (NP) testing can be used to assess cognitive function and help with RTP decisions (1,13)[A].
- Usually, but not always, conducted when the athlete is asymptomatic as a final measure before clearance for RTP (8)[C]
- Cognitive function often resolves after other symptoms, so NP evaluation can add helpful information but sometimes athletes will have normal NP tests despite being symptomatic (1,13)[A].
- Should not be used as the only factor in deciding if an athlete should RTP (1,8,13)[C]
- Consider in the case of a concussion with modifiers/risk factors (1,13)[C].
- Computerized NP tests facilitate administration and interpretation (1,8).
- Most computerized test results include a postconcussion symptom scale, attention, memory, processing speed, and reaction time measures (8).
- Comparing preinjury NP baseline testing with postinjury testing is helpful but not necessary. Using a test that accounts for confounding factors (e.g., a practice effect) that occur with serial tests is critical (1,8,15,25)[C].

- The Reliable Change Index describes test–retest reliability and is a feature available with computerized tests (25).
- A neuropsychologist may administer other formal NP testing if necessary; neuropsychologists are typically the most qualified to interpret NP tests (1,13)[C].
- Vestibular testing may add valuable information, especially when the athlete is showing signs of postural instability (13)[A].
- The BESS evaluates the ability of a person to hold without "error" three positions (legs together, single-leg stance, and tandem stance) with eyes closed and hands on the hips. The test is conducted on a firm and a foam surface and can be performed on the sideline or in the training room (8).
- BESS has been prospectively validated (8)[A].
- BESS has a demonstrated practice effect.
- An m-BESS is one component of the SCAT5.
- More advanced, computer-based vestibular testing can be done in an office setting for more objective data.

TREATMENT

- Base treatment on an individual basis according to the burden, nature, and duration of symptoms and other individual factors (e.g., other preexisting medical and psychological factors, sport, position).
- On-field management as above (1,8,13,19)[C]
- Patient monitoring:
  - A patient should not be left unsupervised following a concussion (1,13)[C]. There is no indication for the need to wake up the patient from sleep, which had been recommended historically.
  - A patient should be monitored for the following: focal neurologic deficit, declining mental status or LOC, and uncontrolled vomiting (8)[C].
  - Emergent medical care should be sought if any of the preceding occur (8)[C].

ONGOING CARE

FOLLOW-UP RECOMMENDATIONS

- After sustaining a concussion, an athlete should be evaluated by a medical professional prior to RTP (19)[C].
- Acetaminophen may be used to treat HA or other pain, but nonsteroidal anti-inflammatory drugs (NSAIDs) and aspirin should be avoided initially.
- Athletes also should avoid sedating medicines or substances such as alcohol that may affect cognitive function. There is currently insufficient evidence that prescribing complete rest achieves the desired objectives. After a brief period of rest during the acute phase (24 to 48 hr) after injury to ease discomfort and to promote recovery by minimizing brain energy demands, patients can be encouraged to become gradually and progressively more active while staying below their cognitive and physical symptom-exacerbation thresholds (i.e., activity level should not bring on or worsen their symptoms). It is reasonable for athletes to avoid vigorous exertion while they are recovering. The exact amount and duration of rest is not yet well defined in the literature and requires further study (21).
- After the symptoms have started to resolve without the use of medicine to mask complaints and an athlete sees a medical provider, a gradual RTP process as well as a return to academics is typically recommended. It is important to be honest about the presence of symptoms because there is some evidence that if someone is incompletely recovered from a concussion and sustains another blow to the head, SIS, a rare yet often fatal process, can occur (9,21,26).
- The 5th International Concussion in Sport Consensus Statement reviews RTP and return to academics (1).
- RTP/return to academics:
  - At present, it is reasonable to conclude that the large majority of injured athletes recover, *from a clinical perspective*, within the 1st mo of injury (1).
  - A six-step graduated RTP protocol is endorsed in the work of the Concussion in Sport Group and by the American College of Sports Medicine (1,13,15,27,28)[C].
  - Athletes progress through each step for a period of at least 24 hr. Before moving forward in the protocol, athletes must be asymptomatic and not taking any drugs that would change or hide their symptoms.
  - If symptoms develop at one stage, the athlete should stop the attempt. Another attempt to progress to the next level can occur the following day.
  - The six steps are as follows: no activity, light aerobic exercise, sport-specific training, noncontact training drills, full contact practice, and RTP.
  - A similar step-by-step protocol should be used to reintroduce academics into the concussed patient's life. One of those protocols could include (each involving no [increased] symptoms for at least 24 hr):
    - Passive participation for a half day, passive participation for a full day, own note taking, taking homework, untimed tests, full participation.

PROGNOSIS

- For most athletes, cognitive deficits, balance, and symptoms improve rapidly during the first 2 wk after injury. There is a sizeable minority of youth, high school, and collegiate athletes who take much longer than 10 days to clinically recover and return to sport.
- 70% of school-aged children show symptom resolution in 28 days (29).

COMPLICATIONS

- Mental illness (depression has been most frequently studied) is reported in retired former professional football players at higher incidence in those with a history of three or more concussions compared with those without (13,30,31,32).
- Mental health issues are common in adolescents and young adults, and often present at this time, despite no involvement in contact or collision sport.
- Chronic traumatic encephalopathy or cognitive impairment is more common in the brains of retired National Football League (NFL) players who donated their brains postmortem (33).
- A small number of patients may develop postconcussion syndrome (PCS) (14,34).
- There are limited data on the incidence and characterization of PCS, especially with respect to sports-related concussions (14,35).
- PCS is characterized by persistent cognitive trouble (concentration deficits, memory difficulty), physical complaints (HA, fatigue), or emotional disturbances (irritability, depression) (22,34).
- NSAIDs and antidepressants are used commonly to treat PCS, and psychological treatment might become necessary (35).
- Athletes should not RTP when still symptomatic (1, 8,9,13,15,27,28).
- No evidenced-based guidelines exist for temporary or permanent disqualification after concussion (21).
- Retirement from sports participation may be considered in the case of continued symptoms or objective exam findings, situations where a lesser impact creates concussion symptoms and the athlete takes longer to recover, or when an athlete sustains multiple concussions (21). These decisions must be individualized.

REFERENCES

1. McCrory P, Meeuwisse W, Dvořák J, et al. Consensus statement on concussion in sport—the 5th international conference on concussion in sport held in Berlin, October 2016. *Br J Sports Med*. 2017;51(11):838–847.
2. Goldberg LD, Dimeff RJ. Sideline management of sport-related concussions. *Sports Med Arthrosc Rev*. 2006;14(4):199–205.
3. Coronado VG, Haileyesus T, Cheng TA, et al. Trends in sports- and recreation-related traumatic brain injuries treated in US emergency departments: the National Electronic Injury Surveillance System-All Injury Program (NEISS-AIP) 2001-2012. *J Head Trauma Rehabil*. 2015;30(3):185–197.
4. Meehan WP III, Mannix R. Pediatric concussions in United States emergency departments in the years 2002-2006. *J Pediatr*. 2010;157(6):889–893.

5. Bakhos LL, Lockhart GR, Myers R, et al. Emergency department visits for concussion in young child athletes. *Pediatrics*. 2010;126(3):e550–e556.
6. Buzzini SR, Guskiewicz KM. Sport-related concussion in the young athlete. *Curr Opin Pediatr*. 2006;18(4):376–382.
7. Karlin AM. Concussion in the pediatric and adolescent population: "different population, different concerns." *PM R*. 2011;3(10 Suppl 2):S369–S379.
8. Meehan WP III, Bachur RG. Sport-related concussion. *Pediatrics*. 2009;123(1):114–123.
9. McCrea M, Hammeke T, Olsen G, et al. Unreported concussion in high school football players: implications for prevention. *Clin J Sport Med*. 2004;14(1):13–17.
10. LaRoche AA, Nelson LD, Connelly PK, et al. Sport-related concussion reporting and state legislative effects. *Clin J Sport Med*. 2016;26(1):33–39.
11. Hootman JM, Dick R, Agel J. Epidemiology of collegiate injuries for 15 sports: summary and recommendations for injury prevention initiatives. *J Athl Train*. 2007;42(2):311–319.
12. McCrory P, Johnston KM, Mohtadi NG, et al. Evidence-based review of sport-related concussion: basic science. *Clin J Sport Med*. 2001;11(3):160–165.
13. Centers for Disease Control and Prevention. Nonfatal traumatic brain injuries from sports and recreation activities—United States, 2001–2005. *MMWR Morb Mortal Wkly Rep*. 2007;56(29):733–737.
14. McIntosh AS, McCrory P, Finch CF, et al. Does padded headgear prevent head injury in rugby union football? *Med Sci Sports Exerc*. 2009;41(2):306–313.
15. Aubry M, Cantu R, Dvorak J, et al. Summary and agreement statement of the First International Conference on Concussion in Sport, Vienna 2001. Recommendations for the improvement of safety and health of athletes who may suffer concussive injuries. *Br J Sports Med*. 2002;36(1):6–10.
16. Iverson GL, Gardner AJ, Terry DP, et al. Predictors of clinical recovery from concussion: a systematic review. *Br J Sports Med*. 2017;51(12):941–948.
17. Sakurai A, Atkins CM, Alonso OF, et al. Mild hyperthermia worsens the neuropathological damage associated with mild traumatic brain injury in rats. *J Neurotrauma*. 2012;29(2):313–321.
18. Concussion (mild traumatic brain injury) and the team physician: a consensus statement. *Med Sci Sports Exerc*. 2006;38(2):395–399.
19. McCrory P, Makdissi M, Davis G, et al. Value of neuropsychological testing after head injuries in football. *Br J Sports Med*. 2005;39(Suppl 1):i58–i63.
20. Inter-Association Task Force for the Appropriate Care of the Spine-Injured Athlete. Prehospital care of the spine-injured athlete. http://www.nata.org/statements/consensus/NATAPreHospital.pdf. Accessed November 14, 2018.
21. Sport concussion assessment tool—5th edition. *Br J Sports Med*. 2017;51(11):851–858.
22. Guskiewicz KM, Marshall SW, Bailes J, et al. Association between recurrent concussion and late-life cognitive impairment in retired professional football players. *Neurosurgery*. 2005;57(4):719–726.
23. McCrea M, Meier T, Huber D, et al. Role of advanced neuroimaging, fluid biomarkers and genetic testing in the assessment of sport-related concussion: a systematic review. *Br J Sports Med*. 2017;51(12):919–929.
24. Lumba-Brown A, Yeates KO, Sarmiento K, et al. Centers for Disease Control and Prevention guideline on the diagnosis and management of mild traumatic brain injury among children. *JAMA Pediatr*. 2018;172(11):e182853.
25. Bailes JE, Cantu RC. Head injury in athletes. *Neurosurgery*. 2001;48(1):26–46.
26. Broglio SP, McCrea M, McAllister T, et al; and CARE Consortium Investigators. A national study on the effects of concussion in collegiate athletes and US Military Service Academy members: the NCAA–DoD Concussion Assessment, Research and Education (CARE) consortium structure and methods. *Sports Med*. 2017;47(7):1437–1451.
27. McCrory P, Johnston K, Meeuwisse W, et al. Summary and agreement statement of the 2nd International Conference on Concussion in Sport, Prague 2004. *Clin J Sport Med*. 2005;15(2):48–55.
28. Wojtys EM, Hovda D, Landry G, et al. Current concepts. Concussion in sports. *Am J Sports Med*. 1999;27(5):676–687.
29. Zemek R, Barrowman N, Freedman SB, et al; for Pediatric Emergency Research Canada (PERC) Concussion Team. Clinical risk score for persistent postconcussion symptoms among children with acute concussion in the ED. *JAMA*. 2016;315(10):1014–1025.
30. Kerr ZY, Marshall SW, Harding HP Jr, et al. Nine-year risk of depression diagnosis increases with increasing self-reported concussions in retired professional football players. *Am J Sports Med*. 2012;40(10):2206–2212.
31. Gouttebarge V, Aoki H, Lambert M, et al. A history of concussions is associated with symptoms of common mental disorders in former male professional athletes across a range of sports. *Phys Sportsmed*. 2017;45(4):443–449.
32. Manley G, Gardner AJ, Schneider KJ, et al. A systematic review of potential long-term effects of sport-related concussion. *Br J Sports Med*. 2017;51(12):969–977.
33. Lee LK. Controversies in the sequelae of pediatric mild traumatic brain injury. *Pediatr Emerg Care*. 2007;23(8):580–586.
34. Ryan LM, Warden DL. Post concussion syndrome. *Int Rev Psychiatry*. 2003;15(4):310–316.
35. Kirkwood MW, Yeates KO, Wilson PE. Pediatric sport-related concussion: a review of the clinical management of an oft-neglected population. *Pediatrics*. 2006;117(4):1359–1371.

ADDITIONAL READING

- SCAT5: http://bjsm.bmj.com/content/bjsports/early/2017/04/26/bjsports-2017-097506SCAT5.full.pdf
- Child SCAT5: http://bjsm.bmj.com/content/bjsports/early/2017/04/28/bjsports-2017-097492childscat5.full.pdf
- Dick RW. Is there a gender difference in concussion incidence and outcomes? *Br J Sports Med*. 2009;43(Suppl 1):i46–i50.

CLINICAL PEARLS

- No RTP while symptomatic
- No RTP the same day
- The younger the patient, the longer the likely recovery
- Receiving a second blow to the head (even a minor one) while still suffering from the effects of the original concussion can lead to SIS, which results in severe brain swelling and often death.
- A stepwise and gradual return to academic and physical activities should occur after the patient is no longer experiencing debilitating symptoms. Developing any symptoms during this program will require additional time before proceeding.
- Sometimes additional testing such as balance testing or formal NP testing may be necessary.
- Evidence exists that three or more concussions are associated with a general increase in injuries, mental illness, slowed and prolonged recovery, substance abuse, early Alzheimer. Athletes should consider this risk of cumulative brain injury from multiple concussions when deciding whether or not to RTP.
- Although helmets cannot prevent concussions, proper headgear for sports should be worn to prevent other head injuries.
- Learning safe fundamentals of a given sport, as well as following the rules, can help to reduce the occurrence and severity of concussions.

CONGENITAL CERVICAL SPINE ANOMALIES

Sara Neal, MD, MA, CAQSM

BASICS

- Congenital cervical spine anomalies (CCSA) are not common.
- They can exist in isolation or as part of a syndrome; 50% are part of the Klippel-Feil syndrome.
- Congenital fusion of two or more cervical vertebrae is the defining characteristic for diagnosis of Klippel-Feil syndrome.
- Many anomalies are asymptomatic but can be associated with other conditions that can be lethal for athletes.
- CCSA can predispose to neurologic injury of the spinal cord during sporting activities.
- CCSA are frequently divided into (i) upper (C1–C3, including the craniovertebral junction and the atlantoaxial interface) and (ii) lower cervical spine abnormalities.
- Upper cervical anomalies: present at a younger age, usually as instability and neurologic problems after minor trauma
- Lower cervical anomalies: commonly present in adults, usually as advanced degenerative changes in hypermobile segments adjacent to fused segments

DESCRIPTION

- CCSA can increase risk for myelopathy from cervical stenosis or instability.
- Specific abnormalities by cervical spine level include craniovertebral junction.
- Atlantoaxial and lower cervical spine vertebral fusions

EPIDEMIOLOGY

- Congenital cervical spine abnormalities are rare but can predispose to myelopathy.
- Often discovered incidentally
- Frequently associated with other congenital defects such as cardiac, retinal, or renal abnormalities

Prevalence

- Unknown because many are asymptomatic
- Prevalence within certain syndromes may be high (e.g., Klippel-Feil, Morquio, and trisomy 21 [Down] syndromes).
- Estimated incidence of CCSA is 1 in 40,000 to 42,000 live births with slight female predominance (1).
- Lower cervical spine fusion is associated with some syndromes (most common is Klippel-Feil syndrome).

ETIOLOGY AND PATHOPHYSIOLOGY

- Abnormalities in the cervical spine cause altered mechanical transfer of axial loading forces, predisposing to neurologic injury.
- Five patterns of CCSA carry especially high risk for neurologic injury, even with minor trauma: (i) fusion of the occiput to C1, (ii) fusion of C1–C2, (iii) fusion of C2–C3, (iv) long cervical fusion (more than three segments fused) plus abnormal junction of the occiput with C1, and (v) two fused segments with a single open interface (two vertebra fused adjacent to one normal vertebra which is then adjacent to two more fused) (2).

Genetics

Teratologic insults (i.e., maternal smoking, alcohol) and mutations in the homeobox (Hox) genes may play a role.

RISK FACTORS

Increased incidence in Klippel-Feil, trisomy 21 (Down), and Morquio syndromes

COMMONLY ASSOCIATED CONDITIONS

- CCSA may be isolated or part of a genetic syndrome.
- Discovery of a cervical spine abnormality should alert the physician to look for associated pathology.
- Klippel-Feil syndrome is defined by the congenital fusion of two or more cervical spine vertebral bodies. Associated abnormalities include:
  - Scoliosis/kyphosis/lordosis (>50%).
  - Hearing impairment (30%).
  - Congenital elevation of the scapula (25–35%).
  - Genitourinary anomalies.
  - Cardiovascular anomalies (more common in females), ventricular septal defect most common.
  - Rib abnormalities.
  - Omovertebral bone (3).
- Lower cervical spine fusion is also seen in fetal alcohol syndrome, Alport syndrome, Crouzon syndrome, and Goldenhar syndrome.
- C1–C2 instability is common in trisomy 21 (Down), Marfan, and Morquio syndromes; juvenile rheumatoid arthritis; and rickets.
- Basilar invagination (narrowing of the foramen magnum) is frequent in achondroplasia.
- Occipitocervical junction anomalies are common in trisomy 21 (Down) syndrome, familial cervical dysplasia, and hyperlaxity syndromes (Ehlers-Danlos and Marfan syndrome).

DIAGNOSIS

HISTORY

CCSA may present with an episode of transient paresis after trauma; more commonly, they are asymptomatic or present with nondescript symptoms such as neck pain or stiffness, headaches, syncope, weakness, numbness, and torticollis.

- Occasionally: symptoms consistent with pyramidal tract or vertebrobasilar insufficiency
- Rarely: cranial nerve or posterior column disturbance
- Those with occipitoatlantal fusion may remain asymptomatic throughout life or present with symptoms after mild trauma; common symptoms (in decreasing frequency): pain in occiput/neck, vertigo, weakness, and ataxia in the lower (and occasionally upper) limbs; occasionally: paresis, paresthesias, hoarseness, dysphagia
- Those with basilar impression and invagination (narrowed foramen magnum) may not have symptoms present until 2nd to 3rd decade.
- Those with occipitoatlantal instability may be symptomatic even in absence of trauma: neck pain, headache, torticollis, weakness, and vertebrobasilar symptoms.
- Those with odontoid anomalies: asymptomatic 50% of the time and average age at diagnosis 19 to 30 yr

PHYSICAL EXAM

- Loss of range of motion (ROM), especially lateral bending, considered a red flag
- Syndromic clinical signs that may be associated with CCSA include:
  - Pterygium colli (webbed neck), shortened neck, torticollis, low posterior hairline
  - Other anomalies that can be associated with CCSA include dwarfism, funnel chest, pes cavus, syndactylies, jaw anomalies, cleft palate, congenital ear deformities, hypospadias, other genitourinary tract defects, and scoliosis (present in 60% of Klippel-Feil syndrome patients) (3).
- Symptoms prompting further evaluation:
  - Radiculopathy: concerning for nerve root irritation from osteophytes at hypermobile segments adjacent to fused vertebrae
  - Upper extremity weakness, numbness, or pain
  - Long-tract signs (spasticity, hyperreflexia, abnormal reflexes) due to pyramidal compression
  - Posterior column signs (altered sensation to deep touch, vibration, and proprioception)
  - Nystagmus, ataxia, and imbalance from cerebellar herniation

DIFFERENTIAL DIAGNOSIS

- Neurologic abnormalities: extensive but include cervical disk disease, congenital spinal stenosis, vascular disease, Arnold-Chiari malformation, and odontoid nonunion
- Torticollis: congenital muscular torticollis (sternocleidomastoid tumor [SMT], muscular torticollis, postural torticollis without SMT mass or tightness), ocular deficiency, hearing deficit, Grisel and Sandifer syndromes, tumor of posterior fossa, syringomyelia/Arnold-Chiari malformation, Klippel-Feil syndrome, rotatory cervical instability, infection, and cervicothoracic scoliosis
- Basilar impression:
  - Secondary basilar impression (owing to softening of osseous skull base): not congenital disease
  - Occasionally, secondary to rickets, osteomalacia, osteogenesis imperfecta, Paget disease, neurofibromatosis, skeletal dysplasia, ankylosing spondylitis, and rheumatoid arthritis
  - Occasionally, erroneously diagnosed as multiple sclerosis, posterior fossa tumors, amyotrophic lateral sclerosis, or traumatic injury

DIAGNOSTIC TESTS & INTERPRETATION

Initial Tests (lab, imaging)

- X-rays: cervical spine anteroposterior (AP) view; open-mouth odontoid view; lateral views in neutral, flexion, and extension ± thoracolumbar posteroanterior and lateral views; abnormalities seen include:
  - AP views: Look for vertebral fusion of facets and spinous processes; AP narrowing of the vertebral bodies (wasp-waist sign); presence of hemivertebrae, omovertebral bone, or spina bifida; condylar dysplasia.
  - On flexion/extension views: Look for decreased movement between fused segments and increased movement between adjacent, nonfused portions.

- Open-mouth view: odontoid anomalies.
- Lateral flexion/extension: Evaluate translational instability (anterior or posterior translation >5 mm) or fusion.
- Basilar impression is difficult to see on x-ray.
- Computed tomography (CT) scan useful for suspected atlanto-occipital fusion, basilar invagination, canal stenosis, and odontoid abnormalities

- Magnetic resonance imaging (MRI): indicated in patients with neurologic deficits; excellent for evaluation of canal stenosis, cord compression, disk bulge/herniation, and craniovertebral junction narrowing; evaluates for associated conditions such as myelomalacia, syringohydromyelia, diastematomyelia, diplomyelia, and Chiari I malformation:
  - Obtain for full evaluation of atlantoaxial instability, basilar invagination, and canal stenosis.

Diagnostic Procedures/Other

Arteriography (or magnetic resonance angiography) if surgery planned or if symptoms warrant (basilar impression, occipitoatlantal fusion, atlas aplasia) because there is increased incidence of vertebral artery anomalies with CCSA

TREATMENT

- Conservative treatment (e.g., activity modification, bracing, and traction) may reduce symptoms. Indications for and timing of surgical stabilization are not clearly defined; consider for significant pain despite conservative measures.
- Spinal stabilization recommended in presence of a neurologic lesion or instability
- If a neurologic process occurs in presence of known canal stenosis, decompression ± stabilization should be considered.

MEDICATION

Analgesics (i.e., acetaminophen, nonsteroidal anti-inflammatory drugs [NSAIDs]) for headache

ISSUES FOR REFERRAL

Generally, all congenital cervical disease should be referred to neurosurgeon and/or neurologist for concurrent observation and management.

SURGERY/OTHER PROCEDURES

- Surgical indication: Posterior column signs and symptoms (most common indication for surgery) require decompression of posterior elements.
- Procedures:
  - Posterior fusion of occiput-atlas complex in occipitoatlantal fusion
  - Suboccipital decompression with decompressive laminectomies of atlas and axis with posterior fusion in basilar impression
- Surgical indication: odontoid abnormalities with any of the following coexisting:
  - Myelopathy, instability of ≥10 mm in flexion and extension, progressive instability, or persistent neck pain with C1–C2 instability
  - Procedure: atlantoaxial arthrodesis (± excision os odontoid)
- Surgical indication: occipitoatlantal instability:
  - Procedure: arthrodesis
- Surgical indication (rarely required): familial cervical dysplasia; procedure: posterior fusion of C1–C2

ONGOING CARE

FOLLOW-UP RECOMMENDATIONS

Patient Monitoring

Return to play recommendations are primarily expert opinions:

- Absolute contraindications to contact/collision sports: odontoid abnormalities, occipitoatlantal fusion, Klippel-Feil syndrome with fusions above C3, and atlantoaxial instability (4,5)[C]
- Caution but no absolute contraindication for Klippel-Feil syndrome with fusion of one or two interspaces below C3; full cervical ROM; and absence of occipital cervical anomalies, instability, disk disease, or degenerative changes (4)[C]

PATIENT EDUCATION

- All congenital cervical diseases: Trauma can be catastrophic (more often with translational instability and with stenotic cervical canal).
- CCSA that carry especially high risk for neurologic injury, even with minor trauma: (i) fusion of the occiput to C1 or C2, (ii) fusion of C2–C3, (iii) long cervical fusion (more than three segments fused) plus abnormal junction of the occiput with C1, and (iv) two fused segments with a single open interface (Two vertebra fused adjacent to one normal vertebra which is then adjacent to two more fused.)

PROGNOSIS

Klippel-Feil syndrome:

- Hypermobility of upper cervical spine: increased risk for neurologic issues
- Lower cervical spine involvement: increased risk for degenerative disease
- Overall prognosis is good, with most patients remaining relatively asymptomatic with occasional mild complaints of headaches, nonradicular weakness, and numbness.

COMPLICATIONS

CCSA may be asymptomatic but can predispose to catastrophic outcomes with minor trauma, including paresis or sudden death.

REFERENCES

1. Tracy MR, Dormans JP, Kusumi K. Klippel-Feil syndrome: clinical features and current understanding of etiology. *Clin Orthop Relat Res*. 2004;424:183–190.
2. Steyaert A. Cervical spine anomalies: a contraindication to sports? *J Sports Sci Med*. 2012;11(1):184–185.
3. Klimo P Jr, Rao G, Brockmeyer D. Congenital anomalies of the cervical spine. *Neurosurg Clin N Am*. 2007;18(3):463–478.
4. Torg JS, Ramsey-Emrhein JA. Management guidelines for participation in collision activities with congenital, developmental, or postinjury lesions involving the cervical spine. *Clin J Sport Med*. 1997;7(4):273–291.
5. Rice SG; for American Academy of Pediatrics Council on Sports Medicine and Fitness. Medical conditions affecting sports participation. *Pediatrics*. 2008;121(4):841–848.

ADDITIONAL READING

- Davis G, Ugokwe K, Roger EP, et al. Clinics in neurology and neurosurgery of sport: asymptomatic cervical canal stenosis and transient quadriparesis. *Br J Sports Med*. 2009;43(14):1154–1158.
- Guille JT, Miller A, Bowen JR, et al. The natural history of Klippel-Feil syndrome: clinical, roentgenographic, and magnetic resonance imaging findings at adulthood. *J Pediatr Orthop*. 1995;15(5):617–626.
- Guille JT, Sherk HH. Congenital osseous anomalies of the upper and lower cervical spine in children. *J Bone Joint Surg Am*. 2002;84-A(2):277–288.
- Hensinger RN. Congenital scoliosis: etiology and associations. *Spine (Phila Pa 1976)*. 2009;34(17):1745–1750.

SEE ALSO

Congenital Cervical Stenosis

CLINICAL PEARLS

- Absolute contraindications to contact/collision sports: odontoid abnormalities, occipitoatlantal fusion, Klippel-Feil syndrome with fusions above C3, and atlantoaxial instability (4,5)[C]
- Caution but no absolute contraindication for Klippel-Feil syndrome with fusion of one or two interspaces below C3; full cervical ROM; and absence of occipital cervical anomalies, instability, disk disease, or degenerative changes (4)[C]
- Discovery of a cervical spine abnormality should alert the physician to look for associated pathology, especially in cardiovascular, renal, and retinal systems.
- X-rays: basic: cervical spine AP view and open-mouth odontoid view; consider: lateral views in neutral, flexion, and extension ± thoracolumbar posteroanterior and lateral
- CT scan useful for suspected atlanto-occipital fusion, basilar invagination, and canal stenosis; also used for flexion/extension evaluation of odontoid abnormalities
- MRI: indicated in patients with neurologic deficits; excellent for evaluation canal stenosis, cord compression, disk bulge/herniation, and craniovertebral junction narrowing; evaluates for associated conditions

CONGENITAL QT SYNDROMES

Chau Bui, DO • Paul Meirick, MD • Suraj A. Achar, MD, FAAFP, CAQSM

BASICS

DESCRIPTION

- Channelopathies refer to a group of inherited arrhythmogenic diseases caused by mutations in genes encoding for ion channel proteins in cardiomyocytes that disrupt the balance of currents in the cardiac action potential. These disruptions may lead to ventricular arrhythmias and sudden cardiac death (SCD).
- The channelopathies include long QT syndrome (LQTS), short QT syndrome (SQTS), Brugada syndrome (see chapter on Brugada Syndrome), and catecholaminergic polymorphic ventricular tachycardia (CPVT) (see supplemental materials for CPVT).
- Congenital QT syndromes:
  - LQTS is a collection of disorders of prolonged myocardial repolarization characterized by a long QT interval:
    - There are two clinical phenotypes of inherited LQTS.
    - Romano-Ward syndrome (autosomal dominant):
      - Characterized by LQTS without other cardiac abnormalities or deafness
      - Most common phenotype
    - Jervell and Lange-Nielsen syndrome (autosomal recessive):
      - Characterized by LQTS and sensorineural deafness
      - Typically has a more malignant course.
  - SQTS is a disorder of accelerated myocardial repolarization characterized by a short QT interval:
    - Mutations of potassium channel genes and loss of function of calcium channel genes
    - Associated with malignant atrial and ventricular arrhythmias and SCD

EPIDEMIOLOGY

Often presents in childhood (mean onset age 14 yr) but may be as early as the newborn period or go undiagnosed into middle age.

Prevalence

- Congenital LQTS:
  - Incidence estimated at 1: 2,000 to 3,000; however, the true incidence of mutations in the population is likely much higher.
  - Congenital LQTS is associated with 3,000 to 4,000 sudden deaths in childhood in the United States per year.
- Congenital SQTS: 1:10,000—uncommon (1)

ETIOLOGY AND PATHOPHYSIOLOGY

- LQTS: >13 genes have been identified that encode for subunits of the potassium, sodium, or calcium voltage dependent ion channels.
- SQTS: Seven genes that encode potassium and calcium channels have been identified.

Genetics

- LQTS: >13 genes identified, with mutations of *KCNQ1* (LQTS1), *KCNH2* (LQTS2), *SCN5A* (LQTS3) accounting for over 90% of cases
- SQTS: Gain of function mutations in potassium channel encoding genes *KCNH2* (SQTS1), *KCNQ1* (SQTS2), *KCNJ2* (SQTS3) (2) and loss of function mutations in several calcium channel encoding genes result in accelerated repolarization.

RISK FACTORS

The primary risk factor for most channelopathies is genetic:

- LQTS:
  - Acquired LQTS can be caused by medications and metabolic or electrolyte abnormalities, particularly hypokalemia and hypomagnesemia.
  - Family history of SCD: first-degree relatives had greater cardiac events than second-degree relatives (26% vs. 10%).
  - Risk factors for precipitating a fatal arrhythmia in a patient with LQTS include swimming (primarily LQTS1) and any strenuous exercise.
  - A corrected QT interval (QTc) >0.46 sec
  - Female gender
- SQTS:
  - SCD most often occurs during rest or sleep (83%), whereas minority occurred during emotional stress or physical effort (3).

GENERAL PREVENTION

SCD resulting from QT syndromes may be prevented by carefully screening and identifying athletes with the condition.

- The preparticipation evaluation is the most important tool for identifying athletes with symptoms that may represent an inherited channelopathy.
- Any athlete with symptoms of palpitations, syncope, presyncope, any collapse, or with a family history of SCD or "accidental" death should be further evaluated with the tools reviewed below.
- Automatic external defibrillators (AEDs) are another important tool in preventing SCD from undiagnosed QT syndrome.

COMMONLY ASSOCIATED CONDITIONS

For certain patients with LQTS only, sensorineural hearing loss is associated.

DIAGNOSIS

- Diagnosis is based mostly on electrocardiogram (ECG) pattern because patients may be symptomatic or asymptomatic.
- Prehospital:
  - In the case that any patient with a QT syndrome converts into a life-threatening arrhythmia in the field, the most useful immediate tool and treatment is an AED.

HISTORY

- Pertinent history in screening athletes:
  - Have you ever passed out, become dizzy, or had chest pain during or after exercise?
  - Do you get tired more quickly than others during exercise?

Antiarrhythmic Drugs	Psychotropic Drugs	Other Drugs
Quinidine	Thioridazine	Diuretics
Procainamide	Phenothiazines	Motility drugs: cisapride, domperidone
Disopyramide	Tricyclic antidepressants	Droperidol
Amiodarone	Haloperidol	HIV protease inhibitors
Sotalol	Selective serotonin reuptake inhibitors (SSRIs)	Vasodilators: prenylamine, bepridil, mibefradil
Dofetilide, ibutilide, azimilide, sematilide	Risperidone	Ketanserin
Antimicrobial drugs	Methadone	Ranolazine
Macrolide antibiotics: erythromycin, telithromycin, clarithromycin, azithromycin (minor)	**Antihistamines**	Organophosphate insecticides
Pentamidine	Terfenadine	Cocaine
Fluoroquinolone: moxifloxacin, gatifloxacin, levofloxacin, sparfloxacin	Astemizole	Papaverine
Spiramycin		Chloral hydrate
Chloroquine, halofantrine, mefloquine		Arsenic trioxide
		Some Chinese herbs

ALERT

Has anyone in the family died suddenly and unexpectedly before the age of 50 yr? *(Remember to ask about family members who died of accidental causes such as sudden infant death syndrome, drownings, and motor vehicle accidents because they may be clues to an undiagnosed family history of channelopathy.)*

- Have you ever had a heart abnormality diagnosed by a doctor?
- Have you ever had an abnormal heart rate (HR), palpitations, or irregular heartbeats?
- Has a physician ever denied or restricted your participation in sports for heart problems?
- Have any of your relatives ever had cardiomyopathy, Marfan syndrome, LQTS, SQTS, or significant heart arrhythmias?

- Pertinent history in potentially affected athletes:
  - LQTS:
    - Most commonly asymptomatic
    - Common symptoms include palpitations, syncope, presyncope, seizures, and cardiac arrest.
    - Hearing loss (occurs in Jervell and Lange-Nielsen phenotype patients only)
    - Arrhythmias are most commonly precipitated by exercise, followed by exercise and emotion together, emotion alone, and less commonly, loud noise or anesthesia.
    - Use of any medications that may cause LQTS or torsade de pointes
    - LQTS1: susceptible to cardiac events with physical exertion (62%) and emotional stress (26%), especially prone during swimming (4)
    - LQTS2: emotional triggers and events occurring during sleep without arousal; auditory events (alarm clocks)
    - LQTS3: susceptible during sleep without arousal
  - SQTS:
    - Most common clinical presentations are cardiac arrest followed by palpitations, syncope, and atrial fibrillation (5).
    - No pattern or association with onset as it has been reported at rest, after startle, and during daily activities
    - Strong family history component

PHYSICAL EXAM

- Because patients with QT syndrome typically have structurally normal hearts, it is not uncommon to observe a completely normal examination when a life-threatening arrhythmia is not present.
- When arrhythmias are present, the examination may be notable for bradycardia or tachycardia, either regular or irregular, depending on the patient's rhythm.

DIFFERENTIAL DIAGNOSIS

Brugada syndrome, CPVT, acquired LQTS with its many reversible metabolic and drug-induced causes, acute coronary syndrome, true right bundle branch block (RBBB), pericarditis, drug-induced ventricular tachycardia (VT) or ventricular fibrillation (VF)

DIAGNOSTIC TESTS & INTERPRETATION

Initial Tests (lab, imaging)

- Genetic testing for identifying the type of LQTS is available:
  - Indications for testing include family history of unexplained early cardiac death, family members with history of LQTS, or clinical suspicion based on patient's personal history.

- In the setting of a life-threatening arrhythmia, it may be indicated to rule out ischemic or metabolic causes with a basic or comprehensive metabolic panel and cardiac enzymes:
  - Hypomagnesemia, hypocalcemia, and hypokalemia may precipitate torsade de pointes in those with a given mutation.

Diagnostic Procedures/Other

ECG is the most important initial diagnostic tool. Holter monitors and echocardiograms may be of use as well:

- LQTS:

ALERT
Prolonged QTc: 440 to 460 ms represent 90 to 95th percentile in general population (>470 ms in men or >480 ms in women (99th percentile) should prompt further evaluation (4).

  - Confirm QTc using Bazett formula ($QTc = QT / \sqrt{RR}$; QT in ms, RR in sec)—although Bazett correction decreases in accuracy with extremes in HR (ensure HR >50 bpm) (4).
  - Common potential ventricular arrhythmias are torsade de pointes (type of polymorphic VT), multiform ventricular premature beats, uniform ventricular premature beats, monomorphic VT.

ALERT
Note: Degree of LQTS penetrance is variable, so some patients may have normal or borderline QTc.

- SQTS: QTc <360 ms in symptomatic patient or with familial history of sudden death at young age. 240 to 330 ms is generally considered affected even if asymptomatic and requires further workup usually with genetic testing (6).

TREATMENT

- Congenital LQTS:
  - All patients with congenital or acquired QT syndrome should be referred to an electrophysiologist or cardiologist.

ALERT
All symptomatic patients should be treated owing to the high risk for SCD. This risk may be up to 50–60% in 10 yr.

  - Treatment of asymptomatic individuals is less clear but may be strongly considered in the following asymptomatic patients: newborns and infants, patients with sensorineural hearing loss, patients with siblings with LQTS and SCD, patients with QTc >0.60 sec.
  - Treatment includes lifestyle modification, medical therapy with β-blockers or other agents, and may include surgical options such as an implantable cardioverter-defibrillator (ICD).
- Congenital SQTS: Mainstay of treatment is ICD, consider medical therapy as adjunct to ICD or if there is a contraindication to ICD placement.

MEDICATION

- LQTS:
  - β-blockers reduce the risk of syncope and SCD (4)[B]; first-line therapy unless contraindicated
  - Propranolol (2 to 3 mg/kg/day) or nadolol (1 to 1.5 mg/kg/day). Atenolol and metoprolol are associated with more clinical failures (4).
  - Efficacy of β-blockers varies by LQTS genotype (maximally effective in LQTS1).
  - Adjunctive treatments include potassium, flecainide, mexiletine, or ranolazine.
- SQTS: Quinidine is effective in prolonging the QT interval (3).

SURGERY/OTHER PROCEDURES

- LQTS:
  - ICD placement or left cardiac sympathetic denervation
  - Recommended for patients who fail β-blockers (syncope or VT), have survived cardiac arrest, or have risk factors for SCD (4)[B]
  - Left cardiac sympathetic denervation:
    - Removal of the first 4 thoracic ganglia
    - Reserved for patients who fail other treatments or ICD contraindicated (4)[C]
- SQTS:
  - ICD placement is first-line treatment (7).
  - Medication is only an adjunct or to be used if contraindication to ICD placement.

ADMISSION, INPATIENT, AND NURSING CONSIDERATIONS

As always, all patients who present with a life-threatening arrhythmia should be treated emergently with cardioversion and/or pharmacotherapy as dictated by standard advanced cardiac life support (ACLS).

ONGOING CARE

All patients with channelopathies should be followed regularly by a cardiologist or electrophysiologist. Education and restrictions regarding exercise are crucial to survival.

FOLLOW-UP RECOMMENDATIONS

Return-to-play decisions:

- Previously, athletes were limited to class IA sports (low static and low dynamic stresses): billiards, bowling, cricket, curling, golf, or riflery.

New American Heart Association/American College of Cardiology (AHA/ACC) 2015 participation guidelines: In a symptomatic athlete, competitive sports participation may be considered following expert consultation from electrophysiologist and cardiologist, initiation of treatment, appropriate precautionary measures, and the athlete has been asymptomatic for at least 3 mo (3)[C].

ALERT

Asymptomatic athlete with genotype-positive/phenotype-negative (concealed channelopathy) may participate in all competitive sports with appropriate precautionary measures (avoidance of QT-prolonging drugs, appropriate electrolyte/hydration replenishment, avoidance of hyperthermic conditions, acquire personal AED, and establish appropriate emergency action plan).

- Athlete with an ICD may be permitted to participate in sports if there have been no shocks for 3 mo.
- Recreational swimming should be avoided by all patients unless proven to be a genotype other than LQTS1.

ALERT

Caution should be used to avoid sports where impaired consciousness would be dangerous or lethal, such as with SCUBA diving, swimming, weight lifting with free weights, and horseback riding.

- Avoid medications that may cause QT prolongation (as listed in table).

REFERENCES

1. Drezner JA, Ackerman MJ, Cannon BC, et al. Abnormal electrocardiographic findings in athletes: recognising changes suggestive of primary electrical disease. *Br J Sports Med*. 2013;47(3):153–167.
2. Brugada R, Hong K, Dumaine R, et al. Sudden death associated with short-QT syndrome linked to mutations in HERG. *Circulation*. 2004;109(1);30–35.
3. Hammond-Haley M, Patel R, Providência R, et al. Exercise restrictions for patients with inherited cardiac conditions: current guidelines, challenges, and limitations. *Int J Cardiol*. 2016;209:234–241.
4. Gomez AT, Prutkin JM, Rao AL. Evaluation and management of athletes with long QT syndrome: an evolved paradigm. *Sports Health*. 2016;8(6):527–535.
5. Giustetto C, Di Monte F, Wolpert C, et al. Short QT syndrome: clinical findings and diagnostic-therapeutic implications. *Eur Heart J*. 2006;27(20):2440–2447.
6. Mazzanti A, O'Rourke S, Ng K, et al. The usual suspects in sudden cardiac death of the young: a focus on inherited arrhythmogenic diseases. *Expert Rev Cardiovasc Ther*. 2014;12(4):499–519.
7. Gaita F, Giustetto C, Bianchi F, et al. Short QT syndrome: a familial cause of sudden death. *Circulation*. 2003;108(8):965–970.

ADDITIONAL READING

- Ackerman MJ, Zipes DP, Kovacs RJ, et al. Eligibility and disqualification recommendations for competitive athletes with cardiovascular abnormalities: Task Force 10: the cardiac channelopathies: a scientific statement from the American Heart Association and American College of Cardiology. *Circulation*. 2015;132(22):e326–e329.
- Maron BJ, Zipes DP, Kovacs RJ. Eligibility and disqualification recommendations for competitive athletes with cardiovascular abnormalities: preamble, principles, and general considerations: a scientific statement from the American Heart Association and American College of Cardiology. *J Am Coll Cardiol*. 2015;66(21):2343–2349.

CLINICAL PEARLS

- Any athlete with symptoms of palpitations, syncope, presyncope, any collapse, or with a family history of SCD or "accidental" death should be further evaluated with the tools reviewed below.
- Asymptomatic athlete with genotype-positive/phenotype-negative (concealed channelopathy) may participate in all competitive sports with appropriate precautionary measures (avoidance of QT-prolonging drugs, appropriate electrolyte/hydration replenishment, avoidance of hyperthermic conditions, acquire personal AED, and establish appropriate emergency action plan).
- Caution should be used to avoid sports where impaired consciousness would be dangerous or lethal, such as with SCUBA diving, swimming, weight lifting with free weights, and horseback riding.
- Treatment of asymptomatic individuals is less clear but may be strongly considered in the following asymptomatic patients: with sensorineural hearing loss, patients with siblings with LQTS and SCD, and patients with QTc >0.60 sec.

CORNEAL ABRASIONS

Nilesh Shah, MD, FAAFP, CAQSM • Mark A. Diamond, MD

BASICS

DESCRIPTION

- Removal or scraping away of the superficial layers of the cornea (stratified squamous epithelium) without penetration of Bowman membrane
- In some cases, the bulbar conjunctiva is also involved.
- In the general population, injury usually results from contact lenses misuse but also can be attributed to foreign bodies, tangential shearing injuries, and contusion to the globe.
- In the workplace, both physical trauma and chemical trauma may be an etiology for corneal abrasions.
- In sports, the mechanism is more commonly direct trauma.
- Severe corneal injuries also can involve the deeper, thicker stromal layer; in this situation, the term *corneal ulcer* may be used.

EPIDEMIOLOGY

- Most common eye injury after soft tissue injuries
- More common in sports with projectiles/balls
- More common in collision sports

RISK FACTORS

- Collision/contact sports
- Contact lenses use, especially soft lenses
- Failure to wear eye protection
- Sports with projectiles/balls

GENERAL PREVENTION

Single-piece construction protective eyewear with 3-mm polycarbonate lenses will reduce the risk of eye injuries.

COMMONLY ASSOCIATED CONDITIONS

- Hyphema (blood in the anterior chamber)
- Scleral rupture: Look for vitreous leak.
- Intraocular foreign body
- Rust ring
- Perforation: Look for vitreous leak.
- Orbital fracture
- Iridodialysis: defect of the iris caused by its separation from the scleral spur
- Superinfection
- Recurrent erosion syndrome

DIAGNOSIS

HISTORY

- Mechanism of injury guides physical exam for associated injuries and delineates the need for further studies.
- History of previous injuries: possible viral keratitis or recurrent erosion syndrome
- Contact lenses history (hard, soft, overuse): Symptoms are usually better with contact in place, acting as a bandage.
- Risk of foreign body: particular sports, windy conditions, etc.

PHYSICAL EXAM

- Signs and symptoms include:
  - Pain.
  - Redness.
  - Lacrimation.
  - Foreign-body sensation.
  - Photophobia.
  - Blepharospasm.
  - Possibly decreased visual acuity.
- Physical examination includes:
  - General bony orbital exam.
  - Cranial nerve assessment.
  - Ocular movements.
  - Topical anesthetic and cycloplegic agents: may be needed to decrease pain and photophobia for optimal exam.
  - Visual acuity.
  - Loupe with good light or slit lamp (preferable).
  - Fluorescein drops/strips: sharply demarcate defects in corneal epithelium and help to differentiate traumatic abrasion (linear or geographic pattern) from herpes keratitis (dendritic pattern with terminal bulbs). Abrasion will appear yellow under normal light and green under cobalt blue light.
  - Anterior chamber and corneal exam: slit lamp preferred to rule out associated injuries (hyphema, perforation).
  - Eversion of upper and lower lids: Identify any foreign bodies under tarsal plate. If discovered, it must be removed by trained individual.
  - Intraocular pressure (IOP): unless perforation/scleral rupture is suspected.
  - Immediate referral if significant vision loss or diplopia, corneal infiltrate/ulcer, hypopyon/hyphema, dilated/nonreactive/irregular pupil, or evidence of penetrating eye injury.

DIFFERENTIAL DIAGNOSIS

- Foreign body
- Corneal laceration
- Perforation
- Infectious keratitis: herpetic, bacterial, fungal
- Conjunctivitis: infectious/allergic
- Iridocyclitis
- Optic neuritis
- Retinal detachment
- Scleritis/episcleritis
- Blepharitis
- Keratoconjunctivitis
- Canaliculitis
- Globe injury
- Orbital fracture
- Photokeratitis/retinitis
- Periorbital cellulitis
- Trichiasis
- Intraocular foreign body
- Dry eye syndrome

DIAGNOSTIC TESTS & INTERPRETATION

- Orbital series: only if history or physical exam suggests fracture
- Ultrasound (US) (brightness [B]-scan)/computed tomography (CT) scan/magnetic resonance imaging (MRI): if occult intraocular foreign body is suspected

TREATMENT

GENERAL MEASURES

- The goal of treatment is to prevent bacterial superinfection, speed healing, and provide symptomatic relief to patients.
- Long-term treatment

ALERT

- Long-term use of topical anesthetics may compromise epithelial healing.
- Acute treatment
- Analgesia:
  - Topical anesthesia (1)[A]: for facilitation of ocular exam only (and only once penetrating injury has been excluded); see warning above. The use of these agents is currently not supported by evidence. In addition, they may block protective corneal reflexes and sensation, potentially increasing the risk of further ocular injury.
  - Oral analgesia as needed

MEDICATION

- Antibiotics:
  - Broad-spectrum topical antibiotics: aid with lubrication and are used for infection prophylaxis (e.g., sulfacetamide/fluoroquinolones)
  - Contact lenses associated: often colonized with *Pseudomonas aeruginosa* and other gram-negative organisms. Therefore, consider a *fluoroquinolone* or *aminoglycoside* (e.g., ciprofloxacin, ofloxacin, gentamicin).
  - Water sport associated: pseudomonal coverage (e.g., fluoroquinolones/aminoglycosides)
- Topical nonsteroidal anti-inflammatory drugs (NSAIDs) (2)[A]: Although traditionally used for pain control, there is a lack of quality evidence to support their use over more cost-effective oral analgesics. Topical NSAIDs may reduce the need for oral analgesia.
- Anticholinergic medications (3)[A]: Cycloplegic agents have traditionally been used for pain control in corneal abrasions. However, they have not been shown to significantly reduce pain. They may be considered for relief of ciliary muscle spasm–related pain, if present. Caution should be used in patients with narrow angles because mydriatic medications can lead to acute angle–closure glaucoma.
- Oral analgesics: Oral anti-inflammatory medications and narcotic pain medications may be used for pain control.

ISSUES FOR REFERRAL

Referral for recurrent abrasions, erosions, larger abrasions, infections, corneal ulcers, or failure to improve 24 to 48 hr after initial treatment

ADDITIONAL THERAPIES

- Most uncomplicated corneal abrasions heal in 24 to 48 hr; daily monitoring until reepithelialization recommended (see "Ongoing Care")
- Topical antibiotics continued for 1 wk after reepithelialization
- Watch for recurrent erosion—sudden pain, redness, tearing—which may lead to recurrent erosion syndrome, possibly requiring débridement and further specialized treatment.
- Pressure patch (4)[A]: Patching is no longer recommended for the treatment of simple, traumatic, corneal abrasions. For small, uncomplicated corneal abrasions, patching has not been shown to decrease pain or increase healing rates. Patching also creates loss of binocular vision.

ONGOING CARE

FOLLOW-UP RECOMMENDATIONS

- If abrasion is small (4 mm or less), vision is normal, and symptoms improving, follow-up is not necessarily needed.
- Follow-up within 24 hr is necessary for those with large abrasions (>4 mm), contact lenses–related abrasions, and those whose visual acuity is affected.
- Contact lenses wearers: daily monitoring until abrasion is healed. Discard contact lenses. New lenses should not be worn until abrasion is healed and symptoms have resolved.
- Hyphema
- Intraocular foreign body/rust ring
- Perforation
- Recurrent erosion syndrome

Patient Monitoring

- Eye rest (i.e., minimize reading or heavy computer work that requires substantial eye movement): This helps to minimize interference with reepithelialization.
- Avoid light or wear sunglasses for comfort if significant photophobia is present.

PATIENT EDUCATION

- Eye protection during the healing process is important, especially in patients whose jobs put them at increased risk of corneal abrasions or ultraviolet (UV) exposure.
- If the patient is unconscious or cannot voluntarily close his or her eyelids (e.g., Bell palsy or other neuropathies), eyelids may be taped closed and use of lubrication considered.

PROGNOSIS

- The prognosis is usually good, with healing and full recovery of vision if prompt evaluation and treatment are initiated.
- Some deep abrasions heal with a scar. If this occurs in the central visual axis (the central area of the cornea directly over the pupil), visual acuity may be permanently lost. Deep abrasions within the central visual axis should be considered for ophthalmologic referral.
- Healing of minor abrasions is expected within 24 to 48 hr. Extensive or deep abrasions may require a week to heal.

COMPLICATIONS

- Deep corneal involvement may result in facet formation in the epithelium or scar formation in the stroma.
- Progression of abrasions into corneal ulcers may lead to devastating outcomes.
- Abrasions involving exposure to vegetable matter are at risk of fungal ulcers.
- Sight-threatening infections
- Abrasions from contact lenses use are at risk for *Pseudomonas* and amoebic keratitis.
- Recurrent erosion syndrome
- Allergic reactions to treatment medications
- Loss of school and work time/productivity
- Use of mydriatics may lead to systemic anticholinergic symptoms or can induce acute angle closure in glaucoma patients.

REFERENCES

1. Puls HA, Cabrera D, Murad MH, et al. Safety and effectiveness of topical anesthetics in corneal abrasions: systematic review and meta-analysis. *J Emerg Med*. 2015;49(5):816–824.
2. Wakai A, Lawrenson JG, Lawrenson AL, et al. Topical non-steroidal anti-inflammatory drugs for analgesia in traumatic corneal abrasions. *Cochrane Database Syst Rev*. 2017;(5):CD009781.
3. Thiel B, Sarau A, Ng D. Efficacy of topical analgesics in pain control for corneal abrasions: a systematic review. *Cureus*. 2017;9(3):e1121.
4. Lim CH, Turner A, Lim BX. Patching for corneal abrasion. *Cochrane Database Syst Rev*. 2016;(7):CD004764.
5. American Academy of Pediatrics Committee on Sports Medicine and Fitness. Protective eyewear for young athletes. *Pediatrics*. 2004;113:619–622.

ADDITIONAL READING

- Ahmed F, House RJ, Feldman BH. Corneal abrasions and corneal foreign bodies. *Prim Care*. 2015;42(3):363–375.
- Aslam SA, Sheth HG, Vaughan AJ. Emergency management of corneal injuries. *Injury*. 2007;38(5):594–597.
- Calder LA, Balasubramanian S, Fergusson D. Topical nonsteroidal anti-inflammatory drugs for corneal abrasions: meta-analysis of randomized trials. *Acad Emerg Med*. 2005;12(5):467–473.
- Heimmel MR, Murphy MA. Ocular injuries in basketball and baseball: what are the risks and how can we prevent them? *Curr Sports Med Rep*. 2008;7(5):284–288.
- Menghini M, Knecht PB, Kaufmann C, et al. Treatment of traumatic corneal abrasions: a three-arm, prospective, randomized study. *Ophthalmic Res*. 2013;50(1):13–18.
- Watson SL, Barker NH. Interventions for recurrent corneal erosions. *Cochrane Database Syst Rev*. 2007;(4):CD001861.
- Wilson SA, Last A. Management of corneal abrasions. *Am Fam Physician*. 2004;70(1):123–128.
- Wipperman JL, Dorsch JN. Evaluation and management of corneal abrasions. *Am Fam Physician*. 2013;87(2):114–120.

CLINICAL PEARLS

- Return to play is based on patient comfort. Once the pain is under control and the patient is not having any visual difficulties, he or she may return to play.
- Patients may wear their contact lenses again when the abrasion has healed fully without complications (usually 3 to 5 days). Furthermore, if the abrasion is related to contact lenses, they need to be replaced and new ones not started until complete healing of the abrasion has occurred.
- There is no increased risk of another corneal abrasion after an initial injury, but anyone in a collision/contact sport or a sport with a projectile/ball should consider wearing protective eyewear.
- Optimal protective eyewear is made of a sturdy frame single-piece construction that will not allow posterior dislocation of the lenses of the eyewear. The lenses should have a 2- to 3-mm center thickness and be made of polycarbonate. Different sports have differing eyewear regulations. They should have American Society for Testing and Materials (ASTM) certification (5).

CUBITAL TUNNEL SYNDROME

Jeremy Schmitz, MD, ABFM • Kenneth P. Barnes, MD, MSc, CAQSM, FACSM

BASICS

- Compression, traction, or irritation of the ulnar nerve as it passes through the cubital tunnel of the medial elbow
- The cubital tunnel is bounded by the medial trochlea, the medial epicondylar groove, and the posterior portion of the ulnar collateral ligament and is roofed by the triangular arcuate ligament.
- Primary complaints are medial elbow and forearm pain.
- Additional complaints are paresthesias in the ring and little fingers.
- Synonym(s): ulnar tunnel syndrome

EPIDEMIOLOGY

Incidence

- The elbow is the most common site of compression of the ulnar nerve.
- Predominant gender: male > female (3 to 8:1)
- The second most common compressive neuropathy (after carpal tunnel syndrome)
- Overhead-throwing athletes are most at risk.

ETIOLOGY AND PATHOPHYSIOLOGY

Possible causes of the compression of the ulnar nerve as it passes the medial elbow include:

- Subluxation of the ulnar nerve over the medial epicondyle.
- Enlarged medial head of the triceps muscle.
- Cubitus valgus.
- Ulnar collateral ligament instability/tears.
- Triangular arcuate ligament tears in baseball pitchers.
- Osteophytes.
- Ganglia or lipomas.
- Tumors.
- Repetitive elbow flexion and extension.
- Anconeus epitrochlearis: anomalous muscle in 70% of population.

RISK FACTORS

- Overhead-throwing athletes
- Repetitive upper extremity activities
- Diabetes
- Obesity
- Peripheral neuropathies

GENERAL PREVENTION

Avoid prolonged pressure on the medial elbow.

COMMONLY ASSOCIATED CONDITIONS

- Ulnar neuritis
- Ulnar collateral ligament instability

DIAGNOSIS

HISTORY

- Vague, aching pain in the region of the elbow, worsening with overhead activities
- Paresthesias over the 4th and 5th digits
- Numbness of the 4th and 5th digits
- Weakness of interosseous and adductor digiti minimi muscles of the hand
- Worsening grip, loss of dexterity, and clumsiness
- Snapping or popping sensation of medial elbow
- Overhead-throwing athletes will complain of loss of control of ball with activity.

PHYSICAL EXAM

- Pain with palpation of cubital tunnel of affected elbow
- Positive Tinel sign: Tapping over the ulnar nerve at the elbow will cause a reproduction of symptoms (1)[B].
- Elbow flexion test: Placing the elbow in full flexion and the wrist in maximal extension will cause pain or paresthesias after 1 min (1)[B].
- Scratch test: Patient faces examiner with arms adducted, elbows flexed, and hands outstretched with wrists in a neutral position. Patient resists adduction/internal rotation to the forearms applied by the examiner. The examiner scratches or wipes fingertips over the cubital tunnel, and resistance to adduction/internal rotation is again applied. In a positive test, the patient has immediate and temporary loss of external resistance tone, which resolves within 5 sec (1)[B].
- Sensory changes in ulnar nerve distribution can be detected with Semmes-Weinstein monofilament testing and, in more advanced cases, with two-point discrimination tests.
- Asymmetric hypothenar atrophy, decreased pinch and grip strength, abducted little finger, or severe claw deformity of little finger only (Wartenberg sign)
- Intrinsic muscle weakness and wasting (especially 1st dorsal interosseous muscle)
- Patient will exhibit decreased sensation in the ulnar nerve distribution.
- Complete medical history and physical exam
- Nerve conduction velocity (NCV) to determine how fast neurologic signals travel down nerve to detect site of compression or constriction. Studies must be performed with elbow at 45 degrees of flexion to lessen chance of erroneous results (2)[C].
- Electromyogram (EMG) to evaluate nerve and muscle function

DIFFERENTIAL DIAGNOSIS

- Systemic: diabetes, renal disease, multiple myeloma, amyloidosis, chronic alcoholism, malnutrition
- Compression: postoperative occupational or recreational activities requiring repetitive flexion and extension, supracondylar process, ligament of Struthers, medial head of triceps, ulnar nerve compression at Guyon canal
- Medial epicondylosis which can coexist with cubital tunnel syndrome
- Ulnar collateral ligament injury
- Cervical radiculopathy
- Thoracic outlet syndrome
- Carpel tunnel syndrome

DIAGNOSTIC TESTS & INTERPRETATION

- Radiograph of elbow to evaluate for bony changes or spurs
- Magnetic resonance imaging (MRI) of elbow to evaluate cubital tunnel for soft tissue masses and continuity of ulnar collateral ligament

- Diagnostic ultrasound (US): ratio of ulnar nerve cross-sectional area at maximal enlargement to cross-sectional area at unaffected site >2.8:1; ratio in control subjects 1.1:1 (3)[B]
- Diagnostic US: Hypoechoic swelling of the ulnar nerve with loss of the fascicular pattern is a sonographic sign of cubital tunnel (4)[B].
- Pathologic findings:
  - At decompression, specific sites of nerve compression usually can be found.
  - Inspect the arcade of Struthers, intermuscular septum, cubital tunnel, and Osborne fascia (between two heads of flexor carpi ulnaris).

TREATMENT

- Conservative treatment is effective in up to 90% of patients irrespective of EMG/NCV results (5,6,7,8)[B].
- The most effective treatment is cessation of activity that is causing the problem.
- A splint or foam elbow pad worn at night (to limit movement and reduce irritation)
- Elbow pad (to protect against chronic irritation from hard surfaces)
- Eccentric exercises to treat associated medial epicondylosis
- Topical or oral nonsteroidal anti-inflammatory drugs (NSAIDs) PRN
- Physical therapy with attention to nerve-gliding exercises

SURGERY/OTHER PROCEDURES

- Consider surgery if symptoms continue after 3 mo of conservative therapy or multiple recurrences in a throwing athlete (9,10,11)[C]:
  - Address ulnar collateral ligament instability if coexisting.
  - Decompression of the nerve in the canal, especially in setting of bone spurs
  - Transposition of the nerve out of the canal in an anterior direction
- Multiple meta-analyses have been inconclusive and differ in results; none specifically for athletes (12,13,14)[A]:
  - No clinical or NCV differences between simple compression and ulnar nerve transposition
- Hypermobile nerve is most frequently treated with epicondylectomy or transposition (15)[B].
- Preference for overhead athlete is transposition of the ulnar nerve to allow for improved movement of the nerve throughout the range of motion (9)[C]:
  - Subcutaneous technique: anterior transposition of nerve without detachment of flexor mass; fascial sling used to prevent subluxation of nerve
  - Submuscular technique: allows inspection and treatment of ligament and osseous pathology; nerve stabilized deep to flexor-pronator muscles but more morbidity and potential for deep scarring

Pediatric Considerations

- Dominant arms of young throwing athletes (15)
- Nonsurgical management only relieves symptoms roughly ~45% of the time (15).
- Anterior transposition should be considered due to the substantial revision rate after decompression (15).

REFERENCES

1. Cheng CJ, Mackinnon-Patterson B, Beck JL, et al. Scratch collapse test for evaluation of carpal and cubital tunnel syndrome. *J Hand Surg Am*. 2008;33(9):1518–1524.
2. Sattari S, Emad M. Changes in ulnar nerve conduction velocity across the elbow in different angles of elbow flexion. *Electromyogr Clin Neurophysiol*. 2007;47(7–8):373–376.
3. Yoon JS, Walker FO, Cartwright MS. Ultrasonographic swelling ratio in the diagnosis of ulnar neuropathy at the elbow. *Muscle Nerve*. 2008;38(4):1231–1235.
4. Draghi F, Bortolotto C. Importance of the ultrasound in cubital tunnel syndrome. *Surg Radiol Anat*. 2016;38(2):265–268.
5. Szabo RM, Kwak C. Natural history and conservative management of cubital tunnel syndrome. *Hand Clin*. 2007;23(3):311–318.
6. Svernlöv B, Larsson M, Rehn K, et al. Conservative treatment of the cubital tunnel syndrome. *J Hand Surg Eur Vol*. 2009;34(2):201–207.
7. Gellman H. Compression of the ulnar nerve at the elbow: cubital tunnel syndrome. *Instr Course Lect*. 2008;57:187–197.
8. Padua L, Aprile I, Caliandro P, et al. Natural history of ulnar entrapment at elbow. *Clin Neurophysiol*. 2002;113(12):1980–1984.
9. Bencardino JT, Rosenberg ZS. Entrapment neuropathies of the shoulder and elbow in the athlete. *Clin Sports Med*. 2006;25(3):465–487.
10. Keefe DT, Lintner DM. Nerve injuries in the throwing elbow. *Clin Sports Med*. 2004;23(4):723–742.
11. Charles YP, Coulet B, Rouzaud JC, et al. Comparative clinical outcomes of submuscular and subcutaneous transposition of the ulnar nerve for cubital tunnel syndrome. *J Hand Surg Am*. 2009;34(5):866–874.
12. Mowlavi A, Andrews K, Lille S, et al. The management of cubital tunnel syndrome: a meta-analysis of clinical studies. *Plast Reconstr Surg*. 2000;106(2):327–334.
13. Zlowodzki M, Chan S, Bhandari M, et al. Anterior transposition compared with simple decompression for treatment of cubital tunnel syndrome. A meta-analysis of randomized, controlled trials. *J Bone Joint Surg Am*. 2007;89(12):2591–2598.
14. Macadam SA, Gandhi R, Bezuhly M, et al. Simple decompression versus anterior subcutaneous and submuscular transposition of the ulnar nerve for cubital tunnel syndrome: a meta-analysis. *J Hand Surg Am*. 2008;33(8):1314.e1–1314.e12.
15. Boone S, Gelberman RH, Calfee RP. The management of cubital tunnel syndrome. *J Hand Surg Am*. 2015;40(9):1897–1904.

ADDITIONAL READING

Cutts S. Cubital tunnel syndrome. *Postgrad Med J*. 2007;83(975):28–31.

CLINICAL PEARLS

- Most important part of treatment is to minimize elbow flexion and pressure on the elbow and to engage in relative rest from repetitive activity.
- Screen overhead athletes for ulnar collateral ligament instability.

C

CUBOID SUBLUXATION AND FRACTURE

Timothy Ryan Draper, DO, ABFM, CAQSM • Karl B. Fields, MD, CAQ

BASICS

DESCRIPTION

- Fracture: can be avulsion fractures, intra-articular, or extra-articular. The majority (48%) are avulsion fractures (1).
- Frequently associated with other fractures, dislocations, or ligamentous injuries
- A "nutcracker" fracture occurs when an axial load is placed on the heel of a plantarflexed fixed foot crushing the cuboid between the calcaneus and the 4th and 5th metatarsals bases. Ballet dancers are a special group at risk for this type of injury due to stresses placed on the midfoot by the en pointe foot position (2).
- Subluxation: poorly understood. Can occur as a result of acute ankle inversion injury or as an overuse syndrome. Noted in patients with hypermobility; most commonly reported in ballet dancers (3)
- Isolated dislocation extremely rare; usually associated with concomitant fractures of the midfoot
- Cuboid stress fractures are extremely rare (4).
- Synonym(s):
  - Subluxation and dislocation: cuboid syndrome; locked cuboid; dropped cuboid; calcaneal cuboid fault syndrome; lateral plantar neuritis
  - Fracture: nutcracker fracture

EPIDEMIOLOGY

Incidence

- Subluxation: Subluxation is considered rare, but some propose that it is underdiagnosed.
- Dislocation: rare
- Fracture: relatively uncommon (1)

RISK FACTORS

- Subluxation:
  - Pronated feet
  - Tight peroneus longus tendon
  - Ballet dancing (3)
  - Trail running or running on uneven surfaces
- Fracture and dislocation:
  - Activities at high risk for foot trauma (e.g., motorsports, equestrian)
  - Long-distance running (stress fracture)

DIAGNOSIS

HISTORY

- Subluxation:
  - May follow inversion ankle injury
  - Subluxation may be precipitated by increased routine activity, increased activity on uneven terrain, or initiation of new activity, especially for patient with excess pronation.
  - Pain in lateral midfoot proximal to and involving the base of the 4th and/or 5th metatarsal, exacerbated with activity
  - Often with symptom-free intervals
  - Associated with foot weakness or difficulty with ambulation
- Fracture and dislocation:
  - Substantial traumatic force needed owing to stable ligamentous attachments
  - Most patients with fractures have difficulty bearing weight, especially walking on their tiptoes.
  - Dislocations often are associated with severe weakness and markedly antalgic gait if patient is able to bear weight.
  - Midfoot deformity may be present with fracture or dislocation.
  - Stress fractures generally present with an insidious onset of lateral midfoot pain

PHYSICAL EXAM

- Subluxation:
  - Tenderness to palpation over cuboid (dorsal and/or plantar surface)
  - Increased mobility to manipulation of the cuboid at the Lisfranc joint
  - Midtarsal adduction test causes pain.
- Dislocation and fracture:
  - Midfoot swelling
  - Tenderness to palpation over cuboid (dorsal and/or plantar surface)
  - With dislocation, abnormal indentation in lateral midfoot may be noted with concomitant fullness in the plantar surface.
  - May be unable to bear weight
  - When fracture is suspected, the foot, ankle, and lower leg need to be carefully inspected because concomitant injury is common.

DIFFERENTIAL DIAGNOSIS

- Peroneus longus tenosynovitis
- Base of 4th and 5th metatarsal fracture
- Calcaneonavicular tarsal coalition
- Peroneus longus tendon subluxation
- Os peroneum fracture
- Other midfoot fractures

DIAGNOSTIC TESTS & INTERPRETATION

- Radiographs: Recommend anteroposterior, lateral, and oblique views. Weight-bearing films should be obtained when possible because subtle injuries to the midtarsal joint complex (i.e., Lisfranc) are often missed on non–weight-bearing views:
  - Oblique view usually demonstrates a cuboid fracture, and dislocation can be seen if medial border of 4th metatarsal is not aligned to medial border of the cuboid.
  - Subluxation is often not seen.
- Computed tomography (CT) scan is often beneficial if fracture is present.
- Magnetic resonance imaging (MRI) is the most sensitive test for stress fracture.

TREATMENT

- Subluxation:
  - Manipulate cuboid back into place.
  - Patient stands with support, affected leg with knee bent to 90 degrees. Examiner grasps forefoot with fingers and places thumbs (one over the other) on plantar aspect of cuboid. Cuboid is manipulated with a quick downward thrust of the thumbs in a dorsal and lateral direction.
  - Alternative manipulation is to perform a "whip maneuver," which involves having the athlete lie prone with the knee flexed to 90 degrees, and the examiner "whips" the cuboid back into place rapid ankle dorsiflexion and plantar flexion (5)[C].
  - Orthotics, use of cuboid pad, and arch straps/taping recommended
  - Strength and proprioception rehabilitation (2)[C]
- Fracture:
  - Avulsion fractures can be managed symptomatically (1); air splint often used
  - Isolated extra-articular fractures can be treated within 6 wk in a controlled ankle motion (CAM) walker boot or short leg walking cast.
  - Most intra-articular fractures require open reduction and internal fixation (ORIF) and should be referred to a surgeon (1).
  - Remember that most cuboid fractures have an association with other more complex foot injuries.
  - Stress fractures heal well with activity modification. Patient may need to be non–weight-bearing or partial weight-bearing on crutches for a couple of weeks if they have pain with walking. A progressive walk to cross-train to running program requires 6 to 12 wk. Evaluate the runner for abnormal supination or pronation.

ONGOING CARE

FOLLOW-UP RECOMMENDATIONS

- Subluxation:
  - Return to play depends on the severity of the athlete's symptoms.
  - Most athletes should be able to return to play almost immediately given proper treatment with orthotics/cuboid pad/arch supports.
  - Some patients may need a period of relative rest with return to play after physical therapy and symptom improvement.
  - Some patients also learn to self-treat in the field after instruction in self-administration of the cuboid whip maneuver.
- Fracture/dislocation:
  - Return to play for cuboid stress fractures is similar to other foot stress fractures.
  - Athletes should follow a slow, incremental, symptom-free return-to-play protocol with rest and regression of intensity if symptoms develop.
  - Return to play for most fractures and dislocations should proceed only after clearance by the orthopedic surgeon and would be slow and incremental.
  - Depending on the severity of the injury, there may be chronic damage ultimately limiting return to play.

COMPLICATIONS

- Subluxation and dislocation: Chronic instability can be a problem for both dislocation and subluxation.
- Fracture: nonunion, particularly if diagnosis/treatment is delayed

REFERENCES

1. Fenton P, Al-Nammari S, Blundell C, et al. The patterns of injury and management of cuboid fractures: a retrospective case series. *Bone Joint J*. 2016;98-B(7):1003–1008.
2. Carsen S, Quinn BJ, Beck E, et al. "Nutcracker fracture" in a ballet dancer performing in The Nutcracker. *J Dance Med Sci*. 2015;19(3):124–127.
3. Macintyre J, Joy E. Foot and ankle injuries in dance. *Clin Sports Med*. 2000;19(2):351–368.
4. Mandell JC, Khurana B, Smith SE. Stress fractures of the foot and ankle, part 2: site-specific etiology, imaging, and treatment, and differential diagnosis. *Skeletal Radiol*. 2017;46(9):1165–1186.
5. Patterson SM. Cuboid syndrome: a review of the literature. *J Sports Sci Med*. 2006;5(4):597–606.

ADDITIONAL READING

- Hunter JC, Sangeorzan BJ. A nutcracker fracture: cuboid fracture with an associated avulsion fracture of the tarsal navicular. *AJR Am J Roentgenol*. 1996;166(4):888.
- Main BJ, Jowett RL. Injuries of the midtarsal joint. *J Bone Joint Surg Br*. 1975;57(1):89–97.
- Omey ML, Micheli LJ. Foot and ankle problems in the young athlete. *Med Sci Sports Exerc*. 1999;31(Suppl 7):S470–S486.

CLINICAL PEARLS

- Frequently associated with other fractures and midfoot injuries
- Weight-bearing foot x-rays should be done if possible because subtle associated injuries to the Lisfranc joint may be missed on non–weight-bearing views.
- Avulsion fractures and isolated extra-articular fractures can be managed conservatively.
- Intra-articular fractures should be referred to an orthopedist for definitive treatment.
- Stress fractures heal well with activity modification.

DE QUERVAIN TENOSYNOVITIS

David A. Wang, MD • Ryan J. Lingor, MD, AT-C, RD, CSCS

BASICS

DESCRIPTION

- First described by Swiss physician Fritz de Quervain in 1895 (1)
- de Quervain tenosynovitis is a stenosing tenosynovitis of the 1st dorsal compartment of the wrist.
- The abductor pollicis longus (APL) and extensor pollicis brevis (EPB) tendons course through this compartment.

ALERT

About 40% of cadavers demonstrate an intracompartmental septum between the APL and EPB tendons, with a higher incidence noted in those who have failed injections or required surgical intervention.

- It is the most frequently encountered tendinosis on the dorsal side of the wrist.
- de Quervain tenosynovitis is typically an overuse injury but may result from direct trauma.
- **Synonym(s)**: de Quervain disease; 1st dorsal compartment tenosynovitis; stenosing tenosynovitis; stenosing tendinitis; peritendinitis; styloid tenovaginitis; stenosing tendovaginitis; texting tenosynovitis; mommy thumb

EPIDEMIOLOGY

- Usually seen in adults aged 30 to 50 yr
- More common in females than males affecting 0.5% of men and 1.3% of women worldwide (2)

ETIOLOGY AND PATHOPHYSIOLOGY

- Repetitive or sustained tension on tendons of the 1st dorsal compartment causes an inflammatory and then fibroblastic response.
- There is thickening and swelling of the extensor tendons and retinaculum.
- Pain is produced from resisted gliding of the APL and EPB tendons in the narrowed fibroosseous canal.
- Histopathology is consistent with collagen disorientation and mucoid changes (tendinosis), not inflammation.

RISK FACTORS

- Pregnancy, postpartum mothers, and caretakers of young infants
- Activities requiring forceful grasp with excessive ulnar wrist deviation or repetitive use of the thumb (e.g., golfing, bowling, wrestling, fly fishing, racquet sports [squash, badminton, tennis], javelin or discus throwing)
- Direct trauma with associated scarring
- Also, can be seen as systemic component of rheumatologic disorders such as rheumatoid arthritis
- Frequent use of electronic devices (e.g., texting, tablets, cell phones)
- Recurrence higher if history of trigger finger (2)

DIAGNOSIS

Clinical diagnosis based on history and physical exam findings

HISTORY

- Gradual onset of pain along the radial styloid of the wrist for several weeks to months but can occur more acutely with high-volume, unaccustomed activity
- Acute onset of pain over the radial styloid after trauma
- Pain is aggravated by moving the wrist or thumb.
- Pain may radiate to the thumb, up the dorsoradial aspect of the forearm, or occasionally into the shoulder.

PHYSICAL EXAM

- Swelling, tenderness, and/or crepitus to palpation of the APL and EPB tendons near the radial styloid process
- Positive Finkelstein test is pathognomonic and the most commonly used test (1)[C].

ALERT

To perform the Finkelstein test, the examining physician grasps the thumb of the patient, and the hand is ulnar deviated sharply. A positive test produces sharp pain along the distal radius.

- A similar test that is often confused with the Finkelstein test was previously described by Eichoff, in which the thumb is placed in the palm of the hand and held with the fingers; the hand is then ulnar deviated, causing intense pain over the radial styloid.
- Other test:
  - Brunelli test (abducting the thumb with the wrist in radial deviation) and wrist hyperflexion and abduction of the thumb (WHAT) test (wrist fully flexed with thumb fully extended and abducted while examiner applies a gradually increasing abduction resistance to the thumb)
- Imaging usually not needed
- Obtain x-rays if patient has history of trauma or to rule out other bone pathology such as osteoarthritis (OA).
- Ultrasound (US) can be helpful as a diagnostic tool:
  - Can demonstrate fluid surrounding the tendons or thickened retinaculum
  - Can identify anatomical variant with intracompartmental septum
  - US-guided injection may help confirm the diagnosis and ensure proper placement of medication, which may increase efficacy and decrease complications and possibly recurrences.
- Magnetic resonance imaging (MRI) is often unnecessary but may be used to rule out concomitant pathologies if considering surgery.

DIFFERENTIAL DIAGNOSIS

- Thumb carpometacarpal joint arthritis
- Intersection syndrome
- Radial styloid fracture
- Scaphoid fracture
- Radial neuritis
- Wartenberg syndrome
- Trigger thumb
- Flexor carpi radialis tendonitis
- Ganglia

TREATMENT

GENERAL MEASURES

- Rest from offending activity
- Ice massage is beneficial when used early.

MEDICATION

- Topical and oral anti-inflammatory agents may benefit some patients especially during an acute onset of symptoms when used in conjunction with rest (3)[C].

ALERT

Corticosteroid injection is effective treatment for most patients (2)[C]:

- Place a rolled-up towel under the wrist to position it in slight ulnar deviation.
- Use a 2-mL mixture of analgesic (lidocaine 1%) and corticosteroid (triamcinolone 10 mg/mL or dexamethasone 10 mg).
- Inject into the 1st dorsal compartment at the radial styloid through a 27-gauge needle at a 45-degree angle to the skin.
- Inject along the axis of the sheath.
- Infiltrate the sheath from distal to proximal.
- Fusiform swelling occurs in the 1st dorsal compartment if properly placed.
- US guidance improves accuracy and outcomes and can be done in the transverse plane.

- Pain relief is often immediate.
- Patient must be cautioned against overuse following an injection.

ALERT

Failure of palpation-guided injection is typically due to an anatomic variant with two tendon sheaths, a septation in the 1st dorsal compartment, or the presence of a ganglion in the 1st compartment. In addition, there can be multiple slips of the APL or EPB tendon. Anatomic variants may be seen in as many as 40–60% of patients who fail injections.

- If palpation-guided injection fails, consider repeat injection under US guidance.
- Consider surgical referral if second injection fails.
- Water-soluble corticosteroid decreases local complications, including subcutaneous atrophy and hypopigmentation.

ALERT

The combination of corticosteroid injection plus temporary splinting may be more effective than either treatment alone (4)[B].

ADDITIONAL THERAPIES

- Using a thumb spica splint may relieve pain, but there is some suggestion that immobilization could increase recovery time.
- There is little research supporting other therapeutic modalities, including stretching, strengthening, iontophoresis, acupuncture, and therapeutic US.
- There is weak evidence to support platelet-rich plasma (PRP) injection and percutaneous needle tenotomy of the 1st dorsal compartment (5)[C].

SURGERY/OTHER PROCEDURES

- If conservative therapy is ineffective with persistent symptoms >3 mo after corticosteroid injection, surgical release of the fibrous 1st dorsal compartment may be considered.
- Surgical intervention has demonstrated a >90% cure rate with relatively low risk of complication (6)[C].

ONGOING CARE

PATIENT EDUCATION

Discussion of the risk factors can lead to insight into what caused the problem and can help reduce recurrence.

PROGNOSIS

Most patients have a very good prognosis; however, recurrence is common, so modification of activities must be a part of the treatment plan.

COMPLICATIONS

ALERT

Complications of injection:

- SC fat atrophy
- Hypopigmentation
- Pain
- Neuritis
- Fat necrosis
- Postinjection flare
- Local infection

Complications of surgery:

- Radial sensory nerve injury
- Incomplete decompression
- Volar subluxation of the APL and EPB tendons

REFERENCES

1. Huisstede BM, Coert JH, Fridén J, et al; for European HANDGUIDE Group. Consensus on a multidisciplinary treatment guideline for de Quervain disease: results from the European HANDGUIDE study. *Phys Ther*. 2014;94(8):1095–110.
2. Earp BE, Han CH, Floyd WE, et al. De Quervain tendinopathy: survivorship and prognostic indicators of recurrence following a single corticosteroid injection. *J Hand Surg Am*. 2015;40(6):1161–1165.
3. Lane LB, Boretz RS, Stuchin SA. Treatment of deQuervain's disease: role of conservative management. *J Hand Surg*. 2001;26(3):258–260.
4. Mardani-Kivi M, Mobarakeh MK, Bahrami F, et al. Corticosteroid injection with or without thumb spica cast for de Quervain tenosynovitis. *J Hand Surg Am*. 2014;39(1):37–41.
5. Peck E, Ely E. Successful treatment of de Quervain tenosynovitis with ultrasound-guided percutaneous needle tenotomy and platelet-rich plasma injection: a case presentation. *PM R*. 2013;5(5):438–441.
6. Lee HJ, Kim PT, Aminata IW, et al. Surgical release of the first extensor compartment for refractory de Quervain's tenosynovitis: surgical findings and functional evaluation using DASH scores. *Clin Orthop Surg*. 2014;6(4):405–409.

ADDITIONAL READING

- Peters-Veluthamaningal C, van der Windt DA, Winters JC, et al. Corticosteroid injection for de Quervain's tenosynovitis. *Cochrane Database Syst Rev*. 2009;(3):CD005616.
- Richie CA III, Briner WW Jr. Corticosteroid injection for treatment of de Quervain's tenosynovitis: a pooled quantitative literature evaluation. *J Am Board Fam Pract*. 2003;16(2):102–106.

CLINICAL PEARLS

- First-line treatment typically involves activity modification, splinting, ice massage, and a topical or oral anti-inflammatory.
- Corticosteroid injection can improve symptoms in a large percentage of patients and can be considered first-line therapy in those with severe or limiting symptoms.
- If a palpation-guided corticosteroid injection fails, consider an anatomical variant and repeating the injection under US guidance.

DENTOALVEOLAR TRAUMA

Christopher Bossart, MD • Christopher McGrew, MD, FACSM, CAQSM

BASICS

DESCRIPTION

Dentoalveolar injuries include dental avulsion, dental luxation, extrusion and intrusion, enamel and crown fractures, root fracture, and alveolar bone fracture.

EPIDEMIOLOGY

- 25% of all respondents in the United States between the ages of 6 and 50 yr reported suffering at least one traumatic dental injury to their anterior teeth (1).
- ~30% of children have experienced dental injuries (2).
- The peak period for trauma to the primary teeth is 18 to 40 mo of age because this is a time of increased mobility for the relatively uncoordinated toddler. Injuries to primary teeth usually result from falls and collisions as the child learns to walk and run (2).
- With the permanent teeth, school-aged boys suffer trauma almost twice as frequently as girls.
- Sports accidents and fights are the most common cause of dental trauma in teenagers.
- Data show that these orofacial injuries occur primarily during recreational sports and organized athletic events. Individuals who incur facial trauma during noncompetitive sporting events go vastly underreported, which skews the reporting. A large retrospective study shows that 69% of the injuries were incurred by males. The age group between 11 and 18 yr was the most commonly affected (3).
- 90.3% of crown fractures or crown-root fractures occur from direct trauma (3).
- The most commonly involved teeth were the central incisors (58.3%), and the second most commonly involved teeth were the maxillary lateral incisors.
- There seems to be a seasonal variation in incidence of orofacial trauma. Many data demonstrate the probable correlation between outdoor activities and predominance of dental trauma during warmer times of the year (in the northern hemisphere) (1).
- 5–35% of the population; 75% <15 yr of age
- Predominant gender: male > female (3:1); equal or higher rates sometimes reported for females than males when corrected for exposure rates

ETIOLOGY AND PATHOPHYSIOLOGY

- Etiology (2):
  - Falls made up 49% of cases (including uncoordinated childhood falls).
  - Traumatic dental injuries account for 18–30% of all oral injuries (4).
  - Sports-related injuries occurred in 18% of cases.
  - Bicycle and scooter accidents accounted for 13% of cases.
  - Assaults made up 7% of cases.
  - Road traffic accidents resulted in 1% of cases.
  - All others 12%
- Pathophysiology:
  - Enamel fracture only (Ellis class I), 15.8%:
    - Roughness of chipped tooth on tongue
    - May go unnoticed by athlete
    - Not a dental emergency
  - Enamel and dentin fracture (Ellis class II), 39.9%:
    - Exposure of yellow dentin
    - Pain with dentin exposure to air, cold drinks, or touch
    - Not a dental emergency
  - Enamel, dentin, pulp exposed (Ellis class III), 25.7%:
    - Dental emergency (within 3 hr)
    - Exposure of red-pink dental pulp
    - Vital with closed root apex: less complex treatment
    - Vital pulp with open root apex: more complex but viable
    - Dental pulp opening appears dry or oozes putrescent exudates and no pain:
      - Nonviable
  - Root fractures (Ellis class IV):
    - Dental emergency (within 3 hr)
    - Middle (1/3) root fractures have a good prognosis depending on time of evaluation and treatment. This root fracture can be identified by its longer visible coronal segment and it being partially extruded compared with other teeth. The tooth is likely to bleed from the gingival sulcus, and with gentle finger pressure, it may be rotated in the socket. As long as the tooth is not visibly markedly loose, the athlete may finish sporting event with mouth guard in place and seek follow-up care in emergency department (ED) within 24 hr (5).
    - Cervical third fractures have the worst prognosis of all root fractures.
    - Apical root fractures have the best prognosis for maintaining viability, especially if lacking segmental mobility.
  - Extrusion, intrusion, lateral luxations:
    - Displacement (not fracture) involving periodontal ligament (i.e., stretch, compress, rupture ligament)
    - Lateral luxation involves movement of tooth in anterior/posterior plane: Follow up with dentist within 24 hr for splinting or immediately if tooth cannot be repositioned.
    - Intrusion involves movement of tooth inward:
      - May be extremely painful, painless, or numb depending on the extent of nerve root injury
      - Dental emergency (within 3 hr)
    - Extrusion is movement of the tooth out of the socket: Follow up with dentist within 24 hr for splinting or immediately if tooth cannot be repositioned.
  - Avulsion (tooth exarticulation): dental emergency (immediate): Time to definitive treatment is inversely related to viability.
  - Associated soft tissue injury (abrasions, lacerations, contusions):
    - Lacerations of the lip: 55.8%
    - Abrasions of face constituted 34.2%.
    - Abrasions of lip constituted 30.2%.
    - Abrasions of mentum constituted 21%.
    - Abrasions of nose constituted 13%.
    - Abrasions of other regions constituted 1.5%.

RISK FACTORS

- Protection: Large meta-analysis showed that athletes are 1.6 to 1.9 times more likely to have orofacial injuries playing sports not traditionally associated with mouth guard use compared to those sports mandating mouth guards (6).
- Sports: baseball, basketball, cycling, hockey, soccer, skiing, rugby, football, wrestling, boxing, and martial arts
- Anatomy: protruding maxillary incisors, lip incompetence, class II malocclusion
- Previous injury

GENERAL PREVENTION

- Face masks, in sports such as hockey and football, provide protection against trauma to the mouth and face.
- Mouth guards reduce oral lacerations and tooth fractures and cushion impacts that could result in condylar displacement and subsequent injury.
- Stock mouth guards are the most inexpensive but lack customized fit. The athlete has to continuously bite down on mouth guard for it to not become loose and free in the mouth. These mouth guards come with the risk that if the patient becomes unconscious, the mouth guard may be extruded from the oral cavity or obstruct the airway. They are often bulky and may interfere with speech and breathing.
- Mouth-formed or boil-and-bite mouth guards are the most commonly commercially sold mouth guards, and many types are available. These mouth guards are best fit by a dentist but may be fit at home. Inconsistent retention, fit, and quality make these mouth guards still not the most desirable option, although they are better option than stock mouth guards. They are molded to the mouth after being placed in boiling water and then are set in cold water after being placed in the athlete's mouth.

- Custom-fitted mouth guards are fit in a two-stage process by a dentist for maxillary (class I or II occlusion) or mandibular (class III occlusion) arches. They provide increased comfort, compliance, and protection. They may last several years but are impractical for children <13 yr of age owing to rapid dental changes. They may be formed by vacuum or pressure lamination (preferred) processes. These mouth guards exhibit the most reliable retention rates and limit the incidence of dental trauma. The high cost of these mouth guards can be easily justifiable economically relative to the cost of cosmetic or restorative dentistry.

COMMONLY ASSOCIATED CONDITIONS

- Facial contusion, laceration, fracture
- Mandible fracture
- Intraoral laceration (tongue, buccal mucosa, gingiva)
- Concussion

DIAGNOSIS

Suspicions for dental trauma:

- Impact to jaw, face, or any part of skull or neck leaving bruising or ecchymosis, diffuse or focal
- Facial swelling, bleeding from mouth or gums
- Patient complains of ear, jaw, or neck pain or headache.
- Patient intolerant of drinking hot or cold fluids ± inability to chew
- Prehospital:
  - Evaluate patient for signs of shock or acute blood loss.
  - Determine the extent of injury because this dictates how quickly action must be taken.
  - Response time is paramount when discussing viability of teeth affected by dental trauma. Better outcomes result from proper interventions done early in the time course.
  - Assess all lacerations for severity and necessity of intervention by dentist or oral maxillofacial surgeon.

HISTORY

- Mechanism of injury and associated injuries (7)
- Force and vector of injury: This is paramount to identify all injuries visible or potentially concealed by soft tissue injury and swelling.
- Time since injury, time tooth was out of mouth, method of storage and transport
- Past dental history, past general medical and surgical history
- Medications and allergies
- Last tetanus shot

PHYSICAL EXAM

- Signs and symptoms include:
  - Pain and tenderness to percussion or palpation.
  - Temperature sensitivity.
  - Color changes.
  - Tooth loosening.
- Physical examination includes:
  - Assess levels of consciousness, and ensure that airway, breathing, and circulation are intact.
  - Begin with general examination of the head and neck, including skull, eyes, ears, nose, cervical spine, and anterior neck.
  - Proceed with extraoral exam. Palpate the mandible, zygoma, temporomandibular joint (TMJ), and mastoid region. Check for any mandibular or maxillary fractures that are present. Find mandibular fractures by feeling the lower border of the mandible for a step-down fracture. Identify any extraoral lacerations, bruises, or swelling. If a laceration is present in the upper or lower lip, the area must be inspected for foreign bodies such as gravel or tooth fragments. Any foreign bodies must be débrided from the soft tissue.
  - The mandibular condyles and maxilla should be carefully palpated. Check jaw movements for normal range of movements. Chin lacerations require careful evaluation of the cervical spine and mandibular condyles. Indications of condylar fractures include an anterior open bite, a malocclusion, or limited mandibular opening. Confirmation of condylar fractures requires a panoramic radiograph with closed- and open-mouth views.
  - Follow this with a detailed intraoral exam. Identify and account for all missing teeth, if possible. Explore oral cavity to identify extent of dental and oral mucosa damage. The labial and buccal mucosa, maxillary frenum, gingival tissues, and tongue should be examined for bruising or lacerations. All intraoral lacerations must be cleaned and explored, looking for any foreign bodies. Palpate the alveolus to detect any fractures. Have the patient clench the teeth so that the dental occlusion can be evaluated. Each tooth should be examined for damage or mobility. Multiple types of injuries to each tooth must be suspected. Excess mobility suggests root and alveolar fractures; this is also seen with luxation injuries to a lesser degree. Malalignment may indicate luxation injury or fracture. Modular movement of adjacent teeth suggests alveolar fractures.

DIFFERENTIAL DIAGNOSIS

- Associated trauma: ruled out by history, physical examination, and radiography
- Mandibular fractures and TMJ damage: Check occlusion, limitation of jaw motion, mobility of multiple teeth or jaw fragments, maxillary/hard palate mobility, anesthesia/paresthesia of the cheek and lip as well as radiography.
- Soft tissue injuries: Include radiographs if not all tooth fragments are accounted for.

DIAGNOSTIC TESTS & INTERPRETATION

- Radiographic examination: For evaluating injuries to the maxillary or mandibular teeth, an occlusal radiograph is the film of choice:
  - Two periapical views at different angles if a root fracture is suspected are required for a definitive diagnosis.
  - For deep tooth structure evaluation (i.e., Ellis class III, root, jaw fractures, intruded teeth), a lateral anterior radiograph provides additional useful information.
  - Chest radiograph if dyspneic, hemoptysis, or missing tooth to evaluate for aspirated tooth fragment
  - Panorex (panoramic radiograph) helps to evaluate suspected mandibular or condylar fractures.
- Routine radiographs may not show root fractures; dental films (panoramic film with selected periapical views at multiple angles) are indicated with a low index of suspicion. Fractures may not be evident initially; negative films may be repeated 1 to 2 days after injury.
- Postreduction views are needed to rule out root or alveolar fractures and confirm placement after reimplantation or splinting of an avulsed tooth.
- Photographic documentation: The use of preoperative and postoperative photography may be useful for documentation purposes.

TREATMENT

- Treatment depends on rapid identification of injury type.
- Initial stabilization:
  - Establish airway, breathing, and circulation.
  - Control soft tissue bleeding: pressure from gauze, fabric, or any other moldable material
  - Provide analgesia:
    - Injection of 1 to 2 mL lidocaine (0.5 to 1 mL for primary teeth) into the buccal gingival mucosa over the injured tooth and root apex, with epinephrine if not contraindicated; less effective with mandibular teeth
    - Inferior alveolar nerve block may be required for pain relief of mandibular teeth, with 2 to 4 mL lidocaine injected just superior to the lingula of the mandible.
    - Orthodontic wax may be applied to protect exposed dentin or pulp and sharp edge.
    - Oral pain medications are not recommended initially owing to the possibility of ingesting blood and fragments of teeth.
- Tooth avulsions (8):
  - Avulsed primary teeth should not be replaced owing to the risk of injury to permanent teeth.
  - Locate all teeth or tooth fragments, and prepare to replace and reposition tooth immediately.
  - Handle the tooth only by the crown. Any contact with the root may render the tooth nonviable.
  - Inspect the tooth to ensure that no foreign material is left on the surface (especially at the root). If any foreign material is present, flush or swish the tooth in a sterile balanced salt solution (Hank balanced salt solution, Earl balanced salt solution) or milk for 10 sec. Do not brush.
  - Replantation should be performed as soon as possible (good prognosis within 20 min but poor after 2 hr) (9). No successful reimplantation has been performed if avulsed tooth has been out of mouth and dry for >60 min (10).
  - Do not attempt to replace tooth in obtunded patient.
  - After exam, flush socket with saline, and prepare to replace tooth.
  - Firmly (but not forcefully) reinsert tooth into the socket after local anesthesia and saline irrigation. Have patient bite gently on gauze to seat tooth in socket. Patient may feel a click or a give and then increased resistance. Once the tooth is firmly implanted in the alveolar socket and is anatomically consistent (labial and lingual surfaces align) with adjacent teeth, place an oversized piece of gauze atop the reimplanted tooth and have the patient bite down firmly on the gauze.
  - Transport immediately to dental office or ED with on-call dentistry, whichever is available at that time.
  - Place nonimplantable teeth or tooth fragments in preserving system such as sterile balanced salt solution (Hank balanced salt solution, Earl balanced salt solution) or milk if available.
  - Tooth may be stored in milk for 3 to 6 hr and even longer in sterile balanced salt solution and in saliva for up to 2 hr. If low risk for aspiration and no other alternatives are available, store sublingually or in buccal vestibule to prevent drying.
  - Do not store in plain water because this causes osmotic lysis of periodontal ligament cells.
  - Do not allow tooth to dry.
  - Dental treatment:
    - 5 to 10 days of antibiotics (penicillin V or alternatives) reduce the risk of root resorption.
    - Because there have been reported treatment failures with oral penicillin, other antibiotics that may be used are ampicillin-sulbactam (intravenous [IV]) or penicillin G (IV) with metronidazole (IV or PO) (11).
    - Splinting/immobilization: Acid-etch resin is used with wire along the labial surface to passively splint the injured tooth.
    - Duration of splinting varies with injury: Semirigid splints should be applied for 7 to 10 days after avulsion.
- Tooth fractures (12):
  - Enamel only (Ellis class I): Locate fragment, if possible. If fragment cannot be reattached or securely replaced, place the fragment in a balanced salt solution. May be reattached up to 48 hr later by a dentist with resin or bonding. If nonviable, smoothing and contouring the rough edge are tactilely therapeutic and aesthetically pleasing; nonurgent referral to smooth rough edges, with cosmetic repair 4 to 8 wk later if needed
  - Enamel and dentin (Ellis class II): Fragment may be reattached with bonding agent or composite resin materials. Transport tooth fragments in tooth-preserving system. Arrange dental referral as soon as possible for best results (same day). Dentist may place composite resin or glass ionomer bandage. Exposed dentin should be sealed as soon as possible; delay may allow bacterial contamination of the pulp via dentinal tubules, especially in immature teeth. Acid-etch composite is used (possibly with tooth fragments) for definitive restoration.
  - Enamel, dentin, and pulp (Ellis class III):
    - Emergent evaluation within 3 hr before proceeding with treatment by dentist. Treatment based on pulp status and dental age of tooth. Direct pulp capping may allow pulp vitality with small pulp exposures. Partial pulpotomy with calcium hydroxide treatment may be indicated in immature teeth to delay root canal treatment until after apex maturation (if pulp remains vital). Teeth with moderate pulp exposure and closed apices necessitate root canal treatment.
  - Crown-root fractures (cleave fractures): Fractures near the alveolar crest rarely heal without either root canal therapy and post/crown placement or extraction and prosthodontic treatment.
  - Root fracture (Ellis class IV): Coronal portion should be repositioned after local anesthesia with radiographic confirmation and rigid immobilization for 2 to 3 mo (shorter for more apical fractures) (13).
  - Root fractures, as mentioned previously, have poorer prognosis the more distal from the apical segment. Apical root fractures may heal by cementum union alone.
  - Middle third fractures require urgent care. Immediate intervention includes using gentle pressure coupled with instructing the athlete to bite down on sterile gauze after repositioning. Subsequent dental evaluation emergently as well as periodically over the next 6 to 8 wk is necessary. The patient may require a root canal if indicated by a dentist.
  - Urgent management remains the same as for middle third injuries, but a dentist's evaluation will determine viability of affected tooth and possible need for extraction and replacement with a dental implant.
- Luxation:
  - For lateral luxation (subluxation of the dentoalveolar joint), if minor, it may be appropriate to attempt reduction if possible.
  - If reduction is possible and successful, provider may approximate and suture any gingival injury; splint for 2 to 4 wk, and follow up with pulp vitality testing, local anesthesia, firm repositioning, and splinting with close follow-up
  - Urgent referral (same day) only if repositioning cannot be done
  - Extrusion injuries: repositioning and splinting with anesthesia as needed
  - Urgent referral (same day) only if repositioning cannot be done
  - Intrusion injuries are dental emergency. Record the distance of intrusion, use local anesthesia, and luxate the tooth with gentle twisting if it is not already slightly mobile. Do not splint. Intrusive luxation with deciduous teeth may need to be extracted or may be left in and may reerupt. Teeth also may ankylose. Urgent repositioning is necessary.
  - Refer within 3 hr to ED or dentist's office for treatment.
- Alveolar fractures:
  - Immediate reduction with manual pressure after clinical diagnosis followed by radiographs and rigid splinting for 1 to 2 mo reduces pulp necrosis.
  - Empirical antibiotic therapy against oral flora is recommended to reduce contamination.

MEDICATION

- Immunizations: tetanus. Consider administration of immunization in cases of lacerations or tooth injuries with exposed pulp or for avulsions in patients for whom immunizations are due (last immunization >5 yr).
- Antibiotic therapy: Consider prophylactic antibiotics in cases of exposed pulp or avulsion. Penicillin VK or clindamycin may be used (14).
- Pain medications: Consider use of nonsteroidal anti-inflammatory drugs (NSAIDs) (ibuprofen) and/or analgesic (acetaminophen, tramadol, codeine, hydrocodone) as needed.

ISSUES FOR REFERRAL

- Patients should be advised to see their dentist in the time frame outlined earlier.
- Urgent oral surgical referral may be necessary owing to associated injuries.

ADDITIONAL THERAPIES

- Photographs and meticulous documentation are particularly important in cases of assault or motor vehicle accidents.
- Aspiration: If an avulsed tooth is not accounted for, a chest film may be indicated. Swallowed teeth rarely require treatment and should not be retrieved unless there is concern for gastrointestinal (GI) obstruction.
- Damage to primary teeth may result in damage to permanent teeth in 25–70% of injuries.

SURGERY/OTHER PROCEDURES

- Dental splinting is used as an initial treatment for subluxed or avulsed teeth that are replaced.
- Root canal might be considered as delayed treatment in cases of injury resulting in damage to the root.

ADMISSION, INPATIENT, AND NURSING CONSIDERATIONS

Hospital admission or observation is rarely required. Criteria may include:

- Multiple, complicated trauma.
- Vital signs instability.
- Abuse or violence suspected in injury history.
- Concern for aspirated tooth.

ONGOING CARE

- Tooth avulsion:
  - Endodontic treatment is usually required at 1 to 2 wk in teeth with a closed apex (after pulpal ischemic necrosis, before infection) to prevent periapical abscess formation and root resorption. Teeth with an open apex may reestablish blood supply; thermal sensitivity testing is performed every 3 to 4 wk, with root canal treatment delayed until clinical or radiographic signs of disease. Calcium hydroxide treatment also may be considered to prevent inflammatory root resorption.
  - Follow-up is essential at least every 6 mo for several years; potential root resorption must be monitored and alveolar bone optimized for prosthetic implantation considerations.
- Tooth fractures:
  - Crown fractures: Definitive restoration should be performed as soon as possible, especially if the arch is crowded, because delay may allow encroachment of adjacent teeth and necessitate orthodontic treatment before restoration. Root canal treatment may be required in 1 to 2 wk in cases of pulp exposure.
  - Root fractures: Monthly clinical and radiographic evaluation should be performed during splinting and then every 3 to 6 mo for at least 2 yr; 20–45% have pulpal necrosis and require pulpotomy, root canal treatment, or prosthesis. Hard tissue union is more likely with pulpal vitality, younger patients, closer fragment opposition, and increased root diameter.
- Tooth luxation:
  - Intrusion: Radiographic monitoring for pulp necrosis or root resorption should occur every 3 wk. Orthodontic extrusion is required if reeruption is not satisfactory after 3 mo. Root canal treatment is required in 2 to 3 wk for 95% of teeth with mature roots and 65% of teeth with immature roots owing to pulp necrosis.
  - Lateral luxation requires follow-up with radiographs every 3 mo for 2 yr to ensure that root resorption or loss of pulp vitality is not evident.

DIET

Soft or liquid diet may be necessary for a time to further protect teeth and allow for healing.

REFERENCES

1. Ranalli DN. Sports dentistry and dental traumatology. *Dent Traumatol*. 2002;18:231–236.
2. Wright G, Bell A, McGlashan G, et al. Dentoalveolar trauma in Glasgow: an audit of mechanism of injury. *Dent Traumatol*. 2007;23(4):226–231. doi:10.1111/j.1600–9657.2006.00430.
3. Castro JC, Poi WR, Manfrin TM, et al. Analysis of the crown fractures and crown root fractures due to dental trauma assisted by the Integrated Clinic from 1992 to 2002. *Dent Traumatol*. 2005;21(3):121–126.
4. Spinas E, Mameli A, Giannetti L. Traumatic dental injuries resulting from sports activities; immediate treatment and five years follow-up: an observational study. *Open Dent J*. 2018;12:1–10.
5. Gould TE, Piland SG, Caswell SV, et al. National Athletic Trainers' Association position statement: preventing and managing sport-related dental and oral injuries. *J Athl Train*. 2016;51(10):821–839.
6. Knapik JJ, Marshall SW, Lee RB, et al. Mouthguards in sport activities: history, physical properties, and injury prevention effectiveness. *Sports Med*. 2007;37(2):117–144.
7. Greenberg MS, Springer PS. Diagnosis and management of oral injuries. In: Torg JS, ed. *Athletic Injuries to the Head, Neck, and Face*. 2nd ed. St. Louis, MO: Mosby-Year Book; 1991:635–649.
8. Dewhurst SN, Mason C, Roberts GJ. Emergency treatment of orodental injuries: a review. *Br J Oral Maxillofac Surg*. 1998;36(3):165–175.
9. Trope M. Clinical management of the avulsed tooth. *Dent Clin North Am*. 1995;39(1):93–112.
10. American Academy of Pediatric Dentistry. Guideline of Management of Acute Dental Trauma. http://aapd.org/media/Policies_Guidelines/G_Trauma.pdf. Adopted 2011. Revised 2011. Accessed 2011.
11. Inouye J, McGrew C. Dental problems in athletes. *Curr Sports Med Rep*. 2015;14(1):27–33.
12. Donly KJ. Management of sports-related crown fractures. *Dent Clin North Am*. 2000;44(1):85–94, vi.
13. Camp JH. Management of sports-related root fractures. *Dent Clin North Am*. 2000;44(1):95–109, vi–vii.
14. Mark DG, Granquist EJ. Are prophylactic oral antibiotics indicated for the treatment of intraoral wounds? *Ann Emerg Med*. 2008;52(4):368–372.

CLINICAL PEARLS

- If the pulp becomes devitalized, the tooth will rapidly change color, along with associated symptoms. If root canal treatment is needed, a slight and gradual darkening may be noticed.
- Depending on the type of injury and promptness of care, chances are good for a successful recovery.

DEVELOPMENTAL DYSPLASIA OF THE HIP

Sunny Gupta, DO

BASICS

Developmental dysplasia of the hip (DDH) is the most common hip disorder in children.

DESCRIPTION

- *Dysplasia* refers to an acetabulum that is shallow or underdeveloped.
- *Subluxation* refers to a femoral head that is not centered within the acetabulum.
- *Dislocation* refers to a femoral head that is completely out of the acetabulum.
- *Teratologic dislocation* refers to a femoral head that is in a fixed dislocated position usually associated with a genetic, developmental, or neuromuscular disorder.
- An *unstable hip* refers to a femoral head that can be subluxed or dislocated on physical examination.
- DDH refers to a wide spectrum of hip disorders from mild underdevelopment of the acetabulum to frank teratologic dislocation of the femoral head from the acetabulum.

EPIDEMIOLOGY

Incidence

- Incidence varies with gender, age, and race.
- Incidence of hip dysplasia is 0.5–2% of live births; however, true dislocation occurs in 0.1–0.2% of live births (1).
- Late dysplasia, subluxation, and dislocation occur in 0.04% of children (2).

ETIOLOGY AND PATHOPHYSIOLOGY

- Caused by any mechanism that prevents femoral head from being positioned correctly within the acetabulum, resulting in a shallow acetabulum
- Firstborn
- Intrauterine factors:
  - Abnormal intrauterine positioning: Breech presentation positions hip in such a way that the femoral head is forced out of the acetabulum.
  - Oligohydramnios
- Underlying ligamentous laxity
- Collagen vascular disorders
- Infection
- Environmental: culture-associated neonatal swaddling
- Congenital:
  - Arthrogryposis
  - Lumbosacral agenesis
  - Spina bifida
  - Neonatal Marfan syndrome
  - Fetal hydantoin syndrome
  - Larsen syndrome

RISK FACTORS

- Predominant race: more common in Caucasians of European descent; rare in African Americans
- Predominant gender: females > males (6:1)
- Birth order: increased risk with firstborns
- Family history: very strong risk factor
- Risk ~13% with one parent with hip dysplasia and 35% with affected parent and sibling
- Intrauterine factors: increased risk with breech presentation and oligohydramnios

GENERAL PREVENTION

- There is no true way to prevent occurrence.
- Early diagnosis is key to management.
- Thorough examination of hips of newborns and infants is the mainstay of early diagnosis.

COMMONLY ASSOCIATED CONDITIONS

Commonly associated with torticollis (20% coexistence) and metatarsus adductus (10% coexistence)

DIAGNOSIS

HISTORY

- Determine risk:
  - Breech delivery?
  - Female?
  - Firstborn?
  - Family history?
  - Race?
- Is the baby moving both lower extremities symmetrically?
- Any abnormal position of lower extremities noticed by parents?

PHYSICAL EXAM

- All infants require clinical screening by primary care provider who has experience in examining the hip.
- Examine patient in supine position.
- Every attempt should be made to examine the infant when he or she is not crying to avoid tensing of lower extremity muscles.
- Observe for signs of asymmetries:
  - Decrease in abduction of hip with adduction contracture
  - Asymmetric gluteal, anterior upper thigh, and popliteal skin folds
  - Galeazzi sign: apparent femoral shortening with hips and knees flexed together
- Ortolani test:
  - Abduction and external rotation of hip with examiner's middle finger over greater trochanter
  - Palpable clunk is positive sign produced by reduction of dislocated hip.
- Barlow test:
  - Adduction and internal rotation of hip
  - Palpable clunk is positive sign as hip dislocates.
- Examination may be normal initially despite the presence of hip dysplasia. Consequently, hip evaluation should be performed as part of neonatal physical examination through 4 mo of age (1).

DIAGNOSTIC TESTS & INTERPRETATION

- False-positive results: Hip clicks will be present in 10% of infants; only a small percentage will have hip dysplasia.
- Overdiagnosis is a problem because avascular necrosis of femur can occur (rarely) as a result of therapeutic interventions (3).
- X-rays:
  - Not useful prior to 4 mo, when the femoral head epiphysis ossifies and acetabular parameters are better defined
  - Various reference lines (Hilgenreiner, Shenton, and Perkin) and angles (acetabular index) are useful to detect frank dislocation (1).

- Ultrasound (US):
  - Most sensitive and effective form of screening
  - Recommended to screen with US starting at age 4 to 6 wk in patients with risk factors, persistent clunk on hip exam, or asymmetric hip exam (3)
  - Static and dynamic imaging (with Barlow and Ortolani maneuvers) to assess femoral head displacement
  - Useful in monitoring progress of therapy
  - Requires experienced ultrasonographer
- Computed tomography (CT) scan and magnetic resonance imaging (MRI) are not useful in diagnosis.

TREATMENT

- Subluxation at birth often resolves spontaneously and therefore may be observed for 3 wk.
- Indication for treatment: Subluxation of hip persists beyond 3 wk, confirmed on physical exam or US. Refer to a pediatric orthopedist (2).
- Pavlik harness:
  - Indicated for infants from ages 3 wk to 6 mo
  - Applied by orthopedist; hips positioned in flexion and abduction
  - Requires weekly evaluation of straps and radiologic confirmation of hip reduction; if hip is stable at 2 wk, reevaluation every 2 wk
  - Gradually weaned as hip stability continues
  - Duration of treatment: 3 mo after hip stability achieved (1)[A]
- Hip spica cast:
  - Indicated for children from ages 6 to 18 mo
  - Applied by orthopedist under general anesthesia; hips positioned in flexion and abduction with cutouts for perineal care
  - Cast changes every 6 wk
  - Duration of treatment: 3 to 4 mo (1)[A]
- Open reduction:
  - Indicated if closed reduction fails or excess abduction (>60 degrees) required for concentric reduction
  - Corrects barriers to reduction and safely increases stability (1)[A]
- Femoral/pelvic osteotomies:
  - Indicated if all prior closed and open reductions fail
  - Usually considered in children from ages 18 to 36 mo (1)[A]

ONGOING CARE

PROGNOSIS

If diagnosed early, prognosis is uniformly excellent.

COMPLICATIONS

- Missed early diagnosis can result in more complicated management and less favorable outcome.
- Failed reduction and redislocation
- Osteonecrosis of femoral head
- Hip labral pathology in adolescence or adulthood
- Osteoarthritis in adulthood

REFERENCES

1. Schwend RM, Shaw BA, Segal LS. Evaluation and treatment of developmental hip dysplasia in the newborn and infant. *Pediatr Clin North Am*. 2014;61(6):1095–1107.
2. Tomlinson J, O'Dowd D, Fernandes JA. Managing developmental dysplasia of the hip. *Indian J Pediatr*. 2016;83(11):1275–1279.
3. Kotlarsky P, Haber R, Bialik V, et al. Developmental dysplasia of the hip: what has changed in the last 20 years? *World J Orthop*. 2015;6(11):886–901.

ADDITIONAL READING

- Beaty JH. Congenital and developmental anomalies of hip and pelvis. In: Canale ST, ed. *Campbell's Operative Orthopaedics*. 10th ed. St. Louis, MO: Mosby; 2003:1079–1117.
- Guille JT, Pizzutillo PD, MacEwen GD. Development dysplasia of the hip from birth to six months. *J Am Acad Orthop Surg*. 2000;8(4):232–242.
- Vitale MG, Skaggs DL. Developmental dysplasia of the hip from six months to four years of age. *J Am Acad Orthop Surg*. 2001;9(6):401–411.

CLINICAL PEARLS

- DDH is the most common hip disorder in children.
- Early diagnosis is key to management. This is accomplished with a thorough examination of hips of newborns and infants.
- US is the most sensitive and effective form of screening; start screening with US at age 4 to 6 wk in patients with risk factors, persistent clunk on hip exam, or asymmetric hip exam.
- Refer to pediatric orthopedist for treatment if subluxation of hip persists beyond 3 wk, confirmed on physical exam or US.

DIABETES IN SPORTS

Marwan A. Bakarman, MBBS, FFCM • Fahad Anwer, FCPS, MRCGP (Int.)

BASICS

DESCRIPTION

Diabetes mellitus (DM) is a chronic disease caused by a genetic and/or acquired deficiency of insulin production due to destruction of the islet cells of the pancreas (type 1) or due to ineffectiveness of the insulin produced (type 2) resulting in elevated blood glucose levels.

EPIDEMIOLOGY

Prevalence

Type 1 and 2: 9.4% of the U.S. population

RISK FACTORS

- Sedentary lifestyle, glucose intolerance, gestational diabetes, and family history are risk factors for DM type 2 because they contribute to weight gain and insulin resistance.
- Exercise in diabetic patients may cause hypo- and/or hyperglycemia, exacerbation of retinopathy, foot injuries due to neuropathy, and injury due to autonomic dysfunction.

GENERAL PREVENTION

- Exercise, including competitive sports, can and should be performed by people with diabetes who have well-controlled blood sugars and, if present, well-managed complications. One notable exception is SCUBA diving, which can be done if the following criteria are met: (i) well-controlled blood sugars, (ii) no diabetic complications, and (iii) no hypoglycemia events or diabetic-related hospitalizations within the past year.
- Aerobic and anaerobic exercises benefit diabetics:
  - May be useful in preventing or delaying the onset of type 2 diabetes
  - May enhance weight loss and, in particular, weight maintenance when used along with an appropriate calorie-controlled meal plan
  - Aerobic exercise benefits include increased insulin sensitivity, oxidative enzymes, compliance and reactivity of blood vessels, lung function, immune and cardiac function, and decreases cardiovascular disease and overall mortality (1).
- Before beginning an exercise program, the individual with DM should undergo a detailed medical evaluation with appropriate diagnostic studies. This examination should carefully screen for the presence of macro- and microvascular complications that may be worsened by the exercise program.
- Avoid exercise if fasting glucose levels are >250 mg/dL and ketosis is present, and use caution if glucose levels are >300 mg/dL and no ketosis is present.

DIAGNOSIS

HISTORY

Known case of diabetes type 1 or type 2

PHYSICAL EXAM

- Body mass index (BMI)
- Vital signs, in particular blood pressure
- Skin and foot examination in diabetic patients looking for ulceration, deformities, and skin infection should be performed. Peripheral pulses and ankle brachial index should be checked to assess for peripheral arterial disease.
- Neurologic examination to assess for signs of neuropathy such as sensory loss
- Eye examination to assess for retinopathy and visual loss

DIAGNOSTIC TESTS & INTERPRETATION

Continuous glucose monitoring for the active person with either DM type 1 or 2:

- Fasting and random plasma glucose
- HbA1C

Follow-Up Tests & Special Considerations

- Unless there is a clear clinical diagnosis (e.g., patient in a hyperglycemic crisis or with classic symptoms of hyperglycemia and a random plasma glucose 200 mg/dL [11.1 mmol/L]), a second test is required for confirmation.
- It is recommended that the same test be repeated or a different test be performed without delay using a new blood sample for confirmation.

Diagnostic Procedures/Other

- Routine laboratory testing should include a fasting lipid profile.
- Electrocardiogram (ECG) in patients age >40 yr
- For patients >30 yr of age or those with DM of >5 yr in duration, screening for microalbuminuria should be performed annually.

Test Interpretation

A person can be diagnosed with diabetes if blood tests show the following results:

- Fasting plasma glucose of 126 mg/dL (7.0 mmol/L). Fasting is defined as no caloric intake for at least 8 hr.
- 2-hr serum glucose ≥200 mg/dL (11.1 mmol/L) during oral glucose tolerance test (OGTT). The test should be performed as described by the World Health Organization (WHO), using a glucose load containing the equivalent of 75-g anhydrous glucose dissolved in water.
- HbA1C of 6.5%
- In a patient with classic symptoms of hyperglycemia or hyperglycemic crisis, a random plasma glucose of ≥200 mg/dL (11.1 mmol/L) (2)[A]

TREATMENT

GENERAL MEASURES

- Exercise:
  - Preexercise medical clearance is generally unnecessary for asymptomatic individuals prior to beginning low- or moderate-intensity physical activity not exceeding the demands of brisk walking or everyday living.
  - Most adults with diabetes should engage in 150 min or more of moderate-to-vigorous intensity activity weekly, spread over at least 3 days/wk, with no >2 consecutive days without activity for type 2 diabetics (1)[B].
  - Children and adolescents with type 1 or type 2 DM should engage in 60 min/day or more of moderate or vigorous intensity aerobic activity, with vigorous, muscle-strengthening, and bone-strengthening activities included at least 3 days/wk (1)[C].
  - Adults with diabetes should engage in two to three sessions per week of resistance exercise on nonconsecutive days.
  - Flexibility training and balance training are recommended 2 times per week for older adults with diabetes. Yoga and tai chi may be included based on individual preferences to increase flexibility, muscular strength, and balance (1)[C].
  - Insulin regimen and carbohydrate intake changes should be used to prevent exercise-related hypoglycemia. Other strategies involve including short sprints, performing resistance exercise before aerobic exercise in the same session, and activity timing (1)[B].
  - Risk of nocturnal hypoglycemia following physical activity may be mitigated with reductions in basal insulin doses, inclusion of bedtime snacks, and/or use of continuous glucose monitoring (1)[C].
  - Physical activity with vascular diseases can be undertaken safely but with appropriate precautions (1)[B].
  - Physical activity done with peripheral neuropathy necessitates proper foot care to prevent and detect problems early to avoid ulceration and amputation (1)[B].
- Reduce sugar and fat intake in diet.
- Weight control
- Quit tobacco use.

MEDICATION

- Type 1 DM: insulin:
  - Insulin infusion pumps are modern, computerized devices, which infuse insulin at a low dose continuously under the skin via a catheter. Continuous subcutaneous insulin infusion (CSII) has become an increasingly important option in the therapy of type 1 diabetes over recent years.
  - Insulin pump treatment involves the insertion of a temporary cannula into the subcutaneous tissue through which rapid-acting insulin is infused continuously using an electronically controlled pump. CSII therapy permits numerous bolus insulin doses to be given without the need for a physical injection each time.
  - The strategies for adjustment of CSII therapy during exercise have focused on the reduction or cessation of insulin infusion during exercise because this should approximate more closely to the physiologic situation and therefore reduce rates of hypoglycemia.
  - Suspending basal insulin at the start of exercise does increase the risk of hyperglycemia but was not observed to increase the risk of ketosis during a short period of exercise.
  - The pump should be removed for contact/collision sports and the catheter site protected. Remove the pump 30 min before exercise lasting <1 hr. An hourly bolus of insulin, approximately 50% of the normal hourly basal rate, may be needed for exercise lasting >1 hr.
- Type 2 DM: Metformin is the first drug to be initiated (2)[A].

ALERT

Glucagon hormone is given to unconscious or semiconscious diabetic patients in acute hypoglycemic state. It can be administered as subcutaneous or intramuscular injection.

- Type 2 DM: If blood sugars are not adequately controlled on metformin alone, combination therapy with one or two of the following hypoglycemic drugs can be added to metformin (2)[A]:
  - Sulfonylureas
  - Thiazolidinediones
  - DPP-4 inhibitor
  - SGLT2 inhibitor
  - GLP-1 receptor agonist
  - Insulin

ISSUES FOR REFERRAL

- Disease complications: Consider annual review—more frequent if disease complications not well managed (2)[B].
- Endocrinologist in cases where management is difficult
- Cardiologist for cardiovascular diseases
- Nephrologist for advanced diabetic nephropathy
- Neurologist for advanced peripheral neuropathy
- Ophthalmologist for advanced diabetic retinopathy
- Vascular surgeon for nonhealing foot wounds/ulcers
- Urologist for erectile dysfunction

ADDITIONAL THERAPIES

- Aspirin 81 mg daily (2)[A]
- Moderate intensity statin therapy for hyperlipidemia (low-density lipoprotein cholesterol [LDL-C] 70 to 189 mg/dL) in diabetics aged 40 to 75 yr old (e.g., simvastatin 20 to 40 mg or atorvastatin 10 to 20 mg at night) (3)[A]
- Angiotensin-converting enzyme (ACE) inhibitors/angiotensin II receptor blockers (ARBs) for hypertension and diabetic nephropathy (e.g., losartan 50 mg daily) (2)[A]
- Gabapentin, pregabalin, or duloxetine oral for neuropathic pain (2)[A]

ADMISSION, INPATIENT, AND NURSING CONSIDERATIONS

- Perform HbA1C for all patients admitted, if not checked in last 3 mo (2)[B].
- Insulin therapy should be initiated for treatment of persistent hyperglycemia starting at a threshold ≥180 mg/dL (10.0 mmol/L) (2)[A].
- A target glucose range of 140 to 180 mg/dL (7.8 to 10.0 mmol/L) is recommended for the majority of critically ill patients (2)[A] and noncritically ill patients (2)[C].

ONGOING CARE

FOLLOW-UP RECOMMENDATIONS

- Two primary techniques are available for clinicians and patients to assess glycemic control: patient self-monitoring of blood glucose (SMBG) levels and HbA1C.
- Continuous glucose monitoring may be a useful adjunct to self-monitoring in selected patients.
- Monitoring the HbA1C every 3 to 6 mo, with a target goal of <7% to prevent microvascular complications (2)[A]
- SMBG frequency and timing should be dictated by patients' specific needs and goals.
- Most patients using intensive insulin regimens (multiple-dose insulin or insulin pump therapy) should perform SMBG prior to meals and snacks, at bedtime, occasionally postprandially, prior to exercise, when they suspect low blood glucose, after treating low blood glucose until they are normoglycemic, and prior to critical tasks such as driving (2)[B].

DIET

- Athlete patients do not need a separate diet from the rest of the family or expensive "diabetes" food products. A diabetic diet is a healthy diet.
- Aim for ≥50% of calorie intake from fiber-rich carbohydrate sources, with minimum fat (especially saturated), refined carbohydrate, and alcohol.
- Adjust total calorie intake according to desired BMI.
- Recommend ≥5 portions of fresh fruit or vegetables per day.
- Spread food intake evenly across the day for athlete patients controlled with oral medications and/or diet.
- Diet sheets should be provided to all athletes with DM.
- Ready-made meals, processed foods, and alcohol are often sources of hidden sugar.
- Snacks may be needed before, during, and after exercise to maintain blood glucose in a normal range.

PATIENT EDUCATION

- It is essential that athletes with DM understand their disorder and learn to handle all aspects of their management as comprehensively and quickly as possible.
- The diabetic athlete should be well-informed about signs, symptoms, prevention, and treatment of hypo-/hyperglycemia.
- It is necessary for diabetics to obtain the approval of a doctor before starting a new sport.
- When a diabetic patient exercises, he or she should take at least 15 g of sugar, such as 1 1/2 cup of fruit juice or five candy bars or glucose cubes, to treat hypoglycemia (4,5).
- Shoes must be appropriate for the chosen sport and have good fit to prevent injuries and cuts in the feet. It is also recommended to wear sports socks made of polystyrene to prevent excessive friction that can cause skin injury.
- Check feet and legs prior to and after exercise to make sure there are no wounds.
- Hydration is important before, during, and after the sport.
- Diabetic patients should have identification and a health alert bracelet or necklace when going out to exercise, in case of needing medical assistance.
- Blood sugar levels should be checked before and after exercise. It is advisable to determine a safe blood glucose range prior to exercise in conjunction with a physician. This is especially important for people who use insulin (5).
- If shivering, anxiousness, dizziness, excessive sweating, or any unusual changes in heart rate develop while exercising, the patient should stop exercising and immediately check a blood sugar level. If low, treat with carbohydrates.
- Start each exercise session with 5 to 10 min of warm-ups, so that the body is ready for sport and is not surprised by difficult and intensive exercise (4).
- Recommended types of exercise for diabetics include aerobic exercise such as walking, jogging, running light, tennis, kayaking, rope jumping, dancing, swimming, cycling, basketball, bicycle, dancing and treadmill (4).
- Resistance exercises are also recommended for patients with DM because they will improve muscle mass and strength, body composition, physical function, bone mineral density, mental well-being, insulin sensitivity, lipid profile, blood pressure, and cardiovascular health. All these lead to better control of HbA1C (1),(5)[A].
- Consider exercising with friends or in a group in order to develop social relationships.
- Vary exercise routines to avoid boredom.
- Home activities and chores are recommended for diabetics.

PROGNOSIS

- DM patients are at 2 to 5 times increased risk of ischemic heart disease and 2 to 3 times increased risk of stroke and peripheral vascular disease. The protective effect of female sex is lost.
- Atherosclerotic disease accounts for most of the excess mortality due to DM.

COMPLICATIONS

- Hypo- and/or hyperglycemia
- Autonomic dysfunction
- Cardiovascular disease
- Renal disease
- Foot problems, including ulcers, deformities, and infections, can manifest from neurologic and microvascular complications.

REFERENCES

1. Colberg SR, Sigal RJ, Yardley JE, et al. Physical activity/exercise and diabetes: a position statement of the American Diabetes Association. *Diabetes Care*. 2016;39(11):2065–2079.
2. American Diabetes Association. 2. Classification and diagnosis of diabetes. *Diabetes Care*. 2017;40 (Suppl 1):S11–S24. doi:10.2337/dc17-S005.
3. Stone NJ, Robinson JG, Lichtenstein AH, et al. 2013 ACC/AHA guideline on the treatment of blood cholesterol to reduce atherosclerotic cardiovascular risk in adults: a report of the American College of Cardiology/American Heart Association Task Force on Practice Guidelines. *Circulation*. 2014;129(25 Suppl 2):S1–S45.
4. Harris GD, White RD. Diabetes in the competitive athlete. *Curr Sports Med Rep*. 2012;11(6):309–315.
5. Shugart C, Jackson J, Fields KB. Diabetes in sports. *Sports Health*. 2010;2(1):29–38.

CLINICAL PEARLS

- Patients with DM should be strongly advised to obtain regular exercise or physical activity as part of their management plan for glycemic control, overall health, and prevention of diabetic complications.
- Exercise plans should be tailored according to the individual's specific needs. Moreover, all diabetic adults should be encouraged to decrease the amount of daily sedentary time and to indulge in regular frequent spells of activity.
- Step counters and pedometers have proven to be useful tools to encourage and guide physical activity. They provide feedback for self-monitoring of physical activity by the diabetic patient. Diabetic patients should set achievable goals for steps per day at the start before progressing toward higher targets. Generally, adult patients should take at least 10,000 steps per day.
- Blood glucose monitoring is a valuable tool for diabetic patients to regulate the intensity and duration of their exercise and sports activities.
- Hyperglycemia and hypoglycemia are the greatest risks to exercising for the diabetic athletes, in particular those with type I DM. Diabetic patients should be educated regarding the symptoms and signs of hypoglycemia. Hypoglycemia can be avoided through reducing the insulin doses and/or increasing consumption of carbohydrates along with having an available source of sugar (15 g) in case of developing hypoglycemia during exercising.
- Diabetic athletes should practice good foot care during and after exercise along with using appropriate footwear during sports activities.

DIP DISLOCATION

Patrick Jenkins III, MD • Tenley Murphy, MD, FAAFP, CAQSM • Jason J. Stacy, MD

BASICS

DESCRIPTION

- Dislocations of distal interphalangeal (DIP) or 1st interphalangeal (IP) joints
- Mechanism is typically a hyperextension injury of the DIP joint.
- Synonym(s): jammed finger

EPIDEMIOLOGY

Incidence

- Pure DIP dislocations are uncommon (1). They are usually accompanied by a fracture or tendon avulsion.
- DIP dislocations are less common than proximal interphalangeal (PIP) dislocations (2).
- Most dislocations occur dorsally, especially when associated with injuries during athletic events. These injuries can lead to volar plate injury.
- Dorsal DIP dislocations are most common in basketball, football, softball, and baseball.

ALERT

Volar dislocations are often associated with crush or twist injuries and with disruption of the terminal extensor tendon at its insertion point, making management more difficult.

- Simultaneous DIP and PIP dislocations are rare but occur most commonly in ring and small fingers.

DIAGNOSIS

HISTORY

- Mechanism of injury (i.e., hyperextension)
- Presence of an obvious deformity (i.e., distal phalanx positioned above or below the plane of the middle phalanx)
- Often self-reduced by the patient on the playing field or before presentation

PHYSICAL EXAM

- Obvious deformity if not already reduced: distal phalanx sitting above (dorsal dislocation) or below (volar dislocation) the plane of the middle phalanx
- Careful examination: With the PIP joint held in extension, check flexor digitorum profundus (FDP) and terminal extensor function and sensation at the tip of the finger.
- Check collateral ligament: Place radial and ulnar stress across DIP joint with joint in full extension and 30 degrees flexion looking for increased laxity compared to the contralateral side. $>$10 degrees of laxity indicates damage (3)[B].
- Check volar plate: Increased hyperextension of the joint is indicative of a volar plate injury.
- Evaluate skin for any signs of open injury. This most commonly seen on palmar surface.
- Evaluate neurovascular status.

DIFFERENTIAL DIAGNOSIS

- Fracture of distal (tuft fracture) or middle phalanx
- FDP rupture (i.e., jersey finger)
- Extensor mechanism rupture (i.e., mallet finger)
- Bony mallet finger (bony avulsion of the insertion of the extensor mechanism at the dorsal base of the distal phalanx)
- Fracture-dislocation
- Collateral ligament disruption
- Chronic instability

DIAGNOSTIC TESTS & INTERPRETATION

- Radiographs: three views preferred (anteroposterior, lateral, and oblique views) pre- and postreduction if it does not significantly delay reduction attempt(s)
- Look carefully for any bony avulsion, especially of the volar plate.
- Other imaging modalities are not typically needed.

TREATMENT

GENERAL MEASURES

- Reduction techniques:
  - On-field reduction should be attempted to reduce pain and usually is easily performed when done immediately (4)[C].
  - Technique for reduction: Maintaining proximal countertraction to the DIP joint, apply a steady longitudinal traction force of the distal finger.
  - Slight hyperextension and volar pressure at the distal phalanx may aid in reduction of dorsal dislocations (4)[C].
  - Sweat can cause the skin to be slick, making reductions attempts difficult. Try using a towel or gauze pad for better grip.
  - Reduction may require a digital block if dislocation is prolonged or associated with significant pain.

ALERT
Postreduction evaluation:
- Careful examination as discussed above, especially checking FDP/extensor function and for skin injury
- Postreduction radiographs from at least two views to ensure joint congruity (3)[C]

- Complications:
  - Dislocation may be irreducible. This is thought to happen for several reasons:
    - Trapped volar plate (5)
    - FDP entrapment behind a single condyle of middle phalanx
    - P2 buttonholed through the volar plate
    - Extensor tendon displacement around the head of P2
- Immobilization:
  - Dorsal dislocations should be placed in a splint with the DIP joint in slight flexion (20 degrees) for 1 to 2 wk (4)[B].
  - Volar dislocations should be treated as a mallet finger injury and placed in a splint with the DIP joint in extension for 8 wk, allowing the extensor tendon to heal.
  - Longer immobilization leads to increased likelihood of long-term joint stiffness (3)[C].
  - When splinting, use caution with regard to the dorsal skin segment between the extensor crease and the nail fold because pressure can cause necrosis.
  - Patient can return to sport once joint stability and range of motion (ROM) are acceptable (5)[C].

ISSUES FOR REFERRAL
- A referral to an orthopedic surgeon or hand specialist should be made when the dislocation is irreducible or an open injury has occurred with joint exposure.
- In addition, chronic dislocations, FDP tendon ruptures, fractures involving >40% of the articular surface, and unstable collateral ligaments should be referred to a specialist (4)[C].

ADDITIONAL THERAPIES
- Start ROM exercises immediately after splint removal.
- Use both active and passive ROM initially.
- Start resisted ROM as soon as active and passive motions are pain free (4)[C].
- Swelling control should be quickly initiated because it can block full ROM. This can be achieved with retrograde massage, elevation, ice, and compression (6)[B].

SURGERY/OTHER PROCEDURES
- Closed reduction and percutaneous pinning (CRPP): Joint instability or associated fracture may require immobilization with use of a Kirschner wire for stabilization.
- Open reduction:
  - May be required in a chronically (>3 wk) dislocated or subluxated joint to remove scar tissue and release tension to facilitate reduction
  - Use of a Kirschner wire depends on degree of stability.

REFERENCES

1. Bielak KM, Kafka J, Terrell T. Treatment of hand and wrist injuries. *Prim Care*. 2013;40(2):431–451.
2. Chen F, Kalainov DM. Phalanx fractures and dislocations in athletes. *Curr Rev Musculoskelet Med*. 2017;10(1):10–16.
3. Carruthers KH, Skie M, Jain M. Jam injuries of the finger: diagnosis and management of injuries to the interphalangeal joints across multiple sports and levels of experience. *Sports Health*. 2016;8(5):469–478.
4. Borchers JR, Best TM. Common finger fractures and dislocations. *Am Fam Physician*. 2012;85(8):805–810.
5. Prucz RB, Friedrich JB. Finger joint injuries. *Clin Sports Med*. 2015;34(1):99–116.
6. Singletary S, Geissler WB. Bracing and rehabilitation for wrist and hand injuries in collegiate athletes. *Hand Clin*. 2009;25(3):443–448.

CLINICAL PEARLS

- Athletes can return to play immediately if dislocation is uncomplicated, successfully reduced, and the athlete is allowed to play in a splint or cast.
- Thumb IP dislocations should be treated exactly the same as DIP dislocations.

DISCOID MENISCUS

Melissa Nayak, MD, CAQSM

BASICS

DESCRIPTION

- Menisci are semilunar fibrocartilaginous structures located between the femoral condyles and tibial plateaus:
  - Medial meniscus is U shaped.
  - Lateral meniscus is C shaped.
- Discoid meniscus lacks C-shaped configuration:
  - Completely filled in center or small void in center with thicker outer rim
  - Decreased collagen fibers, loss of normal collagen orientation, mucoid degeneration
  - Anatomic variation alters normal mechanics and predisposes to tearing.
- Predominantly lateral; may be medial or bilateral
- May be asymptomatic until adolescence or adulthood
- Watanabe classification (1,2,3)[C]:
  - Most widely accepted classification system
  - Type I (complete):
    - Most common
    - Disc-shaped, thickened meniscus with thin center, complete tibial plateau coverage, and normal posterior attachment
  - Type II (incomplete): semilunar-shaped meniscus with partial tibial plateau coverage and normal posterior attachment
  - Type III (Wrisberg type):
    - Least common
    - Hypermobile meniscus resulting from deficient posterior tibial plateau attachment (coronary ligament)
    - Wrisberg ligament present (from posterior horn lateral meniscus to posterior aspect medial femoral condyle)
    - Unstable and may displace

EPIDEMIOLOGY

Incidence

- 1.5–15.5% (lateral discoid meniscus) (1)
- 0.1–0.3% (medial discoid meniscus) (1)
- Bilateral (lateral discoid meniscus) in 20% of patients (1,2,3)
- Increased incidence in Asian populations (2,3)
- True incidence unknown (asymptomatic cases)

Prevalence

- 1.4–15.5% (lateral discoid meniscus) (4)
- 0.06–0.3% (medial discoid meniscus—very rare) (4)
- True prevalence unknown (asymptomatic cases)

ETIOLOGY AND PATHOPHYSIOLOGY

- Exact cause unknown
- May be congenital anomaly or malformation

Genetics

Genetic or familial transmission may play a role.

RISK FACTORS

Asian ancestry

COMMONLY ASSOCIATED CONDITIONS

- Meniscal tears (increased incidence related to structural abnormality, decreased vascularity, and biomechanical stress):
  - Horizontal cleavage tear (most common)
- Osteochondritis dissecans of ipsilateral lateral femoral condyle
- High fibular head
- Fibular muscular defects
- Hypoplasia of lateral femoral condyle with lateral joint space widening
- Hypoplasia of lateral tibial spine
- Abnormal shape of lateral malleolus
- Enlarged inferior lateral geniculate artery

DIAGNOSIS

HISTORY

- Patients may be asymptomatic.
- Signs and symptoms (in absence of trauma):
  - Pain
  - Clunking
  - Giving way
  - Popping
  - Snapping
  - Swelling
  - Locking
  - Decreased knee extension

PHYSICAL EXAM
- Palpable click near complete extension
- Quadriceps atrophy
- Lack of full extension
- Joint line tenderness
- Effusion less common
- Positive McMurray test (with associated meniscal tears)

DIFFERENTIAL DIAGNOSIS
- Meniscal tear
- Osteochondritis dissecans
- Loose body
- Patellar instability
- Snapping of tendons around knee
- Medial plica syndrome

DIAGNOSTIC TESTS & INTERPRETATION
- Radiographs:
  - May be normal
  - Widened lateral joint space
  - Squared-off appearance of lateral femoral condyle
  - Cupping of lateral tibial plateau
  - Flattening of tibial eminence
  - Elevation of fibular head
- Magnetic resonance imaging (MRI):
  - Test of choice
  - May not show abnormal signal intensity
  - Lateral meniscal height greater than medial, with high intrameniscal signal
  - Abnormal, thickened "bow-tie" appearance of meniscus

TREATMENT

No treatment or surgical indications for asymptomatic patients (1,2,3)[C]

ISSUES FOR REFERRAL
Orthopedic surgical consultation is indicated in patients still symptomatic after conservative measures.

SURGERY/OTHER PROCEDURES
- Goal is meniscal preservation (3)[C].
- Arthroscopic partial meniscectomy (saucerization) and repair of unstable or detached peripheral attachments to the capsule (1,2,3,4)[C]
- Arthroscopic total meniscectomy not recommended because it leads to osteoarthrosis; reserved for large or complex tears not amenable to saucerization or repair (2,3)[C]

ONGOING CARE

Postoperative physical therapy for knee range of motion, quadriceps strengthening, hamstring stretching, and gait training

PATIENT EDUCATION
- Asymptomatic discoid meniscus needs no treatment.
- Surgery is recommended if mechanical symptoms present: pain, locking, swelling, giving way, functional limitations, inability to participate in sports.

PROGNOSIS
- Good prognosis when asymptomatic
- Better prognosis in younger patients
- Poorer prognosis when osteochondritis dissecans present

COMPLICATIONS
- Osteochondritis dissecans of lateral femoral condyle
- Postoperative complications:
  - Cartilage remains thickened and more susceptible to developing tear.
  - Osteoarthrosis

REFERENCES

1. Francavilla ML, Restrepo R, Zamora KW, et al. Meniscal pathology in children: differences and similarities with the adult meniscus. *Pediatr Radiol*. 2014;44(8):910–929.
2. Kim JG, Han SW, Lee DH. Diagnosis and treatment of discoid meniscus. *Knee Surg Relat Res*. 2016;28(4):255–262.
3. Yaniv M, Blumberg N. The discoid meniscus. *J Child Orthop*. 2007;1(2):89–96.
4. Kini SG, Walker P, Bruce W. Bilateral symptomatic discoid medial meniscus of the knee: a case report and review of literature. *Arch Trauma Res*. 2015;4(1):e27115.

CLINICAL PEARLS

- Isolated atraumatic lateral meniscal tear in a child <10 yr of age should raise suspicion of a discoid meniscus.
- Horizontal tear is the most common tear pattern associated with a discoid meniscus.
- Discoid meniscus can be asymptomatic.

DISLOCATION, HIP, POSTERIOR

Greg Nakamoto, MD, FACP

BASICS

DESCRIPTION

- Hip dislocations can be congenital or traumatic and can occur in native hips or after total hip arthroplasty.
- The remainder of this topic is dedicated to the evaluation and management of traumatic (posterior) hip dislocations in native hips:
  - Posterior hip dislocation is an orthopedic emergency in which the femoral head is displaced posteriorly relative to the acetabulum.

ALERT
Primary concerns when evaluating the patient with a posterior hip dislocation are the attainment of early reduction (within 6 hr) to prevent long-term sequelae (avascular necrosis [AVN]) and the search for additional injuries (often life- or limb-threatening due to the high forces necessary to create this injury).

EPIDEMIOLOGY

- 46–84% of hip dislocations occur secondary to traffic accidents. The remainders are usually caused by falls, industrial accidents, or high-energy sports injuries (1).
- Posterior dislocations account for ~90% of all hip dislocations.
- More common in young males because these injuries are associated with risk-taking behavior
- Age:
  - Trauma (such as motor vehicle accident) is a more common cause in patients <35 yr than in older patients.
  - Falls are a more common cause in those >65 yr than in younger patients.

RISK FACTORS

- High-energy trauma
- Mechanism is a posteriorly directed force against a flexed knee, with the hip flexed and adducted (2).
- Most common cause is knee striking the dashboard in a head-on motor vehicle accident:
  - Depending on the position of the hip, this can result in either anterior or posterior dislocation.
  - With this mechanism of injury, up to 93% of patients will have magnetic resonance imaging (MRI)-confirmed injuries in the ipsilateral knee (1).
- In athletic competition, low-energy mechanisms of injury include a forward fall onto the knee with a flexed hip or a blow from behind while down on all four limbs.

COMMONLY ASSOCIATED CONDITIONS

- Life-threatening internal organ damage, bleeding, and shock reflect the high energy of the trauma required to dislocate a hip.

ALERT
Ipsilateral sciatic nerve injured in 10–14% of cases; changes a posterior hip dislocation from an orthopedic urgency to a true surgical emergency

- Fractures of the pelvis, acetabulum, femoral head, neck, and shaft

DIAGNOSIS

HISTORY

- Mechanism: can help guide the search for associated visceral and orthopedic injuries
- Position at time of injury: Simple posterior dislocation most commonly occurs with force on a flexed knee with the hip in varying degrees of flexion and adduction. Addition of hip abduction increases the risk of associated acetabular fracture or anterior dislocation.

PHYSICAL EXAM

- Immediate, severe pain, and disability
- Limb shortening with hip flexion, internal rotation, and adduction (1). In the obtunded patient, the examiner may have to recognize the position of posterior hip dislocation if the patient is not able to verbalize.
- Classic position may be absent if there is an associated femoral shaft fracture.
- Vital signs and complete trauma evaluation essential because of the high association with life-threatening injuries
- Pelvic rocking and pubic compression tests to examine for associated pelvic rim fractures
- Distal neurovascular examination to assess for sciatic nerve or vascular injures, which merit more urgent reduction

DIFFERENTIAL DIAGNOSIS

- Anterior dislocation of the hip
- Combined fracture–dislocation
- Fracture of the pelvis, acetabulum, or femur
- Traumatic hip subluxation
- Hip pointer
- Gastrointestinal (GI) or genitoureteral visceral injury

DIAGNOSTIC TESTS & INTERPRETATION

- Lab studies are ordered as needed on the basis of the trauma assessment and for preoperative planning.
- Type and cross of blood products may be necessary.
- Initial x-rays: anteroposterior (AP) and lateral views of the pelvis. AP often reveals the dislocation, but a true lateral may be needed to confirm the direction.
- Search for associated pelvic rim, acetabular, femoral head, neck, and shaft fractures may merit additional x-rays (including 3/4 internal and external obliques of the pelvis as well as femur films) depending on the clinical situation.
- **Role of computed tomography (CT) in the unreduced hip dislocation:**
  - In the case of **suspected nondisplaced femoral neck fracture**, obtain CT before attempted reduction maneuvers so as not to displace an unidentified femoral neck fracture (the presence of a **femoral neck fracture is a contraindication to attempts at closed reduction**; such patients should undergo open reduction) (1,2)[C].
  - In the case of **irreducible dislocations**, obtain CT prior to open surgical reduction (1,2)[C].

TREATMENT

- Prehospital:
  - Patients suffering a high-energy trauma sufficient to cause a hip dislocation commonly have associated injuries that take precedence for overall patient stabilization:
    - Establish airway, breathing, and circulation (ABCs). Stabilize the spine appropriately.
    - Patients with a hip dislocation can be placed on a backboard and allowed to assume the leg position of maximal comfort (i.e., slight hip flexion with leg adducted).
    - Transport to trauma center appropriate for patient's overall clinical status
    - An experienced operator might consider attempt at early reduction in the field if conventional treatment is unavailable in a timely manner (e.g., wilderness or backcountry situations).
- Emergency department (ED) treatment:
  - Rule out and/or stabilize life-threatening injuries. Neurovascular examination to determine if coexisting neurovascular injury; x-rays to confirm the dislocation and evaluate for coexisting fractures

ALERT
Fracture-dislocations and dislocations with associated sciatic nerve injury merit emergent orthopedic consultation.

  - **Indications for primary operative/open reduction**: Dislocations with associated femoral head or shaft fractures, open traumatic hip dislocations, as well as apparently simple dislocations that otherwise defy closed reduction with the methods described below ("irreducible dislocations") are generally treated initially with open reduction (1,2,3)[C].
  - **Closed reduction in the ED** will require analgesics, muscle relaxants, and/or sedation to overcome severe pain and muscular spasm before it can be attempted. Some cases may require spinal or general anesthesia to achieve closed reduction.
  - Reduction of a simple posterior dislocation (i.e., without fracture, or with an insignificant acetabular fracture) is typically treated with closed reduction only (2)[C]:
    - Consider orthopedic consultation if it will not delay relocation beyond a reasonable amount of time, usually within 6 hr, because **reduction under 6 hr reduces the rate of AVN** (4)[A].
    - Some authors advise orthopedic consultation for any hip dislocation and that the orthopedist should be present when attempting closed reduction.
  - For the experienced treating physician, one attempt at reduction of a simple dislocation might be reasonable. However, urgent orthopedic consultation should be obtained for simple dislocations that are not easily reducible with one attempt because **multiple attempts at closed reduction are also associated with poorer outcomes** (4)[A].
  - For posterior dislocations, closed reduction is attempted through hip flexion, internal rotation, and adduction (5). Numerous methods of reduction have been described, with no one method having been proven superior. Three of the more common methods are described below as well as a newer fourth method which has the advantage of improved operator back safety:
    - **Allis method**: An assistant stabilizes the pelvis of the supine patient with downward pressure on the anterior superior iliac spine. The operator applies axial traction in line with the deformity by pulling with his or her hands from behind the flexed knee. While maintaining this traction, the hip is gently flexed to 90 degrees and then gently internally and externally rotated until reduction occurs; requires two operators (1,4,5)
    - **Stimson method**: patient placed prone, with affected hip hanging down over edge of bed. Downward traction is applied to the leg while an assistant applies stabilizing pressure to the pelvis. Requires two operators; might be difficult

to move multiple-injury patient into proper position and difficult to monitor the airway in the prone position (1,4,5)
  - **Whistler method**: patient supine with unaffected knee flexed to 120 degrees such that the unaffected foot is placed firmly on the bed. Standing on the affected side, the operator reaches his hand under the affected knee and places his hand onto the unaffected flexed knee. By straightening his arm and lifting his shoulder, the operator adducts the patient's leg and applies traction until the hip reduces; requires only one operator and airway easily monitored in supine position (5)
  - **Waddell method**: a newer technique, using the principles of the Allis and Bigelow maneuvers but with modifications that lessens the strain on the operator's back. Patient supine, with an assistant stabilizing the patient's pelvis. The operator hovers over the patient and places his forearm behind the knee of the affected hip, which is flexed between 60 degrees and 90 degrees. Keeping the back straight, the operator hugs the knee to his chest, and gently leans back, pulling traction through the femur with minimal strain on the operator's back. The operator can then adduct and internally rotate the leg by leaning and rotating as needed (5).
- **If closed reduction cannot be accomplished**, the dislocated hip should be held in a position of relative extension with the ipsilateral knee in flexion until open reduction can be performed. This position puts the least strain on the sciatic nerve.

ADDITIONAL THERAPIES

- Postreduction considerations include the following:
  - Repeat neurovascular examination of the injured limb.
  - Repeat x-rays, including AP and lateral views, immediately to confirm reduction (1).
  - **After postreduction x-rays confirm a stable and concentric reduction, obtaining CT scan with fine cuts (2 to 3 mm) through the hips should be part of the standard postreduction evaluation of a traumatic posterior hip dislocation** (1,2,4)[A]:
    - To evaluate for presence of osteochondral or intra-articular fragments, femoral head injuries, and acetabular fractures (any of which might make the reduction unstable)
    - Essential in assigning proper classification of posterior fracture-dislocations of the hip, which in turn determines optimal definitive treatment
  - MRI: In children and adolescents, postreduction hip MRI may be better than CT for detecting structural injuries (6)[B].
  - After successful closed reduction, the leg should be extended and externally rotated until further radiographic and orthopedic evaluation is completed; placing the leg in a knee immobilizer helps prevent inadvertent flexion at the hip (3).
  - **Operative versus nonoperative treatment of the reduced hip dislocation (based on postreduction physical examination and CT):**
    - Patients with stable, concentric reductions without associated significant fractures may be treated nonoperatively (4)[A].
    - Patients with unstable reductions, displaced fractures, or acetabular fractures that would likely compromise stability are generally treated operatively (4)[A]. Neurovascular deficit that occurs after closed reduction is also an indication for operative management.
- Dislocation of the prosthetic hip is a special concern:
  - Prostheses are most susceptible to dislocation at 3 to 4 months after initial surgery.
  - Hip prostheses can also deteriorate over time and subsequently dislocate late with minimal force (e.g., crossing of legs, standing up).
  - Reduction of a prosthetic hip dislocation is less urgent than for a native hip if neurovascular status is intact because concern for AVN or osteoarthritis is nonexistent.
  - Reduction is accomplished with same maneuvers as for native hip; however, less force is used so as to avoid iatrogenic fracture.

SURGERY/OTHER PROCEDURES

- Given this injury often occurs in the setting of high-energy trauma, orthopedic evaluation usually occurs in conjunction with the initial trauma evaluation.
- In the case of pure dislocations without other trauma, a single attempt at reduction may be attempted if orthopedic consultation is delayed. However, urgent orthopedic referral should be made for any patient in whom closed reduction does not result in easy reduction because reduction in <6 hr is the goal to reduce the risk of AVN, and multiple attempts at reduction result in poorer long-term outcomes. More urgent reduction is needed if there is associated neurovascular compromise.
- Postreduction, further orthopedic, and radiographic evaluations as above are needed to guide subsequent definitive surgical decision making.

ONGOING CARE

FOLLOW-UP RECOMMENDATIONS

- Given the high-energy mechanism of injury, most patients require admission, often to a trauma service, for continued evaluation and treatment of associated injuries.
- The duration of non–weight-bearing immobilization after reduction of uncomplicated simple hip dislocation is controversial (3)[C]:
  - Many suggest a short period of traction until pain is improved, followed by early gentle range of motion.
  - Recommended period of non–weight-bearing varies from days to months. However, prolonged non–weight-bearing has not been shown to influence incidence of AVN.
- Physical therapy (PT) as directed by the orthopedist often starts with range of motion exercises and progresses to include muscle rehabilitation and strengthening; timing of PT might be influenced by coexisting injuries/fractures at the hip or elsewhere.

COMPLICATIONS

- Complication rate increases directly with time elapsed before relocation.
- **AVN:**
  - AVN risk appears to increase with time to reduction, multiple attempts at reduction, or need for open reduction.
  - In one study, 4% of patients reduced within 6 hr developed AVN, whereas 58% of patients reduced later than 6 hr developed AVN (3).
  - Early weight-bearing after reduction does not appear to increase the incidence of AVN (3).
- **Posttraumatic osteoarthritis** affects 16–24% of patients and up to 89% of patients with an associated femoral head or neck fracture (1,2).
- **Sciatic nerve injury** occurs in up to 10% of adult dislocations (2), either during the initial trauma or during relocation:
  - New neurologic deficits that occur **postreduction** warrant immediate surgical intervention; hence, the importance of a complete neurovascular exam before and after reduction.
- **Myositis ossificans**, **recurrent instability**, and **labral tears** are also noted late complications of posterior hip dislocations.

REFERENCES

1. Beebe MJ, Bauer JM, Mir HR. Treatment of hip dislocations and associated injuries: current state of care. *Orthop Clin North Am*. 2016;47(3):527–549.
2. Mandell JC, Marshall RA, Weaver MJ, et al. Traumatic hip dislocation: what the orthopedic surgeon wants to know. *Radiographics*. 2017;37(7):2181–2201.
3. Foulk DM, Mullis BH. Hip dislocation: evaluation and management. *J Am Acad Orthop Surg*. 2010;18(4):199–209.
4. Yang EC, Cornwall R. Initial treatment of traumatic hip dislocations in the adult. *Clin Orthop Relat Res*. 2000;(337):24–31.
5. Waddell BS, Mohamed S, Glomset JT, et al. A detailed review of hip reduction maneuvers: a focus on physician safety and introduction of the Waddell technique. *Orthop Rev (Pavia)*. 2016;8(1):6253.
6. Thanacharoenpanich S, Bixby S, Breen MA, et al. MRI is better than CT scan for detection of structural pathologies after traumatic posterior hip dislocations in children and adolescents [published online ahead of print January 19, 2018]. *J Pediatr Orthop*. doi:10.1097/BPO.0000000000001127.

ADDITIONAL READING

- Dumont GD. Hip instability: current concepts and treatment options. *Clin Sports Med*. 2016;35(3):435–447.
- Stein MJ, Kang C, Ball V. Emergency department evaluation and treatment of acute hip and thigh pain. *Emerg Med Clin North Am*. 2015;33(2):327–343.

CLINICAL PEARLS

- Of primary concern when evaluating the patient with a posterior hip dislocation is the attainment of early reduction (within 6 hr) to prevent long-term sequelae and the search for additional life- or limb-threatening injury.
- In the case of posterior dislocation without fracture, the experienced physician may perform one attempt at closed reduction. If reduction is not accomplished with ease or if there is an associated fracture of the hip, then, emergent orthopedic consultation is warranted.
- Even postreduction, further orthopedic and radiographic evaluations are needed to guide surgical decision making. CT scan should be part of the standard postreduction evaluation.
- In an isolated posterior dislocation without fracture treated with closed reduction within 6 hr of injury, the managing orthopedist might allow the patient to start weight-bearing as soon as comfort allows. This may be as early as 2 wk after injury.
- Whereas a significant delay between dislocation and reduction may increase the risk of AVN, the overall long-term prognosis is most dependent on the severity of the initial trauma.

DISTAL CLAVICULAR OSTEOLYSIS

Ryan C. Fowler, MD, CAQSM • Keith A. Stuessi, MD, CAQSM

BASICS

DESCRIPTION

- A loss of subchondral bone detail with osteoporosis, cystic changes, osteolysis, and osteophyte formation of the distal clavicle while sparing the acromion
- Most commonly associated with atraumatic mechanism but can be trauma related

EPIDEMIOLOGY

Incidence

- True incidence of distal clavicular osteolysis (DCO) is unknown.
- In teenage population, about 6.5% who present with shoulder pain may have DCO (1)[B].
- In teenage patients, overhead sports were a risk factor for DCO. Weight lifting and overhead sports conferred the biggest risk (1)[C].
- Also in teenage patients, females were affected at 24% (1)[B]. In adult literature, the vast majority of cases are male.
- Associated with repetitive heavy lifting and occasionally as a result of trauma

ETIOLOGY AND PATHOPHYSIOLOGY

- Although the specific pathophysiologic cause has not been determined, atraumatic osteolysis is thought to start as a stress fracture of the distal clavicle from repetitive microtrauma (2).
- Common magnetic resonance imaging (MRI) findings include bone edema and evidence of subchondral injury (2).
- The pathophysiologic process in traumatic injuries is unknown.

RISK FACTORS

- Any activity putting excessive, repetitive force on the acromioclavicular (AC) joint may increase risk.
- Weight lifting appears to be a significant risk factor in nontraumatic cases (3)[B].
- Highest risk factor seen in bench pressers with high frequency (more than once a week), high duration (>5 yr), and with one repetition maximum of >1.5 times the body weight (3)[B]
- Occasionally will result from blunt trauma to the shoulder
- Traumatic injuries include AC joint dislocation and separation as well as clavicle fractures.

GENERAL PREVENTION

- Atraumatic causes are potentially prevented by limiting repetitive lifting, but no studies address this issue.
- Athletes generally are reluctant to decrease training.

DIAGNOSIS

HISTORY

- Insidious onset of aching in the AC joint
- Athletes may have a history of remote trauma.
- Activities placing repetitive stress to the joint may increase the risk.
- In weight lifters, bench press, military press, shoulder shrugs, push-ups, and clean and jerk may cause pain.

PHYSICAL EXAM

- Signs and symptoms:
  - Patient complains of a dull ache over the AC joint.
  - Mild swelling of the joint may be present.
  - Pain usually is worse at the beginning of the exercise period.
  - Any movement of the arm requiring 90 degrees or more of abduction causes pain.
  - Pain can radiate to the adjacent superior trapezius border and deltoid muscles.
- Physical examination:
  - Tenderness over the AC joint
  - Positive cross-arm test: Forward flexion to 90 degrees and adduction of the arm cause pain. This compresses the AC joint.
  - Paxino test: patient's arm at side resting against chest and hand over top of shoulder; examiner's thumb on acromion and fingers on clavicle and compressing them together; pain is a positive test.
  - Sometimes a trapezius spasm will be palpated.
  - Because it is common to have other shoulder pathology in conjunction with DCO, a local anesthetic injection to the AC joint can be helpful in achieving an accurate diagnosis (4)[C].

DIFFERENTIAL DIAGNOSIS

- AC joint trauma, osteoarthritis
- Other shoulder pathology should be considered (e.g., instability, impingement, rotator cuff tears, tendinitis, and labral disease).
- Also includes hyperparathyroidism, rheumatoid arthritis, multiple myeloma, scleroderma, infection (septic arthritis, tuberculosis), rickets, eosinophilic granuloma, and other, more rare diseases including cleidocranial dysplasia, progeria, and pycnodysostosis

DIAGNOSTIC TESTS & INTERPRETATION

Initial Tests (lab, imaging)

- Clavicular or Zanca view: 10 to 35 degrees of cephalic tilt; distal clavicular end will appear frayed; will see bony osteolysis, cystic changes, and translucency of the bone. Bilateral Zanca views are helpful in comparing the involved and uninvolved sides.
- MRI can be used to rule out other pathology and often shows bone edema and evidence of subchondral fracture in the distal clavicle (2)[C].
- MRI is useful, as early plain films may appear normal. Majority of cases, 74–86% had evidence of subchondral fracture (1,2).

Diagnostic Procedures/Other

Diagnostic injection into the AC joint with local anesthetic can be helpful in differentiating the cause of pain (4)[C].

TREATMENT

- Acute treatment:
  - Nonsteroidal anti-inflammatory drugs (NSAIDs) or other pain medications can be used as needed.
  - Cessation of offending activity is often very effective in reducing pain (4,5)[C].
  - Therapeutic corticosteroid injection to the AC joint is often effective at reducing painful symptoms (4,5)[C]. This can also be a predictor of successful distal clavicle resection.
  - Ultrasound guidance is more effective than blind injection (5)[A].
  - Other symptomatic treatment such as ice can be helpful.
- Long-term treatment:
  - Activity modification (4,5)[C]
  - Specific activity modifications are to narrow the hand spacing on the barbell (<1.5 times the biacromial width) and controlling the descent phase to end approximately 4 to 6 cm above the chest (4)[B].
  - Often difficult in athletes
  - Activity modification by weight lifters should include decreased weight with increased repetitions or substitution of exercises.
  - In the teenage population, 93% responded to conservative therapy (1)[B].
  - Physical therapy should be instituted if there is evidence of other shoulder pathology. Rehabilitation also should include range of motion (ROM) therapy and strengthening exercises for the rotator cuff and scapulothoracic stabilizer muscles (5)[C].
  - Surgical resection may be considered for those not responding to conservative therapy.

SURGERY/OTHER PROCEDURES

- Surgery is recommended for those who fail conservative treatment (4,5)[C].
- Surgery may be performed open or arthroscopic.
- Arthroscopic surgery involves less tissue dissection and faster rehabilitation times (2)[C].
- Arthroscopic surgery can be completed directly through the AC joint or indirectly through the subacromial space. It can give the ability to assess for other concomitant conditions. There is controversy as to the best surgical management.

ONGOING CARE

FOLLOW-UP RECOMMENDATIONS

- Referral to an orthopedic surgeon for failure of nonoperative treatment
- Postoperative physical therapy:
  - Active ROM as tolerated
  - Shoulder strengthening
  - Return to sports as soon as symptoms allow; time frame depends on surgical approach.

REFERENCES

1. Roedl JB, Nevalainen M, Gonzalez FM, et al. Frequency, imaging findings, risk factors, and long-term sequelae of distal clavicular osteolysis in young patients. *Skeletal Radiol*. 2015;44(5):659–666.
2. Kassarjian A, Llopis E, Palmer WE. Distal clavicular osteolysis: MR evidence for subchondral fracture. *Skeletal Radiol*. 2006;36(1):17–22.
3. Nevalainen MT, Ciccotti MG, Morrison WB, et al. Distal clavicular osteolysis in adults: association with bench pressing intensity. *Skeletal Radiol*. 2016;45(11):1473–1479.
4. Schwarzkopf R, Ishak C, Elman M, et al. Distal clavicular osteolysis: a review of the literature. *Bull NYU Hosp Jt Dis*. 2008;66(2):94–101.
5. DeFroda SF, Nacca C, Waryasz GR, et al. Diagnosis and management of distal clavicle osteolysis. *Orthopedics*. 2017;40(2):119–124.

CLINICAL PEARLS

- Can resolve without surgery, but only a minority of cases produce satisfactory results, particularly when the athlete does not stop training long enough for the AC joint to heal
- Athletes can return to their former level of competition after surgical resection.

DUPUYTREN CONTRACTURE

Thomas Trojian, MD

BASICS

DESCRIPTION

- Contracture of the palmar fascia owing to fibrous proliferation and resulting in flexion deformities and loss of function. Similar changes rarely may occur in plantar fascia. Dupuytren contracture (DC) usually appears simultaneously.
- Genetics:
  - Autosomal dominant with variable penetrance
  - 10% of patients have a positive family history.
- System(s) affected: musculoskeletal
- Abbreviations: MCP = metacarpophalangeal; PIP = proximal interphalangeal

EPIDEMIOLOGY

Incidence

- Predominant age: 50 yr for males; 60 yr for females
- Predominant gender: male > female (ranges from 2:1 to 10:1)

Prevalence

- Prevalence is about 300/100,000.
- Disease prevalence varies from 2% to 42% depending on population and risk factors.
- Overall prevalence is 8.8% in Northern European population.
- African Americans are less likely to get the disease.
- Japanese and Taiwanese have a prevalence equal to that in Northern Europe. These patients usually present with a less severe form of the disease (1).

ETIOLOGY AND PATHOPHYSIOLOGY

- Unknown
- Ischemia to the fascia with oxygen free-radical formation
- Possibly related to release of angiogenic basic fibroblast growth factor
- Related to microhemorrhage and release of growth factors

Genetics

- Autosomal dominant with variable penetrance; in one family, the gene has been mapped to chromosome 16q.
- >30 unique genes were upregulated, and 6 unique genes were downregulated by 4-fold or greater.
- Upregulated genes include ones that code for fibronectin, tenascin C, transforming growth factor β2 (TGF-β2), collagen III, collagen IV, and collagen VI.
- All three forms of TGF-β are upregulated. TGF-β2 is upregulated 10 to 20 times. As in tendinopathy, it may be a TGF receptor lack of response, so TGF continues to be made.
- Musculoaponeurotic fibrosarcoma oncogene homologue B, or *MafB*, in the family of oncogenes is found in the cord but not paracord fascia of normal control individuals.

RISK FACTORS

- Smoking (mean 16 pack-years; odds ratio = 2.8)
- Alcohol intake
- Using both alcohol and cigarettes combined has a higher risk than individual use alone.
- Increasing age (>40 yr of age)
- Male (increase in androgen receptors in nodules)
- Northern European, Japanese, Taiwanese
- Diabetes mellitus (1/3 affected, increases with time, usually mild; middle and ring fingers involved)
- Epilepsy (may be medications or disease)
- HIV infection (may or may not be associated)
- Vibration work exposure (Some studies show increased risk, whereas other studies show no risk.)
- Rheumatoid arthritis (lower risk) (2)

GENERAL PREVENTION

None known; avoid risk factors when possible.

COMMONLY ASSOCIATED CONDITIONS

- Alcoholism
- Smoking
- Epilepsy
- Diabetes mellitus
- Occupational hand trauma (vibration white finger)

DIAGNOSIS

PHYSICAL EXAM

- Signs and symptoms (2):
  - Typical:
    - Caucasian male aged 50 to 60 yr
    - Bilateral, with greater involvement in one hand
    - Family history positive
    - Unilateral or bilateral (50%)
    - Right hand more frequent
    - Ring finger more frequent
    - Ulnar digits more affected than radial
    - Mild pain early
    - Later painless plaques or nodules in palmar fascia
    - Extends into a cordlike band in the palmar fascia
    - Skin adheres to fascia and becomes puckered.
    - Nodules can be palpated under the skin.
    - Digital fascia becomes involved as disease progresses.
    - Web space contractures
    - Dupuytren diathesis can involve plantar (Ledderhose 10%) and penile (Peyronie 2%) fascia.
    - Knuckle pads
  - Atypical:
    - No age, gender differences
    - No family history
    - May have systemic disease (See "Risk Factors.")
    - May have a history of trauma
    - More common unilateral
    - No ectopic manifestations (Ledderhose or Peyronie)
    - Nonprogressive
- Physical examination:
  - A firm nodule in the palm of the hand proximal to the MCP joint
  - Hueston tabletop test, with positive test if patient is unable to flatten his or her hand on the table

DIFFERENTIAL DIAGNOSIS

- Callus formation
- Nodule on flexor tendon
- Camptodactyly—can occur in early teens, tight facial bands on the ulnar side of small finger
- Soft tissue tumor

DIAGNOSTIC TESTS & INTERPRETATION

Initial Tests (lab, Imaging)

- Not usually needed except in rare cases
- Ultrasound (US) can demonstrate thickening of the palmar fascia as well as the presence of a nodule.
- Magnetic resonance imaging (MRI) can assess cellularity of lesions, which correlate with higher recurrence after surgery.

Diagnostic Procedures/Other

Rarely is a biopsy needed to differentiate Dupuytren nodule from a soft tissue tumor:

- Pathologic findings:
  - Myofibroblasts
  - First stage (proliferative): increased myofibroblasts
  - Second stage (residual): dense fibroblast network
  - Third stage (involutional): Myofibroblasts disappear.

TREATMENT

GENERAL MEASURES

- ~10% of patients will have disease regression without treatment.
- Intralesional steroid injection (triamcinolone) has been shown to reduce the need for surgery.
- With a thickened cord, it may be useful to US prior to intralesional injections in order to identify the underlying tendon, and thus avoid the tendon during the injection.
- Although surgical intervention has been shown to be very helpful in cases of advanced DC, there are inherent risks to surgery, such as nerve injury, hematoma, skin necrosis, and infection.
- Although partial fasciectomy has long been the mainstay of treatment for patients with advanced DC, office procedures such as percutaneous needle aponeurotomy and collagenase injections may represent alternatives to surgery in certain patients.
- Whatever the method selected to treat the contracture, each technique carries with it a significant risk of recurrence.

MEDICATION

First Line

- Collagenase *Clostridium histolyticum* (CCH) at a dose of 0.58 mg per injection for the treatment of DC in a single digit during a 30-day treatment cycle. The collagenase weakens and dissolves the Dupuytren cord. Many patients have a short-term adverse reaction. Treatment is very successful (3,4)[A].
- Steroid injection (triamcinolone) for an acute tender nodule, painful knuckle pad (3)[B]

Second Line

Radiation therapy, 5-fluorouracil, and hyperbaric oxygen have been used (2)[B].

ADDITIONAL THERAPIES

- Steroid injection for acute tender nodule
- Collagenase injections can be used in two nodules at a time. They are very successful.
- Physiotherapy is ineffective alone.
- Isolated involvement of palmar fascia can be followed.
- MCP joint involvement can be followed if flexion contracture is 30 degrees.

SURGERY/OTHER PROCEDURES

- Surgery: partial fasciectomy (2)[A]:
  - Surgical referral should be made when MCP joint contractures reach 30 degrees or any degree of PIP joint contracture develops.
  - May require skin grafts for wound closure with severe cutaneous shrinkage
  - 80% have full range of movement if operated on early.
  - Continuous elongation technique is useful to prepare a severely contracted PIP joint for surgery. The digit frequently can be completely extended but will relapse if surgery is not performed.
  - Amputation of little finger, if severe and deforming (rare)
- Needle aponeurotomy, also called percutaneous needle fasciotomy (PNF), is a minimal invasive technique (5)[B]:
  - Done under local anesthetic
  - Type I DC
  - Done through the skin usually blind with 18-gauge needle or special tool
  - US may be beneficial.
  - Recurrence rates can be high, but recovery is faster and procedure is inexpensive.

ONGOING CARE

FOLLOW-UP RECOMMENDATIONS

- No activity restrictions
- Physical therapy after surgery: started 3 to 5 days after surgery (passive and active exercises, posterior dynamic extension splints)

Patient Monitoring

Follow patient in early stages of disease.

DIET

No special diet

PATIENT EDUCATION

- Avoid risk factors, especially with a strong family history.
- Regular follow-up by physician every 6 mo to 1 yr

PROGNOSIS

- Typical:
  - Unpredictable but usually slowly progressive
  - Patients likely to have aggressive disease (one or more): age 40 yr at onset, knuckle pads, positive family history, bilateral disease involving radial side of hand
  - Reports of clinical regression with continuous passive skeletal traction in extension and under a skin graft
  - Recurrence rate after surgery is 10–34%.
  - Prognosis better for MCP joint versus PIP joint after surgery
- Atypical:
  - Nonprogressive
  - Surgery rarely needed
  - Recurrence unlikely if surgery performed

COMPLICATIONS

- Postoperative stiffness (common)
- Postoperative recurrence or extension 46–80% (common)
- Postoperative development of reflex sympathetic dystrophy (uncommon)
- Postoperative hematoma or infection (rare)
- Intraoperative neurovascular injury (rare)
- Digital infarction (rare)

REFERENCES

1. Lanting R, Broekstra DC, Werker PM, et al. A systematic review and meta-analysis on the prevalence of Dupuytren disease in the general population of Western countries. *Plast Reconstr Surg*. 2014;133(3):593–603.
2. Avery DM, Trojian TH, Rodner CM. Dupuytren contracture. *BMJ Best Practice*. https://bestpractice.bmj.com/topics/en-us/983/pdf/983.pdf. Accessed June 23, 2018.
3. Ball C, Izadi D, Verjee LS, et al. Systematic review of non-surgical treatments for early Dupuytren's disease. *BMC Musculoskelet Disord*. 2016;17(1):345.
4. Brazzelli M, Cruickshank M, Tassie E, et al. Collagenase *Clostridium histolyticum* for the treatment of Dupuytren's contracture: systematic review and economic evaluation. *Health Technol Assess*. 2015;19(90):1–202.
5. Morhart M. Pearls and pitfalls of needle aponeurotomy in Dupuytren's disease. *Plast Reconstr Surg*. 2015;135(3):817–825.

ADDITIONAL READING

Denkler KA, Vaughn CJ, Dolan EL, et al. Evidence-based medicine: options for Dupuytren's contracture: incise, excise, and dissolve. *Plast Reconstr Surg*. 2017;139(1):240e–255e.

CLINICAL PEARLS

- DC is an inherited disease of progressive fibrous tissue contracture of the palmar fascia.
- The disease predominantly affects males of Northern European decent aged >40 yr who are smokers, alcohol drinkers, or diabetics.
- Patients present with a small lump or multiple lumps with pits in the palm of the hand progressing to contractures of the fingers.
- Collagenase is a very successful treatment option U.S. Food and Drug Administration (FDA)-approved in 2010.
- Intralesional steroid injections have been shown to reduce the need for surgery.
- Surgical referral should be made when MCP joint contractures reach 30 degrees or if any degree of PIP joint contracture is present.
- Surgery usually is done in advanced disease in order to restore function of the hand.
- Percutaneous needle aponeurotomy and the emerging therapy of collagenase injections are significant therapeutic alternatives to surgery.

ELBOW DISLOCATION

John Munyak, MD • Yaffa Ilyaguyeva • Stephen R. Paul, MD, CAQSM

BASICS

DESCRIPTION

- Separation/disruption of the articulations between distal humerus, proximal radius, and proximal ulna; typically resulting from trauma and injury to the supporting soft tissue structures
- Subtypes: anterior (rare) versus posterior (common) and simple (soft tissue injury) versus complex (fracture-dislocation)
- Complete (dislocation) or partial (subluxation)
- System(s) affected: musculoskeletal

EPIDEMIOLOGY

- In adults, the elbow is the second most frequently dislocated major joint after the shoulder.
- In the pediatric population, the elbow is the most common dislocated joint.
- Comprises 10–25% of all elbow injuries
- More frequently seen in wrestling, gymnastics, football, falls, and motor vehicle accidents
- Predominate sex: males > females (1)

Incidence

- Adults: 6 to 8/100,000 (1)
- 10–50% sports related
- Usually on the nondominant side

ETIOLOGY AND PATHOPHYSIOLOGY

- Progression of injury from lateral collateral ligament to capsule to medial collateral ligament in posterior dislocation
- Anterior dislocation from trauma to the posterior portion of a flexed elbow
- Fall on outstretched hand
- Axial loading and rotation upon impact

RISK FACTORS

- Anatomical risk factors include a shallow olecranon fossa and a prominent olecranon tip.
- Age and sports activity
- Fall on an outstretched hand

GENERAL PREVENTION

- Sport protective padding may provide a benefit.
- Injury prevention training modalities
- Avoidance of falls

COMMONLY ASSOCIATED CONDITIONS

- Common: radial head/neck fracture, epicondyle avulsion fracture, soft tissue edema, coronoid process fracture
- Wrist and shoulder injuries, which can occur 10–15% should be ruled out (1).
- Rare: neurovascular injury (brachial artery and median nerve), compartment syndrome

DIAGNOSIS

HISTORY

- Mechanism of fall
- Type of activity leading to injury (sports, fall, work, accident)
- Time since injury
- Reduction attempts

PHYSICAL EXAM

- An obvious visual deformity usually is present.
- Note the condition of the skin: Look for wounds indicating an open dislocation.
- Palpation of deformity and effusion:
  - Prominent olecranon: posterior
  - Long extended forearm: anterior
- Neurovascular evaluation, especially brachial artery and ulnar, interosseous and median nerve function
- Consult orthopedics/vascular surgery urgently for any signs of neurovascular injury.
- Rule out additional injuries, especially in contiguous musculoskeletal structures.
- In reduced elbows: Lateral pivot-shift apprehension test is highly sensitive (2)[C]:
  - Sensation of dislocation is a positive test.

DIFFERENTIAL DIAGNOSIS

- Elbow subluxation
- Spontaneous elbow dislocation and reduction
- Be especially cautious in the pediatric age group because supracondylar fractures are common in 5- to 10-yr-olds.
- Nursemaid's elbow (pediatrics)
- Other elbow joint/forearm fracture

DIAGNOSTIC TESTS & INTERPRETATION

Initial Tests (lab, imaging)

- Initial anteroposterior and lateral radiographs: Evaluate relationship between distal humerus and radio-ulnar complex. Identify associated fracture (1)[C].
- Maintain a high index of suspicion for additional injuries and obtain radiographs of the humerus, forearm, or wrist as indicated.
- Exception: On-field reduction by a medical professional can precede initial films (3)[C].
- Postreduction radiographs: all dislocations (3)[C]
- Computed tomography (CT): reserved for complex fracture-dislocations or reconstruction planning

Diagnostic Procedures/Other

Angiography for suspected arterial injury

TREATMENT

GENERAL MEASURES

- In experienced hands, reduction may be performed on the field without analgesia. Otherwise, transport patient to a medical facility that can treat this injury.
- Appropriate monitoring is required, and proper resuscitation equipment should be available.
- In rare instances, general anesthesia in the operating room may be required.
- Postreduction, check elbow stability with range of motion (ROM).
- Obtain postreduction radiographs.
- Immobilize the elbow in a posterior splint as close to 90 degrees of flexion as possible using avoidance of a diminishing radial pulse as a guide.
- Postreduction position is in pronation; check varus, valgus, and rotatory instability (4)[C].
- Perform a postreduction neurovascular examination.
- Closed reduction of dislocation: Goal is atraumatic reduction with minimal attempts. There are several techniques:
  - Option no. 1: supine patient, forearm traction, humeral counter traction, anterior force on olecranon, and forearm supination (1)[C]
  - Option no. 2: prone patient, apply counter traction while extending the arm at the elbow, manipulate the coronoid process past the trochlea (3)[C]
  - Option no. 3 (one-person reduction): patient's arm across the chest, one hand braces the injured distal arm, the other holds the elbow and olecranon while providing traction to allow the coronoid to pass the trochlea (5)[C]
  - Full passive ROM will signify a successful reduction.
- Postreduction evaluation:
  - Postreduction radiographs to confirm position of radial head and ulna in relation to the capitate and distal humerus; also, to exclude iatrogenic fracture
  - Postreduction lateral radiograph demonstrating "drop sign," which conveys a high risk for recurrent instability (Drop sign: Ulnohumeral joint is widened >4 mm.) (4)[C]
  - Neurovascular reassessment to confirm no nerve impingement
  - Assess joint stability:
    - ROM: no locking or crepitation
    - Joint should be examined under gentle stresses (valgus stress/laxity most common following dislocation) (3)[C].
    - Lateral pivot-shift apprehension test for joint stability (1)[C]
  - Stable joint: arm sling for comfort and early mobilization in 3 to 5 days (4)[C]
  - Unstable joint that stabilizes with pronation: Splint in pronation/flexion (1)[C].
  - Joint unstable needs >45 degrees of flexion: Consider surgery (1)[C].

- Issues for referral: initial follow-up with orthopedics/sports medicine for splint removal and early mobilization
- Additional therapies:
  - ROM exercises after initial immobilization for comfort if joint is stable (1)[C]
  - Unstable joints should have a splint that blocks full extension with encouragement of flexion as tolerated (1)[C].
  - Extended therapy required if ROM not improved by 6 to 8 wk postinjury (3)[C]
  - Stability should be confirmed prior to full ROM therapy (6)[C].

MEDICATION
- Analgesia:
  - Reduction can be attempted without analgesia (5)[C].
  - Narcotics:
    - Morphine 0.1 mg/kg intravenous (IV) usually $\sim$10 mg/dose (pediatric 0.1 mg/kg/dose)
    - Fentanyl 25 to 50 μg IV initially, shorter acting, preferred narcotic for conscious sedation (pediatric 2 μg/kg/dose)
    - Reversible with naloxone
    - Multiple oral narcotics available for use
- Postreduction nonsteroidal anti-inflammatory drugs (NSAIDs) are recommended because they also decrease risk of heterotopic ossification (1)[C].
- Anxiolysis:
  - Benzodiazepines:
    - Midazolam 1 mg/dose (pediatric 0.05 mg/kg/dose), short acting, rapid onset, preferred for conscious sedation
    - Lorazepam 0.05 mg/kg/dose (pediatrics 0.05 mg/kg/dose), longer duration not ideal for procedural sedation use
- Conscious/procedural sedation (multiple options): goal of adequate pain control and muscle relaxation:
  - Versed/fentanyl: as above
  - Ketamine: pediatric $>$3 mo 1.5 mg/kg IV with 0.5 mg/kg repeat doses (rarely used in adults due to emergence reactions and agitation)
  - Multiple other options, including propofol, barbiturates, and nitrous oxide
- General sedation:
  - Occasionally required for difficult/painful reductions
- Local anesthesia by joint infiltration can reduce needed analgesic doses (1)[C].
- Precautions:
  - Be aware of respiratory and airway reflex depression with narcotics and benzodiazepines.
  - Thorough preparation required for procedural sedation, including airway management devices, bag-valve mask for ventilation, reversal agents (naloxone/flumazenil) as appropriate, cardiovascular monitoring equipment

ADDITIONAL THERAPIES
- A follow-up radiograph should be obtained 1 and 2 wk after injury. A small percentage of patients will develop recurrent instability, which can be due to insufficiency of the lateral ulnar collateral ligament. These patients may require surgical reconstruction to restore stability.
- Rehabilitation after simple elbow dislocation requires 1 to 3 mo to return to preinjury status. Typically, the outcome is good, with most athletes experiencing little morbidity or loss of function. The most common problem is loss of extension, which is minimized with an active, aggressive, and early rehabilitation program.

SURGERY/OTHER PROCEDURES
- Surgery is limited to select cases because conservative management is preferred (6)[C].
- Open dislocation, compartment syndrome, nerve injury/impingement, unstable fractures, and unstable reductions require operative intervention (1)[C].
- Grossly unstable elbows may require acute ligament repair to confer early stability to allow for ROM and enhanced rehabilitation.
- Complex dislocations with fractures, including significant radial head, olecranon, and coronoid fractures, may require surgical stabilization via open reduction and internal fixation (ORIF) of fracture segments (1)[C].
- Isolated lateral collateral ligament repair in recurrent dislocation has shown success (2)[B]. Chronically unstable elbows may require reconstruction of the lateral ulnar collateral ligament.

ADMISSION, INPATIENT, AND NURSING CONSIDERATIONS
- Admission criteria:
  - Fracture-dislocation requiring operative intervention
  - Nonreducible dislocation
  - Neurovascular injury
  - Edema with concern for compartment syndrome development
- Nursing:
  - Providing ordered medications for patient comfort or sedation as necessary
  - Monitoring of vitals for sedation procedures if needed
  - Reinforcing discharge instructions/plan
- Discharge criteria:
  - Elbow dislocation confirmed by postreduction radiograph
  - Normal postreduction neurovascular exam documented
  - Supply orthopedic follow-up.
  - Reduced elbow splinted for comfort or to maintain stability as needed

ONGOING CARE

FOLLOW-UP RECOMMENDATIONS
Consultation with an orthopedic surgeon should be obtained in most cases.

PATIENT EDUCATION
Avoid activities that specifically stress the elbow joint (e.g., throwing) until ready upon reevaluation.

PROGNOSIS
- Generally full recovery
- Poor outcome related to stiffness/decreased ROM:
  - Early physical therapy/ROM exercises decrease stiffness.

COMPLICATIONS
- Neurovascular compromise
- Stiffness
- Compartment syndrome
- Recurrent dislocation
- Heterotopic ossification

REFERENCES

1. Kuhn MA, Ross G. Acute elbow dislocations. *Orthop Clin North Am*. 2008;39(2):155–161.
2. Burra G, Andrews J. Acute shoulder and elbow dislocations in the athlete. *Orthop Clin North Am*. 2002;33(3):479–495.
3. O'Driscoll SW. Classification and evaluation of recurrent instability of the elbow. *Clin Orthop Relat Res*. 2000;(370):34–43.
4. Parsons BO, Ramsey ML. Acute elbow dislocations in athletes. *Clin Sports Med*. 2010;29(4):599–609.
5. Mehta JA, Bain GI. Elbow dislocations in adults and children. *Clin Sports Med*. 2004;23(4):609–627.
6. Kumar A, Ahmed M. Closed reduction of posterior dislocation of the elbow: a simple technique. *J Orthop Trauma*. 1999;13(1):58–59.

ADDITIONAL READING

- Krul M, van der Wouden JC, van Suijlekom-Smit LW, et al. Manipulative interventions for reducing pulled elbow in young children. *Cochrane Database Syst Rev*. 2009;(4):CD007759.
- Ristic S, Strauch R, Rosenwasser M. The assessment and treatment of nerve dysfunction after trauma around the elbow. *Clin Orthop Relat Res*. 2000;(370):138–153.
- Ross G, McDevitt ER, Chronister R, et al. Treatment of simple elbow dislocation using an immediate motion protocol. *Am J Sports Med*. 1999;27(3):308–311.
- Taylor F, Sims M, Theis JC, et al. Interventions for treating acute elbow dislocations in adults. *Cochrane Database Syst Rev*. 2012;(4):CD007908.
- Work Loss Data Institute. *Elbow (acute & chronic)*. Corpus Christi, TX: Work Loss Data Institute; 2008.

CLINICAL PEARLS
- Recognize neurovascular injury early.
- Confirm relocation with a radiograph.
- Early mobilization reduces postreduction stiffness. The elbow is at risk for stiffness, more rapidly and more often than any other joint—can occur as early as 3 days after immobilization.
- Evaluate for other injuries in all traumas.

EPISTAXIS

Alan Shahtaji, DO, CAQSM • Nicholas Sgrignoli, MD

BASICS

DESCRIPTION

- Bleeding from injured nasal mucosa overlying a blood vessel
- Characterized as either anterior or posterior
- Affected persons usually do not seek medical attention, especially if bleeding is minor or self-limited.
- Synonym(s): nosebleed; nasal bleeding

EPIDEMIOLOGY

- Common problem affecting up to 60% of the general population
- 80–90% of cases occur along the anterior nasal septum at Kiesselbach plexus (little area).
- Bimodal age distribution with incidence peaks at ages <10 yr and >50 yr.
- Severe cases and posterior epistaxis are more common in older adults.
- More frequent in winter months

ETIOLOGY AND PATHOPHYSIOLOGY

- Commonly caused by irritation or trauma to nasal mucosa
- Most common cause is idiopathic followed by trauma.
- Local causes:
  - Local digital trauma
  - Low moisture content in ambient air
  - Facial trauma
  - Allergic or viral rhinitis
  - Medications (e.g., intranasal steroids)
  - Nasal septal deviation
  - Intranasal neoplasm or polyps
  - Chemical irritants (e.g., cigarette smoke)
  - Chronic sinusitis
  - Foreign body
  - Septal perforation
  - Illicit drug use (e.g., cocaine)
  - Aneurysm
  - Hereditary hemorrhagic telangiectasia (Osler-Weber-Rendu disease)
  - Iatrogenic instrumentation
- Systemic causes:
  - Coagulopathies (e.g., von Willebrand disease, hemophilia)
  - Renal failure
  - Platelet dysfunction
  - Thrombocytopenia
  - Hematologic malignancies (e.g., leukemia)
  - Alcoholism
  - Hypertension (may increase length, severity, and risk of recurrence of nosebleeds) (1)
  - Liver disease (e.g., cirrhosis)
  - Medications (e.g., anticoagulants [1,2], selective serotonin reuptake inhibitors [SSRIs] [2], controversial data on correlation with aspirin use, no reported association with nonsteroidal anti-inflammatory drugs [NSAIDs])

DIAGNOSIS

HISTORY

- Determine timing, frequency, laterality, and severity of nosebleed.
- Quantify amount of blood loss.
- Presence of nasal obstruction: may indicate a neoplasm, especially with recurrent bleeding from the same side
- Trauma: Consider other associated injuries.
- Other medical conditions that predispose to bleeding:
  - Tumors and coagulation disorders
  - Cirrhosis
  - HIV infection
  - Intranasal cocaine use
- The presence of chronic medical conditions that can be exacerbated by blood loss:
  - Coronary artery disease/atherosclerosis (1)
  - Chronic obstructive pulmonary disease
- Medications:
  - Aspirin
  - Anticoagulants (1)
  - Intranasal steroids
- Alcohol use
- History of severe nosebleeds or easy bruising
- Family history of bleeding disorders

PHYSICAL EXAM

ALERT
Initial evaluation should focus on airway assessment and cardiovascular stability, looking for signs of airway compromise or hypovolemia.

- Positioning:
  - The examination should take place in a well-lighted room, preferably with a headlamp or mirror.
  - The patient should be seated comfortably in an upright position with head movement restricted in a sniffing position.
- Tools:
  - Wear personal protective equipment including eye protection and gloves.
  - A nasal speculum should be used with blades protracting vertically to better view the nasal mucosa.
  - Basin for patient to spit drainage
- Visualize bleeding:
  - Remove clots and foreign bodies in the anterior nasal cavity by blowing nose, with suction (Frazier suction catheter), irrigation, forceps, or cotton-tipped applicators.
  - If no anterior source is identified on inspection, anterior rhinoscopy may be attempted. Ear, nose, throat (ENT) specialist can perform nasal endoscopy if needed to visualize the remainder of the nasal cavity.
  - Posterior bleeding may be subtle, and the general location of the source of bleeding should be determined (e.g., behind the middle turbinate, roof of the nasal cavity, submucosal masses).
  - Location of bleeding is important because different arteries supply the floor and roof of the posterior nasal cavity.
- Trauma

ALERT
In the case of nasal trauma, be sure to evaluate for concussion, facial fractures, septal hematoma, and dental injury.

  - Assess for deformity with inspection and palpation of bony structures.
  - Evaluate extraocular muscle movements and stability of the teeth to rule out orbital or maxillary fracture. Malocclusion of teeth may indicate maxillary or mandibular fracture.
  - CSF leak should be ruled out using the ring test, if indicated.
- Recurrent nosebleeds:
  - Evaluate for signs of coagulopathy (e.g., ecchymoses, petechiae, telangiectatic lesions).

DIFFERENTIAL DIAGNOSIS

- Pulmonary hemoptysis
- Upper gastrointestinal (GI) bleed such as bleeding esophageal varices
- Tumor bleeding from the pharynx, larynx, or trachea

DIAGNOSTIC TESTS & INTERPRETATION

- Labs are not necessary for majority of patients with epistaxis.
- For severe bleeding, a complete blood count (CBC) should be performed in addition to blood type and crossmatching for possible transfusion.
- In anticoagulated patients, coagulation studies may be required to determine if anticoagulation levels are supratherapeutic.
- Even when testing is done selectively, the results are normal in nearly 80% of patients.
- Radiographic studies are usually not helpful unless a facial fracture is suspected.
- Unexplained recurrent unilateral epistaxis should raise suspicion for neoplasm and warrants consideration of computed tomography (CT) scan or magnetic resonance imaging (MRI) and endoscopic evaluation.

TREATMENT

- Anterior bleed:
  - Minor anterior nosebleeds may resolve without intervention prior to clinical evaluation or with initial tamponade.
- Pretreatment/initial tamponade:
  - The patient should blow his or her nose to remove blood and clots.
  - Local anesthetic and vasoconstrictor should be applied as a topical spray or via saturated cotton pledgets:
    - Drugs commonly used for this purpose are lidocaine with epinephrine and oxymetazoline (Afrin).
    - One small retrospective study found that oxymetazoline spray stopped the bleeding in 65% of consecutive patients with epistaxis presenting to the emergency department (ED).

- The patient should be sitting up and leaning forward to prevent blood from tracking into the pharynx or stomach.
- The patient should tightly pinch the nasal alae (soft cartilaginous part of the nose) against the septum continuously for 10 to 15 min.
- A cold compress applied over the bridge of the nose may help with hemostasis. Sucking ice cubes may decrease nasal blood flow (1)[A],(3)[C].
- Epistaxis that is refractory to pressure and topical vasoconstrictors may require cautery.
- If an anterior bleeding source is visualized, first-line treatment consists of chemical or electrical cautery (4)[B].
- All cautery may be painful, and pretreatment anesthetic is recommended:
  - Chemical cautery is usually performed with silver nitrate:
    - Most useful for minor active bleeds or after active bleeding has stopped and prominent vessels have been identified
    - Apply the cautery for ~10 sec.
    - Begin at the periphery of a small area surrounding the bleeding site and move centrally.
    - Exercise caution with silver nitrate because it cauterizes everything that it touches.

ALERT
Never cauterize both sides of the nasal septum in the same session to reduce the risk of iatrogenic septal perforation.

  - Electrical cautery is useful for more aggressive bleeding or larger vessels of the anterior nasal septum:
    - The nose must first be anesthetized using local anesthetic because electrical cautery can be extremely painful.
    - Anesthetize bilaterally because the electrical current is transmitted through the septum.
    - Electrocautery must be performed cautiously to avoid excessive destruction of healthy tissue.

ALERT
The use of electrocautery on both sides of the septum may increase the risk of septal perforation.

- If cautery is unsuccessful, or if no obvious site of bleeding is seen, nasal packing may be considered to tamponade the epistaxis.

ALERT
Nasal packing may also be used on the sideline for temporary hemostasis enabling return to play.

- A number of absorbable and nonabsorbable packing materials are available for anterior nasal packing.
- Traditional packing products consist of nondegradable materials:
  - Gauze impregnated with petroleum jelly (e.g., Xeroform) may be inserted in layers from the floor of the nasal cavity to tamponade the epistaxis.
  - A preformed nasal tampon made of polyvinyl alcohol that expands when wet (e.g., Merocel) will swell and fill the nasal cavity, applying pressure over the bleeding area.
  - An inflatable carboxymethylcellulose pack consisting of a balloon catheter and hydrocolloid coating (e.g., Rapid Rhino) that forms a lubricant on contact with water and remains in contact with mucosa on balloon deflation may cause less discomfort and be easier to insert and remove.
- Absorbable or degradable materials that do not require formal removal are useful:
  - Oxidized cellulose (e.g., Surgicel) and gelatin foams (e.g., Gelfoam) increase clot formation and provide a degree of tamponade.
  - Bovine-derived thrombin gel (e.g., FloSeal) is conformable to the contours of the nasal cavity, easy to apply, and less painful. Higher costs of its use may be offset by the lack of need for packing removal.
- Packing generally is left in place for 1 to 5 days to ensure adequate clot formation. No benefit has been found with longer duration (4)[B].
- Topical or oral antibiotics typically are used with prolonged nasal packing (>24 hr) because of the possibility of toxic shock syndrome (3)[C].
- Other complications of nasal packing include septal hematomas, abscesses, or pressure necrosis from traumatic packing; sinusitis from blockage of sinus drainage; hypoxia from nasal airway blockage or apneic spells; stimulation of the nasovagal reflex causing syncope during packing; and acute airway obstruction from pack displacement into the oropharynx.
- Failure to control anterior bleeding with cautery or packing may necessitate embolization or surgical ligation of the offending vessels (4)[B].
- Referral to an otolaryngologist is appropriate when bleeding is refractory, complications are present, posterior bleed is suspected, or specialized treatment is required.
- Continued bleeding despite an anterior pack may be due to a posterior bleed.
- Posterior bleed:
  - These bleeds can be difficult to treat and may require either balloon insertion or a formal posterior pack.

ALERT
Referral to specialist and ED would be appropriate.

- Posterior packing usually necessitates hospitalization out of concern for hypoxic complications, cardiopulmonary events, and the risk of asphyxiation should the packing become dislodged.
- Posterior packing can be quite uncomfortable and may require significant anesthesia.
- A posterior pack may be an emergent temporizing measure before surgery or angiographic embolization.

ONGOING CARE

- Once epistaxis is controlled, conservative measures may prevent recurrent bleeding owing to local factors.
- Refrain from activities that may stimulate bleeding:
  - Blowing or picking nose
  - Heavy lifting
  - Strenuous activity
- Patient should abstain from alcohol or hot drinks that may cause vasodilatation of the nasal vessels.
- Nasal saline washes and water-soluble ointments assist in humidification of the nasal mucosa and promote healing.
- Humidified air, especially for patients using oxygen via nasal cannula, may improve local conditions within the nose.

FOLLOW-UP RECOMMENDATIONS

Patients should meet with their primary care physician to investigate for underlying causes and risk factors for epistaxis.

ALERT
All patients with recurrent epistaxis, particularly if unilateral, require formal evaluation with radiographic studies and nasal endoscopy to rule out a neoplastic lesion.

REFERENCES

1. Khan M, Conroy K, Ubayasiri K, et al. Initial assessment in the management of adult epistaxis: systematic review. *J Laryngol Otol*. 2017;131(12):1035–1055.
2. Seidel DU, Jacob L, Kostev K, et al. Risk factors for epistaxis in patients followed in general practices in Germany. *Rhinology*. 2017;55(4):312–318.
3. Barnes M, Spielmann P, White P. Epistaxis: a contemporary evidence based approach. *Otolaryngol Clin North Am*. 2012;45(5):1005–1017.
4. Shargorodsky J, Bleier B, Holbrook E, et al. Outcomes analysis in epistaxis management: development of a therapeutic algorithm. *Otolaryngol Head Neck Surg*. 2013;149(3):390–398.

ADDITIONAL READING

- Kucik CJ, Clenney T. Management of epistaxis. *Am Fam Physician*. 2005;71(2):305–311.
- Schlosser RJ. Clinical practice. Epistaxis. *N Engl J Med*. 2009;360(8):784–789.

CLINICAL PEARLS

- Anterior nosebleeds often are controlled with tamponade, topical medications, and oral ice packs.
- Athletes with an anterior bleed (80–90% of cases) without significant facial trauma, comorbid concussion, and/or underlying condition may return to play during the same event after cessation of bleeding.
- At high-level sports coverage with limited treatment time, consider having topical vasoconstrictors and nasal packing available on the sideline.
- Posterior nosebleeds are more severe and often require specialist involvement and higher level of care.

EXERCISE-ASSOCIATED HYPONATREMIA

Michael K. Seifert, MD, CAQSM • William W. Dexter, MD, FACSM

BASICS

DESCRIPTION

- Decrease in serum sodium concentration to <135 mmol/L during or up to 24 hr after physical activity
- Serum sodium concentration and serum osmolarity are maintained by homeostatic mechanisms involving thirst, antidiuretic hormone (ADH), renal handling of filtered sodium, and perhaps sodium loss through sweat.
- Increased serum osmolarity above normal (280 to 300 mOsmol/kg) stimulates hypothalamic osmoreceptors, which then cause increased thirst and circulating levels of ADH.
- Sodium concentration abnormalities are caused by changes in free water.
- Hyponatremia can be associated with hypervolemia, euvolemia, and hypovolemia.
- Most common form is dilutional hyponatremia. This is true in athletes as well as nonathletes:
  - Excess of water in relation to existing sodium stores
  - Sodium stores can be decreased, normal, or increased. However, the serum concentration of sodium is more reflective of fluid balance.

EPIDEMIOLOGY

- Prevalence varies wildly based on sport/event, athlete level, weather, and race time (1,2)[A].
- Can be seen in up to 51% of ultramarathon participants, 13% of standard marathon finishers, and 25% of Ironman triathletes (1,2)[A].
- After accounting for race time and body mass index, prevalence is equal between men and women (2)[A].
- Many cases are asymptomatic and may never present for medical care (3)[A].

ETIOLOGY AND PATHOPHYSIOLOGY

- Caused by combination of excessive fluid intake and impaired renal excretion of sodium
- Inappropriate secretion of arginine vasopressin (AVP) despite sodium dilution in plasma leads to impaired water clearance:
  - Pain, nausea/vomiting, hypoglycemia, and medication use may play a role.
- Interleukin-6 may be elevated after exercise and also stimulate AVP production.
- Rapid absorption of fluid in stomach immediately after exercise

RISK FACTORS

- Excessive fluid intake, above what is dictated by thirst
- In marathoners, slower runners and finishers who maintain or increase their prerace body weight
- Excess fluid losses (e.g., excessive sweating, vomiting, and diarrhea) that have been replaced primarily by hypotonic fluids
- Inexperienced runner or inadequate training
- Nonsteroidal anti-inflammatory drug (NSAID) medication use before or during activity
- Other disorders that can lead to sodium disturbances:
  - Renal insufficiency, heart failure, cirrhosis, syndrome of inappropriate antidiuretic hormone secretion (SIADH), hypothyroidism, cortisol deficiency, ecstasy use

GENERAL PREVENTION

- Educating participants about dangers of excessive fluid intake
- Instruction to drink as dictated by thirst (rather than perceived exertion, sweating, and distance)
- Reduce availability of fluids along race route.
- Monitor body weights before and after events:
  - If weight is gained, reduce fluid and sodium intake postrace.
- Little data to support that sodium ingestion during event is protective (2).

COMMONLY ASSOCIATED CONDITIONS

Few frequently associated conditions, but several conditions have similar symptoms and can co-occur:

- Exercise-associated collapse—common
- Heat stroke—common
- Hypothermia—common
- Hypoglycemia—common
- Rhabdomyolysis—rare

DIAGNOSIS

HISTORY

- Thorough past medical, surgical, and social history
- Ask about previous episodes of sodium problems or postrace medical issues.
- Attempt to estimate water and food intake during race.
- Inquire about medication use of the following:
  - NSAIDs, selective serotonin reuptake inhibitors (SSRIs), diuretics, antipsychotics, and amiodarone

PHYSICAL EXAM

Signs and symptoms:

- Vary significantly.
- Often asymptomatic
- Vitals signs, including rectal temperature if possible
- Obtain weight and compare to prerace if possible.
- Assess fluid status: blood pressure, skin turgor, edema, pulmonary exam for rales.
- Mental status: confusion, difficulty concentrating, lethargy, lack of responsiveness
- Be cognizant that postrace collapse and dizziness is common and may not be an indication of hyponatremia.
- Coma, obtundation, seizure activity, decorticate or decerebrate posturing, and respiratory arrest are indications of severe disease and should be treated immediately.

DIFFERENTIAL DIAGNOSIS

- Exercise-associated collapse
- Heat stroke
- Hyperthermia
- Hypothermia
- Hypoglycemia
- Myocardial infarction
- Stroke
- Adrenal insufficiency and adrenal crisis
- Congestive heart failure and pulmonary edema
- Gastroenteritis
- Hypothyroidism and myxedema coma
- Renal failure, acute
- Renal failure, chronic
- SIADH
- Cirrhosis
- Nephrotic syndrome
- Psychogenic polydipsia
- Medication related

DIAGNOSTIC TESTS & INTERPRETATION

- If possible, measure blood sodium concentration on site.
- Obtain serum glucose; creatinine if available
- An electrocardiogram (ECG) may allow you to rule out myocardial infarction (MI).
- If serum hyperglycemia is present, then serum sodium must be corrected by a factor of 1.6 mEq/L for each 100 mg/dL increase in serum glucose (4)[A].

TREATMENT

GENERAL MEASURES

- Airway, breathing, and circulation (ABC)
- Obtain rectal temperature (3)[C].
- Consider establishing intravenous (IV) access.
- Place patient in supine position, elevate legs to increase central circulation (1)[A],(3)[C].
- Quickly assess neurologic status (3)[C].
- Assess blood sodium if testing is available (1)[A].
- Consider the differential diagnosis and the possibility of a combination of exercise-associated issues (heat stroke, hypothermia, hyponatremia, collapse, etc.) (3)[C].
- Do not discharge the athlete with suspected exercise-associated hyponatremia until he or she is able to urinate (1)[A],(3)[C].
- For less severe hyponatremia (>130 mEq/L), watchful waiting, with fluid restriction, is appropriate because most will self-correct by diuresis (1)[A],(3)[C]:
  - Fluid restriction would be contraindicated if concerned for comorbid rhabdomyolysis.
  - Oral or IV hypertonic saline would be effective option regardless of fluid status.
- If symptoms do not improve or worsen with the above, IV hypertonic saline would be appropriate.

MEDICATION

- IV and PO hypertonic saline (100 mL 3% saline) have been shown to be equally effective in asymptomatic exercise-associated hyponatremia (5)[A].
- In cases of severe symptomatic exercise-associated hyponatremia, IV hypertonic saline is the best option (6,7)[A]:
  - Use 100 mL bolus of 3% saline with up to two additional boluses at 10 min intervals.
  - 50 mL aliquot of 8.4% sodium bicarbonate can provide a similar sodium load (3)[C].
  - Central pontine demyelination is a theoretical concern but has not been reported in athletes receiving hypertonic saline.

ISSUES FOR REFERRAL

Patients with severe exercise-associated hyponatremia requiring IV hypertonic saline should be considered for transfer to a higher level of care, although immediate treatment should still be initiated if possible.

ADDITIONAL THERAPIES

Athletes with documented hyponatremia and mild to moderate symptoms can be considered good candidates for oral hypertonic solutions (2)[A]:

- 4 bouillon cubes in 125 mL of water
- 100 mL of oral hypertonic saline

ONGOING CARE

PROGNOSIS

- Mild hyponatremia will almost always correct with autodiuresis and have no long-term consequences.
- An episode of exercise-associated hyponatremia may indicate an increase susceptibility to future episodes.
- Untreated severe hyponatremia or hyponatremia worsened with hypotonic saline can lead to cerebral edema, coma, and possibly death.

REFERENCES

1. Urso C, Brucculeri S, Caimi G. Physiopathological, epidemiological, clinical and therapeutic aspects of exercise-associated hyponatremia. *J Clin Med*. 2014;3(4):1258–1275.
2. Hew-Butler T, Rosner MH, Fowkes-Godek S, et al. Statement of the Third International Exercise-Associated Hyponatremia Consensus Development Conference, Carlsbad, California, 2015. *Clin J Sport Med*. 2015;25(4):303–320.
3. Hoffman MD, Joslin J, Rogers IR. Management of suspected fluid balance issues in participants of wilderness endurance events. *Curr Sports Med Rep*. 2017;16(2):98–102.
4. Filippatos TD, Liamis G, Christopoulou F, et al. Ten common pitfalls in the evaluation of patient with hyponatremia. *Eur J Intern Med*. 2016;29:22–25.
5. Owen BE, Rogers IR, Hoffman MD, et al. Efficacy of oral versus intravenous hypertonic saline in runners with hyponatremia. *J Sci Med Sport*. 2014;17(5):457–462.
6. Hew-Butler T, Loi V, Pani A, et al. Exercise-associated hyponatremia: 2017 update. *Front Med (Lausanne)*. 2017;4:21.
7. McGreal K, Budhiraja P, Jain N, et al. Current challenges in the evaluation and management of hyponatremia. *Kidney Dis (Basel)*. 2016;2(2):56–63.

ADDITIONAL READING

- Bennett BL, Hew-Butler T, Hoffman MD, et al. Wilderness Medical Society practice guidelines for treatment of exercise-associated hyponatremia: 2014 update. *Wilderness Environ Med*. 2014;25(Suppl 4):S30–S42.
- Krabak BJ, Lipman GS, Waite BL, et al. Exercise-associated hyponatremia, hypernatremia, and hydration status in multistage ultramarathons. *Wilderness Environ Med*. 2017;28(4):291–298.
- Wharam PC, Speedy DB, Noakes TD, et al. NSAID use increases the risk of developing hyponatremia during an Ironman triathlon. *Med Sci Sports Exerc*. 2006;38(4):618–622.

CLINICAL PEARLS

- Exercise-associated hyponatremia is common in long-distance and endurance events.
- Most cases are asymptomatic.
- Excessive fluid intake beyond what is required by thirst is the primary mechanism.
- Exercise-associated hyponatremia can be associated with other exercise-induced conditions and has overlapping symptoms with them as well.
- Mild hyponatremia will usually self-correct with autodiuresis.
- When in doubt about hydration status, IV or PO hypertonic saline (100 mL 3% saline) is appropriate.

EXERCISE-INDUCED ANAPHYLAXIS

Kimberly Kaiser, MD, CAQSM • Gregory Rubin, DO

BASICS

DESCRIPTION

- Distinct form of physical allergy characterized by a spectrum of exercise-induced symptoms ranging from mild skin symptoms such as pruritus and urticaria to angioedema, hypotension, syncope, and death
- A subgroup may develop food-dependent exercise-induced anaphylaxis (FDEIAn).

EPIDEMIOLOGY

Incidence

- Appears to be increasing (1)
- Predominant gender: female > male (~2:1) (1)

Prevalence

0.03% in study of Japanese adolescents (2)

ETIOLOGY AND PATHOPHYSIOLOGY

No single etiology has been agreed on. Popular theories include (3):

- Release of histamine and tryptase by mast cell degranulation.
- Increased gastrointestinal (GI) permeability.
- Increased activity of tissue transglutaminase in the gut mucosa.
- Increased plasma osmolality causing histamine release by basophils.

RISK FACTORS

- Previous episodes
- Vigorous exercise (2)
- Atopic individuals may be at slightly increased risk.
- Associated factors include:
  - Ingestion of certain foods or medications (particularly aspirin or nonsteroidal anti-inflammatory drugs [NSAIDs]) before exercise may be a predisposing factor. Avoid long-term β-blockers and angiotensin-converting enzyme (ACE) inhibitors.
  - Alcohol consumption (2).
  - Hormonal fluctuations during menstrual cycle may play a role in women (1).
  - Familial variant may exist.
  - Infections or illness.
  - Extremes in temperature.

GENERAL PREVENTION

Preventive medications include (4):

- Nonsedating antihistamines 2 hr prior to exercise or on a daily basis have been shown to be at least partially effective in prevention of symptoms (cetirizine 5 to 10 mg PO daily, loratadine 10 mg PO daily) (4)[C].
- Cromolyn sodium metered-dose inhaler (MDI) 2 to 4 puffs QID may be helpful. High doses 20 min before food ingestion can be useful in FDEIAn (grade 2C).
- Some clinicians advocate for avoiding antihistamines because they may block cutaneous manifestations of exercise-induced anaphylaxis (EIAn) that often serve as a "warning" of impending anaphylaxis (1,5)[C].
- Avoid food/medication triggers. Avoid ingestion of food triggers up to 2 hr before exercise, although FDEIAn has been reported with consumption 6 hr before (rarely when ingested shortly after exercise).

COMMONLY ASSOCIATED CONDITIONS

- Eczema
- Asthma

DIAGNOSIS

HISTORY

- Transient exercise-induced itching and cutaneous erythema ± urticaria
- Other symptoms include generalized itching, dizziness, GI colic, headache, choking sensation, urticaria or angioedema with hypotension or respiratory obstruction, and full anaphylactic shock.
- Occurs within 45 min of starting exercise (6)
- History of previous EIAn
- Identify possible provocative agent: Urticaria with warm shower or anxiety is consistent with cholinergic urticaria. Cold, ultraviolet rays, or water also may induce urticaria. Diagnosis may require an exercise diary.
- Identify any ingestions prior to exercise. Specific food or medication may be a trigger.

PHYSICAL EXAM

Assess airway, breathing, and circulation (ABCs):

- Hypotension or respiratory difficulty may signify impending anaphylactic shock.
- Dermatologic examination may reveal wheals.
- Identifying urticarial size and presence of angioedema aids in diagnosis (7).

DIFFERENTIAL DIAGNOSIS

- Cholinergic urticaria
- Exercise-induced bronchospasm
- Environmental allergy
- Mastocytosis
- Exercise-associated reflux

DIAGNOSTIC TESTS & INTERPRETATION

Initial Tests (lab, imaging)

- Serum tryptase levels are not specific to EIAn/FDEIAn. Elevation at baseline suggests mast cell disorders, kidney failure, and acute myeloid leukemia (2).
- Serum tryptase and histamine levels should be drawn immediately or within 3 hr after the episode and if elevated are suggestive of EIAn (2). A second measurement should be obtained at least 24 hr after resolution of symptoms (8).

Diagnostic Procedures/Other

- Passive warming test (e.g., warm shower or sauna) can be helpful in differentiating cholinergic urticaria from EIAn.
- Exercise challenge test using a treadmill or stationary bike can be performed. A positive test (reproduction of symptoms and urticaria) is helpful in diagnosis, but a negative test does not exclude a diagnosis of EIAn because reproducibility of symptoms is variable. Emergency equipment should be immediately available if exercise test is performed.
- Allergy testing for potential food and common allergen triggers should be done in all patients with EIAn.

TREATMENT

- Prehospital:
  - ABCs
  - Subcutaneous administration of 0.3 to 0.5 mL epinephrine 1:1,000 if systemic symptoms of anaphylaxis are present and then call 911
  - Trendelenburg position
- Emergency department (ED) treatment:
  - Treat symptoms of anaphylactic shock as necessary in appropriate medical setting (e.g., fluid support for hypotension, assisted ventilation for respiratory obstruction).
  - Epinephrine is first-line treatment.
  - Antihistamines may decrease itching and urticaria, but they do not relieve upper and lower airway obstruction or shock.
  - Nebulized albuterol should be given in individuals with severe bronchospasm.
  - Glucocorticoids are not shown to be beneficial in acute management of EIAn or FDEIAn (9).

ONGOING CARE

PROGNOSIS

- Generally favorable prognosis for EIAn and FDEIAn
- Few fatalities have been reported with attacks often becoming less frequent and severe over time.

FOLLOW-UP RECOMMENDATIONS

- Cease physical activity if any symptoms arise.
- Avoid exercise for at least 4 hr after eating (grade 2C).
- Avoid anti-inflammatory drugs before exercise.
- Allow for a period of gradual warm-up.
- Always exercise with a partner and carry injectable epinephrine.
- Possible role for desensitization to physical activity
- Referral to an allergist for identification of possible associated triggers may be beneficial.
- Follow-up to assess recurrence of symptoms and success of drug therapy

PATIENT EDUCATION

- Advise patient on EpiPen use (should have access to one at all times).
- Renew EpiPen annually.
- Advise patient to avoid any known triggers.
- Recommend wearing a medical alert device.

REFERENCES

1. Castells MC, Horan RF, Sheffer AL. Exercise-induced anaphylaxis. *Curr Allergy Asthma Rep*. 2003;3(1):15–21.
2. Feldweg AM. Exercise-induced anaphylaxis. *Immunol Allergy Clin North Am*. 2015;35(2):261–275.
3. Ansley L, Bonini M, Delgado L, et al. Pathophysiological mechanisms of exercise-induced anaphylaxis: an EAACI position statement. *Allergy*. 2015;70(10):1212–1221.
4. Briner WW Jr. Physical allergies and exercise. Clinical implications for those engaged in sports activities. *Sports Med*. 1993;15(6):365–373.
5. Schwartz LB, Delgado L, Craig T, et al. Exercise-induced hypersensitivity syndromes in recreational and competitive athletes: a PRACTALL consensus report (what the general practitioner should know about sports and allergy). *Allergy*. 2008;63(8):953–961.
6. Montgomery SL. Cholinergic urticaria and exercise-induced anaphylaxis. *Curr Sports Med Rep*. 2015;14(1):61–63.
7. Nichols AW. Exercise-induced anaphylaxis and urticaria. *Clin Sports Med*. 1992;11(2):303–312.
8. Simons FE. Anaphylaxis. *J Allergy Clin Immunol*. 2010;125(2 Suppl 2):S161–S181.
9. Choo KJ, Simons FE, Sheikh A. Glucocorticoids for the treatment of anaphylaxis. *Cochrane Database Syst Rev*. 2012;(4):CD007596.

CLINICAL PEARLS

- Epinephrine is first-line treatment.
- Because symptoms may vary significantly from one episode to another and among patients, some patients may not feel comfortable returning to activity knowing that they could have repeat attacks. In addition, patients who have experienced an anaphylactic response to exercise should be cautioned about returning to activity. For those whose symptoms are controlled with medication, it is recommended they continue to carry injectable epinephrine and exercise with a partner.
- EIAn can occur with any level of activity and may be precipitated by the ingestion of foods or medications. Unless a specific trigger is identified, there are no restrictions placed on diet or type of activity. A general rule of thumb is to avoid eating for at least 4 hr before exercise.

EXERCISE-INDUCED BRONCHOCONSTRICTION

Andrea Kussman, MD, CAQSM • Brian Young Kim, MD, MS, CAQSM

BASICS

DESCRIPTION

- A form of airway hyperresponsiveness characterized by a heightened bronchoconstriction response to a variety of stimuli related to exercise
- Characterized by wheezing, coughing, shortness of breath, and/or chest tightness occurring during or after exercise
- Usually within 5 to 15 min of the onset of exercise, an acute episode of airway obstruction begins. This is usually followed by recovery within 30 to 90 min upon completion of the exercise.
- If the athlete has underlying asthma, then it is called *exercise-induced bronchoconstriction (EIB) with asthma;* otherwise, it is *EIB without asthma.*
- Synonym(s): exercise-induced asthma; exercise-induced bronchospasm

EPIDEMIOLOGY

- 10–50% of recreational and elite athletes (1,2)[C]
- Up to 90% of patients with asthma (2)[C]
- 20–50% of cold-weather athletes (1,2)[C]
- A high level of fitness does not confer immunity from either asthma or EIB.
- When controlled, EIB does not restrict exercise performance.

ETIOLOGY AND PATHOPHYSIOLOGY

- The mechanism of EIB has not been established with certainty.
- The hyperosmolarity theory posits that increased airflow, particularly of dehumidified air, causes water loss from the surface liquid of the airways. This causes a hyperosmolar state in the airways, leading to inflammation and bronchoconstriction (1)[C].
- The thermal theory suggests that an increased respiratory rate cools the cells on the surface of the airways. Once exertion subsides, the airways rewarm, causing dilatation of the airway blood vessels, leading to hyperemia and fluid leakage into the bronchioles. This, in turn, causes inflammation and airway constriction. Thermal factors are now thought to be relatively minor compared to hyperosmolarity (1)[C].
- Other theories have associated bronchoconstriction with epithelial cell damage, inflammatory cells, or increased parasympathetic tone.

RISK FACTORS

- Cold-weather sports such as ice hockey, figure skating, and cross-country skiing
- Sports with a long duration of high-intensity exercise such as running, bicycling, swimming, soccer, and rugby
- Environmental factors such as tobacco smoke, chlorine, sulfur dioxide, nitrogen oxide, carbon monoxide, pollens and molds, cold weather, particulate matter, and low humidity

COMMONLY ASSOCIATED CONDITIONS

- Asthma
- Allergic rhinitis and hay fever

DIAGNOSIS

HISTORY

- Personal or family history of allergies or asthma
- Symptoms are often a poor predictor of who has EIB.
- Symptoms occur during or after exercise, typically appearing after 5 to 15 min of exercise.
- Signs and symptoms include:
  - Coughing.
  - Wheezing.
  - Shortness of breath.
  - Chest tightness.
  - Headache.
  - Fatigue.
  - Feeling out of shape.
  - Chest pain or discomfort.

PHYSICAL EXAM

Physical examination should include the following:

- Look for evidence of allergic disease such as pale nasal mucosa or allergic "shiners."
- Cardiac exam to evaluate for cardiac abnormalities
- Lung examination is typically normal; if wheezing is present, consider chronic asthma.
- On the field or after an exercise challenge, physical examination is more likely to reveal wheezing.

DIFFERENTIAL DIAGNOSIS

- Pulmonary:
  - Asthma with exercise exacerbation
  - Vocal cord dysfunction (VCD)
  - Exercise-induced hyperventilation
  - Restrictive lung disease
  - Cystic fibrosis
- Cardiac:
  - Coronary artery disease
  - Congenital/acquired heart defects
  - Arrhythmias
  - Congestive heart failure
  - Cardiomyopathy
- Ear, nose, and throat (ENT):
  - VCD: This represents a frequently missed cause of dyspnea and throat tightness associated with exercise (particularly in young women). Physicians should consider referral to ENT for evaluation of VCD if the patient is not responding as expected to treatment measures for EIB, or if the patient has atypical clinical features such as inspiratory stridor in the absence of wheezing.
  - Laryngeal prolapse
  - Exercise-induced laryngeal dysfunction
  - Laryngomalacia
  - Chronic sinusitis
- Gastrointestinal (GI): gastroesophageal reflux disease
- Allergic: exercise-induced anaphylaxis/urticaria
- Psych: anxiety disorders, panic attacks
- Other: general state of deconditioning

DIAGNOSTIC TESTS & INTERPRETATION

- Direct testing with pulmonary function tests (PFTs) done before and after albuterol should be performed if asthma is suspected (1,2)[A].
- If negative, then move on to testing with one of the following indirect tests.
  - PFTs before and after exercise (2,3)[A]:
    - Spirometry is more accurate than peak expiratory flow rate.
    - 10–15% reduction in preexercise forced expiratory capacity in 1 sec (FEV_1) confirms the diagnosis of EIB.
    - It is best to test athletes during sport-specific exercise or at temperatures of 20–25°C and <50% relative humidity.
    - Exercise at a workload of 80–90% of predicted VO_{2max} for 6 to 8 min during testing
  - Eucapnic voluntary hyperventilation (EVH) (1,2)[A]:
    - Recommended by International Olympic Committee (IOC) Medical Commission for diagnosing athletes
    - Hyperventilation of a gas mixture with 21% O_2 and 5% CO_2 for 6 min at 85% maximum voluntary ventilation
    - FEV_1 is measured prior to the test and 5, 10, and 15 min after the test.
    - Cut off is 10–15% drop in FEV_1.

- Inhaled mannitol testing (1)[A],(4)[C]:
  - A fall in FEV_1 >15% from baseline is diagnostic.
  - Allows for a controlled stepwise increase in stimulus
  - Not available in the United States
- Direct testing with methacholine challenge is third line because it is less sensitive and specific for EIB than indirect testing methods including exercise provocation, EVH, or inhaled mannitol testing (1)[B],(4)[C].
- Ideally, testing should be performed during a period of intense training, as airway responsiveness can normalize with de-escalation of exercise.

TREATMENT

GENERAL MEASURES

- Warm-up of 15 min at moderate exertion 15 to 30 min prior to exercise can induce a refractory period preventing bronchoconstriction (1,3)[A].
- Avoidance of triggers (cold, dry air; exercise close to busy roads; poorly ventilated chlorinated pool environments), if possible
- In cold weather, a mask can be used to warm the air (3)[B].
- Nose breathing can help to warm and moisturize the air.
- Athletes with underlying asthma should be well controlled before beginning a sport/exercise program.

MEDICATION

- Treat as per asthma guidelines (National Heart, Lung, and Blood Institute) for patients with underlying asthma.
- For elite athletes, check the World Anti-Doping Agency (WADA), United States Anti-Doping Agency (USADA), or National Collegiate Athletic Association list of banned substances to be sure that the medications used are in compliance with their rules.

First Line

Prophylactic (preexercise) medication:

- Short-acting β agonist (SABA): 2 to 4 puffs 15 to 30 min before exercise; may repeat during exercise as needed (1,3,5)[A]. If used on a daily basis, tolerance may develop (1)[A].

Second Line

If not responding adequately to a SABA, or requiring daily SABA use, can add:

- Montelukast 10 mg PO 2 hr before exercise (1,3)[A]
- A daily inhaled corticosteroid (3)[A]
- Cromolyn 4 to 10 puffs 10 to 20 min before exercise or nedocromil 2 to 4 puffs 10 to 20 min before exercise (3,5)[A]. Mast cell stabilizing agents are no longer available in the United States but may be prescribed in other countries.
- Long-acting β agonists (LABA) may be used in conjunction with inhaled corticosteroids 30 to 60 min before exercise (5)[A]. However, daily use can contribute to the development of tolerance toward both SABA and LABA (1)[A]. Avoid using LABA without inhaled corticosteroids due to the increased incidence of asthma-related events when used alone (3)[A].
- Consider adding an antihistamine for patients who also have allergies (1)[C],(3)[B]. Inhaled anticholinergic agents may be helpful, but evidence is inconsistent (1)[A].

ONGOING CARE

FOLLOW-UP RECOMMENDATIONS

- If not responding to an inhaled SABA, consider other diagnoses.
- Have the patient return if their use of SABA increases.
- Must continue to monitor because efficacy of medications can differ over time, particularly in different environments or in response to different types of exercise (1)[A]

DIET

There is low-quality evidence for a diet low in salt, high in fish oils, and high in ascorbic acid (1,3)[B].

PATIENT EDUCATION

- All athletes with EIB should have a SABA inhaler with them during practices and games.
- All athletes should be taught the proper use of an inhaler.
- Spacers can help to improve delivery of the inhaler medication.
- The athlete should know the difference between his or her controller and as-needed medication.
- Teach patients to avoid triggers.
- Consider allergy testing.

PROGNOSIS

Good

COMPLICATIONS

Poorly controlled athletes with EIB can progress to airway remodeling that becomes unresponsive to SABA.

REFERENCES

1. Weiler JM, Brannan JD, Randolph CC, et al. Exercise-induced bronchoconstriction update—2016. *J Allergy Clin Immunol*. 2016;138(5):1292–1295.e36.
2. Parsons JP, Mastronarde JG. Exercise-induced bronchoconstriction in athletes. *Chest*. 2005;128(6):3966–3974.
3. Parsons JP, Hallstrand TS, Mastronarde JG, et al. An official American Thoracic Society clinical practice guideline: exercise-induced bronchoconstriction. *Am J Respir Crit Care Med*. 2013;187(9):1016–1027.
4. Schwartz LB, Delgado L, Craig T, et al. Exercise-induced hypersensitivity syndromes in recreational and competitive athletes: a PRACTALL consensus report (what the general practitioner should know about sports and allergy). *Allergy*. 2008;63(8):953–961.
5. Carlsen KH, Anderson SD, Bjermer L, et al. Treatment of exercise-induced asthma, respiratory and allergic disorders in sports and the relationship to doping: part II of the report from the Joint Task Force of European Respiratory Society (ERS) and European Academy of Allergy and Clinical Immunology (EAACI) in cooperation with GA(2)LEN. *Allergy*. 2008;63(5):492–505.

ADDITIONAL READING

- Boulet LP, O'Byrne PM. Asthma and exercise-induced bronchoconstriction in athletes. *N Engl J Med*. 2015;327(7):641–648.
- Smoglia JM, Weiss P, Rundell KW. Exercise induced bronchoconstriction in adults: evidence based diagnosis and management. *BMJ*. 2016;352:h6951.
- Weiler JM, Anderson SD, Randolph C, et al. Pathogenesis, prevalence, diagnosis, and management of exercise-induced bronchoconstriction: a practice parameter. *Ann Allergy Asthma Immunol*. 2010;105(Suppl 6):S1–S47.

CLINICAL PEARLS

- First-line treatment is a SABA before exercise.
- Avoid daily use of a SABA because tachyphylaxis may develop. Have the athlete use this during high-intensity practice and competition.
- If an athlete is requiring daily use of a SABA, consider adding a controller medication.
- Warm-up of 15 min at moderate exertion 15 to 30 min prior to exercise can induce a refractory period preventing bronchoconstriction.
- It is no longer recommended to use LABA without an inhaled corticosteroid.

E

EXERCISE-INDUCED DIARRHEA

Steven K. Poon, MD, CAQSM • Kimberly G. Harmon, MD

BASICS

DESCRIPTION

- Increased stool frequency or volume often accompanied by lower abdominal cramping or urge to defecate associated with strenuous physical activity:
  - Normal physical examination
  - Normal laboratory and diagnostic studies
- Synonym(s): runner's diarrhea; runner's trots

EPIDEMIOLOGY

- Primarily associated with running sports but also common in cycling and reported in swimming, wrestling (1,2,3)
- Difficulty with existing research:
  - Difficult to control all variables (diet, exercise intensity, underlying pathology such as irritable bowel syndrome)
  - Studies often lack a denominator, making a true incidence of symptoms difficult to determine.
  - Many studies are surveys with low response rates, which introduce a selection bias.
  - Subject's dietary recall often is inaccurate.

Prevalence

- Prevalence of diarrhea reported from 8% to 60% in athletes
- Prevalence of diarrhea in control subjects reported up to 40%

ETIOLOGY AND PATHOPHYSIOLOGY

Proposed mechanisms (1,2,3,4):

- Mesenteric ischemia:
  - With strenuous exercise, blood is shifted away from the gut and to the working muscle.
  - Exercising at 70% VO_2 max decreases blood flow to gastrointestinal (GI) tract by 60–70%.
  - May lead to the production of endotoxin
  - Causes a cascade of inflammatory events that can further impair the mucosal integrity
  - Increased activity of the sympathetic nervous system leads to decreased splanchnic blood flow and is caused by:
    - Mental stress.
    - Hyperthermia.
    - Dehydration.
    - Hypoglycemia.
- Increased sympathetic nervous system activity:
  - Suppresses parasympathetic activity
  - Decreased gut tone and resistance
  - Increased colonic transit times
  - Secretion of gastroenteropancreatic hormones
- Reduced GI tract perfusion:
  - Gut barrier dysfunction
  - Damage to intestinal tight junction proteins
  - Increased permeability of gut barrier
- Mechanical stimulation of the colon due to intra-abdominal jostling
- Enteric fluid and electrolyte imbalance

RISK FACTORS

- Underlying bowel pathology may worsen with strenuous exercise.
- Dehydration
- Occurs more frequently with increased exercise intensity
- Occurs more frequently in untrained participants
- Type of exercise (running > cycling, swimming, speed skating, cross-country skiing)
- Meals rich in fat, protein, and fiber taken shortly before exercise worsen symptoms.

DIAGNOSIS

HISTORY

- Increased stool frequency or volume, or loose stools after exercise
- Often accompanied by abdominal cramping and urge to defecate
- May occur just with competition and not with training
- Normal bowel function at other times

PHYSICAL EXAM

- Increased stool frequency
- Increased stool volume
- Loose or explosive stools
- Urge to defecate, often necessitating the athlete to cease exercise
- Abdominal cramping
- Rectal bleeding
- Unremarkable physical examination
- Exercise-associated diarrhea is a diagnosis of exclusion.
- Workup is used to rule out other causes of diarrhea.

DIFFERENTIAL DIAGNOSIS

- Irritable bowel disease
- Inflammatory bowel disease
- Infection
- Colon cancer
- Superior mesenteric or portal venous thrombosis
- Malabsorption
- Microscopic colitis
- Laxative abuse
- Lactose intolerance
- Hyperthyroidism

DIAGNOSTIC TESTS & INTERPRETATION

Initial Tests (lab, imaging)

- Stool cultures, including *Clostridium difficile*
- Consider immunoglobulin A (IgA) antitissue transglutaminase antibodies to rule out celiac sprue.
- Thyroid-stimulating hormone
- Consider stool osmolar gap if eating disorder and/or laxative abuse is suspected:
  - Increased osmotic gap is suspicious for laxative use.
- Imaging studies should be obtained as clinically indicated:
  - Consider barium enema.
  - Contrast-enhanced computed tomography (CT) scan

Diagnostic Procedures/Other

Diagnostic procedures such as sigmoidoscopy or colonoscopy may be considered as clinically indicated.

TREATMENT

GENERAL MEASURES

- Treatment is generally conservative and should include (1,2,3)[C]:
  - Training modification:
    - Increase volume and intensity of training slowly.
  - Try to evacuate prior to exercise.
  - Diet modification.
- Acute symptoms usually rapidly resolve with cessation of activity.

MEDICATION

- All athletes should consult with the governing bodies of their sports regarding banned substances.
- Because symptoms are generally self-limited and typically cease after end of exercise, medications should be used with caution.

First Line

Antispasmodics may be helpful but have anticholinergic side effects and should be used with caution:

- Dicyclomine (Bentyl) 20 mg PO QID
- Hyoscyamine (Levsin) 0.125 to 0.25 mg PO/SL q4h PRN:
  - Sometimes helpful in stopping abdominal cramping after exercise
  - The athlete should remain well hydrated.
  - Use in hot/humid conditions is not ideal.
- Loperamide (Imodium) 2 to 4 mg 30 min before exercise:
  - Decreases intestinal motility and affects water and electrolyte absorption
  - Side effects are rare.

Second Line

- Opiate/atropine combinations (diphenoxylate [Lomotil]) should be used with caution:
  - Opiates are habit forming.
  - May be banned depending on governing body of the sport
  - May adversely affect performance
- Atropine may cause hyperthermia, tachycardia, and heat regulation problems.

ONGOING CARE

DIET

Dietary modification can be helpful (1,2,3,5)[C]:

- Stay well hydrated.
- Avoid caffeine, which is both a diuretic and a cathartic.
- Avoid foods that exacerbate symptoms (e.g., lactose in lactose-intolerant athlete).
- Limit intake of gas-forming foods (broccoli, onions, beans).
- Eat a small, low-fat, low-fiber meal several hours before competition:
  - Use low-osmolar sports drink between meal and competition or training.
- Avoid large doses of vitamin C, sodium bicarbonate, and carbohydrate drink prior to exercise.
- Avoid high fructose–containing foods.
- Caution against the use of nonsteroidal anti-inflammatory drugs (NSAIDs) in prerace or during race settings
- Avoid sugar substitutes or nonabsorbable sugars such as sorbitol.
- If athlete still has difficulty with diarrhea or urge to defecate, try complete nutritional liquid that is low in fiber during the day preceding competition.
- Consider meeting with a registered dietitian to discuss appropriate food, sugar, or allergen elimination nutrition plan or a low-FODMAP (fermentable oligo-, di-, mono-saccharides and polyols) diet.

PROGNOSIS

Most athletes can learn how to manage their symptoms through the use of diet and training.

REFERENCES

1. Casey E, Mistry DJ, MacKnight JM. Training room management of medical conditions: sports gastroenterology. *Clin Sports Med*. 2005;24(3):525–540.
2. Ho GW. Lower gastrointestinal distress in endurance athletes. *Curr Sports Med Rep*. 2009;8(2):85–91.
3. Simons SM, Kennedy RG. Gastrointestinal problems in runners. *Curr Sports Med Rep*. 2004;3(2):112–116.
4. Zuhl M, Schneider S, Lanphere K, et al. Exercise regulation of intestinal tight junction proteins. *Br J Sports Med*. 2014;48(12):980–986.
5. de Oliveira EP, Burini RC, Jeukendrup A. Gastrointestinal complaints during exercise: prevalence, etiology, and nutritional recommendations. *Sports Med*. 2014;44(Suppl 1):S79–S85.

ADDITIONAL READING

- Green GA. Gastrointestinal disorders in the athlete. *Clin Sports Med*. 1992;11(2):453–470.
- Swain RA. Exercise-induced diarrhea: when to wonder. *Med Sci Sports Exerc*. 1994;26(5):523–526.

E

CLINICAL PEARLS

- Exercise-induced diarrhea is associated with strenuous exercise and can worsen with increasing distance or intensity.
- Symptoms are self-limited, and patients are often asymptomatic after cessation of exercise with normal laboratory testing.
- Treatment is usually supportive and focused on dietary modifications, gradual increase in exercise intensity, and managing symptoms.
- The use of antidiarrheals prior to exercise can stop symptoms, making sports participation possible, while dietary modifications are being explored.

EXERCISE-INDUCED URTICARIA

Mark Halstead, MD, FAAP

BASICS

DESCRIPTION

- Spectrum of allergic response to exercise ranging from itching, flushing, and cutaneous warmth to development of well-circumscribed wheals (large papular lesions with pale centers and an erythematous ring) and angioedema to severe anaphylactic shock
- Elevation of serum histamine levels with exercise
- Mast cell degranulation seen in skin biopsies suggesting immunoglobulin E–mediated sensitization
- Described with almost any type of physical exercise
- Distinguishable from cholinergic urticaria, which also has exercise as a possible trigger
- Certain foods in combination with exercise may cause symptoms in susceptible individuals.
- Synonym(s): exercise-induced anaphylaxis; hives

EPIDEMIOLOGY

- Incidence unknown
- Prevalence estimated 0.048% in adolescence (1)
- Predominant gender: male > female
- Predominant age: seen more frequently in young adults but has been described ages 4 to 76 yr (2)
- Exercise-induced anaphylaxis accounts for 5–15% of all anaphylaxis cases; 1/3 to 1/2 of these cases are due to food-dependent exercise-induced anaphylaxis.

RISK FACTORS

- Atopic history (eczema, asthma, allergic rhinitis)
- Other forms of physical allergy
- Food allergy

GENERAL PREVENTION

- Stop exercise with first onset of symptoms.
- Avoid foods 6 to 8 hr before exercise. Exercising first thing in the morning after evening fast is preferable.
- Avoid known problematic food or medication triggers for at least 12 hr before exercise.
- Preventive antihistamine therapy may be useful.
- Patients always should have an epinephrine kit with them while exercising; diphenhydramine (Benadryl) also may be reasonable to have.
- Exercising with a companion knowledgeable in cardiopulmonary resuscitation (CPR) is recommended.
- Recommend wearing medical alert device.

DIAGNOSIS

HISTORY

- Diagnosis usually is made by history.
- Initially, patients describe generalized feeling of tingling, warmth, and itching.
- May start as early as 5 min after initiating exercise or can occur after exercise has been completed
- May have history of food or medication ingestion within previous 6 to 8 hr before exercise
- Patients often (>50%) have atopic history (i.e., eczema, asthma, allergic rhinitis).
- Foods reported to be associated include wheat, alcohol, eggs, lentils, shellfish, peanuts, hazelnuts, tomatoes, peaches, apples, grapes, celery, cereals, cow's milk, mushrooms, beef, pork, poultry, snails, and cheese. Cases have been reported with many other foods.
- Medications: nonsteroidal anti-inflammatory drugs (NSAIDs), aspirin, antibiotics
- Other cofactors reported: menstrual cycle, metal-containing dental amalgams
- Usually resolves within 30 min to 4 hr after exercise
- Headaches may continue for up to 3 to 4 days after a severe reaction.

PHYSICAL EXAM

- Signs and symptoms:
  - Pruritus
  - Urticaria
  - Wheezing
  - Hypotension
  - Flushing
  - Angioedema
  - Headaches
  - Nausea/vomiting
  - Diarrhea
  - Abdominal pain
  - Choking
  - Profuse sweating
- Physical examination:
  - Generally distinguished from cholinergic urticaria because larger (>10 mm) wheals are seen in exercise-induced urticaria, whereas fine punctate (<5 mm) lesions are seen in cholinergic urticaria
  - Wheals are not reproducible with generalized heat application or sweating, which is more characteristic of cholinergic urticaria, or cold application (ice cube) common to cold urticaria.
  - Respiratory examination may demonstrate stridor, wheezing, dyspnea, and retractions during acute attack.
  - Angioedema seen in more severe acute attacks

DIFFERENTIAL DIAGNOSIS

- Physical urticarias (cold, dermographic, delayed pressure, solar, aquagenic, vibratory)
- Cholinergic urticaria (induced by increased body temperature)
- Exercise-induced asthma
- Vocal cord dysfunction

- Insect bites
- Drug eruption
- Urticaria pigmentosa
- Systemic lupus erythematosus
- Erythema multiforme

DIAGNOSTIC TESTS & INTERPRETATION

- Labs not necessary in acute attacks
- May have elevated serum tryptase or histamine following attack but not specific for this disorder
- Allergy testing may be beneficial as an outpatient.
- Positive skin testing does not always mean a cause-and-effect relationship. Suspicious positive skin tests may need to be followed by an exercise challenge because patients with positive food skin tests may not always develop urticaria with exercise and consumption of that food.

TREATMENT

MEDICATION

- Epinephrine (EpiPen) 0.2 to 0.5 mg intramuscular (IM) for severe anaphylactic reaction in adults; 0.01 mg/kg in children
- Diphenhydramine (Benadryl) 25 to 50 mg PO q4–6h (children: 5 mg/kg/day divided q6–8h, not exceeding 300 mg/day)
- Hydroxyzine (Atarax) 25 to 100 mg PO q6h (children: 2 mg/kg/day divided q6–8h)
- During exercise, patients should carry an epinephrine kit (EpiPen) with them at all times.
- H_1 antihistamines as prophylaxis have shown mixed results (fexofenadine 60 mg PO BID, loratadine 10 mg PO daily, and cetirizine 10 mg PO daily).
- Cromolyn taken orally has been reported to be of some benefit.
- H_2 antihistamines may be of help (e.g., cimetidine, ranitidine, and famotidine).
- Doxepin, which has both H_1- and H_2-blocking abilities, may be of value.

ADDITIONAL THERAPIES

- Acutely, care is targeted toward ensuring airway protection if severe anaphylaxis is present.
- Trendelenburg position

ONGOING CARE

FOLLOW-UP RECOMMENDATIONS

- Referral to an allergist may be beneficial for skin testing and controlled exercise challenge testing.
- Preventative medication has been reported to decrease or stabilize attacks in up to 93% of patients (3)[C].

REFERENCES

1. Aihara Y, Takahashi Y, Kotoyori T, et al. Frequency of food-dependent, exercise-induced anaphylaxis in Japanese junior-high-school students. *J Allergy Clin Immunol*. 2001;108(6):1035–1039.
2. Pravettoni V, Incorvaia C. Diagnosis of exercise-induced anaphylaxis: current insights. *J Asthma Allergy*. 2016;9:191–198.
3. Shadick NA, Liang MH, Partridge AJ, et al. The natural history of exercise-induced anaphylaxis: survey results from a 10-year follow-up study. *J Allergy Clin Immunol*. 1999;104(1):123–127.

ADDITIONAL READING

- Chong SU, Worm M, Zuberbier T. Role of adverse reactions to food in urticaria and exercise-induced anaphylaxis. *Int Arch Allergy Immunol*. 2002;129(1):19–26.
- Feldweg AM. Exercise-induced anaphylaxis. *Immunol Allergy Clin North Am*. 2015;35(2):261–275.
- Montgomery SL. Cholinergic urticaria and exercise-induced anaphylaxis. *Curr Sports Med Rep*. 2015;14(1):61–63.

CLINICAL PEARLS

- Exercise may be continued as long as precautions are taken by avoiding all food 6 to 8 hr before exercise and 12 hr after eating food suspected of causing reactions.
- Epinephrine should be carried at all times with the patient when exercising, and a companion who knows CPR ideally would be exercising with the patient.
- Patients who had severe life-threatening reactions likely need counseling to discuss curtailing exercise.
- These reactions are not always preventable. Despite premedication with various antihistamines, patients still can develop urticarial lesions and have anaphylaxis.
- Initiating antihistamine therapy on a daily basis for those who exercise frequently is a worthwhile start to hopefully reduce the number of occurrences of this phenomenon.
- Each individual may react to different foods. Some may react to only a single food but reports of a combination of foods are needed to trigger the reaction.
- Some patients have been reported to react to any food they eat, so avoid eating 4 to 6 hr prior.
- If a food seems to trigger a reaction, it is best to avoid that food for at least 12 hr before exercise.
- It is reasonable to see an allergist for testing and an exercise challenge with suspicious food items.

EXERTIONAL HEADACHE

Nathan Cardoos, MD, CAQSM

BASICS

- There are two types of exertional, or exercise-associated, headaches seen in athletes: (i) primary exercise headache (PEH) and (ii) "weight lifter's headache," a form of primary cough headache.
- These headache syndromes are not associated with intracranial lesions or systemic disorders. They are distinct from migraines, tension headaches, concussion, and cervicogenic headaches—all of which are also seen in athletes—although they may coexist and must be treated accordingly.

DESCRIPTION

- Weight lifter's headache is a short-lasting headache that results abruptly from Valsalva maneuvers, such as with weight lifting, coughing, sneezing, or crying.
- PEH is believed to be distinct from weight lifter's headache because it lasts longer, has a different population profile, results from more sustained intense exercise (such as running, cycling, rowing, swimming, etc.), and is usually not associated with Valsalva maneuvers.

EPIDEMIOLOGY

- PEH occurs typically in younger athletes with an average age of 24 to 40 yr, depending on the case series examined (1).
- Weight lifter's headache is more commonly seen in older individuals, with an average age of 55 to 67 yr (2).

Prevalence

Lifetime prevalence of PEH is 1% of the general population, based on a Danish study; however, other studies have reported a prevalence of up to 26% (3).

ETIOLOGY AND PATHOPHYSIOLOGY

Pathophysiology is largely unknown, but several theories have been postulated:

- Systemic blood pressure (BP) changes or increases in intra-abdominal/intrathoracic pressures during exercise may lead to increased cerebral arterial pressure or cause dilatation of pain-sensitive venous sinuses (2).
- Other theories include inappropriate cerebrovascular dilation with BP changes during exercise or incompetence of the jugular venous valve.

RISK FACTORS

- High altitude (3)
- Hot weather (3)
- Extreme exertion (3)
- Dehydration (3)

GENERAL PREVENTION

Avoidance of physical exertion. It usually takes only a few episodes for the patient to understand what factors precipitate symptoms and to learn to avoid the type of physical exertion that triggers the pain (4).

COMMONLY ASSOCIATED CONDITIONS

- Up to 50% of patients with PEH have a personal or family history of migraine and exercise can be a migraine trigger (3).
- Almost half of cough headache patients have a space-occupying lesion of the posterior fossa, most commonly a Chiari type I malformation (5).

DIAGNOSIS

HISTORY

- All of the defining features below come from a small number of case series and expert opinion (1,3,6).
- PEH:
  - Characterized as bilateral, throbbing, pulsatile
  - Brought on by and occurs only during or after strenuous physical exercise
  - Not associated with head trauma
  - Lasts typically from 5 min to 24 hr but can persist up to 48 hr
  - Not associated with nausea or vomiting, although it should be noted that many patients with migraines experience exercise as a trigger and may have these symptoms
- Weight lifter's headache:
  - Sudden onset brought on by coughing, straining, or other Valsalva maneuver
  - Described as "sharp" or "stabbing"
  - Lasts seconds to minutes
- Thorough history should aim to:
  - Elicit details that may alert to a focal neurologic cause.
  - Rule out history of head trauma.
  - Identify any red flags suggesting other cause of headache, such as confusion, disorientation, fatigue, seizure activity, numbness or focal weakness, memory or speech impairment, aura, phonophobia, photophobia, blurry or double vision, febrile illness, dizziness, ataxia, vomiting, or prolonged duration.
  - Distinguish exertional headache from migraine or tension headache.
  - Identify personal or family history of migraine disorder or other headache disorders.
  - Identify any past history of bleeding disorders or blood clots.
  - Evaluate for cardiac risk factors.

PHYSICAL EXAM

- Check vital signs.
- Perform complete neurologic examination, including strength, coordination, balance, gait, reflexes, sensation, and cranial nerve function. By definition, the neurologic examination will be normal in PEH.
- Conduct funduscopic exam to look for any papilledema. Test visual fields and pupillary reflex.
- Assess mental status, which is normal in PEH.
- Evaluate for signs of meningismus or neck stiffness.
- The rest of the exam should be determined by any red flags or key components of the history.

DIFFERENTIAL DIAGNOSIS

- Concussion
- Cervicogenic headache
- Tension headache
- Migraine disorder
- Systemic disorder, such as a viral illness
- Drug-induced headache
- Central nervous system (CNS) infection
- Intracranial lesion, such as a brain tumor
- Subarachnoid hemorrhage
- Cervical artery dissection
- Reversible cerebral vasoconstriction syndrome
- Cerebral aneurysm or arteriovenous malformation
- Chiari malformation
- Intracranial hypertension
- Cerebral venous thrombosis
- Cardiac cephalgia (cardiac ischemia causing headache without chest pain)
- Pheochromocytoma

DIAGNOSTIC TESTS & INTERPRETATION

Initial Tests (lab, imaging)

- If there are any focal neurologic findings or any concern for a structural lesion or a stroke, then neuroimaging, such as computed tomography (CT) or magnetic resonance imaging (MRI), must be done.
- At younger ages with classic history of PEH, mild symptoms, and normal exam, imaging may not be necessary to make the diagnosis; however, many experts recommend that imaging, including MRI and magnetic resonance angiography (MRA), should be performed for all new or never-evaluated PEH (1,2,6)[C].
- The Ottawa Subarachnoid Hemorrhage (SAH) Rule for headache evaluation states that patients ≥15 yr old with a new, severe, atraumatic headache reaching maximum intensity within 1 hr should be evaluated for SAH if the headache onset occurred with exertion. A patient meeting these criteria should be evaluated acutely for SAH with CT; lumbar puncture should be done if strong suspicion for SAH remains after a normal CT (1)[C].
- For weight lifter's headache to be considered a benign condition, structural lesions, especially in the cerebral posterior fossa, must be ruled out by neuroimaging (6)[C].
- MRI can better evaluate the posterior fossa than CT scan, but CT more quickly evaluates for hemorrhage.
- Consider evaluating for cardiac ischemia in patients >50 yr with known heart disease or risk factors for myocardial infarction.

Diagnostic Procedures/Other

Consider lumbar puncture if there is a suspicion for SAH and the CT scan is normal.

TREATMENT

MEDICATION

- Given the self-limiting nature and short duration of symptoms from weight lifter's headache, avoidance of the provoking activity is the preferred treatment.
- Nonsteroidal anti-inflammatory drugs (NSAIDs) are typically used to treat PEH as well as to prevent recurrence.
- Indomethacin (50 to 100 mg PO 30 to 60 min prior to the headache-causing physical exertion, or 25 to 50 mg TID for long-term prophylaxis) (4)[C] has been used with some success.
- Ergotamine (unspecified dose prior to exercise) can be used for prophylaxis in cases where NSAIDs are not well tolerated (4)[C], but caution needs to be exercised because of its side effects and drug interaction profile.
- Propranolol (20 to 80 mg TID) is another option for prophylactic therapy (4)[C].

ISSUES FOR REFERRAL

Consider referral to a neurologist if headache symptoms are atypical or recalcitrant to treatment, or if assistance is needed in determining the appropriate diagnostic work-up.

ADDITIONAL THERAPIES

- NSAIDs can cause peptic ulcer disease, stomach irritation, nausea, renal dysfunction, and renal failure. They should be taken with food and used sparingly.
- Ergotamine has known complications, including vascular stasis and peripheral vascular constriction, thrombosis, worsening of vascular disease, fibrosis, and increased uterine contractility. It is contraindicated in coronary artery disease, hypertension, liver disease, renal disease, pregnancy, and Raynaud syndrome. It should be used with caution.

ONGOING CARE

PATIENT EDUCATION

- Patients should be advised to avoid exercising in the heat and to stay hydrated.
- Patients with a history of exertional headache should avoid the type of physical exertion that triggers the pain.
- A sudden, severe headache with exercise should lead to evaluation in an emergency room.

PROGNOSIS

- PEH and weight lifter's headache tend to recur with exercise.
- In a study that followed 93 patients, 32% of patients with PEH sustained complete remission within 5 yr, and 78% underwent complete remission or significant improvement in 10 yr (3).
- Primary cough headache is generally self-limited, with 50–90% of patients in remission within 2 yr (3).

REFERENCES

1. Halker RB, Vargas BB. Primary exertional headache: updates in the literature. *Curr Pain Headache Rep*. 2013;17(6):337.
2. Cutrer FM, DeLange J. Cough, exercise, and sex headaches. *Neurol Clin*. 2014;32(2):433–450.
3. Evans RW. Sports and headaches. *Headache*. 2018;58(3):426–437.
4. Allena M, Rossi P, Tassorelli C, et al. Focus on therapy of the chapter IV headaches provoked by exertional factors: primary cough headache, primary exertional headache and primary headache associated with sexual activity. *J Headache Pain*. 2010;11(6):525–530.
5. Alvarez R, Ramón C, Pascual J. Clues in the differential diagnosis of primary vs secondary cough, exercise, and sexual headaches. *Headache*. 2014;54(9):1560–1562.
6. Headache Classification Committee of the International Headache Society. The International Classification of Headache Disorders, 3rd edition (beta version). *Cephalalgia*. 2013;33(9):629–808.

ADDITIONAL READING

Sandoe CH, Kingston W. Exercise headache: a review. *Curr Neurol Neurosci Rep*. 2018;18(6):28.

CLINICAL PEARLS

- PEH occurs during or soon after intense physical activity and can be prevented by avoiding intense exertion. It is typically characterized as bilateral, throbbing, and pulsatile. It lasts 5 min to 48 hr, and the average age of onset is 24 yr.
- Weight lifter's headache is quick in onset, "stabbing," lasts seconds to minutes, and is associated with the Valsalva maneuver. It more commonly affects older individuals.
- Neuroimaging is generally recommended after the initial presentation of either condition, or if there are any signs or symptoms suggestive of intracranial pathology.
- Evidence behind diagnosis and management of exertional headaches is limited.

EXTERNAL EAR CHONDRITIS/ABSCESS

Arturo J. Aguilar, MD, CAQSM

BASICS

DESCRIPTION

- Inflammation and infection of the pinna (1)
- Commonly a complication of otic trauma (1), burns, or neighboring infection
- It may present as a complication of draining a periauricular hematoma (cauliflower ear) in sports such as wrestling and rugby (2).
- Occasionally, chondritis may be a complication of untreated or resistant otitis externa in swimmers (2).
- Cartilage of the external ear is easily damaged and at risk for infection owing to:
  - Lack of overlying subcutaneous tissue.
  - Relative avascularity.
  - Exposed position.

ETIOLOGY AND PATHOPHYSIOLOGY

- Common causes of chondritis include (1,2):
  - Chemical or thermal burns.
  - Otitis externa.
  - Deep abrasions.
  - Frostbite.
  - High piercing of the earlobe.
  - Human bites.
  - Iatrogenic from incision and drainage treatment of hematoma.
  - Mastoid surgery.
- Bacteria involved (2,3):
  - *Pseudomonas aeruginosa*
  - *Staphylococcus* spp

DIAGNOSIS

Typical physical findings in combination with preceding causes

PHYSICAL EXAM

- Initially a dull pain that increases in severity
- Pinna (2):
  - Painful
  - Exquisite tenderness
  - Erythematous
  - Warmth
  - Loss of contours caused by edema often with sparing of the lobule
- Increase in the auriculocephalic angle
- Fluctuant areas develop with eventual breakdown and suppuration.
- Entire ear involvement if untreated: Disfigurement can occur (2).
- Tympanic membrane has normal appearance in the absence of concurrent acute otitis media.
- Auditory canal has normal appearance in the absence of concurrent acute otitis externa.
- Fever/chills

DIFFERENTIAL DIAGNOSIS

- Periauricular hematoma: "cauliflower ear"
- Malignant otitis externa

DIAGNOSTIC TESTS & INTERPRETATION

- Complete blood count (CBC) with differential for systemic symptoms (2)
- Wound culture for signs of localized infection (2)
- Blood culture if systemic signs of infection (2)

TREATMENT

GENERAL MEASURES

- General postinjury preventive measures:
  - Prevention of chondritis is of the utmost importance (4)[C]:
    - Difficult management and disfiguring potential
    - Avoid pressure to the injured ear (unlike the compression treatments used for an auricular hematoma).
    - Minimize active débridement of eschars and crusts.
  - Gentle washing daily with antibacterial soap and water followed by complete drying and application of topical antibiotics (2)
- Complications: disfiguration of the pinna:
  - Occurs without proper treatment
  - Ranges from being shriveled, cauliflower-like ear to complete loss of the external ear and possible stenosis of the auditory meatus

- Ear, nose, and throat (ENT) consult:
  - For treatment of chondritis, abscess, and necrosis of the involved cartilage
  - Early surgical drainage
  - Aggressive early management may prevent gross ear deformity.

MEDICATION

- Oral antibiotics for minor cases of early ear lobe inflammation:
  - Ciprofloxacin preferred (>18 yr old) (1)[A]
  - 1st-generation cephalosporin or dicloxacillin (1)[B]
  - Intravenous (IV) antibiotics for severe infection (1)[B]
  - Apply topical antibacterial when break in skin barrier (3)[C].
- Medications:
  - Ciprofloxacin: 500 mg PO BID or 750 mg BID (adult)
  - Cephalexin: 500 mg (children: 50 mg/kg/day) PO QID
  - Dicloxacillin: 500 mg (children: 25 mg/kg/day) PO QID

ADMISSION, INPATIENT, AND NURSING CONSIDERATIONS

Admission criteria:

- Parenteral antibiotics and early surgical drainage for patients with complicated chondritis
- Toxic patient with fever and chills
- Immunocompromised patient
- Unreliable patient or caretaker

REFERENCES

1. Fisher C, Kacica M, Bennett N. Risk factors for cartilage infections of the ear. *Am J Prev Med*. 2005;29(3):204–209.
2. Thill M, Horoi M, Ostermann K, et al. Acute external ear lesions: clinical aspects, assessment and management. *B-ENT*. 2016;(Suppl 26)(1):155–171.
3. Sosin M, Weissler J, Pulcrano M, et al. Transcartilagenous ear piercing and infectious complications: a systemic review and critical analysis of outcomes. *Laryngoscope*. 2015;125(8):1827–1834.
4. Liu Z, Chokkalingam P. Piercing associated perichondritis of the pinna: are we treating it correctly? *J. Laryngol Otol*. 2013;127(5):505–508.

CLINICAL PEARLS

- Monitor for signs of external ear chondritis/abscess after draining a periauricular hematoma.
- Symptoms include painful, erythematous, warm pinna.
- Most commonly implicated bacteria are *Pseudomonas* and *Staphylococcus*.
- Preferred antibiotic in adults is ciprofloxacin.
- Preferred antibiotic in children are cephalosporins like cephalexin.

E

EXTERNAL GENITAL TRAUMA

David C. Shin, MD • David W. Kruse, MD

BASICS

- Injuries in males:
  - Lacerations, hematomas, avulsions of penis/scrotum
  - Penile fracture
  - Urethral injury
  - Testicular rupture
  - Penetrating injury to penis/scrotum
- Injuries in females:
  - Lacerations, hematomas, avulsions
  - Vaginal impalement injuries
  - Vaginal insufflation injuries
  - Genital trauma from sexual abuse

Pediatric Considerations

- Consider nonaccidental trauma or sexual abuse.
- Sexual abuse is a common etiology in females.
- Urethral damage is frequently caused by traumatic mechanisms similar to those in adults.

DESCRIPTION

- Females:
  - Injuries to the urethra are rare owing to the short, unexposed, and mobile urethra. Most occur at the bladder neck.
  - Risk of associated injuries to neighboring organs after blunt trauma is higher than males
  - Most traumatic injuries are secondary to accidental falls onto objects resulting in impalement or blunt trauma:
    - Blunt trauma:
      - Vulvar lacerations, ecchymosis, hematoma
      - May be associated with voiding problems
      - Can result in crush injury or pelvic fractures
    - Impalement:
      - Physical findings can mimic penetration by blunt forceful trauma, so must evaluate for possible sexual abuse.
      - Vagina, urethra, bladder, anus, rectum, and peritoneal cavity can be pierced by a sharp object.
  - Insufflation with high-pressure water (e.g., falls off jet skis or water skis) can result in vaginal tears.
- Males:
  - Blunt trauma:
    - Penile/soft tissue:
      - Penile fracture results from rupture of the tunica albuginea.
      - Urethral injuries are more common in prostatic urethra versus bulbar or penile urethra.
      - ~95% of posterior urethral injuries are caused by pelvic fractures.
      - Anterior urethral injuries are commonly caused by blunt trauma.
      - As many as 25% of pelvic fractures have concomitant urethral injuries.
      - Laceration, ecchymosis, hematoma, avulsion injuries
    - Scrotal trauma:
      - Most testicular injuries (up to 85%) are from blunt trauma, with majority in athletics.
      - Scrotal ecchymosis, hemorrhage
      - Hematoceles: blood accumulation in space between tunica albuginea and tunica vaginalis
      - Testicular rupture: disruption of the tunica albuginea
      - Traumatically induced hydroceles
      - Traumatically induced testicular torsion
      - Pelvic fracture with significant blunt trauma
  - Penetrating injury: can cause significant injury to soft tissues and scrotum

DIAGNOSIS

Pediatric Considerations

- If an examination of the introitus and perineum cannot be performed easily, examination under anesthesia should occur.
- An examination in the operating room (OR), in addition to being better tolerated by the patient, can help the physician to evaluate for sexual abuse and to confirm that the injury is consistent with the history.
- The workup of male pediatric patients also should include an examination in the OR if an adequate emergency department (ED) examination does not occur or if suspicion of abuse exists.

HISTORY

- Mechanism of injury
- Prior history of trauma
- Pelvic pain, bleeding, inability to void
- Blood at the urethral meatus or hematuria
- History of possible sexual abuse

PHYSICAL EXAM

- Females:
  - Genitourinary (GU) examination to determine extent of injury
  - Vaginal smear to check for spermatozoa and urine and blood analysis (1,2)
  - If injury is minor superficial laceration or hematoma and no history of penetrating injury, normal exam is sufficient.
  - Vaginal lacerations with active bleeding should be repaired by provider with experience to avoid urethra, bladder, and rectal injury.
  - Indications for exam under anesthesia:
    - Young or uncooperative patient
    - Transection of the hymen with inability to see the full extent of injury
    - Vaginal hemorrhage
    - Expanding vulvar or vaginal hematoma
    - History of significant blunt, forceful, or penetrating trauma
    - Significant vaginal laceration or soft tissue injury
    - Complex vaginal and perineal lacerations associated with pelvic fracture or rectal injury
    - Perforation into peritoneal cavity requires exploratory laparotomy/laparoscopy.
- Males:
  - GU examination to determine extent of injury
  - Examine for high-riding prostate, perineal or penile swelling, blood at meatus.
  - Examine testicles for pain or swelling concerning for rupture, hematocele, and torsion.
  - Evaluate for rectal injuries.

DIFFERENTIAL DIAGNOSIS

- Perineal and vaginal trauma
- Bladder trauma
- Ureter or kidney trauma
- Pelvic fracture

DIAGNOSTIC TESTS & INTERPRETATION

- Urinalysis
- Hematocrit
- Blood urea nitrogen (BUN) and creatine (Cr)
- Consider screening for sexually transmitted infections if history or exam is consistent with sexual abuse.

- Scrotal imaging: scrotal ultrasound (SUS):
  - Scrotum exam can be difficult with significant swelling.
  - SUS should be performed because it is sensitive and specific for intrascrotal injury (1,2,3).
  - SUS assesses the integrity and vascularity of the testes.
  - SUS may distinguish testis rupture from hematocele, hydrocele, torsion, and epididymitis (3).
- Urethral injury: retrograde urethrography (RUG):
  - Inability to void, blood at meatus, and any degree of hematuria are absolute indications for RUG (1)[C].
  - Recommended with any penetrating genital injuries (1)[C]
  - Water-soluble contrast material is injected at the urethral meatus.
  - Extravasation of contrast material and location of extravasation can diagnose presence of tear as well as degree of tear.
- Cystography: 40% of urethral injuries have concomitant bladder injuries.
- Proctoscopy: In the female when there is a possibility of impalement injury or pelvic fracture, proctoscopy can aid in evaluating the extent of injury (4).

TREATMENT

- Prehospital:
  - Similar considerations as for major trauma victims
- ED treatment:
  - Initial stabilization, control of bleeding, pain control
  - After appropriate evaluation and workup, urologic or gynecologic consult if warranted
  - Urethral contusions, lacerations, and avulsions are best managed by an experienced urologist.
  - Scrotal hematomas, hydroceles, and contusions can be managed with rest, ice, and elevation.
  - Tetanus immunization if warranted for laceration or avulsion

MEDICATION

Anytime, there is injury to the female mucosal genital surfaces; application of topical estrogen cream can benefit the healing process and decrease scarring (5)[C].

SURGERY/OTHER PROCEDURES

ALERT

- Males:
  - Prompt surgical intervention with closure of the tunica albuginea for penile fractures to prevent erectile dysfunction and penile curvature (1,6)[C]
  - When physical exam findings and mechanism of injury suggest significant testicular injury, operative exploration should be undertaken even with equivocal imaging (2,3)[C].
  - Prompt drainage of large hematoceles is recommended to prevent secondary infection or pressure atrophy (2)[C].
  - Following blunt scrotal trauma, probability of testicular salvage decreases significantly if not explored in 72 hr (3).
  - Posttraumatic testicular torsion and testicular dislocation require immediate surgical intervention.
  - Penetrating trauma to the scrotum or penis warrants prompt surgical exploration (1)[C].
  - Complex avulsions are best managed with initial débridement and delayed reconstruction (3,6)[C].
  - Minor avulsions are managed as simple lacerations with irrigation and primary closure (3)[C].
- Females:
  - Simple perineal and vulvar lacerations usually can be repaired in the ED (5).
  - Large hematoma should be incised and drained (4).
  - See "Physical Exam" for indications for exam under anesthesia.
  - In exam under anesthesia, if peritoneal or rectal cavities are entered, exploratory laparotomy is indicated (3).

ADMISSION, INPATIENT, AND NURSING CONSIDERATIONS

- Initial stabilization:
  - Airway, breathing, and circulation (ABCs) of trauma care take precedence.
- Admission criteria:
  - Concurrent closed head injury, blunt abdominal trauma, or pelvic fracture
  - Need for operative management of urethral, penile, vaginal, pelvic, or bladder injuries
- Discharge criteria:
  - Isolated urethral injuries frequently may be managed in the outpatient setting after appropriate urinary catheterization or suprapubic cystostomy with urologic follow-up.

ONGOING CARE

COMPLICATIONS

- Impotence
- Incontinence
- Strictures
- Infection
- Disfigurement
- Pain
- Scarring
- Infertility

REFERENCES

1. Summerton DJ, Djakovic N, Kitrey ND, et al. Guidelines on urological trauma. http://uroweb.org/guideline/urological-trauma/. Accessed May 2018.
2. Bryk DJ, Zhao LC. Guideline of guidelines: a review of urological trauma guidelines. *BJU Int*. 2016;117(2):226–234.
3. Morey AF, Metro MJ, Carney KJ, et al. Consensus on genitourinary trauma: external genitalia. *BJU Int*. 2004;94(4):507–515.
4. Wessells H, Long L. Penile and genital injuries. *Urol Clin North Am*. 2006;33(1):117–126.
5. Merritt DF. Genital trauma in children and adolescents. *Clin Obstet Gynecol*. 2008;51(2):237–248.
6. Morey AF, Brandes S, Dugi DD III, et al. Urotrauma: AUA guideline. *J Urol*. 2014;192(2):327–335.

ADDITIONAL READING

- Carter CT, Schafer N. Incidence of urethral disruption in females with traumatic pelvic fractures. *Am J Emerg Med*. 1993;11(3):218–220.
- Lee SH, Bak CW, Choi MH, et al. Trauma to male genital organs: a 10-year review of 156 patients, including 118 treated by surgery. *BJU Int*. 2008;101(2):211–215.
- McGeady JB, Breyer BN. Current epidemiology of genitourinary trauma. *Urol Clin North Am*. 2013;40(3):323–334.

CLINICAL PEARLS

- Must rule out a urethral injury if there is blood at the meatus, inability to void, or hemorrhage.
- Increased risk of injury to neighboring organs in females
- Consider nonaccidental trauma or sexual abuse in pediatrics.
- In the setting of significant testicular or scrotal trauma, surgical referral is necessary even if imaging is inconclusive.

E

FEMALE ATHLETE TRIAD

Diana Filtz, MD • Kelsey Logan, MD, MPH, FAAP, FACP

BASICS

DESCRIPTION

A condition of female athletes that refers to low energy availability, with or without disordered eating, menstrual dysfunction, and low bone mineral density (BMD) (1). This condition is a manifestation of the interrelationship of energy availability, menstrual function, and BMD:

- International Olympic Committee (IOC) convened an expert panel to update the 2005 IOC Consensus Statement on the Female Athlete Triad with the purpose of:
  - Replacing and providing guidelines to facilitate risk assessment, treatment, and return-to-play decisions.
  - Introducing a broader, more comprehensive term for the condition known as "female athlete triad."
  - Including the male athletic population.
- Although controversial, this consensus statement coined a new term, relative energy deficiency in sport (RED-S).
- The underlying problem of RED-S is an inadequacy of energy to support the range of body functions involved in optimal health and performance.

EPIDEMIOLOGY

Prevalence

- Female athlete triad: largely unknown; 1–6% in various studies (2)
- Disordered eating: 7–89% depending on sport (2)
- Amenorrhea: 1–60% (secondary amenorrhea) depending on sport (2)
- Osteoporosis: 0–40% (2)

ETIOLOGY AND PATHOPHYSIOLOGY

- Reduced energy availability or an imbalance between intake and output of calories is the ultimate cause of the disorder.
- Restriction of calories may be inadvertent (not taking in enough calories for the demand of the sport) or intentional (trying to lose weight).
- Purging of calories may manifest as vomiting, laxative use, or excess exercise/training with little or no recovery time.
- This energy deficit leads to disruption of normal estrogen production through the hypothalamic–pituitary axis. The pituitary gland does not secrete pulses of luteinizing hormone (LH) at the correct frequency, which decreases bone formation and bone production and, in women, results in a change in menstrual function. Men may demonstrate reduced energy availability and thus a decrease in bone density, also owing to the preceding risk factors.
- The etiology is multifactorial.
- There is a psychological difference between those misusing exercise, laxatives, or calorie restriction to manage/lose weight and those who inadvertently do not match their calories to their sport.
- In many women, the emphasis on leanness in sport, along with the perceived benefits of low body weight (e.g., better fitness, agility, speed), causes increased focus on weight-control measures (3).

RISK FACTORS

- Sports emphasizing leanness or endurance, such as gymnastics, figure skating, cross-country running or skiing, and diving
- Individual sports as opposed to team sports
- Early sport-specific training
- A sudden increase in training volume
- Punitive measures imposed for weight gain
- Unreasonable performance expectations by self or others
- Poor body self-image
- Social isolation

COMMONLY ASSOCIATED CONDITIONS

Psychological disorders such as depression, anxiety, and body dysmorphic disorder

DIAGNOSIS

High index of suspicion required

HISTORY

- Screening questions on menstruation, attitudes about weight, diet, and history of bony injury are recommended and are easily available. The Female Athlete Triad Consensus Statement offers a short screening tool (1).
- One component of the triad raises suspicion for the others.
- Presence of primary (absence of menses by age 15 yr) or secondary amenorrhea (absence of menses for 3 consecutive mo)
- Presence of or history of stress fracture
- Review exercise habits and nutritional history for abnormal weight-control behavior involving food and/or exercise.
- Review life stressors.
- Patient may have fear of weight gain and/or poor body image.
- Patient may have comorbid psychological diagnoses (e.g., depression).
- Symptoms/signs include:
  - Amenorrhea.
  - Stress fracture.
  - Weight-control behaviors and/or weight loss.
  - Cold intolerance.
  - Sore throat/gastroesophageal reflux.
  - Constipation/gastrointestinal (GI) motility problems.
  - Light-headedness.
  - Fatigue.
  - Depression.
  - Introversion.
  - Worsened athletic performance.

PHYSICAL EXAM

- Height, weight, body mass index (BMI <18.5 kg/m^2 considered underweight for women ≥ 18 yr of age)
- Vital signs for evidence of bradycardia and/or orthostatic hypotension
- Observe for fat depletion and muscle wasting.
- Integumentary exam for dry skin, lanugo, brittle hair/nails
- Ocular exam to evaluate for pituitary and thyroid disorders
- Dental examination for evidence of lingual enamel erosion secondary to vomiting
- Parotid gland observation/palpation for hypertrophy secondary to vomiting
- Thyroid palpation
- Cardiac auscultation for evidence of dysrhythmia
- Complete neurologic examination, especially cranial nerves and reflexes
- Tanner staging
- Consider pelvic examination if amenorrheic (rule out uterine pathology, outflow tract obstruction, and disorders of sexual differentiation as causes of primary amenorrhea) (4).
- Careful examination of any musculoskeletal pain, looking for stress fracture
- Laboratory results may be normal, even in very undernourished women.

DIFFERENTIAL DIAGNOSIS

- Pregnancy
- Pituitary disease
- Hyperthyroidism
- Hypogonadism
- Hyperparathyroidism
- Primary ovarian insufficiency
- Polycystic ovarian syndrome
- Adrenal dysfunction
- Autoimmune disease
- Anabolic steroid use/abuse
- Excess glucocorticoid administration
- Malabsorption syndromes

DIAGNOSTIC TESTS & INTERPRETATION

Initial Tests (lab, imaging)

- Pregnancy test
- Urinalysis for specific gravity (should be normal unless dehydration is present)
- Complete blood count (CBC) (normal; possibility of anemia)
- Erythrocyte sedimentation rate (normal)

- Serum electrolytes, blood urea nitrogen, and creatinine (normal, except possibly in the case of bulimia, which may cause electrolyte abnormalities or severe dehydration associated with malnutrition)
- Thyroid function tests (normal)
- LH and follicle-stimulating hormone levels (low or normal)
- Estradiol level (low)
- Serum prolactin (normal)
- Serum cortisol (mildly elevated)
- Serum testosterone and dehydroepiandrosterone sulfate if concern for androgen excess, such as with polycystic ovary syndrome or adrenal tumors
- BMD testing with dual energy x-ray absorptiometry (DEXA) if patient has had stress fracture from mild trauma or two prior stress fractures, 6 mo evidence of hypoestrogenism (oligo- or amenorrhea) and/or disordered eating (1,5)[C]
- Reevaluation on same DEXA machine yearly if chronic
- DEXA of weight-bearing sites (posteroanterior spine, total hip, femoral neck) using lower *Z*-score to base diagnosis of low BMD

Diagnostic Procedures/Other

Progesterone challenge test (e.g., medroxyprogesterone acetate 10 mg PO daily × 10 days): If a period occurs, there is sufficient estrogen to stimulate the endometrium.

TREATMENT

GENERAL MEASURES

- Main goal of treatment is to modify diet and exercise behaviors to increase energy availability, subsequent resumption of menses, and improvement of bone metabolism, bone mass, and strength (3).
- Athlete often resists treatment if negative energy balance is intentional. Treatment discussion requires good patient rapport.
- Requires team approach (i.e., physician, psychologist, athletic trainer, parents, nutritionist, coach) and open communication among all involved
- Counsel athlete that achieving energy balance may require increasing caloric intake and/or decreasing caloric expenditure (through decreased exercise).
- Identify and modify specific behavior triggers or stressors.
- Emphasize performance and injury issues related to negative energy balance (e.g., stress fractures are related to low BMD).
- Monitor progress closely, as indicated by severity and response to treatment.
- May need to restrict patient from sport/training if not making progress or participating in treatment plan
- Prevention is best accomplished through education of athletes, coaches, trainers, and parents.

MEDICATION

- There is no strong evidence to support either hormone replacement therapy or oral contraceptive use to increase or protect BMD in athletes with functional hypothalamic amenorrhea, even if they remain amenorrheic (1).
- Although oral contraceptives may restore regular menses, they do not normalize the underlying metabolic factors impairing bone health and will therefore be unlikely to reverse low BMD (1).
- Bisphosphonates are not recommended for women of reproductive age due to teratogenicity (1).
- Treating comorbid psychiatric conditions is essential, and pharmacotherapy for the specific disorder may be useful here.
- Multivitamin supplements are commonly recommended.
- Supplement calcium between 1,000 and 1,300 mg/day and vitamin D 600 IU for adolescents and children, with higher doses for vitamin D deficiency (1).

ISSUES FOR REFERRAL

- Psychology referral is recommended for cognitive-behavioral therapy; consider family therapy to help identify and cope with stressors.
- Nutrition consultant with disordered-eating experience recommended

ADMISSION, INPATIENT, AND NURSING CONSIDERATIONS

- Electrolyte disturbances
- Severe bradycardia or dysrhythmia
- Severe dehydration
- Significant psychiatric pathology

ONGOING CARE

FOLLOW-UP RECOMMENDATIONS

- Frequent follow-up to gauge compliance with treatment plan
- Monitor weight; address nutritional concerns and goals at each visit.
- Consistent education regarding energy balance and sport performance
- Assess physiologic and psychological functioning, sport performance (if participating).
- Coordinate care with psychology and nutrition consultants.
- Menstruation usually occurs (may take a year or more) with improved nutrition and decreased exercise intensity.

PATIENT EDUCATION

- Body weight and caloric intake below what is necessary for normal physiologic function are detrimental to athletic performance.
- BMD may be *permanently* lowered in adolescents by decreasing bone formation and increasing bone resorption.
- Fertility is decreased with amenorrhea but is not totally impaired; it is possible to conceive without having a period. Fertility issues are not thought to be permanent and may normalize with resumption of menses.

PROGNOSIS

- Diagnosable eating disorders (e.g., anorexia nervosa and bulimia nervosa) are very difficult to treat and rarely are totally resolved. Prognosis is guarded.
- Athletes who have perfectionist-driven tendencies are less likely to comply with treatment and have difficulty recovering.
- Appropriate increase in energy availability has the potential to restore normal estrogenic state, normalize menstrual function, and improve BMD.

COMPLICATIONS

Injury forcing the athlete to take time off from exercising can exacerbate disordered eating practices (e.g., caloric restriction or purging).

REFERENCES

1. De Souza MJ, Nattiv A, Joy E, et al. 2014 Female athlete triad coalition consensus statement on treatment and return to play of the female athlete triad: 1st international conference held in San Francisco, California, May 2012 and 2nd international conference held in Indianapolis, Indiana, May 2013. *Br J Sports Med*. 2014;48(4):289.
2. Gibbs JC, Williams NI, De Souza MJ. Prevalence of individual and combined components of the female athlete triad. *Med Sci Sports Exerc*. 2013;45(5):985–996.
3. Barrack MT, Ackerman KE, Gibbs JC. Update on the female athlete triad. *Curr Rev Musculoskelet Med*. 2013;6(2):195–204.
4. Ranson WA, Patterson DC, Colvin AC. Female athlete triad: past, present, and future directions. *Ann Joint*. 2018;3(4):1–11.
5. Nattiv A, Loucks AB, Manore MM, et al. American College of Sports Medicine position stand. The female athlete triad. *Med Sci Sports Exerc*. 2007;39(10):1867–1882.

SEE ALSO

Eating Disorders; Menstrual Disorders in the Athlete

CLINICAL PEARLS

- Female athlete triad represents a spectrum of low energy availability, with or without disordered eating, menstrual dysfunction, and low BMD (1).
- When one aspect of the triad is found, the others should be investigated (e.g., if a woman presents with a bony stress injury, inquiry about menstrual function and eating habits should ensue).
- Treatment with oral contraceptives or other hormonal agents does not improve BMD in these athletes. The goal of treatment should be positive energy balance, with increased nutritional intake and decreased physical activity, resulting in resumption of normal periods through nonpharmacologic methods.
- Treatment of the triad requires a multidisciplinary approach. Involving a support system, including coaches, teammates, friends, and family, is often helpful.

FEMORO-ACETABULAR IMPINGEMENT (FAI)

Uziel Sauceda, MD, ABFM certified • Fernando Liquido, MD

BASICS

DESCRIPTION

- Femoro-acetabular impingement (FAI) is a condition resulting from a pathologic malformation of the hip.
- The acetabular rim and the proximal femur have excess contact during the end range of motion (ROM) of the hip.
- Leads to pain and restricted hip motion and can lead to chondral or labral injury
- Synonym: hip impingement

EPIDEMIOLOGY

Incidence

- Unknown in general population; estimated range from 10% to 15% incidence in adult population
- Cam-type deformity is more common in young active men.
- Pincer lesions are more common in middle-aged women.

Prevalence

- Young patients with hip pain have high prevalence, up to 85% (1).
- Patients may be asymptomatic with radiologic findings: 37% cam, 67% pincer deformity (2).

ETIOLOGY AND PATHOPHYSIOLOGY

Types of FAI:

- Cam type: malformation of the femoral head resulting in neck widening and asphericity
- Pincer type: malformation of the acetabulum that results in over-coverage of the anterosuperior acetabular wall and abnormal retroversion of the acetabulum
- Mixed type: most common type, combination of cam and pincer lesions
- Theory that repetitive injury to proximal femoral physis during adolescence contributes to development of cam deformity

Genetics

No conclusive evidence FAI is transmitted genetically.

RISK FACTORS

- Idiopathic
- Trauma—malunion of femoral neck fracture, posttraumatic retroversion of the femoral head
- Childhood orthopedic conditions—Legg-Calvé-Perthes disease, slipped capital femoral epiphysis (SCFE), hip dysplasia
- Iatrogenic—femoral osteotomy, overcorrection of retroversion in dysplastic hips
- High-impact sports/activities during bone development (i.e., soccer, basketball, and ice hockey)

GENERAL PREVENTION

Unknown if avoiding high-impact sports during childhood can prevent FAI

DIAGNOSIS

HISTORY

- Anterior or anterolateral hip pain that refers to the groin, associated with activity
- Inability to perform activities such as high hip flexion or internal rotation, including prolonged sitting or squatting
- Painful clicking, locking or instability from a labral tear secondary to undiagnosed FAI
- Past history of developmental dysplasia, trauma or predisposing factors of avascular necrosis
- Insidious onset of symptoms in active young and middle-aged adults
- History limited with children, keep FAI in differential with knee or thigh pain, limp after activity
- Adults may describe a stiffness in the hip.

PHYSICAL EXAM

- Reduced ROM: flexion, adduction, and internal rotation
- Flexion, adduction, and internal rotation (FADDIR)—positive test if pain elicited with adduction of a flexed, internally rotated hip with the patient supine
- Posterior inferior impingement test—positive test if pain elicited with the hip in hyperextension, passively by hanging the leg over the end of the bed; the affected hip is passively externally rotated.
- Flexion, abduction, and external rotation (FABER) test may also produce pain in the affected hip.

DIFFERENTIAL DIAGNOSIS

- Hip dysplasia
- Leg-Calvé-Perthes disease/avascular necrosis femoral head
- SCFE
- Hip subluxation—microinstability
- Labral tear not associated with impingement
- Osteoarthritis
- Muscular pathology of iliopsoas/snapping hip syndrome
- Spinal deformities—scoliosis or kyphosis
- Prior femoral neck fractures or pelvic osteotomy may also cause impingement.

DIAGNOSTIC TESTS & INTERPRETATION

Initial Tests (lab, imaging)

Laboratory tests only helpful if suspect systemic process (infection, autoimmune):

- *Complete blood count (CBC), chemistries, and liver function tests*
- *Plain radiographs:*
  - Anteroposterior (AP) pelvis view: used to assess cam-type deformity, degenerative changes, and a profunda socket
  - Dunn view: AP of hip in neutral rotation, 45 degrees of flexion, and 20 degrees of abduction
  - Cross-table projection in 15 degrees internal rotation
  - Both Dunn and cross-table projection views assess femoral head neck asphericity.
  - Cross-table view more practical for routine use as Dunn view requires an assistant to hold the patient's leg
  - Radiography inadequate to assess for chondral or labral defects
- *Alpha angle usually calculated and helpful to determine amount of cam deformity:*
  - Abnormal if >60 degrees
- *Crossover sign and lateral center edge angle are most commonly used to determine amount of pincer deformity:*
  - Abnormal lateral center edge angle >40 degrees

Follow-Up Tests & Special Considerations

- *Magnetic resonance arthrography (MRA):*
  - Preferred for evaluating labral or chondral pathology
  - May show articular cartilage thinning
- *Position of discomfort (POD) computed tomography (CT) scans:*
  - CT 3D surface reconstruction allows for better mapping of bony pathology, best demonstrating a bony impingement lesion, and helping subsequent planning for surgical resection.

Diagnostic Procedures/Other

- Important to confirm pain origin with a diagnostic hip injection
- Can be done under ultrasound guidance in office or with fluoroscopy guidance by interventional radiology

Test Interpretation

If no pain relief from injection, may need to look for alternate etiology of pain

TREATMENT

GENERAL MEASURES

Nonoperative management (3,4)[C]:

- Modification of activities by avoiding excessive hip end ROM
- Limiting activities and sports are difficult for athletic young individuals.
- Physical therapy can help with movement pattern retraining, muscle flexibility, muscle strengthening.
- Current clinical practice recommendations by the American Physical Therapy Association (APTA) suggest benefits for FAI.

MEDICATION

First Line

- Short course of nonsteroidal anti-inflammatory drugs (NSAIDs) can provide symptomatic relief (3,4)[C]
- Structural defects are not routinely treated with medications.

ISSUES FOR REFERRAL

Best to refer to orthopedic surgeon comfortable with hip arthroscopic or open surgery

SURGERY/OTHER PROCEDURES

- Surgery is the treatment of choice, with the following techniques: arthroscopic, open surgical dislocation (with a trochanteric flip osteotomy), and mini-open (combination of open and arthroscopic procedures) (3,4,5,6)[C]
- Diagnostic imaging was most common criterion in 92% of surgeries reviewed in recent literature, with alpha angle being most commonly reported measure.
- All focus on accessing the area of malformation and correcting the defect.
- Outcomes:
  - Hip arthroscopy was associated with better recovery of function, reduction in nonarthritic hip pain, and a lower reoperation rate.
  - Open surgical dislocation showed more improvement of alpha angle by the Dunn view in patients with cam osteoplasty compared with arthroscopy.

ONGOING CARE

FOLLOW-UP RECOMMENDATIONS

Postoperative care:

- Arthroscopy:
  - Keep patient toe-touch weight-bearing and ambulate with aids for 2 to 4 wk.
  - After 4 wk, low-impact active motion may be resumed.
  - Recovery expected at 4 to 6 mo back to full activity
- Open surgical dislocation:
  - Restriction to toe-touch weight-bearing for 6 to 8 wk
  - Prevent falls with walker or crutches.
  - Physical therapy starts immediately, working on passive ROM for the first 2 wk postoperatively.
  - Early ROM prevents adhesions.
- Mini-open:
  - Keeping patients with toe-touch weight-bearing and use of crutches for first 5 days
  - After 5 days, patients may have full weight-bearing activities without crutches.
  - Patients are also allowed to begin low-impact active exercise, such as cycling.
  - Patients are kept from high-impact or contact sports for a total of 6 mo postoperatively.

PATIENT EDUCATION

- Emphasize activity modification if patient not seeking surgery.
- High-level athletes will likely proceed with surgical consultation.

PROGNOSIS

Common cause for revision surgery is inadequate bony correction of the FAI.

COMPLICATIONS

- Nonsurgical care:
  - Hip degenerative arthritis
  - Labral tears
  - Chondral defects/delamination
- Complications of surgery:
  - Trochanteric nonunion, heterotopic ossification, sciatic nerve palsy, osteonecrosis of the femoral head, femoral neck fracture, injury of the lateral cutaneous femoral nerve, neurapraxia of nerves around the hip joint
  - A meta-analysis by Zhang et al. demonstrated no statistical difference in complications between hip arthroscopy and open surgical dislocation (6).

Geriatric Considerations

Usually, hip pain in elderly is secondary to degenerative arthritis.

Pediatric Considerations

Keep in mind femoral growth plates when evaluating hip pain in pediatric population as well as thinking about SCFE and Legg-Calvé-Perthes disease.

Pregnancy Considerations

- Hip pain in pregnancy may be due to increased laxity.
- Keep in mind transient osteoporosis of hip in 3rd trimester.

REFERENCES

1. Ochoa LM, Dawson L, Patzkowski JC, et al. Radiographic prevalence of femoroacetabular impingement in a young population with hip complaints is high. *Clin Orthop Relat Res*. 2010; 468(10):2710–2714.
2. Frank JM, Harris JD, Erickson BJ, et al. Prevalence of femoroacetabular impingement imaging findings in asymptomatic volunteers: a systematic review. *Arthroscopy*. 2015;31(6):1199–1204.
3. Banerjee P, McLean CR. Femoroacetabular impingement: a review of diagnosis and management. *Curr Rev Musculoskelet Med*. 2011;4(1): 23–32.
4. Griffin DR, Dickenson EJ, O'Donnell J, et al. The Warwick Agreement on femoroacetabular impingement syndrome (FAI syndrome): an international consensus statement. *Br J Sports Med*. 2016;50(19):1169–1176.
5. Peters S, Laing A, Emerson C, et al. Surgical criteria for femoroacetabular impingement syndrome: a scoping review. *Br J Sports Med*. 2017;51(22):1605–1610.
6. Zhang D, Chen L, Wang G. Hip arthroscopy versus open surgical dislocation for femoroacetabular impingement: a systematic review and meta-analysis. *Medicine (Baltimore)*. 2016;95(41):e5122.

ADDITIONAL READING

- Nepple JJ, Clohisy JC; and ANCHOR Study Group Members. Evolution of femoroacetabular impingement treatment: the ANCHOR experience. *Am J Orthop (Belle Mead NJ)*. 2017;46(1):28–34.
- Packer JD, Safran MR. The etiology of primary femoroacetabular impingement: genetics or acquired deformity? *J Hip Preserv Surg*. 2015;2(3):249–257.
- Philippon MJ, Bolia I, Locks R, et al. Treatment of femoroacetabular impingement: labrum, cartilage, osseous deformity, and capsule. *Am J Orthop (Belle Mead NJ)*. 2017;46(1):23–27.
- Rhee C, Le Francois T, Byrd JWT, et al. Radiographic diagnosis of pincer-type femoroacetabular impingement: a systematic review. *Orthop J Sports Med*. 2017;5(5):2325967117708307.
- Wilson AS, Cui Q. Current concepts in management of femoroacetabular impingement. *World J Orthop*. 2012;3(12):204–211.

CLINICAL PEARLS

- Most common type of FAI is combined type.
- Pain at the groin in end ROM is important symptom.
- Surgery is treatment of choice, open surgery may be needed for difficult cases.

F

FLEXOR CARPI ULNARIS AND RADIALIS TENDONITIS

Alicia Chitanand, DO • Kenneth P. Barnes, MD, MSc, CAQSM, FACSM

BASICS

DESCRIPTION

- Flexor carpi radialis (FCR) and flexor carpi ulnaris (FCU) tendons are located on the radial and ulnar aspects of the wrist, respectively.
- Tendonitis of these tendons may occur from trauma or repetitive use.

EPIDEMIOLOGY

- FCU tendonitis is more common than FCR tendonitis.
- FCR tendonitis is considered rare.

ETIOLOGY AND PATHOPHYSIOLOGY

- Anatomy and function:
  - FCR inserts on the volar aspects of the trapezium and 2nd and 3rd metacarpal bases:
    - It is difficult to palpate the insertion point owing to overlying thenar muscles.
    - It palmar flexes and radially deviates the wrist.
  - FCU inserts mainly on the pisiform, with some fibers extending to the hamate hook and bases of the 4th and 5th metacarpals:
    - The pisiform is a sesamoid embedded in the FCU tendon.
    - It palmar flexes and ulnarly deviates the wrist.
- Pathology:
  - With trauma or repetitive use, the synovium of the tendon can become inflamed.
  - Even though the term *tendonitis* is commonly used, *tenosynovitis* is a more appropriate term.
  - Over the long term, trauma and overuse can cause the tendon to degenerate, a condition called *tendinosis*.
- Etiology of tendonitis:
  - Direct injury can trigger tendonitis.
  - A single macrotraumatic event *or*
  - Repeated microtraumatic events (e.g., racquet sports, baseball, golf, hammering, typing, mousing)
  - Improper technique

RISK FACTORS

- Diabetes mellitus
- Sports with grip: tennis, racquetball, golf, cycling, weight lifting, and so forth

COMMONLY ASSOCIATED CONDITIONS

- Other overuse injuries of the wrist and hand
- Median nerve irritation because of close proximity of FCR tendon to the median nerve

DIAGNOSIS

HISTORY

- Pain and possible swelling on volar aspect of wrist
- Increase in pain with activity and gripping
- Limited motion
- Possible crepitus at the site with movement or palpation
- Possible acute or repeated trauma to the area
- Overuse:
  - Repetitive and forceful activity
  - Sudden increase in activity
  - Change in technique or equipment
- FCR tendonitis: pain radially, may radiate into forearm or thumb
- FCU tendonitis: pain ulnarly

PHYSICAL EXAM

- Possible swelling at the volar aspect of wrist
- Tenderness near insertion points:
  - FCR tendonitis:
    - Locate the FCR tendon to the ulnar side of the scaphoid tubercle.
    - Follow the course of tendon about 3 finger-breadths distally to find the approximate insertion point.
  - FCU tendonitis: tenderness at the pisiform or just distal at the 4th and 5th metacarpal bases
- Pain with active contraction:
  - FCR tendonitis: Palmarflex and radially deviate the wrist.
  - FCU tendonitis: Palmarflex and ulnarly deviate the wrist.
- Also may have pain with passive dorsiflexion of the wrist
- Pain with pisotriquetral grind test may suggest osteoarthritis of the pisotriquetral joint.

DIFFERENTIAL DIAGNOSIS

- Radial side of wrist:
  - Fracture of scaphoid, trapezium, or 1st or 2nd metacarpal bases
  - de Quervain tenosynovitis
  - Osteoarthritis at 1st carpometacarpal joint or other joints of the carpus
  - Strain or tendonitis of thenar muscles
  - Ganglion: usually located to the radial side of the FCR tendon
  - Carpal tunnel syndrome
- Ulnar side of wrist:
  - Fracture of pisiform, ulnar styloid, hamate hook, or other carpal bone
  - Triangular fibrocartilage complex tear
  - Osteoarthritis of the pisotriquetral joint or other nearby joints
  - Strain or tendonitis of hypothenar muscles
  - Hypothenar hammer syndrome
  - Ulnar nerve entrapment in Guyon canal
- Miscellaneous:
  - FCR/FCU tendinosis
  - FCR/FCU tendon rupture
  - Tenosynovitis from rheumatologic disorder
  - FCR brevis anomaly

DIAGNOSTIC TESTS & INTERPRETATION

Initial Tests (lab, imaging)

- Radiographs:
  - Usually not needed for diagnosis
  - Views: posteroanterior, lateral, oblique, and lateral in slight supination of wrist
  - Usually normal but may see:
    - Degenerative changes in the pisotriquetral joint.
    - Calcium in the tendon in calcific tendonitis.
- Magnetic resonance imaging (MRI):
  - Use when diagnosis is unclear (especially for ulnar-sided wrist pain).
  - Use when not improving with conservative treatment.

- Findings:
  - High fluid signal within the tendon sheath
  - Tendon sheath thickening
  - Tendon may be enlarged.
- Ultrasound (US):
  - FCR tendonitis: fluid distending the synovial sheath
  - FCU calcific tendonitis: calcium deposition in the tendon proximal to the pisiform
  - Can visualize FCR brevis (1)[C]
  - FCR/FCU tendinosis:
    - Hypoechoic thickening of tendon
    - May show neovascularization on color flow Doppler

Diagnostic Procedures/Other

Pain relief with lidocaine injection into the tendon sheath aids in diagnosis.

TREATMENT

GENERAL MEASURES

- Initial treatment:
  - Avoiding provocative activities
  - Wrist splint in 25 degrees of palmar flexion (2)[C] for 1 to 2 wk or until symptoms improve
  - Icing
  - Nonsteroidal anti-inflammatory drugs (NSAIDs)
- Subsequent treatment as condition improves:
  - Occupational therapy:
    - Stretching and strengthening program
    - Ergonomic improvements
  - Coaching:
    - Improve technique/mechanics.
    - Consider changing racquet grip (3)[C].
- Refractory cases: injection of steroid and local anesthetic into tendon sheath:
  - Resolution of symptoms in 35–40% of patients (4)[C]
  - Calcific tendonitis responds particularly well to steroids.
  - Possibility of tendon rupture after injection (5)[C]

SURGERY/OTHER PROCEDURES

- If symptoms are prominent and not responding to nonoperative treatment, consider surgical consultation.
- Surgical procedure:
  - Surgical release of the tendon
  - Excision of inflamed tenosynovium
  - Tenolysis can be effective (6)[C].
  - Z-plasty lengthening if needed
  - Pisiform excision
- Surgery is usually curative, with return to racquet sports in 6 to 8 wk (4)[C].

ONGOING CARE

PATIENT EDUCATION

- When introducing a new activity or increasing a current activity, do so slowly to help prevent an overuse injury.
- Allow time for recovery between practices and competition.
- Warm up the area well before playing.
- Maintain proper strength, flexibility, and endurance of the forearms, wrists, and hands.
- Use proper technique.

PROGNOSIS

Usually resolves with conservative treatment within 6 wk

REFERENCES

1. Smith J, Kakar S. Combined flexor carpi radialis tear and flexor carpi radialis brevis tendinopathy identified by ultrasound: a case report. *PM R*. 2014;6(10):956–959.
2. Rettig AC. Athletic injuries of the wrist and hand: part II: overuse injuries of the wrist and traumatic injuries to the hand. *Am J Sports Med*. 2004;32(1):262–273.
3. Tagliafico AS, Ameri P, Michaud J, et al. Wrist injuries in nonprofessional tennis players: relationships with different grips. *Am J Sports Med*. 2009;37(4):760–767.
4. Palmieri TJ. Pisiform area pain treatment by pisiform excision. *J Hand Surg Am*. 1982;7(5):477–480.
5. Adams JE, Habbu R. Tendinopathies of the hand and wrist. *J Am Acad Orthop Surg*. 2015;23(12):741–750.
6. Brink PR, Franssen BB, Disseldorp DJ. A simple blind tenolysis for flexor carpi radialis tendinopathy. *Hand (N Y)*. 2015;10(2):323–327.

ADDITIONAL READING

- Bencardino JT, Rosenberg ZS. Sports-related injuries of the wrist: an approach to MRI interpretation. *Clin Sports Med*. 2006;25(3):409–432.
- Osterman AL, Moskow L, Low DW. Soft-tissue injuries of the hand and wrist in racquet sports. *Clin Sports Med*. 1988;7(2):329–348.
- Parellada AJ, Morrison WB, Reiter SB, et al. Flexor carpi radialis tendinopathy: spectrum of imaging findings and association with triscaphe arthritis. *Skeletal Radiol*. 2006;35(8):572–578.
- Young D, Papp S, Giachino A. Physical examination of the wrist. *Orthop Clin North Am*. 2007;38(2):149–165.

F

CLINICAL PEARLS

- FCR and FCU tendonitis usually responds to conservative treatment.
- Steroid/lidocaine injection can be diagnostic as well as therapeutic.
- Surgery is rarely needed.

FLEXOR TENDON AVULSION/JERSEY FINGER

Chau Bui, DO • Suraj A. Achar, MD, FAAFP, CAQSM

BASICS

An acute injury in which there is an avulsion of the flexor digitorum profundus (FDP) tendon off of the volar aspect of the distal phalanx due to forced hyperextension of the distal interphalangeal (DIP) joint while the finger is actively flexed

This injury is often missed by players, trainers, and doctors.

- The Leddy and Packer classification system describes three injury types:
  - Type I: retraction of the tendon into the palm of the hand with nearly complete disruption of the blood supply. The long and short vincula are both ruptured (1).
  - Type II (most common): retraction of the tendon to the proximal interphalangeal (PIP) joint, held in place by the intact vincula longa which helps retain more of its blood supply (1)
  - Type III (unusual): avulsion of a large bony fragment attached to the tendon, remains stuck at the level of the A4 pulley. Both vincula are usually intact maintaining full vascular supply to the tendon (2).
  - Type IV involves a rupture of the FDP tendon insertion with secondary tendon retraction into the finger or palm and a distal phalanx fracture with a large avulsion fragment incarcerated at the A4 pulley (2).

DESCRIPTION

- An avulsion of the FDP tendon from its insertion at the base of the distal phalanx (3)
- Zone I flexor tendon injury (1)
- Synonym(s): jersey finger, rugger finger, FDP avulsion

EPIDEMIOLOGY

- Rare injury seen primarily in contact sports where tackling and grasping of the jersey is probable (rugby, football, hockey, judo)
- Often occurs while grasping the jersey of an opponent who quickly pulls away
- Ring finger is most commonly involved (estimated 75–80% of cases) (4).
- May be misdiagnosed as a jammed or strained finger

ETIOLOGY AND PATHOPHYSIOLOGY

The FDP tendon travels along the volar side of the palm and finger. It passes distally through a split in the flexor digitorum superficialis tendon and inserts at the base of the distal phalanx (palmar aspect of P3). Mesotendons or vincula supply blood and connect the tendon to the underlying phalanges. Jersey finger injury occurs when the FDP tendon is avulsed from its attachment on the distal phalanx (3).

RISK FACTORS

Participation in contact sports such as rugby and football

DIAGNOSIS

HISTORY

- The mechanism of injury involves a sudden forceful extension of a flexed finger which often occurs while grasping another player's jersey (3)[C].
- Typically seen in football and rugby (1)[C]
- Timing of surgical repair varies based on the level of tendon retraction and the presence of a fracture (1).

PHYSICAL EXAM

- Inspection: Swelling and discoloration may be present along the distal phalanx and DIP joint (3)[C].
- Palpation: Tenderness may be present along the length of the flexor tendon, particularly at the site of FDP tendon insertion. A palpable lump may be present at any point along the proximal digit, frequently at the PIP joint or on the palm of the hand at the A1 pulley (1)[C].
- Range of motion: inability to make a full fist and loss of active DIP joint flexion of the involved digit (pathognomonic finding)

ALERT

- Strength: To assess the integrity of the FDP tendon, hold the PIP joint in full extension and ask the patient to actively flex the DIP joint (2) [C]. Active flexion of the PIP joint and metacarpophalangeal (MCP) joint is preserved in the injured digit.
- Neurovascular exam: should always be assessed and should be normal in jersey finger injuries

DIFFERENTIAL DIAGNOSIS

- DIP joint dislocation
- Distal phalanx fracture
- Flexor digitorum superficialis avulsion

DIAGNOSTIC TESTS & INTERPRETATION

- Three view radiographs (anteroposterior, lateral, and oblique) are necessary to determine the presence and degree of bony avulsion and to potentially assess the level of tendon retraction (5)[C].
- Avulsion fractures can be seen on the volar aspect of the distal phalangeal base at the FDP attachment site (3)[C].
- Magnetic resonance imaging (MRI) and ultrasound will show where the tendon has retracted. MRI may show distended tendon "tortuous" or "whirled." Ultrasound offers dynamic imaging to show "asynchronic" movements as well as complete ruptures from focal interruption of fibrillar echo structure of the tendon and posterior acoustic shadowing behind the rupture site.
- Ultrasound is more accurate than physical exam 95% versus 79% (6)[B].

TREATMENT

ALERT

- All FDP avulsion injuries require urgent surgical intervention (3)[C].
- Initial management may include ice, nonsteroidal anti-inflammatory drugs (NSAIDs), and splinting.
- The injured finger should be dorsally splinted to maintain slight flexion at the DIP and PIP joints and avoid DIP extension (1)[C].
- Treatment is influenced by time between injury and treatment, degree of tendon retraction, presence and size of bony avulsion, and level of blood supply to the avulsed tendon (4)[C].

ADDITIONAL THERAPIES

- Treatment options for athletes who present outside the window for primary repair: no treatment, tendon grafting, or terminal interphalangeal joint tenodesis or arthrodesis (3)[C]
- Long palmaris muscle tendon grafting may be offered in certain cases (3)[C].
- Arthrodesis may be offered in cases of DIP instability or articular surface disruption (1)[C].
- Nonoperative treatment generally not recommended unless patient is unable or unwilling to comply with postoperative therapy (4)

SURGERY/OTHER PROCEDURES

- Type I:
  - Surgical repair should be conducted within 7 to 10 days of the injury (4)[C].
- Type II:
  - Early surgical repair within 7 to 10 days is preferred; however, due to the intact vincula longa, surgery can be delayed 6 to 8 wk (1)[C].
- Type III:
  - Early surgical intervention is preferred, but satisfactory results are possible with delayed repair of 2 wk, due to an intact blood supply to the tendon (1)[C].
  - Wires can be removed after 3 to 4 wk postoperatively (4)[C].
- Type IV:
  - The degree of tendon retraction and loss of vascular supply can be similar to a type I injury, requiring surgical intervention within 7 to 10 days (1)[C].

ONGOING CARE

- Following surgery, the affected hand should be placed in a dorsal blocking splint with the wrist in midflexion, the MCP joints at 75 degrees of flexion, and the PIP/DIP joints in extension or near extension (4)[C]. The hand should remain in this splint for 6 wk (1)[C].
- Passive flexion of the PIP and DIP joints can be started within days of the surgery (4)[C].
- Using an experienced hand therapist early in the postoperative period is recommended (1)[C].
- Strengthening activities can usually begin at 12 wk postoperatively (1)[C].
- A mitten-type splint/cast that keeps the wrist slightly flexed with the fingers flexed into the palm may allow an athlete to return to play early, provided no grasping of the hand is required (1)[C].
- Return to play with full grasping capabilities usually takes 4 to 6 mo and is dependent on sport and position (1)[C].

FOLLOW-UP RECOMMENDATIONS

Immediate referral to an orthopedic/hand surgeon is recommended for all types of FDP avulsion injuries.

REFERENCES

1. Elzinga KE, Chung KC. Finger injuries in football and rugby. *Hand Clin*. 2017;33(1):149–160.
2. Tempelaere C, Brun M, Doursounian L, et al. Traumatic avulsion of the flexor digitorum profundus tendon. Jersey finger, a 29 cases report. *Hand Surg Rehabil*. 2017;36(5):368–372.
3. Lapegue F, Andre A, Brun C, et al. Traumatic flexor tendon injuries. *Diagn Interv Imaging*. 2015;96(12):1279–1292.
4. Bachoura A, Ferikes AJ, Lubahn JD. A review of mallet finger and jersey finger injuries in the athlete. *Curr Rev Musculoskelet Med*. 2017;10(1):1–9.
5. Cockenpot E, Lefebvre G, Demondion X, et al. Imaging of sports-related hand and wrist injuries: sports imaging series. *Radiology*. 2016;279(3):674–692.
6. Gilleard O, Silver D, Ahmad Z, et al. The accuracy of ultrasound in evaluating closed flexor tendon ruptures. *Eur J Plast Surg*. 2010;33:71.
7. Kovacic J, Bergfeld J. Return to play issues in upper extremity injuries. *Clin J Sport Med*. 2005;15(6):448–452.

CLINICAL PEARLS

- An acute diagnosis of jersey finger requires urgent surgical treatment (4).
- Return to contact sports may be anticipated 4 to 6 mo after surgery (7).
- Depending on the sport, it may be possible for the patient to return to play early, provided that a playing splint/cast is worn.
- Delaying surgical treatment, particularly for type I injuries, can result in irreparable scarring of the flexor tendon and permanent loss of flexion at the DIP joint. Although delayed surgical intervention may be offered in certain circumstances, favorable results are not guaranteed. Type II and III injuries frequently can be delayed several weeks without significant changes to surgical outcome, but this is not advised (4).

FOLLICULITIS

Timothy Tiu, MD, FAAPMR, CAQSM • Sona Patel, MD, FAAP

BASICS

DESCRIPTION

- Superficial infection of hair follicles
- Usually caused by *Staphylococcus aureus*
- May also be caused by gram-negative organisms (*Pseudomonas*), as in the case of "hot tub" folliculitis

EPIDEMIOLOGY

- Lesions usually occur on areas of skin traumatized by maceration, such as under shoulder pads or sweaty garments.
- May also develop in areas of occlusion, friction and perspiration, such as face, neck, scalp, axillae, groin, extremities and buttocks (1)
- "Hot tub" folliculitis is associated with the use of poorly cleaned hot tubs, whirlpools, jacuzzis, and swimming pools; it can also be spread by sharing sponges or cleaning products (2).
- Infection does not spread in epidemic proportions but may be transmitted through skin trauma.

RISK FACTORS

- Poor hygiene
- Occlusive clothing
- Skin breaks associated with turf burns or trauma (football, soccer) (3)
- Contact sports (football, wrestling, rugby) (3)
- Sharing of equipment or clothing (towels) (3)
- Higher body mass index (BMI) (3)

ALERT

Methicillin-resistant *S. aureus* (MRSA) colonization has been documented on wrestling mats, artificial turf, and football training equipment (3).

GENERAL PREVENTION

- Good personal hygiene, wound care (3)[C]
- Avoid sharing equipment (3)[C].
- Refrain from using common tubs and cosmetic shaving (3)[C].
- Cleaning high-touch surfaces (3)[C]

DIAGNOSIS

HISTORY

Maceration caused by sports equipment is a common cause of folliculitis. This knowledge may lead to a definitive diagnosis.

PHYSICAL EXAM

- Inflammation of the superficial portion of hair follicles (2)
- Small pustules on an erythematous base (2)
- Pus limited to epidermis (4)
- Pseudomonas folliculitis: Lesions usually are pruritic, urticarial, and erythematous; found as clustered lesions under bathing suits on occluded areas (2)

DIFFERENTIAL DIAGNOSIS

- Furuncles appear as inflammatory nodules with pustules, through which hair emerges (4).
- Carbuncle: infection involving several adjacent follicles; a coalescent inflammatory mass with multiple follicular orifices through which pus drains; larger and deeper than furuncles and found commonly on back of neck (4); often with fever and malaise (1)
- Pityrosporum folliculitis: commonly pruritic lesions, found in setting of warmth and sweating; occurs on chest, back, and proximal extremities (1); appear as 2- to 3-mm papules and pustules, perifollicular, erythematous (1)

- Pseudofolliculitis barbae: ("razor bumps") caused by foreign-body reaction to ingrown hair; not truly a bacterial infection; however, often found to have bacterial superinfection at the site; occurs on any shaved area (2)
- Acne vulgaris

TREATMENT

- Localized folliculitis: daily washes with antibacterial soap and topical antibiotics (mupirocin) (1,3)[C]
- Resistant or diffuse cases: Treat with oral antibiotics, directed by culture and sensitivities (1,3)[C]:
  - *S. aureus*: cephalexin, erythromycin, or azithromycin (2,3)[C]
  - Known MRSA carriers or those at high risk: doxycycline or trimethoprim/sulfamethoxazole (2,3)[C].
  - *Pseudomonas*: self-limiting in 5 to 7 days. For recalcitrant cases, some recommend quinolone therapy (ciprofloxacin) (2)[C].
- For recurrent or recalcitrant infections, consider chronic *Staphylococcus* colonization, particularly in the nares, on the skin, or in the vagina (1,2,3,4)[C].

ALERT

Return to play:
- No new skin lesion for 48 hr (3,5)[C]
- Completion of 72 hr of antibiotics (3,5)[C]
- No moist, exudative, or draining lesions (3,5)[C]
- Active lesions shall not be covered to allow participation (3,5)[C].

REFERENCES

1. Cordoro KM, Ganz JE. Training room management of medical conditions: sports dermatology. *Clin Sports Med*. 2005;24(3):565–598.
2. Sedgwick PE, Dexter WW, Smith CT. Bacterial dermatoses in sports. *Clin Sports Med*. 2007;26(3):383–396.
3. Davies HD, Jackson MA, Rice SG; for Committee on Infectious Diseases, Council on Sports Medicine and Fitness. Infectious diseases associated with organized sports and outbreak control. *Pediatrics*. 2017;140(4):e20172477.
4. Stevens DL, Bisno AL, Chambers HF, et al; for Infectious Diseases Society of America. Practice guidelines for the diagnosis and management of skin and soft tissue infections: 2014 update by the Infectious Diseases Society of America. *Clin Infect Dis*. 2014;59(2):e10–e52.
5. Parsons J. *2014–15 NCAA Sports Medicine Handbook*. Indianapolis, IN: National Collegiate Athletic Association; 2014.

CLINICAL PEARLS

- Personal hygiene and cleaning equipment is important to prevent transmission.
- Consider *S. aureus* carriage in recurrent or recalcitrant infections.

FOOT OSTEOCHONDROSES

Alicia Chitanand, DO • Kenneth P. Barnes, MD, MSc, CAQSM, FACSM

BASICS

DESCRIPTION

- Accessory navicular: unfused accessory ossification center at posterior tibialis tendon (PTT) insertion
- Geist classification:
  - Type I: small sesamoid bone in PTT (usually 2 to 3 mm)
  - Type II: synchondrosis between navicular and os naviculare (usually 8 to 12 mm triangular or heart shaped); 70% of symptomatic lesions
  - Type III: cornuate navicular (questionable end stage of type II with ossification across synchondrosis)
- Synonym(s): os tibiale (externum); os naviculare (secundarium); symptomatic accessory tarsal navicular; accessory scaphoid bone; accessory tarsal scaphoid; navicular secundum; prehallux; os scaphoideum accessorium
- Osteonecrosis of tarsal navicular in adults: Mueller-Weiss disease

Pediatric Considerations

- Köhler disease: articular osteochondrosis with secondary involvement of articular and epiphyseal cartilage as a consequence of avascular necrosis of tarsal navicular bone; synonyms: aseptic necrosis of tarsal navicular; avascular necrosis of navicular; Koehler disease; idiopathic osteonecrosis of navicular in children
- Iselin disease: nonarticular osteochondrosis of the 5th metatarsal at site of ligament and tendon attachment and trauma; synonym: traction apophysitis of 5th metatarsal where peroneus brevis inserts

EPIDEMIOLOGY

- Accessory navicular:
  - Most often symptoms found in active children and females in 4th decade
  - Second most common accessory bone of foot
  - Accessory bones in 36% of asymptomatic feet
- Iselin disease:
  - Usually in athletic older children and adolescents (1)

Pediatric Considerations

- Köhler disease: rare:
  - Age of onset 2 to 9 yr
  - Mean age of diagnosis: males 6 yr, females 4.5 yr
- Occasionally bilateral Iselin disease: rarely reported but probably more common than appreciated:
  - Age of onset in late childhood or early adolescence
  - Apophysis appears: males 8 to 11 yr, females 11 to 14 yr
  - Apophysis fuses about 2 yr later.

Prevalence

- Accessory navicular:
  - 4–21% of general population: most asymptomatic
  - 50–90% bilateral
  - In skeletally immature, 64% symptomatic
- Köhler disease: prevalence unknown
- Iselin disease: prevalence unknown

ETIOLOGY AND PATHOPHYSIOLOGY

- Accessory navicular: becomes symptomatic in the following:
  - Adolescent patients from chondroosseous disruption owing to tension and shear forces from PTT and foot dynamics (type II)
  - From pressure of overlying footwear (all types)
  - Older patients owing to posttraumatic disruption of synchondrosis (type II) ± PTT avulsion or rupture
  - Symptomatic type II: microfracture, acute and chronic inflammation, and cellular proliferation
- Köhler disease:
  - Tarsal navicular is last bone to ossify and believed to be more susceptible to compression injury.
  - May be due to ischemia from recurrent cumulative microtrauma or acute macrotrauma
- Iselin disease:
  - Repetitive traction from peroneus brevis
  - Acute avulsion fracture with widening of chondroosseous junction

RISK FACTORS

- Accessory navicular: may be worse with hyperpronation
- Köhler disease: may be more common in late ossification of tarsal navicular
- Iselin disease:
  - May be more common with tight calf muscles
  - Seen most commonly in soccer, basketball, gymnastics, and dance

COMMONLY ASSOCIATED CONDITIONS

Köhler disease: occasionally with other osteochondroses, such as Osgood-Schlatter or Legg-Calvé-Perthes disease

DIAGNOSIS

- Accessory navicular:
  - Symptomatic or asymptomatic
  - Most often clinically relevant accessory navicular is symptomatic type II.
- Köhler disease:
  - Based on history and x-ray findings
  - Does *not* equal asymptomatic feet with abnormal x-ray findings: multiple ossification centers or other process
- Iselin disease: based on history and x-ray findings

HISTORY

- Accessory navicular:
  - Asymptomatic or medial foot pain with navicular bump
  - If painful, onset gradual or acute
  - If painful, onset may be secondary to ankle sprain or contusion.
  - Worse with activity (during or after) and compression with shoes
  - May have limp/antalgic gait
- Köhler disease:
  - Medial foot pain (tenderness at tarsal navicular)
  - Usual gradual in onset
  - Worse with activity
  - Limp/antalgic gait
- Iselin disease:
  - Lateral foot pain (tenderness at proximal 5th metatarsal)
  - Usual insidious onset
  - May be acute after significant trauma; often inversion injury
  - Worse with weight-bearing, lateral movements, cutting, and jumping
  - Limp/antalgic gait

PHYSICAL EXAM

- Accessory navicular:
  - Protuberant tarsal navicular (posteromedial aspect)
  - Normal range of motion (ROM) of foot, ankle, hindfoot
  - Possible overlying swelling
  - Tender to palpation over tarsal navicular ± PTT distally
  - Pain with resisted plantar flexion and inversion
- Köhler disease:
  - Antalgic gait with shifting of weight to lateral aspect of foot
  - Possible overlying swelling
  - Less likely overlying warmth
  - Tender to palpation over tarsal navicular
  - May have pain with resisted plantar flexion and inversion
- Iselin disease:
  - Perhaps prominent proximal 5th metatarsal
  - Very little or no erythema, edema, or ecchymosis
  - May show mild pronation
  - Tender to palpation at peroneus brevis insertion
  - Pain with resisted eversion, extreme inversion, and extreme plantar flexion or dorsiflexion

DIFFERENTIAL DIAGNOSIS

- Accessory navicular:
  - Navicular pathology (stress fracture, tuberosity avulsion fracture)
  - PTT pathology (tendinopathy, tenosynovitis, rupture, dysfunction)
  - Less commonly: deltoid/spring ligament injury, tarsal tunnel syndrome, Köhler disease (in younger patients), tarsal coalition, plantar fasciitis, tight heel cord
  - Systemic: infection, malignancy
- Köhler disease:
  - Accessory navicular, trauma, stress fracture, infection, malignancy
  - If not better with conservative treatment, rarely tarsal coalition (congenital or acquired)
- Iselin disease:
  - Fractures: 5th metatarsal (acute Jones and stress more transverse line), avulsion fracture (more common with lateral ankle sprains and more oblique line)
  - Os vesalianum (incidence 0.1–1%; most often asymptomatic; found within peroneus brevis tendon)

DIAGNOSTIC TESTS & INTERPRETATION

- Accessory navicular:
  - Radiographs:
    - Anteroposterior and lateral foot often miss.
    - Must include external oblique view
    - Findings depend on type (see "Geist classification" in "Description").
  - Ultrasound (US):
    - More for tendinous abnormalities
    - May see heterogeneous synchondrosis (compared with asymptomatic side)
    - May see diastasis in older patient
  - Magnetic resonance imaging (MRI):
    - Rarely needed
    - Short tau inversion recovery (STIR) images show increased signal within accessory navicular at PTT insertion.
  - Bone scan:
    - Increased uptake in region
    - Only 50% specific but 100% sensitive (2)[B]
- Köhler disease:
  - Radiographs:
    - Anteroposterior and lateral foot
    - Commonly, narrowing/flattening of the tarsal navicular and/or loss of trabecular pattern
    - Possibly, apparent fragmentation or diffusely increased density in normal-shaped tarsal navicular
    - Do not confuse with multiple ossification centers without increased density.
  - Bone scan:
    - Decreased uptake, or "cold area"
    - May be present before x-ray changes (3)
  - MRI:
    - Rarely needed
    - Low signal on T1 and high signal on T2
- Iselin disease:
  - Radiographs:
    - Anteroposterior and lateral foot often miss diagnosis.
    - Must include medial oblique view
    - Consider comparing with unaffected side.
    - Apophyseal widening and often fragmentation of ossification center
    - Found almost parallel to long axis of shaft
    - Occasionally, with cystic changes of physis
- Pathologic findings:
  - Accessory navicular: histologically, microfracture, acute and chronic inflammation, and cellular proliferation in symptomatic lesions

TREATMENT

GENERAL MEASURES

- Accessory navicular:
  - Rest, shoe insert/orthotic (soft orthotic initially until pain free and then assess mechanics to see if semirigid orthotic is better for longer term support)
  - Application of doughnut pad over bony prominence
  - Analgesics
  - Physical therapy
  - Occasionally, cast immobilization is warranted.
- Köhler disease:
  - If mild disease, soft arch supports only
  - Short leg cast (10 to 15 degrees of varus, 10 to 20 degrees of equinovarus) for 6 to 8 wk followed by arch support if mild pain persists
  - Casting may lead to shorter length of pain.
  - No significant difference in final outcome between short leg cast and shoe correction, rest, or non–weight-bearing with crutches (4,5)[C]
  - Symptom duration: 8+ wk of casting: 2.5 mo; <8 wk of casting: 4 mo; noncasting: 15.2 mo (5)[C]
- Iselin disease:
  - Rest, ice, calf stretching
  - If severe pain, immobilization for 2 to 4 wk (Aircast, walking cast, or short leg cast with crutches)
  - Physical therapy to improve strength and coordination when pain free

MEDICATION

Analgesics (e.g., acetaminophen and nonsteroidal anti-inflammatory drugs [NSAIDs]) for pain

SURGERY/OTHER PROCEDURES

- Accessory navicular:
  - Indication: no improvement with nonoperative treatment
  - Resection of symptomatic bone with Kidner procedure ± reattachment of PTT (6)[C]
  - Possible percutaneous drilling in young athletes (7)[C]
  - Fixation by screw or tension band wiring has shown improved pain and function (8)[A].
- Iselin disease:
  - Indication: failure of conservative treatment and symptomatic nonunion
  - Very rarely indicated
  - Resection or fixation of symptomatic bone (9)[C]

ONGOING CARE

PROGNOSIS

- Accessory navicular:
  - Most do not become painful.
  - Painful lesions in adolescents often improve with growth.
  - Uncertain prognosis for symptomatic lesion treated nonoperatively
  - Continued symptoms more likely with recurrent stresses of athletics
  - Anecdotally, less likely to improve in physically active youth owing to repeated injury
  - Uncertain if bony union is natural course (10–50% fusion reported)
- Köhler disease:
  - Self-limiting and excellent prognosis
  - Full reconstitution of tarsal navicular (6 to 13 mo, average 8 mo) (4)[C]
  - No evidence of arthritis long term (4,5)[C]
  - Potentially, minor faceting of tarsal navicular (5)[C]
- Iselin disease:
  - Pain resolves with relative rest, immobilization, or eventual bony union.
  - Rare reports of nonunion and prolonged symptoms

REFERENCES

1. Forrester RA, Eyre-Brook AI, Mannan K. Iselin's disease: a systematic review. *J Foot Ankle Surg*. 2017;56(5):1065–1069.
2. Chiu NT, Jou IM, Lee BF, et al. Symptomatic and asymptomatic accessory navicular bones: findings of Tc-99m MDP bone scintigraphy. *Clin Radiol*. 2000;55(5):353–355.
3. Khoury J, Jerushalmi J, Loberant N, et al. Kohler disease: diagnoses and assessment by bone scintigraphy. *Clin Nucl Med*. 2007;32(3):179–181.
4. Ippolito E, Ricciardi Pollini PT, Falez' F. Köhler's disease of the tarsal navicular: long-term follow-up of 12 cases. *J Pediatr Orthop*. 1984;4(4):416–417.
5. Williams GA, Cowell HR. Köhler's disease of the tarsal navicular. *Clin Orthop Relat Res*. 1981;(158):53–58.
6. Ray S, Goldberg VM. Surgical treatment of the accessory navicular. *Clin Orthop Relat Res*. 1983;(177):61–66.
7. Nakayama S, Sugimoto K, Takakura Y, et al. Percutaneous drilling of symptomatic accessory navicular in young athletes. *Am J Sports Med*. 2005;33(4):531–535.
8. Jang HS, Park KH, Park HW. Comparison of outcomes of osteosynthesis in type II accessory navicular by variable fixation methods. *Foot Ankle Surg*. 2017;23(4):243–249.
9. Ralph BG, Barrett J, Kenyhercz C, et al. Iselin's disease: a case presentation of nonunion and review of the differential diagnosis. *J Foot Ankle Surg*. 1999;38(6):409–416.

ADDITIONAL READING

- Canale ST, Williams KD. Iselin's disease. *J Pediatr Orthop*. 1992;12(1):90–93.
- Keles-Celik N, Kose O, Sekerci R, et al. Accessory ossicles of the foot and ankle: disorders and a review of the literature. *Cureus*. 2017;9(11):e1881.
- Sella EJ, Lawson JP, Ogden JA. The accessory navicular synchondrosis. *Clin Orthop Relat Res*. 1986;(209):280–285.
- Ugolini PA, Raikin SM. The accessory navicular. *Foot Ankle Clin*. 2004;9(1):165–180.

CLINICAL PEARLS

- Symptomatic type II accessory navicular may respond less favorably to conservative treatment in adolescent athletes.
- Asymptomatic radiologic abnormalities without pain or antalgic gait are not Köhler disease.
- Avascular necrosis of the tarsal navicular in an adolescent or an adult is not Köhler disease.
- Iselin disease is probably missed often but has a good prognosis.

FRACTURE, AVULSION: ASIS, AIIS, ISCHIAL TUBEROSITY, ILIAC CREST

Andrew Smith, MD, FAAP

BASICS

DESCRIPTION

- Injury that typically occurs at the unfused apophysis (secondary growth center) in an adolescent athlete
- Apophyseal fractures are more common in pediatric patients than muscle tears and strains due to the apophysis being the weakest structure of the musculotendinous junction (1).
- Injury results from sudden, forceful, concentric, or eccentric muscular contraction without external trauma.
- Also may occur from sudden excessive passive lengthening of a muscle
- Chronic injury may occur as a result of repetitive microtrauma or overuse.

EPIDEMIOLOGY

Prevalence

- Occurs almost exclusively in adolescence when secondary ossification centers have not yet fused to pelvic tuberosities (2)
- Accounts for 13–40% of pediatric pelvic fractures
- Occurs more frequently in males than in females with 3:1 ratio (2)
- Anterior inferior iliac spine (AIIS) accounts for 33% of pelvic avulsion fractures (2).
- Ischial tuberosity accounts for 30% of pelvic avulsion fractures (2).
- Anterior superior iliac spine (ASIS) accounts for 28% of pelvic avulsion fractures (2).
- Iliac crest accounts for 7% of pelvic avulsion fractures (2).
- Lesser trochanter and pubic symphysis avulsion fractures are less common (2).
- Bilateral avulsion fractures occur 6% of the time (3).
- More common among adolescents than young children or adults

ETIOLOGY AND PATHOPHYSIOLOGY

- Typically occurs during an athletic event with sudden contracture of lower musculature with jumping, kicking, or sprinting (1)
- AIIS: commonly occurs with contracture of rectus femoris with hip extended and knee flexed (1)
- ASIS:
  - Type I: sudden, forceful contraction of sartorius muscle with hip extended and knee flexed (1)
  - Type II: sudden, forceful contraction of tensor fasciae latae commonly seen in twisting movements with baseball and jumping (1)
- Ischial tuberosity: sudden, forceful contraction of hamstring with knee extended and hip flexed commonly seen with sprinting or kicking (1)
- Iliac crest: avulsion of abdominal muscles seen with forceful turning or lateral flexion (1)

RISK FACTORS

- Adolescent athletes involved in strenuous sporting activities (soccer, football) (3)
- Sprinters (ASIS type I, AIIS) (4)
- Batting in baseball (ASIS type II) (4)
- Gymnasts, dancers, hurdlers, weight lifters (ischial tuberosity) (4)

DIAGNOSIS

HISTORY

- Athlete often reports popping or snapping with immediate onset of severe pain and swelling over fracture site followed by limping or inability to bear weight with associated weakness (4).
- Acute injury may be preceded by prodrome of low-level pain for up to several months owing to chronic apophysitis (5).
- Activity at time of injury helps to define mechanism of injury:
  - Attempting to kick a ball (ASIS)
  - Clearing a hurdle (ischial tuberosity)
  - Being tackled from behind (iliac crest) (5)
- Pattern of pain helps to localize site of avulsion fracture:
  - Ischial tuberosity avulsion fracture may radiate to posterior thigh.
  - AIIS and ASIS avulsion fractures may radiate to anterior thigh.

PHYSICAL EXAM

- Signs and symptoms include:
  - Pain with localized tenderness and swelling at avulsion site.
  - Limitation of motion about the site of avulsion injury.
  - Difficulty (sometimes inability) to bear weight.
- Physical examination includes the following:
  - Palpate regions of suspected avulsion. Acute localized tenderness to palpation is present over involved apophysis; avulsed apophyseal fragment may be palpated.
  - 90% cases with ASIS avulsion fracture have palpable mass with pain just below the iliac crest (4).
  - Assess for strength because it is common to have weakness in affected muscle groups with avulsion fractures (4).
  - Assess active and passive range of motion of involved muscle(s):
    - ASIS type I: pain with passive extension or active flexion of hip; also pain with passive internal rotation and active external rotation of hip
    - ASIS type II: pain with passive extension and active flexion of hip; also pain with passive external rotation and active internal rotation; pain also can be seen with active abduction and passive adduction of hip.
    - AIIS: pain with passive extension and active flexion of hip; also pain with passive knee flexion and active knee extension
    - Ischial tuberosity: pain with passive hip flexion and active hip extension
    - Iliac crest: pain with contraction of abdominal muscles, lateral bending of torso, resisted hip abduction

DIFFERENTIAL DIAGNOSIS

- Apophysitis
- Muscle strain
- Tendon avulsion without fracture
- Malignancy, especially in an adult with nontraumatic pelvic avulsion fracture (5)[B]

DIAGNOSTIC TESTS & INTERPRETATION

- Anteroposterior view of pelvis may demonstrate avulsion of a portion of involved apophysis; fragments may be mildly to severely displaced (4)[C].
- Chronic avulsions may result in prominent bone formation and nonunion. Radiographic appearance of heterotopic ossification may be confused with osseous malignancy or osteomyelitis (4)[C].
- Oblique view of pelvis may better demonstrate avulsions of iliac crest.
- Radiographs demonstrate 99% of avulsion fractures (3)[B].
- Ultrasonography, if available, is also useful tool to help identify avulsion fractures (1)[C].
- When radiographs and ultrasound are negative and there is still a clinical suspicion for fracture, then magnetic resonance imaging (MRI) should be the next diagnostic test (1)[C].

- Ultrasound and MRI can be more useful in younger patient populations who have not developed secondary ossification centers to identify apophyseal injuries because radiographs will be negative (1)[C].
- Computed tomography (CT) scan may be helpful in chronic cases with heterotopic ossification or those without a clear history (4)[C].

TREATMENT

GENERAL MEASURES

- Conservative management indicated for patients with fracture displacement <1.5 to 2.0 cm (2)[A]
- Phased return-to-play protocol guided by pain and function (1)[C]
- Initial period of rest, icing, and non- or partial weight-bearing usually lasting 1 to 3 wk
- Progress to passive range of motion exercises and assisted partial weight-bearing once pain free.
- Progressive resistance training approximately 1 mo after injury
- Aggressive stretching and sport-specific activity 1 to 2 mo following injury if continues to be pain free
- Return to sport at 2 mo if patient with normal motion and strength of involved muscle (1)[C].

MEDICATION

Nonsteroidal anti-inflammatory drugs (NSAIDs) as needed for pain (3)[C]

ADDITIONAL THERAPIES

- Physical therapy and athletic training can guide and assist with phased return to play.
- Sport-specific training followed by return to sport when pain free and with normal motion and strength of involved muscle

SURGERY/OTHER PROCEDURES

- Surgery generally is not needed.
- Open reduction and internal fixation (ORIF) is considered when fragment displacement is >2 cm for most avulsion fractures (1)[B].
- Consider ORIF when fragment displacement is >1.5 cm for ischial tuberosity avulsion fractures (2)[A],(6)[B].
- ORIF may be considered for nonunion or heterotopic ossifications causing pain or functional impairment (2)[A].
- Patients with a high functional demand and avulsion displacement should be counseled on surgical management (2)[A].

ONGOING CARE

FOLLOW-UP RECOMMENDATIONS

- Most fractures heal with conservative treatment.
- Consider repeat radiographs to assess for bony healing if patient has persistent pain or weakness in phased return to play (4)[C].

PROGNOSIS

Athletes typically are able to return to full activity without restrictions or long-term sequelae; however, this may take up to 6 mo.

COMPLICATIONS

- Heterotopic ossification is the most commonly reported complication following nonoperative management.
- Nonunion of fracture fragment
- ASIS fractures may cause meralgia paresthetica owing to associated injury to the lateral femoral cutaneous nerve. This typically resolves spontaneously, but surgical intervention may be considered for severe, persistent symptoms (1)[C].
- Ischial tuberosity fractures may lead to pain with prolonged sitting with radicular pain because sciatic nerve can become entrapped in scarred hamstring fibers (1)[C].
- Chronic muscle weakness and altered gait can be seen with nonunions (4)[C].

REFERENCES

1. Schiller J, Defroda S, Blood T. Lower extremity avulsion fractures in the pediatric and adolescent athlete. *J Am Acad Orthop Surg*. 2017;25(4):251–259.
2. Eberbach H, Hohloch L, Feucht MJ, et al. Operative versus conservative treatment of apophyseal avulsion fractures of the pelvis in the adolescents: a systematical review with meta-analysis of clinical outcome and return to sports. *BMC Musculoskelet Disord*. 2017;18(1):162.
3. Schuett DJ, Bomar JD, Pennock AT. Pelvic apophyseal avulsion fractures: a retrospective review of 228 cases. *J Pediatr Orthop*. 2015; 36(6):617–623.
4. Chang GH, Paz DA, Dwek JR, et al. Lower extremity overuse injuries in pediatric athletes: clinical presentation, imaging findings, and treatment. *Clin Imaging*. 2013;37(5):836–846.
5. Sanders TG, Zlatkin MB. Avulsion injuries of the pelvis. *Semin Musculoskelet Radiol*. 2008;12(1): 42–53.
6. Ferlic PW, Sadoghi P, Singer G, et al. Treatment for ischial tuberosity avulsion fractures in adolescent athletes. *Knee Surg Sports Traumatol Arthrosc*. 2014;22(4):893–897.

ADDITIONAL READING

- Kautzner J, Trc T, Havlas V. Comparison of conservative against surgical treatment of anterior-superior iliac spine avulsion fractures in children and adolescents. *Int Orthop*. 2014;38(7):1495–1498.
- Paletta GA Jr, Andrish JT. Injuries about the hip and pelvis in the young athlete. *Clin Sports Med*. 1995;14(3):591–628.
- Rossi F, Dragoni S. Acute avulsion fractures of the pelvis in adolescent competitive athletes: prevalence, location and sports distribution of 203 cases collected. *Skeletal Radiol*. 2001;30(3): 127–131.
- Steerman JG, Reeder MT, Udermann BE, et al. Avulsion fracture of the iliac crest apophysis in a collegiate wrestler. *Clin J Sport Med*. 2008;18(1):102–103.
- Stevens MA, El-Khoury GY, Kathol MH, et al. Imaging features of avulsion injuries. *Radiographics*. 1999;19(3):655–672.
- Vandervliet EJ, Vanhoenacker FM, Snoeckx A, et al. Sports-related acute and chronic avulsion injuries in children and adolescents with special emphasis on tennis. *Br J Sports Med*. 2007;41(11):827–831.
- White KK, Williams SK, Mubarak SJ. Definition of two types of anterior superior iliac spine avulsion fractures. *J Pediatr Orthop*. 2002;22(5):578–582.

CLINICAL PEARLS

- Pelvic avulsion fractures are common in adolescent athletes.
- The majority of pelvic avulsion fractures can be diagnosed by radiographs.
- Conservative management of pelvic avulsion fractures with phased return to play is appropriate in most patients with fragment displacement <2 cm.
- Surgical management should be considered when displacement of fracture is >1.5 cm in ischial tuberosity avulsion fractures or >2 cm in all other pelvic avulsion fractures. Depending on fracture location, most patients can return to sport within 1 to 3 mo.

FRACTURE, BLOW OUT

Giselle Aerni, MD • Robert L. Howard, MA, ATC

BASICS

DESCRIPTION

Defined as an orbital floor or medial wall fracture without orbital rim involvement owing to blunt trauma to the orbit

EPIDEMIOLOGY

- Sport-related injury accounts for 1/3 of all orbital blowout fractures.
- Observed in any sport that puts the athlete at risk for forceful contact to the face
- Most common: soccer, rugby, boxing, martial arts, baseball, wrestling, basketball, action sports
- Object striking the orbital region is usually larger than orbital rim, such as a baseball or fist.
- Gender differences: more common in males
- Ages: Fractures of orbital floor are relatively rare in children <5 yr old as maxillary sinus pneumatization significantly expands from 6 to 12 yr old.

ETIOLOGY AND PATHOPHYSIOLOGY

- Force transmitted through the orbital structures to the weakest structural point—most commonly the orbital floor or medial wall—resulting in fracture
- Trapdoor fracture is a linear fracture of the orbital bone that reduces spontaneously to original position, entrapping and strangulating infraocular soft tissue:
  - Usually an intraoperative diagnosis
  - Seen almost exclusively in children
- Orbital floor serves as roof to air-filled maxillary and ethmoid sinuses. Communication between the spaces results in orbital emphysema.
- Orbit contains fat, which holds the globe in place:
  - Orbital floor fracture may result in herniation of the fat on the inferior orbital surface into the maxillary or ethmoid sinuses.
  - Leads to enophthalmos owing to orbital volume loss
  - Sinus congestion and fluid collection occur secondary to edema.
- Infraorbital nerve runs through the bony canal 3 mm below the orbital floor:
  - Injury results in hypoesthesia of the ipsilateral cheek.
  - Distinguished from hypoesthesia owing to swelling by testing for decreased sensation on the ipsilateral gingiva, which is within the infraorbital nerve distribution
- Inferior rectus and inferior oblique muscles run along the orbital floor:
  - Restriction of these extraocular muscles (EOM) occurs owing to entrapment within the fracture or contusion or cranial nerve dysfunction.
  - Diplopia on upward gaze
  - Inability to elevate the affected eye normally on examination
- Medial rectus muscle is located above the ethmoid sinus:
  - Less commonly entrapped
  - Diplopia on ipsilateral lateral gaze
- Oculocardiac reflex is defined as an increased vagal tone secondary to soft tissue entrapment. Signs and symptoms include nausea, vomiting, bradycardia, and syncope.

GENERAL PREVENTION

Protective eyewear has been shown to decrease eye injuries, although data is insufficient to demonstrate decrease in orbital blowout fractures specifically.

COMMONLY ASSOCIATED CONDITIONS

- Ocular Injuries:
  - Ruptured globe (incidence 5–10% of blowout fractures) (1)
  - Subconjunctival hemorrhage
  - Corneal abrasion/laceration
  - Hyphema
  - Iridodialysis
  - Traumatic iridocyclitis (uveitis)
  - Traumatic mydriasis
  - Retinal detachment
  - Vitreous hemorrhage
  - Compressive orbital emphysema
  - Retrobulbar hemorrhage
  - Optic nerve injury
  - Central retinal artery occlusion
  - Acute angle glaucoma
- Extraocular muscle (EOM) entrapment:
  - Inferior rectus
  - Inferior oblique
  - Medial rectus (less common)
- Infraorbital nerve injury
- Facial fractures:
  - Nasal bones
  - Zygomatic arch fracture
- Neck injuries
- Intracranial injury

DIAGNOSIS

HISTORY

- Mechanism of injury: significant trauma to the orbit
- Pain
- Swelling
- Bruising
- Double vision with upward gaze

PHYSICAL EXAM

- Periorbital tenderness, swelling, ecchymosis
- Impaired ocular mobility or diplopia:
  - Upward gaze impaired owing to inferior rectus entrapment
  - Ipsilateral lateral gaze impaired with medial rectus entrapment
- Infraorbital hypoesthesia: owing to compression/contusion of infraorbital nerve
- Enophthalmos or hypoophthalmos: owing to herniation of orbital fat through fracture
- Periorbital emphysema
- Normal visual acuity (unless associated ocular injury)
- Epistaxis (indicative of medial wall injury)
- Careful attention not to place pressure on the globe until ruptured globe excluded
- Slit-lamp and funduscopic examination help to identify associated injuries.

DIFFERENTIAL DIAGNOSIS
- Retrobulbar hemorrhage
- Periorbital contusion/ecchymosis
- Cranial nerve palsy
- Ruptured globe
- Orbital cellulitis
- Periorbital cellulitis

DIAGNOSTIC TESTS & INTERPRETATION
- Plain radiographs: limited value
- Computed tomography (CT) scan of orbits: study of choice:
  - Defines involved anatomy
  - Location and extent of fractures
  - Presence of intraorbital hemorrhage
  - Globe injury/rupture
  - EOM entrapment
  - Prolapse of orbital fat
  - CT findings of orbital floor fracture, EOM displacement, and EOM entrapment may predict diplopia (2)[B].
- Forced duction test:
  - Distinguishes nerve dysfunction from entrapment
  - Topical anesthesia is applied to the conjunctiva, and the globe is pulled away from the expected point of entrapment. If the globe is not mobile, the test is positive for entrapment.

TREATMENT

GENERAL MEASURES
- Apply cool compresses for the first 24 to 48 hr to decrease swelling in order to minimize/reverse herniation and avoid surgical intervention.
- Avoid Valsalva maneuvers and nose blowing to prevent compressive orbital emphysema.
- Prophylactic antibiotics (e.g., amoxicillin, cephalexin, or erythromycin) to prevent infection
- Nasal decongestants (e.g., phenylephrine nasal spray)
- Analgesics
- Tetanus prophylaxis

MEDICATION
- Phenylephrine nasal spray: BID × 10 to 14 days
- Amoxicillin: 250 to 500 mg PO TID × 10 to 14 days
- Cephalexin: 250 to 500 mg PO QID × 10 to 14 days
- Erythromycin: 250 to 500 mg PO QID × 10 to 14 days

ISSUES FOR REFERRAL
- Consultation with facial trauma service: Arrange follow-up evaluation within 1 to 2 wk of injury and to determine need for surgery.
- Immediate ophthalmology evaluation if patient has evidence of visual loss or within 24 hr for complete retinal evaluation

SURGERY/OTHER PROCEDURES
- Most resolve without surgical intervention.
- Typically observe for 10 to 14 days until swelling resolves
- Surgery indications:
  - Persistent diplopia
  - Restricted extraocular movements
  - Cosmetically significant enophthalmos or hypoophthalmos
  - Persistent oculocardiac reflex
  - Progressive infraorbital hypesthesia
- Immediate surgical intervention:
  - Trapdoor fractures should be repaired within 24 hr (1)[B].
  - Diplopia with tissue entrapment and nonresolving oculocardiac reflex (3)[B]
- Surgery within 2 wk:
  - Symptomatic diplopia, evidence of entrapped tissue, and minimal improvement (3)[B],(4)[A]
  - Significant enophthalmos (3)[B]
  - Progressive infraorbital hypesthesia (3)[B]
- There is some debate regarding optimal surgical timing:
  - Surgery after 14 days had odds ratio of 3.3 for persistent postoperative diplopia and no significant difference in postoperative enophthalmos (4)[A].

ONGOING CARE

COMPLICATIONS
- Sinusitis
- Orbital infection
- Permanent restriction of extraocular movement
- Enophthalmos
- Decreased visual acuity

REFERENCES

1. Chung SY, Langer PD. Pediatric orbital blowout fractures. *Curr Opin Ophthalmol*. 2017;28(5):470–476.
2. Cellina M, Floridi C, Panzeri M, et al. The role of computed tomography (CT) in predicting diplopia in orbital blowout fractures (BOFs). *Emerg Radiol*. 2018;25(1):13–19.
3. Burnstine MA. Clinical recommendations for repair of isolated orbital floor fractures: an evidence-based analysis. *Ophthalmology*. 2002;109(7):1207–1213.
4. Damgaard OE, Larsen CG, Felding UA, et al. Surgical timing of the orbital "blowout" fracture: a systematic review and meta-analysis. *Otolaryngol Head Neck Surg*. 2016;155(3):387–390.

ADDITIONAL READING

- Aerni GA. Blunt visual trauma. *Clin Sports Med*. 2013;32(2):289–301.
- Jones NP. Orbital blowout fractures in sport. *Br J Sports Med*. 1994;28(4):272–275.
- Lincoln AE, Caswell SV, Almquist JL, et al. Effectiveness of the women's lacrosse protective eyewear mandate in reduction of eye injuries. *Am J Sports Med*. 2012;40(3):611–614.
- Shew M, Carlisle MP, Lu GN, et al. Surgical treatment of orbital blowout fractures: complications and postoperative care patterns. *Craniomaxillofac Trauma Reconstr*. 2016;9(4):299–304

CLINICAL PEARLS

- Pediatric patients >5 yr old are more likely to have trapdoor fractures which require immediate surgical intervention.
- CT scan of the orbits is the diagnostic test of choice.
- Most orbital blowout fractures will resolve without intervention; however, significant diplopia, tissue entrapment, and enophthalmos are main indications for surgery.

FRACTURE, CALCANEUS

Greg Nakamoto, MD, FACP

BASICS

DESCRIPTION

Calcaneus fractures can occur secondary to either acute trauma or recurrent stress (i.e., calcaneal stress fracture). The focus here is on the management of acute traumatic fractures of the calcaneus:

- Of primary concern when evaluating the acute calcaneus fracture is determining whether the fracture is extra- or intra-articular:
  - Most extra-articular fractures can be managed conservatively.
  - Current practice is for most intra-articular fractures to be treated surgically. Such fractures consequently should be referred for orthopedic evaluation.
  - Having said that, no universally accepted guidelines exist as to the optimal treatment of displaced intra-articular calcaneal fractures (1,2,3).
  - It should be noted that most calcaneal fractures (other than stress fractures) are intra-articular.
- Secondarily, one should be aware that many patients with acute calcaneus fractures have other coexisting lower extremity or vertebral injuries.
- Synonyms: Os calcis fracture; heel bone fracture

EPIDEMIOLOGY

Prevalence

- Most commonly seen in young men, representing ~2% of all fractures seen in adults (1,4).
- The calcaneus is the most frequently fractured tarsal bone, accounting for 60% of all tarsal fractures (1,2,4,5).
- Approximately 75% of calcaneal fractures are intra-articular (1,2,4).
- ~2% are open fractures.

RISK FACTORS

- A fall from a height directly onto the heel is the main cause of calcaneal fractures (1,4,5).
- Other mechanisms include a force of impact directly onto the heel (e.g., motor vehicle accident).
- Osteoporosis can predispose to calcaneal fractures despite a seemingly trivial mechanism of injury.
- Extra-articular fractures of the calcaneal body and plantar tuberosity can also be caused by blunt-force trauma or a twisting injury to the hindfoot.
- Avulsion fractures of the calcaneal tuberosity can occur with abrupt contraction of the Achilles.
- Stress fractures of the calcaneus can occur as an overuse injury in athletes.

COMMONLY ASSOCIATED CONDITIONS

- High-energy mechanism of injury usually is required for these fractures, resulting in a high incidence of coexisting lower extremity or spinal injury.
- Calcaneal fractures occur bilaterally in 5–9% of patients (1,4).
- 10% of patients will have sustained a spinal compression fracture as well (4).
- Often associated with significant local soft tissue injury

> **ALERT**
> **Acute compartment syndrome of the foot can occur due to a calcaneal fracture and is a surgical emergency.**

DIAGNOSIS

HISTORY

Mechanism of injury:

- Extra-articular fractures are more commonly due to an indirect mechanism such as a twisting injury or muscular avulsion.
- Intra-articular fractures are due to high-energy accidents.
- History of a fall from a height is particularly concerning for additional lower extremity and lumbar spine injury.

PHYSICAL EXAM

- Signs and symptoms include:
  - Heel pain.
  - Swelling.
  - Ecchymosis.
- Physical examination includes the following:
  - **Look for associated soft tissue injury**. Blisters may occur when swelling is substantial. Excessive soft tissue injury will influence duration of splinting before placing into a cast for those being treated conservatively or may delay definitive surgical treatment in those being treated operatively.
  - **Assess neurovascular function of the foot**. With significant swelling, pulses may be difficult to assess; check capillary refill of the toes.
  - **Pain elicited with gentle squeeze of the heel** in the palm of the examiner's hand is suggestive of calcaneal fracture.
  - **Ecchymosis that tracks distally to the sole of the foot**, known as the *Mondor sign*, is considered pathognomonic for calcaneal fracture.
  - **Check for evidence of lower extremity compartment syndrome**. Significant swelling in the plantar arch may suggest plantar compartment syndrome. This requires emergent surgical referral even if the fracture itself is nonoperative.
  - **Search for associated lower extremity and vertebral fracture** because of high incidence of coexisting injury.

DIFFERENTIAL DIAGNOSIS

- Talar fracture
- Cuboid fracture
- Malleolar fracture
- Ankle dislocation
- Ankle sprain

DIAGNOSTIC TESTS & INTERPRETATION

Whereas standard radiographs are often used to make the initial diagnosis, computed tomography (**CT**) **has become the imaging modality of choice** for visualization and staging of calcaneus fractures:

- Standard initial x-rays: anteroposterior, lateral, and axial calcaneus (Harris) views; usually sufficient for diagnosis of calcaneus fracture but often need to be supplemented for full visualization and staging of the injury (2)
- X-ray criteria for diagnosing calcaneal fractures that are not obvious on initial inspection include assessment of the Böhler tuber joint angle (2):
  - A line is drawn between the posterosuperior aspect of the calcaneus and the highest point of the posterior subtalar articular surface; a second line is drawn from the highest point of the anterior process to the posterior margin of the subtalar surface.
  - The angle of intersection of the two lines measures between 20 degrees and 40 degrees, with a similar angle found in the two calcanei in any one person.
  - In intra-articular fractures, depression of the subtalar joint results in a decrease in Böhler angle.
- Oblique (Broden) views can be helpful in assessing involvement of the articular surfaces.
- Additional x-rays to consider based on history and physical examination include views of the contralateral foot (because of the significant incidence of bilateral injury and to compare Böhler angle with the injured foot), ipsilateral ankle, and lumbar spine and pelvis (because of high frequency of associated fractures).
- **CT scan is the imaging modality of choice for classification of calcaneus fractures** (2,5)[A]:
  - In patients in whom x-rays are inconclusive, CT scan is considered the gold standard for confirming the diagnosis of calcaneal fracture.
  - Additionally, if plain films show articular involvement or if suspicion of articular involvement remains high despite equivocal plain films, then a CT scan is essential for a more specific analysis of the subtalar and calcaneocuboid joints because displacement of either likely will require surgical management.
- The Sanders classification system is based on axial and coronal CT cuts. It is the classification system used most commonly today in treatment decision making and reporting of results (2,5):
  - Type 1—nondisplaced fractures
  - Type 2—fractures that are split into two parts
  - Type 3—depressed fractures and/or fractures that are split into three parts
  - Type 4—comminuted fractures
- Magnetic resonance imaging (MRI): Although not generally used for the evaluation of traumatic calcaneus injuries, MRI may be the preferred imaging modality in patients with suspected stress fractures, particularly in patients with severe osteoporosis, in whom a bone scan may appear falsely negative.
- Follow-up and special considerations: For extra-articular fractures being treated nonoperatively, postreduction imaging involves repeating the standard radiographs to assess adequacy of reduction after closed manipulation. Comparison with the opposite foot often is useful.

TREATMENT

- Ice and oral analgesics are useful in the prehospital setting, and oral analgesics may be required for some time after casting.
- Reduction techniques:
  - Extra-articular calcaneal body fractures with minimal displacement: Mediolateral compression of the heel with the palms of the hands can be applied to reduce displaced extra-articular body fractures being treated nonoperatively.
  - Other extra-articular fractures or any intra-articular fractures: surgical consultation for possible open reduction and internal fixation (ORIF). For details, see "Ongoing Care."
- Postreduction evaluation: Repeat x-rays in 1 wk in any patient being treated nonoperatively.

- Immobilization:
  - Usually begins with splinting or bulky Jones dressing to accommodate changes in soft tissue swelling
  - In patients who require casting (see "Ongoing Care"), the splint can be changed to a short leg cast after the initial soft tissue injury has stabilized after ~3 to 5 days.
  - In patients who require operative treatment, splinting is appropriate until the patient can see an orthopedic surgeon.

SURGERY/OTHER PROCEDURES

- Intra-articular fractures and certain extra-articular fractures as listed below (see "Ongoing Care") should undergo orthopedic evaluation for possible surgical treatment.
- In patients requiring operative treatment, referral should be made promptly so that fixation can occur within 5 to 7 days.
- In patients with significant associated soft tissue injury, prompt orthopedic referral allows for early interventions to reduce edema, which can take 7 to 14 days to accomplish. In such cases, operative treatment within the first 3 wk, before early consolidation of the fracture fragments, is preferred (3)[C].
- All cases of compartment syndrome merit emergent referral.

ONGOING CARE

Optimal management of calcaneal fractures, particularly of intra-articular fractures, remains controversial (1,2,3). New techniques, such as arthroscopically assisted percutaneous pinning, are being developed that may lead to more consistently improved outcomes:

- **Nonoperative treatment of extra-articular fractures:**
  - Consider for minimally displaced extra-articular fractures of the body of the calcaneus (which do not change the weight-bearing surface of the foot and do not alter hindfoot mechanics) (6)[C].
  - A reasonable treatment regimen in such cases would include short-leg casting and no weight-bearing for 2 wk, followed by range of motion exercises. Progressive weight-bearing may start at 8 wk, with full weight-bearing by 12 wk.
- **Operative treatment of extra-articular fractures:**
  - Some extra-articular fractures are still best treated surgically (6)[C]:
    - Fractures of the sustentaculum tali with >2 mm of displacement
    - Displaced avulsions of the Achilles tendon insertion from the calcaneal tuberosity
    - Significant fractures of the calcaneal body
- **Operative versus nonoperative treatment of intra-articular fractures:**
  - Intra-articular fractures and the extra-articular fractures as listed above should be referred for orthopedic consultation (1,2,3)[B].
  - Completely nondisplaced intra-articular fractures (**Sanders type 1**) are still often treated nonoperatively (2,6)[C].
  - Regarding displaced intra-articular fractures, there has been at least one randomized trial that found no symptomatic or functional benefit of operative treatment over nonoperative care (3)[A].
  - Nevertheless, because the trend in the literature has historically been for improved function and satisfaction with operative care, there is general consensus that intra-articular fractures with displacement but minimal comminution (**Sanders type 2**) benefit from operative treatment over nonoperative care (2)[B].
  - There is a particular lack of consistent evidence in the literature, however, for superior outcomes with operative care in **Sanders type 3 and type 4** fractures. Additionally, these fractures are associated with increased risk of wound complication and infection. Consequently, there is lack of consensus as to whether these fractures should be treated operatively (2)[C]. Particularly, patients with type 4 fractures, in whom surgical reduction is considered unlikely to be successful, may also be considered for nonoperative treatment.
  - Despite the aforementioned lack of evidence supporting superior outcomes with initial ORIF of patients with **Sanders type 3 or type 4** fractures, subsequent arthrodesis for posttraumatic arthritis may be more successful in patients who underwent initial ORIF. Consequently, some authors nevertheless recommend ORIF as initial treatment of these fractures if not contraindicated (2)[C].

FOLLOW-UP RECOMMENDATIONS

- Conservative treatment should be reserved for certain extra-articular fractures. All intra-articular fractures and the specific extra-articular fractures listed earlier merit orthopedic evaluation to at least consider surgical fixation.
- In patients treated conservatively, removal from splinting/casting should be followed by referral to physical therapy to restore normal flexibility and strength before allowing return to play.

PATIENT EDUCATION

- Patients should be informed early that treatment can be difficult and that adverse outcomes can be potentially severe and disabling at times.
- Chronic pain and posttraumatic arthritis are not uncommon.

COMPLICATIONS

- In both operatively and nonoperatively treated patients, chronic disability owing to pain from an improperly functioning or arthritic subtalar or calcaneocuboid joint may occur (2).
- Complications specifically seen in patients undergoing ORIF include:
  - Infection.
  - Pain.
  - Swelling.
  - Delayed wound healing.
  - Nonunions of the fracture fragments.
  - Lateral impingement of the peroneal tendon.
  - Sural nerve injury.

REFERENCES

1. Wei N, Yuwen P, Liu W, et al. Operative versus nonoperative treatment of displaced intra-articular calcaneal fractures: a meta-analysis of current evidence base. *Medicine (Baltimore)*. 2017;96(49):e9027.
2. Gotha HE, Zide JR. Current controversies in management of calcaneus fractures. *Orthop Clin North Am*. 2017;48(1):91–103.
3. Griffin D, Parsons N, Shaw E, et al; for UK Heel Fracture Trial Investigators. Operative versus nonoperative treatment for closed, displaced, intra-articular fractures of the calcaneus: randomised controlled trial. *BMJ*. 2014;349:g4483.
4. Renovell-Ferrer P, Bertó-Martí X, Diranzo-García J, et al. Functional outcome after calcaneus fractures: a comparison between polytrauma patients and isolated fractures. *Injury*. 2017;48(Suppl 6):S91–S95.
5. Badillo K, Pacheco J, Padua S, et al. Multidetector CT evaluation of calcaneal fractures. *Radiographics*. 2011;31(1):81–92.
6. Thermann H, Krettek C, Hüfner T, et al. Management of calcaneal fractures in adults. Conservative versus operative treatment. *Clin Orthop Relat Res*. 1998;(353):107–124.

ADDITIONAL READING

- Buckley R, Tough S, McCormack R, et al. Operative compared with nonoperative treatment of displaced intra-articular calcaneal fractures: a prospective, randomized, controlled multicenter trial. *J Bone Joint Surg Am*. 2002;84-A(10):1733–1744.
- Lewis G. Biomechanics as a basis for management of intra-articular fractures of the calcaneus. *J Am Podiatr Med Assoc*. 1999;89(5):234–246.
- Miric A, Patterson B. Pathoanatomy of intra-articular fractures of the calcaneus. *J Bone Joint Surg Am*. 1998;80(2):207–212.
- Randle JA, Kreder HJ, Stephen D, et al. Should calcaneal fractures be treated surgically? A meta-analysis. *Clin Orthop Relat Res*. 2000;(377):217–227.
- Sanders R. Displaced intra-articular fractures of the calcaneus. *J Bone Joint Surg Am*. 2000;82(2):225–250.
- Simpson RB. Fractures of the calcaneus. *Curr Opin Orthop*. 2007;18:124–127.
- Swanson SA, Clare MP, Sanders RW. Management of intra-articular fractures of the calcaneus. *Foot Ankle Clin*. 2008;13(4):659–678.

CLINICAL PEARLS

- During the initial evaluation of a patient with a calcaneus fracture, be aware that many patients will have a coexisting lower extremity or vertebral fracture. Up to 10% will have coexisting compartment syndrome of the foot, which is a surgical emergency.
- Proper management of calcaneus fractures requires determining if the fracture is intra-articular or extra-articular. Intra-articular fractures generally are best treated surgically, whereas extra-articular fractures (with the exceptions noted under "Ongoing Care") are often treated nonoperatively.
- CT scan is the imaging modality of choice in the evaluation of intra-articular calcaneus fractures.
- Optimal treatment of calcaneal fractures is still controversial, with posttraumatic arthritis being the cause of most cases of chronic disability.
- In nonoperative cases, athletes may be ready to return to play in as little as 8 to 12 wk depending on the severity of the original injury. In operative cases, the duration of immobilization and recovery is more variable and depends on the particulars of the fracture.
- Consensus suggests that long-term outcome is determined mainly by the degree of joint destruction at the time of injury.
- There seems to be a subset of calcaneal fractures (Sanders type 3 and 4) that often has a poor outcome regardless of treatment (2).

FRACTURE, CARPAL BONE (OTHER)

Thomas Trojian, MD

BASICS

DESCRIPTION

- Fracture of the carpal bones of the wrist, excluding those of the hamate and scaphoid
- Includes Kienböck disease, a disease of the lunate where the blood supply is compromised, and possible osteonecrosis occurs
- Synonym(s): wrist fracture

EPIDEMIOLOGY

- The carpal bones consist of the scaphoid, lunate, triquetrum, and pisiform in the proximal row and the trapezium, trapezoid, capitate, and hamate in the distal row.
- It is estimated that 8–19% of hand injuries result in a carpal fracture (1).
- Frequency of fracture seen in carpal bones is scaphoid 80%, triquetrum 6%, hamate 5%, trapezium 4%, lunate 3%, capitate 1%, and trapezoid and pisiform, <1% each.
- Carpal fractures are caused by trauma from either a fall on the extended wrist or a direct blow.
- Kienböck disease (osteomalacia of the lunate) in 75% of the cases is preceded by trauma with the wrist in dorsiflexion.

RISK FACTORS

Fractures of the carpal bones other than the scaphoid and lunate bones are often seen in sports using a stick (e.g., hockey, lacrosse).

DIAGNOSIS

HISTORY

- Athletes usually present with a fall on the outstretched hand in the hyperextended position. However, direct trauma or a fall on a flexed wrist can also cause a fracture.
- Pain and restricted motion often are presenting complaints.
- Mechanism of injury can help localize the injury to a specific carpal bone.
- Determine when the wrist began to hurt; recent versus prolonged is important.
- Determine location of pain, whether ulnar or radial, at rest or with motion.
- An occult fracture often will present as a persistent wrist sprain. Carefully examine the patient because Kienböck disease and small chip fractures of the triquetrum can present in this manner (2).

PHYSICAL EXAM

- Pain and tenderness over the dorsum of the wrist
- Localized swelling and limited range of motion (ROM); a prominence may be present.
- Strength testing of the muscles whose tendons insert on or are supported by the injured structure may help localize the injury.
- Neurovascular signs are unusual, except for fracture of the pisiform, which may affect the ulnar nerve and artery.
- Inspect for swelling, deformity, and ecchymosis (the latter usually not seen with carpal fractures).
- Evaluate movement of wrist in flexion, extension, and ulnar and radial deviation.
- Palpate individual carpal bones to determine location of tenderness.
- Test strength of muscles that attach to carpal bones.
- Assess neurovascular integrity (fracture of the pisiform may affect the ulnar nerve, and a lunate dislocation may compress the median nerve).
- Axial loading of metacarpals above the carpal bones may help in diagnosis.

DIFFERENTIAL DIAGNOSIS

- Ligamentous injury (wrist sprain)
- Contusion
- Carpal dislocation
- Metacarpal fracture
- Distal radioulnar fracture
- Osteonecrosis of carpal bones

DIAGNOSTIC TESTS & INTERPRETATION

- Radiographs consisting of six views:
  - Anteroposterior (AP) and lateral, each taken in an exact neutral position; views of maximal radial deviation and maximal ulnar deviation; lateral views in maximal flexion and maximal extension
- Additional radiographic views may be needed if a fracture is suspected for certain carpal bones:
  - Pisiform (carpal tunnel views, oblique view with forearm in 20 degrees supination)
  - Triquetrum (slightly oblique, pronated lateral view)
  - Trapezium (carpal tunnel views and true AP [Robert] view)
  - Trapezoid (oblique views) (3)
- Computed tomography (CT) scanning should be considered if a fracture of the capitate, lunate, pisiform, trapezium, or trapezoid is suspected and negative plain films are seen.
- Postreduction views should be obtained to confirm reduction and correct anatomical alignment.

TREATMENT

- Immobilization of the wrist should eliminate the pain of the fracture.
- Nonsteroidal anti-inflammatory drugs (NSAIDs) and rarely opioids can be added as needed.
- There are theoretical concerns about the adverse effects of NSAIDs on fracture healing; there is not enough clinical evidence to deny patients with simple fractures their analgesic benefits (4)[C].
- Reduction techniques should not be necessary. All displaced or dislocated fractures should be splinted and referred for surgery.
- Lunate dislocation may need immediate reduction if median nerve or artery is involved.
- All treatments are for nondisplaced fractures.
- Triquetrum: short arm cast for 4 to 6 wk for transverse body fracture; short arm cast or splint for 2 to 4 wk for dorsal avulsion
- Trapezium: short arm thumb spica cast for 4 to 6 wk (5)[C]
- Pisiform: short arm cast or splint for 3 to 6 wk
- Trapezoid: short arm thumb spica cast for 4 to 6 wk
- Capitate: short arm thumb spica cast for 6 to 8 wk. Some recommend long arm with finger extension. Consider referral because of possible avascular necrosis (AVN).
- Lunate: short arm cast or at least splint until referred; prolonged immobilization of 12 to 16 wk may need long arm cast with finger extension (4)[C].

ADDITIONAL THERAPIES

ALERT

- Triquetrum:
  - Second most commonly fractured carpal bone
  - Dorsal rim chips of the triquetrum are easily missed on AP view and may be the only sign of a fracture.
  - May have tenderness distal to the ulnar styloid while the hand is in radial deviation
  - Persistent pain after appropriate treatment should alert the treating physician that a concurrent injury (pisiform fracture, triangular fibrocartilage complex injury, and/or lunate-triquetrum ligament tear) was initially not noticed.
- Capitate:
  - Most often fractured with the scaphoid or metacarpal
  - Consider all capitate fractures unstable because of the high likelihood of surrounding carpal instability.
  - Consider serial radiographs in patients with persistent pain.
  - High incidence of delayed nonunion in these fractures
  - Referral to hand specialist is reasonable.
- Trapezium:
  - Easily missed; patients will describe a localized pain at base of the thenar eminence and pain with wrist flexion.
  - Missed fractures cause ongoing pain at base of the thumb.
  - Carpal tunnel view demonstrates fracture of the palmar ridge.
  - When displaced, may affect the integrity of the trapeziometacarpal joint, which is responsible for pinch and grasp motions.
- Pisiform:
  - Sesamoid bone located within the flexor carpi ulnaris tendon, which can be disrupted if a fracture is present
  - Usually caused by direct blow to hand
  - Can compress the ulnar nerve or artery at Guyon canal
  - The pisiform can be excised in chronically symptomatic cases.
- Trapezoid:
  - Least commonly fractured
  - Patients describe pain at the base of the 2nd metacarpal.
  - Axial compression of 2nd metacarpal will elicit tenderness.
- Lunate:
  - Lunate fractures can be occult.
  - AVN is seen in 20% of lunate fractures.
  - Kienböck disease may be secondary to lunate injury.
  - Kienböck disease has a high association with ulna-minus variant.
  - In the early stages of Kienböck disease, plain radiographs are usually not diagnostic; magnetic resonance imaging (MRI) is usually needed for definitive diagnosis.
  - Referral to hand specialist is reasonable.
- Initially, while in cast, the athlete needs to continue fitness training. Constant monitoring of the cast and frequent (weekly) changes may be needed to maintain skin and cast integrity (5)[C].
- Once out of the cast, ROM then strengthening of the wrist need to be done until restoration of a painless, functional arc of wrist motion and near-normal strength are obtained.

SURGERY/OTHER PROCEDURES

Surgery is needed for displaced fracture(s) through the metacarpocarpal joint articulation.

ONGOING CARE

FOLLOW-UP RECOMMENDATIONS

- Any displaced fracture of the carpal bones should be referred to an orthopedic surgeon.
- Lunate fractures may develop AVN (Kienböck disease) and should be considered for referral even if not displaced.
- Return to play varies with the degree of injury and casting. In lunate fractures, it is up to 6 mo; in triquetrum fractures, it is 4 wk, possibly less, in cast. General requirements for returning to play are complete healing of the fracture and any concurrent soft tissue injuries. Thorough rehabilitation with restoration of a painless, functional arc of wrist motion and near-normal strength are essential.
- Wrist stiffness is a common problem after casting, and physical therapy for ROM and strengthening is essential after cast removal. When rehabilitation is done, the wrist is most often free of pain.

REFERENCES

1. Johnson BK, Brou L, Fields SK, et al. Hand and wrist injuries among us high school athletes: 2005/06–2015/16. *Pediatrics*. 2017;140(6):e20171255.
2. Suh N, Ek ET, Wolfe SW. Carpal fractures. *J Hand Surg Am*. 2014;39(4):785–791.
3. Klausmeyer MA, Mudgal CS. Hook of hamate fractures. *J Hand Surg Am*. 2013;38(12):2457–2460.
4. Rettig ME, Dassa GL, Raskin KB, et al. Wrist fractures in the athlete. Distal radius and carpal fractures. *Clin Sports Med*. 1998;17(3):469–489.
5. Papp S. Carpal bone fractures. *Orthop Clin North Am*. 2007;38(2):251–260.

ADDITIONAL READING

- Duckworth AD, Ring D. Carpus fractures and dislocations. In: Court-Brown C, Heckman JD, McKee M, et al, eds. *Rockwood and Green's Fractures in Adults*. 8th ed. Philadelphia, PA: Wolters Kluwer Health; 2014:991–1056.
- Rettig AC. Epidemiology of hand and wrist injuries in sports. *Clin Sports Med*. 1998;17(3):401–406.
- Slade JF III, Milewski MD. Management of carpal instability in athletes. *Hand Clin*. 2009;25(3):395–408.
- Vigler M, Aviles A, Lee SK. Carpal fractures excluding the scaphoid. *Hand Clin*. 2006;22(4):501–516.

CLINICAL PEARLS

- Frequency of fracture seen in carpal bones is scaphoid 80%, triquetrum 6%, hamate 5%, trapezium 4%, lunate 3%, capitate 1%, and trapezoid and pisiform, <1% each.
- Dorsal rim chips of the triquetrum are easily missed on AP view and may only be seen on lateral view.
- Trapezium: easily missed; patients will describe a localized pain at base of the thenar eminence and pain with wrist flexion.
- Pisiform fractures can compress the ulnar nerve or artery at Guyon canal.

FRACTURE, CLAVICLE

Christopher C. Trigger, MD, FACEP, CAQSM

BASICS

- The clavicle is a subcutaneous S-shaped bone.
- First bone to ossify in the human body (5th wk of gestation)
- Functionally acts as a strut that connects the shoulder girdle to the axial skeleton

DESCRIPTION

- Allman classification based on fracture site (1,2)
- Craig further subdivided group II and III fractures:
  - Group I: fracture of the middle third
  - Group II: fracture of the lateral (distal) third:
    - Type I: lateral to coracoclavicular (CC) ligament (typically nondisplaced)
    - Type II: medial to the CC ligaments; causes superior displacement of the medial fragment relative to the lateral fragment
    - Type III: Fracture extends into the acromioclavicular (AC) joint.
    - Type IV: proximal fragment displacement out of periosteal tube (only in children)
    - Type V: comminuted where CC ligaments remain attached to an inferior bone fragment only
  - Group III: fracture of the medial (proximal) third:
    - Type I: nondisplaced
    - Type II: displaced with ligamentous rupture
    - Type III: Fractures extend into the sternoclavicular (SC) joint.
    - Type IV: Fracture causes epiphyseal separation (children and adolescents).
    - Type V: comminuted

EPIDEMIOLOGY

Incidence

- Most commonly fractured bone in children and adolescents
- Bimodal age distribution with peaks in children/adolescents and the elderly
- Predominant gender: male > female (2.5:1)
- 80% are group I, 15% group II, and 5% group III.

RISK FACTORS

- Direct trauma and fall onto the shoulder are the most common mechanisms of injury.
- Highest risk sports in the United States are football, lacrosse, and ice hockey.

COMMONLY ASSOCIATED CONDITIONS

- AC joint injury
- Labral tears
- Rotator cuff injuries
- Proximal humeral fractures
- Rib fractures
- Pneumothorax/hemothorax
- SC joint dislocation
- Brachial plexopathy
- Vascular injuries (uncommon)

DIAGNOSIS

History, physical exam, and appropriate imaging will make the diagnosis.

HISTORY

- Direct trauma or a fall
- Middle-third fractures are frequently seen with fall on an outstretched arm.
- Distal-third fractures most often are associated with loads transmitted to the lateral aspect of the shoulder.

PHYSICAL EXAM

- May have ecchymosis or tenting of the skin over the fracture
- Tenderness to palpation at fracture site
- Pressure along the clavicle may reveal fracture motion or crepitus.
- Careful pulmonary and neurovascular exam must be performed to identify possible associated injury.

DIFFERENTIAL DIAGNOSIS

- AC joint injury
- Glenohumeral dislocation
- Rotator cuff contusion/tear
- Labral injury
- Rib fracture
- Humeral head fracture
- SC joint or physeal injury

DIAGNOSTIC TESTS & INTERPRETATION

Initial Tests (lab, imaging)

- Radiographs:
  - An anteroposterior (AP) view of the clavicle, including the AC and SC joints and the shoulder girdle
  - A 30- to 45-degree cephalic-tilt (Zanca) view is recommended to delineate displacement and comminution in all fracture types.
  - A 40-degree cephalic-tilt view of the SC joint (serendipity view) can rule out SC dislocations.
  - An axillary view can be useful in distal clavicle fractures.
- Computed tomography (CT) scan:
  - Articular fractures of the medial or lateral clavicle may require a CT scan.
  - A CT angiogram or standard angiogram can be used if distal vascular deficit is suspected (1,2).

Diagnostic Procedures/Other

Special considerations: The proximal clavicular epiphysis is the last growth plate in the body to fuse (approximately age 20 yr). Therefore, many injuries involving the SC joint in athletes probably are physeal injuries and are ideally evaluated by thin-cut CT scan.

TREATMENT

- Primary goal in treating clavicular fractures is to obtain bony union and restore shoulder function to preinjury level with little or no residual pain, dysfunction, or cosmetic deformity (1,2).
- Most fractures can be treated nonoperatively (80–90%).

- Most clavicle fractures (when treated nonsurgically) will heal clinically in 6 to 8 wk; radiographic healing takes longer (8 to 12 wk).
- Arm sling and sling and swathe are the most common forms of immobilization (1)[B].
- Figure-of-8 harness is used less frequently because of discomfort, noncompliance, and worse complication rates.
- Range of motion (ROM) and active shoulder flexion (up to 40 degrees) as well as isometric deltoid and rotator cuff strengthening can begin once pain is improved.
- Avoid ROM >45 degrees of forward flexion until clinical evidence of healing is seen.
- As radiographic union progresses, increase ROM and resistive exercises.
- When radiographic union is present, full active use of the arm is allowed.

SURGERY/OTHER PROCEDURES

- Surgery is more commonly performed with varying results.
- Indications for early operative treatment include (3,4,5):
  - Displaced or shortened (>2 cm) and comminuted middle-third fractures of the clavicle.
  - Type II distal clavicle fractures are typically managed surgically owing to the high rate of nonunion; also, operative treatment is recommended in type IV and V fractures.
  - Neurovascular compromise.
  - Any open fractures.
  - Tenting of skin over an irreducible fracture.
  - Concomitant glenoid neck fracture, also known as *floating shoulder*.
  - Posterior fracture dislocations of the medial clavicle should be reduced in the presence of a thoracic surgeon owing to risk of vascular injury.
- Surgical techniques used include open reduction and internal fixation (ORIF) with plates and screws or intramedullary fixation.
- Primary operative fixation is becoming much more common in healthy, young athletes as well as professional athletes with a goal of possibly expediting return to play.
- Secondary operative treatment is considered for:
  - Persistent (>6 wk) displacement and shortening despite immobilization.
  - Malunion or nonunion.

ONGOING CARE

- Follow-up should be scheduled 7 to 10 days after injury to assess clinical symptoms and then every 2 to 4 wk until clinical and radiographic union occur (1).
- Radiographic union progresses more slowly than clinical union.
- Radiographs should be performed at intervals of 4 to 6 wk to assess healing.
- A final radiograph to assess callus formation and clinical union can be useful.
- Athletes should not be allowed to return to play until the fracture is clinically and radiographically healed (typically 6 to 8 wk) (1)[C].
- Noncontact and throwing athletes should have full, painless ROM and at least 90% strength compared with the uninjured arm (usually requires ~6 wk).
- Return to contact/collision sports may take up to 8 to 12 wk.

COMPLICATIONS

- Posttraumatic arthritis
- Nonunion:
  - Degree of displacement and comminution most important factors
  - More common in diabetics, smokers, women, and the elderly
  - Recent studies show a 2% rate of nonunion in patients managed surgically and a 4.5% rate of nonunion in nonoperative patients.
  - Historically, 0.1–1% of nonunions occurred for nonoperative treatment and 3.5–5% for operative treatment. Improved surgical technique and better reporting presumably are the reasons for the change.
  - Rate of nonunion was no different at 6 wk, but at 9 mo, it was significantly reduced with surgical intervention (4)[B].
- Malunion resulting in angulation, shortening, and a poor cosmetic appearance
- Neurovascular injury (uncommon): medial branch (ulnar nerve) of the brachial plexus most commonly affected
- Hardware removal secondary to pain

REFERENCES

1. Pujalte GG, Housner JA. Management of clavicle fractures. *Curr Sports Med Rep.* 2008;7(5):275–280.
2. Kim W, McKee MD. Management of acute clavicle fractures. *Orthop Clin North Am.* 2008;39(4): 491–505.
3. Altamimi SA, McKee MD; and Canadian Orthopaedic Trauma Society. Nonoperative treatment compared with plate fixation of displaced midshaft clavicular fractures. Surgical technique. *J Bone Joint Surg Am.* 2008;90(Suppl 2, Pt 1):1–8.
4. Ahrens PM, Garlick NI, Barber J, et al; and Clavicle Trial Collaborative Group. The clavicle trial: a multicenter randomized controlled trial comparing operative with nonoperative treatment of displaced midshaft clavicle fractures. *J Bone Joint Surg Am.* 2017;99(16):1345–1354.
5. Goudie EB, Clement ND, Murray IR, et al. The influence of shortening on clinical outcome in healed displaced midshaft clavicular fractures after nonoperative treatment. *J Bone Joint Surg Am.* 2017;99(14):1166–1172.

ADDITIONAL READING

- Fanter NJ, Kenny RM, Baker CL III, et al. Surgical treatment of clavicle fractures in the adolescent athlete. *Sports Health*. 2015;7(2):137–141.
- Woltz S, Stegeman SA, Krijnen P, et al. Plate fixation compared with nonoperative treatment for displaced midshaft clavicular fractures: a multicenter randomized controlled trial. *J Bone Joint Surg Am.* 2017;99(2):106–112.

CLINICAL PEARLS

- Most fractures are managed nonoperatively unless displaced and shortened.
- Most patients can return to noncontact sports within 6 to 8 wk.
- Typical return to contact sports is 8 to 12 wk.
- Surgical fixation tends to yield sooner return to play and decreased nonunion rates in the appropriate setting.
- Protective donut pads may be useful in protecting the clavicle from reinjury or pain from a direct blow.

FRACTURE, COCCYX

John Munyak, MD • Yaffa Ilyaguyeva • Amity Tung, MD

BASICS

- The coccyx is the last bony structure at the caudal end of the vertebral column and is triangular in shape.
- Coccygeal fractures can be caused by trauma such as falling and landing on the buttocks (e.g., during ice skating) or in newborns while passing through the vaginal canal.
- Coccyx fractures are also known as a "broken tailbone."
- Although the mechanism may be low impact, immobilization should be considered until other spine injuries are properly evaluated.

DESCRIPTION

- Fall landing in sitting position is most common.
- Also can occur during childbirth (1)
- Surgical procedures performed in area of coccyx
- Fractures of the coccyx are usually transverse.
- More common in women

ETIOLOGY AND PATHOPHYSIOLOGY

- The coccyx is made up of 3 to 5 fused vertebrae with attachments of several important muscles and ligaments. The muscles include the levator ani group, which supports the pelvic floor and aids in maintaining fecal continence, and the gluteus maximus, which aids in thigh extension.
- The coccyx has limited movement at the sacrococcygeal junction and a curvature such that the tip curves into the pelvis.
- Coccyx injuries are often belittled by physicians, but it should be kept in mind that the pain can be extremely severe and debilitating to the patient. Additionally, the coccyx is a weight-bearing structure in the seated position, and an ill-managed coccyx fracture can cause the patient to apply more weight on the ischial tuberosities, causing bursitis.

RISK FACTORS

- Predominantly occur in females because the female pelvis is broader, and the coccyx is more exposed
- Advanced age
- Osteoporosis
- Decreased balance causing more falls
- Congenital bone disorder such as osteogenesis imperfecta
- Involvement in activities such as skating or skateboarding

GENERAL PREVENTION

- Calcium and vitamin D supplements to prevent osteoporosis
- Refraining from activities that would predispose to falling on the buttocks, especially if elderly or if underlying medical conditions such as osteogenesis imperfecta are present

DIAGNOSIS

- Mechanism of injury
- Look for ecchymosis and palpate for tenderness in the gluteal fold.
- Prehospital:
  - Evaluate for other associated injuries (other potential life-threatening injuries such as head injuries may be missed if the focus is on the pain from the coccyx injury).

HISTORY

- Mechanism of injury (fall vs. assault vs. childbirth)
- Factors leading up to the fall (mechanical fall vs. syncope)
- Other associated injuries (other potential life-threatening injuries such as head injuries may be missed if the patient is focusing on the pain from the coccyx injury)
- Use of blood thinners (for ecchymosis out of proportion to the severity of injury)
- Low back pain, buttock pain, rectal bleeding (if associated rectal tear)
- Pain when sitting or defecating—document the PQRST of pain: *P*alliative or *P*recipitating factors, *Q*uality, *R*egion or *R*adiation, *S*everity (1 to 10), and *T*iming
- Risk for cancer (pathologic fracture): bright red blood per rectum (BRBPR), abnormal vaginal bleeding, weight loss

PHYSICAL EXAM

- Palpation of the sacrococcygeal joint for pain
- Digital rectal examination can be diagnostic with mobility and/or crepitus of the coccyx.
- Assess sacrococcygeal joint mobility by palpating the coccyx anteriorly (digital rectal exam) and posteriorly (externally).
- Anoscopy should be performed if gross blood is present to evaluate for possible rectal perforation (very rare).
- Examination of the entire spine is necessary to evaluate for concomitant injury.
- Neurologic exam of the lower extremities to assess radiculopathy
- Radiographs will identify other suspected spinal injuries.
- Displaced coccyx fractures can be seen best on the lateral coccyx view radiograph.
- Radiographs are not necessary if isolated coccyx fracture is apparent on rectal exam.
- Nondisplaced fractures are difficult to see on x-ray.
- When x-rays are used in the diagnosis, three views needed: anteroposterior (AP), lateral, and cone-down (focused) coccyx view
- More extensive diagnostic imaging is unnecessary in traumatic coccyx injuries (2).

DIFFERENTIAL DIAGNOSIS

- Contusion, hematoma
- Coccyx dislocation
- Pilonidal cyst

TREATMENT

Emergency department (ED) treatment:

- Symptomatic treatment
- Rarely, bed rest until ambulation can be tolerated
- Oral analgesics are key; may range from over-the-counter (OTC) acetaminophen or ibuprofen to prescription topical agents based on severity of pain
- Aim for conservative management in the pediatric population given high healing rates (3).
- Attempted manipulation and reduction of the displaced fracture by digital rectal approach is not necessary and futile because the coccyx cannot be stabilized.
- If there is an associated rectal injury, call for a surgical consult immediately. Prescribe antibiotics to cover for enteric pathogens: cefoxitin, cefotetan, and metronidazole.
- Cushions ("doughnuts")
- Sitz baths
- Stool softeners may help to reduce pain during bowel movements.

MEDICATION

- Cefotetan: adult: 2 g intravenous (IV); children: 80 mg/kg/day divided q6–8h (used with rectal injury)
- Cefoxitin: adult: 2 g IV; children: 80 to 160 mg/kg/day divided q6h (used with rectal injury)
- Metronidazole: adult: 0.5 to 1 g IV; children: 30 mg/kg/day divided q12h (used with rectal injury)
- Acetaminophen
- NSAIDS
- Lidoderm 5% patch
- Voltaren 1% gel

ADDITIONAL THERAPIES

Prescription "doughnut pillows" provide comfort until the fracture heals. They are helpful even if only a contusion is present.

SURGERY/OTHER PROCEDURES

Surgery is usually not required. Very rarely, severe trauma results in a comminuted fracture requiring coccygectomy (4).

ADMISSION, INPATIENT, AND NURSING CONSIDERATIONS

- Initial stabilization:
  - Spine immobilization for suspected concomitant cervical, thoracic, or lumbar injuries
  - Pain control with nonsteroidal anti-inflammatory drugs (NSAIDs) or narcotic analgesics
- Admission criteria:
  - Nearly all patients can be managed on an outpatient basis.
  - Only patients with severe pain, an inability to walk or to take care of themselves, other serious injury, or requiring surgery need to be admitted.
- Discharge criteria:
  - Most patients can be managed as outpatients with appropriate follow-up.
  - The patient is discharged home when other conditions are ruled out, and pain is under control.

ONGOING CARE

FOLLOW-UP RECOMMENDATIONS

- Healing is slow.
- Pain may become chronic.
- Orthopedic consultation and possible coccygectomy may be required in severe cases.

PATIENT EDUCATION

- Avoid activities requiring prolonged sitting such as horseback riding, long travel, biking, and so forth.
- Lean forward while sitting to avoid weight-bearing on the coccyx.

PROGNOSIS

Pain usually resolves about a week after callous forms.

COMPLICATIONS

Rarely, chronic pain or instability may require coccygectomy (4).

REFERENCES

1. Kaushal R, Bhanot A, Luthra S, et al. Intrapartum coccygeal fracture, a cause for postpartum coccydynia: a case report. *J Surg Orthop Adv*. 2005;14(3):136–137.
2. Hanna TN, Sadiq M, Ditkofsky N, et al. Sacrum and coccyx radiographs have limited clinical impact in the emergency department. *AJR Am J Roentgenol*. 2016;206(4):681–686.
3. Hamoud K, Abbas J. Fracture dislocation of the sacro-coccygeal joint in a 12-year-old boy. A case report and literature review. *Orthop Traumatol Surg Res*. 2015;101(7):871–873.
4. Ramieri A, Domenicucci M, Cellocco P, et al. Acute traumatic instability of the coccyx: results in 28 consecutive coccygectomies. *Eur Spine J*. 2013;22(Suppl 6):S939–S944.

ADDITIONAL READING

- Rockwood C, Green D, eds. *Fractures in Adults*. 8th ed. Philadelphia, PA: Lippincott-Raven; 2014.
- Simon R, Sherman SC. *Emergency Orthopedics: The Extremities*. 6th ed. Norwalk, CT: Appleton & Lange; 2011.
- Tibble CD, Gibbs M. Pelvic fractures. In: Wolfson AB, Cloutier RL, Hendey GW, et al, eds. *Harwood-Nuss' Clinical Practice of Emergency Medicine*. 6th ed. Philadelphia, PA: Wolters Kluwer; 2015:277–284

CLINICAL PEARLS

- More common in women
- May occur owing to falls or during childbirth (1)
- A self-limited condition
- Treatment includes pain management with oral anti-inflammatory medications, topical agents, and doughnut pillows.
- If there is an associated rectal injury, call for a surgical consult immediately. Prescribe antibiotics to cover for enteric pathogens.

FRACTURE, COMPRESSION

David E.J. Bazzo, MD, FAAFP, CAQSM • Tara Robbins, MD

BASICS

DESCRIPTION

- A compression fracture is defined as failure of the anterior vertebral column of the spine.
- The thoracolumbar spine is divided into three columns:
  - Anterior column (anterior portion of vertebral body, anterior longitudinal ligament, and anterior annulus fibrosus)
  - Middle column (posterior longitudinal ligament, posterior annulus fibrosus, and posterior wall of vertebral body)
  - Posterior column (posterior arch and posterior ligamentous complex)
- Two subtypes: anterior (caused by anterior flexion) and lateral (caused by lateral flexion)
- Three locations: cervical, thoracolumbar (transition between thoracic and lumbar from T10–L2), and lower lumbar vertebrae
- If anterior *and* middle columns are involved, the fracture is termed "burst."
- Synonym(s): wedge fracture

EPIDEMIOLOGY

- Compression fractures make up ~48% of thoracolumbar spinal fractures. L1 is the most commonly fractured vertebrae (1).
- Most common cervical compression fracture is anterior wedge fracture, usually at C5, as a result of axial loading, as might occur in football or diving.
- ~10% of cervical spine fractures have an associated, noncontiguous spinal column fracture.
- 25% of postmenopausal women >50 yr and 40% by 80 yr will suffer a vertebral compression fracture (2).

RISK FACTORS

- Cervical spine injuries are most common in diving, American football (poor tackling technique), and wrestling.
- Vertebral compression fractures are the most common type of fracture secondary to osteoporosis (2).

DIAGNOSIS

HISTORY

- Hyperflexion and axial loading injuries, such as with "spear tackling" in football or striking the forehead on the bottom of the pool, typically cause cervical compression fractures. Hyperextension mechanism suggests a "teardrop" fracture or defect of posterior spinal elements or pars interarticularis.
- Transient or permanent paralysis and/or sensory deficits can occur with compression fractures but are rare. Neurologic deficits imply spinal cord injury due to retropulsion of disk material or the fracture fragment (i.e., burst fracture).

PHYSICAL EXAM

- Sudden, localized pain immediately following direct trauma or axial loading injury
- Palpate the spinal column for "step-off" defect or tenderness.
- Careful neurologic examination, including sensation, motor function, and reflexes. Should be completely intact, but occasionally transient neurologic symptoms occur in an isolated compression fracture.

DIFFERENTIAL DIAGNOSIS

- Burst fracture (anterior and middle column disrupted, with or without posterior involvement)
- Fracture-dislocation (anterior, middle, and posterior columns disrupted)
- "Teardrop" fracture (triangular fracture of anteroinferior vertebral body)
- Transverse process or spinous process fracture
- Lumbar or cervical strain or sprain
- Spondylolysis and/or spondylolisthesis
- Scheuermann disease: kyphosis >50 degrees, wedging of at least three vertebral bodies by at least 5 degrees, disk space narrowing, and irregularity of end-plates
- Spear tackler spine: radiographic evidence of:
  - Developmental narrowing of the cervical spinal canal (<13-mm anteroposterior [AP] diameter of spinal canal on plain film or impedance of contrast medium on myelography)
  - Straightening or reversal of the normal cervical lordotic curve
  - Preexisting minor posttraumatic radiographic evidence of bony or ligamentous injury
  - History of repeated spear tackling. Some authors believe that these findings absolutely prohibit return to contact sports. Others believe that if normal cervical lordosis is restored by treatment and the athlete refrains from further spear tackling, and then there is not a high risk of injury in returning to athletic activity.
- Burning hands syndrome: a variant of central cord syndrome with characteristic complaint of burning paresthesia and dysesthesia in both arms or hands and occasionally legs; associated with bony or ligamentous spine injury in 50% of cases

DIAGNOSTIC TESTS & INTERPRETATION

- AP radiograph: buckling of lateral vertebral cortex next to end plate with decreased interspinous distance; may show lateral wedging with lateral flexion injury
- Lateral radiograph: Height of anterior vertebral body is decreased, whereas posterior height is unchanged, causing increased density of vertebral body from bony impaction and prevertebral swelling; no subluxation of vertebral bodies
- Flexion-extension views: Evaluate cervical ligamentous instability (>3.5 mm horizontal or 11-degree angular displacement between adjacent vertebrae).
- Computed tomography (CT) scan: to confirm intact vertebral ring (posterior wall, pedicles, and lamina). ~25% of compression fractures identified on plain films will be reclassified as burst fractures after CT scanning.
- Myelography: rules out osseous protrusion into spinal canal and better evaluates neural compression than CT
- Magnetic resonance imaging (MRI): recommended to evaluate spinal cord or nerve root compression and intrinsic spinal cord abnormalities if neurologic symptoms persist or plain films are abnormal

TREATMENT

- Prehospital:
  - It is estimated that 3–25% of spinal cord injuries may result from improper stabilization of the spinal column during the transportation period.
  - If spinal cord injury is suspected, then management should be with advanced trauma life support procedures: Airway should be established and protected, breathing maintained, and circulation supported.
  - If the player is wearing a helmet, it should *not* be removed. However, the facemask may be removed for airway access.
- Emergency department (ED) treatment:
  - All suspected spinal cord injuries warrant emergency evaluation as soon as possible. Radiographs should be obtained as soon as possible, and full neurologic exam should be documented.

GENERAL MEASURES

- Cervical compression fractures in the absence of subluxation are treated with a rigid brace for 8 to 12 wk with or without halo (3)[B].
- Thoracic fractures are relatively stable because of surrounding chest cage and strong costovertebral ligaments and can be treated conservatively with relative rest.
- Thoracolumbar injuries (T10–L2) are inherently more unstable and require a longer recumbency and possible immobilization in thoracolumbar spinal orthosis.
- Nonoperative treatment of osteoporotic vertebral compression fractures includes pain control, immobilization with an external orthosis, and administration of nasal calcitonin. Nonoperative treatment is usually continued until the acute pain has subsided, adequate mobilization is achieved, and the absence of progressive deformity is confirmed (2)[B].
- Recent comparative study shows no difference in outcome between soft brace, rigid brace, or no brace (4)[B].

MEDICATION

- Pain control should be achieved with a suitable medication.
- Nonsteroidal anti-inflammatory drug (NSAID) or opioid for acute treatment. If opioids are used, then patient should also be put on a bowel regimen program to prevent constipation.

ADDITIONAL THERAPIES

- Less severe injuries may be managed with bracing and serial imaging to evaluate healing and alignment.
- Unstable injuries mandate urgent surgical treatment.
- A portion of injuries may require delayed surgical intervention.

SURGERY/OTHER PROCEDURES

- Isolated fractures with <25% anterior compression are considered stable and can be treated with thoracic lumbosacral orthosis brace immobilization.
- A >50% loss of anterior vertebral height, multiple adjacent compression fractures, or angulation >20 degrees at the thoracolumbar junction are associated with segmental instability due to posterior ligamentous injury. This requires surgery to prevent formation of chronic instability and possible further kyphotic deformity. The procedure of choice is usually posterior short-segment pedicle screws or interspinous wiring and fusion.
- Kyphotic deformities may be managed with a posterior approach with osteotomies or a combined anterior approach and posterior procedure, although anterior approaches are associated with higher morbidity and complications.
- Vertebroplasty and kyphoplasty are routinely used for pain associated with osteoporotic and pathologic compression fractures. Data has been inconsistent. Two randomized controlled trials comparing vertebroplasty with a sham procedure in patients with acute or chronic vertebral compression fractures found no benefit in pain reduction, function, or quality of life (5)[C].
- Radiofrequency kyphoplasty and polyetheretherketone (PEEK) implants are newer procedures that may prove to be superior to traditional kyphoplasty with better outcomes, less adverse reactions, and more cost-effective (6)[C].

ONGOING CARE

FOLLOW-UP RECOMMENDATIONS

Any patient with unstable radiographic abnormalities should be seen by an orthopedist or neurosurgeon for complete evaluation.

REFERENCES

1. Denis F. The three column spine and its significance in the classification of acute thoracolumbar spinal injuries. *Spine (Phila Pa 1976)*. 1983;8(8):817–831.
2. Goldstein C, Chutkan NB, Choma TJ, et al. Management of the elderly with vertebral compression fractures. *Neurosurgery*. 2015;77(Suppl 4):S33–S45.
3. Khoueir P, Oh BC, Wang MY. Delayed posttraumatic thoracolumbar spinal deformities: diagnosis and management. *Neurosurgery*. 2008;63(Suppl 3):117–124.
4. Kim HJ, Yi JM, Cho HG, et al. Comparative study of the treatment outcomes of osteoporotic compression fractures without neurologic injury using a rigid brace, a soft brace, and no brace: a prospective randomized controlled non-inferiority trial. *J Bone Joint Surg Am*. 2014;96(23):1959–1966.
5. McCarthy J, Davis A. Diagnosis and management of vertebral compression fractures. *Am Fam Physician*. 2016;94(1):44–50.
6. Genev IK, Tobin MK, Zaldi SP, et al. Spinal compression fracture management: a review of current treatment strategies and possible future avenues. *Global Spine J*. 2017;7(1):71–82.

ADDITIONAL READING

- Cantu RC, Bailes JE, Wilberger JE Jr. Guidelines for return to contact or collision sport after a cervical spine injury. *Clin Sports Med*. 1998;17(1):137–146.
- Costa F, Ortolina A, Cardia A, et al. Efficacy of treatment with percutaneous vertebroplasty and kyphoplasty for traumatic fracture of thoracolumbar junction. *J Neurosurg Sci*. 2009;53(1):13–17.
- Maroon JC, Bailes JE. Athletes with cervical spine injury. *Spine (Phila Pa 1976)*. 1996;21(19):2294–2299.
- McGirt MJ, Parker SL, Wolinsky JP, et al. Vertebroplasty and kyphoplasty for the treatment of vertebral compression fractures: an evidenced-based review of the literature. *Spine J*. 2009;9(6):501–508.
- Nicholas J, Herschman E, eds. Thoracic spine injuries in athletes. In: *The Lower Extremity and Spine in Sports Medicine*. St. Louis, MO: Mosby; 1995.
- Oner FC, Dhert WJ, Verlaan JJ. Less invasive anterior column reconstruction in thoracolumbar fractures. *Injury*. 2005;36(Suppl 2):B82–B89.
- Tatsumi RL, Hart RA. Cervical, thoracic and lumbar fractures. In: Trunkey DD, Asensio JA, eds. *Current Therapy of Trauma and Surgical Critical Care*. Philadelphia, PA: Mosby; 2008:513–519.

CLINICAL PEARLS

- Compression fractures without neurologic injuries are considered stable and, once healed completely, should allow the player to return to action when neck pain is gone, range of motion is complete, muscle strength is normal, and fusion is solid (if done).
- Athletes with significant vertebral injury requiring a halo brace or surgical stabilization are considered not to have adequate strength to return to contact sports.

FRACTURE, CORONOID

Delmas Bolin, MD, PhD, FACSM

BASICS

- The coronoid process:
  - An important stabilizer of the elbow to varus stress and posterior ulnar displacement
  - Part of the sigmoid notch, the portion of the proximal ulna that articulates with the humerus
  - Has several important soft tissue insertions:
    - The brachialis muscle inserts anteriorly, distal to the capsule; the anterior joint capsule inserts very close to the tip of the coronoid; the anterior bundle of the medial collateral ligament (MCL) and the lateral collateral ligament (LCL) complex insert at the base of the coronoid.
- When the coronoid is fractured at the base, the ligament insertion sites are often preserved because failure occurs through bone, not the ligament insertions. Smaller fractures are likely to be associated with ligament injury.
- Unusual to see in isolation; usual mechanism of injury is elbow dislocation as a result of a fall on an outstretched hand.

DESCRIPTION

Coronoid fractures are classified based on anatomic location of the fracture based on lateral radiograph (types 1 to 3) and computed tomography (CT) diagnosis of anteromedial (type 4) and anterolateral (type 5) fractures (1); subclassification according to the associated soft tissue injuries and fractures to determine treatment (2,3):

- Type 1: fracture of the tip of the coronoid:
  - Tip subtype 1 fractures involve <2 mm of coronoid and may be isolated or associated with a fracture dislocation.
  - Tip subtype 2 fractures involve >2 mm and generally is associated with "terrible triad" injuries (i.e., elbow dislocation, radial head fracture, and coronoid fractures).
- Type 2: fracture of the anteromedial facet:
  - Anteromedial subtype 1 fractures extend from just medial to the tip of the coronoid to the anterior half of the sublime tubercle (the insertion of the medial band of the MCL).
  - Anteromedial subtype 2 fractures extend to the tip of the coronoid.
  - Anteromedial subtype 3 fractures extend to the anteromedial rim and the entire sublime tubercle but do not always extend to the tip of the coronoid.
- Type 3: fracture of the basal aspect of the coronoid involving >50% of the coronoid:
  - Basal subtype 1 fractures involve the basal coronoid alone.
  - Basal subtype 2 fractures are associated with fractures of the olecranon.
- Type 4 or 5: anteromedial or anterolateral fractures

EPIDEMIOLOGY

- Uncommon, rarely occurring as an isolated injury
- In elbow dislocations, 2–15% of cases have coronoid process fractures.

RISK FACTORS

- Displacement of large coronoid process fracture fragments has been associated with recurrent dislocation.
- No known significant risk factors to date

COMMONLY ASSOCIATED CONDITIONS

- Elbow instability
- Radial head fracture
- Olecranon fracture
- Loss of range of motion (ROM)
- Degenerative joint disease (posttraumatic arthritis)
- Ulnar, median, radial, and anterior interosseous nerve injury
- Brachial artery injury
- Heterotopic ossification

DIAGNOSIS

HISTORY

- Common mechanism is fall on outstretched hand.
- Most patients with coronoid fractures present with elbow dislocations.
- Direct impact is a less common cause.

PHYSICAL EXAM

- Diffuse edema within and around the elbow joint
- Tenderness is usually multifocal. Look for radial head tenderness as well as antecubital fossa tenderness.
- ROM is limited, and crepitus on ROM should be noted.
- Evaluate for anterior/posterior and posterolateral rotatory instability.
- Varus posteromedial instability (with anteromedial coronoid fractures) can be assessed by having patient flex and extend elbow with palm down and shoulder in 90 degrees abduction producing mechanical symptoms (4)[B].
- Neurovascular examination is paramount, especially if there is an elbow deformity.
- If elbow is dislocated, perform neurologic and vascular examinations before reduction. Repeat neurovascular examination after elbow dislocation is reduced, and assess for elbow instability.
- Palpate radial head and olecranon to look for accompanying fractures.

DIFFERENTIAL DIAGNOSIS

- Elbow subluxation
- Posterior lateral rotatory instability
- Acute ulnar collateral ligament sprain
- Radial head fracture
- Hyperextension injuries to joint capsule

DIAGNOSTIC TESTS & INTERPRETATION

- Standard elbow x-ray series (anteroposterior, lateral, and one or both obliques) should be requested at the time of evaluation:
  - Evaluate for comminuted fractures, where reduction may not be advisable.
  - Repeat plain radiographs after elbow relocation.
- If radial head tenderness is present, radial head view should be added to x-ray series.
- Advanced imaging: Small coronoid fractures can be difficult to distinguish from radial head fractures, and both CT scanning (1)[B] and magnetic resonance imaging (MRI) should be considered if radiographs are not definitive.
- Ultrasound imaging, both static and dynamic, can be used to evaluate MCL and LCL structures (5).

TREATMENT

- Acute treatment (1,3)[B]:
  - Elbow dislocations with coronoid fractures should be evaluated for instability and splinted in position of stability.
  - Tip subtype 1 fractures do not involve the insertion of the anterior capsule and can be treated with immobilization for 1 to 2 wk or bracing with protected ROM through the stable range.
  - Prolonged immobilization associated with poor outcomes (6)[B]
  - Tip subtype 2 fractures almost always involve the anterior capsule insertion and are often seen in terrible triad injuries. They should be referred to orthopedics; they often will require suture fixation because the fragments are too small to be secured with screws.
  - Anteromedial subtype fractures are associated with incongruent articulation of the ulnohumeral joint and may lead to posttraumatic degenerative joint disease. These fractures require surgical stabilization.
  - Basal coronoid fractures generally have less soft tissue disruption than tip or anteromedial fractures but require stabilization to prevent recurrent instability and traumatic degenerative joint disease.
- Special considerations:
  - Posttraumatic degenerative joint disease correlates with patient age.
  - Ulnar nerve injuries occur from handling of nerve and do not always resolve.
  - Subluxation or repeat dislocation usually requires repeat surgery.
  - Contractures and heterotopic ossification are common after treatment.
- Rehabilitation:
  - Early mobilization with active and active assistive ROM should begin as soon as comfort allows, generally after 1 wk (6)[B].
  - A hinged brace to protect the elbow from varus and valgus stress generally is prescribed for the 1st mo, and blocking of the terminal 30 degrees of extension during early rehabilitation is common.
  - Prophylaxis for heterotopic ossification is not routine (e.g., indomethacin or naproxen).
  - Resistive exercises generally are delayed for 6 wk.
  - Serial radiographs are commonly obtained to confirm maintenance of concentric reduction.

SURGERY/OTHER PROCEDURES

Surgery to repair soft tissue injuries associated with coronoid fractures is being performed increasingly.

ONGOING CARE

PROGNOSIS

- Joint stiffness and limited ROM are common with prolonged immobilization.
- Presence of posttraumatic arthritis correlates with patient age.
- Pain is a common complaint in at least half of all patients after treatment.

COMPLICATIONS

- Vascular and neurologic injuries associated with elbow dislocations
- Complex dislocations with loss of ROM and stability
- Persistent pain and loss of ROM after treatment

REFERENCES

1. Adams JE, Sanchez-Sotelo J, Kallina CF IV, et al. Fractures of the coronoid: morphology based upon computer tomography scanning. *J Shoulder Elbow Surg*. 2012;21(6):782–788.
2. Ring D. Fractures of the coronoid process of the ulna. *J Hand Surg AM*. 2006;31(10):1679–1689.
3. Doornberg JN, Ring D. Coronoid fracture patterns. *J Hand Surg AM*. 2006;31(1):45–52.
4. Ramirez MA, Stein JA, Murthi AM. Varus posteromedial instability. *Hand Clin*. 2015;31(4):557–563.
5. Tagliafico AS, Bignotti B, Martinoli C. Elbow US: anatomy, variants, and scanning technique. *Radiology*. 2015;275(3):636–650.
6. Regan W, Morrey B. Fractures of the coronoid process of the ulna. *J Bone Joint Surg Am*. 1989;71(9):1348–1354.

CLINICAL PEARLS

- Coronoid fractures can be managed conservatively with meticulous diagnosis.
- Athletes with associated soft tissue injuries or instabilities should be referred early for orthopedic evaluation.
- Athletes return to play when fractures are healed and when they have restored painless ROM with full strength and flexibility.
- Recovery can be prolonged, and careful follow-up is important.
- Patients with type 1 tip fractures generally can return to play within 6 to 8 wk; surgical patients frequently require longer rehabilitation prior to return to play.
- Lockout elbow bracing should be considered to stabilize the elbow and can be an important adjuvant to healing and rehabilitation.

FRACTURE, DISTAL FEMUR

James C. Ritchey, MD, MS, FAAFP

BASICS

DESCRIPTION

- Fracture involves the distal 15 cm of the femur.
- Fractures may be:
  - Supracondylar: Zone is from the femoral condyles to the junction of the metaphysis and femoral shaft.
  - Intracondylar.
  - Condylar.

EPIDEMIOLOGY

- Bimodal distribution: young, healthy males, elderly osteopenic females
- Distal femur fractures represent 4–6% of all fractures of the femur (1).
- Predominantly women and in the elderly with >50% of patients who are >65 yr (2)
- No data on the incidence in the athletic population

Pediatric Considerations

- Up to 60% of femoral fractures in children 3 yr old or younger may be the result of nonaccidental trauma (3).
- Spiral fractures of the femur strongly suggest child abuse (3).

ETIOLOGY AND PATHOPHYSIOLOGY

- Fractures generally occur from significant axial loading with associated varus, valgus, or rotation force.
- May occur from direct trauma as well
- In young adults, fractures are usually associated with high-energy trauma such as:
  - Motor vehicle accidents, falls from heights, direct impact.
  - Motor sports, downhill skiing.
- In older individuals, especially those with osteoporosis, a slip and fall may be enough force to cause injury.
- Muscle attachments, quadriceps, hamstring, and gastrocnemius cause the observed deformity in distal femur fractures.

RISK FACTORS

- High-energy sports such as motor sports and downhill skiing
- Osteoporosis

COMMONLY ASSOCIATED CONDITIONS

- Fractures are generally from high-energy mechanism, so a full trauma survey should be performed.
- Complications may include:
  - Proximal or shaft fractures of the femur.
  - Ligament and cartilage injuries of the knee.
  - Proximal tibia fractures.
  - Open fractures: 5–10% of all supracondylar fractures.
  - Quadriceps tendon injury.
  - Vascular injuries are relatively uncommon.

DIAGNOSIS

Pediatric Considerations

- Cartilaginous components of the proximal and distal ends of the developing femur alter the fracture patterns seen in hip and knee injuries in children.
- Essential workup:
  - Radiographs
  - Assess distal pulses, palpate compartments, and evaluate sensation and motor function:
    - If pulses are not equal or palpable, bedside Doppler may be necessary.
  - Search for associated injuries.
  - In suspected child abuse, obtain skeletal survey or bone scan.

HISTORY

- History will help to guide examination and workup.
- High-energy injuries require full examination and search for associated injuries.
- Direct trauma and low-energy mechanism do not necessarily require a more comprehensive evaluation.

PHYSICAL EXAM

- Tenderness on examination, deformity, thigh shortening, swelling (secondary to hematoma), and crepitus with movement
- Limited movement of hips and knees
- Commonly presents with associated injuries: chest or abdominal trauma, hip or knee injury, direct blow to the extremity
- Vascular compromise (arterial injury): expanding hematoma, absent or diminished pulses, progressive neurologic deficits in a closed fracture (1)
- Hypotension and tachycardia secondary to significant blood loss
- Radiographs:
  - Anteroposterior (AP) view of pelvis, true lateral of hip, AP and lateral views of femur, and complete knee series
  - Other imaging as indicated by trauma protocols
- Computed tomography (CT) scan: Complex intra-articular injuries generally necessitate CT scan for operative planning:
  - CT scan is recommended because 55% of these fractures are intra-articular (2).
- Arteriography: should be performed for evidence or suspicion of vascular compromise

DIFFERENTIAL DIAGNOSIS

- Hip fracture or dislocation
- Knee dislocation
- Proximal tibia fracture
- Thigh contusion or hematoma

DIAGNOSTIC TESTS & INTERPRETATION

If surgery is planned, complete blood count (CBC), type, and crossmatch

TREATMENT

Pediatric Considerations

- Assess markers for nonaccidental trauma:
  - Delay in presentation; history of mechanism inconsistent with the injury
  - Isolated trauma to the thigh; associated burns, bruises, or linear abrasions
- Assess for dislocation of the femoral capital epiphysis.
- Depending on the age of the patient and the fracture type, pediatric femoral fractures may not require operative treatment.

- Prehospital:
  - Long-leg splint should be applied to the extremity in the position it was found.
  - If signs of neurovascular compromise, reduce limb with in-line traction.
  - Use analgesia when possible.
  - Do not attempt to reduce open fractures in the field.
  - Apply wet sterile dressing over an open fracture.
  - If wound is grossly contaminated, use sterile saline irrigation.
- Emergency department (ED) treatment:
  - Primary and secondary trauma surveys
  - If surgical treatment will be delayed or for selected patients in whom nonoperative management is the treatment of choice, consider fracture reduction.
  - Reduce fractures to near-anatomic alignment by using in-line traction (Hare, Buck, or long posterior splint): reduces pain and helps to prevent hematoma formation
  - Pain management: parenteral or IV opiate-type analgesia
  - Infection prophylaxis: with open fractures, tetanus toxoid if indicated, cefazolin with gentamicin
  - For injuries with highly contaminated wounds, add penicillin G to cover *Clostridium* spp.
  - Emergently consult an orthopedic surgeon.
  - Femur fractures with vascular (expanding hematoma, absent or diminished pulses) or progressing neurologic compromise require immediate angiography or vascular consultation for femoral artery exploration.
  - Consider transferring patients with a femur fracture if:
    - Necessary orthopedic consults are not available.
    - There are associated serious injuries that may require a trauma center for management.

MEDICATION

For open fractures:

- Cefazolin: adult: 2 g IM/IV; children: 20 mg/kg IM/IV
- Gentamicin: 1.5 mg/kg IV
- Penicillin G: adult: 2 million IU IV; children: 25,000 IU/kg/day IV divided q8h

SURGERY/OTHER PROCEDURES

- Surgical reconstruction should be performed as soon as possible (1)[B],(4)[C].
- If surgery will be delayed >24 hr (closed fractures), tibial pin traction should be applied to maintain limb length (5)[C].
- Multiple surgical techniques can be performed to obtain reduction and fixation and depend on both surgeon experience and the specific fracture (2)[C].
- Anatomic reduction of the fracture with particular attention to the articular surface is more closely related to positive outcomes than the actual surgical technique.
- Children aged 6 mo to 5 yr with a diaphyseal fracture and <2 cm of shortening may be treated with early spica casting or traction and delayed spica casting (6)[B].
- There is unclear benefit of surgery versus casting in fractures with >2 cm shortening or varying degrees or rotation and angulation (6)[C].

ADMISSION, INPATIENT, AND NURSING CONSIDERATIONS

- Monitor heart rate and blood pressure (BP) continuously because large volumes of blood (i.e., 4 to 6 units) may be contained within the thigh.
- Most femur fracture patients should be admitted.
- Conservatively treated fractures in a pediatric patient may not require hospitalization.

ONGOING CARE

PROGNOSIS

- Depends on multiple factors:
  - Fracture type
  - Associated injuries
  - Patient comorbidities
- Fracture with intra-articular involvement carries a high risk of posttraumatic arthritis.

COMPLICATIONS

- Hemorrhagic shock secondary to significant blood loss
- Neurovascular injury
- Infection secondary to open fractures
- Fat embolism and adult respiratory distress syndrome can cause respiratory failure.
- High mortality rate in elderly populations

REFERENCES

1. Lupescu O, Nagea M, Patru C, et al. Treatment options for distal femoral fractures. *Maedica (Buchar)*. 2015;10(2):117–122.
2. Ehlinger M, Ducrot G, Adam P, et al. Distal femur fractures. Surgical techniques and a review of the literature. *Orthop Traumatol Surg Res*. 2013;99(3):353–360.
3. Hui C, Joughin E, Goldstein S, et al. Femoral fractures in children younger than three years: the role of nonaccidental injury. *J Pediatr Orthop*. 2008;28(3):297–302.
4. Weinberg DS, Scarcella NR, Napora JK, et al. Can vascular injury be appropriately assessed with physical examination after knee dislocation? *Clin Orthop Relat Res*. 2016;474(6):1453–1458.
5. Albert MJ. Supracondylar fractures of the femur. *J Am Acad Orthop Surg*. 1997;5(3):163–171.
6. Kocher MS, Sink EL, Blasier RD, et al. Treatment of pediatric diaphyseal femur fractures. *J Am Acad Orthop Surg*. 2009;17(11):718–725.

ADDITIONAL READING

- Macnicol MF. Fracture of the femur in children. *J Bone Joint Surg Br*. 1997;79(6):891–892.
- Starr AJ, Hunt JL, Reinert CM. Treatment of femur fracture with associated vascular injury. *J Trauma*. 1996;40(1):17–21.

CLINICAL PEARLS

- Be aware of potential associated injuries in all femur fractures.
- Fractures of the distal femur are severe, and medical management and treatment are difficult.
- Evaluate for signs of child abuse in children <3 yr.
- It is imperative to achieve anatomical reduction, restoration of functional anatomy, and stable fixation to ensure optimal function and reduce recovery time.

FRACTURE, DISTAL PHALANX

Thomas L. Pommering, DO, FAAFP

BASICS

- Fractures of the distal tip (tuft fracture):
  - Open
  - Closed
- Fractures of the shaft:
  - Longitudinal
  - Transverse
- Fractures of the base:
  - Mallet fracture
  - Reverse mallet fracture (jersey finger)
  - Pediatric epiphyseal fractures:
    - Salter-Harris (SH) type I or type II
    - Seymour fracture (pediatric mallet finger)

DESCRIPTION

- *Mallet finger*: a pure tendon injury where there is disruption of the extensor tendon caused by forced flexion of the fingertip while the distal interphalangeal (DIP) joint is in extension. This causes loss of DIP extension, leaving the fingertip in slight flexion.
- *Mallet fracture*: a disruption of the terminal extensor tendon from its insertion onto the proximal aspect of the distal phalanx dorsally *with* a bony avulsion
- *Jersey finger*: flexor digitorum profundus (FDP) rupture from its insertion onto the palmar distal phalanx; can be a pure tendinous injury or be a bony avulsion fracture
- *Seymour fracture*: extra-articular transverse fracture of the base of the distal phalanx usually involving the distal physis (SH I or II) or 1 to 2 mm distal to the physis; this fracture mimics mallet finger deformities but does not involve the articular surface. The FDP tends to pull the distal metaphyseal fragment volarly, whereas the extensor tendon insertion onto the proximal aspect of the distal phalanx pulls the epiphysis dorsally in the opposing direction.
- *Tuft fracture*: a fracture of the distal tip of the distal phalanx; usually from a crush injury and associated with a subungual hematoma and/or a nail bed injury; can be an open or closed injury. This is the most common hand injury in toddlers and preschool-aged children.

EPIDEMIOLOGY

Incidence

- Most common peak incidence is during early teenage years, followed by a second peak during toddler years (crush injury in doors).
- In the pediatric population, physeal fractures of the phalanges account for 37% of all physeal fractures, with the small finger being affected most often (30%), followed by the thumb (20%).
- Hand injuries, in general, account for 9% of all sports injuries.
- Seen more often with contact sports, where direct trauma is more likely (e.g., football), or with sports where the hand is exposed to projectiles (e.g., baseball, softball, or basketball)

ETIOLOGY AND PATHOPHYSIOLOGY

- The tip of the distal phalanx ends with broad, spade-like ungual tuberosity that provides a stable and protective base for the distal digital pulp.
- On the palmar surface, the FDP inserts onto the midportion of the distal phalanx.
- On the dorsal side, the terminal extensor tendon attaches to the proximal aspect of the distal phalanx (or the epiphyseal plate in children), blending with the joint capsule and periosteum.
- Collateral ligaments span the DIP joint (or the epiphyseal plate in children) and insert onto the metaphysis of the distal phalanx.
- Lateral interosseous ligaments originate on and span the distance of the distal phalanx, protecting the neurovascular bundle as they pass dorsally from the pulp to the nail bed.

RISK FACTORS

- Crush injury to tip of finger (e.g., getting stepped on by opponent's spiked shoes or finger slammed in a door) results in comminuted fracture or *tuft injury*.
- Acute flexion of an extended DIP joint (e.g., catching a ball on the tip of the finger or striking an object with the finger extended) results in *mallet finger*.
- Forced extension while actively flexing the DIP joint (e.g., grabbing a jersey of a ball carrier in football or catching the rim while dunking a basketball) results in *jersey finger*.

GENERAL PREVENTION

- Proper catching technique ("soft hands")
- Buddy taping to the adjacent digit or interphalangeal joint taping for high-risk athletes

DIAGNOSIS

HISTORY

- Crush: *tuft or Seymour fracture*
- Direct trauma, torsional, or hyperflexion/hyperextension mechanism: shaft or base of phalanx fracture
- Blunt trauma or projectile force against the fingertip resulting in forced flexion: *mallet finger/fracture*
- Forced extension on a flexed distal phalanx (e.g., grabbing a jersey during a tackle): jersey finger

PHYSICAL EXAM

- Signs and symptoms include:
  - Pain, swelling, and ecchymosis.
  - Loss of range of motion (ROM), malalignment, or angular deformities noted with flexion.
  - Obvious deformity, especially if associated with dislocation.
  - Subungual hematomas.
  - Traumatic swelling and tenderness over the volar aspect of the distal phalanx with additional palmar pain is a *rupture of the FDP* until proven otherwise.
- Physical examination should include the following:
  - Sites of tenderness, loss of active ROM, evidence of instability, and neurovascular examination
  - Radiographs should be obtained before any manipulative examination.
  - *Mallet finger*: 40- to 45-degree loss of extension at the DIP joint with inability to extend the distal phalanx; there is also pain and swelling over the dorsal aspect of the joint.
  - *Jersey finger*: inability to flex the distal phalanx, with tenderness over the volar aspect of the joint. Pain in the palm or proximal to the proximal interphalangeal (PIP) could indicate retraction of the tendon proximally.

DIFFERENTIAL DIAGNOSIS

- Fracture
- Sprain
- Volar plate rupture
- Tendon rupture or avulsion
- Interphalangeal dislocations

DIAGNOSTIC TESTS & INTERPRETATION

- Imaging should be obtained before any manual reduction attempts.
- Three views of the affected digit: anteroposterior (AP), lateral, and oblique views
- Consider comparison views of the unaffected side if skeletal immaturity and unaccustomed to pediatric radiology.
- Magnetic resonance imaging (MRI), computed tomography (CT) scan, or ultrasound (US) are usually not indicated in the initial evaluation of distal phalanx injuries unless physical exam is equivocal or x-rays are nondiagnostic:
  - MRI and/or US can be used to delineate soft tissue ligamentous or tendon injury.
  - CT scan is occasionally useful to delineate osseous injury for preoperative planning or to evaluate suspicious bone lesions.

TREATMENT

- *Distal phalanx or tuft fractures*:
  - *Closed with minimal to no displacement*:
    - Inherently stable
    - Often have an associated subungual hematoma that may need evacuated (see "Surgery/Other Procedures") for pain control
    - Ice for swelling and pain control
    - Protective splint covering the tip of the finger for support and protection; usually not needed for >2 to 3 wk, leaving the PIP joint free (1,2)[C]
    - Nonunion is rare, but radiographic union can take up to 6 mo.
    - The tip of the finger can remain sensitive for up to 6 mo after the injury (2)[C].
  - *Open*:
    - Inherently unstable because of disruption of the supporting pulp and nail bed
    - Require careful débridement, irrigation, and soft tissue repair often with loop magnification
    - Oral antibiotics and tetanus prophylaxis
    - Consider surgical consultation.
- *Shaft fractures*:
  - *Closed longitudinal or transverse shaft*:
    - Usually inherently stable
    - Longitudinal fractures: heal within 3 to 4 wk; splint for protection
    - Transverse fractures: take longer, requiring slightly longer support until clinical discomfort abates or radiographic union is evident
  - *Open shaft fractures*:
    - Unstable
    - Proper alignment is necessary.
    - Surgical consultation is recommended.
- *Base-of-phalanx fractures*:
  - Tend to be unstable regardless of the overlying soft tissue involvement owing to the deforming traction of the extensor or flexor tendons (3)[C]
  - Lack the intrinsic support of the overlying nail and nail plate
  - Tend to angulate with the apex pointing dorsally
  - If >1/3 to 1/2 of the articular surface is involved or if displaced, consider surgical consultation.
- *Mallet fracture*:
  - Continuous 24 hr/day splinting with the DIP joint in extension using a molded thermoplast splint or properly fitted polythene (Stack) splint for 6 to 8 wk; followed by an additional 2 to 4 wk of night splinting (4,5)[C]

  - Hyperextension of the DIP joint should be avoided.
  - PIP joint is always left free.
  - Any momentary loss of extension (e.g., during changing or removal of splint for hygiene) mandates restarting back at day 1 of immobilization.
  - Some extension lag after treatment is expected.
  - The goal is to prevent a hyperextension PIP joint deformity (swan neck deformity).
  - Because the surgery often is deceptively difficult to perform and is associated with several complications, operative management is reserved for injuries with volar subluxation of the distal phalanx or if displaced and involving >30% of the joint surface (5)[C].
  - Surgical consultation is advised for failed conservative treatments and those with subluxation/dislocation complications.
- *Mallet finger*:
  - Pure tendon injury; 8 to 12 wk of continuous splinting of DIP joint followed by 2 to 4 wk of night splinting (5,6)[C]
  - Continuous splinting should be resumed if failed or interrupted treatment because the prognosis for healing is still very good.
  - Chronic mallet fingers can be treated as far out as 3 mo from injury with a good prognosis for recovery.
  - Generally, conservative treatment is preferred owing to the complication risks of surgical treatment.

ALERT

Closed nondisplaced fracture of the volar surface in adults (jersey finger with avulsion fracture):
- Ring finger involved 75% of the time
- Avulsed fragment from the volar surface is attached to the FDP, which tends to promote displacement.
- Prompt surgical referral (within 7 to 10 days) should be the rule to optimize full functional outcome and avoid late complications (5)[C].

Pediatric Considerations

- Seymour fracture:
  - Children <5 yr of age often have a SH I or II fracture.
  - The FDP tendon is attached to the distal shaft, pulling it in the volar direction, whereas the epiphysis remains extended owing to the traction of the extensor tendon.
  - Extra-articular fracture of the base of the distal phalanx before closure of the epiphysis
  - Clinically, mimics mallet fracture or DIP joint dislocation (although is not an intra-articular injury) (1,2)[C]
  - Splint application for up to 6 wk in slight hyperextension
  - Close follow-up with weekly lateral radiographs for the first 2 wk to confirm alignment and stability to prevent permanent deformity (2)[C]
  - Surgical referral for open fractures, those not amenable to closed reduction, or if unfamiliar with treatment of this injury in children
- *Reduction techniques*:
  - *Transverse or comminuted distal phalanx fractures*: No reduction usually is required, only protective splinting for 3 to 4 wk, elevation, and analgesics. Treat associated subungual hematomas.
  - *Displaced distal phalanx fractures with AP displacement*: Apply traction to the distal aspect, and mold the fragments by squeezing the end of the finger between your thumb and index finger. Lateral displacement is corrected by compressing the lateral borders of the terminal phalanx with your thumb and index finger. Be aware that these can be difficult to reduce when soft tissues become interposed between fragments. If uncorrected, this may lead to nonunion.
- Postreduction evaluation:
  - Repeat radiographs.
  - Neurovascular examination
- Prehospital:
  - Protect and splint.

MEDICATION

- If reduction is needed or repair of associated soft tissue injuries (e.g., nail bed laceration), a hematoma block, digital block, or wrist block can be used.
- Conscious sedation or reduction under general anesthesia may be needed.

Second Line

Chronic pain control usually can be achieved with splinting alone or with adjunctive nonnarcotic analgesics or mild narcotic pain medication.

ISSUES FOR REFERRAL

- Displaced fractures not responsive to manual reduction
- Suspected flexor tendon rupture or avulsion fracture
- Open fracture of the shaft or intra-articular fracture
- Open tuft fractures are often unstable and involve complex injuries to the nail bed requiring skilled repair under loop magnification.
- Suspected neurovascular injury or secondary infection

ADDITIONAL THERAPIES

- Hematoma evacuation from the nail bed when >30–50% of the nail is involved or there is a need for pain control
- Usually accomplished using either a heated paper clip or electric cautery device. Take care not to damage the nail bed.

ALERT

With fractures associated with subungual hematomas involving >30–50% of the nail, concomitant nail bed lacerations should be suspected and repaired if present. This is usually done using 5–0 or 6–0 dissolvable sutures and replacing the nail plate if possible. This is treated as an open fracture in the sense that it should be done under sterile conditions followed by antibiotic coverage for 7 to 10 days.

- Physical therapy with a qualified hand therapist is recommended in postoperative cases, after prolonged immobilization, and after splinting mallet finger if return to full ROM is not progressing.

SURGERY/OTHER PROCEDURES

- FDP tear (jersey finger) or avulsion fracture
- Mallet finger with volar subluxation of the distal phalanx
- Comminuted distal phalanx fracture with significant displacement (tuft fracture)
- Any distal phalanx fracture with malalignment that is not reducible by closed methods

ADMISSION, INPATIENT, AND NURSING CONSIDERATIONS

Generally reserved for severe, infected, or complicated injuries requiring surgical intervention

ONGOING CARE

FOLLOW-UP RECOMMENDATIONS

Repeat radiographs:
- *Mallet fractures*: 1 to 2 wk to document stability (x-ray in splint) and at 4 to 6 wk if there is any evidence of extension lag
- *Pediatric epiphyseal fractures (including Seymour fracture)*: at 1 to 2 wk to document stability; optional at 4 wk depending on clinical progress
- *Longitudinal and transverse shaft fractures*: at 2 wk

PROGNOSIS

In general, distal phalanx fractures are usually stable and heal with an uneventful course.

COMPLICATIONS

- Nonunion or malunion
- Infection for open fractures or Seymour fractures
- Joint stiffness or arthrofibrosis
- Permanent loss of flexor tendon function or dysfunction with undiagnosed or delayed treatment for flexor tendon avulsions or disruptions
- Physeal arrest in children
- Avascular necrosis with displaced unicondylar fractures, especially in children
- Swan neck deformity especially with mallet finger
- Neurovascular injury
- Skin necrosis from splints applied too tightly
- Skin hypersensitivity with distal injuries
- Osteoarthritis for late, undiagnosed, or inadequately healed intra-articular fractures

REFERENCES

1. Nellans KW, Chung KC. Pediatric hand fractures. *Hand Clin*. 2013;29(4):569–578.
2. Abzug JM, Dua K, Bauer AS, et al. Pediatric phalanx fractures. *J Am Acad Orthop Surg*. 2016;24(11):e174–e183.
3. Carpenter S, Rohde RS. Treatment of phalangeal fractures. *Hand Clin*. 2013;29(4):519–534.
4. Bloom JM, Khouri JS, Hammert WC. Current concepts in the evaluation and treatment of mallet finger injury. *Plast Reconstr Surg*. 2013;132(4):e560–e566.
5. Bachoura A, Ferikes AJ, Lubahn JD. A review of mallet finger and jersey finger injuries in the athlete. *Curr Rev Musculoskelet Med*. 2017;10(1):1–9.
6. Alla SR, Deal ND, Dempsey IJ. Current concepts: mallet finger. *Hand (N Y)*. 2014;9(2):138–144.

CLINICAL PEARLS

- *Mallet finger*: Patients who remove their splint even for a brief moment must start treatment over at day 1. Monitoring of skin care should be a priority because splinting for this injury is continuous and prolonged. Delayed injuries as old as 3 mo may be amenable to standard conservative treatment.
- *Jersey finger*: FDP ruptures should be identified early so that primary repair can occur within 7 to 10 days.
- *Tuft fracture*: often associated with subungual hematoma which may need to be drained
- *Seymour fracture*: pediatric SH fracture in young children mimicking mallet fracture or dislocation injury
- All open fractures need antibiotic and tetanus prophylaxis.

FRACTURE, DISTAL RADIUS

Kevin B. Gebke, MD • Dina Elnaggar, MD, MS

BASICS

DESCRIPTION

- Classically, the fractured distal portion will be dorsally displaced and angulated ("silver-fork deformity"); commonly referred to as Colles fracture
- Other variations include:
  - Smith fracture (volar displacement and angulation).
  - Dorsal Barton fracture: dorsal fracture-dislocation involving displacement of carpus with distal fragment.
  - Volar Barton (also known as reverse Barton): fracture with volar displacement.
  - Hutchinson fracture (also known as chauffeur's fracture): lateral-oriented fracture through radial styloid process extending into radiocarpal articulation.
  - Galeazzi fracture-dislocation: fracture of distal third of radius with associated dislocation of distal radioulnar joint.
  - Die-punch fracture: a depressed fracture of the lunate fossa on the articular surface of the distal radius.
- Synonym(s): Colles fracture; Smith fracture; Barton fracture; dorsal Barton; reverse Barton fracture; volar Barton; Hutchinson fracture; chauffeur's fracture; Galeazzi fracture-dislocation; die-punch fracture

EPIDEMIOLOGY

- Most common fracture of the upper extremity (1)
- Most common fracture in children <16 yr old and most common during the metaphysical growth spurt (1)
- Incidence also peaks in patients 60 and 69 yr of age. 60–70% of all Colles fractures occur in postmenopausal women (1).
- Distal radius fractures represent 12.5% of fractures caused by sporting activity in one study (2): percentages of total fractures by sport that were distal radius: snowboarding 34.8%, ice skating 36.4%, soccer 19.1%, rugby 14.7%, mountain biking 14%

ETIOLOGY AND PATHOPHYSIOLOGY

Commonly sustained by falling onto an outstretched hand with the wrist in extension

RISK FACTORS

- In general, decreased bone mineral density and unsteady gait
- In sports activities: high risk of falls and impact: snowboarding, football, ice skating, etc.

GENERAL PREVENTION

Wrist guards can decrease the rates of wrist injury, including distal radius fractures in snowboarders (3)[B]:

- Beginner snowboarders get the most benefit from wrist guards.

COMMONLY ASSOCIATED CONDITIONS

- Arthrosis secondary to poor joint approximation at radioulnar or radiocarpal joint
- Joint stiffness or weakness
- Median nerve dysfunction—the median nerve and flexor tendons run volar to the distal radius.
- Triangular fibrocartilage complex (TFCC) injury

DIAGNOSIS

HISTORY

- Elicit specific details regarding fall or trauma involved in high- or low-energy mechanism.
- Comorbid conditions such as osteoporosis or malignancy

PHYSICAL EXAM

- Key is to always describe fracture location, angulation, displacement, and involvement of either radiocarpal or radioulnar joints.
- Gross visualization of the involved extremity for bony deformity and evidence of open injury
- Pain, swelling, and limitation of movement of distal upper extremity
- Tenderness to the dorsal aspect of the wrist
- Paresthesias, weakness, or coolness to touch (associated neurologic or vascular injury)
- Neurologic evaluation, including radial, median, and ulnar nerve testing
- Vascular evaluation, including capillary refill, radial and ulnar pulses
- In addition to fracture, one must evaluate for associated injuries at the scapholunate joint, distal radioulnar joint, ulnar styloid, and elbow injuries.
- Multiple classification systems have been described: Fernandez is based on mechanism of injury, Frykman is based on joint involvement, Melone divides intra-articular fractures into four types based on displacement, AO/OTA is a more comprehensive classification system, Lafontaine criteria and the McQueen equation predict secondary displacement after reduction.

DIFFERENTIAL DIAGNOSIS

- Carpal fracture
- Ulnar fracture
- Radiocarpal sprain
- Radioulnar sprain
- Soft tissue/bony contusion

DIAGNOSTIC TESTS & INTERPRETATION

- Consider obtaining bilateral x-rays to compare angulation.
- Anteroposterior (AP)/lateral views of wrist, forearm, and elbow
- AP view of the wrist: measures radial height (normal 13 mm, note shortening >5 mm), radial inclination (normal 22 degrees, note change >5 degrees), articular step-off (note >2 mm step-off), and ulnar variance:
  - Decreased radial height and inclination result in a hand that appears radially deviated with increased prominence of the ulnar head.
- Lateral view of the wrist: measures lateral tilt (normal 11 degrees volar, note dorsal angulation >5 degrees or within 20 degrees of contralateral distal radius):
  - Altered lateral tilt of the articular surface may cause midcarpal instability.
- AP and lateral view of the forearm and elbow: useful for identifying a Galeazzi fracture-dislocation (Loss of radius length producing an ulnar positive wrist increases the chance of symptomatic ulnar impaction syndrome.)
- Computed tomography (CT) scan: important to evaluate intra-articular involvement and for surgical planning
- Magnetic resonance imaging (MRI): useful to evaluate for soft tissue injuries such as TFCC injuries, scapholunate ligament injuries, and lunotriquetral injuries
- In a recent study, sports ultrasound has been found to have a sensitivity of 97.1% specificity of 100%, and a positive predictive value of 100% in diagnosing distal radius fractures in the pediatric population (4)[C].

TREATMENT

Treatment of the fractures may vary significantly based on the type of fracture, patient demands, and physician experience:

- Analgesia:
  - Adequate pain relief using oral and/or intravenous (IV) narcotics
  - For pediatric fractures, ibuprofen is equal to acetaminophen (Tylenol) with codeine (5)[A].
  - Hematoma blocks can provide pain relief for closed reductions (may be less effective than IV regional anesthesia).
- Nondisplaced/minimally displaced fractures:
  - Can be initially immobilized in a sugar tong splint or radial gutter splint until follow-up
- Pediatric torus fracture can be treated safely with a wrist immobilizer. Displaced fractures/unstable fractures warrant orthopedic referral.
- Reduction techniques:
  - Goal is to achieve anatomical alignment to allow proper healing of the fragments and eventual restoration of normal function.
  - Reduction should always be accomplished in a timely manner before soft tissue inflammatory changes progress, especially if signs of neurovascular compromise are present.
  - Finger trap reduction method is most common:
    - Finger traps are applied to thumb, index, and middle fingers with manual traction or by finger traps hanging from an IV pole with the patient's arm at 90 degrees.
    - Reduction may be achieved by distal manual reduction methods or by a weighted stockinette.
  - More than two attempts at closed reduction in pediatric fractures involving the physis increases the risk of growth arrest (6)[B].

- Postreduction evaluation:
  - Repeat neurovascular examination.
  - Post reduction x-rays (AP and lateral) after application of immobilizing device to assure maintenance of reduction

MEDICATION

- Acetaminophen is preferred for mild to moderate pain due to theoretical concern about nonsteroidal anti-inflammatory drugs (NSAIDs) inhibiting bone healing.
- Narcotic pain medications are commonly used in the first few weeks following injury.

ISSUES FOR REFERRAL

- Emergent orthopedic referral:
  - Open fractures
  - Acute neuromuscular compromise
  - Tenting of the skin
  - Compartment syndrome
- Nonemergent orthopedic referral:
  - Unstable fractures
  - Intra-articular involvement
  - Comminution
  - Fractures involving the physis
  - Severe osteoporosis
  - Displacement involving >2/3 the width of the radius
  - Dorsal angulation >5 degrees or >20 degrees of contralateral distal radius
  - >5 mm radial shortening or ulnar variance >5 mm
  - Progressive loss of volar tilt and loss of radial length following closed reduction and casting

ADDITIONAL THERAPIES

There is limited evidence to suggest a short-term benefit of physical therapy after distal radius fracture.

COMPLEMENTARY & ALTERNATIVE MEDICINE

Vitamin C 500 mg 1 × day for 50 days decreased the incidence of complex regional pain syndrome (CRPS) (7)[A].

SURGERY/OTHER PROCEDURES

- Surgery is indicated for unstable and significantly displaced fractures (1)[C].
- Multiple surgical techniques, percutaneous pinning, external fixation, volar or dorsal plating, and so forth, are used in the treatment of distal radius fractures.
- Nonoperative management is generally preferred in the geriatric population in appropriate circumstances.
- Operative treatment may allow athletes to return to play faster than nonoperative treatment (8)[C].
- Depending on where the athlete is in the season, and if their performance is not substantially limited by pain or being in a cast, a displaced fracture requiring surgery may be delayed by waiting 1 to 2 wk until the end of the season (8)[C].

ONGOING CARE

FOLLOW-UP RECOMMENDATIONS

- Most patients should be reexamined and x-rays repeated in 3 to 5 days for nondisplaced and 2 to 3 days for displaced fractures to ensure fracture stability.
- Splint removed and short arm cast for 4 to 6 wk for nondisplaced fractures and long arm cast for reduced fractures for 3 to 4 wk and then a short arm cast for a total of 6 to 8 wk
- Repeat x-rays every 2 to 3 wk for nondisplaced and every week for reduced fractures.
- Healing time is generally 6 to 8 wk in adults and 3 to 4 wk in children.
- Range of motion (ROM) exercises (8)[C]:
  - Immediately: without resistance for fingers, elbow, and shoulder
  - 3 wk: forearm rotation within the confines of a short arm cast
  - After removal of cast: wrist ROM
  - After resolution of tenderness: strengthening exercises
- Step-wise return to play is recommended after at least 80% of baseline ROM and strength is regained as well as radiographic healing if use of wrist is required. If use or wrist is not required, the athlete may return to play in a cast (9)[C].

PROGNOSIS

Generally good, with most patients regaining full function and motion at the wrist

COMPLICATIONS

- Severe acute complications, such as neurovascular injuries and compartment syndrome, are associated with high-energy trauma and are, fortunately, rare (1).
- TFCC injuries
- Median nerve neuropathy (carpal tunnel syndrome):
  - Most frequent neurologic complication
  - 1–12% in low-energy fractures and 30% in high-energy fractures
  - Prevent by avoiding immobilization in excessive wrist flexion and ulnar deviation (Cotton-Loder position).
- Ulnar nerve neuropathy: seen with distal radioulnar joint injuries
- Extensor pollicis longus tendon rupture (9):
  - Most common in nondisplaced or minimally displaced distal radius fractures (incidence from 0.3% to 5%)
  - Usually between 6.6 wk after distal radius fracture
- Degenerative changes, stiffness, and pain are more common in intra-articular fractures (1).
- Malunion and nonunion may occur. Malunion is the most common complication in pediatric patients.
- Radial physeal arrest in pediatric fractures is relatively common (up to 7%) but generally asymptomatic (6):
  - Risk increases with more than two attempts at closed reduction.
  - Ulnocarpal impaction may also occur from continued growth of the ulna after radial arrest.
- CRPS is an uncommon complication and may be associated with fibromyalgia (10)[B].

REFERENCES

1. Wulf CA, Ackerman DB, Rizzo M. Contemporary evaluation and treatment of distal radius fractures. *Hand Clin*. 2007;23(2):209–226, vi.
2. Court-Brown CM, Wood AM, Aitken S. The epidemiology of acute sports-related fractures in adults. *Injury*. 2008;39(12):1365–1372.
3. Russell K, Hagel B, Francescutti LH. The effect of wrist guards on wrist and arm injuries among snowboarders: a systematic review. *Clin J Sport Med*. 2007;17(2):145–150.
4. Ko C, Baird M, Close M, et al. The diagnostic accuracy of ultrasound in detecting distal radius fractures in a pediatric population [published ahead of print November 15, 2017]. *Clin J Sport Med*. doi:10.1097/JSM.0000000000000547.
5. Drendel AL, Gorelick MH, Weisman SJ, et al. A randomized clinical trial of ibuprofen versus acetaminophen with codeine for acute pediatric arm fracture pain. *Ann Emerg Med*. 2009;54(4):553–560.
6. Lee BS, Esterhai JL Jr, Das M. Fracture of the distal radial epiphysis. Characteristics and surgical treatment of premature, post-traumatic epiphyseal closure. *Clin Orthop Relat Res*. 1984;(185):90–96.
7. Zollinger PE, Tuinebreijer WE, Breederveld RS, et al. Can vitamin C prevent complex regional pain syndrome in patients with wrist fractures? A randomized, controlled, multicenter dose-response study. *J Bone Joint Surg Am*. 2007;89(7):1424–1431.
8. Crijns TJ, van der Gronde BATD, Ring D, et al. Complex regional pain syndrome after distal radius fracture is uncommon and is often associated with fibromyalgia. *Clin Orthop Relat Res*. 2018;476(4):744–750.
9. Romano N, Fischetti A, Mussetto I, et al. Extensor pollicis longus (EPL) tendon rupture as a complication of distal radius fracture: the role of ultrasound examination. *Med Ultrason*. 2018;1(1):114–115.
10. Beleckas C, Calfee R. Distal radius fractures in the athlete. *Curr Rev Musculoskelet Med*. 2017;10(1):62–71.

ADDITIONAL READING

LaMartina J, Jawa A, Stucken C, et al. Predicting alignment after closed reduction and casting of distal radius fractures. *J Hand Surg Am*. 2015;40(4):934–939.

CLINICAL PEARLS

- Swelling and pain over the physis may indicate a physeal injury even with normal radiographs.
- Physical exam and radiographic analysis are key to determining management of distal radius fractures.

F

FRACTURE, FIBULA

Anna L. Waterbrook, MD, FACEP, CAQSM

BASICS

DESCRIPTION

- Isolated fracture of the shaft of the fibula without evidence of associated ligamentous injury
- Synonym(s): fibula shaft fracture; fibula diaphyseal fracture

EPIDEMIOLOGY

Isolated fibula shaft fractures are rare.

RISK FACTORS

- Direct blow or trauma to the lateral leg leading to injury of the fibular shaft
- Contact sports or sports that require high repetitive axial loading may make some athletes more susceptible (1,2,3)[C].

DIAGNOSIS

HISTORY

Patients usually will describe direct trauma to the lateral leg and complain of pain and swelling in that area. They may be able to bear weight with minimal or no pain.

PHYSICAL EXAM

- Tenderness to palpation over the fracture site with evidence of swelling and possible ecchymosis
- It is important to examine the ankle and the knee for concomitant injuries, including proximal fibula fracture, distal fibula or tibia fracture, or injury to the syndesmosis.
- Detailed neurovascular exam with particular attention to the peroneal nerve

DIFFERENTIAL DIAGNOSIS

Fracture or injury to the knee, ankle, tibia, proximal or distal fibula, peroneal nerve, and/or anterior syndesmosis

DIAGNOSTIC TESTS & INTERPRETATION

- Radiographs of the tibia/fibula with anteroposterior and lateral views
- Stress views or radiographs of the knee and ankle if suspicion for associated injuries exists.
- No further imaging is necessary for isolated fibular shaft fractures.
- High-resolution ultrasound imaging may be useful when radiographs are not immediately available or when evaluating for stress or occult fracture if not seen on initial radiographs (4)[C].

TREATMENT

GENERAL MEASURES

- Treatment is based on patient comfort.
- If patient is having pain with ambulation, then a splint, cast, or walking boot should be used.
- Otherwise, a compression dressing is sufficient.
- Immobilization for 3 to 4 wk generally is recommended, followed by graded progression back to sport.
- Healing time usually takes about 6 to 8 wk but may be prolonged in some athletes (3)[C].

ISSUES FOR REFERRAL

Patient should be referred to an orthopedic surgeon if fracture is comminuted, significantly displaced, there is an associated fracture of the tibia, or there is evidence of neurovascular injury or painful nonunion.

ALERT

Special attention should be given to evaluation of the syndesmosis and peroneal nerve (1,5,6)[C].

REFERENCES

1. Al-Kashmiri A, Delaney JS. Case report: fatigue fracture of the proximal fibula with secondary common peroneal nerve injury. *Clin Orthop Relat Res*. 2007;463:225–228.
2. King WD, Wiss DA, Ting A. Isolated fibular shaft fracture in a sprinter. *Am J Sports Med*. 1990;18(2):209–210.
3. Slauterbeck JR, Shapiro MS, Liu S, et al. Traumatic fibular shaft fractures in athletes. *Am J Sports Med*. 1995;23(6):751–754.
4. Hoffman DF, Adams E, Bianchi S. Ultrasonography of fractures in sports medicine. *Br J Sports Med*. 2015;49(3):152–160.
5. Cheung Y, Perrich KD, Gui J, et al. MRI of isolated distal fibular fractures with widened medial clear space on stressed radiographs: which ligaments are interrupted? *AJR Am J Roentgenol*. 2009;192(1):W7–W12.
6. Mino DE, Hughes EC Jr. Bony entrapment of the superficial peroneal nerve. *Clin Orthop Relat Res*. 1984;(185):203–206.

CLINICAL PEARLS

- Patients should generally be immobilized for 3 to 4 wk.
- The fracture will heal in 6 to 8 wk.
- Depending on symptoms, rehabilitation may begin at 4 to 6 wk and training at 6 to 8 wk. Return to contact activities may take longer and has increased risk of refracture (3)[C].
- Usually there are no complications, but a small percentage may result in nonunion, peroneal nerve injury, or associated damage to the interosseus membrane (1,2,3,5,6)[C].
- Careful evaluation of the mechanism of injury should be made to avoid missing pronation–external rotation injuries that often have associated ligamentous injury (Weber C fractures). Such fractures may be unstable, and prompt orthopedic referral should be made if they are suspected.

F

FRACTURE, FIFTH METATARSAL (AVULSION, JONES FRACTURES)

Ryan Reese, DO • Mark E. Lavallee, MD, CSCS, FACSM

BASICS

DESCRIPTION

- Fractures of the proximal 5th metatarsal of the foot occur at different locations, often with different etiologies. Prognosis and treatment differ vastly, and there is potential to have chronic pain and instability of the foot if not treated properly. Proximal 5th metatarsal fractures are classified into three types by region, especially in relation to the joint at the base of the 4th/5th metatarsals (1,2,3,4):
  - Avulsion fracture of the tuberosity:
    - Near splayed insertion of the peroneus brevis tendon (within 0.5 cm from proximal tip of 5th metatarsal)
    - Located extra-articular and do not extend into the joint between the 4th and 5th metatarsal. These fractures intersect cubometatarsal joint
  - Jones fracture (metaphyseal–diaphyseal junction):
    - Fracture line extends into or toward the articulation between the bases of the 4th and 5th metatarsals (measuring usually between 0.5 cm and 1.5 cm from the proximal tip of the 5th metatarsal).
    - They heal more slowly and are prone to delayed union and nonunion because they have a relatively poor blood supply and have increased stresses across intertarsal ligament and fracture site.
  - Diaphyseal stress fractures:
    - Most commonly occur just distal to the 4th and 5th intermetatarsal articulation to midshaft
    - Result of chronic, repetitive microtrauma, especially in younger athletes
    - Heal most slowly and have greatest risk of delayed union, nonunion, and recurrence.
  - Torg classification according to healing potential (2):
    - **Type I** (acute): acute without prior fracture. X-rays show clean fracture without sclerosis.
    - **Type II** (delayed union): involves prior symptoms or a known stress fracture. X-rays show medullary sclerosis and a widened fracture line.
    - **Type III** (nonunion): involves prior symptoms or a known stress fracture. X-rays show evidence of repeated trauma, widened fracture line, and exuberant sclerosis (suggesting fracture nonunion).
- Synonym(s): dancer's, tennis, or pseudo-Jones fracture: avulsion fracture of base of the 5th metatarsal

EPIDEMIOLOGY

- 5th metatarsal fractures account for 68% of metatarsal fractures (2).
- **Avulsion fractures** are the most common type of fracture (93% of fractures).
- **Diaphyseal stress fractures** are the least common type of fracture (3% of fractures).

ETIOLOGY AND PATHOPHYSIOLOGY

- Avulsion fracture of the tuberosity: inversion ankle injuries
- Jones fracture: twisting injuries of the forefoot, vertical forces over the lateral aspect of forefoot while foot is plantarflexed, trauma to the area
- Stress fracture: repetitive impact to the lateral foot (3)

RISK FACTORS

- Previous fracture to the proximal 5th metatarsal
- Lateral ankle instability
- Static forefoot adduction

COMMONLY ASSOCIATED CONDITIONS

Associated injuries and complications:

- Lateral ankle sprain: Tuberosity avulsion fractures are commonly associated with ankle sprains with the foot inverted and plantarflexed. The anterior talofibular and calcaneofibular ligaments often are injured, and there may be swelling and ecchymosis just anterior and distal to the lateral malleolus.
- Proximal 5th metatarsal stress fracture: Patient may have had a previously undiagnosed and slightly symptomatic stress fracture of the proximal 5th metatarsal.
- There is a high incidence of delayed union, nonunion, and refracture with Jones and diaphyseal stress fractures.

DIAGNOSIS

HISTORY

- Q: How and when did it occur?
- A: Mechanism of injury is important to determine.
- Q: Did athlete injure this foot previously?
- A: Determine presence of previous fracture of the 5th metatarsal.
- Q: Was there a recent history of ankle sprain prior to this injury?
- A: Loss of proprioception and reflex inhibition may have predisposed athlete to this injury.
- Q: History of other medical conditions?
- A: Osteoporosis, multiple stress fractures, diabetes or other causes of peripheral neuropathy

PHYSICAL EXAM

- Signs and symptoms:
  - Patient may complain of pain over the lateral aspect of foot, especially when weight-bearing on plantarflexed foot.
  - Jones fractures often occur due to a pivot in the direction opposite the planted foot.
  - Often, there may be swelling or ecchymosis of the proximal 5th metatarsal and lateral foot.
- Physical examination:
  - Patient is tender to palpation over the proximal 5th metatarsal.
  - Palpate the peroneus brevis tendon to assess its integrity.
  - Check neurovascular status: posterior tibial and dorsalis pedis pulses and normal capillary refill.
  - Resisted eversion/external rotation of foot activates the peroneus brevis muscle and checks its strength; will typically reproduce pain at fracture site with activation
  - Full examination of the distal fibular, lateral ligaments, and foot helps identify associated ankle or foot injury.
  - Check sensation: If decreased around lateral aspect of foot, the lateral dorsal cutaneous nerve, a branch off the sural nerve, may be injured.

DIFFERENTIAL DIAGNOSIS

- Peroneus brevis or peroneus longus tendon injury
- Anterior process calcaneus fracture
- Apophysis (Secondary ossification center closes between ages 9 and 11 yr in girls, 11 and 14 yr in boys.)
- Apophysitis (Iselin disease) or apophyseal avulsion fracture
- Accessory ossicles
- Hematoma of lateral proximal foot
- Midshaft diaphyseal fracture of the 5th metatarsal
- Sprain of the cubometatarsal joint

DIAGNOSTIC TESTS & INTERPRETATION

- Standard x-ray films: anteroposterior (AP), lateral, and oblique views of the foot. If findings are suggestive of ankle trauma meeting the Ottawa criteria (patient between ages of 15 and 55 yr old with inability to walk five steps after injury *or* tender over posterior third of distal fibula), ankle films (AP, lateral, and oblique views) should also be taken.
- Acute stress fractures may not be detected on initial radiographs. Repeat radiographs recommended in 10 to 14 days if clinically suspected (2).

TREATMENT

Acute treatment:

- **ANALGESIA:**
  - Apply ice, rest, and elevate foot.
  - Oral pain relief (acetaminophen or tramadol) or topical lidocaine are often sufficient if reduction not necessary.
  - If reduction is needed, performing a hematoma block (2 to 5 mL of 1% lidocaine)
  - Significantly displaced fracture warrants an orthopedic referral for possible surgery.
- **REDUCTION TECHNIQUES:**
  - Generally, not recommended if surgical fixation is an option
  - Grab the 5th toe and distract in a longitudinal plane. Apply plantar or dorsal pressure to the proximal portion of the 5th metatarsal.
- **POSTREDUCTION EVALUATION:**
  - Check alignment via postreduction radiographs.
- **IMMOBILIZATION:**
  - Avulsion fractures:
    - Place in a hard-soled shoe or postoperative shoe for 3 to 4 wk (1)[A].
    - Can place in a walking boot or walking cast if can't ambulate without pain in shoe, or if worried about patient compliance. Will reduce plantar flexion thus forefoot load; may weight-bear as tolerated (1,3)[A].
  - Jones (metaphyseal–diaphyseal) fractures and diaphyseal stress fractures:
    - *Type I* (acute): For nondisplaced or minimally displaced fractures (<2 mm), can place patient in short leg cast and make strict non–weight-bearing for 6 to 8 wk (or longer). Otherwise, consider surgical fixation (1,3)[A]. Nonsurgical fracture healing rates approach 75%.
    - *Type II* (delayed union/stress): Consider surgical fixation because of better prognosis and quicker return to activity. Occasionally can consider prolonged immobilization (up to 16 wk) with non–weight-bearing for selective patients (1,2)[A].
    - *Type III* (nonunion): Consider surgical fixation (1,3)[A].

ADDITIONAL THERAPIES

- Special considerations: When deciding on treatment for type II fractures, consider the athlete's timetable and previous medical history.
- Operative treatment is preferred for elite athletes who wish to avoid the prolonged immobilization of conservative treatment.
- Occasionally after conservative treatment, a nonunion develops secondary to "distal to proximal" vascular supply to the bone.
- Bone stimulation (electrical or ultrasound) has shown in some cases to improve healing for delayed union and nonunion fractures (1)[B]. Progression to surgery may be indicated instead of using bone stimulation or if there is inadequate healing with bone stimulation.
- **REHABILITATION:**
  - Avulsion fractures: Start with range of motion and progress to strengthening of the peroneus brevis (external rotation and pronation of the foot). Patient may return to play after 3 to 4 wk and when no longer symptomatic.
  - Jones fractures: Once no longer immobilized, start with range of motion and progress to strengthening. Electrical stimulation may help patient initially learn to reactivate musculature. Resume weight-bearing activities slowly after radiographic and clinical healing progressive rehab for strength and proprioception.

SURGERY/OTHER PROCEDURES

- Avulsion fractures rarely require surgery (3)[A].
- Jones (metaphyseal–diaphyseal) and diaphyseal stress fractures:
  - Type I: Consider surgical fixation (open reduction, internal fixation with a cannulated screw) for athletes and active patients who wish quicker return to play (1,2,3,5)[A].
  - Type II (delayed union) and type III (nonunion): Refer for surgical evaluation (1,3)[A].

ONGOING CARE

FOLLOW-UP RECOMMENDATIONS

Referral/disposition:

- Orthopedic referral for surgery as indicated above and for avulsion fractures that are displaced (rare), comminuted (rare), or involve >30% of the cubo-metatarsal articulation
- Patients not responding to home exercise programs after immobilization is complete may benefit from referral to physical therapy.
- *Type I* Jones or diaphyseal stress fractures should be referred to an orthopedist if patient prefers surgery in order to return to play quicker or the fracture is displaced or comminuted.

REFERENCES

1. Bowes J, Buckley R. Fifth metatarsal fractures and current treatment. *World J Orthop*. 2016;7(12):793–800.
2. Cheung CN, Lui TH. Proximal fifth metatarsal fractures: anatomy, classification, treatment and complications. *Arch Trauma Res*. 2016;5(4):e33298.
3. Fetzer GB, Wright RW. Metatarsal shaft fractures and fractures of the proximal fifth metatarsal. *Clin Sports Med*. 2006;25(1):139–150.
4. Hatch RL, Alsobrook JA, Clugston JR. Diagnosis and management of metatarsal fractures. *Am Fam Physician*. 2007;76(6):817–826.
5. Yates J, Feeley I, Sasikumar S, et al. Jones fracture of the fifth metatarsal: is operative intervention justified? A systematic review of the literature and meta-analysis of results. *Foot (Edinb)*. 2015;25(4):251–257.

ADDITIONAL READING

Porter DA. Fifth metatarsal jones fractures in the athlete. *Foot Ankle Int*. 2007;39(2):250–258.

CLINICAL PEARLS

Physician responses to common patient questions:

- Q: How long until I can play again?
- A: Avulsion fractures and diaphyseal stress fractures: up to 20 wk with conservative therapy. Type 1: ≥8 wk. Types 2 and 3: if casted, 3 to 5 mo and 8 wk for surgery

F

FRACTURE, FRONTAL SINUS

Andrew Smith, MD, FAAP

BASICS

Pediatric Considerations

- Frontal sinuses are not present at birth and begin to develop around 7 yr of age (last of sinuses), continuing to develop until puberty (1).
- Ethmoid and maxillary sinuses are present at birth.
- Sphenoid sinuses develop around 5 yr of age.

DESCRIPTION

- Typically owing to high-velocity blunt trauma localized to the face/head/frontal sinus area
- The most common mechanisms of injury are motor vehicle collisions, assaults, falls, and other accidents.
- Because the anterior table is thick, it requires 800 to 2,200 lb of force to cause frontal sinus fracture (twice the force required to fracture other facial bones).
- Most common classification identifies involved frontal sinus anatomy:
  - Anterior wall/table
  - Posterior wall/table
  - Anterior and posterior walls/table
  - Nasofrontal duct (NFD) involvement

EPIDEMIOLOGY

- Frontal sinus fractures account for 5–15% of all facial fractures (2).
- 35% have concomitant orbital fractures.
- 17% have zygomatic fractures.
- 15% have nasoorbitoethmoid fractures.
- 0.7–2.1% have involvement of both anterior and posterior walls of the frontal sinus
- More common in males

RISK FACTORS

- High-velocity trauma to the face, especially in presence of other facial bone fractures
- Motor vehicle collisions, assaults, and falls are the most common causes of mechanisms of injury (3).
- Acromegaly: size and extension of frontal sinuses enlarged

GENERAL PREVENTION

- Avoidance of motor vehicle collisions
- Proper use of vehicle safety restraints (4)

COMMONLY ASSOCIATED CONDITIONS

- Due to high amount of force required, concomitant facial and bodily injuries are common.
- Laceration of the supraorbital ridge, glabella, or lower forehead
- Frontal ecchymosis
- Disruption of the NFD
- Intracranial injuries in 12–17% of patients with frontal sinus fractures
- Associated cerebrospinal fluid (CSF) leak in ~15% of patients with frontal sinus fractures
- Ocular injuries are present in up to 59%.
- Periorbital fractures
- Traumatic subcutaneous emphysema (TSE)
- Pneumothorax is present in up to 24% (5).
- Upper and lower extremity fractures are present in up to 25% (5).
- Concussion

DIAGNOSIS

- Evaluate and treat life-threatening injuries first.
- Carefully palpate the frontal area for crepitus or depression.
- Lacerations over the frontal sinus area should raise suspicion of frontal sinus fracture and mandate digital palpation for a fracture.
- Perform a nasal speculum examination looking for blood, septal hematoma, or CSF high in the nasal cavity.
- Perform otoscopic exam looking for otorrhea and/or hemotympanum (indicating more serious cranial injury).
- Perform a careful neurologic examination to look for central nervous system (CNS) injury, including concussion.
- Perform a careful ophthalmologic exam.

HISTORY

- Victim of motor vehicle collision, assault to head/face, fall, or other high-velocity trauma
- May or may not have loss of consciousness

PHYSICAL EXAM

Failure to diagnose a frontal sinus fracture can lead to abscess formation, meningitis, mucocele formation, osteomyelitis of the calvarium, or permanent cosmetic deformity. Findings to raise concern for frontal sinus fracture are:

- Laceration on the supraorbital ridge, glabella, or lower forehead.
- Ecchymosis of periorbital region.
- Periorbital edema.
- Depression or step-off identified on palpation of frontal sinus area.
- Crepitus over the frontal sinus area.
- Subcutaneous emphysema of periorbital region.
- Associated facial trauma with supraorbital, orbital, nasal, frontonasoethmoid, or maxillary fractures.
- Associated ocular trauma may be present.
- Bloody discharge from the nose without visible nasal source.
- Clear rhinorrhea or otorrhea indicative of CSF leak.
- Absent tearing that may be indicative of NFD injury.
- Diplopia with upward or downward gaze.
- Supraorbital ridge anesthesia.
- Loss of consciousness or altered mental status secondary to associated brain injury or posterior table fracture.
- Diplopia, anesthesia to skin surrounding eye, "postnasal drip" sensation (owing to CSF leak).
- May present with facial subcutaneous emphysema following Valsalva maneuver owing to previously undiagnosed paranasal fracture following facial trauma

DIFFERENTIAL DIAGNOSIS

- Nasofrontoethmoid fractures
- Cribriform plate fractures
- Facial fractures, including the orbits, maxilla, nasal, and zygomatic bones
- Frontal bone fractures not involving the frontal sinus (may have a similar presentation)

DIAGNOSTIC TESTS & INTERPRETATION

- Halo sign test on filter paper to identify CSF leak. Confirmatory test for CSF leak is the β_2-transferrin test.
- Requires acute examination and imaging:
  - Computed tomography (CT) scanning is the imaging modality of choice:
    - Serial 1.5-mm cuts in both the axial and coronal planes
    - Identification of frontal sinus fractures and concomitant paranasal and facial fractures
    - Anterior table fracture, displaced or non-displaced; *displacement* is defined as bony displacement more than or equal to the width of the outer table.
    - Posterior table fracture identification: Associated intracranial injuries on CT scan may include subdural hemorrhage or pneumocephalus.
    - Frontonasal duct integrity
  - Caldwell and lateral radiographic views are good for preliminary evaluation, but frontal sinus fractures can be subtle on these films. Sinus pathology is strongly suspected when the x-rays show air-fluid levels, a diffusely cloudy sinus, or pneumocephalus.

TREATMENT

- Prehospital:
  - Physical examination, including complete neurologic exam
  - High suspicion for fracture given nature of trauma and physical findings
  - Airway, breathing, and circulation (ABCs)
  - Identify concomitant life-threatening injuries (5)[B].
  - Cervical immobilization as needed

- Emergency department (ED) treatment:
  - If during frontal scalp laceration irrigation, the patient can taste the irrigating solution or notes the irrigating fluid in the nose, the frontal sinus is disrupted.
  - Lacerations overlying frontal sinus fractures involving only the anterior table may be sutured in the ED. Ear, nose, and throat (ENT) or plastic surgery should evaluate lacerations associated with more complex sinus injuries.
  - If an isolated simple anterior table fracture is noted without a posterior table fracture and intracranial injuries are ruled out, the presence of a frontonasal duct injury should be evaluated by instilling fluorescein into the frontal sinus. Lack of visualization of the fluorescein in the nose is indicative of disruption of the duct.
  - Perioperative antibiotics are indicated in patients requiring surgical management. The use of antibiotics prophylactically and postoperatively is controversial (6)[A].
  - Nondisplaced frontal sinus fracture with a patent NFD and *no* neurologic involvement usually can be managed nonsurgically.
  - All displaced anterior wall fractures, all posterior wall fractures, all frontal sinus fractures with involvement/obstruction of the NFD, and all frontal sinus fractures with neurologic involvement require further surgical evaluation and probable surgical repair.

MEDICATION

- Cefotaxime: adult: 2 g intravenous (IV); children: 50 mg/kg IV single dose
- Cephalexin: adult: 250 to 500 mg PO QID.; children: 25 to 50 mg/kg/day divided QID

ADDITIONAL THERAPIES

The approach to each patient should be individualized but, in general, is based on three clinical factors:

- Fracture location and displacement
- Dural and cerebral involvement
- Damage to the frontal sinus drainage system

ADMISSION, INPATIENT, AND NURSING CONSIDERATIONS

- Initial stabilization:
  - ABCs of trauma care: Attend to the airway as the first priority:
    - Rapid sequence intubation (RSI) is the initial airway management of choice.
    - Massive facial injuries may require a surgical airway if RSI is unsuccessful.
  - If associated injuries are present, protect the cervical spine until cleared.
  - Other major injuries and life threats take precedence over the frontal sinus fracture.
- Admission criteria:
  - Patients with other significant associated trauma
  - Patients with posterior table fractures (neurosurgery or ENT evaluation)
  - Patients with associated intracranial injuries (neurosurgery)
  - Patients with CSF leak
- Discharge criteria:
  - Patients with frontal sinus fractures who may be discharged are those with isolated frontal sinus fracture and those who have no involvement of the posterior table or evidence of an intracranial injury on CT scan.
  - Referral to ENT in 24 to 36 hr is appropriate.
  - Patients with complex fractures may be discharged when cleared by neurosurgery and/or ENT.

ONGOING CARE

PATIENT EDUCATION

- Avoid Valsalva maneuver (e.g., sneezing, nose blowing, etc.) to minimize risk of subcutaneous emphysema.
- Avoid air travel for a period (individualize for each patient) after frontal sinus fracture.

COMPLICATIONS

- Early complications:
  - Contour deformity postoperatively
  - Sinusitis: Treat with antibiotics and decongestants. If swelling and/or pain to periorbital region persists, may need to refer for surgical sinus mucosal obliteration.
  - Hematoma (1)[C]
  - Wound infection (1)[C]
  - Meningitis
- Late complications:
  - Thrombosis of cavernous sinus
  - Hypoesthesia/anesthesia (1)[C]
  - Encephalitis
  - Mucocele
  - Mucopyocele
  - Osteomyelitis
  - Brain abscess
  - Surgical referral for any of these

REFERENCES

1. Guy WM, Brissett AE. Contemporary management of traumatic fractures of the frontal sinus. *Otolaryngol Clin North Am*. 2013;46(5):733–748.
2. Kim IA, Boahene KD, Byrne PJ. Trauma in facial plastic surgery: frontal sinus fractures. *Facial Plast Surg Clin North Am*. 2017;25(4):503–511.
3. Fox PM, Garza R, Dusch M, et al. Management of frontal sinus fractures: treatment modality changes at a level 1 trauma center. *J Craniofac Surg*. 2014;25(6):2038–2042.
4. Chouake RJ, Miles BA. Current opinion in otolaryngology and head and neck surgery: frontal sinus fractures. *Curr Opin Otolaryngol Head Neck Surg*. 2017;25(4):326–331.
5. Rodriguez ED, Stanwix MG, Nam AJ, et al. Twenty-six-year experience treating frontal sinus fractures: a novel algorithm based on anatomical fracture pattern and failure of conventional techniques. *Plastic Reconstr Surg*. 2008;122(6):1850–1866.
6. Gerhard GS, Borsuk DE, Okhah Z, et al. Antibiotics and facial fractures: evidence-based recommendations compared with experience-based practice. *Craniomaxillofac Trauma Reconstr*. 2015;8(1):64–78.

ADDITIONAL READING

- Bell RB. Management of frontal sinus fractures. *Oral Maxillofac Surg Clin North Am*. 2009;21(2):227–242.
- Bell RB, Dierks EJ, Brar P, et al. A protocol for the management of frontal sinus fractures emphasizing sinus preservation. *J Oral Maxillofac Surg*. 2007;65(5):825–839.
- Brasileiro BF, Cortez AL, Asprino L, et al. Traumatic subcutaneous emphysema of the face associated with paranasal sinus fractures: a prospective study. *J Oral Maxillofac Surg*. 2005;63(8):1080–1087.
- Eirale C, Lockhart R, Chalabi H. Conservative treatment in an isolated anterior wall frontal bone fracture in an elite soccer player. *Clin J Sport Med*. 2010;20(2):125–127.
- Kalavrezos N. Current trends in the management of frontal sinus fractures. *Injury*. 2004;35(4):340–346.
- Kaufman BR, Heckler FR. Sports-related facial injuries. *Clin Sports Med*. 1997;16(3):543–562.
- Keefe SO, et al. Frontal sinus fractures. In: English GM, ed. *Otolaryngology*. Vol 4. Rev ed. Philadelphia, PA: JB Lippincott; 1994:342–364.
- Lauder A, Jalisi S, Spiegel J, et al. Antibiotic prophylaxis in the management of complex midface and frontal sinus trauma. *Laryngoscope*. 2010;120(10):1940–1945.
- Manson PN. Maxillofacial injuries. *Emerg Med Clin North Am*. 1984;2(4):761–782.
- Rohrich RJ, Hollier LH. Management of frontal sinus fractures. Changing concepts. *Clin Plast Surg*. 1992;19(1):219–232.
- Tiwari P, Higuera S, Thornton J, et al. The management of frontal sinus fractures. *J Oral Maxillofac Surg*. 2005;63(9):1354–1360.

CLINICAL PEARLS

For lacerations, ecchymosis, and/or edema to frontal sinus region following trauma, consider and evaluate with CT scan for frontal sinus fracture.

F

FRACTURE, HAMATE: HOOK, BODY

Mark Stovak, MD

BASICS

DESCRIPTION

A fracture through the hook or the body of the hamate

EPIDEMIOLOGY

Hamate fractures occur in three patterns:

- Type 1: hook
- Type 2a: coronal (dorsal oblique and splitting)
- Type 2b: transverse (1)

Incidence

- Hook fracture:
  - Hook of the hamate fractures account for <2% of all carpal bone fractures (2).
  - The number of hook of the hamate fractures reported in the literature is low because routine x-rays usually are normal, and symptoms are nonspecific. Standard radiographs are often inconclusive and only identify 31% of fractures (2,3).
  - Average length of time from injury to correct diagnosis was 27 days with advanced imaging (4).
  - Fractures most commonly occur at the base of the hook (1).
- Body fracture: Body of the hamate fracture is rare and much less common than hook fractures.

ETIOLOGY AND PATHOPHYSIOLOGY

- Acute traumatic injury
- Repetitive stress leads to a stress fracture.

RISK FACTORS

Hook fracture: sporting activities that involve a bat, club, or racquet (2)

GENERAL PREVENTION

Avoid holding the handle end of the bat, club, or stick in the palm to prevent it from creating pressure on the hook of the hamate.

DIAGNOSIS

HISTORY

- Hook fracture:
  - Hook of the hamate fracture occurs in athletes who use equipment with a handle (e.g., golf clubs, baseball bats, and racquets) (2).
  - Athlete grips the handle of the club, bat, or racquet over the distal ulnar aspect of the palm, placing the handle in close proximity to the hook of the hamate (2).
  - In golf, the fracture often occurs when the club head accidentally strikes too much ground and a large divot is taken. In baseball, most fractures occur at the end of forceful check swings as opposed to swings that make contact with the ball (2).
  - A less common mechanism of injury is a fall on an outstretched hand (2).
  - Stress fractures are also possible of the hook and are likely if no traumatic event can be identified in the history.
- Body fracture:
  - Body fractures often result from punching a hard stationary object, such as a wall, with a closed fist (type 2a). The 4th and 5th metacarpals are driven back into the hamate, leading to a fracture. Body fractures may accompany a boxer's fracture (1).
  - 4th and 5th metacarpal dislocations are also common findings with body fractures.
  - They also may occur when the hamate is smashed between two objects in a dorsopalmar fashion (type 2b) (1).
- Stress fractures have been described from repetitive military-style knuckle push-ups (5).

PHYSICAL EXAM

- Point tenderness occurs in the palm over the hook of the hamate. The hook is located by projecting a line from the pisiform to the center of the head of the index metacarpal. Rarely, if the fracture is at the base of the hook, pain may be greater over the dorsal hamate than over the hook in the palm (because the hamate is covered on the volar aspect with thick skin, subcutaneous fibrofatty tissue, and parts of the palmaris brevis muscle and transverse carpal ligament, making palpation difficult) (2).
- Painful and weak grasp (2)
- Positive "pull test" may elicit pain on resisted flexion of the ulnar two digits with the wrist held in ulnar deviation (2). This test places force against the injured hamate as the flexor tendons lever against it during finger flexion and ulnar deviation (6).
- Check pulses: An Allen test will help to rule out ulnar artery thrombosis (2).
- Signs of partial or complete 4th/5th flexor digitorum profundus (FDP) tendon rupture may be present. Pain with grip; decreased grip strength; crepitance with 4th/5th finger motion; and, eventually, loss of active flexion at the 4th/5th finger distal interphalangeal joints may indicate FDP injury; a small percentage of all hook fractures are correctly diagnosed only after FDP tendon rupture (2,3).
- Decreased sensation or weakness may be due to ulnar or median nerve injury. The fracture fragments may injure the nerves directly, or swelling and inflammation may injure them indirectly (2).

DIFFERENTIAL DIAGNOSIS

- Flexor/extensor carpi ulnaris tendon injury
- Metacarpal/carpal bone fracture or contusion
- Ulnocarpal ligament sprain
- Triangular fibrocartilaginous complex tear
- Ulnar artery thrombosis
- Ulnar nerve entrapment/neuropathy
- Carpal tunnel syndrome

DIAGNOSTIC TESTS AND INTERPRETATION

- Hook fracture:
  - The routine wrist series (anteroposterior [AP], lateral, and oblique views) usually are inconclusive, only identifying 31% of fractures and often delaying diagnosis (2).
  - Ring of the hook can be visualized on AP view; if it is not present, this may be a clue to a hook fracture (3).
  - Carpal tunnel view often will aid in making the diagnosis. However, to obtain this view, the wrist must be forcefully hyperextended. During the acute phase of the injury, pain and limited range of motion may not allow proper positioning to make this x-ray possible. The carpal tunnel view is 40–50% sensitive (2).
  - Another useful view is the supinated oblique thumb–abducted view (2).
  - An additional view is the hamate hook lateral view with the hook in the first web space with the wrist ulnar deviated and the thumb opposed (2).
  - Computed tomography (CT) scanning is the gold standard for diagnosis but often is unnecessary if plain films show the fracture. CT scans are useful if plain films are negative and a fracture is highly suspected. CT scanning has the advantage of visualizing both hamates at the same time and can be used to evaluate the extremely rare case of a bipartite hamate, which usually is bilateral and is a normal variant. CT scan is performed with both hands in the praying position (palm to palm). CT scanning has a 100% sensitivity, a 98.4% specificity, and a 97.2% accuracy in the diagnosis of acute fractures (2,6).
  - Magnetic resonance imaging (MRI) may be useful to evaluate for tendon or nerve injury (6).
- Body fracture:
  - The routine wrist series (AP, lateral, and oblique views) is more useful for the diagnosis of body fractures than for hook fractures. The oblique and lateral views are the most useful. However, many fractures are still missed by plain films (1).
  - CT scan may be needed to delineate further the exact fracture pattern and degree of fragment displacement. CT scan should be considered when routine films are negative but a fracture is highly suspected (1).

TREATMENT

- Hook fracture:
  - Acute treatment (<2 wk):
    - *Conservative management:*
      - Conservative option for nondisplaced fractures is a short arm cast. The cast should immobilize the metacarpophalangeal joints of the 4th/5th fingers and be a thumb spica to decrease micromotion at the hook. Cast should be worn for 6 to 12 wk to prevent nonunion, but nonunion is common with nonoperative management. If pain is still present after cast removal, then excision for nonunion is the treatment of choice (2)[C].
    - Decision between casting and surgery is based on the lifestyle demands of the patient. The athlete who does not want to risk having a nonunion after casting may opt for surgery to minimize the time away from sport. Similarly, a patient with a job that requires repetitive grabbing, gripping, or lifting may elect for excision to reduce the risk of an extended period of time away from work (2)[C].
  - Delayed treatment (>2 wk):
    - Nonunion of the hook of the hamate is very common. Nonunion is related to micromotion from the soft tissue attachments to the hook but also may be related to a tenuous blood supply similar to the scaphoid (2,4)[C].
    - Excision of the hook is the treatment of choice for these injuries to prevent a nonunion. The sooner the fragment is removed and the base smoothed, the less likely is the chance for tendon rupture and/or neurovascular damage. There is a 15–17% incidence of flexor tendon ruptures in untreated hook fractures (2)[C].
    - An alternative approach is open reduction and internal fixation (ORIF); the goal is to maintain maximal grip strength by preserving the pulley system for the 4th/5th FDP tendons. Although this seems logical, the loss of grip strength associated with excision has been minimal, resulting in excision being the most popular surgical treatment method. Owing to the risk of nonunion and the potential for symptomatic hardware, ORIF is not recommended in athletes (2)[C].
    - Treatment for painless nonunion is excision to reduce the risk of tendon rupture and/or neurovascular injury (2)[C].
    - Ultrasound therapy has some reported success. A case study of two baseball players with hook of hamate fracture nonunion 5 and 3.5 mo postinjury were successfully treated with ultrasound therapy. The patients received therapy for 20 min a day for 4 mo and were limited to daily activities during this time. Bone union was confirmed with a CT scan, and neither patient reported any pain nor complications at a 1-yr follow-up. However, these athletes were 15 and 16 yr of age and began treatment many months after their injury (3).
- Body fracture:
  - Coronal fractures are often associated with 4th and 5th metacarpal dislocations that require reduction. Once reduced, stability must be assessed. If the reduction is stable and the fracture nondisplaced, then a short arm cast can be used for 4 to 6 wk. If the fracture is displaced, then ORIF or closed reduction with pinning must be used to obtain congruent joint surfaces to prevent degenerative joint disease (1)[C].
  - Transverse fractures, if not displaced, can be treated in a short arm cast for 4 to 6 wk or by ORIF or closed reduction and pinning if displacement has occurred (1)[C].

SURGERY/OTHER PROCEDURES

Hook fracture:

- Acute treatment (<2 wk):
  - One option is excision of the hook distal to the fracture. Most patients return to their previous level of functioning in their sport or occupation, and return to activity is symptom dependent.
  - Immobilization lasts 2 wk with light motion and throwing at 4 wk and return to bat or club sports at 6 wk. The palmar incision may demonstrate prolonged sensitivity for 3 mo, but a glove with padding may be used until scar sensitivity resolves. Excision has been the favored approach for both displaced and nondisplaced fractures (2)[C].

ONGOING CARE

PROGNOSIS

- Prognosis of hook fractures is generally good if they are diagnosed and treated (cast, excision, ORIF) early before tendon injury/rupture occurs (2).
- Prognosis for hamate body fractures is generally good if they are diagnosed and treated (cast, ORIF, closed reduction and pinned) early enough to maintain congruent joint surfaces (6).

COMPLICATIONS

- Complete rupture of the FDP tendon is reported to occur in 14–17% of cases of nonunion. The FDP of the little finger ruptures more commonly than that of the ring finger (2).
- Hamate hook fractures, when left untreated, reliably progress to nonunion with reported rates of 90–100% (6).
- Complications related to fragment excision have been self-reported at a rate of 3% and include injury to the motor branch of the ulnar nerve or the superficial palmar arch intraoperatively and transient median or ulnar nerve neuropathy and decreased grip strength postoperatively (6).

REFERENCES

1. Hirano K, Inoue G. Classification and treatment of hamate fractures. *Hand Surg*. 2005;10(2–3):151–157.
2. Ivy A, Stern P. Hamate hook and pisiform fractures. *Operative Techniques in Sports Medicine*. 2016;24(2):94–99.
3. Bachoura A, Wroblewski A, Jacoby SM, et al. Hook of hamate fractures in competitive baseball players. *Hand (N Y)*. 2013;8(3):302–307.
4. Kadar A, Bishop AT, Suchyta MA, et al. Diagnosis and management of hook of hamate fractures. *J Hand Surg Eur Vol*. 2018;43(5):539–545.
5. Busche MN, Knobloch K, Rosenthal H, et al. Stress fracture of the hamate body and fourth metacarpal base following military style push-ups: an unusual trauma mechanism. *Knee Surg Sports Traumatol Arthrosc*. 2008;16(12):1158–1160.
6. Pan T, Lögters TT, Windolf J, et al. Uncommon carpal fractures. *Eur J Trauma Emerg Surg*. 2016;42(1):15–27.

CLINICAL PEARLS

- The treatment option that will allow the quickest return to play with the least amount of residual symptoms is excision of the hook of the hamate.
- Routine plain-film radiographs are not sensitive for identifying hook of the hamate fractures. A specialized view (e.g., carpal tunnel; radial-deviated, supinated oblique with thumb abduction; or hamate hook lateral) or a CT scan is usually needed for identification.
- Surgery is recommended to prevent tendon rupture even in the absence of pain related to fracture.

FRACTURE, HUMERAL HEAD

Julie Chuan, MD, FAAFP, CAQSM

BASICS

- *Caution*: Excessive movement of the arm may produce further neurovascular injury.
- *Controversy*: Prehospital reduction is not recommended because manipulation may lead to neurovascular compromise or further displacement of a fracture.

DESCRIPTION

- Proximal humeral fractures involve fractures of the humeral head, greater and lesser tuberosities, and anatomic and surgical neck.
- Mechanisms of injury:
  - Fall onto an outstretched hand
  - High-energy trauma in younger patients is often associated with soft tissue and neurovascular injury.
  - Low-energy trauma leads to fractures in the elderly due to osteoporotic bone.
  - Excessive rotation of the arm in the abducted position
  - Electrical shock or seizure
  - Pathologic fracture from metastatic disease

EPIDEMIOLOGY

Incidence

- Proximal humeral fractures account for 5% of all fractures.
- Typically seen in adults >65 yr old
- Female > male, 2:1
- In children, boys are 3 to 4 times more likely than girls.

Prevalence

- Proximal humerus fractures are the second most common upper extremity fractures (1)[C].
- In patients >65 yr, they are the third most common fracture after distal radius and hip fractures.

RISK FACTORS

- Highest risk factors for humeral head fractures are low bone mineral density and falls.
- Other risk factors include age, history of fracture, family history, smoking, heavy drinking, steroids, and rheumatoid arthritis.
- Indirect risk factors for falls include depression, epilepsy, diabetes with neuropathy, balance disorders, muscle weakness, and visual and hearing impairment (1)[C].

GENERAL PREVENTION

Increased moderate physical activity, calcium supplementation to optimize bone density, minimize psychotropic medications, and fall prevention (nonslip shoes) minimize the risk of proximal humerus fractures (1)[C].

DIAGNOSIS

Pediatric Considerations

- In children, proximal humeral fractures consist of metaphyseal fractures and physeal separations. Three fracture patterns tend to vary depending on the age group:
  - Children <5 yr: Salter-Harris type I fractures are seen:
    - Neonatal fractures occur from obstetric trauma, and pseudoparalysis is seen often.
    - Risk factors include vaginal delivery, breech, prolonged labor, and macrosomia (>4.5 kg).

ALERT
Physeal separation in an infant also may be the result of physical abuse, but a careful history should be performed before calling child protective services.

  - Children 5 to 10 yr: Metaphyseal fractures tend to occur in this age group because rapid growth causes thinning of the metaphyseal cortex. Most fractures are transverse or short oblique.
  - Children >11 yr: Salter-Harris type II fractures tend to be seen in adolescents (2)[C].
- Careful history and physical examination to localize the injury and to rule out any other significant injuries
- Assessment of neurovascular status:
  - Assess function of radial, median, ulnar, axillary (sensation to the lateral aspect of the shoulder), and musculocutaneous nerves (sensation to the extensor aspect of the forearm).
  - Presence of radial, ulnar, and brachial pulses and good capillary refill in all digits
- Shoulder radiographs: anteroposterior (AP), scapula Y, and axillary. Surgery is considered based on angulation, displacement, and age (2)[C].
- Consider "Little League shoulder":
  - Months of progressive pain with throwing
  - Tenderness over the anterolateral proximal humerus
  - Weakness with resisted shoulder abduction, internal and external rotation
  - X-rays show widening of the proximal humerus growth plate (2)[C].

PHYSICAL EXAM

- Signs and symptoms include:
  - Pain, swelling, and tenderness about the shoulder, especially around the greater tuberosity.
  - Difficulty in initiating active motion.
  - Position of the arm is often adducted and held closely against the chest.
  - Crepitus may be present.
  - Shoulder effusion owing to hemarthrosis developing into ecchymoses within 24 to 48 hr at the area of fracture and may spread to chest wall, flank, and distal extremity.
  - Diminished peripheral pulses or decreased sensation, especially over the deltoid muscle (axillary nerve).
  - Disruption of the deltoid contour or prominent subacromial sulcus suggests concurrent dislocation, often associated with high impact mechanism of injury.
- Remember to examine:

ALERT
Nerve: sensation over the deltoid muscle (axillary nerve) and distal motor and sensory function in the hand and fingers. 45% risk of nerve injury, axillary is the most common.

  - Vascular: radial and ulnar pulse, capillary refill time
  - Associated injuries: clavicle, scapula, wrist, and elbow for range of motion and tenderness for concomitant injury (1)[C]

DIFFERENTIAL DIAGNOSIS

- Shoulder dislocation
- Acute hemorrhagic bursitis
- Traumatic rotator cuff tear
- Acromioclavicular separation
- Calcific tendinitis
- Pathologic fracture

DIAGNOSTIC TESTS & INTERPRETATION

- Standard radiographs should be taken while in sling include AP, scapular Y, and axillary views:
  - True AP view, taken 35 to 40 degrees from the sagittal plane, shows the articular surface of the humeral head and glenohumeral joint space.
  - Scapular Y view, taken 90 degrees from the true AP and 40 degrees from the coronal plane, shows the scapular contour and position of the humeral head in the glenoid.
  - Axillary view, taken with the shoulder abducted 70 to 90 degrees with the beam cephalad, shows shoulder dislocations, humeral head compression fractures, and glenoid and lesser tuberosity fractures; may need to use trauma axillary view or Velpeau view
- Computed tomography (CT) scan: Consider CT scan if articular involvement is suspected to evaluate the glenoid and humeral head:
  - Intra-articular fractures
  - Suspected occult fractures
  - Posterolateral compression fractures
  - Evaluate for multipart fractures of humeral head (3)[A].

TREATMENT

Pediatric Considerations

- Birth fractures heal rapidly with only 2 to 3 wk of immobilization (2)[C].
- Pediatric patients are often less compliant with immobilization and less able to verbalize complaints and may benefit from admission to the hospital for observation and neurovascular checks.

ALERT

In children nearing skeletal maturity, determining the degree of displacement or separation of the proximal humeral epiphysis is essential because exact reduction is important to prevent later growth disturbance.

GENERAL MEASURES

Emergency department (ED) treatment:

- Proper immobilization, orthopedic consultation, and pain management
- Operative versus nonoperative treatment is decided in conjunction with orthopedics.
- Neer classification: This system identifies the number of fragments, displacement, and their location, 1 to 4 parts. The fractures consist of 2- to 4-part fractures, and the locations include the anatomic neck, the surgical neck, the greater tuberosity, and the lesser tuberosity:
  - Displacement is defined as >1 cm of separation or >45 degrees of angulation between fragments.
  - In general, the higher the number of fragments in the fracture and the greater the degree of displacement, the more difficult it is to manage the patient with a closed reduction (4)[C].
- AO (Arbeitsgemeinschaft für Osteosynthesefragen) classification:
  - A: unifocal, extra-articular, 2-part fracture with an intact blood supply
  - B: bifocal, extra-articular, 2-part fracture with possible injury to the blood supply
  - C: articular fracture involving the anatomic neck, high likelihood of injury to the blood supply, and risk of avascular necrosis of the humeral head (4)[C]
- Nonoperative treatment:
  - Initial immobilization and early motion: succeeds in many cases because most proximal humeral fractures are minimally displaced
  - Use a sling, swathe, and axillary pad to immobilize up to 2 wk and early physical therapy (4)[C].
  - Closed reduction should be performed with consultation of an orthopedic surgeon.
  - Conscious sedation should be used for all closed reductions.
  - Following reduction, the stability of the fracture can be tested in different positions to ascertain that significant displacement requiring surgical intervention will not occur.
- Surgical referral:
  - 1- and 2-part fractures are often treated successfully with closed reduction, but 3- and 4-part fractures are unstable and may need open reduction and internal fixation (ORIF) unless contraindicated.
  - Any open fractures, vascular or neurologic injuries require urgent surgical intervention.
- Surgical interventions:
  - Closed reduction percutaneous pinning
  - ORIF
  - Intramedullary nail
  - Hemi or total arthroplasty (4,5)[C]

MEDICATION

- Pain medications are indicated for comfort.
- Conscious sedation should be used if attempting a closed reduction.

ADDITIONAL THERAPIES

- A fracture is considered a nonunion if it is not clinically healed after 3 mo diagnosed on two consecutive x-rays taken 6 to 8 wk apart.
- Surgical management for nonunion is considered at 3 to 6 mo after injury (5)[C].
- Risk factors for nonunions include:
  - Displacement of the fracture.
  - Inadequate immobilization.
  - Aggressive rehabilitation.
  - Patient noncompliance.
- Comorbidities that can be a risk factor for nonunions include:
  - Disrupted blood supply.
  - Osteoporosis.
  - Alcoholism.
  - Tobacco usage.
  - Mental illness.
  - Systemic corticosteroids.
  - Rheumatologic disease.

ADMISSION, INPATIENT, AND NURSING CONSIDERATIONS

- Initial stabilization:
  - Airway, breathing, and circulation (ABCs) and secondary survey for associated injuries
  - Immediate immobilization is important to prevent further fracture displacement or neurovascular injury:
    - Sling with arm supported at the side or in the Velpeau position
    - Axillary pad also may be used for comfort.
    - After immobilization, perform another neurovascular examination.
- Admission criteria:
  - Open fractures for operative management and parenteral antibiotic therapy for open fractures
  - Displaced fracture that cannot be treated through closed reduction and therefore requires operation
  - Significant associated injuries that require admission and observation
- Discharge criteria:
  - Patients with either a nondisplaced fracture or a fracture that is treated successfully through closed reduction and who have no associated injuries

ONGOING CARE

The proximal humerus is supplied by the axillary artery, which is often disrupted with displaced fractures resulting in avascular necrosis of the humeral head.

PROGNOSIS

- About 90% are treated nonsurgically.
- Nonunions can be treated nonoperatively if pain is minimal with adequate range of motion and function.
- Nonunions can be surgically reduced with internal fixation if the glenohumeral articular surface is preserved.
- Arthroplasty is preferred when the articular surface is disrupted (5)[C].

REFERENCES

1. Tsuda T. Epidemiology of fragility fractures and fall prevention in the elderly: a systematic review of the literature. *Curr Orthop Pract*. 2017;28(6):580–585.
2. Popkin CA, Levine WN, Ahmad CS. Evaluation and management of pediatric proximal humerus fractures. *J Am Acad Orthop Surg*. 2015;23(2):77–86.
3. Robinson BC, Athwal GS, Sanchez-Sotelo J, et al. Classification and imaging of proximal humerus fractures. *Orthop Clin North Am*. 2008;39(4):393–403, v.
4. Kancherla VK, Singh A, Anakwenze OA. Management of acute proximal humeral fractures. *J Am Acad Orthop Surg*. 2017;25(1):42–52.
5. Cadet ER, Yin B, Schulz B, et al. Proximal humerus and humeral shaft nonunions. *J Am Acad Orthop Surg*. 2013;21(9):538–547.

ADDITIONAL READING

- Hawkins RJ, Angelo RL. Displaced proximal humeral fractures. Selecting treatment, avoiding pitfalls. *Orthop Clin North Am*. 1987;18(3):421–431.
- Neer CS II. Displaced proximal humeral fractures. I. Classification and evaluation. *J Bone Joint Surg Am*. 1970;52(6):1077–1089.
- Rasmussen S, Hvass I, Dalsgaard J, et al. Displaced proximal humeral fractures: results of conservative treatment. *Injury*. 1992;23(1):41–43.

CLINICAL PEARLS

- Axillary artery is the most common neurovascular injury and can result in avascular necrosis of the humeral head.
- When evaluating shoulder dislocations, consider associated humeral head fractures.
- When the fracture is stable with evidence of callus on radiograph, consider initiating gentle range of motion exercises as early as tolerated.

FRACTURE, HUMERAL SHAFT

Julie Chuan, MD, FAAFP, CAQSM

BASICS

- Direct trauma from a fall
- Direct blow to the upper arm
- Fall on elbow or outstretched arm (FOOSH injury)
- Motor vehicle or industrial accident
- Pitching a ball (Torque causes a spiral fracture.)
- Bone malignancy (pathologic fracture) (1)[B]

DESCRIPTION

- Transverse fractures occur from a bending force.
- Spiral fractures occur from torsion.
- Oblique fractures occur from bending and torsion and may have an associated butterfly fragment.
- Proximal or distal comminuted fractures occur from compressive forces.

Pediatric Considerations

Spiral fractures in children are concerning for child abuse.

EPIDEMIOLOGY

- Bimodal distribution in the 3rd and 7th decades
- 3rd decade male predominance owing to sports and vehicular trauma
- 7th decade female predominance owing to simple falls (1)[B]
- 90% are due to trauma.
- Risk factors include trauma, increasing age, and osteoporosis.
- Types:
  - Midshaft: 60%
  - Proximal shaft: 25%
  - Distal shaft: 10% (1)[B]

DIAGNOSIS

- History and physical examination with special attention to a thorough neurovascular and skin examination
- Consider associated injuries such as ipsilateral shoulder, elbow, wrist, or hand fractures or dislocations.
- Diagnosis is confirmed by x-ray.
- Prehospital:
  - Immobilize with sling and swath for transport.
  - Evaluate for open fracture.
  - Evaluate for distal neurologic and vascular deficit.
  - Rapid transport in presence of neurologic or vascular deficits

HISTORY

- History of fall: Simple trip and fall, a low-impact force, is often associated with older (70+ yr), osteoporotic women.
- Collision or direct blow: higher impact, occurring more commonly in younger men
- Pain after throwing or pitching
- History of malignancy
- *Consider as pathologic fractures any humerus fracture produced by low-energy mechanism; the humerus can be a common site of metastatic disease.*

Pediatric Considerations

- "Falls" in toddlers or infants are concerning for abuse.
- Check for other bruises and injuries suggesting abuse.
- Examine the elbow in children who are guarding their arm.
- Elbow dislocations are more common in toddlers (nursemaid's elbow).
- Supracondylar fractures are more common in children when they sustain a fall.

PHYSICAL EXAM

- Pain and swelling over the area of the humeral shaft
- Shortening, deformity, or decreased mobility
- Crepitus on gentle passive range of motion (ROM)
- Neurologic deficit (2)[C],(3)[B]:
  - Radial nerve is most commonly injured, occurring in 15% of humeral shaft fractures:
    - It is tethered down and emerges through the intermuscular septum at the middle to distal shaft.
    - Injury will affect active extension in the wrist, hand, and fingers.
    - Motor function can be tested by giving the "thumbs-up" sign.
    - Occurs most frequently in middle and distal shaft fractures and spiral fractures
    - Usually a neurapraxia or axonotmesis (perineurium and epineurium intact)
  - Ulnar nerve injury will affect finger abduction (spreading the fingers apart).
  - Median nerve injury will affect thumb opposition (thumb and small finger pinch), loss of sensation on the palmar surface of the thumb, and the index and middle fingers.
  - Injury to the largest branch of the median nerve is the anterior interosseous nerve. Damage will result in loss of hand and finger flexion.
- Vascular injury: presenting as decreased pulse, slow distal capillary refill, and/or cool extremity:
  - Brachial artery
  - Cephalic and basilic veins
- Open fracture: If the skin is disrupted over the site of the fracture, there is a high risk of infection and need for surgical evaluation.

DIFFERENTIAL DIAGNOSIS

- Bone contusion
- Muscle contusion: primarily the biceps, triceps, or deltoid
- Hematoma
- Tendon rupture: primarily the biceps
- Neurapraxia: primarily the radial nerve
- Abscess

DIAGNOSTIC TESTS & INTERPRETATION

- Anteroposterior (AP) and lateral views of the entire humerus are mandatory to assess for fracture pattern:
  - Displacement, including angulation and shortening type of fracture: transverse, spiral, oblique
  - Location of the fracture on the humeral shaft in relation to muscle attachments
  - Number of fracture segments (butterfly fragments) and comminution
- Include shoulder and elbow views to exclude associated joint involvement.
- The AO/ASIF system defines humeral shaft fractures as follows (3)[B]:
  - Type A: simple fractures:
    - A1: simple spiral
    - A2: simple short oblique
    - A3: simple transverse
  - Type B: wedge fractures:
    - B1: spiral wedge
    - B2: bending wedge
    - B3: fragmented wedge
  - Type C: complex pattern fractures:
    - C1: complex spiral
    - C2: segmental fracture
    - C3: irregular comminuted fracture
- Pathologic findings:
  - Pathologic fractures of the humeral shaft are associated with the following malignancies (1)[B]:
    - Women:
      - Breast 40%
      - Myeloma 23%
      - Lung 9%
      - Kidney 9%
    - Men:
      - Prostate 33%
      - Kidney 25%
      - Myeloma 8%
      - Lung 8%

TREATMENT

GENERAL MEASURES

- These fractures usually do not require elaborate reduction or immobilization.
- Fractures without neurovascular compromise can be treated conservatively; see immobilization options below.
- Immobilize for 4 to 6 wk until clinically and radiographically healed.
- Prehospital:
  - With the introduction of functional (Sarmiento) bracing, conservative treatment has become more popular and can be managed in the office.
  - Conservative care can be undertaken with 80% healing rates for adults with low to moderate functional demands. The degree of displacement accepted in these studies was up to 20 degrees and 2 cm of shortening:
    - Fractures can displace further after injury owing to contraction of the surrounding muscles (see below).
    - No randomized, controlled trials support these recommendations, so they are class C recommendations.
  - Open fractures or fractures associated with neurovascular compromise require immediate orthopedic consultation.
  - Children remodel well and usually are able to compensate with overgrowth for fractures up to 1.5 cm shortening and 20 degrees of angulation.
  - Anyone with high functional demands such as elite athletes, mechanics, and carpenters should be considered for surgical fixation for optimal anatomic alignment.
  - Of the nonunions, 90% ultimately heal with surgical intervention.
  - The carrying angle (valgus angle at the elbow when the arm is fully extended) is most often affected in displaced humeral shaft fractures (4)[C].

MEDICATION

- Immobilization: Immobilize to limit movement at the site of the fracture, which is one of the most effective methods of pain control.
- Ice: Icing the fracture site intermittently (15 min QID) for the first few days will reduce swelling and help to control pain.

- Elevation: After immobilization, try to elevate the arm above the level of the heart as much as possible to minimize swelling.
- Analgesic medications:
  - Narcotic analgesics: initially may be needed for adequate pain control
  - Nonnarcotic analgesics: After the fracture stabilizes (about 1 wk), nonsteroidal anti-inflammatory drugs (NSAIDs) and/or acetaminophen should provide sufficient pain relief.

ISSUES FOR REFERRAL

Surgical indications (4)[B]:

- Unacceptable alignment after closed reduction
- Radial nerve palsy at any evaluation, including after closed reduction
- Multisite trauma
- Open or segmental fractures
- Floating elbow: occurs when there is a fracture above and below the elbow and is considered an "unstable" injury
- Ipsilateral arm injuries
- Pathologic fractures
- Fracture with significant gap between segments usually represents muscle or fat separating the bone fragments and is unlikely to heal.
- Vascular injury: Refer for urgent vascular surgery evaluation.

ADDITIONAL THERAPIES

Consider displacing forces of the contracted muscles around the site of fracture when immobilizing the injury:

- Supraspinatus, infraspinatus, and teres minor externally rotate the humeral head.
- Subscapularis internally rotates the humeral head.
- Pectoralis pulls fragments toward the chest (medially) and forward (anteriorly).
- Latissimus and teres major pull fragments inward toward the chest.
- Deltoid displaces the fracture outward (abducts) away from the chest.

SURGERY/OTHER PROCEDURES

- Surgical options:
  - Intermedullary nailing
  - External fixation
  - Plate fixation
- Immobilization options for conservative management (3)[C]:
  - Sling immobilization: best for nondisplaced fractures that do not need distraction but can predispose to further shortening
  - Sugar-tong, coaptation, or U-shaped splint: best for limitation of transverse fracture displacement; limits shoulder and elbow motion, predisposing to stiffness after prolonged immobilization
  - Hanging cast: better for displaced or comminuted fractures needing distraction:
    - Elbow is placed in 90 degrees of flexion and the forearm in a neutral position.
    - Needs closer follow-up after injury to evaluate for signs of compartment syndrome
    - Cannot keep arm elevated to minimize swelling because gravity aids with distraction of the fracture
  - Functional bracing:
    - Preferred definitive treatment of transverse humerus shaft fractures and most other mid-shaft fractures
    - Allows for elbow mobility and earlier ROM; applied after initial swelling subsides and fracture starts to stabilize, usually 2 wk after injury
  - *Always repeat the vascular and neurologic examination after splint or cast application.*
- Surgical treatment:
  - Benefits:
    - More predictable alignment
    - Immediate stability
  - Risks:
    - Infection
    - Nerve and vascular injury
    - Nonunion
    - Anesthesia risks
- Conservative treatment (5)[B]:
  - Benefits:
    - Functional bracing usually allows for full or nearly full shoulder and elbow mobility.
    - Less infection and neurovascular injury risk
  - Risks:
    - Skin breakdown
    - Angular or translational malalignment/deformity
    - Nonunion (higher in simple fractures or type 1)
    - Shoulder or elbow stiffness

ONGOING CARE

- Immobilize until clinical healing and pain free, with bony callus on radiographs, usually 4 to 6 wk.
- Begin pendulum exercises within 1 wk.
- Start passive ROM after 2 wk to minimize shoulder and elbow stiffness.

FOLLOW-UP RECOMMENDATIONS

Nonunion risk factors:

- Open fracture
- Segmental (more than two fragments)
- Transverse (tend to displace into varus owing to displacing forces)
- Highly comminuted (unable to hold alignment)
- Associations: smoking, use of NSAIDs
- Comorbidities: diabetes, hypothyroid, infection, metabolic bone disease (2)[C]

Patient Monitoring

- Weekly follow-up: initially, every week to assess for displacement of the fracture
- Every other week: Once the fracture is stable on consecutive radiographs (usually 2 to 3 wk after injury), follow every 2 wk:
  - Once callus is noted on radiograph and no pain on examination, splint can be removed, and shoulder and elbow should be mobilized with gentle ROM exercises.
  - Continue to follow clinically until ROM is restored and healing noted on radiographs (usually 8 to 12 wk).
- At 12 to 14 wk, if union is not complete clinically and radiographically, consider referral to surgery for intervention.

PATIENT EDUCATION

- Compartment syndrome signs and symptoms if casted
- Monitor for new neurologic deficit.
- Monitor for new vascular deficit.
- Encourage wrist, hand, and shoulder ROM exercises.
- Sleep upright (recliner) if in a hanging cast until fracture is stable to minimize displacement.

COMPLICATIONS

- The most common complications are neurovascular compromise and nonunion.
- Neurovascular; radial nerve injury
- Nonunion; occurring in 2–10% of all humeral shaft fractures treated nonoperatively
- Varus angulation is most common in transverse fractures.
- Compartment syndrome

REFERENCES

1. Ekholm R, Adami J, Tidermark J, et al. Fractures of the shaft of the humerus. An epidemiological study of 401 fractures. *J Bone Joint Surg Br*. 2006;88(11):1469–1473.
2. Anglen JO, Archdeacon MT, Cannada LK, et al. Avoiding complications in the treatment of humeral fractures. *Instr Course Lect*. 2009;58:3–11.
3. Papasoulis E, Drosos GI, Ververidis AN, et al. Functional bracing of humeral shaft fractures. A review of clinical studies. *Injury*. 2010;41(7):e21–e27.
4. Ekholm R, Tidermark J, Törnkvist H, et al. Outcome after closed functional treatment of humeral shaft fractures. *J Orthop Trauma*. 2006;20(9):591–596.
5. Jawa A, McCarty P, Doornberg J, et al. Extra-articular distal-third diaphyseal fractures of the humerus. A comparison of functional bracing and plate fixation. *J Bone Joint Surg Am*. 2006;88(11):2343–2347.

ADDITIONAL READING

Simon R, Koenigsknecht S. *Emergency Orthopedics: the Extremities*. 3rd ed. Norwalk, CT: Appleton & Lange; 1995.

CLINICAL PEARLS

- Radial nerve injury is the most common neurovascular injury, occurring in about 15% of humeral shaft fractures.
- 10 to 20 degrees of angulation and 1 to 2 cm of shortening generally are well tolerated owing to compensated overgrowth and the surrounding muscles.
- Contraction of the muscles around the humerus can displace the fracture after the initial injury and should be considered when immobilizing the fracture.
- Consider close weekly follow-up after immobilization to monitor for fracture displacement.

FRACTURE, LATERAL AND MEDIAL MALLEOLI

Jeremy Schmitz, MD, ABFM • Kenneth P. Barnes, MD, MSc, CAQSM, FACSM

BASICS

DESCRIPTION

- Any fracture involving the most distal portions of the fibula or tibia, commonly known as the lateral and medial malleoli, respectively
- Synonyms: ankle fracture

EPIDEMIOLOGY

- Very common: ~170 ankle fractures per 100,000 people each year (1)
- Fractures to ankle or midfoot occur in <15% of ankle sprains.
- Most ankle fractures are malleolar fractures: 70% are unimalleolar (lateral being most common), 20% are bimalleolar, and 10% are trimalleolar (medial, lateral, and posterior malleoli) (1).

RISK FACTORS

- History of prior ankle injury
- Inadequate rehabilitation of injury
- Skeletal immaturity
- Weakness in dynamic (muscles) and/or static (ligamentous) stabilizers of the ankle
- Abnormal gait and/or foot biomechanics
- Foot and ankle proprioceptive dysfunction (dysfunction in the ability of the foot and ankle to adapt to uneven terrain)
- Cigarette smoking
- Obesity

COMMONLY ASSOCIATED CONDITIONS

- Pilon fracture
- Maisonneuve fracture

DIAGNOSIS

HISTORY

- Elicit mechanism: inversion versus eversion and external versus internal rotation of the ankle and foot
- Most frequent injury is inversion.
- Occasionally caused by direct blow to the affected malleolus
- Patient may hear or feel a "pop."
- Immediate, disabling pain and difficulty bearing weight
- Acute onset of swelling
- Development of ecchymosis
- Assess for neurovascular symptoms.

PHYSICAL EXAM

- Swelling and/or deformity about the ankle
- Ecchymosis
- Limited range of motion of the ankle
- Tenderness to palpation over the affected malleolus
- Difficulty or inability to bear weight and/or ambulate
- May note instability of the ankle joint on examination
- Check for signs of neurovascular compromise (pulses/sensation in the foot).

DIFFERENTIAL DIAGNOSIS

- Contusion
- Ankle sprain
- Tear of ankle retinacular structures
- Syndesmosis injury ("high ankle sprain")
- Foot fracture
- Posttraumatic subluxation of peroneal tibialis posterior tendons

DIAGNOSTIC TESTS & INTERPRETATION

- Ottawa Ankle Rules are used to determine whether x-rays are necessary. Obtain x-rays for pain in the malleolar zone associated with any of the following:
  - Bony tenderness along distal 6 cm of posterior tibia or fibula or at medial or lateral malleolar tip
  - Inability to bear weight (four steps) on ankle immediately after injury and at time of evaluation
- The Ottawa Ankle Rules have a sensitivity for fracture near 100% and a modest specificity (2)[A].
- Ottawa Ankle Rules have been validated for children 10 yr and older (3)[A].
- X-rays include anteroposterior (AP), lateral, and mortise (AP with foot in 15 degrees of adduction) views.
- Some ankle fractures may not be initially seen. Presence of a large ankle effusion on the lateral radiograph may indicate an occult fracture and the need for further evaluation (4)[C].
- On the mortise view, the joint space between the talus and lateral malleolus and the distal tibia and medial malleolus should be equal. Inequality should raise suspicion of an unstable ankle injury.
- Computed tomography (CT) not indicated in most ankle fractures; however, it is performed when an occult fracture is suspected or to further evaluate pilon (comminuted distal tibial fracture), triplane (tibial fracture in sagittal, coronal, and axial planes), or suspected talar fractures.
- When performed, order thin-cut CT in case coronal or sagittal reconstructions are required.

TREATMENT

GENERAL MEASURES

- Acetaminophen at recommended age- or weight-based dosages every 6 to 8 hr as needed
- Consider nonsteroidal anti-inflammatory drugs (NSAIDs), although controversy exists as to their effect on bone healing.
- Narcotics as needed for severe pain only
- Cryotherapy applied 20 to 30 min every 2 to 4 hr for the first 24 to 48 hr after injury. Use caution to avoid thermal injury to the skin.
- Relative rest and elevation of affected limb for first 48 to 72 hr
- Isolated lateral malleolar fractures with 2 mm or less of displacement do not need reduction. Refer to orthopedist for >2 mm displacement (5)[C].
- Isolated medial malleolar fractures with any displacement other than small avulsion injuries should be referred to an orthopedist. Do not attempt to reduce.
- Check neurovascular status of foot postreduction.
- Postreduction x-rays are same views as initial films.
- Non–weight-bearing in stirrup or posterior splint, with ankle in neutral position, for 3 to 5 days
- Isolated, minimally displaced lateral malleolar fracture: short leg walking cast with ankle in a neutral position or fracture boot with (e.g., controlled ankle motion [CAM] walker) or without adjustable ankle range of motion for 4 to 6 wk

- Isolated simple avulsion fracture of the medial malleolus: Stirrup splint or CAM walker can be used short term for comfort, typically 2 to 4 wk.

ISSUES FOR REFERRAL

- Any open fracture or fracture associated with neurologic or vascular deficits requires emergent surgical evaluation.
- Ankle injuries that are unstable or incongruent should be evaluated by an orthopedic surgeon.

ADDITIONAL THERAPIES

- Patients should seek attention immediately for pain that is increasing, new or worsening numbness, or skin pallor/duskiness distal to the fracture or splint/cast.
- Repeat x-rays at 2 wk to ensure maintained alignment and at 6 wk to assess bony healing (6)[C].
- Repeat x-rays every 2 wk if not healing.
- Total healing time: 6 to 8 wk; may take months to see complete radiographic healing
- Athletes should cross-train while healing to maintain fitness.
- Proper rehabilitation of these injuries with a home instructional program or with formal physical therapy guidance is crucial to successful healing and return to full function.
- After period of immobilization is complete, start standard ankle rehabilitation range of motion exercises, strengthening exercises, and proprioceptive training.
- The shorter the period of immobilization, the easier it should be for the patient to regain ankle motion and strength.
- Follow up every 2 to 3 wk to assess progress of rehabilitation.

SURGERY/OTHER PROCEDURES

The following injuries are frequently managed with surgical intervention:

- Disrupted mortise joint
- Fracture-dislocations
- Bimalleolar fractures
- Trimalleolar fractures
- Unimalleolar fracture with contralateral ligament rupture
- Lateral malleolar fractures with >2 mm displacement
- Lateral malleolar fractures above the tibiotalar joint line (as they are frequently associated with syndesmotic disruption)
- Medial malleolar fractures with >2 mm displacement (5)[C]
- Posterior malleolus fractures involving >25% of the articular surface or >2 mm displacement (5)[C]

Pediatric Considerations

- 5% of all fractures in pediatrics with a higher incidence in children with an increased body mass (7)
- Physis are vulnerable, and ligamentous structures are robust (7).
- Salter-Harris (SH) type II is the most common (7).
- SH III and IV may damage the reserve zone and are at a higher risk of causing physeal growth disturbance (7).
- Long-term treatment is to minimize angular deformity and leg length discrepancy, to achieve normal ankle function, and to avoid posttraumatic arthritis (7).

ADMISSION, INPATIENT, AND NURSING CONSIDERATIONS

Admission criteria:

- Open fracture
- Fracture-dislocations in which adequate reduction is not achieved with manual manipulation
- Evidence of or concern for neurovascular compromise (severely comminuted pilon fracture, compartment syndrome)

REFERENCES

1. Elsoe R, Ostgaard SE, Larsen P. Population-based epidemiology of 9767 ankle fractures. *Foot Ankle Surg*. 2018;24(1):34–39.
2. Derksen RJ, Knijnenberg LM, Fransen G, et al. Diagnostic performance of the Bernese versus Ottawa Ankle Rules: results of a randomised controlled trial. *Injury*. 2015;46(8):1645–1649.
3. Halai M, Jamal B, Rea P, et al. Acute fractures of the pediatric foot and ankle. *World J Pediatr*. 2015;11(1):14–20.
4. Clark TW, Janzen DL, Ho K, et al. Detection of radiographically occult ankle fractures following acute trauma: positive predictive value of an ankle effusion. *AJR Am J Roentgenol*. 1995;164(5):1185–1189.
5. Michelson JD. Fractures about the ankle. *J Bone Joint Surg Am*. 1995;77(1):142–152.
6. Goost H, Wimmer MD, Barg A, et al. Fractures of the ankle joint: investigation and treatment options. *Dtsch Arztebl Int*. 2014;111(21):377–388.
7. Su AW, Larson AN. Pediatric ankle fractures: concepts and treatment principles. *Foot Ankle Clin*. 2015;20(4):704–719.

ADDITIONAL READING

- Eiff MP, Hatch RL. *Fracture Management for Primary Care*. 3rd ed. Philadelphia, PA: WB Saunders; 2011.
- Rockwood CA, Green DP, Bucholz RW, et al, eds. *Rockwood and Green's Fractures in Adults*. 4th ed. Philadelphia, PA: JB Lippincott; 1996.

CLINICAL PEARLS

- 70% are unimalleolar with lateral being the most common.
- Ottawa Ankle Rules have been validated for 10-yr-olds and older.
- Any open fracture or fracture with neurologic or vascular compromise requires emergent surgical evaluation.
- In pediatrics, ligamentous structures are more robust than the physis.

FRACTURE, LE FORT

Amy Leu, DO, FAAFP, CAQSM

BASICS

Le Fort fractures are midface maxillary fractures involving the maxilla; the maxilla, orbital bones, and nasal bones; or the maxilla, orbital bones, nasal bones, and zygoma.

Pediatric Considerations

- Maxillofacial fractures occur less frequently in children:
  - Because of the smaller facial skeleton, there is a higher incidence of skull fractures and head trauma compared with midface injuries.
  - Le Fort fractures are particularly uncommon in young children. By ages 10 to 12 yr, as facial morphology becomes adult-like, more mid- and lower facial fractures are seen.
  - Be suspicious of child abuse or family violence as possible causes of midfacial injuries, especially in children age <6 yr.
- Cautions:
  - Airway management:
    - Airway compromise is common.
    - Bag-valve-mask (BVM) ventilation may be difficult.
    - Avoid nasotracheal intubation.
  - Strict cervical spine precautions
  - Multisystem injury is likely with high-energy trauma.

DESCRIPTION

- Maxillofacial fractures caused by high-energy blunt trauma to the midface: The most common causes include motor vehicle accidents (including motorcycle accidents and all-terrain vehicles), physical assault, sports injuries (football, baseball, hockey among others), and domestic violence. Among combat victims, mechanisms can include gunshot wounds and explosive or incendiary devices. Head and cervical spine injuries are commonly seen in patients with high-velocity facial trauma.
- Le Fort fractures are separated in three categories based on the facial bones that are involved. Identification can be made with initial physical exam. On traction of the maxillary arch/hard palate, you should find:
  - Le Fort I (horizontal): movement of the hard palate and maxillary dentition only; can arise from a blow low on the maxillary alveolar rim; involves only the maxillary bone.
  - Le Fort II (pyramidal): movement of the hard palate, maxillary dentition, and the nose; can arise from a blow to the lower to middle maxilla; involves the maxilla and nasal bones.
  - Le Fort III (transverse): movement of the entire midface, including orbital rims (inferior and lateral aspects); can arise from a blow to the nasal bridge or upper maxilla; involves the maxilla, nasal bones, and zygoma.

EPIDEMIOLOGY

Prevalence

Midface fractures have been reported to make up ~30% of all facial fractures.

COMMONLY ASSOCIATED CONDITIONS

- Higher velocity injuries are commonly associated with head and cervical spine injuries.
- Le Fort III fractures are commonly associated with lateral rim and zygomatic fractures.
- Visual changes may signify a disturbance of the optic canal, problems within the globe or retina, or other neurologic lesions.
- Disturbances of extraocular motion or enophthalmos may signify a blowout in the orbital floor.
- Consultation with an ophthalmologist is appropriate when extensive involvement of the orbit or globe is suspected.
- Le Fort III fractures also can extend to the base of the sphenoid and can result in a cerebrospinal fluid (CSF) leak.

DIAGNOSIS

Pediatric Considerations

- Young children are often frightened and in pain. Through kindness, patience, and distraction, cooperation can be gained.
- Sedation may be required to perform a thorough exam after ruling out head injury.
- Incomplete (greenstick) fractures with minimal or no displacement can occur.
- Be cognizant of possible child abuse, and evaluate for prior nonaccidental trauma, if appropriate.
- Evaluate the patency of the airway and need for immediate airway control.
- There is a high incidence of cervical spine injuries associated with facial trauma; thus, cervical spine precautions always must be taken (1)[C].
- Le Fort fractures can be diagnosed by careful intraoral examination and the pattern of facial movement:
  - If fracture fragments are impacted, there may be little or no midface mobility.
  - Carefully evaluate the patient for CSF rhinorrhea and malocclusion.
  - If any disturbance of vision or extraocular motion is suspected, consider the presence of a blowout fracture and/or ophthalmologic involvement.
- Prehospital:
  - Establishing airway patency is of utmost importance. Orotracheal intubation is preferred over blind nasotracheal intubation.
  - Bleeding from facial wounds may complicate endotracheal intubation.
  - If a ruptured globe is suspected, use of an eye cup or noncontact shielding should be used to prevent compression of the eye while establishing an airway.
  - Avulsed tissue (ears, skin flaps) should be transported with the patient in saline-soaked gauze.
  - Avulsed teeth should also be transported with the patient in their mouth (in between the buccal mucosal and gum) if they have normal mental status and can protect their airway. If they are intoxicated, have altered mental status, are immobilized and cannot sit upright, or are complaining of nausea or vomiting, their teeth should be transported in sterile saline.
  - In severe Le Fort II and III cases, the maxillary plate can be displaced posteriorly and inferiorly, possibly occluding the airway.
  - There is a high incidence of cervical spine injuries associated with facial trauma; thus, cervical spine precautions always must be taken (1)[C].

HISTORY

History may be difficult to obtain directly from the patient, but these types of fractures typically arise from a high-energy force directed at different aspects of the face. Situations can include motor vehicle accidents, altercations, sports injuries, and falls.

PHYSICAL EXAM

- Facial injury with massive swelling and ecchymosis
- Facial hemorrhage/epistaxis
- Airway obstruction may be present.
- Dyspnea (especially when supine)
- Malocclusion
- Vision disturbance (diplopia)
- Facial lengthening or flattening, periorbital ecchymosis (raccoon's eyes), periorbital swelling
- CSF rhinorrhea
- Facial anesthesia, midface mobility on traction, open bite
- Frequently associated with multisystem injury (especially head and cervical spine)

DIFFERENTIAL DIAGNOSIS

- Le Fort fracture classification:
  - Le Fort I: transverse (horizontal) through the maxilla above the roots of the teeth; can be unilateral or bilateral
  - Le Fort II: pyramidal dysjunction, including the nasal bridge, maxilla, lacrimal bones, and orbital floor and rim; typically bilateral
  - Le Fort III: craniofacial dysjunction; rare
  - Le Fort IV: involves the frontal bone in addition to a Le Fort III maxillary fracture
- Different grade Le Fort fractures may be found on opposite sides of the face.

DIAGNOSTIC TESTS & INTERPRETATION

- Facial imaging may be delayed for 24 to 72 hr in patients requiring care of other life-threatening conditions.
- Computed tomography (CT) scanning is the diagnostic standard for defining midface fractures with thin (2 mm) cuts in the coronal and axial planes.
- Conventional radiographs may be used as a screening test. The occipitomental (Waters) and lateral views of the skull may reveal bony fracture/asymmetry, subcutaneous emphysema, or layering of blood in the maxillary sinuses. Sinus films and cervical spine films usually are included as part of the screening examination.
- Ultrasound of the eye can be used in patients with suspected ocular injuries for the detection of vitreous hemorrhage, retinal detachment, and globe rupture if urgent operative management of nonfacial injuries is planned and there is not time for a facial CT.

TREATMENT

Pediatric Considerations

- Surgical cricothyroidotomy should not be considered in children age <10 yr.
- Needle cricothyroidotomy with jet ventilation may be attempted if intubation attempts fail.
- There is a higher incidence of multiple injuries in children, especially head trauma, skull fractures, and orthopedic injuries.
- Cervical spine injuries tend to involve upper levels more commonly in children. Also, spinal cord injury without radiographic abnormality (SCIWORA) syndrome may be seen.
- Definitive repair of pediatric facial fractures should not be delayed for more than 3 to 4 days. The facial bones heal rapidly, and delayed repair may result in malunion and cosmetic deformity.

GENERAL MEASURES

Emergency department (ED) treatment:

- Cervical spine: Owing to the risk of cervical spine injury in patients with head and maxillofacial trauma, it is imperative that radiographic clearance of the cervical spine is obtained.
- Hemorrhage control: Direct pressure should be applied to areas of bleeding, and nasal packing (anterior and posterior) may be necessary for epistaxis. In some cases, manual reduction of the midface may be required to control intractable hemorrhage. Although blood loss from facial bleeding may be significant, it is rarely a primary cause of hemorrhagic shock.
- Early consultation with oral maxillofacial or plastic surgeon
- Analgesics, antibiotics, and tetanus prophylaxis

MEDICATION

	Adult Dose (mg/kg IV)	Pediatric Dose (mg/kg IV)
Sedative/analgesics[a]		
Diazepam	0.1–0.2	0.1–0.2
Droperidol	2.5-mg aliquots	1- to 1.5-mg aliquots
Etomidate	0.2–0.3	0.2–0.3
Fentanyl	2–10 μg	2–3 μg
Ketamine	2	1–2
Meperidine	1–2	1–2
Midazolam	0.1	0.15
Morphine sulfate	0.1–0.2	0.1–0.2
Defasciculating drug		
Vecuronium	0.01	0.01
Paralytic agents		
Pancuronium	0.1–0.15	0.1–0.15
Rocuronium	0.6	0.6
Succinylcholine	1.5	1.5–2
Vecuronium	0.1–0.3	0.1–0.3

[a]All these sedatives/analgesics should be titrated to effect.
IV, intravenous.

SURGERY/OTHER PROCEDURES

- Often, maxillomandibular fixation (MMF) is used in conjunction with open reduction and internal fixation (ORIF) of maxillofacial injuries to maintain optimal immobilization.
- In the pediatric population, several considerations are taken into account, including duration of MMF, use of smaller hardware, and avoiding injury to developing teeth.

ADMISSION, INPATIENT, AND NURSING CONSIDERATIONS

- Initial stabilization:
  - Aggressive airway control is paramount.
  - Orally suction patients to minimize aspiration of blood, saliva, and stomach contents.
  - Remove any foreign matter or teeth from the airway.
  - After cervical spine clearance, stable and alert patients may be allowed to sit up and suction themselves.
  - When airway management is needed, rapid-sequence induction is recommended to maximize airway control and minimize rise of intracranial pressure (ICP) in patients with head injuries (2)[B].
  - If there is concern that paralysis will result in loss of airway tone and inability to intubate because of subsequent distortion of airway anatomy in patients with severe facial injuries, oral intubation under sedation with midazolam, etomidate, droperidol, or ketamine is an option.
  - Emergency cricothyroidotomy may be necessary if orotracheal intubation is unsuccessful. Recall that BVM ventilation may be difficult owing to loss of bony support and altered anatomy.
  - Nasotracheal intubation is not recommended in patients with midface trauma because of the lack of success and danger of intracranial placement (2)[B],(3)[C],(4)[B].
- Admission criteria:
  - All patients are admitted for ORIF of maxillofacial injuries.
  - Patients should be admitted to an intensive care unit (ICU) setting.

ONGOING CARE

COMPLICATIONS

- Infection can emerge from multiple stages during the treatment process, particularly if there is extensive soft tissue involvement.
- Scarring can occur depending on the suturing technique used as well as the patient's ability to keep the repaired area immobilized.
- Nerve damage can arise from the original trauma as well as a result of the type of surgery used to repair the fractures.
- Malunion and, less commonly, nonunion also can result if adequate immobilization is not achieved.

REFERENCES

1. Rajkumar GC, Ashwin DP, Singh R, et al. Ocular injuries associated with midface fractures: a 5 year survey. *J Maxillofac Oral Surg*. 2015;14(4):925–929.
2. Septa D, Newaskar VP, Agrawal D, et al. Etiology, incidence and patterns of mid-face fractures and associated ocular injuries. *J Maxillofac Oral Surg*. 2014;13(2):115–119.
3. American Academy of Otolaryngology—Head and Neck Surgery. Upper facial trauma. In: *Resident Manual of Trauma to the Face, Head, and Neck*. Alexandria, VA: American Academy of Otolaryngology—Head and Neck Surgery; 2012:41–73.
4. Mithani SK, St-Hilaire H, Brooke BS, et al. Predictable patterns of intracranial and cervical spine injury in craniomaxillofacial trauma: analysis of 4786 patients. *Plast Reconstr Surg*. 2009;123(4):1293–1301.

ADDITIONAL READING

- Colucciello SA, Sternbach G, Walker SB. The treacherous and complex spectrum of maxillofacial trauma: etiologies, evaluation, and emergency stabilization. *Emerg Med Rep*. 1995;16(7):59–69.
- Hehmann RJ, Sargent LA. Maxillary fractures. *Trauma Q*. 1992;9:67–75.
- Hunter JG. Pediatric maxillofacial trauma. *Pediatr Clin North Am*. 1992;39(5):1127–1143.
- Rosen CL, Wolfe RE, Chew SE, et al. Blind nasotracheal intubation in the presence of facial trauma. *J Emerg Med*. 1997;15(2):141–145.
- Sargent LA, Rogers GF. Nasoethmoid orbital fractures: diagnosis and management. *J Craniomaxillofac Trauma*. 1999;5(1):19–27.
- Shimoyama T, Kaneko T, Horie N. Initial management of massive oral bleeding after midfacial fracture. *J Trauma*. 2003;54(2):332–336.
- Subhashraj K, Nandakumar N, Ravindran C. Review of maxillofacial injuries in Chennai, India: a study of 2748 cases. *Br J Oral Maxillofac Surg*. 2007;45(8):637–639.
- Tessier P. The classic reprint: experimental study of fractures of the upper jaw. 3. René Le Fort, M.D., Lille, France. *Plast Reconstr Surg*. 1972;50(6):600–607.

CLINICAL PEARLS

- Le Fort fractures are typically the result of high-velocity blunt force trauma to the midface, thus evaluation for concurrent cervical spine injury and intracranial trauma must be considered.
- True Le Fort fractures rarely happen in children <12 yr given their smaller facial skeleton. Head trauma and skull fractures are more likely.
- Be suspicious for child abuse/family violence for pediatric patients that present with a midface fracture, especially in those <6 yr of age.
- Airway management is of utmost importance during evaluation, and if an airway is needed, orotracheal intubation is preferred over blind nasotracheal intubation due to risk of intracranial displacement.

F

FRACTURE, LISFRANC

William H. West, MD • Kenneth Bielak, MD, FACSM, FAAFP, CAQSM

BASICS

DESCRIPTION

- Injury may occur from direct or indirect mechanisms.
- Direct injury occurs with crush injury to the tarsometatarsal joint.
- Causes of indirect injury:
  - Hindfoot placed in a fixed position with forefoot forcefully abducted in sports such as equestrian and windsurfing produces lateral displacement of the metatarsals with associated fracture of 2nd metatarsal base.
  - An axially applied force to a plantarflexed foot (tiptoe position) causing disruption of the dorsal ligament complex
  - A force applied to the heel and the axis of the foot with the toes fixed in plantar position
- Recent American football study showed that 90% of injuries occurred while player was engaged with or by another player. Injury occurred most with the foot plantarflexed and toes dorsiflexed. The majority of these injuries were due to external rotation of the midfoot (1).
- Synonyms: Lisfranc fracture; tarsometatarsal fracture; first–second metatarsal–cuneiform fracture

EPIDEMIOLOGY

- 1 case/50,000 to 60,000 patients per year
- A review of 2,000 reported cases reported that 43% occurred from motor vehicle accident; 10% during sport activity; 13% due to crush injuries; 24% from falls, jumps, and twisting injuries (2).
- 0.2% of all fractures per year
- Estimated that 20% are missed on initial presentation.

ALERT

- Males 4 times more likely than females due to high impact sports
- Majority is closed (87.6%).
- 2nd tarsometatarsal joint is most frequently injured.

RISK FACTORS

- Slips, falls, motor vehicle accidents, high energy sports
- Positional injury may also occur by using high heels because foot is continually plantarflexed.
- Axial load on a plantarflexed foot (i.e., tackled from behind)
- Horseback riding also common source of injury in the event of a fall due to foot being plantarflexed in a stirrup
- Although these injuries are associated with a low mortality rate, prompt assessment and treatment is required to limit long-term morbidity and disability.

COMMONLY ASSOCIATED CONDITIONS

- Cuneiform and cuboid fracture dislocations
- Compartment syndrome of the foot
- Late recognition and treatment: posttraumatic arthritis with resulting pes planus and forefoot abduction, which may require tarsometatarsal arthrodesis

DIAGNOSIS

HISTORY

- Determine the mechanism of injury as outlined above.
- May present with diffuse foot pain:
  - High index of suspicion needed. Up to 20% of subtle injuries may be missed on initial exam.
- Was the injury associated with a low- or high-velocity trauma?:
  - High velocity, usually has an obvious deformity, whereas low velocity may cause only minor discomfort in the midfoot.

PHYSICAL EXAM

- Signs and symptoms:
  - Midfoot pain and swelling

ALERT

Pain with weight-bearing on involved foot or inability to bear weight, particularly to walk on tiptoes

  - Plantar ecchymosis
  - Possible deformity of foot if injury was sustained and high energy of physical examination.
  - Gap sign between the 1st and 2nd metatarsals
- Physical examination should include:
  - Evaluation of the integrity of the soft tissue and performing a neurovascular examination.
  - Palpation of each articulation for tenderness and swelling. Medial cuneiform and 1st metatarsal joint is the most frequent site of pain and swelling.
  - Stressing 2nd metatarsal joint by elevating and depressing the 2nd metatarsal head relative to the 1st metatarsal head; elicits pain in Lisfranc joint
  - Compression of midfoot from side to side reproduces pain in interval between the bases of the 1st and 2nd metatarsals.
  - Flexion at Lisfranc joint may demonstrate instability and dorsal subluxation of the metatarsals.
  - Marked swelling, redness, and deformity may indicate complete dislocation and risk for compartment syndrome; maybe misdiagnosed as cellulitis
  - Medial or lateral stress force applied to the metatarsals may reveal more specifically which part of the joint is unstable.

DIFFERENTIAL DIAGNOSIS

- Lisfranc fracture dislocation
- Tarsometatarsal sprain
- Metatarsal fracture
- Cuboid fracture
- Cuneiform fracture

DIAGNOSTIC TESTS & INTERPRETATION

Initial Tests (lab, imaging)

Plain radiograph (3):

- Unilateral non–weight-bearing radiograph may be the initial study:
  - Anteroposterior (AP), internal oblique, and lateral views should be taken.
  - This is often sufficient to see *obvious* Lisfranc injuries but may miss up to 50% of subtle injuries. Therefore, weight-bearing radiograph should be performed next.

ALERT

- Bilateral weight-bearing radiograph:
  - AP, internal oblique, and lateral views should be taken.
  - Subtle differences between the feet may be more easily seen if bilateral.
  - May be too painful. If that is the case, regional anesthesia with ankle block or general anesthesia may be rarely necessary.
  - Craniocaudal angulation during AP view can give very good visualization of Lisfranc joint.

- Look for the following relationships (4):
  - Good alignment of medial margins of 2nd metatarsal and middle cuneiform
  - Lateral margin of 1st metatarsal should be aligned with lateral margin of medial cuneiform.
  - Medial margins of 4th metatarsal and cuboid should be well aligned (oblique view).
  - Any malalignment indicates Lisfranc dislocation.
- Any small fractures in and around the Lisfranc joint should cause suspicion of significant injury in that area.
- Diastasis >1 to 2 mm between 1st and 2nd metatarsal bases indicates rupture of Lisfranc ligament (best seen in AP view).
- "Fleck sign" avulsion fracture in medial cuneiform 2nd metatarsal space represents rupture of Lisfranc ligament.
- Compression fracture of cuboid ("nutcracker injury") may be apparent.

• Computed tomography (CT) scan
  - Used to help identify subtle injuries, especially superimposed bone fragments and tendon damage
  - A good modality overall for verifying radiographic findings and locating subtle fractures
• Magnetic resonance imaging (MRI):
  - Allows optimal evaluation of malalignment of the midfoot and is superior modality to detect injury to ligaments
  - T1- and T2-weighted sequences most helpful in detection
• Ultrasound:
  - In office testing available
  - Can distract and look for abnormal motion
  - Can see small fleck avulsions and can see ligament tears
• Bone scintigraphy
  - Most helpful for diagnosis of low-grade injuries when other imaging modalities do not depict abnormalities (5)

Test Interpretation

Multiple classification systems used describe level of diastasis as well as dislocation of metatarsals.

TREATMENT

• Nonoperative management for those with stable injury with no diastasis (6):
  - Immobilization in short walker boot with protected weight-bearing for 2 wk and then reexamination:
    - If tenderness has resolved and no evidence of diastasis on repeat imaging, weight-bearing as tolerated in boot
    - Weight-bearing out of boot after 6 wk
    - No high-impact activity for first 3 to 4 mo after injury
• Single leg hop test pain-free before activity permitted
• Any evidence of dynamic instability or clear diastasis at Lisfranc joint complex requires operative management:
  - Returning to sport is variable. Studies have shown a range of 3 to 8 wk of non–weight-bearing and a range of 12 to 24 wk before returning to sport.
  - Open reduction and internal fixation (ORIF) and primary arthrodesis are usually successful and have high likelihood for successful return to play, although some may experience a decrease in level of performance, and residual pain is not uncommon in some (7).
• Prehospital: Immobilize with posterior splint, non–weight-bearing, elevation, and ice/compression.

SURGERY/OTHER PROCEDURES

ALERT

Any diastasis (>1 mm) or fracture may require operative reduction and screw fixation:

• Primary treatment by ORIF is the most common surgical intervention for athletes.
• Functional improvement and earlier return to work and activity have been seen with ORIF; however, some injury patterns have shown to improve better with primary arthrodesis (8).

ONGOING CARE

FOLLOW-UP RECOMMENDATIONS

Early orthopedic referral is indicated for any fracture, dislocation, or instability of the Lisfranc joint.

REFERENCES

1. Kent RW, Lievers WB, Riley PO, et al. Etiology and biomechanics of tarsometatarsal injuries in professional football players: a video analysis. *Orthop J Sports Med*. 2014;2(3):2325967114525347.
2. Lewis JS Jr, Anderson RB. Lisfranc injuries in the athlete. *Foot Ankle Int*. 2016;37(12):1374–1380.
3. Welck MJ, Zinchenko R, Rudge B. Lisfranc injuries. *Injury*. 2015;46(4):536–541.
4. Welck MJ, Zinchenko R, Tudor F. A painful foot: Lisfranc fracture-dislocations. *BMJ*. 2016;352:i882.
5. Siddiqui NA, Galizia MS, Almusa E, et al. Evaluation of the tarsometatarsal joint using conventional radiography, CT, and MR imaging. *Radiographics*. 2014;34(2):514–531.
6. Seybold JD, Coetzee JC. Lisfranc injuries: when to observe, fix, or fuse. *Clin Sports Med*. 2015;34(4):705–723.
7. Shakked RJ. Lisfranc injury in the athlete. *JBJS Rev*. 2017;5(9):e4.
8. Weatherford BM, Bohay DR, Anderson JG. Open reduction and internal fixation versus primary arthrodesis for Lisfranc injuries. *Foot Ankle Clin*. 2017;22(1):1–14.

ADDITIONAL READING

• Coetzee JC. Making sense of Lisfranc injuries. *Foot Ankle Clin*. 2008;13(4):695–704.
• Eleftheriou K, Rosenfeld P. Lisfranc injury in the athlete: evidence supporting management from sprain to fracture dislocation. *Foot Ankle Clin*. 2013;18(2):219–236.
• Lau S, Bozin M, Thillainadesan T. Lisfranc fracture dislocation: a review of a commonly missed injury of the midfoot. *Emerg Med J*. 2017;34(1):52–56.
• OrthopaedicsOne. Lisfranc fracture dislocation (Version 24). https://www.orthopaedicsone.com/x/GAsCAg. Accessed March 10, 2018.

CLINICAL PEARLS

• Have high index of suspicion for Lisfranc injuries with high-energy trauma, plantar ecchymosis, or inability to bear weight.
• Instability requires prompt referral to orthopedic surgeon for evaluation.
• Postsurgery recovery includes non–weight-bearing cast for 6 wk, followed by progressive weight-bearing in a cast or range of motion boot for 3 to 6 wk.

FRACTURE, LUNATE/KIENBÖCK DISEASE

Kevin E. Burroughs, MD, CAQSM • Z. Victor Ratajczak, MD

BASICS

DESCRIPTION

- Kienböck (pronounced "Keen-bock") disease, or lunatomalacia, is a painful disorder of the wrist, in which there are histologic and radiologic changes showing avascular necrosis of the lunate.
- First described in 1910 by Robert Kienböck
- Synonym(s): lunatomalacia; lunate avascular necrosis

EPIDEMIOLOGY

- Most commonly seen between the ages 20 and 40 yr (1)
- Predilection for the right hand in manual laborers
- Bilateral changes occur less frequently than unilateral changes.
- A 0.1–2% incidence of asymptomatic cases has been reported (2).

ETIOLOGY AND PATHOPHYSIOLOGY

- A true etiology of Kienböck disease is unknown; however, the end result of lunate fragmentation and collapse is definitively osteonecrosis.
- Essentially, two theories exist: vascular and mechanical.
- Increased intraosseous pressures have been recorded in Kienböck disease, supporting impaired venous outflow as a potential etiology. Revascularization success with vascular pedicle grafts also supports the circulatory etiology.
- Mechanical theory describes necrosis secondary to progressive trabecular collapse of the lunate owing to excessive loads and repetitive microfractures. Anatomic factors that would lead to abnormal pressure on the lunate would include negative ulnar variance, uncovering of the lunate by the distal radius, the shape of the lunate (trapezoidal), the existence of a midcarpal facet on the lunate to articulate with the hamate, and radial inclination of the distal radius.

RISK FACTORS

- Previous wrist trauma including lunate fracture
- Negative ulnar variance
- Repetitive trauma (manual labor)
- Anatomic and biomechanical features, including vulnerable blood supply or fixed position of the wrist (loss of range of motion)

DIAGNOSIS

Lichtman classification of staging for Kienböck disease (via x-ray) (1):

- Stage I: normal architecture and bone density; may be either a linear or a compression fracture
- Stage II: definite density changes, but size, shape, and anatomic relationship of the bones not altered; later in this stage, anteroposterior (AP) view shows loss of height on radial side of lunate.
- Stage IIIA: Entire lunate collapses, but the carpal height is relatively unchanged.
- Stage IIIB: There is additionally proximal migration of the capitate and disruption of the carpal architecture, including a fixed hyperflexion of the scaphoid (cortical ring sign). On lateral view, a dorsovolar ribbon-like elongation of the lunate is seen.
- Stage IV: in addition to stage III changes, generalized degenerative changes in the carpus

HISTORY

- Longer duration of pain increases probability.
- Both an inciting traumatic event and repetitive trauma have been linked with the occurrence of Kienböck disease.

PHYSICAL EXAM

- Painful, stiff, and often swollen wrist joint
- Usually >1 mo of pain at presentation
- Pain most often mild to moderate in severity
- Asymptomatic presentation can occur.
- Look for swelling, erythema, and calor at the radio-ulnar joint. Erythema and calor are not associated with Kienböck disease.
- Evaluate range of motion; decreased in Kienböck disease, especially dorsiflexion

DIFFERENTIAL DIAGNOSIS

- On physical examination:
  - Triangular fibrocartilage complex tear (more lateral)
  - Scapholunate ligament instability
  - Distal radioulnar joint complex ligament instability
  - Monoarticular arthritides (multiple)
  - Intraosseous cyst
- On x-ray:
  - Lunate fracture
  - Ulnar abutment
  - Degenerative joint disease carpals

DIAGNOSTIC TESTS & INTERPRETATION

Initial Tests (lab, imaging)

- Laboratory tests for the diagnosis of inflammatory and erosive arthritides (i.e., sedimentation rate, C-reactive protein, rheumatoid factor, anti–cyclic citrullinated peptide [CCP] antibodies, etc.) can be used in those with wrist symptoms to evaluate for other conditions.
- Standard AP, lateral and oblique radiographs with attention to changes in lunate morphology and density
- Initially, the lunate may have normal architecture and density.
- Subsequently, there is increasing density of the lunate and then altered shape and diminished size.
- Adjacent arthritic changes and carpal row collapse can ultimately occur.
- Computed tomography (CT) scan may be useful to detect early changes, including fracture lines.
- Radiographic measures such as a smaller lunate diameter and height, a more radially inclined lunate tilting angle, and a flatter radial inclination have been shown in those with Kienböck disease (3)[B].
- Magnetic resonance imaging (MRI):
  - T1-weighted images show loss of signal intensity (corresponding to osteonecrosis).
  - T2-weighted images initially may show hyperintensity (early signs of osteonecrosis).
  - If negative, unlikely Kienböck disease in a patient with wrist symptoms; may show alternative diagnosis better than plain films

Diagnostic Procedures/Other

- Wrist arthroscopy has been used to assess and classify Kienböck disease.
- Assessment of the surfaces of the lunate is used to stage disease and plan appropriate surgical interventions.

TREATMENT

- Acute treatment

ALERT

Immobilization:
- In initial stages, immobilization for 7 days is a reasonable first step because synovitis and tenosynovitis usually resolve, and examination may become more focused.
- After classification is established, in stage I, initial treatment consists of up to 3 mo of casting or similar form of immobilization

- Arthroscopy with synovectomy also can be used for intervention in stages I and II.

ADDITIONAL THERAPIES

Over time, it has become evident that immobilization will not prevent long-term collapse of the lunate. Some studies showed similar pain relief in conservative versus surgical treatment.

SURGERY/OTHER PROCEDURES

- If the patient still has pain after conservative measures or has more advanced disease, there are a few other options.
- Hand therapy with fluidotherapy and ultrasound protocol to unload wrist and increase blood flow supply to lunate (4)[C]
- In stages II and IIIA: Revascularization procedure can be considered. One such procedure is called a keyhole vascularization, where a vascularized bone graft from the distal radius employing the 4th and 5th extra-compartmental artery pedicles is used as a mechanical support to enable fracture union (5)[C].
- In stage II or IIIA *with positive ulnar variance*: direct revascularization plus external fixation or temporary scaphotrapeziotrapezoid pinning (stage II only), radial wedge or dome osteotomy, capitate shortening with or without capitohamate fusion, combination of joint leveling, and direct revascularization procedures
- In stages II and IIIA with *negative or neutral ulnar variance*: radius-shortening osteotomy, ulnar lengthening, capitate shortening
- In stage IIIA: distal radius metaphyseal core decompression with cancellous bone impaction without shortening procedure leading to improved vascularization (6)[B]
- In stages II, IIIA, IIIB: bone marrow transfusion, low intensity pulsed ultrasound, and external fixation (7)[B]
- In stages IIIA, IIIB, IV: tendon ball arthroplasty using a palmaris longus tendon to fill the defect (8)[B]
- In stage IIIB: scaphotrapeziotrapezoid or scaphocapitate fusion with or without lunate excision with palmaris longus autograft, radius-shortening osteotomy, proximal row carpectomy
- In stage IV: proximal row carpectomy, wrist arthrodesis, wrist denervation
- Lunate excision can reduce symptoms but does not prevent carpal collapse.

ONGOING CARE

FOLLOW-UP RECOMMENDATIONS

Prompt referral to an orthopedist after detection to evaluate, accurately stage, and discuss with the patient available current treatments

COMPLICATIONS

- A continuum from wrist stiffness to a fused and immovable wrist
- Persistent pain
- Nonunion in attempted arthrodesis

REFERENCES

1. Allan CH, Joshi A, Lichtman DM. Kienbock's disease: diagnosis and treatment. *J Am Acad Orthop Surg*. 2001;9(2):128–136.
2. van Leeuwen WF, Janssen SJ, ter Meulen DP, et al. What is the radiographic prevalence of incidental Kienböck disease? *Clin Orthop Relat Res*. 2016;474(3):808–813.
3. Thienpont E, Mulier T, Rega F, et al. Radiographic analysis of anatomical risk factors for Kienböck's disease. *Acta Orthop Belg*. 2004;70(5):406–409.
4. Wollstein R, Wollstein A, Rodgers J, et al. A hand therapy protocol for the treatment of lunate overload or early Kienbock's disease. *J Hand Ther*. 2013;26(3):255–260.
5. Havulinna J, Jokihaara J, Paavilainen P, et al. Keyhole revascularization for treatment of coronal plane fracture of the lunate in Kienböck disease. *J Hand Surg Am*. 2016;41(11):e441–e445.
6. De Carli P, Zaidenberg EE, Alfie V, et al. Radius core decompression for Kienböck disease stage IIIA: outcomes at 13 years follow-up. *J Hand Surg Am*. 2017;42(9):752.e1–752.e6.
7. Ogawa T, Ochiai N, Nishiura Y, et al. A new treatment strategy for Kienböck's disease: combination of bone marrow transfusion, low-intensity pulsed ultrasound therapy, and external fixation. *J Ortho Sci*. 2013;18(2):230–237.
8. Mariconda M, Soscia E, Sirignano C, et al. Long-term clinical results and MRI changes after tendon ball arthroplasty for advanced Kienböck's disease. *J Hand Surg Eur Vol*. 2013;38(5):508–514.

ADDITIONAL READING

- Bain GI, Begg M. Arthroscopic assessment and classification of Kienböck's disease. *Tech Hand Up Extrem Surg*. 2006;10(1):8–13.
- Bonzar M, Firrell JC, Hainer M, et al. Kienböck disease and negative ulnar variance. *J Bone Joint Surg Am*. 1998;80(8):1154–1157.
- Luo J, Diao E. Kienböck's disease: an approach to treatment. *Hand Clin*. 2006;22(4):465–473.
- Mennen U, Sithebe H. The incidence of asymptomatic Kienböck's disease. *J Hand Surg Eur Vol*. 2009;34(3):348–350.
- Peltier LF. The classic. Concerning traumatic malacia of the lunate and its consequences: degeneration and compression fractures. Privatdozent Dr. Robert Kienböck. *Clin Orthop Relat Res*. 1980;(149):4–8.
- Schuind F, Eslami S, Ledoux P. Kienböck's disease. *J Bone Joint Surg Br*. 2008;90(2):133–139.

CLINICAL PEARLS

- Most commonly seen in ages 20 to 40 yr with a predilection to the right hand
- Previous wrist trauma, repetitive trauma, and negative ulnar variance are predisposing factors.
- X-ray shows sclerosis initially and then lucency, but MRI can show changes at an earlier stage.
- Casting is the initial therapy and then orthopedic referral for other treatment considerations.

F

FRACTURE, MANDIBULAR

Giselle Aerni, MD • David Cole, MD

BASICS

DESCRIPTION

- Fracture of the mandible is usually due to a direct force.
- The most common area fractured is the angle, followed by the condyle, molar, and mental regions.
- Because of its thickness, the mandibular symphysis is rarely fractured.
- Mandibular fractures typically occur at more than one site.

EPIDEMIOLOGY

Incidence

Incidence is lowest in children >5 yr of age and highest in males in their 20s.

Prevalence

- Frequently injured because of the mandible's prominence and relative lack of support
- The mandible is the second most common facial fracture following nasal fractures. They account for 40% of all pediatric facial fractures.
- Fractures of the mandible have been reported to account for 36–70% of all maxillofacial fractures.

ETIOLOGY AND PATHOPHYSIOLOGY

- Leading cause of mandible fractures in the Western Hemisphere is interpersonal violence, whereas vehicular accidents are primary etiology in Africa and Asia.
- Remaining etiologies include contact sports, falls, work accidents, and pathologic/iatrogenic factors.

RISK FACTORS

- Drug and alcohol use
- Male between the ages of 21 and 30 yr

COMMONLY ASSOCIATED CONDITIONS

- Additional traumatic facial fractures, other facial injuries, and dentoalveolar trauma
- Patients may be intoxicated and unable to give a complete history of the injury.

DIAGNOSIS

- The first priority in evaluating a possible mandible fracture is to protect the airway. Severe fractures of facial structures may result in airway obstruction from lack of glossal supporting structures, blood clots, loose teeth, dentures, or bony fragments.
- Depending on the trauma, C-spine stabilization may be required during the evaluation process.

HISTORY

- The source, size, and direction of traumatic force are helpful in diagnosis.
- Patients involved in motor vehicle accidents tend to sustain compound, comminuted fractures.
- Localized trauma (e.g., pipe, stick, hammer, fist) tends to cause a single comminuted fracture because the force is concentrated in a small area.
- Trauma distributed to a larger surface area may cause several fractures (e.g., symphysis and condyle) secondary to distribution of the force throughout the mandible. More than 50% of patients have multiple fractures.
- Direction of the force can help in making the diagnosis of concomitant fractures. Trauma directed to the chin often results in a symphyseal fracture with concomitant unilateral or bilateral condylar fractures.
- Patient complaints include:
  - Facial asymmetry, deformity, dysphagia, and mandibular pain.
  - Malocclusion, decreased range of motion of the temporomandibular joint, or a grating sound conducted to the ear with movement of the mandible.

PHYSICAL EXAM

- Inspect the maxillofacial area for obvious deformity:
  - Note facial lacerations, swelling, and hematomas.
  - A common site for a laceration is under the chin and is associated with subcondylar or symphysis fracture.
- Look for loose, fractured, or missing teeth; gross malalignment of teeth; separation of tooth interspaces; and ecchymosis or hematoma of the floor of the mouth.
- Look for intraoral mucosal or gingival tears:
  - Floor of the mouth ecchymosis may indicate a mandibular body or symphyseal fracture.
- Palpate the inferior border of the mandible from the symphysis to the angle on each side. Note areas of swelling, step-off deformity, or tenderness.
- Palpate the movement of the condyle through the external auditory meatus. Pain elicited through palpation of the preauricular region should alert the clinician to a possible condylar fracture.
- Inability of the examiner to note motion of the mandibular condyles when palpated through the external ear canals with motion of the jaw is highly suggestive of a mandibular fracture.
- Observe any deviation on opening of the mouth, or for an inability to chew or open mouth:
  - Deviation on opening is typically toward the side of the mandibular condyle fracture.
  - Note any limited opening and trismus that may be a result of reflex muscle spasm, temporomandibular effusion, or mechanical obstruction to the coronoid process resulting from depression of the zygomatic bone or arch.
- Evaluate for protrusion or lateral excursion of the jaw and any interference with normal mandibular function, including decreased range of motion or deviation of the mandible with opening:
  - The examiner should be able to insert three fingers between the mandible and maxilla.
  - Suggested by inability of the patient to break a tongue depressor placed between the teeth and forced downward
- Changes in occlusion are highly suggestive of a mandibular fracture.
- Paresthesia of the lower lip or gums strongly indicates a mandibular fracture with secondary damage to the inferior alveolar nerve.

DIFFERENTIAL DIAGNOSIS

- Dislocation of the mandible
- Contusions
- Isolated dental trauma

DIAGNOSTIC TESTS & INTERPRETATION

- The following types of radiographs are helpful in diagnosis of mandibular fractures:
  - Panoramic radiograph
  - Bilateral oblique radiographs
  - Posteroanterior mandibular view
  - Reverse Towne view
  - Mandibular occlusal view
- Mandibular views are best for evaluating the condyles and neck of the mandible.
- Dental panoramic views are best for evaluating the symphysis and body as well as dentition.
- Computed tomography (CT) has become a primary modality for diagnosis of mandibular fracture with 3D digitally reconstructed views helping to best visualize complex mandibular fracture (1)[A].
- CT, however, may not be adequate in characterizing dental trauma, and a Panorex view may still be needed in the case of dental concerns.

TREATMENT

GENERAL MEASURES

- 20–40% of patients have associated injuries, and treatment should address the most lethal concerns from airway obstruction, aspiration, major hemorrhage, cervical spine or cord injury, and/or intracranial injury.
- Airway compromise can occur from intraoral edema and hematoma, bony fragments, loose teeth, and loss of tongue support.

- C-spine precautions should be maintained.
- If intubation is needed, an oral trachea tube should be placed.
- Nasotracheal or cricothyrotomy may be indicated, depending on the extent of the injuries.

MEDICATION

- Use of preoperative and perioperative antibiotics in mandible fractures with dentate involvement is well established to reduce the risk of infection. Evidence for postsurgical antibiotics shows no improvement in infection rates (2,3)[A].
- Diazepam: adult: 10 mg intravenous (IV); pediatrics: 0.1 to 0.2 mg/kg/dose IV
- Midazolam: adult: 2 to 5 mg IV; pediatrics: safety not established but 0.02 to 0.05 mg/kg/dose have been used
- Clindamycin: adult: 600 to 900 mg IV prior to surgical intervention; pediatrics: 20 mg/kg 30 to 60 min prior to procedure
- Cefazolin: adult: 1 g IV prior to surgery; pediatrics: 50 mg/kg
- Metronidazole: adult: 500 mg IV prior to surgery; pediatrics: 15 mg/kg IV prior to surgery

SURGERY/OTHER PROCEDURES

- Definitive care usually consists of reduction and fixation by wiring upper and lower teeth in occlusion for 4 to 6 wk (4)[A].
- Linear, nondisplaced, or greenstick fractures may be treated with a soft/liquid diet without wiring.
- With the exception of condylar fractures, many mandibular fractures are associated with mucosal, gingival, or tooth socket disruption and should be treated as open fractures.
- Preoperatively, patients should receive antibiotics: Penicillins, cefazolin, metronidazole, and clindamycin are most often used to cover oral flora.
- Patients should have their tetanus updated if needed.
- If mandible dislocation is present, reduction may be necessary to free the condyle from its anterior position to the eminence:
  - The operator's thumbs are placed on the external oblique line of the mandible (lateral to the 3rd molar area) or, after wrapping the thumbs in gauze, on the occlusal surface of the lower molars. The other fingers are curled under the mandible.
  - The patient is asked to open wide, as if yawning, and the operator then applies downward force on the molars while applying upward force over the chin until the mandible reduces.
  - Once reduced, the patient should be placed in a Barton bandage for temporary immobilization until he or she receives definitive care.
  - Reduction is facilitated by muscle relaxants (diazepam or midazolam) or anesthetic injection of mastication muscles.
  - A bite block should be used or examiner's fingers should be wrapped in gauze to prevent injury to the treating provider.

Pediatric Considerations

Mandibular fractures are uncommon in children <5 yr of age. When they do occur, they are usually greenstick fractures and can be managed with soft diet alone. Parents should be informed that any fracture of the mandible has the potential to damage permanent teeth and cause facial asymmetry; long-term follow-up with a specialist is advisable.

ADMISSION, INPATIENT, AND NURSING CONSIDERATIONS

- Those fractures in which there is significant displacement or associated dental trauma, or those fractures that are thought to be open, require urgent specialty consultation for admission.
- The severity of associated trauma may indicate admission.
- Any patient with the potential for airway compromise, including oropharyngeal edema or bilateral mandibular body fractures, should be admitted.
- An unreliable patient with nondisplaced fractures should be admitted for definitive fixation.
- In the pediatric population, if the mechanism of injury is not appropriate to the injuries seen, evaluate for child abuse.

ONGOING CARE

PATIENT EDUCATION

- Smokers and patients with systemic medical conditions may have an increased incidence of complications, and it is important to maintain adherence to prescribed regimens.
- Alcohol often plays a role in the etiology of mandibular fractures, and evaluation for abuse should be discussed.
- Parents of children should be informed that any fracture of the mandible has the potential to damage permanent teeth and cause facial asymmetry; long-term specialist follow-up should be recommended.

PROGNOSIS

- Patients will usually be immobilized for 4 to 6 wk and can resume contact sports within 1 to 2 mo after treatment with appropriate protective equipment (e.g., customized headgear to provide protection).
- A better prognosis is achieved with removal of grossly diseased teeth.
- Physical therapy is also recommended to improve jaw opening.

COMPLICATIONS

- Treatment should occur as soon as possible. Prolonged delay in treatment contributes to infection.
- Immobilization of the fracture segments is perhaps the most important aspect in avoiding delayed union, nonunion, and infection.
- Potential complications include malocclusion, infection, chronic pain, neurosensory disturbances, tooth loss, and inability to chew hard food.

REFERENCES

1. Pickrell BB, Hollier LH Jr. Evidence-based medicine: mandibular fractures. *Plast Reconstr Surg*. 2017;140(1):192e–200e.
2. Adalarasan S, Mohan A, Pasupathy S. Prophylactic antibiotics in maxillofacial fractures: a requisite? *J Craniofac Surg*. 2010;21(4):1009–1011.
3. Morris LM, Kellman RM. Are prophylactic antibiotics useful in the management of facial fractures? *Laryngoscope*. 2014;124(6):1282–1284.
4. Pickrell BB, Serebrakian AT, Maricevich RS. Mandible fractures. *Semin Plast Surg*. 2017;31(2):100–107.

ADDITIONAL READING

- Koshy JC, Feldman EM, Chike-Obi CJ, et al. Pearls of mandibular trauma management. *Semin Plast Surg*. 2010;24(4):357–374.
- Miles BA, Potter JK, Ellis E III. The efficacy of postoperative antibiotic regimens in the open treatment of mandibular fractures: a prospective randomized trial. *J Oral Maxillofac Surg*. 2006;64(4):576–582.
- Shorey CW, Campbell JH. Dislocation of the temporomandibular joint. *Oral Surg Oral Med Oral Pathol Oral Radiol Endod*. 2000;89(6):662–668.

CLINICAL PEARLS

- Consider a mandibular fracture for any athlete that has facial deformity, dysphagia, and mandibular pain after direct trauma to the face.
- The first priority is to maintain the airway and the C-spine.

FRACTURE, METACARPAL BASE/SHAFT: I-V

Tara Robbins, MD

BASICS

DESCRIPTION

- Metacarpal shaft and base fractures are defined by their location, pattern, and displacement:
  - Three types of metacarpal shaft fractures: transverse, oblique or spiral, and comminuted
  - Two types of metacarpal base fractures: intra-articular and extra-articular
- Metacarpal fractures involving the 1st metacarpal (thumb) are considered separately from those involving the 2nd to 5th metacarpals.
- Two intra-articular fractures of the thumb deserve special mention:
  - Bennett fracture: fracture combined with a subluxation or dislocation of the metacarpal joint
  - Rolando fracture: T- or Y-shaped fracture involving the joint surface

EPIDEMIOLOGY

- Metacarpal fractures account for up to 50% of all hand fractures.
- Small finger is the most commonly injured (50%), followed by the thumb, index, long finger, and ring finger (1).
- Fractures of metacarpal base occur most commonly in the 4th and 5th metacarpals.
- Metacarpal fractures account for 10–39% of pediatric hand injuries.

Incidence

Lifetime incidence of metacarpal fracture is 2.5%.

ETIOLOGY AND PATHOPHYSIOLOGY

- Transverse and comminuted metacarpal shaft fractures usually result from a direct blow:
  - Dorsal angulation is common.
- Spiral metacarpal fractures result from indirect trauma or rotational torque applied to a digit:
  - Fracture fragments tend to shorten and rotate, especially in the index and small fingers.
- Intra-articular metacarpal base fractures are high-energy injuries and usually result from a direct blow over the base of the metacarpal or a significant axial force or torque applied to the digit:
  - Associated with carpometacarpal (CMC) dislocations
  - Most frequently occur in ring and small fingers
  - Uncommon in index and middle fingers
  - Avulsion fractures usually occur due to tractional forces from tendons that insert into the base of the metacarpals.
- Extra-articular metacarpal base fractures occur from same forces as intra-articular metacarpal base fractures:
  - Most are stabilized by intermetacarpal ligament, resulting in only minimal displacement.
  - Can be associated with CMC dislocation of adjacent digit

RISK FACTORS

Gymnastics, contact sports, racquet sports, boxing, karate

DIAGNOSIS

HISTORY

- Direct blow versus indirect blow with rotational torque: Rotational torque often leads to spiral fractures.
- Nerve injury or damage to the extensor tendon frequently is associated with crush injuries.

PHYSICAL EXAM

- Tenderness and swelling over the dorsal hand
- Pain with motion
- Inability to make a fist
- All patients require a thorough neurovascular examination distal to the fracture site. 4th and 5th metacarpal base fractures may cause injury to the motor branch of the ulnar nerve, resulting in paralysis of the intrinsic hand muscles.

ALERT

Evaluate for rotational malalignment:

- All the fingers of a semiclenched fist should point to the scaphoid tubercle.
- In comparison to the asymptomatic hand, no crowding or digital overlap should be present when the digits are fully flexed.
- With metacarpophalangeal (MCP) at 90 degrees flexion and digits in extension, the plane of the fingernails should be parallel on the injured and normal hand.

- Function of each flexor and extensor tendon must be documented.

DIFFERENTIAL DIAGNOSIS

- Metacarpal head and neck fractures
- MCP collateral ligament injuries
- CMC fracture dislocation

DIAGNOSTIC TESTS & INTERPRETATION

- Radiographic evaluation with three views is mandatory because many fractures are overlooked or misinterpreted.
- Standard anteroposterior and lateral views: Pronation of 10 to 30 degrees in lateral view facilitates visualization of the 2nd and 3rd metacarpals; supination of 10 to 30 degrees in lateral view aids in viewing the ring and small fingers.
- Oblique views allow better visualization of intra-articular fractures, spiral fractures, and epiphyseal plate injuries.
- Robert view with the hand in maximal pronation is helpful for differentiating between intra-articular and extra-articular fractures of the thumb because it allows for visualizing intra-articular extension of an epibasilar fracture.
- Tomograms or computed axial tomographic scans help define CMC relationships and are of benefit for defining comminuted intra-articular fractures (1)[B].

ALERT

Malrotation should be suspected if there is metacarpal shortening or a discrepancy in the shaft diameter.

TREATMENT

GENERAL MEASURES

- Once thorough neurovascular examination is complete, wrist or hematoma block may facilitate reduction if necessary.
- Impaction fractures of the metacarpal bases that are not significantly displaced can be treated with splinting, followed by early mobilization.
- Fractures amenable to closed manipulative reduction are transverse fractures, isolated spiral/oblique fractures with <3 mm of shortening, and extra-articular fractures of the thumb.
- Closed reduction of metacarpal shaft fractures is performed with longitudinal traction, dorsal pressure at the fracture site, and rotation as needed.
- Closed reduction of extra-articular base fractures typically requires only longitudinal traction.
- Postreduction films are mandatory. Limits of angular deformity depend on mobility of different metacarpals at base: <0 degrees for 2nd and 3rd metacarpals, <20 degrees for 4th and <30 degrees for the 5th metacarpals (2)[C], and <25 degrees of both angulation and rotation are acceptable for the thumb. The more proximal the fracture, the more pronounced the deformity and the less angulation that can be accepted.
- Orthopedic referral is required if satisfactory reduction cannot be performed or maintained.
- Radiographs should be repeated 1 wk after injury to reevaluate for angulation, rotation, and shortening.
- Dorsal and volar splints must include all metacarpal shafts and wrist while avoiding immobilization of the interphalangeal joint. Splint should be left in place for 3 to 4 wk (1)[B].
- Ulnar gutter splint for 3 to 4 wk for extra-articular metacarpal base fractures if ring and/or little finger(s) are involved

- Volar or radial gutter for 3 to 4 wk for extra-articular metacarpal base fractures of index and long finger
- Functional brace (Galveston) if fracture requires significant reduction
- Thumb spica cast for extra-articular fractures of the thumb for 4 to 6 wk
- Bulky compressive dressing for unstable fractures
- For angulated fractures, closed reduction with local block or conscious sedation and immobilization is generally effective for children (1)[B].
- Referral is needed for unstable or unsatisfactory reductions in children.
- Long oblique and spiral fractures typically require closed reduction and percutaneous pinning in children (1)[B].
- Fractures involving the physis and epiphysis are uncommon in children:
  - Usually Salter-Harris type II, which almost always are treatable with closed reduction and immobilization
  - Salter-Harris type III fractures are rare. These require open reduction because osteonecrosis of the metacarpal head can result if inadequately reduced.
- Children can be immobilized longer due to additional flexibility.

ISSUES FOR REFERRAL

ALERT
- Any rotational deformity
- >5 mm of shortening
- >10 degrees angulation for 2nd and 3rd metacarpals, >20 degrees angulation for 4th and 5th metacarpals, >25 degrees angulation of the thumb
- >25% articular surface involvement (3)[C], >1 mm step-off (2)[C]
- Intra-articular base fractures
- Inability to perform or maintain satisfactory closed reduction
- All surgical cases, including special situations such as multiple fractures, nerve or tendon injury, and open fractures

ADDITIONAL THERAPIES

- Field management: Splint immobilization provides comfort and minimizes soft tissue injury.
- Ice packs should be used proximal to the metacarpals to prevent digital injuries.
- Active motion as soon as 3 wk for fractures treated with immobilization and closed reduction if non-tender (i.e., clinical healing) (4)[C]
- Buddy taping may provide stability when mobilization begins.
- Clinical union is manifested by absence of tenderness at the fracture site with palpation and range of motion (ROM). Radiographic union will lag behind clinical union by several weeks.

SURGERY/OTHER PROCEDURES

Open reduction and internal fixation or closed reduction with percutaneous pinning is advocated for patients with malunion or unstable fractures (Bennett, Rolando, comminuted, intra-articular, spiral/oblique with shortening, and rotation).

ONGOING CARE

FOLLOW-UP RECOMMENDATIONS

- Follow up 1 wk after injury with radiographs to evaluate for angulation, rotation, and shortening.
- Splint/cast should remain in place for 3 to 4 wk minimum.
- Rehabilitation should be delayed until 3 to 4 wk postinjury for distal metacarpal shaft fractures (5)[C].
- Both active and passive ROM at interphalangeal joints can be started immediately for metacarpal base and proximal shaft fractures (5)[C].
- Gentle active ROM at the MCP joint is allowed in most proximal stable shaft fractures 3 to 4 wk after injury (5)[C].
- Passive ROM at MCP joint can be added when there are signs of clinical union, usually 5 to 6 wk after the injury (5)[C].
- Strengthening exercises should be added at 8 wk (5)[C].

COMPLICATIONS

- Stiffness can develop after prolonged immobilization or delayed rehabilitation.
- Chronic CMC joint stiffness is associated with intra-articular fractures.
- Malunion usually manifests as malrotation or dorsal angulation, so confirm that the patient's fingertips point toward the scaphoid tuberosity in flexion at each visit:
  - 5 degrees of malrotation can result in 1.5 cm of digital overlap and cause a decrease in grip strength.
  - Function is more likely to be affected if the malunion is proximal, involves either the 2nd or the 3rd metacarpal, or is rotational.
- Nonunion is uncommon in metacarpal fractures.
- Surgical complications can also arise. Plates and other prominent hardware frequently cause tendon adhesions and stiffness. Metal may become tender to palpation. Treatment includes hardware removal and extensor tendon tenolysis (6)[C].

REFERENCES

1. Chin SH, Vedder NB. MOC-PSSM CME article: metacarpal fractures. *Plast Reconstr Surg*. 2008;121(Suppl 1):1–13.
2. Wong VW, Higgins JP. Evidence-based medicine: management of metacarpal fractures. *Plast Reconstr Surg*. 2017;140(1):140e–151e.
3. Diaz-Garcia R, Waljee JF. Current management of metacarpal fractures. *Hand Clin*. 2013;29(4):507–518.
4. Ben-Amotz O, Sammer DM. Practical management of metacarpal fractures. *Plast Reconstr Surg*. 2015;136(3):370e–379e.
5. Weinstein L, Hanel D. Metacarpal fractures. *J Am Soc Surg Hand*. 2002;2(4):168–180.
6. Kollitz KM, Hammert WC, Vedder NB, et al. Metacarpal fractures: treatment and complications. *Hand (N Y)*. 2014;9(1):16–23.

ADDITIONAL READING

- Capo JT, Hastings H. Metacarpal and phalangeal fractures in athletes. *Clin Sports Med*. 1998;17(3):491–511.
- Harrison BP, Hilliard MW. Emergency department evaluation and treatment of hand injuries. *Emerg Med Clin North Am*. 1999;17(4):793–822, v.
- Lyn E, Antosia R. Hand. In: Marx JA, Hockberger R, Walls RM, et al, eds. *Marx: Rosen's Emergency Medicine: Concepts and Clinical Practice*. 6th ed. Philadelphia, PA: Mosby; 2006.
- Mastey RD, Weiss AP, Akelman E. Primary care of hand and wrist athletic injuries. *Clin Sports Med*. 1997;16(4):705–724.
- Peterson JJ, Bancroft LW. Injuries of the fingers and thumb in the athlete. *Clin Sports Med*. 2006;25(3):527–542, vii–viii.
- Simon RR, Koenigsknecht SJ, eds. *Emergency Orthopedics*. Stamford, CT: Appleton Lange; 1996.

CLINICAL PEARLS

- Metacarpal fractures that are more distal and ulnar are better tolerated and are more amendable to nonoperative treatment.
- Boxer's fractures are metacarpal neck fractures involving the small finger.
- Return to play needs to be individualized, depending on the type of fracture, mobility, and clinical healing.

FRACTURE, METACARPAL NECK: I-V

Chris Koutures, MD, FAAP

BASICS

DESCRIPTION

- The metacarpal neck (distal metaphysis) is the aspect of the metacarpal shaft immediately underneath the metacarpal head.
- The weakest point of the metacarpal is located at the distal metaphysis, so metacarpal fractures frequently involve the neck (1).
- The mechanism of injury is usually an axial load on the metacarpophalangeal (MCP) joint while in a flexed position, such as when throwing a punch.
- Fractures about the metacarpal neck must be scrutinized for malrotation and angulation.
- As 2nd and 3rd metacarpals are necessary for handgrip power, much less angulation is tolerated in these injuries.
- Synonym(s): boxer's fracture; 5th metacarpal neck fracture

EPIDEMIOLOGY

- 5th metacarpal neck fractures (boxer's fractures) are the most common hand fracture, accounting for 20% of all hand fractures (1).
- Fractures of the 1st metacarpal neck are uncommon.

ETIOLOGY AND PATHOPHYSIOLOGY

- Due to the action of the interosseous muscles, the distal fracture fragment (metacarpal head) displaces volarly, resulting in an apex dorsal angulation.
- The index and long fingers cannot tolerate angulation deformities given their relatively fixed articulations with the distal carpal bones.
- The ring and small fingers, however, have limited flexion and extension, so angular deformities are better tolerated and they heal with minimal loss of function.

RISK FACTORS

"Out-of-control tempers": Boxer's fractures usually are due to striking an opponent or a wall with a clenched fist.

DIAGNOSIS

HISTORY

- Axial load or direct trauma, often to clenched fist or dorsum of the hand
- Immediate pain and swelling noted

PHYSICAL EXAM

- Swelling and tenderness on the dorsum of the hand, often accompanied by MCP joint depression
- Extreme angulation may lead to pseudoclawing, which is hyperextension of the MCP joint along with proximal interphalangeal (PIP) joint flexion as the patient attempts to extend the finger.
- Tenderness and swelling about the dorsal aspect of the distal metacarpals. Examine skin closely for teeth marks, redness, warmth, or streaking suggesting infection, or other injuries.
- Evaluate the digits for malrotation, which occurs more in 4th and 5th metacarpal neck fractures. Have the patient bring all the fingernails into the palm and compare with the noninjured hand. All the nails should point toward the base of the 1st metacarpal. If the injured finger is out of this alignment, strongly suspect significant fracture malrotation.

DIAGNOSTIC TESTS & INTERPRETATION

- Anteroposterior, oblique, and true lateral radiographic views of the hand usually are sufficient.
- Normally, the metacarpal neck is situated with a baseline of 15 degrees of volar angulation. Ensure adequate visualization on the lateral view to evaluate the degree of fracture angulation.
- A conservative rule for limits of acceptable angulation of the 2nd through 5th digits is 10 to 30. Thus, the 2nd digit can only tolerate 10 degrees of angulation (in addition to the baseline 15 degrees); the 5th metacarpal can accept 30 degrees above the baseline. Many other experts will tolerate a greater degree of angulation of the 5th metacarpal; this decision often is influenced by the particular activity, hobbies, work requirements, or sport of the patient.
- Degrees of acceptable angulation vary in current literature. For the index or long finger, some authors report that angulations of >15 degrees above baseline are not tolerated due to the lack of carpal metacarpal motion (1)[C]. Others report that for the ring finger, up to 30 degrees of excessive angulation (above baseline) at the metacarpal neck is acceptable, and for the small finger, up to 40 degrees of excessive angulation (above baseline) at the 5th metacarpal neck is acceptable (2)[B],(3)[C].

DIFFERENTIAL DIAGNOSIS

- Metacarpal head fracture
- Metacarpal shaft fracture
- Open fracture
- MCP joint dislocation
- MCP joint sprain

TREATMENT

GENERAL MEASURES

- Nonsteroidal anti-inflammatory drugs (NSAIDs) can be used along with ice for immediate analgesia.
- Teeth marks can represent entry pathway for infection, especially if noted adjacent to MCP joint. Any sign of deeper infection (including fever, redness, streaking, or focal discharge) requires immediate evaluation by a hand surgical specialist.
- Closed reduction is considered in cases of significant angulation of 4th (>20 degrees above baseline) and 5th (>30 degrees above baseline) metacarpal neck fractures.
- Anesthesia can be obtained by hematoma block or ulnar nerve block.
- Flex the MCP, PIP, and distal PIP joints all to 90 degrees. Apply dorsally directed pressure along the proximal phalanx shaft through the flexed PIP joint while simultaneously applying volarly directed pressure over the proximal fracture fragment (3)[C].
- Obtain a postreduction lateral view of the hand to ensure adequate reduction and immobilization.
- Nondisplaced and nonangulated fractures of the 2nd or 3rd metacarpal necks can be immobilized in a radial gutter splint with the wrist in 30 degrees extension, MCP joint in 70 to 90 degrees of flexion, and PIP/distal interphalangeal (DIP) joints near full extension.
- Mildly angulated 4th (<20 degrees above baseline) and 5th (<30 degrees) metacarpal neck fractures can be immobilized in ulnar gutter splints with the same positions.
- Alternatively, some literature recommends functional treatment by casting (glove cast) or by taping with pressure bandage (2)[B],(3)[C]. For functional casting, the cast is applied circularly around the metacarpals, and it starts distal to the palmar crease of the wrist and ends just proximal to the MCP joint. This allows maximal range of motion of the finger and wrist while providing immobilization and protection of the fracture fragment.
- Elevate the hand and consider application of ice for 20-min intervals on a regular basis over the first 24 to 48 hr after injury.
- Splints should be applied to injuries requiring orthopedic referral (see below), unless that consultant is immediately available.
- There are variable recommendations regarding the optimal management for metacarpal neck fractures, particularly for fracture of the 5th metacarpal neck.

- Points of discussion include:
  - How much angulation is acceptable (recommendations in literature vary from 20 to 70 degrees for the 5th metacarpal)?
  - Which splinting method is most optimal, and if splinting is absolutely necessary?
  - What length of immobilization is optimal (literature varies anywhere from no immobilization to 1 wk of immobilization followed by functional treatment to pure immobilization ranging from 2 to 4 wk)?
- No differences in functional outcome were found between boxer's fractures treated with immobilization in an ulnar gutter cast for 3 wk and those treated with functional taping for 1 wk. Furthermore, range of motion of the 5th MCP joint was not affected in fractures with angulation <70 degrees that were not reduced (2)[B].
- A randomized controlled trial supported the use of soft wrap and buddy taping for treatment of boxer's fracture with palmar angulation ≤70 degrees and no rotational deformity. Although there was no statistical difference in satisfaction with the aesthetic appearance, the patient must be willing to accept the loss of the "knuckle" with this treatment method (4)[B].
- A 2005 Cochrane Review concluded that there is no single nonsurgical treatment method that can be recommended as superior to another (5)[B].

ISSUES FOR REFERRAL

Open reduction and internal fixation is indicated for:

- Significant angulation of 2nd (>10 degrees above baseline) and 3rd (>10 degrees above baseline) metacarpal neck fractures or those with any displacement.
- Failure to achieve acceptable angles after reduction of the 4th and 5th metacarpals.
- A retrospective study found that closed reduction and splint immobilization of 5th metacarpal neck fractures was not an effective means of maintaining a significant improvement in fracture alignment upon healing. Other means, such as closed reduction with pin fixation or open reduction internal fixation, should be considered when maintenance of reduction is desired (6)[B].
- Any metacarpal neck fracture with rotational malalignment or comminution
- Any potential open fracture
- Degree of residual angulation that is unacceptable to the patient
- Inability to hold reduction position
- Athlete who desires immediate return to play in cast orthosis

ONGOING CARE

- If splint used, fractures should remain splinted for a minimum of 3 to 4 wk.
- Clinical healing is defined as no tenderness with palpation of the fracture site.
- Once the splints are removed, begin range of motion work with emphasis on handgrip and manipulation strength: key to prevent stiffness of the MCP joint.

FOLLOW-UP RECOMMENDATIONS

- Follow-up radiographs may not be indicated for most 5th metacarpal base and neck fractures. Follow-up radiographs should be performed at the discretion of the treating physician on an as-needed basis for fractures at risk for displacement (7).
- For 2nd and 3rd metacarpal neck fractures, follow-up radiographs should be obtained in 5 to 7 days to monitor fracture alignment.
- For 4th and 5th metacarpal neck fractures, follow-up radiographs should be considered at 7 to 10 days.
- Perform follow-up visits at 2-wk intervals to monitor for malalignment, rotational deformity, angulation, and progress of healing.

Patient Monitoring

- Return to sports participation recommended when there is pain-free range of motion and when strength approaches that of the contralateral hand
- In general, conservative guideline for return to contact sports with splint/orthotic protection is after 2 to 4 wk of immobilization. Some experts may allow immediate return to play with a protective cast or splint.
- Use of orthotic protection during contact sports should continue for 8 to 10 wk after the initial injury.

PATIENT EDUCATION

- Patients should be warned that despite reduction and splinting, loss of knuckle prominence may result.
- After splint removal, educate patient on range of motion exercises to prevent MCP joint stiffness.

COMPLICATIONS

- MCP joint stiffness due to prolonged immobilization, interosseous muscle contractures, or tendon adhesions
- Cosmetic deformity without functional loss still may ensue.
- Although uncommon, delayed union or nonunion of the fracture site may occur.
- Pseudoclawing

REFERENCES

1. Capo J, Hastings H II. Metacarpal and phalangeal fractures in athletes. *Clin Sports Med*. 1998;17(3):491–511.
2. Statius Muller MG, Poolman RW, van Hoogstraten MJ, et al. Immediate mobilization gives good results in boxer's fractures with volar angulation up to 70 degrees: a prospective randomized trial comparing immediate mobilization with cast immobilization. *Arch Orthop Trauma Surg*. 2003;123(10):534–537.
3. Leggit JC, Meko CJ. Acute finger injuries: part II. Fractures, dislocations, and thumb injuries. *Am Fam Physician*. 2006;73(5):827–834.
4. van Aaken J, Fusetti C, Luchina S, et al. Fifth metacarpal neck fractures treated with soft wrap/buddy taping compared to reduction and casting: results of a prospective, multicenter, randomized trial. *Arch Orthop Trauma Surg*. 2016;136(1):135–142.
5. Poolman RW, Goslings JC, Lee JB, et al. Conservative treatment for closed fifth (small finger) metacarpal neck fractures. *Cochrane Database Syst Rev*. 2005;(3):CD003210.
6. Pace GI, Gendelberg D, Taylor KF. The effect of closed reduction of small finger metacarpal neck fractures on the ultimate angular deformity. *J Hand Surg Am*. 2015;40(8):1582–1585.
7. Heckmann N, Dusch MN, Pannell WC, et al. The utility of plain films for nonoperative fifth metacarpal fractures: are follow-up radiographs necessary? *Hand (N Y)*. 2017;1558944717733278.

CLINICAL PEARLS

- Must consider metacarpal neck fractures in any punching, striking, or axial load injury mechanism
- Common complications include open bite wounds, malrotation, and significant fracture angulation.
- Patient's opinion may help dictate treatment in cases of angulation that may result in cosmetic concerns or functional impact on sport choice (using racquets, ball placement in hand).

FRACTURE, METATARSAL

Adam T. Chrusch, MD, CAQSM

BASICS

The anatomy of the foot is divided into the hindfoot, the midfoot, and the forefoot:

- The hindfoot includes the calcaneus and talus.
- The midfoot includes the navicular, cuboid, and cuneiform bones.
- The forefoot includes the metatarsals and phalanges:
  - The forefoot functions to transmit ground reaction forces to the midfoot with weight-bearing activities.
  - Fractures in the forefoot, specifically to the metatarsals, can alter the normal distribution of weight and lead to secondary metatarsalgia (pain) as well as transfer lesions such as plantar callouses and stress lesions.

DESCRIPTION

- A metatarsal fracture can be described as being extra-articular, partial intra-articular, or articular, depending on where on the metatarsal the fracture occurs. Extra-articular fractures may be transverse (straight across the long axis), oblique, or spiral. An articular or partial intra-articular may be a simple isolated fracture extending into the joint, comminuted, or an avulsion fracture.
- A stress injury with normal radiographs but a positive exam (pain to palpation) may be categorized as macrotrabecular (visible fracture lines on magnetic resonance imaging [MRI]) or stress reaction (T2 signal change on MRI without visible fracture lines).

EPIDEMIOLOGY

- Metatarsal fractures are likely more common in athletes involved in weight-bearing exercise such as dancers, runners, or contact sport athletes.
- Any direct trauma, however, can cause fracture, and lower risk athletes such as swimmers or bikers still may present with this injury.

Incidence

- Metatarsal fractures are common with the 5th metatarsal constituting >50% of all metatarsal fractures (1)[A].
- Incidence peaks in men in their 30s and in women in their 60s (1)[A].

ETIOLOGY AND PATHOPHYSIOLOGY

- When the cortical bone's mechanical strength is exceeded acutely by direct trauma, such as a heavy object falling on the foot, it will fracture.
- A fracture may also occur when the bone-tendon interface is acutely stressed past its mechanical failure point.
- An additional mechanism for fracture occurs when repetitive subthreshold forces are incompletely healed, and the additive damage eventually causes an overt fracture.

RISK FACTORS

- Those with osteopenia or osteoporosis have a greater risk.
- Any activity that increases the likelihood of direct trauma to the foot increases the risk of metatarsal injury.
- Twisting mechanism is associated with 5th metatarsal fractures (1)[A].
- Excessively rapid progressions of training volume and/or stress on the foot can also increase the risk of metatarsal stress injury.
- Alcohol abuse may increase the risk for nonunion complicating this fracture (2)[A].

GENERAL PREVENTION

- Gradual increases in workload allow a bone to adapt to mechanical stress and become stronger.
- Bone is a dynamic organ that is subject to anabolic forces tending to build it up as well as to catabolic forces tending to break it down.
- This balance allows a bone to remodel and adapt to stress but may also cause progressive weakening if catabolic forces outweigh the anabolic ones, such as with too-rapid progression of training load.

COMMONLY ASSOCIATED CONDITIONS

- The same forces that cause fracturing of the metatarsals may also injure adjacent structures such as the midfoot joint (between the row of cuneiform bones articulating with the 1st through 4th metatarsals and the cuboid articulating with the 4th and 5th metatarsal). At the other end, the metatarsophalangeal (MTP) joints may be involved when a fracture extends into the joint or when the joint capsule or ligamentous structures are disrupted.
- Other injuries to consider:
  - Midtarsal joint injury (calcaneocuboid or talonavicular): can include lateral process of talus or anterior process of calcaneus
  - Navicular or cuboid contusion/fracture
  - Metatarsocuneiform (MTC)/cuboid injury: Lisfranc joint injury may include ligamentous disruption and/or fracture of surrounding bone.
  - MTP injury: can include capsular or ligamentous sprain (turf toe) or fracture of adjacent bone
  - Phalangeal fracture
  - Sesamoid contusion or fracture
- Predisposing conditions:
  - Hallux valgus/hallux rigidus: Altered mechanics at the 1st MTP joint leads body weight shifting laterally over the lesser caliber 2nd metatarsal.
  - Osteopenia/osteoporosis: Decreased mechanical strength of the bone increases susceptibility to stress fracture and acute fracture.
  - Diabetes mellitus puts one at risk for a poorer outcome (3)[C].

DIAGNOSIS

- Diagnosis of overt metatarsal fracture is by radiograph.
- Standard views include the anteroposterior (AP), lateral, and oblique views.
- Addition of weight-bearing views may help identify subtle lesions as well as Lisfranc injuries if the patient tolerates them.
- Point of care ultrasound may be an alternative imaging modality because it is quick and sometimes more readily available. Radiography is still the standard of care (4)[A].
- Diagnosis of radiographically negative stress injury is via a technetium-99 bone scan or by MRI:
  - Advantages of MRI over bone scan include differentiation of stress reaction without fracture lines versus macrotrabecular fracture.
- Prehospital:
  - Prehospital/on-field care includes minimizing weight-bearing on the affected extremity as well as icing to reduce swelling and inflammation.
  - If there is no evidence for open fracture or vascular compromise, plain radiographs may be obtained at the patient's convenience.
  - If there is visible bone penetrating the skin or the extremity is cool indicative of vascular compromise, immediate transport to the emergency room is advisable.

HISTORY

- With acute injury, the patient will usually be able to point to the area of direct trauma to the foot or a twisting injury causing pain.
- More subtle stress injuries will typically have a history of recent increases in training volume or impact load and possibly a prior history of other stress fractures, disordered eating, or menstrual irregularities.

PHYSICAL EXAM

- Point-tenderness directly over the metatarsal is the typical finding on exam.
- The foot will usually show some swelling in comparison to the unaffected foot and possibly some bruising as well.
- Gross displacement is not common. Open fractures will present with bone penetrating through the skin.
- Focal tenderness and/or swelling over the metatarsals after an injury is a clear indication for plain radiographs to rule out a fracture.
- Chronic symptoms of foot pain with weight-bearing and negative radiographs warrant further imaging such as bone scan or MRI.
- An urgent need for a clear diagnosis after an acute injury and negative radiographs also suggests the need for further imaging.
- Tuning fork testing is a quick and easy sideline/clinic test which can provide some reassurance if negative but is widely variable for accuracy and specificity.

DIFFERENTIAL DIAGNOSIS

- MTP joint synovitis: inflammation of the joint rather than stress reaction in the bone itself. Bone scan will show distal uptake around MTP joint. MRI is diagnostic. Claw toe may also cause synovitis with plantar displacement of metatarsal head or a metatarsal stress reaction.
- MTP capsular strain and/or chip fracture of 1st metatarsal head (turf toe)
- Lisfranc sprain/fracture: injury to the 2nd MTC articulation. Any pain at the proximal 2nd metatarsal in association with a twisting injury in plantar flexion should raise concern for this injury.
- Midfoot sprain: injury to MTC ligamentous structures
- Forefoot mass (ganglion or tumor)
- Metatarsalgia
- Morton neuroma (interdigital neuroma)
- Freiberg infarction: osteonecrosis of 2nd metatarsal head; more common in adolescent athletes with unilateral (usually) pain in 2nd metatarsal head

DIAGNOSTIC TESTS & INTERPRETATION

- Plain radiographs will show cortical disruption if a significant fracture has occurred.
- The findings may be subtle with mild injury.
- A stress fracture may show subtle sclerotic borders/periosteal elevation or be entirely normal.
- Plain films only become positive once healing has progressed enough to produce visible bony callus. In the interim, an MRI should show changes on T2 images, and a bone scan should be positive for focal hot spot over the painful area.
- A computed tomography (CT) scan may be indicated for an intra-articular fracture to delineate any articular step-off.
- Ultrasound will show a cortical irregularity and fracture hematoma (4)[A].

TREATMENT

The goal of treatment is to stabilize the fracture such that normal length, rotation, and declination of the metatarsal is maintained, and the area is protected from further injury until healing has occurred:

- Prehospital:
  - If possible, the foot should be elevated and cooled with ice as soon as possible after injury.
  - Limited or crutch-assist weight-bearing is advisable until emergency department (ED) or physician evaluation has occurred.
  - Chronic complaints can be evaluated in a physician's office rather than an ED.
- ED treatment:
  - Evaluation of acute injury to the foot in the ED includes AP, lateral, and oblique plain radiographs. Good neurovascular status must be verified, as compartment syndrome can occur with a forefoot crush injury. The need for closed or open reduction is then assessed. Multiple metatarsal fractures with >4 mm of displacement or an apical angulation of the metatarsal head of >10 degrees on the lateral view could require open/closed reduction to ensure a normal weight-bearing position of the metatarsal head.
  - Open reduction of metatarsal, phalangeal, and MTP joint injuries can cause scarring and stiffness in addition to the original trauma. It is used largely to maintain a plantigrade foot for normal weight-bearing. An open fracture requires surgical intervention for débridement and stabilization.
  - Nondisplaced fractures of the metatarsal neck and shaft may be treated with a short leg cast, fracture brace, or a cast shoe. Weight-bearing is permitted as tolerated on discharge from ED. The minimum amount of immobilization necessary for comfort should be used. Fractures at the base of the 5th metatarsal may be treated with an ankle stirrup brace, cast shoe, or fracture brace to maintain comfort.

MEDICATION

- Depending on the severity of the injury, nonsteroidal anti-inflammatory drugs (NSAIDs) are first-line drugs to treat pain.
- Acetaminophen is also used.
- More severe pain may require narcotic pain relief.

First Line

- NSAIDs
- Acetaminophen

Second Line

- Oral low- to mid-potency narcotics such as hydrocodone
- Tramadol and codeine are also options but should be avoided in patients age <12 yr as well as breast feeding women (5).
- Tramadol should also be avoided in patients taking selective serotonin reuptake inhibitors (SSRIs) due to the risk of serotonin syndrome.

ISSUES FOR REFERRAL

- Multiple metatarsal fractures
- Single metatarsal fracture with >4 mm of displacement
- Single metatarsal fracture with >10 degrees of dorsal angulation of distal segment
- Possible compartment syndrome
- Displaced/comminuted fracture of the 1st metatarsal
- Open fracture
- Proximal 5th metatarsal fracture nonunion after 12 wk of conservative care

ADDITIONAL THERAPIES

- Proximal 5th metatarsal avulsion fracture (pseudo-Jones fracture):
  - Mechanism is usually due to an acute inversion injury to the ankle in plantar flexion. This can cause avulsion of the peroneus brevis or lateral plantar aponeurosis at the metatarsal tuberosity. May be a stress injury. They tend to be nondisplaced and experience relatively rapid union with symptomatic treatment. More distal injuries (without being a Jones fracture) may require short leg casting with non–weight-bearing (NWB) status for up to 6 to 8 wk. Use open reduction and internal fixation (ORIF) for delayed union or nonunion, significant displacement, or if cuboid 5th metatarsal joint involved.
- Jones fracture (proximal shaft of 5th metatarsal):
  - The metaphyseal/diaphyseal junction is a watershed zone for blood flow and is susceptible to delayed union or nonunion. Consider ORIF in higher level athletes primarily and if nonunion occurs as well as displaced acute Jones fractures. Treat initially with short leg cast/fracture brace with no weight-bearing until evidence of bony callus formation is seen. Progress to weight-bearing at that point; may present with preinjury symptoms similar to stress fracture exacerbated by inversion injury
- Spiral fracture of 5th metatarsal (dancer's fracture):
  - This is typically treated nonsurgically with a fracture brace or cast shoe. Weight-bearing is allowed as tolerated. Radiographic healing may take up to 12 wk.

SURGERY/OTHER PROCEDURES

- Proximal 5th metatarsal fracture/Jones fracture: ORIF with malleolar screw Kirschner wires
- Bone grafting may be required with a nonunion.
- Lisfranc fracture/dislocation: involves 2nd through 5th MTC joints; ORIF with cortical screws and Kirschner wires

ADMISSION, INPATIENT, AND NURSING CONSIDERATIONS

- Metatarsal fractures rarely require inpatient care.
- Open fractures and multiple traumatic injuries that include a metatarsal likely require intravenous (IV) antibiotics and observed care.

ONGOING CARE

- Upon discharge from the ED or after initial diagnosis, a patient with a metatarsal fracture should be seen in the office for follow-up radiographs in 1 wk to document correct bony alignment and adequacy of the treatment mode. Assuming radiographs show stability, follow-up films can be obtained at 6 wk, when full healing should be expected.
- The least-limiting form of immobilization should be considered. With the exception of a Jones fracture, most metatarsal fractures tolerate weight-bearing with use of a cast shoe/wooden-soled shoe fairly quickly, if not at the time of diagnosis. If fracture brace/controlled ankle motion (CAM) boot use is required initially, transition to a stiff-soled or cast shoe should be considered when tolerated. A steel shank insert into a gym shoe may also be used.
- Restriction from full weight-bearing stress without protection should continue for at least 4 wk for a stress fracture and for 4 to 6 wk for a nondisplaced metatarsal fracture. Pain to palpation and forefoot swelling should subside as the fracture heals. Evidence for radiographic healing, resolution of edema, and pain-free direct palpation are needed for return to sports.
- Jones fracture:
  - Once diagnosis is made, an NWB fracture brace/cast is used for 6 wk to allow for healing to occur. Repeat radiographs are done at this point to assess progress, but up to 12 wk may be needed. Nonunion at 12 wk may require ORIF. The decision to pursue ORIF for a Jones fracture in a competitive athlete may occur at the time of initial diagnosis.

PATIENT EDUCATION

The patient should be advised to:

- Elevate the leg frequently to minimize forefoot edema.
- Use ice up to 20 min/hr to control swelling.
- Notify the physician if there is any significant increase in pain/swelling during the recovery process.
- Reduce activity level to remain pain free and use stiff-soled shoe for all weight-bearing activity until healing is complete.

PROGNOSIS

Good

COMPLICATIONS

- Nonunion
- Malunion with painful plantar calluses under the metatarsal head
- Dorsal corns secondary to friction over prominent metatarsal head

REFERENCES

1. Kane JM, Sandrowski K, Saffel H, et al. The epidemiology of fifth metatarsal fracture. *Foot Ankle Spec*. 2015;8(5):354–359.
2. Thorud JC, Mortensen S, Thorud JL, et al. Effect of obesity on bone healing after foot and ankle long bone fractures. *J Foot Ankle Surg*. 2017;56(2):258–262.
3. Bowes J, Buckley R. Fifth metatarsal fractures and current treatment. *World J Orthop*. 2016;7(12):793–800.
4. Kozaci N, Ay MO, Avci M, et al. The comparison of radiology and point-of-care ultrasonography in the diagnosis and management of metatarsal fractures. *Injury*. 2017;48(2):542–547.
5. Jin J. Risks of codeine and tramadol in children. *JAMA*. 2017;318(15):1514.

CLINICAL PEARLS

- The 1st metatarsal carries a large amount of load, and fractures of it are often surgical.
- Fracture-dislocations involving the Lisfranc joint are often missed on NWB films.
- Dancer's fractures, even displaced, will usually heal with conservative nonoperative management, whereas Jones fracture has a higher rate of nonunion and more often needs surgical fixation.

FRACTURE, MIDDLE PHALANX

Michael M. Linder, MD, CAQSM • Andrew M. Warner, MD

BASICS

DESCRIPTION

- Represents ~5% of all metacarpal and phalangeal fractures (1)
- Shaft is the most common location for fracture.
- Physeal fractures often occur in skeletally immature individuals.

ETIOLOGY AND PATHOPHYSIOLOGY

- The nature of deformation is unpredictable when compared to proximal and distal phalangeal bones (1).
- The flexor digitorum superficialis (FDS) and the central extensor slip (CES) insert onto the middle phalanx and account for the primary deforming forces on shaft fractures.
- Fractures proximal to the insertion of the FDS result in volar angulation of the distal fragment.
- Fractures distal to the insertion of the FDS will result in volar angulation of the proximal fragment.
- The CES may also pull the proximal fragment in dorsal angulation if the fracture is proximal to the FDS insertion.
- Interphalangeal collateral ligament injuries may result in avulsion fractures affecting articular surfaces.

COMMONLY ASSOCIATED CONDITIONS

- Distal interphalangeal (DIP) or proximal interphalangeal (PIP) joint dislocations
- Distal artery or nerve injury
- Extensor mechanism injuries
- Volar plate injuries and resulting swan neck deformities

DIAGNOSIS

HISTORY

Mechanism of injury:

- Grabbing a jersey, jammed finger, crush, traction, or twisting
- Document occupation and hand dominance.
- Probe for initial deformity or excessive blood loss.

PHYSICAL EXAM

- Inspect for deformity, ecchymosis, swelling, and open wound.
- Assess joint range of motion proximal and distal to the bony injury.
- Assess integrity of all joint structures.
- Assess rotational alignment (all digits should point to scaphoid tuberosity when flexed).
- Assess sensation (touch, pinprick, and two-point discrimination).
- Assess capillary refill. All should be compared either to contralateral side or adjacent finger.

DIFFERENTIAL DIAGNOSIS

- PIP dislocation
- DIP joint dislocation
- Tendon rupture
- Volar plate disruption
- CES separation
- Bone contusion
- Soft tissue contusion
- Capsular sprain

DIAGNOSTIC TESTS & INTERPRETATION

ALERT

All fractures require anteroposterior (AP), true lateral, and oblique with affected finger in isolation.

May require preimaging anesthesia (e.g., digital block)

TREATMENT

- Open, unstable, spiral, comminuted, or those that fail to maintain reduction require orthopedic referral (2).
- Fractures at the base (2):
  - Axial load injury common inciting mechanism
  - Nondisplaced fractures should be splinted for 2 wk with a dorsal extension block splint and then buddy taped for weeks 2 to 4.
  - Nondisplaced volar fractures, secondary to dorsal extension forces or dislocation, involving <30% of the articular surface are considered stable and may be splinted for 4 to 6 wk.
  - Fractures affecting the dorsum are frequently associated with central slip attachment and may result in a boutonnière deformity; treatment of these requires 6 wk in extension splinting.
- Transverse fractures of the shaft (2):
  - Nondisplaced: may be treated with buddy taping for 2 to 4 wk
  - Displaced: Attempt reduction under anesthesia (recommend orthopedic referral); with longitudinal traction and manipulation of distal fragment. Tape splint may be necessary for postreduction radiography; generally 15-degree angulation in plane of motion is tolerated; if postreduction films show adequate alignment, splint 4 to 6 wk.
- Condylar fractures (3):
  - Nondisplaced: managed with buddy taping for 2 to 4 wk
  - Displaced: require orthopedic consultation
- Open fractures necessitate careful management (2,3):
  - Will require orthopedic evaluation and intervention
  - Appropriate antibiotic coverage, sterile dressing, elevation, and splinting may be necessary until definitive operative treatment obtained.

ONGOING CARE

FOLLOW-UP RECOMMENDATIONS

- Repeat radiographs at 2 wk may add to follow-up.
- Deformity may result from no treatment, improper reduction, or poor splint compliance.
- Stiffness may result from overtreatment.
- Hand or occupational therapy is indicated for loss of function, or following surgical intervention (4).
- Return to play may be as early as 2 wk for nondisplaced simple transverse fracture but as long as 6 wk for more complicated fractures (4).
- A goal of lifelong function should take precedence when making return-to-play decisions.
- Pediatric injuries may require close attention throughout growth and play.

REFERENCES

1. Koval KJ, Zuckerman JD. *Handbook of Fractures*. 5th ed. Philadelphia, PA: Lippincott Williams & Wilkins; 2015.
2. Eiff MP, Hatch RL. *Fracture Management for Primary Care*. 3rd ed. Philadelphia, PA: WB Saunders; 2011.
3. Browner BD, Levine AM, Jupiter JB, et al. *Skeletal Trauma*. 5th ed. Philadelphia, PA: WB Saunders; 2015.
4. DeLee JC, Drez D. *Orthopaedic Sports Medicine*. 2nd ed. Philadelphia, PA: WB Saunders; 2003.

ADDITIONAL READING

Birrer RB, Griesemer BA, Cataletto MB, eds. *Pediatric Sports Medicine for Primary Care*. Philadelphia, PA: Lippincott Williams & Wilkins; 2002.

CLINICAL PEARLS

- All fractures require AP, lateral, and oblique views in isolation of affected digit.
- Splinting and buddy taping remain mainstay of nondisplaced, closed, middle phalangeal fractures, with follow-up 2 to 4 wk following injury.
- Hand/occupational therapy only indicated for functional impairment or following surgical intervention
- Open, unstable, spiral, comminuted or those with failure to maintain stability/reduction require orthopedic intervention.
- In pediatric and high-performance athlete patients, lifelong function is precedent to return-to-play consideration, requiring close follow-up throughout healing process.

F

FRACTURE, NASAL

Brandon M. Bockewitz, MD, CAQSM

BASICS

EPIDEMIOLOGY

- Most frequently injured and fractured facial structure due to its prominence:
  - Third most commonly fractured structure of the skeleton
- Most fractures occur in the lower half of the nasal bones, where they are thinner and broader.
- Annual incidence in the United States is 53.2/100,000.
- Occurs twice as often in males, most frequently between 15 and 25 yr of age and age >60 yr

ETIOLOGY AND PATHOPHYSIOLOGY

- The upper third of the nose is a bony tripod formed by a pair of nasal bones that meet in the midline, with the thin perpendicular plate of the ethmoid as a weak center strut.
- A pair of upper and lower lateral cartilages supported by the central quadrangular septal cartilage makes up the lower 2/3.
- Most common cause of injury by age group:
  - <20 yr: accident and sports related
  - 21 to 40 yr: assault related
  - 41 and older: accident related

COMMONLY ASSOCIATED CONDITIONS

- Fracture of other facial bones
- Septal hematoma
- Septal dislocation
- Cribriform plate injury with leakage of cerebrospinal fluid (CSF)
- Laceration
- Orbital fracture
- Concussion
- Cervical spine injury

DIAGNOSIS

HISTORY

- Force: Low-velocity trauma, such as a blow from an elbow, usually causes a simple fracture pattern. High-velocity trauma from a stick or fast-moving ball/puck more likely causes a complex comminuted fracture as well as associated injuries to the face, head, and cervical spine.
- Direction of blow: Lateral is most common and can cause fracture displacement and dislocation of the septum. Direct blows can lead to nasal obstruction. Inferior blows can disrupt the septal cartilage and nasal tip.

PHYSICAL EXAM

- Nasal deformity
- Epistaxis
- Nasal airway obstruction
- Periorbital swelling and ecchymosis
- Nasal bone reduction: best if done either immediately after the injury or 3 to 5 days later when swelling will not interfere with assessment
- Palpate nasal bones for deformity and crepitus.
- Ring test to rule out CSF leak by collecting fluid from the nose onto filter paper to see if a clear ring of CSF diffuses out beyond the central area of blood
- Intranasal examination must be performed on each side to evaluate for a bulging septal hematoma or septal dislocation. Use suction and a topical decongestant to control bleeding and then a nasal speculum, otoscope, or rigid nasal endoscope along with a light source for adequate visualization.
- Palpate all bony structures of the face, including teeth, to assess for associated trauma.
- It is imperative to establish that the airway is not compromised, and there is no other concomitant injury such as a concussion.

DIAGNOSTIC TESTS & INTERPRETATION

- Diagnosis is clinical because radiographs have not been shown to be helpful for diagnosis or management (1)[A].
- If suspicious for fracture of other facial bones, computed tomography (CT) is study of choice.
- Ultrasonography is more accurate than radiography for diagnosis. It also has a higher sensitivity than CT, especially for fractures that involve separation without depression (2)[B].

TREATMENT

GENERAL MEASURES

- Head-up position; lean forward to aid expectoration of blood.
- Direct pressure, ice
- Topical decongestant
- Cautery of visible bleeding sites in Kiesselbach plexus using silver nitrate sticks
- For refractory epistaxis, may have to pack both sides of the anterior nose with a tampon or antibiotic-soaked petrolatum gauze
- Posterior epistaxis can require inflation of a Foley bulb within the nasal fossa in addition to anterior packing to achieve hemostasis.

ADMISSION, INPATIENT, AND NURSING CONSIDERATIONS

- Can consider immediate closed reduction before swelling develops if the nose is severely displaced and health care provider is well trained
- In most cases, simply provide analgesics and re-examine in 2 to 5 days.
- Adults with nondisplaced fractures that cause minimal deformity may not require reduction.
- Persistent rhinorrhea that is clear and watery should raise suspicion for potential cribriform damage and CSF leak, in which case the patient needs to be transferred to the hospital for a CT scan and acute consultation with otolaryngology (3)[C].

ONGOING CARE

- Generally, nasal fractures should be managed within 2 to 3 wk after injury, and manipulation should occur within 10 days for adults and 7 days for children (4)[B].
- Closed reduction (5)[B]:
  - Ideally performed in first 3 to 6 hr after injury, before significant swelling occurs
  - If delayed, should be done within 10 to 14 days of the injury, before significant bone healing occurs
  - Indications for adult population:
    - Unilateral or bilateral nasal bone fracture
    - Nasal deviation <1/2 the width of the nasal bridge
  - Local anesthesia using a 5% or 10% topical cocaine solution is highly effective for both analgesia and vasoconstriction but rarely available.
  - Topical nasal sprays, including lidocaine, bupivacaine, and Pontocaine, are alternatives for adequate anesthesia.
  - Topical vasoconstrictors, such as phenylephrine hydrochloride and oxymetazoline, provide adequate hemostasis and decrease edema.
  - A 1:1 mixture of topical oxymetazoline or phenylephrine and 4% topical lidocaine has been cited as an equally efficacious alternative to topical cocaine (6).
  - Blunt probe is placed within the nose and used to elevate the depressed nasal bone. Forceps are used to reduce septal deformity.
  - External splint and packing for 1 to 2 wk
- Open reduction (5)[B]:
  - Indications for adult population:
    - Extensive/complicated fracture-dislocation of nasal bones and septum
    - Nasal deviation >50% the width of the nasal bridge
    - Open fracture
    - Persistent nasal deformity after closed reduction
    - Involvement of the caudal septum

REFERENCES

1. Nigam A, Goni A, Benjamin A, et al. The value of radiographs in the management of the fractured nose. *Arch Emerg Med*. 1993;10(4):293–297.
2. Dogan S, Kalafat UM, Yüksel B, et al. Use of radiography and ultrasonography for nasal fracture identification in children under 18 years of age presenting to the ED. *Am J Emerg Med*. 2017;35(3):465–468.
3. Patel Y, Goljan P, Pierce TP, et al. Management of nasal fractures in sports. *Sports Med*. 2017;47(10):1919–1923.
4. Basheeth N, Donnelly M, David S, et al. Acute nasal fracture management: a prospective study and literature review. *Laryngoscope*. 2015;125(12):2677–2684.
5. Mondin V, Rinaldo A, Ferlito A. Management of nasal bone fractures. *Am J Otolaryngol*. 2005;26(3):181–185.
6. Kucik CJ, Clenney T, Phelan J. Management of acute nasal fractures. *Am Fam Physician*. 2004;70(7):1315–1320.

ADDITIONAL READING

- Procacci P, Ferrari F, Bettini G, et al. Soccer-related facial fractures: postoperative management with facial protective shields. *J Craniofac Surg*. 2009;20(1):15–20.
- Rubinstein B, Strong EB. Management of nasal fractures. *Arch Fam Med*. 2000;9(8):738–742.

CLINICAL PEARLS

Return to play following a nasal fracture:

- It can take 6 wk for a nasal fracture to completely heal. An athlete should be advised that returning to competition before complete healing means that even minor contact could disrupt a minimally displaced or previously reduced fracture and require additional intervention. A general guideline is no contact for 1 to 2 wk followed by return to play while wearing a nasal protective device for another 4 wk following the initial insult. This is extended to 6 wk should operative intervention be required.
- If the patient participates in combat sports such as boxing or mixed martial arts, operative intervention is more common and 10 to 12 wk is recommended.
- 92% of athletes eventually return to play (3)[C].
- Case reports have been published of return to play within 7 to 10 days with nasal protective device worn for 4 wk postreduction with encouraging results.

F

FRACTURE, OLECRANON

Greg Nakamoto, MD, FACP

BASICS

The issue of fundamental concern when evaluating fractures of the olecranon is determining whether the fracture is displaced or nondisplaced:

- Nondisplaced fractures can be managed with immobilization.
- Displaced fractures should be referred to an orthopedic surgeon for consideration of fixation

DESCRIPTION

- The olecranon is the curved process extending from the posterior proximal surface of the ulna. It forms a large portion of the articulating surface between the ulna and the trochlea of the humerus. The triceps inserts into the posterior third of the olecranon.
- For a fracture of the olecranon to be considered nondisplaced and stable, it must be displaced <2 mm, must not change in position with gentle flexion to 90 degrees, and must not change in position with extension against gravity (1).

EPIDEMIOLOGY

- Account for ~10% of fractures of the adult elbow (1,2)
- Olecranon fractures can range from simple nondisplaced fractures to complex fracture dislocations of the elbow (1).
- Olecranon fractures are uncommon in children because early in life the olecranon process is short, thick, and relatively stronger than the distal humerus. When they do occur, they are often associated with radial head subluxation or dislocation.

RISK FACTORS

- Direct trauma, such as a fall onto the tip of the elbow, may cause a fracture directly and is most often associated with isolated injuries (1):
  - In one series, fall from a standing height was the mechanism for 70% of olecranon fractures (2).
- Indirect trauma, such as a fall onto the hand with the elbow partially flexed, may cause an avulsion owing to eccentric contraction of the triceps (1).
- Fracture-dislocation also is possible with a high-energy mechanism of injury. The olecranon fragment usually displaces posteriorly (1).

COMMONLY ASSOCIATED CONDITIONS

ALERT

The evaluating physician should be aware of the following conditions which can complicate the evaluation and treatment of olecranon fractures:

- **Ipsilateral upper extremity fracture**: In the series noted above, 22% of all olecranon fractures were associated with an ipsilateral upper extremity injury, the most common being fractures of the radial head and neck (2).
- Due to its superficial position at the medial elbow, **ulnar nerve injury** is reported in 2–5% of cases.
- **Discontinuity of the triceps mechanism**
- **Fracture-dislocation** of the elbow
- **Open fracture**
- Although rare, the forearm should be evaluated for **compartment syndrome.**

DIAGNOSIS

HISTORY

Mechanism of injury (1,2,3):

- A fall, often from standing height, or blunt trauma to the posterior elbow may cause the fracture directly.
- A fall onto an outstretched hand may cause a fracture indirectly, often through avulsion by the triceps.
- A high-energy mechanism of injury increases the likelihood of fracture dislocation.

PHYSICAL EXAM

- Pain and swelling over the posterior elbow
- Elbow effusion owing to the intra-articular component of the fracture
- Painful and limited motion at the elbow
- Determine if patient can extend the elbow against gravity. Inability to extend suggests either discontinuity of the triceps mechanism or a mechanical block. Either problem merits surgical consultation (1)[C].
- Perform distal neurovascular examination. The ulnar nerve may be injured; more common in comminuted fractures (1)
- Excessive soft tissue injury, swelling, or ecchymosis may influence the timing of surgery (1)

DIFFERENTIAL DIAGNOSIS

- Radial head fracture
- Coronoid process fracture
- Olecranon bursitis

DIAGNOSTIC TESTS & INTERPRETATION

- Standard radiographs: Anteroposterior (AP) and lateral views are traditionally considered sufficient for the evaluation of isolated olecranon fractures; some authors also advocate obtaining oblique views (1)[C].
- A true lateral view is necessary to evaluate for fracture displacement and articular disruption; slightly oblique views are inadequate substitutes for a true lateral.
- Fat pad signs: Collection of intra-articular fluid (e.g., caused by intra-articular fracture) causes displacement and, hence, visualization of the fat pads around the elbow. The anterior fat pad sometimes may be visible in the normal elbow; the posterior fat pad usually is not visible on a normal lateral radiograph and may be the only radiographic evidence of occult fracture.
- Children: often helpful to obtain radiographs of the contralateral elbow for comparison
- Computed tomography (CT) scan:
  - Traditional teaching is that good-quality standard radiographs as just listed are essential for accurate diagnosis, classification, and operative planning. In cases of isolated olecranon fracture, they also should be sufficient, and CT scan in such cases rarely provides additional information that alters decision making. CT scan generally is reserved for more complex fracture combinations (1)[C].
  - However, in one study of surgical plating of olecranon fractures, six of the seven fractures thought to be simple on plain film analysis were found to have occult comminution on CT. The authors concluded that comminution should consequently be considered in all cases of olecranon fractures, even when plain film displays simple patterns, because it may affect choice of surgical fixation (see Wellman et al. in "Additional Reading")

TREATMENT

- Radiographic classification and staging of olecranon fractures can help guide decisions regarding operative versus nonoperative treatment:
  - There are several systems used for classification of olecranon fractures, including the AO classification, the Schatzker classification, the Mayo classification, and the Colton classification. No single classification is used universally (4).
  - The Mayo classification is useful in determining whether an olecranon fracture should be treated surgically (1)[C]. Classification is based on stability, displacement, and comminution (4):
    - Mayo type I fractures (undisplaced [<2 mm] ± comminution) can be treated nonoperatively.
    - Mayo type II (stable fractures with >3 mm displacement) and type III fractures (unstable, displaced fracture-dislocations) should be treated surgically.
  - The Colton classification is based on the degree of displacement and fracture pattern. In one comparative study of classification systems, it had high interobserver agreement, presumably because of its simplicity (4):
    - Type I—undisplaced (<2 mm of separation and no increase in displacement with flexion of 90 degrees, and the patient can actively extend the elbow against gravity)
    - Type II—displaced (including IIA, avulsions; IIB, transverse and oblique; IIC, comminuted; and IID, fracture-dislocations)
  - The AO classification considers olecranon fractures as a subset of elbow fractures (4):
    - Type A—extra-articular fractures of the metaphysis of the radius or ulna (thus, olecranon fractures are not included in type A fractures)
    - Type B—intra-articular fractures of the radius or ulna (Olecranon fractures are subclassified as type B1 fractures.)
    - Type C—intra-articular fractures of both the olecranon and radial head
  - The Schatzker classification considers fracture morphology as it relates to biomechanical considerations for each type of surgical fixation (4):
    - Type A—simple transverse fracture
    - Type B—transverse impacted fracture
    - Type C—oblique fracture
    - Type D—comminuted fracture
    - Type E—oblique fracture that begins and ends distal to the midpoint of the trochlear notch (and as such, is actually extra-articular)
    - Type F—fracture-dislocations
  - As no single classification system is considered superior or used universally, achieving familiarity with the system used most commonly in your institution may be more practical than trying to learn all of them.
  - In the specific case of avulsion fractures, treatment is generally operative (1)[C].
- Reduction techniques:
  - Nondisplaced fractures: unnecessary
  - Displaced fractures: surgical reduction and fixation
  - Fracture-dislocation: See "Elbow Dislocation."

- Nonoperative treatment:
  - Patients with nondisplaced fractures (<2 mm displacement) with intact extensor mechanism (active extension against gravity) are good candidates for nonoperative management.
  - Immobilization of nondisplaced fractures can be done at any degree of flexion. Displacement is generally reduced by keeping the elbow in more extension. However, immobilization at 90 degrees is often more convenient.
  - Traditionally, a more **conservative approach** treated all nondisplaced olecranon fractures in a long arm cast with the elbow in 90 degrees of flexion for 3 to 4 wk, followed by protected range of motion exercises (1)[C]:
    - Follow-up x-rays are obtained 5 to 7 days after cast application to ensure that displacement has not occurred.
    - Flexion past 90 degrees is avoided until complete radiographic bony healing at 6 to 8 wk.
    - To avoid excessive stiffness, elderly patients are allowed to start range of motion before 3 wk if pain allows.
  - Other authors advocate an approach allowing for **early motion**, with immobilization for as little as 7 to 10 days. In such cases, treatment might proceed as follows:
    - Patient is immobilized at 90 degrees in a splint or cast for 7 to 10 days.
    - After 7 to 10 days, the patient starts gentle motion, beginning with pronation and supination.
    - At 2 to 3 wk, limited flexion and extension exercises can begin.
    - Flexion past 90 degrees can occur when radiographs show complete bone healing.
    - Repeat standard x-rays weekly until evidence of healing to ensure that there is no displacement requiring surgical referral.
    - Lifting can usually be allowed at 6 to 8 wk.
  - **Elderly patients with nondisplaced olecranon fractures**: Because of their propensity to develop stiffness at the elbow, elderly patients should spend much less time immobilized. In patients most prone to stiffness, joint immobilization can be achieved with a sling initially, and careful range of motion can begin once the patient is comfortable as soon as a few days later.
  - **Nonoperative treatment of displaced olecranon fractures in elderly patients** (5)[B]:
    - Recent retrospective studies of elderly patients (mean ages ranged from 76 to 82 yr depending on the study) revealed good to excellent functional and satisfaction outcomes.
    - In one study, nonunion occurred in 85% of patients but did not significantly impact satisfaction scores.
    - On the basis of such data, the nonoperative treatment of displaced olecranon fractures in low-demand elderly patients is consequently increasing in practice and is increasingly seen as an acceptable treatment option for such patients (5)[B].

ADDITIONAL THERAPIES

- Splinting: If there is a delay until definitive treatment can be accomplished, then temporary splinting may be done for patient comfort and protection:
  - Undisplaced fractures should be splinted with the elbow flexed at 90 degrees and hand in neutral position.
  - Displaced fractures should be splinted in a comfortable position with the elbow between 45 and 90 degrees and hand in neutral position; prompt orthopedic consultation should be obtained.
- Ice and oral analgesics are useful in the prehospital setting. Oral analgesics may be required for several days after casting.
- Nondisplaced fractures: Protected range of motion advanced as described earlier. If the patient still has stiffness, then dynamic splinting and physical therapy referral for elbow range of motion may be of benefit.
- Displaced fractures: range of motion to be initiated as determined by the operating surgeon

SURGERY/OTHER PROCEDURES

Indications for operative treatment include (1)[A]:

- Displaced or unstable fractures.
- Avulsion fractures and/or extensor mechanism disruption.
- Fracture-dislocations.

ONGOING CARE

FOLLOW-UP RECOMMENDATIONS

- Nondisplaced fractures (Mayo type I): can be released to home in a splint or cast with follow-up x-rays in 1 wk
- Displaced fractures: disposition determined in consultation with an orthopedic surgeon

COMPLICATIONS

ALERT

- **Loss of motion**:
  - Typically, 10 to 15 degrees of extension in isolated olecranon fractures (1)
  - Motion may improve somewhat for up to 2 yr after injury.
- **Nonunion** is reported in 1–5% of patients (1).
- **Heterotopic calcification** occurs in 13–14% of patients.
- For surgical patients, **painful hardware**, sometimes requiring subsequent removal, is one of the most common complications after internal fixation; reported in up to 80% of patients (1)

REFERENCES

1. Veillette CJ, Steinmann SP. Olecranon fractures. *Orthop Clin North Am*. 2008;39(2):229–236.
2. Brolin TJ, Throckmorton T. Olecranon fractures. *Hand Clin*. 2015;31(4):581–590.
3. Ali M, Hatzantonis C, Aspros D, et al. Management of type IIB and IIIB olecranon fractures. Case series. *Int J Surg Case Rep*. 2017;41:296–300.
4. Benetton CA, Casa G, El-Kouba Junior G, et al. Agreement of olecranon fractures before and after the exposure to four classification systems. *J Shoulder Elbow Surg*. 2015;24(3):358–363.
5. Motisi M, Kurowicki J, Berglund DD, et al. Trends in management of radial head and olecranon fractures. *Open Orthop J*. 2017;11:239–247.

ADDITIONAL READING

- Duckworth AD, Bugler KE, Clement ND, et al. Nonoperative management of displaced olecranon fractures in low-demand elderly patients. *J Bone Joint Surg Am*. 2014;96(1):67–72.
- Duckworth AD, Clement ND, McEachan JE, et al. Prospective randomised trial of non-operative versus operative management of olecranon fractures in the elderly. *Bone Joint J*. 2017;99-B(7):964–972.
- Gallucci GL, Piuzzi NS, Slullitel PA, et al. Non-surgical functional treatment for displaced olecranon fractures in the elderly. *Bone Joint J*. 2014;96-B(4):530–534.
- Kubik J, Schneider P, Buckley R, et al. Evaluating the utility of the lateral elbow radiography in central articular olecranon reduction: an anatomic and radiographic study. *J Orthop Trauma*. 2018;32(3):e81–e85.
- Marot V, Bayle-Iniguez X, Cavaignac E, et al. Results of non-operative treatment of olecranon fracture in over 75-year-olds. *Orthop Traumatol Surg Res*. 2018;104(1):79–82.
- Veras Del Monte L, Sirera Vercher M, Busquets Net R, et al. Conservative treatment of displaced fractures of the olecranon in the elderly. *Injury*. 1999;30(2):105–110.
- Wellman DS, Lazaro LE, Cymerman RM, et al. Treatment of olecranon fractures with 2.4- and 2.7-mm plating techniques. *J Orthop Trauma*. 2015;29(1):36–43.

CLINICAL PEARLS

- The goal when evaluating fractures of the olecranon is determining whether the fracture is nondisplaced and stable versus displaced and/or unstable.
- For a fracture of the olecranon to be considered nondisplaced and stable, it must be displaced <2 mm, must not change in position with gentle flexion to 90 degrees, and must not change in position with extension against gravity.
- The assessment of stability and displacement usually can be made with standard radiographs and clinical examination. CT scan is usually reserved for the evaluation of clearly more complex fracture patterns; however, there is some limited data to suggest that comminution should be considered in all olecranon fractures.
- Stable, nondisplaced fractures (Mayo type I) can be treated nonoperatively. Additionally, low-demand elderly patients with displaced fractures may also be candidates for nonoperative treatment. All other fractures merit orthopedic consultation for consideration of surgical treatment.
- Physician response to common patient questions:
  - How long do I need to wear this cast/sling?
    - Nondisplaced fractures: In the case of a stable fracture in a reliable patient, immobilization is for comfort and can be discontinued after initial pain and swelling have resolved in 7 to 10 days (even less in the elderly patient prone to stiffness). If the patient is at particular risk for displacing an otherwise stable fracture, immobilization in a long-arm cast for up to 3 wk may be required.
    - Displaced fractures: depends on the extent of injury and type of repair required

FRACTURE, ORBITAL

Jennifer J. Mitchell, MD, FAAFP, CAQSM • Kelly T. Mitchell, MD

BASICS

DESCRIPTION

- Fracture of the osseous walls of the orbit
- Orbital anatomy:
  - Bony orbit is a conical structure:
    - Base faces anterolaterally.
    - Apex originates posteromedially.
    - Seven bones: frontal, maxilla, zygoma, ethmoid, lacrimal, palatine, sphenoid
  - Orbital roof:
    - Forms floor of frontal sinus
  - Orbital floor:
    - Forms roof of maxillary sinus
    - Most commonly fractured area of orbit
  - Medial wall:
    - Forms walls of ethmoid sinus, sphenoid sinus, and nasal cavity
    - Second most frequently fractured area of orbit
  - Lateral wall:
    - Not bordered by a sinus
    - Thickest and strongest of the orbital walls (1)
- Types of orbital fractures:
  - Orbital rim: caused by direct blow to bony orbit
  - Orbital wall: caused by blunt trauma to globe:
    - Blowout fracture: most common; fracture fragment is directed away from the bony orbit.
    - Blow-in fracture: trauma typically directed against frontal bone or maxilla; fracture fragment(s) is displaced toward the orbital space, decreasing the orbital volume (2).
- Trapdoor orbital fracture
- Pure orbital floor fracture, typically in pediatric patient
- Bony fragment displaces into maxillary sinus.
- Extraocular muscle(s) can become entrapped (inferior oblique or inferior rectus, most commonly).
- Usually, restriction of upward gaze occurs.
- Also called white-eyed blowout fracture due to minimal outward signs of trauma
- Significant oculocardiac reflex can occur (3,4).

EPIDEMIOLOGY

- ~1/3 of orbital blowout fractures are sustained during sport. Other causes include motor vehicle accidents, assaults, and falls.
- Eye injury is the second leading cause of visual impairment after cataract.
- 40% of monocular blindness is due to eye trauma.
- 57% of eye injuries were sustained by individuals <30 yr of age.
- Males sustain around 80% of eye injuries.
- 13% of serious eye injuries are related to sports and recreation.
- Estimated 1,400 of every 100,000 U.S. citizens will sustain an eye injury in their lives (5).

Incidence

Trauma to the eye represents ~3% of all emergency department (ED) visits in the United States.

Prevalence

- Around 2.5 million new eye injuries occur annually.
- Eye trauma is the cause of 40,000 to 60,000 new cases of blindness each year.
- Annually, ~11,000 eye injuries sustained by children are caused by toys or home playground equipment (5).

ETIOLOGY AND PATHOPHYSIOLOGY

- Blowout fractures:
  - Occur along medial wall and/or orbital floor
  - Orbital rims are intact.
- Two proposed theories (3):
  - Hydraulic theory:
    - Blunt object of larger than diameter of the orbital entrance strikes the eye.
    - Compresses globe, resulting in sudden increase in intraorbital hydraulic pressure
    - Globe does not rupture.
    - Increased intraocular pressure dissipates via soft tissues to weakest portions of orbit: posteromedial orbital floor, lamina papyracea of ethmoid bone, or medial orbital wall.
  - Buckling theory:
    - Fractures occur as a result of direct trauma to the inferior orbital rim.
    - Causes buckling of the orbital floor
    - Thinnest area fractures

RISK FACTORS

- Most common causes of orbital fracture:
  - Sporting events/falls/assaults
- Sports most commonly associated with orbital fracture in the United States:
  - Baseball, football, basketball, racquetball

GENERAL PREVENTION

- Use of eye protection for any sport where an object or another participant may impact the globe
- Monocular athlete should always wear polycarbonate eye protection in American Society for Testing and Materials (ASTM)-approved frames (1).

COMMONLY ASSOCIATED CONDITIONS

- Ocular injury is associated with blowout fracture 14–40% of the time.
- Potential associated injuries:
  - Mild ocular injuries:
    - Subconjunctival hemorrhage
    - Conjunctival laceration
    - Corneal abrasion
  - Vision-threatening injuries:
    - Corneal laceration
    - Globe rupture
    - Hyphema
    - Traumatic iridocyclitis
    - Acute glaucoma
    - Lens subluxation/dislocation
    - Posttraumatic cataract
    - Vitreous hemorrhage
    - Retinal detachment/tear
    - Commotio retinae, traumatic retinal swelling
    - Foreign body: intraocular or intraorbital
    - Optic nerve injury
    - Orbital emphysema with ocular vascular compromise
    - Retrobulbar hemorrhage
  - Injuries to ocular adnexa:
    - Eyelid contusion ± ecchymosis
    - Eyelid laceration ± margin involvement
    - Canthal injury, laceration, or avulsion
    - Traumatic ptosis
  - Intracranial injuries:
    - Pneumocephalus
    - Cerebral injury
    - Cerebrospinal fluid leak
  - Delayed complications:
    - Enophthalmos
    - Hypoglobus

DIAGNOSIS

HISTORY

- Timing
- Mechanism:
  - Penetrating trauma:
    - Energy/velocity
    - Type of material
    - Size of object
  - Nonpenetrating trauma
- Location
- Protective eyewear in use
- Visual symptoms:
  - Change in vision
  - Diplopia
  - Discharge
  - Flashing lights
  - Floaters
  - Pain
  - Photophobia
- Prior ocular history:
  - Contact lens use
  - Previous visual impairment/visual correction
  - Prior trauma
  - Surgical history
- Tetanus status

PHYSICAL EXAM

- Signs and symptoms include (3)[A]:
  - Decreased vision.
  - Diplopia.
  - Enophthalmos.
  - Exophthalmos.
  - Hypoesthesia in V2 distribution:
    - Infraorbital, cheek, lateral nose, upper lip
  - Intraorbital emphysema.
  - Nosebleed.
  - Periorbital ecchymosis.
  - Step-off abnormality of bony structures.
- Systematic physical examination includes the following (3)[A],(4)[C]:
  - Neurologic survey first
  - If neurologically intact, then initial visual acuity (VA) to evaluate for emergent visual changes
  - Avoid placing pressure on globe; risk of vitreous herniation if globe is ruptured
  - VA before manipulation of eye
  - Near vision (near-reading card or other readily available reading material)
  - Far vision (Snellen chart)
  - Patient should use his or her corrective lenses (not contacts).
  - Patient unable to see well enough to read:
    - Display number of fingers
    - Detection of hand motion
    - Light perception
  - Pupil exam:
    - Size, shape, symmetry
    - Reaction to light
  - Swinging flashlight test: Afferent pupillary defect is present if the pupil of the affected eye dilates when exposed to the light source.
  - Examine head, scalp, face, and periorbital tissues.
  - Lacerations: location, depth, length
  - Lid edema
  - Foreign body
  - Sensory deficit
  - Bony tenderness to palpation around orbital rim
  - Orbital rim fracture
  - Step-offs: blowout fracture

- Exophthalmos
- Enophthalmos
- External eye structures:
  - Conjunctiva:
    - Blood (subconjunctival hemorrhage)
    - Chemosis (swelling)
    - Foreign bodies
  - Cornea:
    - Fluorescein stain/cobalt blue light
    - Irregularities (abrasion, laceration, ulceration)
    - Foreign bodies
- Extraocular motility: Generally, decreased motility may be due to edema.
- Impaired upward gaze: orbital floor fracture
- Impaired downward gaze: inferior rectus or oblique muscle entrapment
- Intraocular pressure: Use Tono-Pen; do not use Schiötz tonometer or manual pressure.
- Funduscopic exam:
  - Defer if vision is near normal and ophthalmology will perform indirect exam less urgently.
  - If vision with significant abnormality, defer as ophthalmology evaluation is imminent.
  - Red reflex presence or absence
  - Decreased intensity can imply vitreous hemorrhage or large retinal detachment.
  - Central retinal artery pulsations
- Slit-lamp exam:
  - If available: anterior chamber, cornea, iris, lens, or defer to ophthalmology
  - If not available, use penlight to look for:
    - Hyphema.
    - Obvious laceration.
    - Shrunken-appearing globe.

DIAGNOSTIC TESTS & INTERPRETATION

- Plain-film radiographs:
  - Rarely used for diagnosis in orbital trauma
  - High false-negative rate: 50%
  - Nondiagnostic rate: 30%
- If plain films ordered:
  - Waters view best displays inferior orbital rims, nasoethmoid bones, and maxillary sinuses.
  - Teardrop sign represents orbital contents herniated into maxillary sinuses.
  - Air–fluid levels/opacifications of sinuses that may indicate fracture
  - Orbital emphysema: medial wall blowout fracture
- Computed tomography (CT) scan, standard imaging modality (4)[C]:
  - Thin-sliced helical CT with coronal reconstructions:
    - Improved image quality
    - Reduced radiation to lens
  - If helical CT scan not available (4)[C]:
    - CT scan with slices of 3 mm or less
    - Axial plane *and* coronal plane
    - Only way to assess orbital floor and roof
    - Sagittal reconstruction helpful
  - Sensitivity 79–96%
  - May help distinguish between orbital edema and entrapment of extraocular muscles
  - Findings may predict future enophthalmos or diplopia: may play a role in prompting surgery.
- Ultrasound:
  - Contraindicated if high suspicion of globe rupture
- Magnetic resonance imaging (MRI):
  - Limited usefulness in acute stages of ocular trauma
  - Do not perform if metallic intraocular foreign body may be present.
  - Helpful if suspicion of optic nerve injury
  - May identify organic foreign body

TREATMENT

Not emergent unless:

- Visual impairment
- Globe injury
- Immediate referral to ophthalmology for open globe injury, facial fracture, symptomatic orbital emphysema, orbital compartment syndrome, retrobulbar hemorrhage, child with trapdoor fracture, optic neuropathy, and to rule out other ophthalmologic injuries
- Prehospital:
  - Airway, breathing, and circulation (ABCs) first priorities
  - Cervical spine immobilization and neurologic evaluation
  - Control active bleeding with direct pressure.
  - No direct pressure to orbit if open globe is possible or suspected.
  - Cover with a protective shield, and refer to ophthalmologist immediately.

MEDICATION

- Antibiotics may be prudent when fracture communicates with sinus.
- Pain control to include acetaminophen, nonsteroidal anti-inflammatory drugs (NSAIDs), narcotics, and local anesthetics. Avoid aspirin.

ADDITIONAL THERAPIES

- Cold packs for at least 48 hr
- Nasal decongestants
- Elevate head of bed.
- Avoid nose blowing; increased risk of orbital cellulitis
- Avoid Valsalva maneuvers such as coughing.
- Sneeze with mouth open.
- Tetanus booster, if not current (3)[A]

SURGERY/OTHER PROCEDURES

- Surgical goal (4)[C]:
  - Reconstruct the defect area of the fractured wall
  - Does not attempt to achieve bone healing
- Strong surgical indications (3)[A]:
  - Diplopia, not improving
  - Enophthalmos >2 mm
  - Fracture >50% of floor
  - Increase in orbital volume >1 cm^3
  - Lack of ocular motility
  - Significant hypoglobus
- Lesser degrees of trauma indications controversial
- Timing of surgery is controversial:
  - Rarely urgent, except when:
    - Oculocardiac reflex present (bradycardia, nausea/vomiting)
    - Ocular motility lesions in children
    - Muscle entrapment in trapdoor fracture:
      - In pediatrics, early surgery (within 24 to 48 hr) appears to be associated with better outcomes (4)[C].
    - Penetrating craniocerebral injuries
    - Concern for optic nerve compression
  - Appropriate timing important for achieving good results:
    - Delay allows for:
      - Orbital swelling resolution.
      - Assisting in ensuring accurate diagnosis.
      - Strengthening indications for surgery.
- No consensus on best material for repair
- If not emergent indications, conservative management may be considered with close follow-up because spontaneous improvement is possible and may be an emerging paradigm (6)[B].

ONGOING CARE

Return to play:

- Based on significance of ocular injury and associated findings
- Fracture only:
  - Noncontact sport: 2 wk
  - Contact sport: 4 to 6 wk
- Surgery for fracture:
  - Return will vary.
  - Depends on specific repair required
- Return to activities with proper eye protection

PATIENT EDUCATION

Return sooner than planned follow-up for:

- Intense eye pain.
- Change in vision.
- Proptosis.
- Tense globe.

REFERENCES

1. Micieli JA, Easterbrook M. Eye and orbital injuries in sports. *Clin Sports Med*. 2017;36(2):299–314.
2. Uzelac A, Gean A. Orbital and facial fractures. *Neuroimaging Clin N Am*. 2014;24(3):407–424.
3. Gart MS, Gosain AK. Evidence-based medicine: orbital floor fractures. *Plast Reconstr Surg*. 2014; 134(6):1345–1355.
4. Chung SY, Langer PD. Pediatric orbital blowout fractures. *Curr Opin Ophthalmol*. 2017;28(5): 470–476.
5. May DR, Kuhn FP, Morris RE, et al. The epidemiology of serious eye injuries from the United States Eye Injury Registry. *Graefes Arch Clin Exp Ophthalmol*. 2000;238(2):153–157.
6. Young SM, Kim YD, Kim SW, et al. Conservatively treated orbital blowout fractures: spontaneous radiologic improvement. *Ophthalmology*. 2018; 125(6):938–944.

ADDITIONAL READING

- American Society for Testing and Materials: http://www.astm.org/Standards/F803.htm
- Kontio R, Lindqvist C. Management of orbital fractures. *Oral Maxillofac Surg Clin North Am*. 2009; 21(2):209–220.
- Petrigliano FA, Williams RJ III. Orbital fractures in sport: a review. *Sports Med*. 2003;33(4):317–322.

CLINICAL PEARLS

- Significant changes in VA or vision loss: possible optic nerve compromise:
  - Ophthalmic emergency
  - Immediate ophthalmology consultation
- Significant other exam abnormality: immediate ophthalmology consultation
- All other abnormalities: ophthalmology consultation within 48 hr
- To diagnose orbital fracture, helical CT scan with coronal reconstructions or CT scan with 3-mm or smaller slices in both axial and coronal planes to assess orbit floor and roof is essential
- Most orbital fractures will resolve without significant visual sequelae or need for surgical intervention.

FRACTURE, PATELLA

Aaron J. Provance, MD, FAAP, CAQSM

BASICS

Mechanisms of injury:

- Direct trauma: often comminuted but minimally displaced; associated with fractures of the tibia, femur, and hip as well as posterior hip dislocation
- Indirect trauma: exertional loading of the extensor mechanism beyond the tensile strength of the patella; often with unexpected knee flexion; frequently transverse with significant displacement and disruption of the extensor retinaculum

ALERT
Pediatric sleeve fractures: Cartilage of the inferior pole of the patella is pulled off, often with a small avulsed bone fragment. This occurs with a vigorous contraction of the quadriceps muscle group when the knee is in a flexed position.

- Patellar subluxation or dislocation: associated with osteochondral fractures of the medial facet of the patella; avulsion fractures of the medial aspect of the patella can occur at the attachment of the medial retinaculum.

EPIDEMIOLOGY

Incidence

- 1% of all fractures
- Usually 20 to 50 yr of age

Pediatric Considerations

- Patellar sleeve fractures occur between 8 and 12 yr of age and are the most common form of patella fracture <16 yr of age.
- Osteochondral fractures are common in the adolescent years.
- Incidence of osteochondral fractures (patellar and femoral) in patients with first-time traumatic patellar dislocations can be as high as 24%.
- Predominant gender: male > female (2:1); patellar sleeve fractures: male > female (3:1).

DIAGNOSIS

- Transverse (50–80%): Usually displaced, of the middle and lower thirds in the adult population, most patellar fractures sustained during sports participation are of the transverse type (1)[C]. They often result from a strong quadriceps contraction, such as in a partial fall or in jumping sports, also with associated direct trauma.
- Stellate (30%): usually comminuted and nondisplaced; often secondary to high-impact direct trauma in sport or motor vehicle accidents
- Longitudinal (12–25%): due either to trauma (especially of the lateral facet) or to subluxation/dislocation of the patella; often in adolescents with resulting osteochondral fragments

ALERT
- Sleeve fractures: significant articular cartilage and a small bony fragment avulsed from the distal pole; often difficult to see on plain films; may have an ipsilateral patella alta
- Stress fractures: Majority have been documented in weight lifters and gymnasts.

HISTORY

- Activity (partial fall, exertional strain, etc.)
- Trauma (object, direction, force)
- Subluxation or dislocation
- Popping or snapping
- Locking or joint instability
- Loss of range of motion (ROM)
- Difficulty weight-bearing
- Speed and extent of swelling
- Characterization of pain
- Constitutional symptoms, especially with delayed presentation or evidence of infection
- Previous knee injuries
- Past medical and surgical history
- Medications and allergies

PHYSICAL EXAM

- Signs and symptoms include:
  - Tenderness to palpation and pain with passive motion of the patella.
  - Hemarthrosis or diffuse soft tissue swelling of the knee.
  - Limited range of active leg extension owing to disruption of soft tissues.
- Physical examination includes the following:
  - Pain and tenderness with palpation
  - Pain with passive motion
  - Palpable step-off defect
  - Effusion or soft tissue swelling
  - Distal neurovascular status
  - Full range of active knee extension implies preservation of extensor mechanism.
  - Rule out associated injuries, especially hip, femur, leg, and ankle.
  - Soft tissue injuries, contamination, or signs of infection

Pediatric Considerations

Stress testing of ligaments should be delayed until after radiographic evaluation, if there are concerns of growth plate injury in children.

ALERT
- Open fractures should be ruled out owing to the risk of osteomyelitis and septic arthritis.
- Patellar apprehension test is used to help identify acute patellar dislocation.

DIFFERENTIAL DIAGNOSIS

Bipartite patella: usually bilateral and not associated with point tenderness, with rounded edges at the superior and lateral corners of the patellae

Pediatric Considerations

- Sinding-Larsen-Johansson syndrome: Overuse injury of the inferior pole of the patella typically occurring between 10 and 14 yr of age may be misdiagnosed as a patellar fracture.
- Acute patellar dislocation: moderate to large hemarthrosis and positive apprehension sign; may or may not have underlying osteochondral defect
- Proximal tibia or distal femur fractures: should be ruled out radiographically with plain films
- Occult physeal injuries: may require magnetic resonance imaging (MRI) if not apparent on plain films
- Anterior cruciate ligament tears: may present with moderate to large hemarthrosis; can have similar mechanism of injury as patellar dislocation; meniscal tears: may present with hemarthrosis and lack of ROM; tenderness usually along medial or lateral joint line

DIAGNOSTIC TESTS & INTERPRETATION

- Anteroposterior (AP) and lateral radiographs: used to evaluate patella, distal femur, proximal tibia, and soft tissues. The AP view can help to determine fracture lines, and the lateral view can help to determine the number of fragments and combination (1)[C].
- Axial (sunrise, merchant) views: help to identify osteochondral medial patellar avulsion and other longitudinal fractures. Comparison views of the contralateral side should be used to help determine fractures. Sunrise view (90 degrees of flexion) can be very difficult to obtain with lack of ROM and pain. Merchant view (30 to 60 degrees of flexion) may be easier to obtain acutely.
- Computed tomography (CT) scan: used to detect suspected occult fractures
- Bone scan: used to evaluate stress reactions, stress fractures, and osteomyelitis
- MRI: used to evaluate suspected soft tissue injuries and patellar sleeve and osteochondral fractures. MRI is a critical tool for evaluating the severity of an osteochondral defect and assessing the true extent of injury to the extensor mechanism with patellar sleeve fractures (2)[C].

ALERT
All patients with first-time traumatic dislocations should be suspected of having an osteochondral injury until proven otherwise by MRI, CT scan, or continued clinical examination (3)[C].

- Osteochondral fractures have been reported to be missed on 30–40% of initial radiographs based on MRI studies and surgical findings (4)[A].

TREATMENT

- Acute management:
  - Analgesia
  - Aspiration of hemarthrosis may be followed by injection of local anesthesia to facilitate assessment of the extensor mechanism. Presence of fatty globules is indicative of an osteochondral defect or occult patellar fracture (4)[A].
  - Consider aspiration of tense anterior hematomas.
  - Ice and elevation to control swelling (avoiding prolonged, direct application)
  - Nonsteroidal anti-inflammatory drugs (NSAIDs) PRN only for pain control
- Immobilization: splinting and support in position of comfort (usually slight flexion) to minimize quadriceps contraction and fracture distraction

- Nonoperative treatment:
  - Displacement of <3 mm in any plane or <2 mm at the articular surface
  - Full range with active knee extension as compared to the contralateral side

ALERT

The athlete's ability to straight-leg raise against gravity is crucial when selecting treatment options (2)[C]:

  - Compressive dressings and aspiration of hemarthrosis (if present) before cast application may help to control edema and discomfort.
  - Immobilization in full extension in a locked knee brace with early weight-bearing as tolerated for initial 2 to 3 wk (5)[C]
  - Early active ROM with hinged knee brace with progression in flexion after 2 to 3 wk
  - Weekly radiographs should be obtained to evaluate for possible fracture displacement and appropriate healing (2)[C].
  - Progressive ROM and strengthening are used until the patient can perform a straight-leg raise against gravity without extension lag (2)[C].

ADDITIONAL THERAPIES

Special considerations: open fractures: intravenous (IV) antibiotics and emergent referral for extensive irrigation and débridement, usually followed by internal fixation

SURGERY/OTHER PROCEDURES

- Displacement of >2 mm of articular step-off or >3 mm in any plane of fracture separation
- Disruption of extensor mechanism is indicated by lack of full extension against gravity.
- Open reduction and internal fixation (ORIF): modified tension-band wiring with either circumferential wire loops or in fragmentary wires or screws (depending on fragment configuration) in conjunction with repair of medial and lateral retinaculum; small fragments might not be amenable to surgical fixation and need to be resected (6)[A].
- Partial patellectomy: indicated with severe patellar comminution or inability to restore a smooth articular surface; involves repair of retinaculum and reinsertion of patellar or quadriceps tendon into remaining patellar fragment near its articular surface
- Total patellectomy: reserved for severe comminution precluding retention of any significant (>25%) patellar fragments; involves soft tissue repair with shortening of the quadriceps tendon; loss of knee extension strength (up to 40%) is frequently reported.
- Inferior pole avulsion fractures: The normal height of the patella can be maintained by preserving the patellar pole.
- Osteochondral fractures: difficult to detect on plain films; usually heal if nondisplaced but require arthroscopic removal or screw fixation if displaced; associated patellar instability may be surgically corrected at the same time (3)[C].
- Surgery may be delayed with extensive or contaminated soft tissue injury.

ONGOING CARE

- Immobilization: long leg cast for nonoperative treatment and for 3 to 6 wk after partial or total patellectomy; immediate joint motion if intraoperative fracture stability is achieved (1)[C]
- Weight-bearing as tolerated in a cast or locked brace: reduces quadriceps contraction and fragment distraction
- Isometric exercises and straight-leg raises: started within days of cast application or surgical fixation
- ROM exercises such as continuous passive motion may be started immediately after stable internal fixation with a delay of 3 to 6 wk for immobilization in nonoperative treatment and after unstable fracture repair. Exercises should be delayed no more than 6 wk to reduce pain and improve ROM. Active flexion and passive extension are performed until the fracture is healed and then progress with resistance exercises (1)[C].
- Resistance exercises: Several months of resistance exercises may be required to achieve full strength and ROM.
- Return to play when bony healing is demonstrated on AP, lateral, and merchant radiographs; complete and painless ROM are achieved; 90% of quadriceps strength is achieved; and balance and proprioception are restored (1)[C].

FOLLOW-UP RECOMMENDATIONS

- Check ROM and strength as compared with the contralateral side.
- Repeat plain films (AP, lateral, and merchant) to document signs of healing with callus formation and periosteal reaction.
- Functional testing prior to return to sport
- Orthopedic referral whenever criteria for nonoperative treatment are not met

COMPLICATIONS

- Patellofemoral arthritis is the most common complication. Risk factors include incongruence of the articular surface and damage to articular cartilage. Treatment includes physical therapy, with patellectomy and tibial tubercle elevation reserved for severe cases.
- A slight decrease in flexion is common but not usually clinically significant. Early postoperative motion and physical therapy help to maintain ROM, with manipulation under anesthesia and arthroscopic lysis of adhesions required if unsuccessful.
- Painful hardware: common complication; managed by removal after fracture union (minimum 6 mo) or tendon healing (minimum 3 mo). In a recent study, patients reported quality of life and pain outcomes improved significantly after removal of hardware ($p = .001$ and $p = .002$, respectively). Functional outcome scores did not improve significantly after hardware removal (6)[A].
- Infection: local care for superficial infections; osteomyelitis or septic osteoarthritis often requires IV antibiotics with surgical irrigation and débridement, removal of loose hardware, and delayed closure.
- Radiographic evidence of avascular necrosis consists of a sclerotic area evident 1 to 2 mo after injury, usually of the proximal fragment; mostly asymptomatic, resolving spontaneously
- Loss of fixation: often owing to unrecognized comminution; requires surgery if fragments are significantly displaced
- Nonunion: very uncommon; repeat surgery indicated if symptomatic.
- Periosteal sleeve overgrowth: Patellar sleeve can continue to form new, excess bone which may need to be surgically removed.

REFERENCES

1. Bharam S, Vrahas MS, Fu FH. Knee fractures in the athlete. *Orthop Clin North Am*. 2002;33(3):565–574.
2. Dupuis CS, Westra SJ, Makris J, et al. Injuries and conditions of the extensor mechanism of the pediatric knee. *Radiographics*. 2009;29(3):877–886.
3. Bauer KL. Osteochondral injuries of the knee in pediatric patients. *J Knee Surg*. 2018;31(5):382–391.
4. Stefancin JJ, Parker RD. First-time traumatic patellar dislocation: a systematic review. *Clin Orthop Relat Res*. 2007;455:93–101.
5. Tříska Z, Urban J, Látal P, et al. Treatment of displaced patellar fractures with multiple circular cerclage. *Acta Chir Orthop Traumatol Cech*. 2017;84(3):202–207.
6. Greenberg A, Kadar A, Drexler M, et al. Functional outcomes after removal of hardware in patellar fracture: are we helping our patients? *Arch Orthop Trauma Surg*. 2018;138(3):325–330.

ADDITIONAL READING

Safran M, Zachazewski JE, Stone DA, (eds). Patellar fracture. In: *Instructions for Sports Medicine Patients*. 2nd ed. Philadelphia, PA: Elsevier; 2012:755–760.

CLINICAL PEARLS

- Most athletes with patellar fractures return to play the following season (3 to 6 mo) with little residual deficit. Return of function is more limited with comminuted, high-impact mechanisms of injury. Strength of terminal knee extension will be reduced by ~15–30% if patellectomy is required.
- If criteria for nonoperative treatment are met, studies have shown a failure rate of <5% for fractures managed nonoperatively.
- MRI is essential for evaluating associated soft tissue injury when there is concern for extensor mechanism disruption, and the results may influence the decision to proceed with surgical intervention.
- Many patients have some residual complaints, but most report good to excellent results overall after ORIF. Slightly fewer achieve this level of satisfaction after partial patellectomy, and fewer still after total patellectomy.

FRACTURE, PELVIC

David Carfagno, DO, CAQSM • Timothy Perdue, DO

BASICS

DESCRIPTION

- Most common mechanism of injury is motor vehicle accidents.
- 3% of skeletal injuries, mortality between 5% and 16%, higher in elderly populations
- The most widely used classification scheme is the Young-Burgess system, which focuses on the mechanism of injury.
- Fracture types:
  - *Lateral compression (LC)*: anterior injury—rami fractures:
    - The most common mechanism of pelvic fractures
    - This usually involves rami fractures anteriorly with a sacral impaction iliac wing fracture. This type of injury is rotationally unstable but usually vertically stable. LC I: sacral fracture on side of impact; LC II: crescent fracture on side of impact (iliac wing fracture); LC III: type I or II injury on side of impact with contralateral open book injury
    - Fracture of individual pelvic bone with no break in ring continuity
    - Isolated rami fractures: commonly seen in falls in the elderly
    - Iliac wing fractures (Duverney fractures) due to direct trauma or LC
    - Sacral fractures
    - Coccygeal fractures
  - *Anterior–posterior compression (APC)*: anterior injury = symphysis diastasis/rami fractures:
    - The first point of failure is the symphysis pubis. As increasing external rotation is applied, the sacrotuberous, sacrospinous, and anterior sacroiliac (SI) ligaments fail under tension. APC I: minor opening of symphysis and SI joint anteriorly; APC II: opening of anterior SI, intact posterior SI ligaments; APC III: complete disruption of SI joint
    - Significant urogenital, vascular, and neurologic injuries are accompanied by the APC and vertical shear (VS) injuries due to the stretch and traction placed on these structures as the injuring forces are applied.
    - Open book fracture:
      - Wide separation of symphysis pubis (often >2.5 cm) associated with SI joint disruption from anterior/posterior pelvic compression
    - Two ipsilateral ischiopubic rami fractures; most common type II fracture
    - Symphysis pubis fracture: often associated with genitourinary injury
    - VS type: vertical displacement of hemipelvis with symphysis diastasis or rami fractures anteriorly, iliac wing, sacral facture, or SI dislocation posteriorly
    - Combination (CM type): any combination of above injuries:
      - Multiple breaks in pelvic ring continuity
      - High risk for associated injuries and pelvic hemorrhage
      - Malgaigne fracture
      - Anterior and posterior break in the ring on the same side
      - Straddle fracture: fractures of all four pubic rami or ipsilateral fracture of two pubic rami with dislocation of symphysis pubis; due to LC or straddle injury (i.e., fall on object)
      - Severe multiple fractures and crush injuries or falls resulting in multiple fractures and gross instability
  - *Avulsion fractures*:
    - The ischial tuberosity is the most common location for apophyseal avulsion injury in the pelvis and usually results from a forceful contraction of the hamstring muscles.
    - Avulsion of the ischial tuberosity is most often associated with intense athletic activity, such as sprinting, or with excessive passive lengthening of the hamstring muscles, as often occurs during cheerleading or gymnastics.
    - The patient may experience a popping sensation at the time of injury and typically presents with severe posterior thigh or gluteal pain and complains of difficulty walking.

ETIOLOGY AND PATHOPHYSIOLOGY

- The incidence of pelvic fractures in the United States is estimated to be >100,000 per year.
- 60% of pelvic fractures occur from motor vehicle accidents, most commonly pedestrians struck by automobiles.
- 30% are due to falls from heights.
- Represent the third most common cause of death in motor vehicle accidents
- Mortality rate from pelvic fractures reported is 5–42%.
- Increases to nearly 50% with hemorrhagic shock
- Significant pelvic hemorrhage can occur in unstable pelvic fractures, particularly type III fractures:
  - Bleeding most commonly arises from the venous plexuses.
  - Significant hemorrhage results in retroperitoneal hematoma formation that may tamponade in the enclosed pelvic space.

RISK FACTORS

Etiologies of pelvic fractures in descending order of frequency:

- Motorcycle crash
- Vehicle–pedestrian collision
- Side-impact motor vehicle collision
- Fall >15 feet
- Motor vehicle crash

DIAGNOSIS

- In awake patients, pain on palpation of the sacrum and SI joints has the highest sensitivity (98%) for posterior pelvic ring fractures (1)[A].
- Multidetector computer tomography (MDCT) is the gold standard for diagnosing pelvic injuries. It has high sensitivity for fractures and can determine additional areas of injury and hemorrhage (2,3)[A].
- In hospitals without MDCT capabilities or in hemodynamically unstable patients, a single anteroposterior (AP) view of the pelvis should be obtained as early as possible:
  - Most significant unstable pelvic fractures will be seen on the single AP view.
  - Once the patient is stable, specialized radiographs (inlet/outlet, Judet) can be obtained.

PHYSICAL EXAM

- Does the patient have pelvic pain?
- Are there neurologic deficits involving sciatic, femoral, or obturator nerves?
- Are there contusions, ecchymoses, or abrasions at or near the bony prominences of the pelvis?
- Are there ecchymoses of the scrotum or perineum?
- Is there blood at the urethral meatus?
- Is there blood in or around the rectum, and is the prostate normal?
- Are there open wounds of the groin, buttock, or perineum?
- Is there a leg length difference, or is the resting position of one leg different from the other?
- Is there pain or abnormal pelvic motion on compression of the anterior iliac spines, LC of the iliac crests, rotation of the lower extremity, or hip flexion–extension?

DIFFERENTIAL DIAGNOSIS

- Normal variants (i.e., os acetabuli epiphyseal line can mimic type I fracture on x-ray)
- Ligamentous injury
- Spinal injury
- Intra-abdominal injury and hemorrhage

DIAGNOSTIC TESTS & INTERPRETATION

- Type and crossmatch
- Hemoglobin/hematocrit, platelet count, and coagulation studies (prothrombin time/partial thromboplastin time)
- *Diagnostic studies*:
  - Prioritization of studies: computed tomography (CT), angiography, or surgery
  - *Imaging*:
    - In the hemodynamically stable patient, the patient can go to CT scan for evaluation of the abdomen, pelvis, and retroperitoneum (4)[C].
    - In the hemodynamically *unstable* patient, a rapidly performed AP radiograph or focused assessment with sonography in trauma (FAST) exam can determine treatment course.
    - Abdominal US (FAST exam) is highly specific for retroperitoneal bleeding, not very sensitive.
    - FAST exam has largely replaced diagnostic peritoneal aspirate (DPA) or DPL as the initial diagnostic exam of choice in trauma patients. However, DPA is still used in certain circumstances, such as determining if intraperitoneal fluid in the unstable patient is blood or urine:
      - If the FAST is positive, the patient should go for celiotomy with external pelvic fixation and peritoneal packing.
      - If the FAST is negative, DPA should be performed. If DPA is positive for hemorrhage, the patient should go for celiotomy with external pelvic fixation and peritoneal packing.
      - If the FAST and DPA are negative, pelvic stabilization, peritoneal packing should be performed.
      - The majority of patients will need pelvic angiography, but peritoneal packing controls bleeding more rapidly.
      - In the hemodynamically stable patient, the patient can go to CT scan for evaluation of the abdomen, pelvis, and retroperitoneum (4)[C].

  - MRI is indicated when there is evidence of neurologic injury.
- *Angiography*:
  - Angiography may be necessary in complicated pelvic fractures where vascular concern is an issue.
  - According to the Pelvic Injury Symposium in 2000, physicians can determine when interventional radiology may be needed based on certain scenarios:
    - Hemodynamic instability, poorly responsive to fluid challenge, no hemoperitoneum, pelvic fracture
    - Hemodynamic stability, little hemoperitoneum, pelvic fracture, >4 to 6 U transfusion over 24 to 48 hr, respectively
    - Large or expanding retroperitoneal hematoma encountered at laparotomy or active bleed on CT scan
    - Angiography is usually used in these above scenarios within the first 3 hr with a 90% rate of finding extravasation.
- *Red flags*:
  - Clinical signs that suggest an increased risk of ongoing pelvic fracture bleeding:
    - Prehospital hypotension
    - Admission base deficit >5
    - Persistent tachycardia in face of normal oxygenation and adequate pain control
    - Recurrent hypotension during resuscitation
    - Requirement for 6 U blood during first 24 hr

TREATMENT

GENERAL MEASURES

- LC I/AP I:
  - Protected weight-bearing on the affected side and treated conservatively with bed rest, analgesics, and comfort measures
  - Further surgical treatment may be needed if displacement of the fracture occurs after the patient starts to bear weight.
  - Follow-up x-rays can determine displacement after 2 to 5 days of physical therapy.
- AP II/LC I:
  - Marked displacement of the anterior ring without complete ring disruption. Consult orthopedic surgery.
- LC II, LC III, AP III, and VS:
  - Complete disruption of the posterior ring, and in general, require stabilization of both the anterior and posterior rings. Consult orthopedic surgery; patient should remain nothing per orem (NPO).
  - May require emergency department (ED) pelvic stabilization measures
  - Assess for pelvic hemorrhage (see below).
- Pelvic hemorrhage:
  - Angiography and selective vessel embolization
  - Direct operative control of pelvic bleeding
- *ED course*:
  - Determine which pelvic fractures are stable and unstable (see "Treatment").
  - *Initial stabilization*:
    - Airway, breathing, and circulation (ABCs) of trauma care:
      - Avoid using lower extremity intravenous (IV) sites.
      - Aggressive resuscitation with blood or crystalloid, 0-negative or type-specific blood if hemodynamically unstable
      - Immobilize the pelvis to prevent further injury and decrease bleeding.
      - Pneumatic antishock garment (PASG): Use in ED is controversial but allows rapid pelvic immobilization and pelvic compression to slow bleeding.

ALERT
PASG is an option, particularly when faced with a prolonged transport time or hemodynamically instability.

ALERT
Aggressive fluid resuscitation must occur before deflation of the PASG.

      - External fixator requires more time to place than PASG but "splints" pelvis in a similar manner; contraindicated in severely comminuted pelvic fracture
    - Placement of a stabilization device should not interfere with further workup and care (diagnostic peritoneal lavage [DPL], etc.).

MEDICATION

- Crystalloid fluids: normal saline or lactated Ringer, IV bolus 2 L; pediatrics: 20 cc/kg
- Blood products: crossmatched, type specific, or 0-negative 4 to 6 IU; pediatrics: 10 cc/kg
- Broad-spectrum IV antibiotics should be used in open fractures as prophylaxis against tetanus.

SURGERY/OTHER PROCEDURES

- Several factors play into the initial approach to bony stabilization, including hemodynamic status and response to resuscitation, fracture pattern, associated injury, and inflammatory status.
- Hemodynamic status is of particular concern because the pelvis may be the primary source of bleeding or may be contributing very little to bleeding. In the presence of ongoing thoracic or abdominal hemorrhage, orthopedic management beyond placement of a pelvic binder is delayed. Associated long bone fractures should be immediately splinted with coverage of open wounds.

ADMISSION, INPATIENT, AND NURSING CONSIDERATIONS

- *Hospital admission criteria*:
  - Hemodynamic instability and pelvic hemorrhage to the ICU
  - "Triad of death" is a term coined to describe patient decompensation in the presence of acute blood loss, resulting in hypothermia, coagulopathy, and acidosis.
  - Type III or IV pelvic fracture
  - Other related injuries (genitourinary, intra-abdominal, neurologic, etc.)
  - Intractable pain
  - Most elderly patients will require hospitalization.
- *ED discharge criteria*:
  - Type I or II fractures; hemodynamically stable with no evidence of other injuries
  - Patient able to ambulate and pain is adequately controlled

ONGOING CARE

COMPLICATIONS

- Vascular injury leading to blood loss
- Closed head injuries
- Visceral injury (bladder and urethral, small bowel, diaphragm)
- Nerve injury
- Deep venous thrombosis
- Atelectasis/pneumonia
- Musculoskeletal back pain
- Sexual dysfunction
- Malunion/nonunion of pelvic fracture

Pediatric Considerations

- Children can have proportionately greater hemorrhage.
- Nonaccidental trauma is a concern.

REFERENCES

1. McCormick JP, Morgan SJ, Smith WR. Clinical effectiveness of the physical examination in diagnosis of posterior pelvic ring injuries. *J Orthop Trauma*. 2003;17(4):257–261.
2. Mohseni S, Talving P, Kobayashi L, et al. The diagnostic accuracy of 64-slice computed tomography in detecting clinically significant arterial bleeding after pelvic fractures. *Am Surg*. 2011;77(9):1176–1182.
3. Dormagen JB, Tötterman A, Røise O, et al. Efficacy of plain radiography and computer tomography in localizing the site of pelvic arterial bleeding in trauma patients. *Acta Radiol*. 2010;51(1):107–116.
4. Magnone S, Coccolini F, Manfredi R, et al. Management of hemodynamically unstable pelvic trauma: results of the first Italian consensus conference (cooperative guidelines of the Italian Society of Surgery, the Italian Association of Hospital Surgeons, the Multi-specialist Italian Society of Young Surgeons, the Italian Society of Emergency Surgery and Trauma, the Italian Society of Anesthesia, Analgesia, Resuscitation and Intensive Care, the Italian Society of Orthopaedics and Traumatology, the Italian Society of Emergency Medicine, the Italian Society of Medical Radiology—Section of Vascular and Interventional Radiology—and the World Society of Emergency Surgery). *World J Emerg Surg*. 2014; 9(1):18.

CLINICAL PEARLS

- Most common mechanism of injury is motor vehicle accidents, so assess the pelvis in victims of such accidents.
- Significant vascular injury can accompany pelvic fractures, so rapid diagnosis and intervention are necessary. MDCT is the gold standard, but one AP radiograph should be used in unstable patients.
- Minor fractures can be managed conservatively; fractures with significant displacement will require surgical intervention.

FRACTURE, POSTERIOR MALLEOLUS

Kristina Quirolgico, MD

BASICS

DESCRIPTION

- Ankle fracture involving the posterior aspect of the distal tibial articular surface
- Also known as posterior pilon fracture

EPIDEMIOLOGY

- Isolated posterior malleolus fractures are rare—about 0.5–1% of all ankle fractures.
- Posterior malleolus fractures are present in 44% of all ankle fractures and 71% of spiral distal tibia fractures.

ETIOLOGY AND PATHOPHYSIOLOGY

Pronation or supination external rotation injury, posterior displacement of the talus, vertical loading during plantar hyperflexion, or a combination of these forces causes fracture of the posterior malleolus.

RISK FACTORS

- Repetitive vertical loading
- Osteoporosis

COMMONLY ASSOCIATED CONDITIONS

- Associated soft tissue and ligamentous ankle injuries (lateral, deltoid, and syndesmosis injuries)
- Bimalleolar or trimalleolar (posterior malleolus fractures in conjunction with lateral malleolus fractures, medial malleolus fractures, or both)
- Fracture patterns can be suggestive of posterior malleolar involvement:
  - Tibial spiral fractures are often associated with occult posterior malleolar involvement.

DIAGNOSIS

Diagnosis of posterior malleolar fractures relies on a high degree of clinical suspicion.

HISTORY

- Very important to obtain exact mechanism of injury:
  - Posterior malleolus fracture has been described in association with supination external rotation-abduction injuries, fall from great height, or motor vehicle accident (MVA).
- History should address chronic versus acute injury.
- Chronic presentation: ankle "sprain" that persists in being painful but is not unstable

PHYSICAL EXAM

- Observe for obvious deformity, ecchymosis, and swelling.
- Palpate for pain, starting away from area of maximal tenderness, and compare to uninvolved foot and ankle.
- Check for ligamentous laxity with anterior drawer and talar tilt tests.
- Assess neurovascular status.
- Assess gait and ability to bear weight.
- Consider a fracture if patient is unable to bear weight or has significant swelling or ecchymosis in an acute setting.

DIFFERENTIAL DIAGNOSIS

- Acute setting:
  - High-grade ankle sprain
  - Lateral/medial malleolus fractures
  - Achilles tendon injury
  - Peroneal tendon subluxation and dislocation
- Chronic setting:
  - Posterior ankle impingement (os trigonum syndrome or prominent posterior process of the talus)
  - Retrocalcaneal bursitis
  - Achilles tendinopathy

DIAGNOSTIC TESTS & INTERPRETATION

Use Ottawa Ankle Rules to decide on getting ankle x-rays to confirm diagnosis (1)[C]:

- Anteroposterior (AP), lateral, and mortise views should be obtained.
- Computed tomography (CT) and magnetic resonance imaging (MRI) are used to evaluate complex ankle fractures including tibial spiral fractures because they are often associated with occult posterior malleolar involvement (1)[C]:
  - CT recommended if high clinical suspicion and negative plain films
  - Addition of 3D reconstruction is preferable, especially for preoperative planning.

TREATMENT

Isolated posterior malleolus fractures and nondisplaced posterior malleolus fractures (<25% of distal tibial articular surface) in bimalleolar/trimalleolar ankle fractures are treated nonoperatively (2)[A]:

- Posterior ankle splint with compression wrap
- Ice, elevation
- Non–weight-bearing on crutches for 1 wk then follow-up
- Apply cast for total of 6 wk if fracture is nondisplaced on plain films.
- If fracture is displaced (>2 mm or >25% of distal tibial articular surface), then refer to orthopedic surgeon for evaluation (see "Surgery/Other Procedures").

MEDICATION

Pain management with nonsteroidal anti-inflammatory drugs (NSAIDs) versus opioids:

- Although animal studies have shown NSAIDs delay fracture union, human studies have not definitively shown an association between NSAIDs and fracture nonunion (3,4)[C].
- NSAIDs are acceptable to use in absolute stability (primary bone healing) and during the first week of healing via callous formation (secondary bone healing) (3,4)[C].
- Prolonged NSAID use may interfere with successful bone healing (3)[C].
- Opioids are associated with negatively impacting fracture healing, but there is no human study that can determine direct causality (4)[C].

ADDITIONAL THERAPIES

Physical therapy after both operative and nonoperative care (1)[C]:

- Goal is to regain ankle full range of motion, strength, and proprioception.

SURGERY/OTHER PROCEDURES

- If >25% of the articular surface of the distal tibia is involved, or if the fracture is displaced >2 mm, then open reduction and internal fixation (ORIF) is recommended (2)[A],(5)[B],(6)[A].
- When associated with syndesmosis injury, stabilization of the posterior malleolus fracture with posterolateral plating may be preferred over syndesmotic screw (5)[B],(6)[A].
- Postoperative care (1)[C]:
  - Active, compliant patients are treated in boot or walker with partial weight-bearing of 15 to 20 kg for 6 wk.
  - Older, noncompliant patients are offloaded in a wheelchair and below-knee cast.
  - Those with poor bone quality (osteoporosis, poorly controlled diabetes with neuropathy) are offloaded up to 12 wk.
  - Gradual increase of weight-bearing and activity once there is radiographic evidence of bony consolidation

ONGOING CARE

FOLLOW-UP RECOMMENDATIONS

Orthopedic referral should be considered for any isolated fractures of the posterior malleolus because they often are complicated by other injuries.

PATIENT EDUCATION

- It is important to discuss that ankle sprains and fractures often are difficult to differentiate.
- If diagnosed with ankle sprain, persistent symptoms (pain, swelling, limp) warrant follow-up and further workup.
- Many different outcomes exist depending on the severity and type of ankle fracture: Compliance is critical.
- Advise patients to avoid smoking because this can affect fracture healing.

PROGNOSIS

- Isolated posterior malleolar fractures have an excellent prognosis.
- Posterior malleolar fractures associated with significant comorbid fractures and/or syndesmotic injuries are much more likely to have long-term issues (see "Complications").

COMPLICATIONS

Variable depending on nonoperative versus operative management and patient comorbidities and compliance:

- Posttraumatic osteoarthritis
- Loss of normal range of motion
- Wound infection postoperative
- Postoperative pain due to hardware
- Persistent intra-articular step-off of >2 mm
- Nonunion
- Posttraumatic chronic regional pain syndrome
- Persistent talar subluxation

REFERENCES

1. Bartoníček J, Rammelt S, Tuček M. Posterior malleolar fractures: changing concepts and recent developments. *Foot Ankle Clin*. 2017;22(1):125–145.
2. Odak S, Ahluwalia R, Unnikrishnan P, et al. Management of posterior malleolar fractures: a systematic review. *J Foot Ankle Surg*. 2016;55(1):140–145.
3. Giannoudis PV, Hak D, Sanders D, et al. Inflammation, bone healing, and anti-inflammatory drugs: an update. *J Orthop Trauma*. 2015;29(Suppl 12):S6–S9.
4. Richards CJ, Graf KW Jr, Mashru RP. The effect of opioids, alcohol, and nonsteroidal anti-inflammatory drugs on fracture union. *Orthop Clin North Am*. 2017;48(4):433–443.
5. Li M, Collier RC, Hill BW, et al. Comparing different surgical techniques for addressing the posterior malleolus in supination external rotation ankle fractures and the need for syndesmotic screw fixation. *J Foot Ankle Surg*. 2017;56(4):730–734.
6. Veltman ES, Halma JJ, de Gast A. Longterm outcome of 886 posterior malleolar fractures: a systematic review of the literature. *Foot Ankle Surg*. 2016;22(2):73–77.

ADDITIONAL READING

- Barelds I, Krijnen WP, van de Leur JP, et al. Diagnostic accuracy of clinical decision rules to exclude fractures in acute ankle injuries: systematic review and meta-analysis. *J Emerg Med*. 2017;53(3):353–368.
- Boyd AS, Benjamin HJ, Asplund C. Splints and casts: indications and methods. *Am Fam Physician*. 2009;80(5):491–499.
- Donken CC, Goorden AJ, Verhofstad MH, et al. The outcome at 20 years of conservatively treated 'isolated' posterior malleolar fractures of the ankle: a case series. *J Bone Joint Surg Br*. 2011;93(12):1621–1625.
- Prasam ML, Lorich DG. Posterior malleolus fractures in athletes. *Oper Tech Sports Med*. 2017;25:82–86.
- Tenenbaum S, Shazar N, Bruck N, et al. Posterior malleolus fractures. *Orthop Clin North Am*. 2017;48(1):81–89.

CLINICAL PEARLS

- Posterior malleolar fractures rarely occur in isolation, so a high index of suspicion is necessary when lateral or medial malleolar fractures and/or syndesmotic injuries are diagnosed.
- An undiagnosed posterior malleolus fracture can be the source of chronic pain in the setting of ongoing pain associated with an ankle "sprain."
- Apply the Ottawa Ankle Rules to catch these on x-ray; posterior malleolar fractures are usually seen on lateral view. If not seen on x-ray, consider CT scan if there is a high clinical suspicion.
- Treat nonoperatively with splint/cast and non–weight-bearing for at least 6 wk for isolate, nondisplaced posterior malleolar fractures. Consider orthopedic surgery referral if posterior malleolar fracture involves >25% articular surface or >2 mm displacement.

FRACTURE, PROXIMAL PHALANX

James H. Lynch, MD, MS, FACSM • Gary Means, MD

BASICS

EPIDEMIOLOGY

- The most common fracture of the hand in adults
- Base of proximal phalanx fracture is most common pediatric hand fracture.
- Little finger is the most common ray involved, followed by the thumb.
- Males affected 3 times as often as females
- Crush or direct blow to the finger accounts for >80% of injuries.

ETIOLOGY AND PATHOPHYSIOLOGY

- Intrinsic muscles of the hand (interossei) insert into the extensor expansion on the dorsum of the proximal phalanx.
- Proximal phalangeal fractures usually angulate volarly due to the proximal fragment flexed by interossei and the distal fragment extended by the central slip's insertion on the base of the middle phalanx.
- Metacarpophalangeal (MCP) joint collateral ligaments are taut in 70 to 90 degrees of flexion and provide stabilization of the MCP joint.

COMMONLY ASSOCIATED CONDITIONS

- Digital nerve injury: contusion, transection
- Digital artery injury: open or closed fracture; usually does not require treatment
- Tendon injury: complete or partial rupture; infrequent with proximal phalangeal fracture
- Thumb avulsion fracture common with ulnar collateral ligament injury (See "MCP (Metacarpophalangeal) Collateral Ligament Sprain.")

DIAGNOSIS

HISTORY

- Mechanism of injury: direct blow, axial load, axial traction, twisting/torque, or "grabbing a jersey"
- History of previous injury, surgery, or deformity

PHYSICAL EXAM

- Pain, swelling, bruising, tenderness, loss of motion, and function are typical findings.
- Gross deformity in some cases
- Open (compound) fractures usually are obvious and require emergent care.
- May be mistaken for MCP or proximal interphalangeal (PIP) joint dislocation
- Malrotation is common with spiral and oblique shaft fractures and must be detected and corrected early.
- Inspection/observation: location and degree of deformity, swelling, and ecchymosis
- Rotational malalignment: With MCP and PIP flexed to 90 degrees, all fingers should point toward the scaphoid. When viewed "end on," the plane of all fingernails should be symmetrical.
- Range of motion (ROM): usually decreased. Compare with contralateral side.
- Palpation: Feel for crepitus. Determine point of maximal tenderness.
- Provocation: Axial loading or distraction often results in pain at the fracture site (nonspecific).
- Adjacent structures: MCP and PIP joints, tendon function, and soft tissues
- Neurocirculatory function: sensation, capillary refill, skin color, and temperature

DIFFERENTIAL DIAGNOSIS

- MCP joint dislocation
- PIP joint dislocation
- Soft tissue contusion, sprain, strain, or rupture

DIAGNOSTIC TESTS & INTERPRETATION

- Radiographs should be obtained before any manipulative examination.
- Anteroposterior (AP), true lateral, and oblique views are diagnostic.
- Describe rotation of fragments, angulation, and intra-articular versus extra-articular.
- Differences in diameter of fragments suggest rotation.
- Skilled ultrasonographers can detect phalangeal fractures with moderate sensitivity and specificity (1)[B].

TREATMENT

- Open (compound) fractures: irrigation, sterile wet dressing, ice, elevate, splint, refer to orthopedic surgeon:
  - Prophylactic antibiotics should be administered (2)[A].
  - Empiric antibiotics to cover *Staphylococcus aureus*: cephalosporin, penicillin (methicillin-susceptible *Staphylococcus epidermidis* [MSSE]), or clindamycin, cotrimoxazole (methicillin-resistant *Staphylococcus aureus* [MRSA])
  - Tetanus toxoid and/or immunoglobulin if indicated
- Reduction of fracture fragments to anatomical positions is desired to speed healing and maximize hand function. Closed reduction is often successful and should usually be attempted.
- After reduction, immobilization should be applied, and postreduction imaging should be obtained.
- Prehospital:
  - Apply sterile dressing over any open wounds.
  - Splint in a position of comfort, apply ice if available, and transport for radiographs and definitive treatment.
- Emergency department (ED) treatment:
  - Stable, nondisplaced without angulation or rotational deformity:
    - Dynamic splinting ("buddy taping") to an adjacent normal digit
    - Use absorbent material between digits for padding and to prevent maceration.
    - Early ROM: Patient should use the hand normally as comfort allows.
  - Nondisplaced and impacted fractures:
    - Some degree of intrinsic stability; do not require surgery
    - Splint with MCP joint flexed 70 to 90 degrees, interphalangeal (IP) joints extended, and buddy taping to adjacent finger to control rotation for 3 wk. Wrist and distal interphalangeal joint (DIP) need not be immobilized (3)[B]. This position of function shifts the extensor aponeurosis distally to cover the majority of the proximal phalanx dorsally, which compresses and stabilizes the fracture.
  - Displaced or angulated transverse midshaft:
    - Volar angulation common, generally unstable, with variable response to closed reduction, which should be attempted
    - Technique:
      - Metacarpal or digital block
      - Longitudinal traction and flexion of the MCP joint with manual realignment of fracture fragments
      - If reduction achieved/maintained, apply gutter splint or Burkhalter splint (dorsal slab of stabilizing material placed from the end of a short arm cast to just proximal to the PIP, with MCP joints flexed 70 to 90 degrees).
      - If reduction not achieved after splinting, refer to ortho/hand.

- Oblique fractures:
  - Attempt reduction and splinting (3)[B].
  - If reduction not achieved after splinting, refer to ortho/hand.
- Displaced fractures of the base:
  - Significant volar angulation requires reduction.
  - Technique:
    - Metacarpal or digital block
    - Longitudinal traction and flexion of the MCP joint and correct volar angulation with direct pressure
    - If reduction achieved/maintained, apply gutter or Burkhalter splint; if not, refer to ortho/hand.
- Unstable: condylar (lateral or medial aspect of base) and displaced intra-articular fractures:
  - Refer to ortho/hand for pin fixation or open reduction and internal fixation (ORIF).
- AP, true lateral, oblique to confirm reduction
- Unacceptable, unstable, or unsure alignment: early consultation with orthopedic surgeon advised
- Persistence of significant displacement, angulation of >15 degrees, intra-articular component, or any degree of rotational malalignment necessitates an orthopedic surgeon consultation (4)[C].

MEDICATION
- Oral analgesics may be used if needed.
- Digital or metacarpal block with local anesthetics may be used if reduction or repair of associated soft tissue injury is required.

ISSUES FOR REFERRAL
The following phalangeal fractures in children warrant prompt orthopedic consultation because many will require immediate surgery (5)[C]:
- Displaced phalangeal neck or condyle fractures: Failure to treat this injury with pin stabilization can result in a malunion that limits digital flexion.
- Malrotation fractures
- Widely displaced, irreducible proximal phalanx base fractures (due to entrapment of soft tissue)
- Avulsion fractures of the thumb MCP ulnar collateral ligament insertion (pediatric equivalent of skier's thumb, usually a displaced Salter-Harris type III intra-articular fracture)

ONGOING CARE

FOLLOW-UP RECOMMENDATIONS
On follow-up x-rays, any malalignment should prompt an orthopedic surgeon consultation.

Patient Monitoring
Monitor specific fractures as follows (6)[B]:
- Stable, nondisplaced without angulation or rotational deformity:
  - Treated with buddy taping
  - Dynamic splinting for 3 wk; x-ray at 7 to 10 days to check alignment and stability
  - Daily ROM exercises after 1 wk as comfort allows
  - Continued dynamic splinting for athletic activities for another 4 to 6 wk
- Nondisplaced and impacted fractures treated with splint or cast:
  - Recheck radiographs in 7 to 10 days to assess healing.
  - After 3 wk, early protected mobilization with buddy taping
- Displaced or angulated transverse midshaft treated with closed reduction and splint or cast:
  - X-ray at 5 and 10 days to assure reduction is maintained; if not, refer to ortho/hand.
  - If reduction maintained, continue splint for 3 to 4 wk; if reduction fails, refer to ortho/hand for ORIF or percutaneous fixation.
- Displaced fractures of the base:
  - X-ray at 5 and 10 days to assure reduction is maintained; if not, refer to ortho/hand.

COMPLICATIONS
- Joint stiffness and subsequent functional disability. Adhesions between extensor mechanism and periosteum may result in loss of motion requiring surgical intervention. Adhesions between flexor superficialis and flexor profundus may follow prolonged immobilization and require surgical intervention to restore function.
- Arthritis can result from intra-articular fractures.
- Nonunion is rare; however, risk of nonunion is greater when improperly immobilized, patient is noncompliant, or open fractures.

REFERENCES

1. Aksay E, Kilic TY, Yesilaras M, et al. Accuracy of bedside ultrasonography for the diagnosis of finger fractures. *Am J Emerg Med*. 2016;34(5):809–812.
2. Gosselin RA, Roberts I, Gillespie WJ. Antibiotics for preventing infection in open limb fractures. *Cochrane Database Syst Rev*. 2004;(1):CD003764.
3. Verver D, Timmermans L, Klaassen RA, et al. Treatment of extra-articular proximal and middle phalangeal fractures of the hand: a systematic review. *Strategies Trauma Limb Reconstr*. 2017;12(2):63–76.
4. Held M, Jordaan P, Laubscher M, et al. Conservative treatment of fractures of the proximal phalanx: an option even for unstable fracture patterns. *Hand Surg*. 2013;18(2):229–234.
5. Abzug J, Dua K, Bauer A, et al. Pediatric phalanx fractures. *J Am Acad Orthop Surg*. 2016;24(11):e174–e183.
6. Stanton JS, Dias JJ, Burke FD. Fractures of the tubular bones of the hand. *J Hand Surg Eur Vol*. 2007;32(6):626–636.

ADDITIONAL READING

- Cornwall R, Ricchetti ET. Pediatric phalanx fractures: unique challenges and pitfalls. *Clin Orthop Relat Res*. 2006;445:146–156.
- Giddins G. The nonoperative management of hand fractures in United Kingdom. *Hand Clin*. 2017;33(3):473–487.

CLINICAL PEARLS
- Return-to-play decision based on stability, ROM, current clinical and radiographic healing status, and specific demands of sport
- Most athletes with stable fractures are able to return as early as 2 wk after the injury with protection such as buddy taping.
- For unstable fractures, early surgical intervention may be desirable for better outcome and earlier return.
- Begin mobilization at 3 wk to prevent finger stiffness.

FRACTURE, PROXIMAL TIBIAL PLATEAU

Holly J. Benjamin, MD, FAAP, FACSM • Spencer Kirk, MD, MS

BASICS

- Tibial plateau fractures occur as a result of trauma:
  - Force directed either medially (valgus deformity) or laterally (varus deformity)
  - Axial compressive force
  - Combination of both
- An axial compressive force, a fall from a height onto an extended knee, usually results in a bicondylar fracture.
- Associated ligamentous injuries occur due to continued deforming force after the fracture has been sustained:
  - 68% of tibial plateau fractures have posterolateral ligamentous corner injury (1).
  - These ligamentous injuries may not always occur after the fracture but may be coincident with the tibial plateau fracture.
  - Medial plateau fractures are considered a knee dislocation variant.

DESCRIPTION

- Fracture that includes the articular surface of the medial and/or lateral tibial condyles
- Synonym(s): tibial plateau fracture
- First coined a "fender fracture" by Cotton in 1929:
  - 40–60% of tibial plateau fractures involve an automobile hitting a pedestrian. Fracture results from a medially directed force.

EPIDEMIOLOGY

- Tibial plateau fractures account for ~1% of all fractures and 8% of fractures in the elderly. Elderly are less likely to have meniscal or ligamentous injury.
- Lateral tibial plateau is smaller and weaker. Fractures of the lateral plateau account for 55–70%.
- Bilateral plateau fractures account for 11–31%.
- Medial plateau fractures account for 10–23%.
- In both sexes, the highest frequency was between the ages of 40 and 60 yr.

RISK FACTORS

- Osteoporosis
- Perioperative fracture associated with total or unicompartmental knee arthroplasty (2)
- Sports: skiing, football

COMMONLY ASSOCIATED CONDITIONS

- Tibial plateau fractures often accompany a predictable pattern of associated soft tissue knee injury:
  - Medial tibial plateau fracture: lateral collateral ligament and medial meniscus injuries
  - Lateral tibial plateau fracture: medial collateral ligament and lateral meniscus injuries
  - Anterior cruciate ligament (ACL) injuries can be seen with either medial or lateral plateau fractures. Also see intracondylar eminence fractures.
- Owing to brisk hemorrhage and swelling, tibial plateau fractures can be associated with acute compartment syndrome.

DIAGNOSIS

- X-ray: anteroposterior (AP), lateral, oblique; possible tunnel view
- Magnetic resonance imaging (MRI): indicated for assessment of associated ligamentous or cartilaginous injury
- Computed tomography (CT) scan: best to assess bone deformity
- Schatzker classification system for tibial plateau fractures (3,4):
  - Type I: lateral split
  - Type II: lateral split with depression
  - Type III: pure lateral depression
  - Type IV: pure medial depression
  - Type V: bicondylar
  - Type VI: metaphyseal-diaphyseal dissociation
- Ancillary studies: Knee aspirate may help to reveal the presence of fat globules (indicating osteochondral injury) and to reduce pain.

HISTORY

- An accurate history will help to determine the direction of the force, velocity (high vs. low), and initial deformity produced.
- Swelling can be immediate or delayed, often indicating osteochondral fracture or internal derangement.

PHYSICAL EXAM

- Signs and symptoms:
  - Painful swollen knee
  - Unable to bear weight
  - May have compartment syndrome signs and symptoms (see below)
- Physical examination:
  - Most accurate way to evaluate the extent of the soft tissue injuries
  - Allows for evaluation of the vascular and neurologic status of the extremity
  - Gives insight into any associated ligamentous injuries and subsequent stability of the extremity
  - Pain and swelling about the knee may be associated with varus or valgus knee deformity.
  - Visible knee deformity indicates a severe injury.
  - Tenderness to palpation is noted over the medial and/or lateral tibial plateau.
  - Associated ligamentous injuries may show tenderness to palpation and instability of the collateral or cruciate ligaments.
  - Key finding is excursion of endpoint movement.
  - Large hemarthrosis usually is present.
  - If not present, it may indicate a torn capsule if the plateau is depressed.
  - Document distal pulses.
  - Check neurologic status with focus on the peroneal nerve and tendon function.
  - Check for abrasions or possible open fracture.
  - Watch for compartment syndrome findings:
    - Pain out of proportion to the physical examination findings
    - Pressure or tightness in the compartment
    - Pallor
    - Paresthesias
    - Paralysis: sign of cell death and need for immediate compartment release

DIFFERENTIAL DIAGNOSIS

- Intercondylar eminence fracture ± ACL tear: Segond sign on plain film indicates lateral capsule avulsion.
- Collateral ligament avulsion
- Tibial tubercle avulsion
- Proximal fibular fracture
- Patella fracture
- Hemarthrosis from patellar dislocation, ACL tear, or meniscal tear (if in the red or red-white zone)
- Stress fracture
- Physeal injury (pediatric)

DIAGNOSTIC TESTS & INTERPRETATION

- Standard radiographs in AP, lateral, and two oblique views:
  - Initial x-rays may miss a small tibial plateau fracture.
  - High index of suspicion must be maintained based on mechanism of injury, presence/absence of an effusion, and joint instability.
  - Series provides information allowing for accurate assessment of the fracture pattern:
    - Internal oblique view best assesses the lateral plateau.
    - External oblique view best assesses the medial plateau.
    - Tunnel view helpful if suspicious for intercondylar eminence fractures
    - Lateral view demonstrates presence of depression:
      - Medial side is concave.
      - Lateral side is convex.
  - Posterior collateral ligament injury may show avulsion fracture.
- CT scan:
  - Image of choice if negative films but high index of suspicion for fracture

ALERT
Bicondylar tibial plateau fracture all need CT imaging.

  - Provides cross-sectional and sagittal assessment of the fracture pattern
  - Reveals extent and position of the fracture lines
  - Allows visualization of areas of depression (AP and lateral planes)
  - If necessary, three-dimensional reconstructions can be provided to enhance the understanding of the fracture.
- MRI: allows for assessment of associated ligamentous injuries; may not show fracture well
- Arteriography:
  - Should be considered in any tibial plateau fracture where the stability of the joint is in question
  - Also may use ankle brachial index (ABI); if <0.8, then indicates arterial insult
  - Medial plateau fractures have a high incidence of vascular insult (owing to greater energy injuring force).
  - Arteriography/ABI should be performed and documented in most instances.
  - Presence of a palpable pulse does not exclude the possibility of intimal tear.
  - May lead to intraoperative occlusive thrombosis that could jeopardize the extremity

TREATMENT

- No more than 5 mm (0.5 cm) of depression/displacement is acceptable for conservative treatment.
- Emergency department (ED) treatment:
  - Acute treatment:
    - Non–weight-bearing or toe-touch weight-bearing
    - Long leg splint with knee in full extension, ankle splinted at 90 degrees if instability or dislocation present

  - Hinged knee brace with 0 to 90 degrees of motion preferred for stable fracture
  - Ice, elevation
  - Pain management as needed. Acetaminophen, ice, and elevation are first line with limited use of narcotics and nonsteroidal anti-inflammatory drugs (NSAIDs).
  - If plain films show <5 mm of displacement, then nonoperative management is acceptable.

MEDICATION

- Conflicting evidence regarding safety of NSAIDs for pain management. Use caution if high risk for nonunion (5).
- Use total range of motion (TROM) brace locked in extension, and make the patient non–weight-bearing if pain control is difficult and to promote fracture healing.

ADDITIONAL THERAPIES

- Patient's age, medical condition, history of osteoporosis, and expected level of activity should be taken into consideration on a case-by-case basis in terms of operative versus nonoperative management.
- There are no specific recommendations regarding patient age or comorbid arthritis to dictate operative versus nonoperative management.
- Nonoperative treatment is possible with hinged TROM-style bracing and strict non–weight-bearing for 4 to 6 wk if:
  - Under adequate sedation, there is no varus/valgus instability through a full arc of motion.
  - The fracture shows no elements of depression or <5 mm of displacement.

ISSUES FOR REFERRAL

- Emergent referral and treatment if there is associated acute compartment syndrome and/or vascular injury
- Referral recommended within 48 hr if fracture is depressed or displaced (≥5 mm) or associated with significant ligament/meniscal injuries
- Key to good outcome is early range of motion (ROM) and non–weight-bearing compliance.
- Important to encourage quadriceps strengthening after bracing discontinued
- Physical therapy: warranted once evidence of fracture healing (4 to 6 wk); vital if <90 degrees flexion by 4 wk

SURGERY/OTHER PROCEDURES

- The goals of treating an intra-articular fracture of the tibia are to preserve pain-free joint mobility, stability, axial alignment, and articular cartilage congruity and avoid posttraumatic osteoarthritis.
- Best accomplished by anatomic reduction of the joint surface and restoration of axial alignment
- Intra-articular fractures, regardless of open or closed treatment, must be mobilized quickly to achieve the best ROM.
- Only percutaneous or open reduction and stable fixation allow early motion without loss of articular cartilage.
- Fractures treated initially by closed reduction often will show persistent displacement of articular cartilage fragments.
- If open reduction cannot be achieved owing to mitigating circumstances, then treatment should consist of skeletal traction and early mobilization.
- Bicondylar tibial plateau fractures are best managed with locked plating in favor of external fixation (6).
- Absolute surgical indications:
  - Open fractures
  - Acute compartment syndrome
  - Acute vascular injury
- Total knee replacement may be necessary in complex patterns in specific patient populations.
- Timing of surgery: immediate if open fractures, associated compartment syndrome, and fractures with associated vascular injuries
- Careful evaluation of fractures with tomography/CT scan/MRI is recommended:
  - Delay of 24 to 48 hr will not compromise the outcome.
  - Evaluation for soft tissue injury is important.
- Patients delayed >48 hr can be placed in skeletal traction.
- Postoperative management:
  - Depends on the degree of stability achieved with fixation and the findings at surgery
  - If stable, early motion by continuous passive motion (CPM) is beneficial.
  - Motion from full extension to 40 to 60 degrees of flexion on postoperative night 1.
  - CPM is increased to 90 degrees as quickly as possible.
  - If CPM is not available, immobilization of the knee in 60 to 90 degrees of flexion is recommended for the first 48 to 72 hr, followed by active motion.
  - Immobilization in flexion greatly affects postoperative motion.
  - Non–weight-bearing ambulation is encouraged postoperatively.
  - Stable type I to V fractures may start partial weight-bearing at 8 wk.
  - More comminuted fractures should be held non–weight-bearing for 10 to 12 wk.
  - *Early motion and non–weight-bearing are critical keys to long-term success.*

ONGOING CARE

PROGNOSIS

- High rate of osteoarthritis associated with tibial plateau fractures (7)
- Prognosis for full return of motion in the presence of osteoarthritis is poor.
- Outcomes are generally better in younger patients.

COMPLICATIONS

- Compartment syndrome (preoperative and postoperative); most common significant short-term complication
- Posttraumatic osteoarthritis
- Infection
- Wound slough
- Loss of ROM
- Loss of normal gait pattern
- Fixation failure
- Loss of articular reduction
- Malunion
- Nonunion (rare)
- Deep vein thrombosis
- Pseudoarthrosis

REFERENCES

1. Gardner MJ, Yacoubian S, Geller D, et al. The incidence of soft tissue injury in operative tibial plateau fractures: a magnetic resonance imaging analysis of 103 patients. *J Orthop Trauma*. 2005;19(2):79–84.
2. Kim KI, Egol KA, Hozack WJ, et al. Periprosthetic fractures after total knee arthroplasties. *Clin Orthop Relat Res*. 2006;446:167–175.
3. Schatzker J. Tibial plateau fractures. In: Browner B, Jupiter JB, Levine AM, et al, eds. *Skeletal Trauma*. Philadelphia, PA: WB Saunders; 1992:1745–1769.
4. Eiff MP, Hatch R. Patellar, tibial, and fibular fractures. In: *Fracture Management for Primary Care*. 3rd ed. Philadelphia, PA: Elsevier; 2012:234–243.
5. Marquez-Lara A, Hutchinson ID, Nuñez F Jr, et al. Nonsteroidal anti-inflammatory drugs and bone-healing: a systematic review of research quality. *JBJS Rev*. 2016;4(3). doi:10.2106/JBJS.RVW.O.0005.
6. Krupp RJ, Malkani AL, Roberts CS, et al. Treatment of bicondylar tibia plateau fractures using locked plating versus external fixation. *Orthopedics*. 2009;32(8). doi:10.3928/01477447-20090624-11.
7. Ding C, Cicuttini F, Jones G. Tibial subchondral bone size and knee cartilage defects: relevance to knee osteoarthritis. *Osteoarthritis Cartilage*. 2007;15(5):479–486.

ADDITIONAL READING

- Elsoe R, Larsen P, Nielsen NP, et al. Population-based epidemiology of tibial plateau fractures. *Orthopedics*. 2015;38(9):e780–e786.
- Prat-Fabregat S, Camacho-Carrasco P. Treatment strategy for tibial plateau fractures: an update. *EFORT Open Rev*. 2017;1(5):225–232.
- Stanitski CL, Harvell JC, Fu F. Observations on acute knee hemarthrosis in children and adolescents. *J Pediatr Orthop*. 1993;13(4):506–510.

CLINICAL PEARLS

- Need to have a high index of suspicion with ligamentous injury, especially in the setting of large swelling shortly after injury
- Although tibial plateau fractures have a low overall incidence, these injury patterns must be thought of in trauma owing to the risk of associated vascular insult (see discussion on arteriography under "Diagnostic Tests & Interpretation").
- Liberal use of advanced imaging is encouraged for full understanding of the extent of the injury, although x-ray evaluation is still considered the "gold standard" for imaging assessment.
- Consider compartment syndrome both pre- and postoperatively as a potential complication.
- The keys—both for early treatment and for long-term reasonable prognosis—lie in compliance with non–weight-bearing and ROM.
- Anticipate the development of osteoarthritis, and educate these patients accordingly.

F

FRACTURE, RADIAL HEAD

Ryan C. Fowler, MD, CAQSM • Keith A. Stuessi, MD, CAQSM

BASICS

As classified by modified Mason classification (Johnston adding type IV, Morey adding displacement and percentage affected for type II, and Rineer trying to establish stability for type II):

- Type I: nondisplaced or minimally displaced fracture of head or neck:
  - Intra-articular displacement of the fracture <2 mm and fragment size $\leq 30\%$ of articular surface
  - Forearm rotation (pronation/supination limited only by acute pain and swelling)
- Type II: displaced fracture of the head or neck:
  - Fracture displaced 2 to 5 mm with fragment size $>30\%$ of articular surface
  - Motion may be mechanically limited.
  - Rineer suggests if the fragments have cortical contact, they are more likely to be stable versus if no cortical contact more likely to be unstable.
- Type III: severely comminuted fracture of the radial head and neck
- Type IV (added to Mason's classifications by Johnston):
  - Radial head fracture with an associated elbow dislocation (1)

DESCRIPTION

- Fracture of the head of the radius, most often caused by direct axial loading, as with a fall on outstretched hand (FOOSH) injury
- Can also be caused by posterior lateral rotary force, any injury causing posterior dislocation to the elbow that may result in radial head fracture (such as Monteggia fracture or coronoid fracture-dislocation), or rarely, a direct blow

EPIDEMIOLOGY

Radial head fractures are the most common fracture about the elbow, accounting for about 1/3 of all elbow fractures in adults, with an estimated incidence of 2.5 to 2.8 per 10,000 inhabitants per year (1); uncommon in children, accounting for only 1% of all fractures

COMMONLY ASSOCIATED CONDITIONS

- 1/3 of patients will have a concomitant injury.
- Essex-Lopresti lesion: disruption of triangular fibrocartilage complex of the wrist and interosseous membrane of the forearm, resulting in instability of the forearm and subluxation of the distal radioulnar joint
- Concomitant capitellar, olecranon, and coronoid fractures (often associated with elbow dislocation)
- Posterior Monteggia fractures: proximal 1/3 ulna fracture with radial head dislocation
- The "terrible triad" includes posterior dislocation of the elbow with radial head fracture and associated coronoid process fracture.
- Medial collateral ligament tear
- Lateral collateral ligament tear
- Presence or absence of mechanical block with rotation. Examination achieved after aspiration of hematoma, with or without intra-articular injection of anesthetic; mechanical block associated with displaced fragment of radial head and affects surgical treatment
- Neurologic injuries can occur rarely with isolated radial head fracture but are more commonly associated with dislocation. Ulnar and median nerve are more commonly injured than the radial and posterior interosseous nerve.
- Brachial artery injuries can occur but are rare.

DIAGNOSIS

HISTORY

Determining the mechanism of injury is extremely helpful in differentiating from other elbow fractures. The typical mechanism of injury is a fall onto an outstretched hand in a pronated position, thus creating an axial load to the elbow (2).

PHYSICAL EXAM

- Patient usually holds injured arm gently against the chest with elbow flexed.
- Typically, there is pain and moderate swelling over the lateral side of the elbow.
- Any attempt to flex or extend the elbow or rotate the forearm may accentuate pain.
- Preservation of active elbow range of motion (ROM) was 97% specific for absence of a fracture.
- Focal tenderness over the radial head (located just distal to the lateral epicondyle)
- Palpation of radial head with passive rotation of the forearm typically elicits pain and occasionally, crepitation.
- Forearm and wrist examination required to rule out associated injuries such as acute radioulnar dissociation and/or injury to the interosseous ligament of the forearm
- Palpation of medial ligament necessary for signs of possible disruption
- Neurovascular status checked distally, especially with history of elbow dislocation

DIFFERENTIAL DIAGNOSIS

- Other fractures of the elbow, including capitellar, olecranon, and coronoid
- Supracondylar fractures (much more prevalent in children)
- Radial head or other bone contusion
- Elbow sprain
- Elbow effusion

DIAGNOSTIC TESTS & INTERPRETATION

Initial Tests (lab, imaging)

- Anteroposterior and lateral radiographs of the elbow are usually sufficient.
- If fat pad sign present (either anterior "sail sign" or posterior fat pad sign) and fracture not apparent, radiocapitellar views are helpful, taken with forearm in neutral rotation and x-ray beam angled 45 degrees cephalad.
- Computed tomography (CT) scan considered for estimating fracture size, degree of fragmentation, and displacement
- If wrist or forearm pain present, x-rays of the forearm and/or wrist in neutral rotation view should be taken.
- Magnetic resonance imaging (MRI) is helpful if there is concern for other soft tissue injury.

Diagnostic Procedures/Other

- Patient may have limited ROM due to pain and effusion.
- Joint aspiration for pain control is performed at the lateral elbow in the soft spot at the center of the dorsal olecranon, radial head, and lateral epicondyle (3)[A].
- If arthrocentesis is avoided, serial exams may be helpful (3)[A].
- Concerns for fracture orientation, severity, or healing should be referred to orthopedics (3)[A].

TREATMENT

GENERAL MEASURES

- Aspiration alone may provide some pain relief versus aspiration with local anesthetic instillation (3)[A].
- Type I:
  - Treated nonoperatively (4)[A]
  - Sling for pain control for 48 hr and followed by active mobilization. Mobilization should be supported by physical therapy as needed (4)[A].
  - Active ROM can begin as soon as pain permits. Flexion and extension of the elbow and supination and pronation of the forearm should be taken to the point where mild pain begins.
  - If required, hematoma aspiration is safe and effective for pain relief (3)[A].
  - Cast immobilization should be avoided (4)[A].
  - Ice therapy for 2 to 5 days
  - Acetaminophen and oral narcotics as necessary for pain control
- Type II:
  - Orthopedic consultation should be obtained with any type II fracture. There is still considerable controversy on proper treatment and no specific criteria for surgical versus nonsurgical treatment. A randomized controlled trial (RCT) is awaiting publication Radial Head Amsterdam Amphia Boston Others (RAMBO trial).
  - Without associated injuries and moderate displacement (2 to 5 mm), can be treated nonoperatively such as type I. Recent retrospective study in athletes showed good outcomes with nonsurgical treatment (5)[A]. Another retrospective study showed no difference in open reduction and internal fixation (ORIF) versus nonoperative (6)[A].
  - Associated injuries, especially causing elbow instability or mechanical block, should be referred for orthopedic consultation and possible ORIF.
- Type III:
  - ORIF versus resection and arthroplasty versus resection alone
  - Best treatment strategy for types III and IV is controversial. However, many studies are attempting to address this as new techniques become available.
- Type IV:
  - Treated as above, with obvious attention paid to reduction of dislocation and surgical repair of both fractures and associated ligamentous injuries

ADDITIONAL THERAPIES

- Initiate ROM exercises early.
- More aggressive strength and flexibility exercises added progressively as tolerated
- If ROM does not improve on a weekly basis, a mechanical block should be excluded. Once excluded, formal therapy may be needed.
- Only mild restriction of extension and rotation should be expected at 6 wk.

ONGOING CARE

- Contractures and loss of motion may develop if early active ROM is not initiated.
- Increased sensitivity to cold, which may persist for up to 1 yr
- Long-term pain is rarely a complication.
- Nonunion is possible but is frequently asymptomatic.
- Nerve injuries in the form of partial ulnar nerve and posterior interosseous nerve injury have been documented, mainly associated with surgical exploration.

FOLLOW-UP RECOMMENDATIONS

Early orthopedic input is essential in all but type I fractures due to potential need for surgical correction and controversy surrounding treatment.

REFERENCES

1. Kodde IF, Kaas L, Flipsen M, et al. Current concepts in the management of radial head fractures. *World J Orthop*. 2015;6(11):954–960.
2. Jordan RW, Jones AD. Radial head fractures. *Open Orthop J*. 2017;11:1405–1416.
3. Chalidis BE, Papadopoulos PP, Sachinis NC, et al. Aspiration alone versus aspiration and bupivacaine injection in the treatment of undisplaced radial head fractures: a prospective randomized study. *J Shoulder Elbow Surg*. 2009;18(5):676–679.
4. de Muinck Keizer RJ, Walenkamp MM, Goslings JC, et al. Mason type I fractures of the radial head. *Orthopedics*. 2015;38(12):e1147–e1154.
5. Guzzini M, Vadalà A, Agrò A, et al. Nonsurgical treatment of Mason type II radial head fractures in athletes. A retrospective study. *G Chir*. 2017;37(5):200–205.
6. Yoon A, King GJ, Grewal R. Is ORIF superior to nonoperative treatment in isolated displaced partial articular fractures of the radial head? *Clin Orthop Relat Res*. 2014;472(7):2105–2112.

ADDITIONAL READING

- Akesson T, Herbertsson P, Josefsson PO, et al. Primary nonoperative treatment of moderately displaced two-part fractures of the radial head. *J Bone Joint Surg Am*. 2006;88(9):1909–1914.
- Darracq MA, Vinson DR, Panacek EA. Preservation of active range of motion after acute elbow trauma predicts absence of elbow fracture. *Am J Emerg Med*. 2008;26(7):779–782.
- Herbertsson P, Josefsson PO, Hasserius R, et al. Uncomplicated Mason type-II and III fractures of the radial head and neck in adults. A long-term follow-up study. *J Bone Joint Surg Am*. 2004;86-A(3):569–574.
- Kaas L, van Riet RP, Vroemen JP, et al. The incidence of associated fractures of the upper limb in fractures of the radial head. *Strategies Trauma Limb Reconstr*. 2008;3(2):71–74.
- Pike JM, Athwal GS, Faber KJ, et al. Radial head fractures—an update. *J Hand Surg Am*. 2009;34(3):557–565.
- Ring D. Fractures and dislocations of the elbow: radial head fractures. In: Rockwood CA, Green DP, Bucholz RW, eds. *Rockwood and Green's Fractures in Adults*. 6th ed. Philadelphia, PA: Lippincott Williams & Wilkins; 2006:1011–1019.
- Rosenblatt Y, Athwal GS, Faber KJ. Current recommendations for the treatment of radial head fractures. *Orthop Clin North Am*. 2008;39(2):173–185.

CLINICAL PEARLS

- In type I fractures, typically, athletes can return to play as early as 6 to 8 wk, depending on pain, ROM, and strength.
- Protection of the elbow may be needed if returning to contact sports. In types II to IV fractures, return to play is based on extent of associated injuries and surgical correction.

FRACTURE, RIB

Robert J. Baker, MD, PhD, FAAFP, FACSM

BASICS

DESCRIPTION

- Usually the result of acute blunt trauma, especially in contact sports
- Rib fractures can also result from rowing, swinging golf clubs, and throwing.
- Stress fractures can occur as a result of chronic overuse of the upper body.
- Fractures may be complete, incomplete, or stress related.
- Rib fractures may often be associated with other fractures, soft tissue injuries, and deep organ trauma.

EPIDEMIOLOGY

- Isolated fractures of the upper four ribs are rare because they are well protected by the shoulder complex (1,2)[B].

ALERT

When injury occurs, trauma can be significant enough to fracture other bones of the shoulder, and injury to the deep organs such as lungs, heart, bronchus, blood vessels, and/or esophagus must be considered (2)[C].

- Blunt trauma to the lower eight ribs commonly results in fractures, most commonly in contact sports, such as football, hockey, and rugby (2,3)[C].
- Forceful contraction, usually against a significant amount of resistance, of muscles with an attachment to the ribs may result in incomplete, complete, or avulsion fractures of the ribs (2,3)[B].
- Chronic stress of upper body muscles, which attach to the ribs, can result in stress fractures of the ribs; commonly seen in rowing, tennis, golf, gymnastics, and baseball (2,3)[B]
- 1st rib fractures have been reported as a result of falling on an outstretched arm as well as direct trauma; 1st rib stress fractures also reported in the literature (1,2,4,5)[B]
- Avulsion fractures of the lower three floating ribs often occur at the attachment of the external oblique muscles; known to occur in baseball pitchers and batters (6)[B]
- Multiple rib fractures occur in high-impact trauma such as automobile, motorcycle, mountain biking, and bicycle racing (2,6)[B].
- Rib fractures are more common in adults compared to children due to the relative inelasticity of the adult chest wall compared to children (1,7)[C].

ETIOLOGY AND PATHOPHYSIOLOGY

- There are 12 pairs of ribs, the first 7 of which articulate both posteriorly with the spine and anteriorly with the sternum.
- Ribs 8 to 10 attach anteriorly to the costal cartilage.
- The lowest two ribs are "floating" and do not connect anteriorly.
- Immediately below each rib travels its neurovascular bundle, including the intercostal vein, artery, and nerve.
- Most acute rib fractures occur as a result of direct trauma, either blunt or penetrating missile (i.e., ball, gunshot) (6)[C].
- Relative long, thin shape of the rib predisposes to fractures. Common specific location is posterior lateral bend (8,9)[C].
- Because of the rib's thin bony structure compared to other long bones, fracture may occur earlier due to pathologic causes (8,9,10)[C].
- Because there are multiple muscle attachments of the rib to the neck and upper extremities, stress can lead to fatigue fractures of the ribs (8,9)[B]. The 1st rib is unique in that the scaleni insert onto it, and it therefore is exposed to stresses from the action of these neck muscles.
- Superior three pairs of ribs protected by the scapula, clavicle, and soft tissue less likely have isolated fractures. This significant force increases the potential for injury to major vessels and lung parenchyma.
- The inferior "floating" ribs are relatively mobile and more susceptible to injury from blunt trauma.
- The ribs act as a unit during respiration, moving in the anteroposterior (AP) and coronal planes. This concerted rib motion, in addition to the actions of the diaphragm and the intercostal muscles, enables inspiration (by increasing intrathoracic volume and decreasing intrathoracic pressure) and expiration (by decreasing intrathoracic volume and increasing intrathoracic pressure).

RISK FACTORS

- Contact and collision sports such as football, hockey, boxing, wrestling, rugby, and soccer (1,8,9)[A]
- As with any trauma, injuries can be more severe in athletes unprepared, either from lack of conditioning or contact from the back or blind side.
- Stress fractures of the ribs more likely to occur in sports with increased upper body demands such as golf, rowing, gymnastics, baseball, tennis, racquet sports, and weight lifting. Overuse and poor technique can contribute to rib stress fractures (8,9)[B].
- Other predisposing factors include a history of bone or joint disease, bone tumors, metastatic cancer, poor nutrition, and calcium deficiency (1,2,6,7)[C].

COMMONLY ASSOCIATED CONDITIONS

Organ injuries that may occur with acute rib fractures include:

- Pulmonary contusion.
- Pneumothorax.
- Tension pneumothorax.
- Hemothorax.
- Liver laceration, especially with lower rib fractures.
- Spleen laceration, especially with lower rib fractures.
- Esophageal rupture.
- Great vessel injury, aorta, and superior vena cava with upper and middle rib fractures (1,2)[C].

DIAGNOSIS

HISTORY

- Acute rib fracture usually presents after chest trauma; can result from a fall on an outstretched arm
- Often, the pain may be localized to one or two ribs (3)[C].
- The patient can frequently reproduce or exacerbate the pain by taking a deep breath.
- Athletes may experience the sensation of having "the wind knocked out of them."
- Athlete may recall feeling a "pop" when the trauma occurred.
- Athlete may complain of abdominal pain if the lower (11th and 12th) ribs are involved.
- Stress fractures usually occur in elite athletes who train intensely. These fractures tend to be more gradual in onset (7,8)[C].
- Rib stress fractures present with a gradual onset of activity-related chest wall pain, similar to stress fractures of other bones. Often the pain first occurs only with the inciting activity (e.g., rowing, swinging a golf club, throwing), then progresses to pain with deep breathing or simple movements, such as rolling over in bed or reaching overhead (7,8)[B].

PHYSICAL EXAM

- Localized pain, swelling, or ecchymosis may be present over the involved rib(s).
- Palpable deformity may be present in complete displaced fracture.
- Pain generally exacerbated by deep inspiration and may result in shallow, rapid breathing
- An auscultated click caused by movement of the rib fracture and can be heard with a stethoscope placed over the fracture site.
- Pain aggravated by coughing and sneezing
- Other symptoms, such as increasing shortness of breath, increasing pain, cyanosis, and subcutaneous emphysema, may indicate serious life-threatening conditions requiring emergent attention.
- With significant chest trauma, a thorough cardiopulmonary examination must be performed to evaluate for complications or associated injuries (1,2)[B].
- If trauma occurred to the upper chest, special attention should be given to the neck, shoulders, and major vessels (2,3)[B].
- If trauma occurred to the lower chest, a thorough abdominal examination should be performed to rule out injury to the liver, spleen, gastrointestinal (GI) tract, and kidneys (1,2)[C].
- Diminished breath sounds may reflect splinting from the pain of a simple chest wall contusion or the presence of significant injury (e.g., pneumothorax, hemothorax, or pulmonary contusion).

DIFFERENTIAL DIAGNOSIS

- Rib/chest wall contusion
- Muscle strain
- Rupture of pectoralis major
- Costochondral separation/sprain
- Sternal fracture (anterior)
- Intervertebral joint/disc injury
- Apophyseal joint sprain
- Costovertebral joint sprain
- Scheuermann disease (posterior)
- Other causes of chest pain, such as cardiac causes, peptic ulcer disease, gastroesophageal reflux disorder, pneumothorax, pulmonary embolism, asthma, pleurisy, herpes zoster

DIAGNOSTIC TESTS & INTERPRETATION

- Standard posteroanterior (PA) and lateral chest radiographs are adequate to identify some rib fractures, but overall sensitivity is poor (1,2,7)[C].
- Dedicated rib series includes oblique views of the chest wall not included with a standard chest series.
- Clinicians can base their diagnosis and management on plain radiographs and clinical findings, and a rib series is unnecessary (1,2)[C].
- In the case of pathologic fractures, other blood work, such as complete blood count (CBC), comprehensive metabolic panel, and isoenzymes of alkaline phosphatase, may be directed by history and physical exam (1,2,3)[B].

- Other than in cases of complications, continued pain, and poor healing, routine repeat films are not necessary.
- A bone scan of the chest wall is the preferred study to diagnose rib stress fractures early in the pathologic process (8,9)[C].
- Magnetic resonance imaging (MRI): Oblique orientation of the ribs and the difficulty with numbering them on axial or coronal scanning can make MRI more difficult to interpret (9,10)[C].
- With upper thoracic rib fractures, arteriography is indicated if there is evidence of vascular insufficiency, hemorrhage, or concomitant brachial plexus injury; marked displacement of the rib fragments; fractures of the scapula, vertebrae, or sternum; widening of the mediastinum; left apical cupping; or downward displacement of the left main stem bronchus (1,2,3)[B].

TREATMENT

GENERAL MEASURES

- Treatment is generally supportive.
- Pain control is the cornerstone of treatment and may be required for up to 3 to 6 wk after injury.
- Ice and nonsteroidal anti-inflammatory drugs (NSAIDs) may control symptoms, but stronger oral pain medications may be rarely indicated.
- Local intercostal nerve blocks remain an option if other pain control techniques fail (1,2)[B].
- Epidural anesthesia is also an option for pain control (1,2)[C].

ALERT

Strapping or a chest binder has been advocated to help with pain. Caution should be exercised because immobilization techniques may result in inhibition of deep breathing, leading to atelectasis and possibly pneumonia (1,6)[C].

- If immobilization is deemed necessary for comfort, its use should be minimized.
- Rib stress fractures are treated similarly to other low-risk stress fractures: with restriction of the inciting activity for 4 to 6 wk, followed by a gradual return to the activity as tolerated.
- Rehabilitation should include proper mechanics and eliminating training errors to avoid recurrence of rib stress fractures (9,10)[C].

MEDICATION

- For isolated injuries, generally begin treatment with NSAIDs without opioids (1,2)[B].
- For more severe injuries, and if ventilation is compromised, admission and invasive treatments such as intercostal nerve blocks may be indicated (1,2,3)[C].

ADDITIONAL THERAPIES

- For stress fractures, biomechanics of their upper thoracic and shoulder areas based on sport should be evaluated and corrected if necessary (2)[C].
- Use of incentive spirometry can prevent atelectasis and its complications.
- Rib belts or binders are not recommended because they compromise respiratory function.

SURGERY/OTHER PROCEDURES

- Need for surgery is rare in cases of isolated rib fractures (1)[C].
- Exception is in the case of flail chest. Open reduction and internal fixation may be required (1,2,3)[C].
- Surgical fixation may be of benefit with chest wall deformity, flail chest, or symptomatic nonunion.
- Suspected internal injuries associated with rib fractures should be referred for possible surgical repair.
- Chronic pain due to recurrent stress fracture, nonunion, or recurrent dislocation or subluxation may improve with surgical excision of the involved rib (10)[B].

ONGOING CARE

FOLLOW-UP RECOMMENDATIONS

- Pain from rib fractures can be severe for several days following the injury.
- The athlete should be encouraged to continue activities as tolerated, except for contact sports (7)[C].
- Contact should be limited for the first 3 wk following injury. Consider rib protection in contact sports after return (8)[C].
- Most rib fractures heal within 6 to 8 wk.
- Monitor regularly for signs of delayed complications (8)[B].
- Delayed injuries from isolated rib fractures sustained during blunt trauma occur infrequently.
- A follow-up examination 6 to 8 wk after the injury is reasonable to assess the patient, if they are unable to return to sports or work by that time.

PATIENT EDUCATION

- Athletes should be educated when to follow up, especially if they experience fever, chills, worsening pain, dizziness, light-headedness, fatigue, persistent cough, or respiratory distress.
- Athletes should be educated that it is common to have significant pain. They should not be reluctant to take pain medication early on. This allows for more normal breathing and less chance of complications like pneumonia (8)[C].

ALERT

Signs of injuries due to rib fractures (e.g., pneumothorax, pulmonary contusion) may be delayed for hours or days, and all discharged patients must be given precise instructions about signs of injury to watch for and told to return to the emergency department (ED) immediately should any such sign appear (1,2)[B].

- Educate the athlete in the role and use of "incentive spirometry."
- For a stress fracture, avoid the activity that caused your stress fracture for 4 to 6 wk and slowly restart that activity.
- Avoid smoking. A fracture can take longer to heal if you smoke.

PROGNOSIS

- Intensive training for athletes with stress fractures is not recommended for at least the first 3 wk.
- Athletes can gradually increase activity as pain permits for isolated rib fractures.
- Full healing usually takes 6 to 8 wk; however, athletes may return to participation in noncontact sports when pain free.
- Early return to contact sports may be possible prior to 6 wk if pain is controlled, and the area can be protected adequately until full healing occurs (10)[C].

COMPLICATIONS

- Nonunion of the ribs is rare in general. Symptomatic nonunion can occur and would be an indication for surgery (4,8)[B].
- Pseudoarthrosis of the 1st rib is described in the literature and has been a cause for discontinued participation (4,8,10)[B].
- Early and adequate pain relief is essential to avoid complications from splinting and atelectasis, primarily pneumonia.
- Significant complications may include pneumothorax, pulmonary contusion, pneumonia, and intercostal hemorrhage.

REFERENCES

1. Sirmali M, Türüt H, Topçu S, et al. A comprehensive analysis of traumatic rib fractures: morbidity, mortality and management. *Eur J Cardiothorac Surg*. 2003;24(1):133–138.
2. Brasel KJ, Moore EE, Albrecht RA, et al. Western trauma association critical decisions in trauma: management of rib fractures. *J Trauma Acute Care Surg*. 2017;82(1):200–203.
3. Chien CY, Chen YH, Han ST, et al. The number of displaced rib fractures is more predictive for complications in chest trauma patients. *Scand J Trauma Resusc Emerg Med*. 2017;25(1):19.
4. Khadavi MJ, Fredericson M. Chest pain in athletes from personal history section (musculoskeletal causes). *Curr Sports Med Rep*. 2015;14(3):252–254.
5. Shulzhenko NO, Zens TJ, Beems MV, et al. Number of rib fractures thresholds independently predict worse outcomes in older patients with blunt trauma. *Surgery*. 2017;161(4):1083–1089.
6. Murphy CE IV, Raja AS, Baumann BM, et al. Rib fracture diagnosis in the Panscan era. *Ann Emerg Med*. 2017;70(6):904–909.
7. Reissig A, Copetti R, Kroegel C. Current role of emergency ultrasound of the chest. *Crit Care Med*. 2011;39(4):839–845.
8. Chapman BC, Overbey DM, Tesfalidet F, et al. Clinical utility of chest computed tomography in patients with rib fractures CT chest and rib fractures. *Arch Trauma Res*. 2016;5(4):e37070.
9. Sakellaridis T, Stamatelopoulos A, Andrianopoulos E, et al. Isolated first rib fracture in athletes. *Br J Sports Med*. 2004;38(3):e5.
10. D'Ailly PN, Sluiter JK, Kuijer PP. Rib stress fractures among rowers: a systematic review on return to sports, risk factors and prevention. *J Sports Med Phys Fitness*. 2016;56(6):744–753.

CLINICAL PEARLS

- In most cases of isolated rib fractures, simple chest films are all that are required. Dedicated rib series may also be obtained based on clinical findings.
- Patients should continue to be as active as they can tolerate and may use NSAIDs or acetaminophen for pain for isolated fractures.
- Multiple rib fractures correlate more closely with serious intrathoracic and intra-abdominal injuries. Fractures of superior ribs (numbers 1 to 3) reflect trauma involving significant force and the potential for injury to major blood vessels and lung parenchyma.
- Displaced fractures increase the risk of internal injury and delayed bleeding and generally warrant admission.
- Rib stress fractures are treated with restriction of the inciting activity for 4 to 6 wk, followed by a gradual return to the activity as tolerated.
- Virtually, all rib fractures heal well with conservative management, and follow-up chest radiographs are unnecessary, unless indicated by clinical symptoms.

FRACTURE, SACRAL

Rebecca Bacharach, DO

BASICS

- Sacral injuries are rare, but most authors believe that sacral fractures are generally underrecognized.
- A high degree of suspicion is required to make the diagnosis:
  - Only 10–30% of sacral fractures are seen on standard radiographs (1).
  - Advanced imaging is often required to appreciate sacral injury.

DESCRIPTION

- Traumatic fractures of the sacrum are most commonly described using the Denis system of fracture orientation:
  - Zone 1:
    - Fracture line usually vertically through the sacral ala
    - Entirely lateral to foramina
    - Typically, strength of sacroiliac (SI) ligaments spares SI joint from injury, but fractures that enter SI joint at greater risk for instability
    - Neural elements typically spared; <10% with neurologic involvement
  - Zone 2:
    - Fracture line through the neural foramina, but sparing the central spinal canal
    - 20–30% with neurologic injury
  - Zone 3:
    - Fracture line medial to neural foramina; typically includes transverse fractures
    - >50% with neurologic injury
- Atraumatic injuries result from a mismatch between bone stress and bone strength:
  - Stress fractures in athletes
  - Insufficiency fractures in elderly:
    - Typically, bilateral in those with normal gait and unilateral in those with altered gait mechanics

EPIDEMIOLOGY

Sacral fractures need to be considered in several clinical scenarios:

- Multitrauma patients with other pelvic or thoracolumbar injury:
  - Sacral fractures rarely occur as isolated injury (<5%).
- Osteoporotic patients with low back or gluteal pain:
  - Atraumatic or trivial injury
- Athletes with activity-related pain of low back/SI region:
  - 1.6% of sports-related low back pain (2)
  - Usually in running-based sports:
    - Often after increases in training intensity
  - May produce thigh pain as well

ETIOLOGY AND PATHOPHYSIOLOGY

Sacral fractures may occur by the following mechanisms:

- Posttraumatic injuries:
  - Producing large forces and fracture across healthy bone:
    - Typically, motor vehicle accidents or falls from a height
- Atraumatic injuries:
  - Normal stresses (or trivial injury) producing fractures across relatively weakened bone:
    - Insufficiency fractures in the elderly/ill
    - Fractures often bilateral
  - Increased stress or overuse, producing fracture across relatively normal bone:
    - Stress fractures in the younger, athletic population
    - Fractures often unilateral

RISK FACTORS

- Insufficiency fractures are most common in elderly osteoporotic females:
  - May occur in others at risk for poor bone density, including the following:
    - Chronic corticosteroid use
    - History of pelvic irradiation
- Stress fractures occur most commonly in running athletes:
  - As with other stress fractures, risk probably increases with the following:
    - Training errors (inadequate recovery, increasing training, etc.)
    - Biomechanical factors (leg length discrepancy, poor core, and pelvic stabilization)
    - Increased impact forces (footwear, training surface)
    - Nutritional/hormonal impacts on bone density (relative energy deficiency in sport [RED-S], inadequate calcium [Ca]/vitamin D)

COMMONLY ASSOCIATED CONDITIONS

Acute sacral fractures may be seen in conjunction with:

- Other bony injury:
  - Other pelvic ring disruptions
  - Other spinal fractures:
    - May be noncontiguous
  - Fracture-dislocations of lower facet joints or disruption of lumbosacral junction
- Neurologic injury:
  - Should be described according to the Gibbons grading system:
    - Grade 1: no neurologic deficit
    - Grade 2: paresthesias/sensory changes only
    - Grade 3: motor deficit but gastrointestinal (GI)/genitourinary (GU) function normal
    - Grade 4: loss of GI/GU function
- Injury to other pelvic contents:
  - Rectal perforation most common
- Atraumatic sacral fractures
- Osteoporosis
- RED-S

DIAGNOSIS

Prehospital:

- Traumatic sacral fractures typically occur in the multitrauma patient.
- Initial assessment and treatment should proceed as per Advanced Trauma Life Support for patients with suspected spine injury:
  - Airway, breathing, and circulation (ABCs)/resuscitation
  - Spine precautions/backboard
  - Transport

HISTORY

- Injury to sacrum is suggested by pain in lower back or pelvic pain and can radiate to the leg, groin, buttocks, or thigh (3).
- Pain is often worse with weight-bearing activity; improved with rest
- Important to inquire about possible nerve root involvement:
  - Incontinence of bowel or bladder, sexual dysfunction
  - Sciatica
  - Paresthesias, especially of saddle region
- Patients without history of trauma should be asked about:
  - Change in activity or footwear, especially in running-based sports.
  - Risk factors for poor bone density:
    - Osteopenia/osteoporosis in patient or family members
    - Past or present disordered eating pattern
    - Oligo- or amenorrhea in females

PHYSICAL EXAM

- Trauma patient:
  - Inspect for ecchymosis/bruising over sacral prominence.
  - Palpate entire spinal column and bony pelvis in addition to the sacrum.
  - Neurologic testing of L5–S5 nerve root function should be completely assessed initially then periodically reevaluated:
    - Pinprick sensation, rectal sphincter contraction and tone as well as cremasteric, bulbocavernosus, perianal wink reflexes
    - L5 injuries most common with zone 2 injuries
    - Sacral roots have bilateral input, and unilateral injuries to S2–S5 are difficult to detect.
  - Digital rectal and vaginal evaluation to exclude open fractures
- Atraumatic patient with possible insufficiency or stress fracture:
  - No pathognomonic findings
  - Typically with tenderness over sacrum, paraspinal, or over region of SI joint
  - FABER test (with hip in flexion, abduction, external rotation) often positive
  - Tenderness with lateral compression
  - Squish test—patient supine, palpate anterior superior iliac spine (ASIS) bilaterally
  - Distal neurovascular assessment typically normal
  - Gait may be antalgic and may have pain with a hop test.

DIFFERENTIAL DIAGNOSIS

- Differential diagnosis for acute fractures:
  - Contusion
  - Other pelvic or lumbar fractures
  - Nerve root injuries
- Differential diagnosis for atraumatic/stress fractures:
  - Lumbar disc disease
  - Mechanical low back pain
  - SI dysfunction
  - Spondylolysis

DIAGNOSTIC TESTS & INTERPRETATION

- Trauma patients should have stool assessed for occult blood.
- Consider secondary osteoporosis such as hyperthyroidism, hyperparathyroidism, and osteomalacia (thyroid-stimulating hormone [TSH], parathyroid hormone [PTH], Ca, phosphate [Phos], albumin, 25-hydroxyvitamin D, urinary Ca, complete blood count [CBC], liver function test [LFT], C-reactive protein [CRP], erythrocyte sedimentation rate [ESR]).
- Traumatic injury:
  - Although radiographs typically only reveal about 30% of sacral fractures, they may be useful for initial assessment of suspected sacral injury:
    - Anteroposterior (AP) views of the pelvis are standard in multitrauma patients.
    - Visualization of suspected sacral injuries may be enhanced with the addition of pelvic inlet view: 35 to 40 degree caudal tilt of radiograph

tube; pelvic outlet view: 45-degree cranial tilt of radiograph tube; lateral view of sacrum
  - Look for transverse L5 fractures, which can be seen in up to half of pelvic and sacral fractures.
- Computed tomography (CT) scanning is now standard for definitive assessment of suspected acute sacral fracture:
  - Routine CT scans often not satisfactory
  - Close consultation with radiologist on gantry alignment recommended
  - Thin section (1.0 to 1.5 mm cuts) with coronal and sagittal reconstructions; relatively high radiation exposure: 10 to 20 mSV
- Magnetic resonance imaging (MRI) may help delineate neural compression or injury:
  - Multiplanar nature may also better assess fracture alignment.

- Atraumatic injury:
  - Initial lumbar spine series as well as AP views of the pelvis are often obtained:
    - Usually unremarkable
  - MRI of sacrum appropriate for diagnosis:
    - Gold standard for sacral stress fracture
    - Most bony stress injuries will have high signal on T2-weighted images, low signal on T1-weighted images.
    - Fracture line may or may not be present.
  - CT is an alternative to MRI:
    - Increased radiation
    - Can see sclerotic healing or fresh fracture line
  - Bone scan most sensitive but not specific for bony stress injury:
    - Stress fractures in athletes; typically with unilateral uptake sacral ala
    - Insufficiency fractures; often with multiple sites of injury; classic "H" sign seen in about 40% of patients; bilateral vertical fractures with horizontal component
    - Uptake can be obscured by residual in bladder; outlet views in addition to standard anterior and posterior projections

TREATMENT

- Acute fracture:
  - See below for surgical indications.
  - Stable injuries without neurologic involvement treated with initial bed rest and gradual ambulation and activity advancement as tolerated:
    - Fractures through S3 and distally often require protection with sitting until pain free.
- Stress fracture: average ±6 wk for return to sport (but some may take up to 3 mo):
  - Protected weight-bearing if limp or pain with ambulation:
    - Advance weight-bearing as tolerated
  - Discontinue painful activity/relative rest.
  - Maintain cardiovascular conditioning with pain-free activity:
    - May need to begin with non–weight-bearing activity (typically swimming or cycling)
  - Begin progressive rehabilitation typically after 3- to 5-day pain-free interval:
    - Core/pelvic stabilization; address underlying biomechanical deficiencies.
    - Cardiovascular cross-training progression through following sequence when activity is pain free: non–weight-bearing (i.e., pool running, bicycling), weight-bearing/nonimpact (i.e., elliptical-type trainer), impact (i.e., running), sports-specific functional progression
- Insufficiency fractures in elderly may have prolonged symptoms (up to 9 mo):
  - Initial treatment is usually nonoperative, even for patients with neurologic deficit:
    - Many authors recommend initial period bed rest followed by progressive ambulation.
    - Neurologic symptoms appear to improve as pain resolves.
  - Consider surgery if severe pain after 3-mo trial conservative treatment.

MEDICATION

- Analgesics should be titrated for symptom relief:
  - Should not be used specifically to allow for progression of activity or sport participation
  - Scheduled doses for first several days of diagnosis may allow for pain-free rest:
    - Over-the-counter analgesics often sufficient for stress fractures: acetaminophen up to 1,000 mg q4h PRN; pediatric dosage 10 to 15 mg/kg up to q4h nonsteroidal drugs often beneficial. Theoretically may impair bony healing, but no consensus on effect on clinical outcomes. Naproxen 500 mg q12h; pediatric dosage 10 to 20 mg/kg/day divided BID
  - Patients with severe pain may need stronger medications for first several days:
    - Hydrocodone/acetaminophen 5/500 1 to 2 PO q4–6h PRN; pediatric suspension 7.5/500/15 mL; patient weight 32 to 45 kg: 10 mL q4–6h PRN
    - Tramadol 50 mg 1 to 2 tabs q4–6h PRN; maximum dose 400 mg/day; caution in elderly and with renal or hepatic impairment
- Supplemental vitamin D and Ca for stress or insufficiency fractures:
  - 1 g Ca daily
  - 800 to 1,000 IU vitamin D daily

SURGERY/OTHER PROCEDURES

- Surgical consideration for traumatic sacral fractures:
  - Unstable injuries
  - Severe disruption of sagittal or coronal alignment:
    - In AP plane displacement, >1 cm generally recognized as unstable
  - Neurologic impairment
  - Injuries with persistent pain after about 6 mo
- Insufficiency fractures considered for surgery if with persistent, severe pain after 3 mo conservative treatment

ADMISSION, INPATIENT, AND NURSING CONSIDERATIONS

- Acute traumatic sacral fractures often require hospitalization for additional injury:
  - Isolated and stable zone 1 or 2 fractures with no neurologic deficit and adequate pain control may be considered for outpatient treatment.
- Stress fractures and insufficiency fractures are generally managed in outpatient setting.

ONGOING CARE

Sacral stress or insufficiency fractures may be a bellwether for underlying metabolic bone disease:

- Bone density testing or other laboratory evaluation should be considered.

DIET

Patients with insufficiency or stress fractures should be counseled on appropriate intake of Ca and vitamin D.

PATIENT EDUCATION

Education should focus on biomechanical issues and training errors predisposing to injury:

- Importance of maintaining adequate strength and flexibility of core and pelvic musculature
- Advance training volume by ~10% per week to minimize risk of additional overuse injury.
- Especially in the running athlete, the importance of appropriate footwear selection:
  - Effective life span of most running shoes is 300 to 400 miles.

PROGNOSIS

- Healthy athletes with sacral stress injury:
  - Usually able to return to normal activity 4 to 6 wk
  - Usually able to return to sport 6 to 10 wk
- Elderly patients with insufficiency fractures may have pain for many months.
- Fractures requiring surgery often with instrumentation:
  - Up to 1/3 may have hardware failure.

COMPLICATIONS

- Deformity or bony callus formation after acute injury may lead to nerve root entrapment.
- Prolonged pain common in elderly with insufficiency fractures

F

REFERENCES

1. Beckmann NM, Chinapuvvula NR. Sacral fractures: classification and management. *Emerg Radiol*. 2017;24(6):605–617.
2. Kaneko H, Murakami M, Nishizawa K. Prevalence and clinical features of sports-related lumbosacral stress injuries in the young. *Arch Orthop Trauma Surg*. 2017;137(5):685–691.
3. Longhino V, Bonora C, Sansone V. The management of sacral stress fractures: current concepts. *Clin Cases Miner Bone Metab*. 2011;8(3):19–23.

ADDITIONAL READING

- Kuklo TR, Potter BK, Ludwig SC, et al. Radiographic measurement techniques for sacral fractures consensus statement of the Spine Trauma Study Group. *Spine (Phila Pa 1976)*. 2006;31(9):1047–1055.
- Levine AM. Fractures of the sacrum. In: Browner BD, Levine AM, Jupiter JB, et al, eds. *Skeletal Trauma*. 4th ed. Philadelphia, PA: Saunders; 2008.
- Micheli LJ, Curtis C. Stress fractures in the spine and sacrum. *Clin Sports Med*. 2006;25(1):75–88.
- Shah MK, Stewart GW. Sacral stress fractures: an unusual cause of low back pain in an athlete. *Spine (Phila Pa 1976)*. 2002;27(4):E104–E108.
- White JH, Hague C, Nicolaou S, et al. Imaging of sacral fractures. *Clin Radiol*. 2003;58(12):914–921.

CLINICAL PEARLS

- Consider sacral injury in any acute injury resulting in other pelvic or spinal injury.
- Consider sacral injury in chronic cases of low back, thigh, or buttock pain.
- Sacral fractures are typically occult on plain radiographs and often require advanced imaging for definitive diagnosis.

FRACTURE, SCAPHOID

Jason A. Krystofiak, MD

BASICS

DESCRIPTION

- Most commonly fractured carpal bone
- Fractures occur in three anatomic sections: proximal, waist, and distal.
- Mechanism of injury is normally a fall onto an outstretched hand.
- Proximal pole fractures have an increased risk of nonunion.
- Synonym: fracture, carpal navicular

EPIDEMIOLOGY

- Carpal bone fractures account for 5% of all fractures.
- The scaphoid is the most commonly fractured carpal bone, accounting for 70% of carpal fractures:
  - 60% at the waist
  - 20% at the proximal pole
  - 20% at the distal pole
- Increased rate in males ages 20 to 24 yr and less common in children and older adults (In children, distal radial physeal injuries occur more often than scaphoid [Salter-Harris fracture types 1 and 2]; in older adults, distal radius metaphyseal fractures occur before scaphoid fractures.)

Incidence

- Varying incidence but overall greater in men compared to women
- Estimated to occur in 1 out of 100 college football athletes (1,2)

ETIOLOGY AND PATHOPHYSIOLOGY

- Classic injury: Mechanism is an axial load of a hyperextended, radially deviated wrist.
- Normally associated with falls, athletic injuries, or motor vehicle trauma
- Increased risk of nonunion in proximal pole fractures due to a retrograde blood supply

DIAGNOSIS

HISTORY

- Patients report falling on an outstretched hand or a forced wrist extension.
- Pain and swelling at the radial wrist near the 1st metacarpal base
- Characterized as a deep and dull pain made worse with gripping or squeezing

PHYSICAL EXAM

- Tenderness at the anatomic snuffbox:
  - Bordered by the extensor pollicis longus tendon medially and extensor pollicis brevis and abductor pollicis longus tendons laterally
  - Sensitivity 90%, specificity 40% (3)
  - False positives may occur by compression of the radial nerve sensory branch as it passes through the snuffbox.
- Tenderness of scaphoid tubercle:
  - Extend patient's wrist and apply pressure to the tuberosity at the proximal wrist crease.
  - Sensitivity 87%, specificity 57% (3)
- Scaphoid compression test:
  - Axially/longitudinally compressing patient's thumb along the 1st metacarpal
  - Some studies show a poor predictive value (3).
- Diminished grip strength:
  - Compared to contralateral side
  - Increases the positive predictive value for the presence of a scaphoid fracture (3)

DIFFERENTIAL DIAGNOSIS

- Scapholunate dissociation
- Distal radius fracture
- Extensor carpi radialis sprain
- 1st metacarpal fracture
- Flexor carpi radialis sprain
- Carpometacarpal or radiocarpal arthritis

DIAGNOSTIC TESTS & INTERPRETATION

- Plain radiographs of the wrist:
  - Obtain posteroanterior (PA), true lateral, and oblique views. Also, include a scaphoid specific view: PA of the wrist in full pronation and ulnar deviation.
  - May request additional views: PA wrist with clenched fist in radial and ulnar deviation
  - Plain radiographs may be normal immediately after injury, with a false-negative rate near 20% (4).
  - Fracture may become apparent 10 to 14 days after injury (immobilization allows demineralization of the fracture line).
  - Examine radiographs for evidence of scapholunate widening (Terry Thomas sign) evidenced by >3 mm between the scaphoid and the lunate:
    - Indicates ligamentous injury to the scapholunate ligament
- Magnetic resonance imaging (MRI):
  - Consider when initial radiographs are negative and/or other ligamentous injury is suspected.
  - Sensitivity 88%, specificity 100% (4)
  - MRI shows diminished signal in T1-weighted and increased signal in T2-weighted images.
  - Cost-effective when compared to immobilization followed by repeat radiographs (5)
- Bone scan:
  - Consider in patients with persistent tenderness but negative plain radiographs.
  - Excellent sensitivity (99%), but specificity (86%) is less than MRI and computed tomography (CT) (4)
  - Positive scan shows focal increased uptake at the scaphoid 72 hr after the injury.
  - Highest radiation dose of imaging modalities for evaluation of scaphoid (4)
- CT scan:
  - Can be used to accurately help diagnose, characterize displacement, and assess for fracture union
  - Sensitivity 72%, specificity 99% (4)

TREATMENT

GENERAL MEASURES

Scaphoid fractures or suspected fractures with negative radiographs (3)[C]:

- Immobilize in a thumb spica.
- Sling for comfort
- Ice and elevation

MEDICATION

- Tylenol or nonsteroidal anti-inflammatory drugs (NSAIDs) as needed
- Narcotics for breakthrough pain

ADDITIONAL THERAPIES

- Classification systems exist (Herbert, Russe, etc.); however, these classifications are not prognostic.
- <1 mm separation of the fracture is considered nondisplaced (1).
- Most nondisplaced fractures can be treated successfully with cast immobilization (1,3,6)[B].
- Time to fracture union with cast immobilization varies by location:
  - Distal pole (6 to 8 wk) < waist (8 to 12 wk) < proximal pole (3 to 6 mo) (1,2)
- Thumb immobilization does not appear to affect the rate of nonunion (2,3)[B].
- Long-arm cast (vs. short-arm cast) does not improve nonunion rates (1,2,3,6)[C].
- Displaced fractures and proximal pole fractures (prone to nonunion and avascular necrosis) should be referred for surgical fixation (1,2,3)[B].
- Postoperative or postcasting hand therapy
- Management of associated injuries: fracture of the distal radius, radial head, and lunate; ligamentous injury leading to scapholunate dissociation; and possible injury to the median nerve

SURGERY/OTHER PROCEDURES

- Operative fixation is recommended for displaced fractures and proximal pole fractures (1,3,6)[B].
- Consider surgery for nondisplaced fractures in high-demand athletes/patients where the necessary length of casting would interfere significantly with competition, training, or work (1,2)[C].
- Multiple surgical techniques can be used (dorsal open reduction internal fixation [ORIF], volar ORIF, percutaneous, arthroscopic assisted):
  - Each has advantages and disadvantages.
  - Surgeon preference and experience is often the deciding factor in operative technique.

ONGOING CARE

FOLLOW-UP RECOMMENDATIONS

- Nondisplaced waist or distal pole fractures can be managed closely by a primary care physician.
- Refer patients with displaced fractures and proximal pole fractures.
- Patients with a delayed presentation, carpal ligament instability, and evidence of nonunion should also be referred.
- Consider referring high-demand athletes/patients with nondisplaced fractures.

COMPLICATIONS

- Avascular necrosis of the proximal fracture fragment, leading to wrist dysfunction and early osteoarthritis
- High incidence of fibrous nonunion (~10%)
- Frequent malunion
- Chronic scapholunate advanced collapse (SLAC)
- Posttraumatic arthritis

REFERENCES

1. Winston MJ, Weiland AJ. Scaphoid fractures in the athlete. *Curr Rev Musculoskelet Med*. 2017;10(1):38–44.
2. Fowler JR, Hughes TB. Scaphoid fractures. *Clin Sports Med*. 2015;34(1):37–50.
3. Phillips TG, Reibach AM, Slomiany WP. Diagnosis and management of scaphoid fractures. *Am Fam Physician*. 2004;70(5):879–884.
4. Mallee WH, Wang J, Poolman RW, et al. Computed tomography versus magnetic resonance imaging versus bone scintigraphy for clinically suspected scaphoid fractures in patients with negative plain radiographs. *Cochrane Database Syst Rev*. 2015;(6):CD010023.
5. Yin ZG, Zhang JB, Gong KT. Cost-effectiveness of diagnostic strategies for suspected scaphoid fractures. *J Orthop Trauma*. 2015;29(8):e245–e252.
6. Grewal R, King GJ. An evidence-based approach to the management of acute scaphoid fractures. *J Hand Surg Am*. 2009;34(4):732–734.

ADDITIONAL READING

- Ram AN, Chung KC. Evidence-based management of acute nondisplaced scaphoid waist fractures. *J Hand Surg Am*. 2009;34(4):735–738.
- Shehab R, Mirabelli MH. Evaluation and diagnosis of wrist pain: a case-based approach. *Am Fam Physician*. 2013;87(8):568–573.

F

CLINICAL PEARLS

- A scaphoid fracture is unlikely in the absence of tenderness in the anatomic snuffbox and at the scaphoid tubercle.
- High-demand athletes may do better with early surgical fixation of even nondisplaced fractures because this allows earlier return to activity.

FRACTURE, SPINOUS AND TRANSVERSE PROCESSES

David E.J. Bazzo, MD, FAAFP, CAQSM • Tara Robbins, MD

BASICS

DESCRIPTION

- Transverse and spinous process fractures are considered minor spine injuries and usually are stable and benign. Both types can be markers of considerable trauma and should encourage the physician to look for additional injury.
- Fractures of the spinous process typically occur at C7 or any of the lower cervical or upper thoracic vertebrae. They are commonly avulsion-type injuries resulting from contraction of the trapezius, rhomboid minor, and/or serratus posterior.
- Traditionally referred to as "clay shoveler injuries" but now are found mostly after sudden deceleration in motor vehicle accidents or forced flexion of the neck, often in football players and weight lifters
- Synonym(s): minor spinal fracture

EPIDEMIOLOGY

- Spinous process fractures are relatively rare since mechanization replaced clay shovelers.
- "Sentinel spinous process fractures" are associated with fractures of lamina and facets, which can lead to instability.

ALERT

Up to 21% of transverse process fractures resulting from high-energy trauma (e.g., motor vehicle accidents) are associated with visceral injuries, most commonly to the spleen and liver (1).

- A recent study has shown an overall incidence of nonspinal-associated orthopedic injuries of 68.9% in trauma patients with isolated thoracic or lumbar transverse process fractures (2).
- Up to 11% have other spine injuries not detected by plain radiographs but identified on computed tomography (CT) scanning (1).
- L2 is the most frequently fractured level followed by L3 in high-energy trauma (2).
- Transverse process fractures resulting from low-energy trauma (e.g., playing football) do not generally have associated spinal, nerve root, or visceral injuries.

RISK FACTORS

Growth spurts, training errors, improper technique, and repetitive trauma predispose the athlete to spine fractures.

DIAGNOSIS

HISTORY

- Forceful hyperflexion of the neck (e.g., spearing in football) is associated with lower cervical spinous process fractures. Lumbar transverse process fractures usually result from direct trauma.
- Pain with hip flexion indicates possible lumbar transverse process fracture. Pain with neck flexion suggests cervical spinous process fracture.

PHYSICAL EXAM

- Localized pain over injured area without radiation
- Pain increased with neck flexion (lower cervical spinous process fracture) or hip flexion (lumbar transverse process fracture)
- Careful neurologic examination for weakness, reflex changes, or sensory changes in a dermatomal distribution. Because neurologic injuries are not commonly associated with minor fractures, abnormal results should raise suspicion of additional spinal injury.
- Pain worse with hip flexion (site of iliopsoas origin) seen in lumbar transverse process fractures
- Benign abdominal examination does not exclude coexistent intra-abdominal injury.

DIFFERENTIAL DIAGNOSIS

- "Burst" fracture
- Cervical or lumbar strain
- Ligamentous spinal injury
- Disc herniation
- Spondylolysis and/or spondylolisthesis

DIAGNOSTIC TESTS & INTERPRETATION

- CT scan: superior to plain films to evaluate extent of spinal fractures and rule out serious spine injury but has limited field of view and high radiation dose
- Magnetic resonance imaging (MRI): only necessary if neurologic symptoms are present to evaluate extrinsic spinal cord compression or intrinsic cord injury
- Radiographic appearance often lags behind clinical healing and should not be used as the primary criterion for return to play.
- Cervical lateral radiograph:
  - Very important to visualize C7 spinous process, which often is obscured by the shoulders
  - Obtain "swimmer's view" if necessary to visualize C7–T1 junction.
  - Anteroposterior (AP) radiograph may show double shadow of spinous process due to avulsion.
  - Flexion-extension films to rule out ligamentous instability and lamina or facet injury
- Thoracolumbar AP radiograph:
  - Relatively insensitive at identifying transverse process fractures
  - May show double shadow of spinous process due to avulsion
  - Hematoma may obscure evidence of transverse process fracture. Loss of normal psoas shadow may be most prominent finding.

TREATMENT

GENERAL MEASURES

- Short-term rest is often the most effective treatment for isolated injury.
- Cryotherapy repeated frequently within initial 36 to 48 hr may help prevent muscle spasm.
- Nonopioid medication (e.g., nonsteroidal anti-inflammatory drugs [NSAIDs]) and gentle range of motion exercises may be helpful in lumbar transverse process fractures.
- In all cases of suspected spine injury, immobilization with a backboard and rigid cervical collar is mandatory until the patient can be cleared radiographically.

ADDITIONAL THERAPIES

- If transverse process fractures result from high-energy trauma, there should be a high index of suspicion for associated visceral and orthopedic injuries.
- Urinalysis should be performed; if >8 red blood cells (RBCs) per high-power field are seen, perform cystogram and intravenous (IV) pyelogram to evaluate for possible urinary tract injury (1)[B].
- Recent research has found an association with L4 transverse process fracture with acetabular fractures and L5 transverse process fracture with pelvic ring injuries (2)[B].

ALERT

If transverse process fractures are identified on plain radiographs, abdominal CT should be performed due to possible associated visceral, abdominal, and orthopedic injuries (1,2)[B].

ALERT

- With cervical injury, protection against flexion with an orthosis should be provided for 4 to 6 wk:
  - Obtain flexion/extension radiographs at end of immobilization period.
  - Return to play once fracture is healed and patient has full, painless range of motion and no neurologic deficits (3)[B].
- There is controversy whether bracing is beneficial in thoracolumbar fractures without associated spinal injury. Some authors have suggested the use of bracing for symptomatic relief. Others have shown that it is not effective in immobilization and can result in complications such as skin breakdown. At the time of publication, there is no evidence for the effectiveness of bracing in patients with thoracolumbar fractures (4)[C],(5)[B].
- If there is associated spinal injury, a rigid orthosis is needed. The patient should be limited to isometric exercises, with restricted upper extremity exercises, until full range of motion and no tenderness to palpation are present.
- Isolated fractures of the transverse process usually cause disability for a few weeks and carry a very low likelihood of long-term sequelae. Early mobilization and physical therapy is important in rehabilitation:
  - Healing of the transverse process often does not occur because of distraction of the fracture fragment from muscle pull. Healing is often determined by radiographs and palpation at site of injury.
  - Return to play once range of motion is painless and the trunk has been strengthened
  - Likely, no equipment changes will be needed in noncontact sports, but padded equipment modification may be helpful in reducing the risk for reinjury in contact sports.
- Contiguous transverse process fractures should be observed carefully for development of pseudoarthrosis or myositis ossificans.

Pediatric Considerations

There is an association between transverse process fractures and spinous process fractures, with chest injury being common with higher thoracic injuries and abdominal injuries with lower thoracic or lumbar fractures. Pediatric patients benefit from conservative management and aggressive treatment of their comorbidities (6)[C].

SURGERY/OTHER PROCEDURES

Nonunion of fractured fragments is common in both injuries, but most authors advocate avoiding excision of fragments unless pain persists beyond the period of immobilization.

ONGOING CARE

FOLLOW-UP RECOMMENDATIONS

Patients with isolated fractures do not need orthopedic or neurosurgical referral.

REFERENCES

1. Patten RM, Gunberg SR, Brandenburger DK. Frequency and importance of transverse process fractures in the lumbar vertebrae at helical abdominal CT in patients with trauma. *Radiology*. 2000;215(3):831–834.
2. Acree J, Schlechter J. Level-specific thoracic and lumbar transverse process fractures and concomitant orthopedic injuries: is there an association? *Curr Orthop Pract*. 2015;26(4):411–413.
3. Boden BP, Jarvis CG. Spinal injuries in sports. *Neurol Clin*. 2008;26(1):63–78.
4. Boulter JH, Lovasik BP, Baum GR, et al. Implications of isolated transverse process fractures: is spine service consultation necessary? *World Neurosurg*. 2016;95:285–291.
5. Giele BM, Wiertsema SH, Beelen A, et al. No evidence for the effectiveness of bracing in patients with thoracolumbar fractures. *Acta Orthop*. 2009;80(2):226–232.
6. Akinpelu BJ, Zuckerman SL, Gannon SR, et al. Pediatric isolated thoracic and/or lumbar transverse and spinous process fractures. *J Neurosurg Pediatr*. 2016;17(6):639–644.

ADDITIONAL READING

- Homnick A, Lavery R, Nicastro O, et al. Isolated thoracolumbar transverse process fractures: call physical therapy, not spine. *J Trauma*. 2007;63(6):1292–1295.
- Krueger M, Green D, Hoyt D, et al. Overlooked spine injuries associated with lumbar transverse process fractures. *Clin Orthop Relat Res*. 1996;327:191–195.
- Nicholas J, Hershman E. *The Lower Extremity and Spine in Sports Medicine*. St. Louis, MO: Mosby; 1995.
- Sturm JT, Perry JF Jr. Injuries associated with fractures of the transverse processes of the thoracic and lumbar vertebrae. *J Trauma*. 1984;24(7):597–599.
- Tewes DP, Fischer DA, Quick DC, et al. Lumbar transverse process fractures in professional football players. *Am J Sports Med*. 1995;23(4):507–509.

CLINICAL PEARLS

- Isolated transverse process fractures can be treated conservatively without concern for long-term outcome sequelae such as pain, neurologic deficits, or ambulatory difficulties (4).
- Athletes involved in contact sports may feel more comfortable in a flak jacket, although there is no evidence that they prevent reinjury or accelerate return to competition.

FRACTURE, STERNUM

Steven Cuff, MD, FAAP, CAQSM • Thomas L. Pommering, DO, FAAFP

BASICS

DESCRIPTION

- Direct:
  - Results from direct force applied to the sternum, most often from a blow to the body of the sternum in the lower part
  - Fracture typically occurs near manubrium.
- Indirect:
  - Results from an indirect flexion-compression injury of the cervicothoracic spine, usually a forced flexion of the cervical spine that causes the upper two ribs to pull the manubrium posteriorly (downward and posterior force on the manubrium and upper two ribs)
  - May be exacerbated by chin striking the manubrium
  - Always involves the upper two segments of the sternum
- Stress fracture:
  - Results from repetitive motion of chest wall muscles, ribs, and clavicles with associated stress transmitted to sternum
- Muscular:
  - Results from violent muscular action that causes fracture through opposing muscle groups (i.e., tetanus)
  - Extremely rare

EPIDEMIOLOGY

- Sternal fractures are not common, especially in children and adolescents, due to elasticity of sternum and costal cartilage.
- Accounts for about 3–8% of all blunt trauma
- More common in men (60–80%) (1,2)

ETIOLOGY AND PATHOPHYSIOLOGY

- In adults, most commonly related to automobile accidents (68–84%) (1,2), typically from a direct mechanism
- Striking the steering wheel or dashboard
- Flexion of the sternum across the diagonal part of the seat belt, which acts as a fulcrum
- Although seatbelts decrease the risk of serious injury, they do not seem to decrease the risk of sternal fractures during motor vehicle accidents (MVAs); however, they do decrease the risk of internal injury, likely because of the fracture mechanism.
- Other causes from direct trauma include auto versus pedestrian, cardiopulmonary resuscitation (CPR), direct impact sports, falls, and assaults (2,3,4).
- In children, more likely related to a fall off a bicycle (direct) or from a height (indirect)
- Indirect forces more likely to result in pathologic or insufficiency fractures (3)

RISK FACTORS

- Insufficiency fractures caused by decreased bone density or weakened bone can occur spontaneously in patients with underlying bone density problems (esp. women), those on long-term steroids, and those with severe thoracic kyphosis (3).
- Repetitive upper body exercise transmitting force to the sternum, such as in golf, wrestling, and weight lifting, can lead to stress fracture (3).

COMMONLY ASSOCIATED CONDITIONS

ALERT

The overall mortality from isolated sternal fractures is low (0.7%); however, because of the high energy associated with these injuries, 2/3 of sternal fractures will have secondary injuries that have a mortality of 25–45%.

- Trauma to heart, mediastinum, great vessels, tracheobronchial tree, lung parenchyma, or liver: mediastinal injury much less common with an indirect mechanism. Always consider cardiac contusion, especially with double or comminuted fracture and in fracture involving the sternal angle.
- Pulmonary contusion
- Myocardial laceration
- Bone marrow embolization
- Pneumothorax
- Hemothorax
- Pericardial tamponade
- Sternoclavicular dislocation
- Rib fractures: can cause flail chest
- Vertebral fracture: most commonly thoracic vertebrae, but also may occur in lower cervical or upper lumbar vertebrae
- Head injury
- Limb fracture

DIAGNOSIS

HISTORY

- Mechanism of injury: direct blow to chest wall
- Forced flexion of cervical spine (heavy blow to back of head or fall onto head or upper back)
- Pain with inspiration
- Crepitus with respiratory excursion
- Dyspnea, usually transient. If persistent, consider more severe underlying injury like cardiopulmonary contusions.
- Symptoms in patients with spontaneous insufficiency or stress fracture may create a greater diagnostic challenge, because the symptoms may resemble other serious conditions.

PHYSICAL EXAM

- Pain
- Localized tenderness over the fracture site that is readily reproducible
- Bruising
- Swelling
- Deformity
- Possible dyspnea
- Palpable or visible step-off (deformity present only with displaced fracture)
- Palpable crepitus with respirations (more rare)
- Edema, ecchymosis
- Screen for associated rib fracture, clinical evidence of pulmonary contusion, vascular injury, pneumothorax, and pericardial friction rub.

DIFFERENTIAL DIAGNOSIS

- Costochondral dislocation
- Sternoclavicular dislocation
- Sternal contusion
- Costochondritis/Tietze syndrome
- Rib fracture/dislocation
- Cardiac causes: contusion, laceration, ischemia, myocarditis
- Aortic dissection
- Pleurisy
- Sickle cell crisis
- Osteomyelitis

DIAGNOSTIC TESTS & INTERPRETATION

- Chest posteroanterior (PA) and lateral radiographs gold standard (3)[C] (fracture missed in >80% of anteroposterior views); possible pneumothorax or mediastinal injury. Widened mediastinum could indicate hematoma due to underlying vascular injury until ruled out. Sternal fracture displacement and sternal dislocation occur in the sagittal plane.
- Care must be taken not to confuse nonossified intrasternal cartilage in young patients with fractures.
- Ultrasound has higher sensitivity but lower specificity (5)[A],(6)[C].
- Chest computed tomography (CT) scanning is less sensitive than plain radiographs because the fracture may be positioned between image cuts.

ALERT

Electrocardiogram (ECG): may see ECG changes in >50%, especially if from a direct mechanism. No single test is consistently reliable for diagnosis of myocardial contusion. If initial ECG is normal, consider repeat in 24 hr. May see ST or T-wave abnormalities or bundle branch block; may see major arrhythmia in first 24 hr (rare)

- Cervical, thoracic, lumbar spine radiographs: especially if from an indirect mechanism
- Consider other studies (echocardiogram, CT, aortography, serial troponins) if underlying injury is suspected.

TREATMENT

- Evaluate and treat any associated life-threatening injuries.
- Most nondisplaced fractures are treated conservatively with rest and analgesia until symptoms subside.
- Consider hematoma block using ultrasound if reduction is necessary.
- Some displaced fractures can be reduced by having the patient lay supine and hyperextending the thoracic spine by placing a sandbag transversely under the shoulders, slightly below the level of the spines of the scapulae. Extension can be maintained by bracing or bed rest.
- For simple displaced fractures, some authors recommend having the patient lay supine and simultaneously lifting the head and the extended lower extremities, thus separating the upper and lower parts of the sternum. Use thumb to place pressure on the anteriorly displaced fragment (should infiltrate with local anesthetic first, or can use intravenous [IV] procedural sedation).
- Open reduction internal fixation: Primary indication is pain with respiration that limits respiratory excursion; also flail chest; if not stabilized, can have pseudoarthrosis that can be source of ongoing pain or instability
- Consider 24-hr inpatient observation and monitoring due to the relatively high likelihood of associated underlying injuries.
- Immobilization typically is not necessary with nondisplaced fractures.
- Short-term immobilization may be necessary after surgical repair.

ADDITIONAL THERAPIES

- Consider cardiac monitoring while performing reduction if available.
- Avoid aggravating activities and contact sports.
- May start general conditioning within the limits of discomfort

SURGERY/OTHER PROCEDURES

- Surgical treatment for displaced fractures as above
- Consider surgical repair if nonunion (rare).

ONGOING CARE

FOLLOW-UP RECOMMENDATIONS

- Usually heals without any sequelae
- Consider early orthopedic referral if displaced fracture, open fracture, or flail chest.
- Early consultation as appropriate if there are associated underlying thoracic injuries (pneumothorax, cardiac contusion, etc.)
- Patients should know that sternal pain will last for 8 to 12 wk for all age groups.
- *Precautions*:
  - Brace the chest when coughing, sneezing, or turning. You may need a pillow or to cross your arms over your chest (splinting). This may help to prevent pneumonia.
  - Do not lift, push, or pull anything >10 lb.
  - Avoid any maneuvers that cause you pain such as repetitive overhead reaching.
  - Do not reach back with both arms at the same time.
  - Do not push or pull with your arms when moving or getting out of bed. Use your legs to change position in bed; lower yourself to the side and bring your feet onto the bed.

REFERENCES

1. Yeh DD, Hwabejire JO, DeMoya MA, et al. Sternal fracture—an analysis of the National Trauma Data Bank. *J Surg Res*. 2014;186(1):39–43.
2. Recinos G, Inaba K, Dubose J, et al. Epidemiology of sternal fractures. *Am Surg*. 2009;75(5):401–404.
3. Khoriati A, Rajakulasingam R, Shah R. Sternal fractures and their management. *J Emerg Trauma Shock*. 2013;6(2):113–116.
4. Miller AC, Rosati SF, Suffredini AF, et al. A systematic review and pooled analysis of CPR-associated cardiovascular and thoracic injuries. *Resuscitation*. 2014;85(6):724–731.
5. Yousefifard M, Baikpour M, Ghelichkhani P, et al. Comparison of ultrasonography and radiography in detection of thoracic bone fractures; a systematic review and meta-analysis. *Emerg (Tehran)*. 2016;4(2):55–64.
6. Lahham S, Patane J, Lane N. Ultrasound of sternal fracture. *West J Emerg Med*. 2015;16(7):1057–1058.

ADDITIONAL READING

- Athanassiadi K, Gerazounis M, Moustardas M, et al. Sternal fractures: retrospective analysis of 100 cases. *World J Surg*. 2002;26(10):1243–1246.
- Baker JC, Demertzis JL. Manubrial stress fractures diagnosed on MRI: report of two cases and review of the literature. *Skeletal Radiol*. 2016;45(6):833–837.
- Celik B, Sahin E, Nadir A, et al. Sternum fractures and effects of associated injuries. *Thorac Cardiovasc Surg*. 2009;57(8):468–471.
- Dixit S, Chang C. Sternal fracture. In: Madden C, Putukian M, McCarty E, et al, eds. *Netter's Sports Medicine*. 2nd ed. Philadelphia, PA: Elsevier; 2018:403.
- Ferguson LP, Wilkinson AG, Beattie TF. Fracture of the sternum in children. *Emerg Med J*. 2003;20(6):518–520.

CLINICAL PEARLS

- Contact sports should be avoided until symptoms subside, typically 6 to 12 wk.
- General conditioning or training program permitted within the limits of discomfort posed by the injury
- When returning to play, should consider chest protector if likelihood of reinjury

FRACTURE, STRESS: METATARSAL, NAVICULAR

Stephen M. Simons, MD, FACSM • Christopher Jordan, MD, ATC, CAQSM

BASICS

DESCRIPTION

- Overload, repetitive stress injury to bone
- Manifest as fatigue fractures to otherwise normal bone

EPIDEMIOLOGY

- Stress fractures account for 10% of overuse injuries in sports (1). Stress fractures of the 2nd and 3rd metatarsals are most common in running and dancing (1,2).
- Tarsal navicular stress fractures are rare in the general population but relatively common in sprinting and jumping athletes (3).
- Tarsal navicular stress fractures have been reported in athletes as young as 13 yr old (4).
- High-risk stress fractures include the proximal 5th metatarsal and tarsal navicular due to high-tensile load and diminished blood flow (1).
- 5th metatarsal is the most frequently fractured metatarsal bone (5).

RISK FACTORS

- Training errors: number, frequency, intensity, and duration of strain cycles
- Impact attenuation: muscle fatigue, training surfaces, footwear
- Gait mechanics: foot type, lower extremity alignment, altered gait
- Bone health: nutrition, genetics, hormones, bone disease

DIAGNOSIS

HISTORY

- Pain onset acute or insidious? Usually insidious
- Pain location? Site of fracture; forefoot for metatarsal stress fractures and dorsomedial midfoot for tarsal navicular stress fractures. Some patients may report ankle pain related to the tarsal navicular stress fractures.
- Associated findings? There is usually minimal or no swelling with stress fractures.
- Does pain improve or worsen during the activity?

Tendinitis pain often improves as the injured tissue warms up, but stress fracture pain persists or worsens during the activity.

PHYSICAL EXAM

- Metatarsals: forefoot pain that progressively worsens with activity
- Tarsal navicular: vague, dorsal midfoot pain sometimes radiating along the medial arch or into the ankle
- Minimal or no forefoot swelling
- Tenderness at the base, head, or midshaft of the metatarsal
- Axial load applied to head of the metatarsal causes pain at the fracture site (shaft), even though the examiners pressure is applied distal on the metatarsal.
- Examine callous patterns, which may clue the examiner to excessive loads to individual metatarsals.
- Tender over the dorsum of the navicular at the "N" spot in the space between the anterior tibial tendon and the extensor hallucis longus tendon
- Biomechanical examination, joint range of motion, strength, and flexibility to assess predisposing conditions

DIFFERENTIAL DIAGNOSIS

- Tendinitis
- Tendon rupture, partial or complete
- Metatarsalgia
- Symptomatic accessory ossicle
- 5th metatarsal apophyseal injury

DIAGNOSTIC TESTS & INTERPRETATION

- Radiographs:
  - Metatarsals: Anteroposterior and lateral radiographs are often initially normal; 2 to 3 wk following symptom onset, periosteal thickening and sometimes a radiolucent line can be appreciated; initial imaging modality due to low cost and wide availability (6)[C]
  - Tarsal navicular: Plain radiographs often are normal throughout the course of a navicular stress fracture (3)[B].
- Bone scan:
  - Metatarsals: very sensitive, but necessary only if a diagnosis is needed quickly, as with a competitive athlete; not specific and must be correlated with clinical history and examination (1)
  - Navicular: no longer preferred due to poor specificity (6)[C]
- Computed tomography (CT) scan:
  - Metatarsals: not helpful
  - Navicular: Thin-sliced cuts in the plane of the talonavicular joint reveal the curvilinear fracture extending from the dorsal cortex surrounded by exuberant bony sclerosis. CT is helpful to determine an incomplete fracture versus a complete dorsoplantar transection of the navicular. CT scan can also help differentiate between navicular stress fracture and a stress reaction (3)[B].
- Magnetic resonance imaging (MRI):
  - Although generally not necessary, metatarsals will demonstrate intramedullary edema.
  - Edema seen on short TI inversion recovery (STIR) or T2-weighted MRI images may help distinguish an active tarsal navicular stress fracture from a persistent, chronic mature fracture as sometimes seen on CT (1)[C].
- Pathologic findings:
  - Navicular fracture types (3):
    - Type 0.5: stress reaction; signal change on MRI but no fracture on CT scan
    - Type I fractures involve only the dorsal cortex.
    - Type II fractures are fractures that extend into the navicular body.
    - Type III fractures traverse the entire navicular and extend into the plantar cortex.
  - 5th metatarsal high-risk fracture zones (1):
    - Zone 1—metatarsal tuberosity; avulsion fracture
    - Zone 2—metaphyseal/diaphyseal junction; Jones fracture (high-risk area)
    - Zone 3—proximal diaphyseal junction (high-risk area)

TREATMENT

GENERAL MEASURES

- Metatarsals:
  - Cease sporting activities.
  - Non–weight-bearing only needed for pain control
  - Rest period, average 6 wk
- Navicular:
  - Non–weight-bearing on crutches with below-the-knee cast or removable brace for 6 to 8 wk; high failure rate with weight-bearing rest (1)[C],(2)[A]
  - Studies continue to show poorer outcomes with early weight-bearing (1)[B].
  - Follow-up clinical assessment for tenderness at the "N" spot. Radiographic assessment not helpful. Continued tenderness should extend non–weight-bearing another 2 to 3 wk.

SURGERY/OTHER PROCEDURES

- Surgery is rarely required for metatarsal stress fractures.
- 90% of navicular stress fractures can be managed with non–weight-bearing cast. However, type III fractures should be referred for surgical management (3)[C].
- Surgical fixation with internal screw, bone grafting, or both is necessary for fractures not clinically healed by nonoperative means.
- Recent studies show comparative long-term outcomes between conservative non–weight-bearing and surgery.

ONGOING CARE

- Metatarsals (6)[C]:
  - Modify activity level and training activities to provide relative rest.
  - Address abnormal biomechanics.
  - Consider calcium and vitamin D supplementation.
  - Return to progressive gradual training only after pain-free walking and no local tenderness at the fracture site.
  - Orthotics may be used, although there is only anecdotal evidence of benefit.
  - Proximal 5th metatarsal: Surgical fixation may result in quicker return to sport (7)[B].
- Navicular (3,6)[C]:
  - Time to full recovery may take >4 mo.
  - May benefit from formal physical therapy
  - Reexamine patient every 2 to 3 wk to ensure adequate recovery.
  - First 2 wk following cast removal: activities of daily living, swimming, water running
  - Second 2 wk: Assess "N" spot; if nontender, then 5-min jogging on grass every other day. Gradually increase to 10 min per session.
  - Third 2 wk: Assess "N" spot; if nontender, then faster running for short distances, that is, 50 m on alternate days; gradual speed increase
  - Fourth 2 wk: Assess "N" spot; if nontender, then gradual return to full training over several weeks. Average time to return to sport is 5 to 6 mo from diagnosis.
  - Attention throughout the rehabilitation time to soft-tissue massage and joint mobilization to the talocrural, subtalar, and midtarsal joints
  - Strength training to reverse the atrophy acquired during immobilization

FOLLOW-UP RECOMMENDATIONS

- Metatarsal stress fractures not healing in a reasonably expected period should be referred to orthopedic surgery or podiatry. Consider referring for biomechanical evaluation for recurrent stress fractures.
- Navicular: Refer the persistently symptomatic navicular stress fracture that does not heal by the above outlined protocol.
- Consider early referral to orthopedic surgeon or podiatrist for zone 2 or 3 fractures of the 5th metatarsal.

REFERENCES

1. McInnis KC, Ramey LN. High-risk stress fractures: diagnosis and management. *PM R*. 2016;8(Suppl 3):S113–S124.
2. Welck MJ, Hayes T, Pastides P, et al. Stress fractures of the foot and ankle. *Injury*. 2017;48(8):1722–1726.
3. Saxena A, Behan SA, Valerio DL, et al. Navicular stress fracture outcomes in athletes: analysis of 62 injuries. *J Foot Ankle Surg*. 2017;56(5):943–948.
4. Ostlie DK, Simons SM. Tarsal navicular stress fracture in a young athlete: case report with clinical, radiologic, and pathophysiologic correlations. *J Am Board Fam Pract*. 2001;14(5):381–385.
5. Yates J, Feeley I, Sasikumar S, et al. Jones fracture of the fifth metatarsal: is operative intervention justified? A systematic review of the literature and meta-analysis of results. *Foot (Edinb)*. 2015;25(4):251–257.
6. Patel DS, Roth M, Kapil N. Stress fractures: diagnosis, treatment, and prevention. *Am Fam Physician*. 2011;83(1):39–46.
7. Mallee WH, Weel H, van Dijk CN, et al. Surgical versus conservative treatment for high-risk stress fractures of the lower leg (anterior tibial cortex, navicular and fifth metatarsal base): a systematic review. *Br J Sports Med*. 2015;49(6):370–376.

ADDITIONAL READING

- Cheung CN, Lui TH. Proximal fifth metatarsal fractures: anatomy, classification, treatment and complications. *Arch Trauma Res*. 2016;5(4):e33298.
- Thompson P, Patel V, Fallat LM, et al. Surgical management of fifth metatarsal diaphyseal fractures: a retrospective outcomes study. *J Foot Ankle Surg*. 2017;56(3):463–467.
- Toren AJ, Hahn DB, Brown WC, et al. Vascularized scapular free bone graft after nonunion of a tarsal navicular stress fracture: a case report. *J Foot Ankle Surg*. 2013;52(2):221–226.
- Torg JS, Moyer J, Gaughan JP, et al. Management of tarsal navicular stress fractures: conservative versus surgical treatment: a meta-analysis. *Am J Sports Med*. 2010;38(5):1048–1053.

CLINICAL PEARLS

- Risk factors for stress fractures include overuse or training errors, biomechanical factors, choice and/or age of shoe, nutrition, and menstrual issues for women.
- Careful attention to the risk factors, particularly training errors, will minimize the risk of reinjury.
- Surgery is rarely indicated for metatarsal and tarsal navicular stress fractures.
- High-risk stress fractures of the foot include the tarsal navicular and proximal 5th metatarsal.

FRACTURE, TALUS

Timothy Ryan Draper, DO, ABFM, CAQSM • Karl B. Fields, MD, CAQ

BASICS

DESCRIPTION

- Relatively uncommon fracture usually involving the talar neck, lateral process, or osteochondral fracture of talar dome
- Excluding smaller osteochondral fractures, talar neck fractures account for 50% of talar fractures, talar body fractures 40%, and talar head fractures 5–10%.
- Osteochondral fractures (a subset of talar body fractures) can occur in up to 6.5% of acute ankle sprains.
- Shepherd fracture (posterior tubercle fracture) represents the largest single group of talar body fractures.
- "Snowboarder's ankle," a lateral process fracture, is the second most common type of talar body fracture.
- Stress fractures of the talus have been reported but are rare (1).

EPIDEMIOLOGY

- Talar fractures constitute 3–6% of all foot fractures and are estimated at 1% of all fractures in the entire human body.
- "Snowboarder's ankle" (lateral process fracture) appears to be increasing in frequency.

ETIOLOGY AND PATHOPHYSIOLOGY

- 60–70% of the talar surface consists of cartilage, accommodating seven different articulations.
- The talus has no muscular insertions or origins and is held in place by its osseous neighbors and constraining ligamentous attachments.
- The talar neck is the only section of the talus that is primarily extra-articular.
- The tibiotalar articulation is responsible for hindfoot motion in the plantar/dorsiflexion plane; the subtalar joint provides hindfoot inversion/eversion motion.
- The talus transmits axial force.
- The tibiotalar joint has more loads per unit area than any other joint in the body (2).
- Only 40% of the talus can be perfused by blood vessels. The other 60% is covered by articular cartilage. As a result, talus fractures are at a high risk of avascular necrosis.

RISK FACTORS

- In general, fractures of the talar head and neck are the result of high-energy trauma.
- Snowboarding is associated with acute dorsiflexion/inversion injuries to the ankle, which can cause lateral process fractures.

DIAGNOSIS

HISTORY

- Fractures of the talar head and neck usually are found after high-velocity trauma (e.g., motorcycle accidents).
- Fractures of the talar neck occur as a result of hyperdorsiflexion and axial loading of the foot against a stationary tibia.
- Crush fractures of the talar head occur via a compressive load through the calcaneus sustentaculum tali.
- Shear fractures of the talar head occur via an axial load through the navicular (3).
- Anterolateral osteochondral fractures are associated with an inversion-dorsiflexion injury of the ankle.
- Posterolateral osteochondral fractures are associated with plantar flexion, inversion, and external rotation of the ankle.
- Historically, lateral process fractures involved dorsiflexion and inversion with an axial load, but more recent cadaveric studies have suggested that eversion can also be involved (4).
- Chronic osteochondral fractures present with pain following an adequate healing time for ligamentous injury, complaints of ankle "giving out," catching, or locking up.

PHYSICAL EXAM

- Talar head fractures cause swelling and tenderness at the talonavicular joint.
- Talar neck fractures present with swelling and tenderness of the proximal dorsal foot. With displaced fractures, the normal ankle contours will be changed.
- Acute inversion injuries of the ankle that remain painful after conservative treatment should make the clinician suspicious for osteochondral lesion of the talus or a lateral process fracture.

ALERT

Thoracolumbar spinal fractures have been found in association with fractures of the talar neck and talar body (5).

ALERT

Lateral talar process fractures have the same symptoms as an acute sprain of the anterior talofibular ligament. Findings may include tenderness inferior and anterior to the tip of the lateral malleolus associated with pain on active and passive range of motion of the ankle and subtalar joints.

- Acute osteochondral fractures present with edema, ecchymosis, range of motion limited by guarding, and pain to palpation.
- Displaced talar neck fractures can lead to skin necrosis due to significant stretching of the soft tissues (5).

DIFFERENTIAL DIAGNOSIS

Conditions that can mimic osteochondral fractures of the talar dome include osteochondritis dissecans, degenerative joint disease, and/or loose bodies.

DIAGNOSTIC TESTS & INTERPRETATION

- Initial radiographic workup of most talar fractures should include ankle mortise views with routine anteroposterior (AP) and lateral views.
- The Canale view (foot internally rotated 15 degrees with x-ray angled at 75 degrees from the plane of the table) gives a direct AP view of the talus and is very useful in evaluating talar neck fractures.

- To best view lateral osteochondral lesions with plain x-rays, films should be obtained with 10 to 35 degrees of internal rotation and maximal plantar flexion.
- Lateral osteochondral fractures have a thin, wafer-like appearance; medial osteochondral lesions have a deep, cup-shaped appearance.
- If plain x-rays show abnormalities of the talar dome, computed tomography (CT) scan should be performed to determine size and nature of lesion, essential in preoperative planning.

ALERT
If an injury to the talar dome is suspected but plain radiographs are unremarkable, further imaging, ideally with a magnetic resonance imaging (MRI) or CT, is indicated.

- Fractures of the posterolateral process can be potentially mistaken as an os trigonum (6).
- Ultrasound can be used as a screen in minor injuries and recurrent ankle pain. Studies correlate excellent ability to determine articular cartilage thickness at the talar dome. The authors have noted a number of talar dome fractures in scans for chronic ankle pain (7).

TREATMENT

- Displaced talar fractures require anatomical reduction to prevent arthrosis and avascular necrosis and usually require surgical fixation.
- Reduction of a displaced talar neck fracture can be attempted by plantar flexion of the foot, bringing the head and body into line. This is an orthopedic emergency if there are signs of skin necrosis.
- Clinical signs and symptoms correlated with repeated radiographic examination are important during conservative treatment to assure proper healing.
- Although nondisplaced talar fractures may be treated in a short, non–weight-bearing leg cast for 6 to 12 wk, it is recommended only for nonambulatory patients or those medically unable to tolerate surgery (8)[C].
- Stress fractures are treated with 3 to 6 wk of non–weight-bearing immobilization with a controlled ankle motion (CAM) walker, followed by progressive mobilization, rehabilitation, and return to activity based on case reports.

ADDITIONAL THERAPIES

- 50% of talar neck fractures go on to avascular necrosis, as do 25–50% of talar body fractures.
- Treatment of osteonecrosis is primarily conservative, and patient can begin weight-bearing once there is evidence of stable changes on x-ray. Failure of conservative measures to allow weight-bearing may require surgery (5).
- Talar head fracture complications include midtarsal instability, talonavicular arthritis, and avascular necrosis of the talar head.
- Standard range of motion, strengthening, and proprioceptive rehabilitation are appropriate after the fracture has healed.

SURGERY/OTHER PROCEDURES

ALERT
Any talar fracture that is displaced, even minimally, requires surgical treatment, given the risks of avascular necrosis and future arthritis.

- Nondisplaced osteochondral fractures can be managed conservatively for up to 12 mo without compromising subsequent surgical outcomes.
- Any loose body associated with a fracture may require arthroscopic removal.

REFERENCES

1. Ahmad J, Raikin SM. Current concepts review: talar fractures. *Foot Ankle Int*. 2006;27(6):475–482.
2. Boon AJ, Smith J, Zobitz ME, et al. Snowboarder's talus fracture. Mechanism of injury. *Am J Sports Med*. 2001;29(3):333–338.
3. Grossman JP, Lyons MC II. A review of osteochondral lesions of the talus. *Clin Podiatr Med Surg*. 2009;26(2):205–226.
4. Grear BJ. Review of talus fractures and surgical timing. *Orthop Clin North Am*. 2016;47(3):625–637.
5. Fortin PT, Balazsy JE. Talus fractures: evaluation and treatment. *J Am Acad Orthop Surg*. 2001;9(2):114–127.
6. Majeed H, McBride DJ. Talar process fractures: an overview and update of the literature. *EFORT Open Rev*. 2018;3(3):85–92.
7. Onat ŞŞ, Ata AM, Serrano S, et al. Ultrasonographic measurements of the metacarpophalangeal and talar cartilage thicknesses: a reliability study in healthy subjects. *J Back Musculoskelet Rehabil*. 2018;31(2):253–257.
8. Vallier HA. Fractures of the talus: state of the art. *J Orthop Trauma*. 2015;29(9):385–392.

ADDITIONAL READING

- Mandracchia VJ, Buddecke DE Jr, Giesking JL. Osteochondral lesions of the talar dome. A comprehensive review with retrospective study. *Clin Podiatr Med Surg*. 1999;16(4):725–742.
- Mayer D. Isolated talus fractures: description of a new clinical sign. *Am J Emerg Med*. 1997;15(4):412–414.
- Schachter AK, Chen AL, Reddy PD, et al. Osteochondral lesions of the talus. *J Am Acad Orthop Surg*. 2005;13(3):152–158.
- Sormaala MJ, Niva MH, Kiuru MJ, et al. Outcomes of stress fractures of the talus. *Am J Sports Med*. 2006;34(11):1809–1814.

CLINICAL PEARLS

- "Snowboarder's fracture" is becoming more common with the increasing popularity of the sport.
- If ankle pain persists after adequate time for a simple ankle sprain to heal, be suspicious of a possible osteochondral fracture.
- Most talar fractures need referral to orthopedic surgery. Even nondisplaced fractures may require open reduction and internal fixation (ORIF).

FRACTURE, TIBIAL PLATEAU

Ramon Ylanan, MD, CAQSM • Larry Balle II, MD, MPH

BASICS

DESCRIPTION

- Fracture and/or depression of the proximal tibial articulating surface (1)
- Largest and most kinematically complex joint (2)
- Also referred to as *tibial condylar fractures*
- Mechanism of injury: axial loading force and coronal plane (varus/valgus) force (3) resulting in articular shear, depression, and mechanical axis malalignment (2)
- Most commonly used classification: Schatzker (1):
  - Type I—pure cleavage, lateral femoral condyle driven into articular surface of tibial plateau, wedge-shaped split-off fracture of the lateral tibial plateau displaced outward and down (1):
    - Best prognosis

Pediatric Considerations

Occurs in patients with higher demand and good bone stock, the tibial plateau resists depression (2).

- Type II—cleavage combined with depression, lateral wedge is split with varying portions of remaining lateral plateau and articular surface area comminuted and depressed downwards into metaphysis (1):
  - Commonly occurs in patients with osteopenia (2)
- Type III—pure central depression, articular surface of the lateral plateau is depressed and driven into lateral tibial condyle, no lateral wedge split-off and lateral cortex is intact (1)
- Type IV—medial condyle fracture (1), most commonly posteromedial aspect (2):
  - A—split-off wedge fragment of medial plateau (1)
  - B—medial fragment depressed or comminuted
  - Either may be combined with fracture of tibial spine
- Type V—bicondylar fracture, both plateaus fractured, appearance of inverted Y, may be associated with fracture of intercondylar eminence, metaphysis and diaphysis intact (1)
- Type VI—tibial plateau fracture with dissociation of tibial metaphyseal-diaphyseal junction via oblique or transverse fracture, with varying degrees of comminution of one or both tibial condyles and articular surface (1)

ALERT

- With high-energy mechanisms, associated major life-threatening injuries take precedence.
- Immobilize early to prevent further neurologic or vascular injury.

EPIDEMIOLOGY

Incidence

- ~1.2% of all fractures (2)
- Highest frequency in both sexes between ages 40 and 60 yr
- 55–70% are lateral tibial plateau in isolation.
- 10–25% are medial tibial plateau in isolation.
- ~15% are bicondylar.
- In as many as 90%, some degree of soft tissue injury occurs with 1–3% presenting as open fractures.

COMMONLY ASSOCIATED CONDITIONS

- *Lateral* plateau fractures commonly associated with medial collateral ligament:
  - According to Porrino et al. in a retrospective review, anterior cruciate ligament injuries (8 of 9 although not statistically significant in small sample size) (4)
- *Medial* plateau fractures (type IV, V, VI) are less common overall (3) but more common in younger patients with high-energy injuries and associated soft tissue injuries (2):
  - Associated injuries include posterior lateral corner injuries, lateral collateral ligament, posterior cruciate ligament, medial meniscus, and neurovascular injury to peroneal nerve (1% incidence) and popliteal vessels.

ALERT

Isolated medial plateau fractures (type IV) may be associated with knee dislocation-relocation injury with neurovascular injury in posterior knee.

- Compartment syndrome is most common in Schatzker types IV to VI (up to 18% in Schatzker VI injuries and 53% in medial plateau fractures) (2).

DIAGNOSIS

HISTORY

- Mechanism of injury important in diagnosis
- *High-energy injuries* (5):
  - Pedestrian struck in the lower leg by an automobile
  - Passenger in motor vehicle collision
  - Fall from a height resulting in femoral condyles impacting tibial surface
  - Violent twisting force (e.g., skiing or dancing)

Geriatric Considerations

Elderly patients present more often with low-energy lateral tibial plateau fractures without insult to soft tissue often radiographically occult (2).

PHYSICAL EXAM

- Painful, swollen knee
- Inability to bear weight on the injured leg
- Knee effusion (hemarthrosis)
- Decreased (both active and passive) range of motion (ROM) of the knee
- Tenderness along the proximal tibia (either medial or lateral tibial plateau)
- Possible varus or valgus deformity of the knee
- Possible joint instability associated with ligamentous injury
- Neurovascular examination (2)[A]:
  - Evaluate for neurovascular damage and compartment syndrome.
  - Check popliteal, posterior tibial, and dorsalis pedis arterial pulse (consider ankle brachial index if knee dislocation in the differential normal >0.9).
  - Check integrity of peroneal nerve, ankle and toe dorsiflexion, and sensation in the web space between the great and 2nd toes.

DIFFERENTIAL DIAGNOSIS

- Knee dislocation
- Cruciate ligament tears/avulsion
- Collateral ligament tears/avulsion
- Meniscal tears
- Quadriceps tendon rupture
- Patellar fracture
- Patellar dislocation

DIAGNOSTIC TESTS & INTERPRETATION

Initial Tests (lab, imaging)

- Plain radiography—initial investigation of choice (2)[A]
- Anteroposterior (AP) and lateral views of the knee and proximal tibia—79% sensitivity for predominantly lateral plateau fractures (2)
- Tibial plateau view—AP view with the knee in 10 to 15 degrees of flexion helps to visualize depressions (5).
- Oblique views increase sensitivity to approximately 85% (2):
  - Oblique internal and external views: determine the location and degree of depression that may not apparent on other films (5)
- Caudal tilt plateau view—determines the degree of articular step off
- Subtle fractures—if lipohemarthrosis (fat-fluid level) seen on lateral view and no obvious fracture seen on x-ray, a computed tomography (CT) should be performed to avoid missing covert fracture (2).

- Cross-sectional imaging: CT and magnetic resonance imaging (MRI):
  - More detailed image of fracture (1)
  - Helpful in preoperative planning and identification of associated injuries (2)
  - CT coupled with angiography quantifies magnitude of fracture or depression and evaluates vascular involvement (2,5).
  - CT/MRI angiography is indicated if (5):
    - High-energy mechanism.
    - Schatzker type IV, V, or VI fracture.
    - Alteration in distal pulses.
    - Expanding hematoma.
    - Bruit on exam.
    - Injury to anatomically related nerves.
- MRI can be used to better identify soft tissue (ligamentous, chondral, meniscus, and neurovascular) injuries (2) and classify fracture using the Schatzker system, especially in the pediatric population (5).

Diagnostic Procedures/Other

- Compartment pressures if compartment syndrome clinically suspected:
  - Pain not over fracture site
  - Pain on passive stretch
  - Paresthesia
  - Abnormality of pulses
  - Pressures >30 mm Hg—indication for fasciotomy
- Arthrocentesis to look for fat globules if effusion present and mechanism strongly suggests that fracture present without x-ray findings (2)

TREATMENT

GENERAL MEASURES

- Airway, breathing, and circulation (ABCs)/advanced trauma life support (ATLS) protocol in multiple trauma victim
- Long-leg splint
- Ice
- Elevation
- Emergency department (ED)/clinic management:
  - Nonoperative management:
    - Schatzker type I—undisplaced fractures in low-demand patients (2)
  - Coronal plane stabilizing brace (2), hinged knee brace (3)
  - Restricted weight-bearing
  - Permit full ROM.
  - Rest, ice, compression, and elevation

ALERT
Non–weight-bearing and early ROM are critical (3).

- Average time to heal is 12 to 20 wk (3).
- Consider aspiration of hemarthrosis and injection of local anesthetic.
- Timetables (3):
  - Non–weight-bearing for 4 to 6 wk or until radiographic evidence of healing is noted and then may proceed with partial weight-bearing with crutch assistance
  - Initial 10 to 14 days in brace with full extension
  - Begin gradual ROM, with goal of 90 degrees of flexion by 4 wk.
  - Follow-up with repeat x-rays every 2 to 3 wk
- Pain control
- Early orthopedic follow-up if knee is unstable

ISSUES FOR REFERRAL

- Indications for orthopedic consultation for closed fractures (2)[A]:
  - Lateral plateau fracture with:
    - Articular step off >3 mm
    - Condylar widening >5 mm
    - Coronal plane instability
  - Displaced medial plateau fracture (60% of weight-bearing through medial plateau)
  - Bicondylar fractures
- Fracture dislocations, vascular injuries, and compartment syndrome (2)[A]:
  - Emergent orthopedic consultation
- Open fractures:
  - Emergent orthopedic consultation
  - Remove contaminants.
  - Apply moist sterile dressing.
  - Assess tetanus immunity.
  - Consider empiric antibiotics.

SURGERY/OTHER PROCEDURES

- Depending on severity of injury, may require staged management due to compromise of soft tissue and physiology (2).
- Operative options:
  - Standard plating
  - Minimally invasive and percutaneous techniques
  - Definitive external fixation
  - Primary arthroplasty

ADMISSION, INPATIENT, AND NURSING CONSIDERATIONS

Admission criteria:

- Open fractures for débridement, irrigation, and intravenous (IV) antibiotics (6)
- Comminuted bicondylar fractures for traction
- High-energy mechanism for observation of neurovascular status
- Suspected compartment syndrome
- Pain control

ONGOING CARE

FOLLOW-UP RECOMMENDATIONS

Patient Monitoring

- Nonoperative treatment: biweekly follow-up initially with x-rays to evaluate fracture
- If knee is unstable, early follow-up with orthopedics to evaluate ligamentous injury

PATIENT EDUCATION

Formal physical therapy early can help to restore function (3).

COMPLICATIONS

Posttraumatic osteoarthritis common sequelae (2)

REFERENCES

1. Millar SC, Arnold JB, Thewlis D, et al. A systematic literature review of tibial plateau fractures: what classifications are used and how reliable and useful are they? *Injury*. 2018;49(3):473–490.
2. Mthethwa J, Chikate A. A review of the management of tibial plateau fractures. *Musculoskelet Surg*. 2018;102(2):119–127.
3. Eiff MP, Hatch RL. *Fracture Management for Primary Care*. 2nd ed. Philadelphia, PA: Saunders; 2003.
4. Porrino J, Richardson ML, Hovis K, et al. Association of tibial plateau fracture morphology with ligament disruption in the context of multiligament knee injury [published online ahead of print September 12, 2017]. *Curr Probl Diagn Radiol*. doi:10.1067/j.cpradiol.2017.09.001.
5. Markhardt BK, Gross JM, Monu JU. Schatzker classification of tibial plateau fractures: use of CT and MR imaging improves assessment. *Radiographics*. 2009;29(2):585–597.
6. Torrey SB. Lower extremity and pelvis trauma. In: Barkin, ed. *Pediatric Emergency Medicine*. St. Louis, MO: CV Mosby; 1992:357–365.

ADDITIONAL READING

- Blokker CP, Rorabeck CH, Bourne RB. Tibial plateau fractures. An analysis of the results of treatment in 60 patients. *Clin Orthop Relat Res*. 1984;(182):193–199.
- Rang M. *Children's Fractures*. 2nd ed. Philadelphia, PA: JB Lippincott; 1984.
- Simon RR, Sherman SC, Koenigsknecht SJ. Proximal tibia fractures. In: Simon RR, Sherman SC, Koenigsknecht SJ, eds. *Emergency Orthopedics: The Extremities*. 5th ed. Norwalk, CT: Appleton & Lange; 2007:396–403.
- Wiss DA, Watson JT, Johnson EE. Fractures of the knee. In: Rockwood CA, Green DP, Bucholz RW, et al, eds. *Rockwood and Green's Fractures in Adults*. 4th ed. Philadelphia, PA: Lippincott-Raven; 1996:1593–1652.

CLINICAL PEARLS

- Mechanism of injury important in diagnosis: high-energy axial force with coronal force component
- Lateral tibial plateau more commonly injured
- X-rays—AP, lateral, and obliques
- Schatzker type I may be treated nonoperatively.
- Schatzker type IV associated with dislocation-relocation injury (check ankle/brachial index)
- In Schatzker types IV to VI, neurovascular compromise is high risk, emergent orthopedic consultation.

FRACTURE, TIBIAL SPINE AVULSION

Chris Koutures, MD, FAAP • Alana Ryan, DO

BASICS

DESCRIPTION

- Tibial spine avulsion fractures occur when the anterior cruciate ligament (ACL)–tibial spine bone interface is ruptured by undue stress.
- In children, the weaker, incompletely ossified bone will fail before the ligament is injured resulting in fracture.
- Thus, an injury that typically would result in an ACL tear in an adult instead would cause a fracture through the anterior tibial spine via pull of the ACL.
- Fracture through the posterior tibial spine (where the posterior cruciate ligament attaches) is rare and generally occurs in skeletally mature patients.
- Mechanism of injury:
  - Hyperextension ± valgus stress or rotation about the knee
  - Fracture also can occur with a direct blow to the distal end of the femur with the knee flexed.
- Synonym(s): tibial eminence fracture; intercondylar eminence fracture

EPIDEMIOLOGY

- Avulsion fractures of the ACL attachment to the tibial spine are relatively rare, accounting for three fractures per 100,000 children annually and approximately 2% of all knee injuries in children (1)[C].
- Most prevalent in children 8 to 14 yr of age but are also seen in adults >35 yr of age who have low bone density.
- ACL avulsion from the femoral attachment is less common, as is posterior cruciate ligament avulsion from the posterior tibial eminence.
- Tibial spine fractures classically have been associated with a fall from a bicycle or motorcycle on an outstretched leg (1)[C].
- The injury is now also commonly seen in sporting activities (1)[C].

RISK FACTORS

- Children <16 yr of age
- Adults >35 yr of age who are osteopenic or undergo high-energy trauma (1)[C]

COMMONLY ASSOCIATED CONDITIONS

- In adolescents and adults, tibial spine avulsion fractures are commonly associated with concomitant knee injury.
- These most commonly include meniscal entrapment or tear, chondral injury, bone contusion, intrinsic ACL injury, and collateral ligament pathology (1)[C],(2)[B].

DIAGNOSIS

HISTORY

- In children aged 8 to 11 yr, often due to hyperextension injury
- Above this age, owing to either hyperextension injury or single-leg landing from a jump, both associated with a rotational or twisting stress to the knee
- Audible "pop" at the time of injury
- Immediate (within 1 to 2 hr) prominent swelling of the knee (acute hemarthrosis)
- Frequently unable to bear weight after injury

PHYSICAL EXAM

- Signs and symptoms:
  - Presence of a large, tense knee effusion (especially in a child <16 yr of age) should raise concern for a potential ACL avulsion fracture.
  - Examination findings of an ACL tear should raise suspicion.
- Physical examination:
  - Large, tense effusion noted with loss of range of motion (ROM)
  - ACL stress tests (Lachman, anterior drawer, and pivot shift) show more forward translation of the tibia compared with the noninjured side.
  - A positive posterior drawer sign or if the tibia is displaced posteriorly relative to the femur when compared with the noninjured knee may suggest posterior cruciate ligament avulsion from the tibial spine.
  - Evaluate other ligamentous and meniscal structures, particularly the menisci and collateral ligaments, for concomitant pathology.

DIFFERENTIAL DIAGNOSIS

- Midsubstance ACL tear
- Congenital absence or deficiency of the ACL
- Midsubstance tear of the posterior cruciate ligament
- Tibial plateau fracture
- Patellar dislocation or subluxation
- Osteochondral fracture of the femoral condyle

DIAGNOSTIC TESTS & INTERPRETATION

- Plain radiographs should include anteroposterior (AP), lateral, and tunnel views. The latter outlines the femoral notch and tibial eminence.
- The lateral view is most helpful to assess fracture position and degree of displacement.
- Radiographs should be obtained on an urgent basis at the first evaluation.
- Types of anterior tibial spine avulsion fractures are based on degree of displacement. The Meyers and McKeever classification scheme is the most widely accepted:
  - Type I: minimal displacement of the anterior eminence
  - Type II: elevation of the anterior third to half of the eminence with hinging on posterior eminence
  - Type IIIA: complete displacement and separation of fragment without rotational malalignment
  - Type IIIB: complete displacement and separation of fragment with rotational malalignment
- Types II and III are of equal incidence, are more common than type I, and more likely to be associated with concomitant knee injury (2,3)[B].
- Consideration for computed tomography (CT) or magnetic resonance imaging (MRI) to evaluate degree of displacement and surrounding injury may be important in clinical decision making (1)[C].
- With negative plain radiographs, nondisplaced fracture or ligament injury still must be suspected in patients with acute hemarthrosis. MRI should be obtained in these instances to further evaluate extent of injury.

TREATMENT

- Acute treatment
- Analgesia:
  - Nonsteroidal anti-inflammatory drugs (NSAIDs) are used initially for pain control.
  - Frequent application of ice for 20-min periods as tolerated by patient
- Aspiration of the joint may enhance comfort and allow further knee extension. Lack of full knee extension may imply a mechanical block (i.e., fracture fragment or meniscal entrapment).
- Immobilization:
  - Initial care includes complete knee immobilization with minimal knee flexion for 2 to 3 days until effusion begins to resolve.
  - Crutch ambulation is recommended in this initial stage.

ISSUES FOR REFERRAL

- All suspected ACL avulsion fractures should promptly be referred to an orthopedic surgeon.
- Tibial spine avulsions in patients with open growth plates would benefit from urgent consultation with a pediatric orthopedic specialist.

ADDITIONAL THERAPIES

- Type I fracture: After effusion resolves, type I fractures are best managed by long leg cast immobilization with knee flexed at ~0 to 20 degrees (degree of confirmed fragment reduction) for 6 wk (1)[C].
- Type II and III fractures:
  - Controversy exists regarding optimal treatment for fractures with greater degrees of displacement.
  - Type II tibial spine fractures can be managed by either closed reduction with the knee immobilized as in type I fractures or surgically with arthroscopy or open reduction and internal fixation (1)[C].
- Type III fractures generally require open or arthroscopic reduction with fragment fixation with either suture or metal fixation (1)[C].
- Special considerations:
  - The knee should be immobilized while awaiting surgical consultation.
- After completion of cast immobilization, focus should be on recovering knee ROM followed by strengthening of knee extensors.
- Aggressive rehabilitation and early achievement of ROM is predictive of successful functional outcomes (1)[C].
- Proprioception is another key part of the rehabilitation process.

SURGERY/OTHER PROCEDURES

- Arthroscopic or open reduction with internal fixation should be performed for displaced type II fractures if closed methods fail to obtain or maintain reduction of fracture fragment.
- Many authors prefer arthroscopic reduction owing to less surgical trauma and prompt initiation of the postoperative rehabilitation course.

ONGOING CARE

FOLLOW-UP RECOMMENDATIONS

- In the immediate postinjury or postoperative period, follow-up radiographs are necessary to evaluate for loss of fracture reduction.
- Radiographic demonstration of proper fracture union should be obtained before discontinuing knee immobilization and allowing knee mobilization.

PROGNOSIS

- Tibial spine fractures generally have an excellent prognosis, even when the fracture fragment is completely displaced.
- Despite true anatomic reduction, about 50% of pediatric patients may have mild objective, measurable ACL laxity owing to interstitial ligament damage that occurs before the avulsion. However, it generally does not result in functional instability.
- Fewer data on treatment outcome are available for skeletally mature patients, with one study reported symptomatic knee instability as the main complication of nonoperative treatment of tibial spine fractures (4)[C].

COMPLICATIONS

Although overall prognosis is remarkably good, some complications may include:

- Patients >18 yr old are more likely to experience loss of motion and joint stiffness due to arthrofibrosis than those <18 yr old.
- Meniscal entrapment may represent significant blocks to anatomic reduction resulting in nonunion (2).
- Some cases of residual ACL laxity require ACL reconstruction.
- Physeal arrest is a rare complication of surgical reduction (1)[C].

REFERENCES

1. Shin YW, Uppstrom TJ, Haskel JD, et al. The tibial eminence fracture in skeletally immature patients. *Curr Opin Pediatr*. 2015;27(1):50–57.
2. Rhodes JT, Cannamela PC, Cruz AI, et al. Incidence of meniscal entrapment and associated knee injuries in tibial spine avulsions. *J Pediatr Orthop*. 2018;38(2):e38–e42.
3. Mayo MH, Mitchell JJ, Axibal DP, et al. Anterior cruciate ligament injury at the time of anterior tibial spine fracture in young patients: an observational cohort study [published online ahead of print May 17, 2017]. *J Pediatr Orthop*. doi:10.1097/BPO.0000000000001011.
4. Aderinto J, Walmsley P, Keating JF. Fractures of the tibial spine: epidemiology and outcome. *Knee*. 2008;15(3):164–167.

ADDITIONAL READING

Accousti WK, Willis RB. Tibial eminence fractures. *Orthop Clin North Am*. 2003;34(3):365–375.

CLINICAL PEARLS

- History of either hyperextension or rotational stress to the knee (e.g., landing single legged from a jump)
- Similar mechanism of injury for a midsubstance ACL injury
- Thus, in any case of a suspected ACL injury, obtain urgent radiographs at the first evaluation to look for a potential tibial spine avulsion fracture. Images should include AP, tunnel, and lateral (most helpful to assess fracture position and degree of displacement) views.
- Initial care includes complete knee immobilization with minimal knee flexion for 2 to 3 days until effusion begins to resolve.
- All suspected ACL avulsion fractures should be urgently referred to an orthopedic surgeon.
- Tibial spine fractures generally have an excellent prognosis, even when the fracture fragment is completely displaced.

FRACTURE, VOLKMANN (POSTEROLATERAL MALLEOLUS)

Holly J. Benjamin, MD, FAAP, FACSM • David J. Pohl, DO

BASICS

Pediatric Considerations

- Volkmann fracture is a rare injury in children <14 yr of age, given the relative weak physis of the tibia.
- Salter-Harris fractures occur during external rotation and abduction injuries, which only occasionally involve the posterior tubercle. The fracture fragment usually is contiguous with the medial malleolar fragment.

DESCRIPTION

- Ankle fracture involving avulsion of the posterior lip of the tibia at its articular surface (Volkmann tubercle or posterior malleolus)
- The name is confusing because there is also a Volkmann contracture, which is a flexion contracture of the upper extremity.
- Fracture occurs via a force through the posterior inferior tibiofibular ligament (PITFL) at its tibial attachment.
- The Lauge-Hansen (L-H), Danis-Weber, and Orthopaedic Trauma Association/Arbeitsgemeinschaft für Osteosynthesefragen systems have been used to describe ankle injury patterns. The L-H system can aid in closed reduction maneuvers.
- Volkmann fracture is classified by the L-H system as supination external rotation (SER) stage III, pronation external rotation (PER) stage IV, or pronation abduction (PA) stage II.
- In SER injuries, anterior inferior tibiofibular ligament (AITFL) rupture and spiral/oblique fracture of the fibula precede Volkmann fracture.
- In PER injuries, deltoid ligament rupture, medial malleolar fracture, AITFL disruption, and spiral/oblique fibular fracture precede Volkmann fracture.
- In PA injuries, deltoid ligament rupture or avulsion of the medial malleolus occurs first.

EPIDEMIOLOGY

- The prevalence of isolated posterior malleolar fracture is low, accounting for 1–4% of all ankle fractures.
- Volkmann fracture more commonly occurs concurrently with other malleolar fractures, spiral fibular fractures, and deltoid ligament and syndesmotic membrane injuries.
- Posterior malleolus fractures occur in up to 44% of all ankle fractures (1)[C].
- Fracture usually involved a significant portion of the articular surface or fibular displacement.

ETIOLOGY AND PATHOPHYSIOLOGY

- Volkmann tubercle or triangle is part of the posterior aspect of the distal tibia and is commonly referred to as the posterior malleolus.
- The posterior malleolus extends from the fibular notch of the tibia to the medial malleolus.
- The PITFL's attachment to the posterior malleolus resists posterior translation of the talus.
- The PITFL is also referred to as the posterior tibiofibular ligament and is one of four syndesmotic ligaments that maintain integrity between the tibia and fibula.
- The PITFL provides >40% of ankle syndesmotic stability (1)[B].
- Given that the PITFL is markedly stronger than the AITFL, the torsional/rotational forces rupture the AITFL but avulse the posterior tibial tubercle through an intact PITFL.

DIAGNOSIS

HISTORY

- Ankle injury involving a Volkmann fracture is rarely subtle, given typical concomitant fractures and ligament tears.
- A mechanism of injury involving a significant external rotation or abduction force and the presence of associated injuries should evoke suspicion.
- Any floor or field sport, particularly contact sports, can result in a posterior malleolar fracture.
- Patients should be questioned for specific injury mechanism, associated sounds such as "pops" or "cracks," and weight-bearing ability.

PHYSICAL EXAM

- Emergent examination:
  - Should focus on neurovascular compromise secondary to joint dislocation or leg compartment syndrome and skin integrity
  - Doppler ultrasound (US) should be used if pulses are nonpalpable, and a detailed sensorimotor examination of the foot should be done.
  - Concern for early compartment syndrome should prompt measurement of leg compartment pressures.
- Nonemergent examination:
  - Systematic ankle, foot, leg, and knee examination should be performed, including soft tissues and neurovascular assessment.
  - Observation, palpation, and careful range of motion should be done, followed by stability testing.
  - Acute examination will reveal a painful, tender, and swollen ankle with limited or inability to bear weight consistent with a moderate or severe injury.
  - Possible findings include an increased posterior drawer test, increased internal rotation, and, with associated syndesmotic instability, a positive squeeze and external rotation tests.

DIAGNOSTIC TESTS & INTERPRETATION

- Radiographs: anteroposterior, lateral, and mortise views are standard (1)[C]. Weight-bearing films unless otherwise contraindicated or too painful; typically, that may help to show any tibiofibular diastasis if there is syndesmotic disruption.
- Lateral films generally show the posterior malleolar fracture but do not reliably estimate the size of the avulsion or the articular surface involvement (2)[B].
- Some authors recommend an external rotation lateral view (45 to 50 degrees) to estimate fragment size (3)[C].
- Standard views will help diagnose associated injuries that are almost always present.
- Stress radiographs are controversial and not routinely indicated.
- If Volkmann fracture is seen on plain film evaluation, computed tomography (CT) is recommended to elucidate the extent of articular involvement, size of the fragment, and integrity of the anterior tibiofibular joint and syndesmosis, which are often used in determining treatment (1)[C].
- Magnetic resonance imaging (MRI) is used for evaluation of soft tissues, including the syndesmosis, but is generally not indicated unless CT films are inadequate for detailing the injury characteristics. Both CT and MRI can help with surgical decisions.

TREATMENT

GENERAL MEASURES

- Closed reduction is generally not indicated prior to definitive treatment, unless the neurovascular structures or skin are compromised.
- If compromised, reduction of dislocation or deformity should be accomplished immediately by closed reduction using the L-H classification to reverse the order of injury or, if on the field, carefully attempt to restore anatomic alignment.
- Isolated, nondisplaced fractures can be considered for conservative treatment in a short-leg walking cast (1)[C],(4)[A].
- Use of a modified Jones compression dressing and posterior splint is important to reduce swelling. Severe or untreated swelling is associated with a poor surgical outcome.
- Compression dressing with frequent icing and elevation can allow for operative intervention in the first 2 to 3 days.

SURGERY/OTHER PROCEDURES

- Indications for surgical fixation are debated and varied.
- Most prominent indications are >25% of articular surface involvement, fragment displacement >2 mm, or joint instability (5)[C].
- If factors such as displacement of malleoli, talar subluxation, plafond articular incongruity, or syndesmotic instability exist, internal fixation is recommended.
- Surgical fixation of the posterior malleolus can restore up to 70% of syndesmotic stability compared to 40% from syndesmotic screw fixation without fracture fragment reduction (1)[B].
- Operative approaches, methods of fixation, and recovery times are similarly varied based on fracture characteristics and associated injuries.

ONGOING CARE

PROGNOSIS

- Posterior tubercle fractures adversely affect the prognosis of ankle fractures compared to single or bimalleolar fractures (1)[C],(4)[A],(6)[B].
- Although often used as an indication for surgery, the size of the posterior malleolar fragment is not strongly correlated to outcomes (4)[A].
- Factors such as fracture displacement, congruency of the articular surface, and residual tibiotalar subluxation are related to outcomes (4)[A].
- Overall incidence of posttraumatic osteoarthritis, including surgical and nonoperative management, is 33% (4)[A].

REFERENCES

1. Irwin TA, Lien J, Kadakia AR. Posterior malleolus fracture. *J Am Acad Orthop Surg*. 2013;21(1):32–40.
2. Haraguchi N, Haruyama H, Toga H, et al. Pathoanatomy of posterior malleolar fractures of the ankle. *J Bone Joint Surg Am*. 2006;88(5):1085–1092.
3. Ebraheim NA, Mekhail AO, Haman SP. External rotation-lateral view of the ankle in the assessment of the posterior malleolus. *Foot Ankle Int*. 1999;20(6):379–383.
4. Odak S, Ahluwalia R, Unnikrishnan P, et al. Management of posterior malleolar fractures: a systematic review. *J Foot Ankle Surg*. 2016;55(1):140–145.
5. Bartoníček J, Rammelt S, Tuček M, et al. Posterior malleolar fractures of the ankle. *Eur J Trauma Emerg Surg*. 2015;41(6):587–600.
6. Fitzpatrick DC, Otto JK, McKinley TO, et al. Kinematic and contact stress analysis of posterior malleolus fractures of the ankle. *J Orthop Trauma*. 2004;18(5):271–278.

ADDITIONAL READING

- Clare MP. A rational approach to ankle fractures. *Foot Ankle Clin*. 2008;13(4):593–610.
- Donken CC, Goorden AJ, Verhofstad MH, et al. The outcome at 20 years of conservatively treated 'isolated' posterior malleolar fractures of the ankle: a case series. *J Bone Joint Surg Br*. 2011;93(12):1621–1625.
- Mandracchia DM, Mandracchia VJ, Buddecke DE Jr. Malleolar fractures of the ankle. A comprehensive review. *Clin Podiatr Med Surg*. 1999;16(4):679–723.
- Stanitski CL. Pediatric and adolescent sports injuries. *Clin Sports Med*. 1997;16(4):613–633.
- van den Bekerom MP, Haverkamp D, Kloen P. Biomechanical and clinical evaluation of posterior malleolar fractures. A systematic review of the literature. *J Trauma*. 2009;66(1):279–284.
- Vander Griend RA, Michelson JD, Bone LB. Fractures of the ankle and the distal part of the tibia. *Instr Course Lect*. 1997;46:311–321.
- Vander Griend RA, Savoie FH, Hughes JL. Fractures of the ankle. In: Rockwood CA Jr, Green DP, Bucholz RW, eds. *Rockwood and Green's Fractures in Adults*. Vol 2. 3rd ed. Philadelphia, PA: JB Lippincott; 1991:1983–2039.

CLINICAL PEARLS

- Volkmann fractures are avulsion fractures of the posterior lip of the tibia at its articular surface via a significant external rotation or abduction force through the PITFL.
- Lateral ankle radiographs generally show the posterior malleolar fracture best and when found should prompt CT evaluation to assess the extent of articular involvement, size of the fragment, and integrity of the anterior tibiofibular joint.
- Indications for surgical fixation are debated, but most prominent indications are >25% of articular surface involvement, fragment displacement >2 mm, or joint instability.
- Because the PITFL accounts for 40% of syndesmotic stability, significant (>2 mm) displacement of the Volkmann fragment causes some syndesmotic instability and should prompt surgical evaluation and fixation. This is also why only isolated, nondisplaced posterior malleolus fractures should be considered for nonoperative management.

FRACTURE, ZYGOMA (ZF)

Tarek S. Hadla, MD, CAQSM • Holly J. Benjamin, MD, FAAP, FACSM

BASICS

- Zygoma: main support between the maxilla and the skull (1)
- Composes the lateral wall and floor of the orbit as well as the zygomatic arch
- Zygoma fracture (ZF) results from blunt trauma to the *side of the face*: fist, object, accident, and so forth (2).

EPIDEMIOLOGY

- In United States, second most common fracture of the face after nasal bone fractures
- Outside United States, most common maxillofacial trauma
- Males > females, 20s and 30s mainly (3)
- Accidental falls more in older patients (3)
- Professionals > amateurs

ETIOLOGY AND PATHOPHYSIOLOGY

- Any blow to the cheek potentially causes a ZF.
- Most common causes are:
  - Motor vehicle collisions.
  - Falls.
  - Physical assault.
  - Sports:
    - Combat sports (boxing, taekwondo, kickboxing, and Muay Thai) (4)
    - Kickboxing caused the most maxillofacial injuries (4).
    - Skiing, soccer, biking, and rugby has also shown to have high traumatic injury rates, including facial fractures (4).
    - Blunt-force trauma from athletic equipment, including ball(s)
- Known as "cheek bone" or "malar bone"
- Found on anterior-lateral aspect of the face
- Posteriorly is the "zygomatic arch"—part of the temporal bone.
- Zygomatic bone and arch contain:
  - Zygomaticofacial and zygomaticotemporal arteries.
  - Second division of the trigeminal nerve providing sensation to check and anterior temple
  - Infraorbital nerve.
  - Muscle attachments: the masseter, the zygomaticus major, and temporalis fascia.
  - The Whitnall tubercle: maintains the eyelid contour (2).
- The *direction* and *magnitude* of force are important factors:
  - A side blow directed posteriorly and medially causes a zygomatic body (tripod) fracture.
  - A lateral blow often results in an isolated zygomatic arch fracture.

Pediatric Considerations

- Facial trauma is rarely seen in the pediatric population.
- Children have a relatively larger cranium to facial skeleton, thus higher incidence of head trauma.
- Falls and motor vehicle accidents account for the majority of facial trauma in children.
- Consider *abuse* in nonaccidental trauma, particularly in children under age 6 yr.

GENERAL PREVENTION

- Appropriate use of athletic helmet/face shield
- Safety apparel and protective guards during combat sports if facial injury is to be prevented (4)
- Seatbelts and improvements in safety mechanisms such as airbags (5)
- Public/athletes education

DIAGNOSIS

HISTORY

- Trauma: accident, physical assault, sports (see above)
- Vision issues:
  - Direct ocular injury or intraorbital hemorrhage
  - Binocular diplopia: 30%
- Paresthesia of face in equivalent dermatome
- Periorbital edema
- Trismus—difficulty with mastication
- Flattening of the cheek
- Ipsilateral epistaxis could occur as a result of lacerated maxillary sinus mucosa (6).

PHYSICAL EXAM

- Evaluation for associated injuries (cervical spine, head, globe, other maxillofacial bones, etc.)
- Pain with palpation: 70% of patients
- Ophthalmic evaluation:
  - Proptosis
  - Periorbital edema
  - Subconjunctival ecchymosis
  - Enophthalmos—sunken eyes
  - Diplopia
  - Scleral show
- Crepitus from subcutaneous emphysema
- Proptosis and visual loss may occur with forceful nose blowing due to emphysema.
- Paresthesias: in distribution of infraorbital, zygomaticofacial, or zygomaticotemporal nerves
- Associated skull base fractures: Watch out for rhinorrhea or otorrhea (7).
- Paranasal sinus fractures
- Limited ocular mobility
- Trismus
- Flattened cheekbone: depression of malar eminence
- "Step off" palpable defect along the infraorbital
- "Scleral flame": result of the tendon of the lateral canthal being depressed and disrupted
- Evaluate for other globe injuries.

Pediatric Considerations

- Consider child abuse if <6 yr and nontraumatic cause.
- Sedation may be required to properly examine some children.
- If a head injury is suspected, sedation is not recommended.

DIFFERENTIAL DIAGNOSIS

- Other maxillary facial bone fractures and injuries
- Enophthalmos
- Floor orbital fracture
- Globe retraction
- Medial wall orbital fracture
- Facial contusions
- "Le Fort" fractures: transfacial fracture of the midface
- Classification:
  - Several classifications but none universally accepted
  - Based on the degree of comminution, whether simple or compound, and the site of the fractures
  - In 75% of cases, these fractures are displaced inferiorly, medially, and posteriorly.

DIAGNOSTIC TEST & INTERPRETATION

- *X-ray*: first line (8); radiographic facial series consists of four views:
  - Waters (occipitomental projection): single most useful
  - Caldwell (occipitofrontal projection)
  - Lateral
  - Submentovertex
- *Computed tomography (CT) scan*: imaging modality of choice
- *Ultrasonography*: could be useful as a screening

TREATMENT

- Airway, breathing, circulation (ABCs)
- 10–50% require no surgical intervention (5).
- Stable, nondisplaced fractures may be observed weekly for healing.
- Treat within 10 days if displaced fractures.
- Avoidance of nose blowing is *mandatory* because air can be forced between the disrupted orbital walls into the retrobulbar space causing pain and permanent visual loss.
- Goal is restoration of:
  - Normal facial contour.
  - Normal sensory nerve function.
  - Normal globe position.
  - Normal masticatory function.
- Indications for surgical repair include:
  - Displacement or instability of the fracture.
  - Mechanical restriction of mandibular movement (chewing).
  - Alteration in facial contour.
  - Globe dystopia.
  - Enophthalmos.
  - Diplopia.
  - Sensory nerve deficit.

Pediatric Considerations

- Multiple injuries are often seen: head trauma, skull fracture, and orthopedic injuries.
- Definitive repair of facial fractures should not be delayed beyond 3 or 4 days.
- Facial bones heal rapidly in children.
- Delays >3 to 4 days can lead to malunion and cosmetic defect.
- Consult social services and local child welfare agency if needed.

MEDICATION

- The treatment of zygomatic complex fractures is primarily surgical.
- Supportive treatment may include analgesics and nasal decongestants.
- The routine use of systemic antibiotics is not recommended.
- The efficacy and safety of perioperative intravenous corticosteroids are inconclusive.

ONGOING CARE

PATIENT EDUCATION

- Avoid nose blowing for fear of orbital emphysema and potential blindness.
- Warn about signs and symptoms of orbital/retrobulbar hemorrhage.
- Advise patients to call the surgeon at any time if orbital bleeding is suspected.

PROGNOSIS

Favorable outcome includes:

- Early intervention especially in children.
- Bony union.
- Absence of skeletal or soft tissue deformity.
- Normal range of mandibular movement.

COMPLICATIONS

- Associated ophthalmic or intracranial trauma
- Ectropion
- Epiphora
- Cosmetic deformities
- Hypoesthesia of face
- Postoperative orbital hemorrhage: rare but may lead to permanent blindness

REFERENCES

1. Gruss JS, Van Wyck L, Phillips JH, et al. The importance of the zygomatic arch in complex midfacial fracture repair and correction of posttraumatic orbitozygomatic deformities. *Plast Reconstr Surg.* 1990;85(6):878–890.
2. Song WC, Choi HG, Kim SH, et al. Topographic anatomy of the zygomatic arch and temporal fossa: a cadaveric study. *J Plast Reconstr Aesthet Surg.* 2008;62(11):1375–1378.
3. Motamedi MH. An assessment of maxillofacial fractures: a 5-year study of 237 patients. *J Oral Maxillofac Surg.* 2003;61(1):61–64.
4. Shirani G, Kalantar Motamedi MH, Ashuri A, et al. Prevalence and patterns of combat sport related maxillofacial injuries. *J Emerg Trauma Shock.* 2010;3(4):314–317.
5. Salentijn EG, Boffano P, Boverhoff J, et al. The epidemiological characteristics of zygomatic complex fractures: a comparison between the surgically and non-surgically treated patients. *Natl J Maxillofac Surg.* 2013;4(2):214–218.
6. Barry C, Coyle M, Idrees Z, et al. Ocular findings in patients with orbitozygomatic complex fractures: a retrospective study. *J Oral Maxillofac Surg.* 2008;66(5):888–892.
7. Hasheminia D, Kalantar Motamedi MR, Hashemzehi H, et al. A 7-year study of 1,278 patients with maxillofacial trauma and cerebrospinal fluid leak. *J Maxillofac Oral Surg.* 2015;14(2):258–262.
8. Druelinger L, Guenther M, Marchand EG. Radiographic evaluation of the facial complex. *Emerg Med Clin North Am.* 2000;18(3):393–410.

CLINICAL PEARLS

- Suspect a ZF if blow to side of the face.
- Consider coexisting ocular, head, and cervical spine injury.
- X-ray is used first, but CT is the modality of choice.
- Tell the patient not to blow their nose for 10 days.
- Close follow-up within 10 to 14 days
- Consider child abuse if <6 yr and no traumatic cause.
- Consult surgery if unstable ZF, worsening symptoms or simply if in doubt.

FREIBERG DISEASE

Christopher McGrew, MD, FACSM, CAQSM • Margaret Pusateri, MD

BASICS

DESCRIPTION

- Osteonecrosis of the superior portion of the metatarsal head of unknown etiology
- Freiberg first described this entity in 1914, in six patients as an infraction (incomplete fracture without displacement of the fragments).
- Fourth most common osteochondrosis
- Affects women more commonly than men
- Synonym(s): Freiberg infraction; eggshell fracture; Koehler second disease; metatarsal flat-head; metatarsal epiphysitis; osteochondritis deformans metatarsojuvenilis; peculiar metatarsal disease; malakopathie

EPIDEMIOLOGY

- Incidence unknown
- Male:female ratio is 1:5.
- Peak onset around 11 to 17 yr, but reported age range of 10 to 77 yr
- Has been hypothesized that the condition is progressive, beginning in adolescence and remaining asymptomatic until later in life when symptoms occurs secondary to joint arthrosis
- Most common involvement is the 2nd metatarsal head, approximately 2/3 of cases
- Second most common involvement is the 3rd metatarsal head, involved in 27% of cases
- 4th and 5th metatarsal heads rarely involved
- Bilateral involvement is seen in <10% of cases.
- Usually affects the longest metatarsal
- Occasionally seen in sports requiring sprinting and jumping

ETIOLOGY AND PATHOPHYSIOLOGY

- No single clear etiologic factor exists.
- Several theories have been postulated:
  - Traumatic factors include metatarsal stress during normal activity and/or abnormal biomechanics of the forefoot intrinsically or as a result of footwear, causing repetitive microtrauma on the dorsal aspect of the distal metatarsal head.
  - Vascular factors include abnormal metatarsal head vascular variations as well as trauma-induced vessel damage, spasm, and eventual ischemia.
  - Mechanical factors include immobility of the 2nd metatarsal due to its "keystone" position at its articulation with the midfoot, a longer 2nd metatarsal, a short 1st metatarsal, a hypermobile 1st metatarsal, hallux abducto valgus, use of high-heeled shoes, and rapid weight gain.
  - Systemic factors are thought to be possible contributors including infection, endocrine disturbance, hormonal changes, osteopenia, steroid use, inflammatory diseases such as systemic lupus erythematous, and hypercoagulable states.

Genetics

Unknown

RISK FACTORS

- No known risk factors
- May be related to repetitive microtrauma versus vascular deficiency or both

GENERAL PREVENTION

None

COMMONLY ASSOCIATED CONDITIONS

None known

DIAGNOSIS

HISTORY

- Slow development of significant, dull, aching pain over affected metatarsal head
- Patient may notice loss of range of motion.
- Pain increases with activity and motion.
- Pain worsens with weight bearing, especially barefoot or in high-heeled footwear.
- Pain often relieved by rest, but pain may awaken patient from sleep

PHYSICAL EXAM

- Surrounding soft tissue swelling
- Tenderness over affected metatarsal head
- May be painful with motion
- May be limited motion of metatarsophalangeal (MTP) joint
- Palpable bony prominences and crepitus possible in advanced disease
- Other foot deformities may be present such as hallux valgus.

DIFFERENTIAL DIAGNOSIS

- Fracture: acute or stress
- Tendonitis
- Capsulitis
- Septic joint
- Neuroma
- Gout
- Metatarsalgia

DIAGNOSTIC TESTS & INTERPRETATION

ALERT

Radiography normal in early stages:

- Asymmetric joint space widening may be seen 3 to 6 wk following symptom onset, differentiating it from other arthritides whose characteristic finding involves joint space narrowing.
- As the disease progresses, osteonecrotic changes are seen on the superior/central head.
- Eventually, the superior/central head collapses and flattens.
- Medial and lateral dorsal osteophytes develop.
- Osteophytes may break free, becoming loose bodies, best seen on lateral oblique radiographs.
- Cystic changes may be seen in the head.
- The inferior portion of the metatarsal head is usually not involved.
- Radiographic staging of disease, based on correlation with Smillie classification:
  - Stage I: MTP joint space widening, with increased subchondral bone density
  - Stage II: metatarsal head flattening (anteroposterior view)
  - Stage III: collapse of the central portion of the dorsal part of the distal metatarsal head

- Stage IV: medial and lateral fractures of the projections of the remaining metatarsal head (multiple loose bodies in the joint)
- Stage V: complete loss of joint anatomy and integrity

- Three-phase bone scan in the early stages will reveal a photopenic area surrounded by a focal uptake. Later stages show generalized increased uptake of the entire affected metatarsal head (1)[C].
- Magnetic resonance imaging (MRI) has been purported to be the gold standard in early diagnosis of Freiberg as radiographs are often normal in the early stages (2)[C].
- Early stages of Freiberg will have a hypointense signal on T1-weighted images and heterogeneous increased on T2-weighted images.
- In addition to MRI, 3D computed tomography (CT) scans have also been used to determine the exact Smillie stage and aid in preoperative planning.

TREATMENT

GENERAL MEASURES

- Nonoperative management should be the first line of treatment regardless of stage at time of presentation.

ALERT
Goal is to restrict weight-bearing for a sufficient time to allow healing to take place.

- Immediate cessation of sports and high-impact activities
- Use of crutches to restrict weight-bearing may be indicated in early stages when most painful.
- As symptoms subside, may progressively bear weight with use of metatarsal pads, bars, and/or a custom orthosis
- Occasionally may need a walking boot or short-leg walking cast with a toe plate
- By restricting weight-bearing, the lesion may heal over a period of 6 to 12 wk.
- Return to sports when asymptomatic with custom foot orthosis.
- Operative treatment indicated if nonoperative treatment fails or if disease is advanced
- Smillie stages I to III have a good chance of success with nonoperative, conservative management.
- Smillie stages IV to V are more likely to require operative management.
- There is a wide range of surgical procedures described in the literature for management of Freiberg.
- Joint-preserving procedures are typically performed in the early stages of disease, whereas joint-destructive procedures are reserved for advanced stages.

MEDICATION

Symptomatic treatment with acetaminophen or nonsteroidal anti-inflammatory drugs (NSAIDs) as indicated (3)[C]

ISSUES FOR REFERRAL

Orthopedic surgery or podiatry referral indicated if nonoperative treatment fails or if disease is advanced

SURGERY/OTHER PROCEDURES

- Surgery is reserved for those patients who fail conservative therapies or those with late stage and demonstrated degenerative joint progression.
- Examples of joint-sparing procedures include core decompression, bone grafting, metatarsal osteotomies, joint débridement, and microfracture surgery.
- Examples of joint-destructive procedures include arthroplasty, implant arthroplasty, interpositional arthroplasty, metatarsal head resection, and osteochondral distal metatarsal allograft replacement.

COMPLEMENTARY & ALTERNATIVE MEDICINE

None

ONGOING CARE

FOLLOW-UP RECOMMENDATIONS

No standard return to participation protocol has been established. Protocol should be individualized and based on radiographic confirmation of healing as well as symptom resolution.

PATIENT EDUCATION

Patient education should focus on the need for activity modification and a functional symptom-based rehabilitation program.

PROGNOSIS

- For most nondegenerative lesions, conservative therapy is likely to lead to healing and resolution of symptoms.
- Current surgical procedures are demonstrating satisfactory results but continue to be an investigative topic.

COMPLICATIONS

Joint degeneration or destruction with resultant chronic pain and/or loss of function

REFERENCES

1. Talusan PG, Diaz-Collado PJ, Reach JS Jr. Freiberg's infraction: diagnosis and treatment. *Foot Ankle Spec*. 2014;7(1):52–56.
2. Schade VL. Surgical management of Freiberg's infraction: a systematic review. *Foot Ankle Spec*. 2015;8(6):498–519.
3. Seybold JD, Zide JR. Treatment of Freiberg disease. *Foot Ankle Clin*. 2018;23(1):157–169.

ADDITIONAL READING

- Ishimatsu T, Yoshimura I, Kanazawa K, et al. Return to sporting activity after osteochondral autograft transplantation for Freiberg disease in young athletes. *Arch Orthop Trauma Surg*. 2017;137(7):959–965.
- Pereira B, Frada T, Freitas D, et al. Long-term follow-up of dorsal wedge osteotomy for pediatric Freiberg disease. *Foot Ankle Int*. 2016;37(1):90–95.
- Shane A, Reeves C, Wobst G, et al. Second metatarsophalangeal joint pathology and Freiberg disease. *Clin Podiatr Med Surg*. 2013;30(3):313–325.

CLINICAL PEARLS

Typical presentation is an adolescent female in a growth spurt who presents with forefoot pain with walking or activity.

GANGLION CYST

Jean Pierre Valette, MD • David E.J. Bazzo, MD, FAAFP, CAQSM

BASICS

DESCRIPTION

- Benign fluid-filled cysts overlying a joint or tendon sheath that contains a mucinous, gelatinous fluid
- Unlike synovial cysts, ganglion cysts do not have a layer of synovium in their capsule.
- Previously known as "bible cysts" as an early form of treatment was closed rupture of the cyst by hitting them with a large book such as the bible (1)
- Most commonly arise in the wrist and hand but can occur less commonly at other joints such as the knee and foot or arise from tendon sheaths, again most commonly in the hand.
- Sites:
  - 60–70% are found on dorsum of the wrist.
  - 13–20% are found on volar aspect of the wrist.
  - 10% are found arising from the tendon sheath of the hand.
  - 10% are found elsewhere.
- Ganglion cysts arising from the distal interphalangeal (DIP) joints of the fingers are also called mucous cysts and are associated with Heberden nodules. They are most commonly found in women ages 40 to 70 yr with osteoarthritis.

EPIDEMIOLOGY

- Most common soft tissue mass found within the hand or wrist (accounts for 60–70% total) (2)
- Usually arises between 2nd and 5th decades of life
- Female > male predominance with reported ratio ranging from 2:1 to 3:1

ETIOLOGY AND PATHOPHYSIOLOGY

- Unproven as yet, although thought to occur from mucoid degeneration of periarticular structures from repetitive microtrauma
- A one-way valve mechanism has been postulated based on studies where contrast injected into the communicating joint traveled into the ganglion cyst and contrast injected into cysts did not travel back into the communicating joint.
- Ganglion cysts are often attached to joint capsules or tendon sheaths via a pedicle with a small tortuous lumen.
- The theory that ganglion cysts are simply herniations from joint capsules or tendon sheaths, however, is not supported by the fact that ganglion cysts do not have a synovial lining.

RISK FACTORS

Sports with repetitive microtrauma and strain of the hands and wrists such as gymnastics

DIAGNOSIS

HISTORY

- Typically presents with a painless cyst over a joint or tendon sheath in a typical location
- If compression of local structures such as nerves or arteries is occurring can present with pain, numbness, or rarely weakness
- If pain is present, most patients rate it as mild and report that it is bothersome rather than debilitating
- Patients often report concern about the cosmetic appearance or concern that it is a malignant tumor.
- Ganglion cysts can enlarge over time or remain stable in size.

PHYSICAL EXAM

- Firm, smooth, well-circumscribed mass usually 1 to 2 cm in size
- Typically fixed to deeper structures as opposed to the skin
- Ganglion cysts associated with joints can be made more prominent with flexion of the joint away from cyst.
- Readily transilluminates
- No warmth or erythema

DIFFERENTIAL DIAGNOSIS

- Epidermal inclusion cyst
- Lipoma
- Rheumatoid nodule
- Tophus
- Infectious tenosynovitis
- Tenosynovial giant cell tumor
- Synovial sarcoma

DIAGNOSTIC TESTS & INTERPRETATION

- Diagnosis is clinical and imaging is not typically necessary.
- Radiographs are generally unremarkable but can be used to rule out any underlying related osseous abnormality.
- Ganglion cyst appearance on magnetic resonance imaging (MRI): well-circumscribed mass with uniform fluid intensity on T2-weighted imaging (2)
- Ganglion cyst appearance on ultrasound:
  - Partitioned, anechoic structure with nonvascularized walls on Doppler (3)
  - Communication with joint capsule via small pinhole can sometimes be visualized with ultrasound.
  - Ultrasound can also be used during aspiration to assist in avoiding nearby structures.

TREATMENT

GENERAL MEASURES

- Reassure patient on benign nature of cyst as many will have concern of malignancy.
- Explain that spontaneous resolution of untreated ganglion cysts ranges from 40% to 58% (4) and that often will correlate with the volume of activity (resolve with decreased repetitive activity).

MEDICATION

No medications have shown any efficacy in treating ganglion cysts.

SURGERY/OTHER PROCEDURES

- Aspiration:
  - Aspiration should be performed with a larger bore needle as the mucinous contents are thick and may not easily be aspirated through a small gauge needle.
  - Local anesthetic infiltration should be used at designated aspiration site prior to large gauge needle insertion.
  - Aspiration of ganglion cysts will cause resolution in the short term, however recurrence rate is high ranging from 39% to 69% (4).
  - Multiple punctures of ganglion cysts during aspiration has not been shown to reduce recurrence rate (5).
  - Complications other than recurrence from aspiration include infection and damage to nearby structures (most commonly median nerve and radial artery injury for volar wrist ganglion cysts).
  - Ultrasound-guided aspiration can be used to reduce but not eliminate the risk of damaging nearby structures.
- Injection:
  - There are many of studies investigating effectiveness of subsequently injecting ganglion cysts after aspiration with multiple different substances such as alcohol, antibiotics, hypertonic saline, anesthetic agents, phenol, corticosteroids, hyaluronidase, sodium tetradecyl sulfate, but none of them show improved outcomes, and many had higher risks of complications (6).
- Thread technique:
  - Threading of a ganglion cyst with suture at right angles whose ends are tied together then subsequently massaging the area at different intervals has been tried as an alternative treatment method (7).
  - Although the original study using this technique reported a recurrence rate of 4.8%, there was a high rate of infection.
  - Additionally, subsequent studies found a recurrence rate approaching 50% which is similar to conservative treatment.
- Surgery:
  - Surgical removal of ganglion cysts has the lowest rate of recurrence but has slightly higher complication risk than aspiration.
  - Technique developed by Angelides and Wallace is considered the gold standard and involves removing the entire cyst, it's stalk and pedicle, any attachments to nearby structures or joints as well as a small segment of an associated joint capsule.
  - Recurrence rates using the Angelides and Wallace technique range from 1% to 31% (4).
  - Arthroscopic approach is preferred over open excision as it has a lower rate of complication 0–28% versus 0–8.5% (4).
  - Complications from surgery include wound infection, neuroma formation, scar, keloid, and damage to nearby structures such as median nerve or radial artery for volar ganglion cysts.
  - Complication rates for volar wrist ganglion cysts are higher than dorsal wrist ganglion cysts because of the proximity of the median nerve and radial artery.

REFERENCES

1. Meena S, Gupta A. Dorsal wrist ganglion: current review of literature. *J Clin Orthop Trauma*. 2014;5(2):59–64.
2. Gregush RE, Habusta SF. *Cyst, Ganglion*. Treasure Island, FL: StatPearls; 2018. https://www.ncbi.nlm.nih.gov/books/NBK470168/. Accessed September 22, 2018.
3. Vuillemin V, Guerini H, Morvan G. Musculoskeletal interventional ultrasonography: the upper limb. *Diagn Interv Imaging*. 2012;93(9):665–673.
4. Suen M, Fung B, Lung CP. Treatment of ganglion cysts. *ISRN Orthop*. 2013;2013:940615.
5. Stephen AB, Lyons AR, Davis TR. A prospective study of two conservative treatments for ganglia of the wrist. *J Hand Surg Br*. 1999;24(1):104–105.
6. Kuliński S, Gutkowaska O, Gosk J. Chemical substances used in the treatment of ganglions located in the hand and wrist. *Polim Med*. 2016;46(1):95–100.
7. Gang RK, Makhlouf S. Treatment of ganglia by a thread technique. *J Hand Surg Br*. 1988;13(2):184–186.

CLINICAL PEARLS

- Ganglion cysts are benign fluid-filled cysts overlying a joint or tendon sheath, most commonly the wrist or hand that contain a mucinous, gelatinous fluid.
- Diagnosis is clinical and imaging is typically only needed to rule out other potentially concerning diagnoses.
- Spontaneous resolution of untreated ganglion cysts ranges from 40% to 58%.
- Aspiration of ganglion cysts will cause resolution in the short term; however, recurrence rate is high ranging from 39% to 69%.
- Surgical removal of ganglion cysts has the lowest rate of recurrence but has slightly higher complication risk than aspiration.

GLENOHUMERAL DISLOCATION, ANTERIOR

Kamel Azhar, MD, MAS • Johnnie Faircloth, MD, CAQSM

BASICS

DESCRIPTION

- Humeral head is displaced anteriorly beyond the glenoid fossa due to external rotation while arm is in abduction (1,2,3).
- Sometimes (less commonly) caused by direct contact to the posterior aspect of the shoulder (traumatic) (3,4)

EPIDEMIOLOGY

- Most commonly dislocated diarthrodial joint; 50% of all dislocations are of the shoulder with an incidence rate of 23.9 per 100,000 person-years(1,4,5).
- Bimodal incidence with peaks in the 2nd and 6th decades of life (1,2)
- 96% of glenohumeral dislocations are anterior (2,3,4).

RISK FACTORS

- History of previous dislocation (1,5)
- Generalized ligamentous laxity (5)
- Sports such as wrestling, football, rugby, skiing, and skateboarding

COMMONLY ASSOCIATED CONDITIONS

- Bankart lesions: detachment of inferior glenohumeral ligament-labral complex from anterior glenoid rim. Very common in younger patients; strongly associated with dislocation recurrence (1,2,3,5)
- Rotator cuff tears: Between 14% and 63% of anterior dislocations are associated with rotator cuff tears, often subscapularis, with increasing frequency in older individuals (1,2,3).
- Fractures: Humeral head and neck (significant displacement may be a contraindication to closed reduction), glenoid rim (bony Bankart), and greater tuberosity avulsions; seen especially with traumatic etiology (2,3,4,5)
- Hill-Sachs lesion: depression fracture of posterolateral humeral head. In patients <40 yr old, >50% of anterior dislocations are associated with this type of lesion (1,2,3,5).
- Neurologic injury: common complication with 10% suffering injury to the axillary nerve. Less frequently injured are the brachial plexus or musculocutaneous nerve (2,3). Most often these injuries recover spontaneously.
- Vascular injury: infrequent complication (1–2%), axillary artery most frequently injured in anterior dislocation, higher incidence in older individuals given the loss of arterial elasticity secondary to atherosclerosis (2,3)

DIAGNOSIS

HISTORY

- Often occurs after a fall on the outstretched arm or with reaching (making a tackle) and having arm forcibly abducted (1)[A]
- First time event versus recurrence (may affect ease of reduction and long-term treatment plan) (1)[A],(4)[C]
- Amount of trauma involved (traumatic vs. atraumatic) can give clues as to whether there is a component of ligamentous instability (3,4)[C].
- Duration shoulder has been dislocated (helps in decision concerning analgesia) (3)[C].

PHYSICAL EXAM

- Anterior fullness of the shoulder (1,2)[A],(3)[C]
- Forearm of affected arm often cradled with shoulder in an externally rotated, partially adducted position (2)[A],(3)[C]
- Perform distal neurovascular exam, both before and after reduction, to check for previously mentioned neurovascular injuries (2)[A],(3)[C].
- Check deltoid muscle strength and lateral shoulder sensation to assess axillary nerve function (former not always practical prior to reduction of dislocated shoulder) (3,4)[C].
- Check proximal and distal muscle function and (if no obvious deformity is present) range of motion (active and passive) before and after relocation (1)[A],(3,4)[C].
- No crepitus should be felt or heard during relocation.

Some special exam maneuvers such as a sulcus sign, load and shift, and apprehension test may not be appropriate to perform in the acute setting.

DIFFERENTIAL DIAGNOSIS

- Acute subluxation
- Acromioclavicular joint separation
- Fractures of humeral head, coracoid, acromion, proximal humerus, clavicle, rib (4)[C]
- Rotator cuff injury
- Posterior dislocation

DIAGNOSTIC TESTS & INTERPRETATION

- Acute traumatic shoulder dislocations are evaluated with a trauma series that includes an axillary view, a trans-scapular (Y) lateral view, and a true shoulder anterior-posterior view (1,2)[A],(3,4)[C].
- Standard anteroposterior: head of humerus displaced medially on glenoid; difficult to distinguish anterior from posterior dislocations (3)[C]
- True lateral (trans-scapular, Y) view: humeral head displaced toward coracoid process
- Axillary view: allows easier visualization of associated injuries but requires movement of an already uncomfortable patient. A velpeau view is an alternative if axillary view cannot be accomplished.
- West Point view (reverse axillary lateral) helps in showing bony Bankart lesions (1)[A].
- Stryker notch view (anteroposterior internal rotation of humerus) good to demonstrate Hill-Sachs deformity
- Computed tomography (CT) scan can be used to evaluate for glenoid and humeral head abnormalities.
- Magnetic resonance imaging (MRI) can evaluate for soft tissue injuries but can miss bony abnormalities. MRI arthrogram may further evaluate the surrounding ligaments (labrum ligamentous complex).
- There is a paucity of evidence which advanced imaging test (CT vs. MRI) to recommend.

TREATMENT

- Analgesia often not needed if reduction is performed immediately after dislocation (1,2)[A],(3,4)[C].
- Verbal coaching to relax the patient is helpful.
- Analgesic and benzodiazepine medications may be required, if reductions are not performed early, to relax spasm and ease relocation (1)[A],(4)[C].
- Some sources recommend local glenohumeral joint anesthesia using 10 to 20 mL of 1% lidocaine (2)[A],(4)[C].

ALERT

Intra-articular lidocaine has been shown to have similar relocation success rates versus intravenous (IV) analgesia and sedation, and a significant decrease in cost and length of stay in the emergency department, although patient satisfaction tends to be higher with the use of IV agents (2)[A],(3,4)[C].

- Reduction techniques:
  - Traction methods: Stimson (prone traction with weight applied to arm hanging down). Success rate: not reported; supine traction/countertraction (gentle traction at 45 degrees of abduction while countertraction applied with folded sheet under axilla); success rate: not reported
  - Leverage methods: Kocher (with patient supine, flex elbow to 90 degrees, adduction, externally rotate arm, and forward flexion of the shoulder); success rate: 81–100%
  - Axillary pressure by assistant's hand may help guide the humeral head over the glenoid.
  - Combination methods: Milch: Stabilize the humeral head, fully abduct the arm, apply traction,

and push humeral head over glenoid rim. Success rate: 70–100%; scapular manipulation: patient prone or seated with arm at 90 degrees of flexion with mild traction applied (10 to 15 lb), apply medially directed force to inferolateral border of scapula; may also do when patient is supine to assist with other techniques; success rate: 79–96%
  - Self-reduction techniques are also available and are highly successful if used early and for recurrent dislocations. Manual assist can also help. The best technique described is to have the patient lock hands in front of ipsilateral knee and relax backwards allowing gentle traction with the relaxation of shoulder muscles.
  - Experience, familiarity, and available resources (time and help) are important considerations when deciding which technique to use (3)[C].
- Postreduction:
  - Recheck neurovascular exam and rotator cuff; postreduction radiographs (3)[C]
  - Controversy exists as to best approach to post dislocation management, but many authors at this time would recommend immobilization in a sling for comfort about 1 wk, followed by range of motion exercises and then progression to strengthening exercises, with an emphasis placed on periscapular muscle strengthening. Shorter immobilization period decreases the risk of adhesive capsulitis in the older patient (age >30 yr) (1,2)[A].
  - Recent reports have suggested that immobilization in external rotation for 3 wk instead of traditional internal rotation may be associated with a lower rate of recurrence. In clinical practice, patients may find it difficult to function with their arm immobilized in external rotation (1,2)[A].
  - Immobilization theoretically allows time for "scarring" of injured anterior structures and healing of pathologic lesions (3)[C].
  - Contraindications to closed reduction:
    - Humeral head and neck fractures
    - Significantly displaced (<1 cm) greater tuberosity fractures
    - Severe scapula fractures
    - Intrathoracic humeral head fractures

ADDITIONAL THERAPIES

- Early range of motion in older patients (age >30 yr) to prevent adhesive capsulitis (2)[A],(3)[C]
- Strengthening of rotator cuff muscles and scapular stabilizers help in maintaining dynamic stability (1,2)[A].
- Most helpful in nontraumatic dislocations in patients who have multidirectional instability or generalized ligamentous laxity (traumatic unilateral Bankart lesions, surgery [TUBS] vs. atraumatic, multidirectional, bilateral shoulders, rehabilitation, inferior capsular shift [AMBRI]).
- Glenohumeral joint stability braces aid in return to play and prevention of recurrence (1)[A].

SURGERY/OTHER PROCEDURES

- Surgical stabilization recommended for many athletic first-time dislocators, especially if "throwing shoulder, younger athletes, or participation in high-risk sports" (1)[A],(3)[C]
- Surgery recommended for those with recurrent dislocations, especially if the episodes appear to require less "trauma" than prior episodes (1)[A],(3)[C]

ONGOING CARE

- Little data exist as to when it is safe for an athlete to return to play after sustaining a dislocation (2)[A],(4)[C].
- Most experts would recommend waiting until athlete has full range of motion and strength before their return (2)[A],(4)[C].
- Recurrence:
  - Risk factors for recurrent instability: male, age ≤40 and hyperlaxity (1)[A]

ALERT

Athletes returning to play with history of instability are at risk for recurrence, with one study showing 37% incidence of repeat dislocation during the ongoing season (2)[A],(4)[C].

- There is 39% chance of recurrent instability after sustaining a traumatic shoulder dislocation, but recurrence rate varies inversely with age.
- Up to 95% recurrence in athletic patients with initial dislocation at <20 yr old without surgical intervention (1,2)[A],(3)[C]
- Presence of a Hills-Sachs lesion associated with recurrent dislocation (1)[A]

FOLLOW-UP RECOMMENDATIONS

- Growing consensus for early arthroscopic stabilization after primary anterior shoulder dislocation in young athletic patients unwilling to modify their risk factors because numerous studies have shown a high rate of recurrence in nonoperative treated subjects in this group
- When surgically stabilized, athletes show significant decreased rates or dislocation recurrence (4)[C].
- Recurrent instability patients likely to benefit from orthopedic referral for arthroscopic or open surgical repair as warranted
- Patients with multidirectional instability should be treated with traditional methods, although surgical repair may be necessary with recurrences.
- Early sports medicine referral indicated for all except uncomplicated, recurrent anterior dislocations
- Orthopedic referral with humeral head or neck fractures and irreducible dislocations

REFERENCES

1. Alkaduhimi H, van der Linde JA, Flipsen M, et al. A systematic and technical guide on how to reduce a shoulder dislocation. *Turk J Emerg Med*. 2016;16(4):155–168.
2. Eljabu W, Klinger HM, von Knoch M. The natural course of shoulder instability and treatment trends: a systematic review. *J Orthop Traumatol*. 2017;18(1):1–8.
3. Youm T, Takemoto R, Park BK. Acute management of shoulder dislocations. *J Am Acad Orthop Surg*. 2014;22(12):761–771.
4. Cutts S, Prempeh M, Drew S. Anterior shoulder dislocation. *Ann R Coll Surg Engl*. 2009;91(1):2–7.
5. Olds M, Ellis R, Donaldson K, et al. Risk factors which predispose first-time traumatic anterior shoulder dislocations to recurrent instability in adults: a systematic review and meta-analysis. *Br J Sports Med*. 2015;49(14):913–922.

ADDITIONAL READING

Dodson CC, Cordasco FA. Anterior glenohumeral joint dislocations. *Orthop Clin North Am*. 2008;39(4):507–518.

CLINICAL PEARLS

- TUBS usually responds better to surgical fixation.
- AMBRI: rehabilitation for 3 to 6 mo or more (patient needs to perform exercises independently), if fails, prolonged exercise program may benefit from inferior capsular shift.
- There is high risk of recurrence in young male athletes.
- Look for signs of associated conditions and do not attempt closed reduction if a fracture is suspected.
- No reduction technique is necessarily superior to the others. Use the technique that is most familiar and comfortable.

GLENOHUMERAL DISLOCATION, POSTERIOR

Benjamin Boswell, DO • Tracy Ray, MD, FACSM, CAQSM

BASICS

DESCRIPTION

- A posterior glenohumeral dislocation (PGHD) occurs when the humeral head disarticulates from the glenoid and rests posteriorly to its normally seated position on the glenoid.
- Glenohumeral (GH) instability is classified by:
  - Mechanism (traumatic or atraumatic).
  - Direction (anterior, posterior, superior, inferior, or multidirectional).
  - Circumstance (acute, chronic, or recurrent).
  - Degree (subluxation or dislocation).
- Other names:
  - Posterior shoulder dislocation
  - Shoulder instability

EPIDEMIOLOGY

- Glenohumeral dislocation (GHD) is frequent, but PGHD is rare, with an incidence of 1–4% of all GHD (1)[C]. Approximately 15% of these cases involve bilateral shoulders.
- The highest incidence is in males ages 35 to 55 yr.
- Diagnosis can be a challenge: Sometimes, it can be omitted due to incorrect diagnosis, absence of consideration in differential diagnosis, suboptimal radiographic evaluation, and absence of characteristic signs and symptoms; missed diagnosis reaches 60–79%, and the diagnosis can delay from 24 hr to a year (1)[C].
- Extremely rare in pediatrics because force necessary to cause a dislocation will instead cause a proximal humerus fracture.

ETIOLOGY AND PATHOPHYSIOLOGY

- In the absence of trauma, posterior dislocations occur most often as a result of a seizure (contraction of the internal rotators) or electrocution.
- Traumatic dislocation can occur when an axial load is applied to the upper extremity in the "at-risk" position: forward flexion, adduction, and internal rotation.
- Injury can occur in athletes with a fall on a flexed elbow and adducted arm or by a direct axial load to the humerus.

RISK FACTORS

- The "E"s of posterior shoulder dislocation: epilepsy, electrocution, or extreme trauma
- History of posterior shoulder dislocation or instability
- Disorders such as Charcot shoulder and Ehlers-Danlos syndrome have been well documented.
- Congenital anomalies, such as scapular aplasia, increase the risk of dislocation.
- Glenoid hypoplasia and excessive glenoid retroversion increase risk.
- At-risk sports/positions for posterior instability and/or dislocation include offensive linemen in American football with arms in blocking position, backhand stroke in racquet sports, pull-through phase of swimming, and follow-through phase in golf or throwing motion (2)[C].
- The group aged 15 to 19 yr was at the highest risk for recurrent dislocations and instability (3)[C].
- Gender was not a significant predictor of instability (3)[C].

GENERAL PREVENTION

- Rotator-cuff strength and control
- General muscle strength
- Overall core stability

COMMONLY ASSOCIATED CONDITIONS

- Multiple trauma
- Epilepsy
- Connective tissue disorders
- Scapular dysplasia
- Scapular dyskinesia

DIAGNOSIS

HISTORY

- Traumatic mechanism of injury is generally direct trauma to anterior aspect of shoulder.
- Epileptic or electrocution event with complaint of shoulder pain and inability to range GH joint
- Direction of applied force and position of the arm (the "at-risk" position)
- Can be acute or chronic
- History of previous injury or pain in affected shoulder
- Previous or present description of pain, including location, intensity, and duration
- Previous or present history of tingling, weakness, catching, and locking
- Any aggravating or alleviating factors

PHYSICAL EXAM

- Severe shoulder pain that increases with movement
- An arm held in internal rotation and adduction
- Key feature: External rotation is blocked, a critical feature of the examination that should raise suspicion.
- Prominence in the posterior aspect of the shoulder with flattening of the normal anterior contour of the deltoid
- There may be prominence of the coracoid process and squaring off of the anterolateral acromion.
- The humeral head may be visible or palpable posteriorly.
- Routine observation, gentle palpation, range of motion, and strength of the affected extremity should be performed.
- Limitation with passive external rotation and abduction may be noted.

ALERT

It is of utmost importance to monitor the neurovascular status of the affected arm. Injury to the axillary vessels is rare but potentially catastrophic.

- Although neurovascular compromise is less common than with anterior shoulder dislocation, the axillary nerve is most commonly injured and results in shoulder badge weakness and numbness. This usually resolves without intervention.
- Evaluate for atrophy of posterior rotator cuff muscles as an indication of chronic posterior instability.
- Assess for generalized ligamentous laxity.
- Scapulothoracic mechanics and rhythm should be observed, if position not "fixed."

DIFFERENTIAL DIAGNOSIS

- Acute subluxation
- Anterior shoulder dislocation
- Fractures (clavicle, scapula, and humerus)
- Rotator cuff pathology (strain, partial or complete tear)
- Adhesive capsulitis/frozen shoulder
- Acromioclavicular joint pathology
- Intra-articular pathology (labral, glenoid, or ligamentous)
- Scapular winging/instability

DIAGNOSTIC TESTS & INTERPRETATION

Initial Tests (lab, imaging)

- Plain radiographs for a suspected posterior shoulder dislocation should include an anteroposterior (AP) view, a transscapular lateral view (Y view), and a modified axillary view.

ALERT

Evidence of posterior dislocation on a standard AP view is subtle and may be undiagnosed in 50% of cases.

- The normal lateral projection of the greater tuberosity in the AP view is lost in a posterior shoulder dislocation.
- The anterior aspect of the humeral head becomes impacted against the posterior rim of the glenoid, causing a compression fracture on the anterior aspect of the humeral head. This causes a reverse Hill-Sachs lesion that gives the appearing of a "trough sign" on the radiographic AP view.
- With disarticulation of the humeral head posteriorly, the anterior rim of the glenoid is void of the humeral head, which is displaced medial to the glenoid convexity. This is visualized best with the radiographic axillary view.
- Axillary view is helpful for evaluating for glenoid rim fracture and morphology (hypoplasia, retroversion).
- Bedside ultrasound (US) has shown a sensitivity and specificity of 100% respectively for diagnosis of shoulder dislocation (4)[B]. This is a valuable tool to use for both initial diagnosis and to evaluate for proper postreduction alignment.

Follow-Up Tests and Considerations

Advanced imaging (computed tomography [CT], magnetic resonance imaging [MRI], or arthrography) should be reserved for evaluating the extent of associated humeral head fractures/impression defect, glenoid fractures, rotator cuff tears, labral pathologies, morphology of the glenoid, and articular surface integrity. However, if surgery is warranted, CT scan for preoperative planning is acceptable (2)[B].

TREATMENT

GENERAL MEASURES

- Expedited reduction is key. Delay in reduction leads to worsening muscle spasm and tightness, making reduction attempts more difficult.
- Generally, closed reduction attempts should only be attempted if posterior dislocation has been present for 3 wk or less.
- Multiple factors influence the choice of anesthesia. For example, a patient with multiple dislocations and shoulder instability may only require pain management with opioids, whereas a first-time dislocation with delayed time to reduction attempt may require procedural sedation.

- At times, reduction may be delayed due to multiple trauma, hemodynamic instability, or other comorbidities.
- On-field or sideline reduction attempts are associated with risk because there may be an associated fracture.
- Procedural sedation or general anesthesia may be necessary if a gentle and atraumatic reduction cannot be obtained.
- Early attempts at reduction should be performed in all cases, except if associated fractures of the anatomic or surgical neck of the humerus.
- With the patient supine, gentle longitudinal traction is applied to the affected arm while the elbow is flexed at 90 degrees. Countertraction used with a sheet wrapped around patient's chest by an assistant is often necessary. While traction is applied, gentle internal rotation of the arm often unlocks the humeral head from the rim of the glenoid. It may be necessary to also use direct anterolateral pressure on the humeral head to unlock it from the glenoid rim.
- An alternative technique is to apply gentle internal rotation and lateral traction to disimpact the humeral head.
- If this dislocation is seen hours or even days after occurring, it may be impossible to reduce nonsurgically.
- If an atraumatic reduction cannot be achieved, reduction in the operating room under general anesthesia should be considered.
- Open reduction should also be considered for persistent dislocation (>6 wk), chronic dislocations, and humeral head compression fracture with involvement >25%.
- Associated fractures also may require operative intervention, and open reduction may be necessary.
- Confirm intact neurovascular status after any reduction attempt.
- Obtain postreduction radiographs to confirm reduction and to evaluate humeral or glenoid fractures.
- Consider repeat physical exam, taking care not to cause repeat dislocation.

ALERT
Immobilization should not include the use of a sling and swathe because internal rotation should be avoided.

- Immobilize in neutral to external rotation, allowing for healing of the posterior capsulolabral complex.
- A shoulder spica cast or commercial brace for posterior shoulder dislocation; arm held in 20 degrees of external rotation and 0 to 20 degrees of abduction
- Duration of immobilization depends on age, chronicity, associated fractures, and operative intervention.
- For first-time, uncomplicated dislocations: 7 to 14 days of immobilization for patients >45 yr of age to avoid shoulder stiffness

Pediatric Considerations

Younger patients are immobilized 4 to 6 wk to allow capsular scarring to occur.

MEDICATION

Postreduction pain management can be at provider's discretion, but some avoid nonsteroidal anti-inflammatory drugs (NSAIDs) due to theoretical increased malunion rate if a fracture is present.

ISSUES FOR REFERRAL

If unable to perform closed reduction, patient should be referred to orthopedic surgery urgently for operative management.

ADDITIONAL THERAPIES

- Independent of the duration of immobilization, aggressive physical therapy should be completed.
- Isometric external rotation strengthening can occur during the immobilization stage in the brace.
- Progressive range of motion with strengthening of the internal and external rotators
- Advanced rehabilitation program for athletes concentrating on sport-specific activities and proprioception
- Return to athletics for first-time nonoperative dislocators is not fully understood due to limited data. It should be individually based on GH functionality and strength.
- Repeat nonoperative dislocators may return to activity once pain free and full strength has been recovered. These patients are likely to have recurrent dislocations.

SURGERY/OTHER PROCEDURES

- A conservative nonoperative trial of physical therapy may allow an individual with an uncomplicated dislocation to resume pain-free daily activities.
- Patients with a defect size <25% of the articular surface are generally treated conservatively with a favorable outcome (5)[B].

ALERT
Athletes (specifically overhead athletes) may continue to have disability that is not amenable to an extended conservative trial of rehabilitation (3 to 6 mo). In these patients, operative intervention should be considered following the initial dislocation.

- Surgical intervention is indicated with associated injuries, such as fractures, rotator cuff tears, and suspected labral pathology.
- Although the posterior capsulolabral complex often heals with nonoperative management, recurrent instability may necessitate the need for surgical repair and possibly additional soft tissue repair for improved posterior stability.
- Operative interventions often include examination under anesthesia, diagnostic arthroscopy, and arthroscopic or open stabilization procedures.
- Recent advances in arthroscopic stabilization procedures have documented recurrence rates at approximately 5%. Long-term results are still unavailable on arthroscopic stabilizations (6)[B].

ADMISSION, INPATIENT, AND NURSING CONSIDERATIONS

Consider admission for patients that have failed initial closed reduction attempts.

ONGOING CARE

FOLLOW-UP RECOMMENDATIONS

Orthopedic referral should be considered for all PGHD. Potential associated injuries of fractures, rotator cuff tears, and labral pathology require evaluation and long-term management.

PROGNOSIS

Prognosis is generally favorable when managed properly. There is limited data on recurrence rate specifically for PGHD, although general recurrence rates for all GHDs are higher in the population ages 15 to 19 yr with no difference between genders (3)[C].

COMPLICATIONS

ALERT
- Although neurovascular injury is less common in posterior GH dislocation, it can occur. Axillary nerve injury is most common, causing shoulder badge weakness and numbness. This generally resolves without intervention. Always evaluate neurovascular bundle with any shoulder dislocation.
- Reverse Hill-Sachs lesion, compression fracture of the anterior humeral head, leading to joint instability
- Reverse Bankart lesion, detachment of the posteroinferior capsular periosteum, leading to laxity of the posterior band of the inferior GH ligament and a labral tear, resulting in joint instability

REFERENCES

1. Rosas-Medina JA. Undetected traumatic posterior glenohumeral dislocation [in Spanish]. *Acta Ortop Mex*. 2017;31(4):196–201.
2. Bradley JP, Forsythe B, Mascarenhas R. Arthroscopic management of posterior shoulder instability: diagnosis, indications, and technique. *Clin Sports Med*. 2008;27(4):649–670.
3. Shields DW, Jefferies JG, Brooksbank AJ, et al. Epidemiology of glenohumeral dislocation and subsequent instability in an urban population. *J Shoulder Elbow Surg*. 2018;27(2):189–195.
4. Abbasi S, Molaie H, Hafezimoghadam P, et al. Diagnostic accuracy of ultrasonographic examination in the management of shoulder dislocation in the emergency department. *Ann Emerg Med*. 2013;62(2):170–175.
5. Guehring M, Lambert S, Stoeckle U, et al. Posterior shoulder dislocation with associated reverse Hill-Sachs lesion: treatment options and functional outcome after a 5-year follow up. *BMC Musculoskelet Disord*. 2017;18(1):442.
6. Savoie FH III, Holt MS, Field LD, et al. Arthroscopic management of posterior instability: evolution of technique and results. *Arthroscopy*. 2008;24(4):389–396.

ADDITIONAL READING

- Andrews JR, Wilk KE. *The Athlete's Shoulder*. New York, NY: Churchill Livingstone; 1994.
- Canale TS. *Campbell's Operative Orthopaedics: Fractures and Dislocations*. St. Louis, MO: Mosby; 1998.
- Dee R, Mango E, Hurst LC. *Principles of Orthopaedic Practice*. New York, NY: McGraw-Hill; 1989.
- Miller MD, Thompson SR. *DeLee and Drez's Orthopaedic Sports Medicine Principles and Practice*. Vol 1. 4th ed. New York, NY: Saunders; 2014.

CLINICAL PEARLS

- Due to the high rate of missed posterior shoulder dislocations, one must include an axillary view to the standard series of shoulder radiographs. Have a low threshold to check advanced imaging such as CT or MRI if the diagnosis is suspected and initial radiographs are negative. US shows promise in diagnosis of shoulder dislocation and can be used as a dynamic imaging tool.
- Early reduction attempts increase rate of successful closed reduction.
- All PGHDs should be referred to orthopedics for long-term management.

GLENOID LABRAL TEARS/SLAP LESIONS

Brian Lowell, MD, CAQSM

BASICS

DESCRIPTION

- The anatomy of the glenohumeral (GH) joint is complex, and stability is provided from combination of the capsule, tendons, muscles, bones, and the labrum:
  - Labrum acts by increasing surface area for humeral head contact.
  - Provides attachment site for GH ligament and the tendon of the long head of the biceps
  - Composed of fibrocartilage and dense fibrous collagenous tissue
  - The superior aspect is more mobile than the inferior portion that is tightly attached to the glenoid rim.
  - Multiple anatomic variations exist: congenitally absent portions of the labrum, different anchor sites for the GH ligament, different biceps tendon origins, and superior labral recesses (1).
- There are currently 10 described SLAP lesions (superior labrum anterior-to-posterior), of which the four originally described by Snyder are the most common:
  - Type I is degenerative fraying of the labrum.
  - Type II is a detached labral/biceps complex.
  - Type III is a bucket-handle tear.
  - Type IV is a bucket-handle tear with extension into the biceps tendon (2).
- SLAP lesions occur as acute injuries or with chronic degradation.

EPIDEMIOLOGY

- Incidence of SLAP lesions is relatively low, occurring in approximately 3–6% of all arthroscopic shoulder cases.
- Reported to occur in up to 25% of patient with symptomatic shoulder instability
- More common in men than women
- Most commonly seen in individuals in their mid-20s

ETIOLOGY AND PATHOPHYSIOLOGY

- SLAP lesion development consists of an internal rotation deficit, tightening of the posterior capsule, posterior superior GH shift, maximization of external rotation forces at the biceps anchor and superior labral attachment, and "peel back" of the labrum. Alterations in scapular movements (dyskinesis) exacerbate this mechanism (1).
- Mechanisms of injury to the glenoid labrum occur via acute trauma or repetitive microtrauma from overhead motions:
  - Acute mechanism of injury:
    - Compression due to a fall on an outstretched arm or onto an adducted shoulder
    - Traction injury from a swift pull
    - Humeral head shearing such as during vehicle accidents from seat belt restraint
  - Chronic mechanism of injury:
    - Secondary to repetitive motions that result in micro trauma accumulation
    - Chronic instability

RISK FACTORS

- Repetitive overhead motions (sports or occupational):
  - Baseball (commonly pitchers)
  - Football (quarterbacks)
  - Weight lifters (military press)
  - Swimmers
  - Tennis (serving)
  - Volleyball (serving)
- Shoulder instability/trauma
- Anatomic variation or underlying generalized laxity/instability

GENERAL PREVENTION

- There are no definitive guidelines for prevention of SLAP lesions. Generally, physical therapy practices are followed:
  - Rotator cuff strengthening
  - Scapular stabilizer strengthening
  - Posterior capsule stretching
  - Limiting internal rotation deficits
  - Ensuring proper overhead mechanics
- Additionally, monitoring pitch counts in the youth has been implemented as a preventative technique.

COMMONLY ASSOCIATED CONDITIONS

Labral tears are commonly associated with other underlying shoulder problems, as forces that cause labral injuries can cause other pathology. Thus, a high index of suspicion is required when evaluating for SLAP lesion, as other shoulder pathology coexist in approximately 85% of cases (Bankart lesions, GH instability, rotator cuff, and bicipital tendon pathology). This can significantly confound the diagnosis.

DIAGNOSIS

Labral tear diagnosis is made by history, physical, and appropriate imaging. The gold standard for diagnosis of a SLAP lesion is direct visualization via arthroscopy.

HISTORY

- Most individuals complain of nonspecific shoulder pain. Commonly anterior/superior in nature. Patient's experience is extremely variable.
- Other pertinent positives in the history may include:
  - Acute injury or repetitive overhead motion (sport, hobby, occupational).
  - Mechanical symptoms: catching, clicking, or popping deep within the shoulder with overhead movements.
  - Decrease in athletic performance (strength, velocity, accuracy, precision).
  - Weakness in the upper extremity.
  - Sense of instability.

PHYSICAL EXAM

- Examination maneuvers are generally inaccurate; there is no gold standard clinical test.
- Combinations of clinical tests provide higher accuracy. Combining two tests from a group with relatively high sensitivity (compression rotation test, anterior apprehension test, or O'Brien test) with one test from a group with relatively high specificity (Yergason test, biceps load test II, or Speed test) results in sensitivity and specificity of nearly 75% and 90% respectively (3).
- Relatively high-sensitivity tests:
  - Compression rotation test: With patient supine, the patient's arm is abducted to 90 degrees and the elbow is flexed to 90 degrees while the examiner applies axial force to the humerus; positive if pain or clicking is noted
  - Anterior apprehension test: With patient supine, examiner passively abducts and externally rotates the humerus; positive if pain or sensation of instability is noted
  - O'Brien test: With patient standing, the arm is forward flexed to 90 degrees with the elbow in full extension. With an adducted arm to 10 degrees and an internally rotated humerus, the examiner applies downward force to the arm as the patient resists. Patient then fully supinates the arm and repeats resistance; positive if pain is elicited with internal rotation and reduced with external rotation (supination)
- Relatively high-specificity tests:
  - Yergason test: With patient standing with elbow at 90 degrees of flexion, patient supinates forearm against examiner's resistance while examiner palpates long head of biceps tendon; positive if pain at biceps tendon
  - Biceps load II test: With patient supine, examiner grasps patient's wrist and elbow. The arm is abducted 120 degrees and fully externally rotated (apprehension position), with elbow held in 90 degrees of flexion and forearm supinated. Examiner then resists elbow flexion by patient; positive if pain is noted
  - Speed test: With patient seated, elbow extended and forearm in full supination, the clinician resists active forward flexion from 0 to 60 degrees; positive if pain is increased in the shoulder and the patient localizes the pain to the bicipital groove (3)[C]

DIFFERENTIAL DIAGNOSIS

- GH arthritis
- Rotator cuff impingement, tendinopathy or tear
- Biceps tendinopathy, tear or subluxation
- Shoulder instability
- Acromioclavicular (AC) joint disorder
- Cervical radiculopathy or other referred pain
- Paralabral ganglion cyst
- Pain syndromes (complex regional pain or Parsonage-Turner syndrome)

DIAGNOSTIC TESTS & INTERPRETATION

Initial Tests (lab, imaging)

- Plain radiographs are useful in identifying bony pathology such as fracture, GH arthritis, AC joint arthritis, and calcific deposits.
- Ultrasound is useful in evaluating for coexistent injuries (biceps tendon, rotator cuff tendons, joint capsule, and AC joint) but is insensitive for labral pathology. Joint effusion, bicipital sheath effusion, and paralabral cysts are secondary findings that suggest intra-articular pathology, which may include SLAP lesion.
- Magnetic resonance imaging (MRI) and magnetic resonance arthrography (MRA) are the mainstays in imaging for SLAP lesions.
- Arthrography with contrast medium improves imaging by outlining the intra-articular and synovial surfaces through slight distension of the capsule:
  - Direct (intra-articular) MRA is superior to plain MRI and vascular contrast-enhanced MRI for detecting SLAP lesions with respect to both sensitivity and specificity (4)[A].

Diagnostic Procedures/Other

GH arthroscopy:

- Gold standard
- Most sensitive and specific test for labral pathology
- Evaluation of the biceps labral complex should be done with a probe because it may appear normal with just visualization.

TREATMENT

GENERAL MEASURES

- Ideal treatment of SLAP injuries remains unclear. Current recommendations support an initial nonsurgical approach prior to surgical intervention.
- Initial therapy (nonoperative):
  - Relative rest from aggravating activities
  - Physical therapy with a focus on endurance and strengthening of the rotator cuff and scapular stabilizers and posterior capsule stretching to assist with limitations on internal rotation (2)[C]
  - A history of trauma or participation in overhead activities is strongly associated with failure of nonoperative treatment.

MEDICATION

- Oral pain control should be considered with nonsteroidal anti-inflammatory drugs (NSAIDs) or acetaminophen.
- With minimal pain relief from oral pharmacologics, subacromial or intra-articular corticosteroid injection can be considered.

ISSUES FOR REFERRAL

- Referral to a surgical specialist should be made if a patient is experiencing persistent symptoms despite 3 to 6 mo of adequate physical therapy.
- Consider early referral in elite and overhead athletes for possible faster return to sport.

SURGERY/OTHER PROCEDURES

- Evaluation with diagnostic arthroscopy and treatment is indicated if initial treatment interventions do not appropriately manage symptoms.
- Although there is no uniform approach to SLAP lesion surgical repair, several options are available (débridement, SLAP repair/fixation, subacromial decompression, tenotomy of the long head of the biceps tendon, and tenodesis of the long head of the biceps) (5)[C].
- Due to discouraging surgical results (poor outcomes with respect to return to previous level of play and surgical complications) with SLAP repair, biceps tenodesis is becoming more prevalent (5)[C].
- Other surgical intervention may be required depending on associated conditions such as rotator cuff tears or instability.

ONGOING CARE

- Postoperative care varies among individuals and depends on overall surgical intervention. Therapy is largely patient directed.
- Example of postoperative therapy are as follows:
  - Sling immobilization to protect shoulder for first 4 wk
  - Shoulder, elbow, and hand ROM for first 4 wk; full ROM typically achieved by 10 wk
  - Restore strength/balance and begin isotonic rotator cuff strengthening 8 to 12 wk postoperatively.
  - Plyometric training at approximately 20 wk
  - Throwing exercises between 24 and 28 wk
  - Return to activity 6 to 9 mo (2)[C]

FOLLOW-UP RECOMMENDATIONS

Rigorous follow-up is recommended with nonsurgical and surgical management of SLAP lesions.

PROGNOSIS

- Contact athletes typically return to sport quicker than overhead athletes and had a greater percentage of athletes return to their prior level of play. The evidence is rather unfavorable for overhead athletes returning to prior level of play status post SLAP repair (40–70%).
- Return to play and return to previous level was limited in pitchers compared to other positional players in baseball.
- Individuals with isolated SLAP lesions (rare) return to activity much quicker (2.6 mo) than individuals with concomitant shoulder pathology (6 mo).
- Age appears to affect outcomes because younger athletes appear to do better overall (6)[C].

COMPLICATIONS

Complications associated with surgical intervention include infection, hemarthrosis, failed surgical intervention, instability, adhesive capsulitis, and chondral injury.

REFERENCES

1. Abrams G, Safran M. Diagnosis and management of superior labrum anterior posterior lesions in overhead athletes. *Br J Sports Med*. 2010;44(5):311–318.
2. Manske R, Prohaska D. Superior labrum anterior to posterior (SLAP) rehabilitation in the overhead athlete. *Phys Ther Sport*. 2010;11(4):110–121.
3. Oh JH, Kim JY, Kim WS, et al. The evaluation of various physical examinations for the diagnosis of type II superior labrum anterior to posterior lesion. *Am J Sports Med*. 2008;36(2):353–359.
4. Symanski JS, Subhas N, Babb J, et al. Diagnosis of superior labrum anterior-to-posterior tears by using MR imaging and MR arthrography: a systemic review and meta-analysis. *Radiology*. 2017;285(1):101–113.
5. Popp D, Schöffl V. Superior labral anterior posterior lesions of the shoulder: current diagnostic and therapeutic standards. *World J Orthop*. 2015;6(9):660–671.
6. Rangavajjula A, Hyatt A, Raneses E, et al. Return to play after treatment of shoulder labral tears in professional hockey players. *Phys Sportsmed*. 2016;44(2):119–125.

G

CLINICAL PEARLS

- Glenoid labral tears are relatively uncommon shoulder injuries but are more commonly seen in overhead athletes and those who participate in contact sports.
- Labral injuries typically cause vague pain, decreased performance, and mechanical symptoms. Physical exam, although helpful, is unreliable for definitive diagnosis, so have a low threshold for imaging in appropriate cases.
- Generally, nonsurgical treatment is indicated prior to surgical intervention.
- Evaluation with diagnostic arthroscopy and treatment is appropriate if nonsurgical therapy does not manage symptoms.
- Consider early referral in elite and overhead athletes for possible faster return to sport.
- The evidence is rather unfavorable for overhead athletes returning to prior level of play status post SLAP surgical repair. If no labral pathology is identified, broaden differential to include cervical or brachial plexus pathology.

GOUT

Kenneth S. Taylor, MD, FAAFP, CAQSM • Natalie Voskanian, MD • Suraj A. Achar, MD, FAAFP, CAQSM

BASICS

- Gout is an acute disease that can progress to a chronic state.
- The most common inflammatory arthropathy, affecting >8 million Americans (1)
- Consists of painful inflammatory deposition of monosodium urate crystals into joints and may also form at the joint space and soft tissues (tophaceous gout)
- Pseudogout is a similar but distinct entity in which the inflammatory process is instigated by calcium pyrophosphate dihydrate (CPPD) crystal deposition instead of monosodium urate.

DESCRIPTION

- Gout has three stages:
  - Acute phase: inflammatory monarthritis; resolves within several days to just over a week
  - Interval phase: The patient is asymptomatic.
  - Chronic phase: intermittent repeated flairs of monarticular or polyarticular gout and soft tissue deposition of tophi
- Common joints affected by gout: 1st metatarsophalangeal (MTP) joint (most common site of initial presentation; also known as *podagra*), olecranon, ankle, wrist, knee, tarsal joints, and interphalangeal joints of the hand
- Much less commonly affected joints include shoulder, sternoclavicular joint, spine, and sacroiliac joints.
- Tophaceous gout can extend to periarticular structures (tendons, skin, and soft tissue) and rarely can affect visceral organs.
- Up to 20% of gout patients may present with polyarticular or tophaceous gout at initial presentation.

EPIDEMIOLOGY

Incidence

- Commonly presents in middle-aged men (30 to 50 yr old)
- Also commonly seen in elderly men and postmenopausal women, typically in those with multiple medical comorbidities
- Predominant gender: male > female (2 to 4:1)

Prevalence

- Prevalence of gout in United States is ~3% and increases with increasing age (2).
- Others have found a prevalence of 8.4 per 1,000 (3).

ETIOLOGY AND PATHOPHYSIOLOGY

- Precipitation of monosodium urate crystals in a joint space or soft tissue
- This triggers immune activation with the release of cytokines and neutrophil recruitment.
- This inflammatory process results in localized pain, swelling, and erythema of the affected joint.
- This disease process closely resembles infection.

RISK FACTORS

- Male
- Pacific islander
- Excessive alcohol intake (especially beer and liquor)
- Hypertension and cardiovascular disease
- Chronic diuretic use (thiazide and loop)
- Organ transplant recipients treated with calcineurin inhibitors
- Recent surgery
- Hyperuricemic state (from either overproduction or underexcretion of uric acid)
- Rapid changes in uric acid level
- Diets high in purine-containing products
- Diets low in dairy or high in meat or fish (hazard ratio up to 1.41 in high-quantity meat eaters and 1.51 in high-quantity fish eaters) (4); total protein intake is not correlated with risk for gout.
- Risk factors for the presence of tophaceous gout at initial diagnosis:
  - Postmenopausal women
  - Coexisting chronic renal disease
  - Diuretic therapy
- Dehydration (a very important risk factor)

GENERAL PREVENTION

- Factors that can reduce risk of gout:
  - High-quantity dairy product intake (hazard ratio of 0.56) (4)
  - Minimizing diuretic use and dose
  - Minimizing alcohol intake
- Urate-lowering agents are used for the prevention of chronic gout. See "Medication."

COMMONLY ASSOCIATED CONDITIONS

- Hypertension
- Chronic diuretic therapy
- Obesity
- Hyperlipidemia
- Chronic renal disease
- Cardiovascular disease
- Hyperuricemic syndromes such as myeloproliferative or lymphoproliferative disorders, psoriasis, cyclosporine A use (in organ transplant patients), and inherited defects in purine metabolism
- Patients with gout are at increased risk for uric acid nephrolithiasis.

DIAGNOSIS

HISTORY

- Initially a severely painful, erythematous, and swollen joint (noninfectious monarthritis)
- There is no significant trauma of the joint preceding the attack.
- Rarely, there may be polyarticular involvement at first onset.
- Maximal pain reaches peak at 24 to 48 hr (1,5).

PHYSICAL EXAM

- Gout:
  - Swelling, erythema, warmth, and tenderness of affected joint
  - 80% of flares involve a single joint (1st MTP, knee, ankle, and other joints).
  - Sometimes overlying skin can be erythematous and desquamated, resembling cellulitis.
- Tophi:
  - Subcutaneous nodules (resembling rheumatoid arthritis) or a bulky mass overlying a joint
  - ± Tenderness or erythema of tophi
  - Aspirated tophi contents appear as white pasty or chalky material.

DIFFERENTIAL DIAGNOSIS

- Pseudogout
- Rheumatoid arthritis
- Septic arthritis
- Osteoarthritis
- Reactive arthritis
- Osteomyelitis
- Malignancy
- Joint trauma

DIAGNOSTIC TESTS & INTERPRETATION

Initial Tests (lab, imaging)

- Distinction from an infectious process may be difficult.
- Complete blood count (CBC): Leukocytosis may be extremely high.
- C-reactive protein (CRP) and erythrocyte sedimentation rate (ESR) are often elevated as well.
- Chemistry panel to assess renal function: Not only is renal impairment associated with gout, but chronic hyperuricemia can lead to urate nephropathy.
- Uric acid level often will be high during an acute gout attack but may be normal:
  - Incidence of gout in patients with uric acid levels >9 mg/dL is 6 times greater than in patients at 7 to 8.9 mg/dL (5).
  - In a group of 339 patients with acute gout, 14% had uric acid levels ≤6 mg/dL and 32% were ≤8 mg/dL (6).
  - Thus, uric acid level on its own cannot be used to diagnose or rule out gout, but a high uric acid level in the appropriate clinical context can be suggestive of gout (6)[B].
- Although sometimes helpful, imaging is not necessary to make a diagnosis of gout (7)[A].
- Can be used to evaluate for an alternate diagnoses such as rheumatoid arthritis
- Chronic gout is often characterized by subcortical cysts, bony erosions, overhanging edges, and diffuse soft tissue calcifications on x-ray or magnetic resonance imaging (MRI) (7).
- Large tophi can be identified on MRI but often will need to be aspirated to confirm the diagnosis (7)[A].
- Pseudogout, on the other hand, does not typically have bony abnormalities but instead consists of chondrocalcinosis (calcification of fibrocartilage).

Diagnostic Procedures/Other

- The "gold standard" diagnosis of gout is made by aspiration (arthrocentesis) of the affected joint's synovial fluid (8)[A].
- Characteristic needle-shaped, negatively birefringent monosodium urate crystals are seen under polarized light microscopy.
- In contrast, pseudogout consists of rhomboid-shaped crystals with weakly positive birefringence.
- Aspirate: Check cell count, Gram stain, and bacterial culture to evaluate for infection (with a negative Gram stain and negative culture).
- Aspirate white blood cell (WBC) count: 2,000 to 50,000 seen in gout (also pseudogout or rheumatoid arthritis); >50,000 is suspicious for septic arthritis.
- It is important to look for septic arthritis, which can mimic gout (and rarely may coexist with gout).
- Ultrasound-guided aspiration can improve accuracy.

TREATMENT

GENERAL MEASURES

- See "Risk Factors" for what to avoid.
- Therapy for gout includes diet modification (see "Risk Factors"), using medications that reduce overall uric acid levels (such as losartan, calcium channel blockers, and fenofibrate), and minimizing medications that are known to increase gout flairs (such as diuretics and aspirin) when appropriate.

MEDICATION

- Acute treatment:
  - Nonsteroidal anti-inflammatory drugs (NSAIDs) are first-line therapy; typically naproxen (500 mg BID) or indomethacin (50 mg TID) is used (9)[A]; should be given within 24 to 48 hr of symptom onset for best results (5)[B]
  - Cyclooxygenase-2 (COX-2) inhibitors are equally effective according to recent studies (10)[B].
  - Duration of treatment varies, often ranging from 3 to 10 days until the attack subsides.
  - Within several days of treatment, the dosing can be decreased if clinical improvement (1)[B].
  - Corticosteroids (intravenous [IV], oral, or intra-articular) are an effective alternative first-line agent if NSAIDs are contraindicated (2,11)[A]:
    - Begin oral prednisone at 30 to 40 mg/day or prednisolone 30 mg/day × 2 to 3 days, then taper over total of 5 to 10 days (5,8)[C].
    - Intra-articular injections; can use:
      - Betamethasone 3 to 6 mg
      - Dexamethasone 5 to 10 mg
      - Methylprednisolone 20 to 40 mg
      - Triamcinolone 20 to 40 mg
  - Septic arthritis is an absolute contraindication to intra-articular corticosteroid treatment.
  - Colchicine is very effective for treatment of acute gout (12)[A].
  - Use oral colchicine 0.6 mg 2 to 3 times per day or 1 to 2 times per day in patients with renal impairment or elderly patients:
    - For best results, colchicine should be given within 24 to 48 hr of symptom onset (12)[B].
  - IV colchicines should not be used and are no longer approved by the U.S. Food and Drug Administration (FDA) owing to the high level of toxicity (12)[A].
- Preventive treatment:
  - Dietary modifications:
    - Reduce or eliminate:
      - Beer and liquor (no increased risk with wine).
      - High-fructose products/sweetened beverages.
      - Meat/seafood (4).
    - Increase/beneficial:
      - Dairy/skim milk
      - Coffee (Tea does not reduce risk.)
      - Vitamin C 500 mg/day
      - Cherry/cherry extract (possible) (4)
- Indications for chronic preventative therapy include (13)[B]:
  - Recurrent or disabling gout attacks (specifically >2 gout attacks per year).
  - Persistent tophi.
  - Joint damage noted on imaging.
  - Uric acid nephropathy or nephrolithiasis.
- The symptom-free period required prior to starting prophylactic therapy once the acute attack has resolved is unclear:
  - Some advocate using concomitant colchicine or NSAID treatment the first 3 to 6 mo of urate-lowering treatment (14)[C].
  - Some suggest waiting about 2 to 6 wk after the acute attack before starting prophylactic medication, although recent evidence shows it is safe in conjunction with NSAIDs (1),(5)[C].
- If a gout attack occurs while on urate-lowering treatment, the urate-lowering medication should *not* be stopped (1,5)[B].
- Uric acid level should be monitored for a goal of <6 mg/dL (355 μmol/L) because this is associated with a significantly lower incidence of gout (5)[B].
- Allopurinol is a xanthine oxidase inhibitor that decreases uric acid production:
  - Used most commonly
  - Therapeutic dose is 100 to 300 mg/day: Start at a lower dose (50 or 100 mg/day), and titrate up slowly over several weeks (e.g., by 100 mg every 2 to 4 wk) to target uric acid goal of <6 mg/dL (8)[C].
  - Patients with renal insufficiency require lower doses.
  - Periodic laboratory testing (liver enzymes and CBC) should be considered.
  - Chinese, Thai, or Korean descent has a higher risk of hypersensitivity skin reactions—genetic testing is available (1).
- Febuxostat is a newer medication:
  - Cleared through the liver and therefore an appropriate alternative in renal disease
- Probenecid is a uricosuric agent that increases uric acid secretion:
  - Second-line medication for prophylaxis (9)
  - Ineffective in patients with impaired creatinine clearance
  - Avoid in patients with nephrolithiasis.
  - Caution for multiple medication interactions
- NSAIDs (naproxen 250 mg 2 times per day) or colchicine (≤0.6 mg 1 to 2 times per day) can be used as chronic suppression therapy in the place of or in addition to urate-lowering agents (5)[B].
- Low-dose prednisone (≤10 mg) also can be considered, but it has long-term side effects (5)[B].
- Recently approved drug Leisured is being studied as an adjunct to allopurinol to improve efficacy. Lesinurad: Uric acid reabsorption inhibitor combined with allopurinol in 200 mg or 300 mg increments is superior to allopurinol alone in lowering uric acid levels.

ISSUES FOR REFERRAL

- Rheumatology if refractory condition, multiple comorbidities, or unusual presentation
- Orthopedics if suspected septic arthritis

ADMISSION, INPATIENT, AND NURSING CONSIDERATIONS

- Consider for severe cases of gout, especially if needed for pain control or for diagnostic confirmation.
- Suspected septic arthritis requires IV antibiotics and orthopedic referral.

ONGOING CARE

PROGNOSIS

Prior to advent of preventative therapy up to 2/3 patients undergoing a gout attack will have another one within 12 mo.

COMPLICATIONS

- It takes, on average, about 10 yr for chronic tophaceous gout to develop after the initial attack (5).
- Chronic gout can lead to joint damage and destruction.
- Frequent attacks can be very painful and disabling and have a negative impact on quality of life.
- Chronic urate nephropathy

REFERENCES

1. Hainer BL, Matheson E, Wilkes RT. Diagnosis, treatment, and prevention of gout. *Am Fam Physician*. 2014;90(12):831–836.
2. Rainer TH, Cheng CH, Janssens HJ, et al. Oral prednisolone in the treatment of acute gout: a pragmatic, multicenter, double-blind, randomized trial. *Ann Intern Med*. 2016;164(7):464–471.
3. Lawrence RC, Felson DT, Helmick CG, et al. Estimates of the prevalence of arthritis and other rheumatic conditions in the United States. Part II. *Arthritis Rheum*. 2008;58(1):26–35.
4. Beyl RN Jr, Hughes L, Morgan S. Update on importance of diet in gout. *Am J Med*. 2016;129(11):1153–1158.
5. Keith MP, Gilliland WR. Updates in the management of gout. *Am J Med*. 2007;120(3):221–224.
6. Schlesinger N, Norquist JM, Watson DJ. Serum urate during acute gout. *J Rheumatol*. 2009;36(6):1287–1289.
7. Schumacher HR Jr, Becker MA, Edwards NL, et al. Magnetic resonance imaging in the quantitative assessment of gouty tophi. *Int J Clin Pract*. 2006;60(4):408–414.
8. Terkeltaub RA. Clinical practice. Gout. *N Engl J Med*. 2003;349(17):1647–1655.
9. Zhang W, Doherty M, Bardin T, et al. EULAR evidence based recommendations for gout. Part II: management. Report of a task force of the EULAR Standing Committee for International Clinical Studies Including Therapeutics (ESCISIT). *Ann Rheum Dis*. 2006;65(10):1312–1324.
10. Wortmann RL. Recent advances in the management of gout and hyperuricemia. *Curr Opin Rheumatol*. 2005;17(3):319–324.
11. Janssens HJ, Janssen M, van de Lisdonk EH, et al. Use of oral prednisolone or naproxen for the treatment of gout arthritis: a double-blind, randomised equivalence trial. *Lancet*. 2008;371(9627):1854–1860.
12. Terkeltaub RA. Colchicine update: 2008. *Semin Arthritis Rheum*. 2009;38(6):411–419.
13. Shoji A, Yamanaka H, Kamatani N. A retrospective study of the relationship between serum urate level and recurrent attacks of gouty arthritis: evidence for reduction of recurrent gouty arthritis with antihyperuricemic therapy. *Arthritis Rheum*. 2004;51(3):321–325.
14. Borstad GC, Bryant LR, Abel MP, et al. Colchicine for prophylaxis of acute flares when initiating allopurinol for chronic gouty arthritis. *J Rheumatol*. 2004;31(12):2429–2432.

CLINICAL PEARLS

- Gout is an acute inflammatory arthritis of rapid onset that can mimic infection.
- A painful, warm, erythematous, swollen joint should be aspirated to evaluate for septic arthritis versus gout.
- Tophaceous gout is the chronic form of gout that, in rare cases, can present acutely.
- Prophylactic treatment should be considered in recurrent patients because it has been shown to reduce chronic flairs and joint damage.
- Dietary modifications and losing weight can greatly reduce the risks of gout
- Pseudogout is a disease that is distinct from gout but has various similarities, is generally less debilitating, and less common.

GREENSTICK FRACTURE

Greg Canty, MD

BASICS

DESCRIPTION

Greenstick fractures are incomplete fractures that occur when a bone is exposed to angulation and rotational bending forces. The bending forces are strong enough that the bone begins to fracture on tension side, but the force is not sufficient enough to result in a complete fracture:

- The fracture appears on the tension (convex) side of the bone as a break in the periosteum and the cortex.
- The compression side of the bone, or the concave surface, remains intact and appears as a hinge.
- This fracture pattern is most commonly described in forearm fractures of growing children.
- Greenstick fractures may be isolated or may coexist with other complete fractures in forearm injuries.

EPIDEMIOLOGY

- Studies suggest up to 5% of childhood and adolescent fractures are of the greenstick variety (1)[B].
- Some studies suggest an even greater percentage of childhood fractures may be of the greenstick variety.
- Although extremely rare, there have actually been a few case reports of greenstick fractures in the young adult population (2)[B].
- Forearm (radius or ulna) = most common
- Proximal humerus
- Tibia

ETIOLOGY AND PATHOPHYSIOLOGY

Greenstick fractures occur in children and adolescents because the bone is more:

- Porous.
- Compliant.
- Resilient.
- Soft.

COMMONLY ASSOCIATED CONDITIONS

- Complete fracture of an accompanying bone (common)
- Fracture/dislocation like a Monteggia variant (proximal 3rd ulna fracture with anterior disruption of radial head) (rare)

DIAGNOSIS

Prehospital:

- Suspect with any forearm injury having a mild angular deformity, swelling, and pain.

HISTORY

- Establish mechanism of injury, which is often a fall on outstretched hand with some rotational force.
- Inquire about any numbness, tingling, or pain out of proportion to exam findings.

PHYSICAL EXAM

- Pain and localized tenderness to palpation
- Unwillingness to use or mobilize the affected extremity
- Mild to moderate angular deformity
- Swelling
- Ecchymosis
- Palpation of bony deformities
- Crepitus
- Assess the distal portion of the affected extremity for:
  - Circulation (capillary refill and pulses).
  - Motor function.
  - Sensation.
- Assess proximal and distal joints/bones for related injuries.

DIFFERENTIAL DIAGNOSIS

- Complete fracture
- Compound fracture
- Plastic deformation/bowing deformity
- Torus (buckle) fracture
- Contusion
- Sprain

DIAGNOSTIC TESTS & INTERPRETATION

- Anteroposterior and lateral radiographs required for diagnosis
- Look for tearing of the periosteum and cortex on the convex side of affected bone.
- Concave surface of affected bone should have intact periosteum.
- Plastic deformation of bone may also be apparent.
- Oblique views may occasionally be helpful.
- Radius crossover sign may be helpful in determining rotational malalignment after reduction (3)[B]. The typical radiographs, where the radius crossover sign is present, demonstrate a pronated appearance of the proximal forearm with a neutral position of the distal forearm.
- Repeat radiographs after reduction.

TREATMENT

GENERAL MEASURES

- Prehospital:
  - Ice to affected region for pain control and swelling
  - Splint in comfortable position using:
    - Air splint or board.
    - Tape.
    - Rolled towels.
- Emergency department (ED) treatment:
  - Pain control (see "Medication")
  - Fracture reduction (4)[C]:
    - Most greenstick fractures of the forearm are reduced by rotating the palm toward the apex of the fracture.
    - Greenstick fractures are incomplete fractures and may require completing the fracture in order to obtain adequate reduction.
  - Immobilize the injury with either a cast or splint:
    - Immobilize in reduced position.
    - Long-arm cast/splint with elbow at 90 degrees if fracture of proximal or middle third of forearm
    - May consider below-the-elbow cast or removable splint if fracture is in distal third of forearm (5)[B]
    - Ensure proper three-point molding to maintain any reduction.
    - Postreduction films after casting/splinting (Look for radius crossover sign discussed in imaging.)
  - Ensure reduction is maintained with immobilization prior to discharge from ED.

MEDICATION

First Line

- Ibuprofen (10 mg/kg) with maximum of 800 mg every 6 to 8 hr (6)[B]
- Oxycodone (available as an elixir containing 1 mg/1 mL) (7)[B]:
  - 0.05 to 0.15 mg/kg every 4 to 6 hr

Second Line

- Fentanyl 1 to 2 μg/kg IV every 1 to 4 hr (maximum dose 50 μg); may also consider intranasal 1.5 μg/kg (maximum 100 μg)
- Morphine 0.1 to 0.2 mg/kg every 2 to 4 hr (maximum 10 mg)

ISSUES FOR REFERRAL

- Refer if unable to maintain reduction.
- Refer for any signs of median nerve or tendon entrapment.
- Refer for any progressive deformity.

SURGERY/OTHER PROCEDURES

Rarely indicated unless nerve/tendon entrapment or inability to maintain reduction

ADMISSION, INPATIENT, AND NURSING CONSIDERATIONS

- Admission criteria:
  - Any suspicion of a nonaccidental injury (NAI):
    - History is best predictor of NAI.
    - Best predictor of NAI is whether history is consistent with injury pattern/severity.
- Discharge criteria:
  - Pain is well controlled.
  - Orthopedic referral available within 1 wk
  - Splint/cast care/pain management instructions:
    - Ice/cold pack application
    - Elevation of the injured limb
    - Analgesic plans for mild, moderate, and severe pain
    - Return precautions

ONGOING CARE

FOLLOW-UP RECOMMENDATIONS

Patient Monitoring

- With greenstick fractures of the forearm, clinical follow-up and radiographs obtained at 2 to 6 wk postinjury reduce overall care costs and radiation exposure without compromising clinical results (8)[B].
- Greenstick fractures of the tibia are at risk for valgus deformity and may be followed for 1 to 2 yr.
- Loss of reduction or progression of any deformity warrants surgical consideration, although younger patients have excellent capability of remodeling and rarely require surgery.

PROGNOSIS

- Greenstick fractures are expected to heal completely.
- Complications are rare.
- Remodeling capabilities are tremendous in young patients.
- Excellent prognosis

COMPLICATIONS

- 10–15% of greenstick fractures may lose reduction after immobilization.
- Nerve or tendon sheath entrapment
- Unrecognized accompanying injuries

REFERENCES

1. Cheng JC, Shen WY. Limb fracture pattern in different pediatric age groups: a study of 3,350 children. *J Orthop Trauma*. 1993;7(1):15–22.
2. Casey PJ, Moed BR. Greenstick fractures of the radius in adults: a report of two cases. *J Orthop Trauma*. 1996;10(3):209–212.
3. Wright PB, Crepeau AE, Herrera-Soto JA, et al. Radius crossover sign: an indication of malreduced radius shaft greenstick fractures. *J Pediatr Orthop*. 2012;32(4):e15–e19.
4. Noonan KJ, Price CT. Forearm and distal radius fractures in children. *J Am Acad Orthop Surg*. 1998;6(3):146–156.
5. Boutis K, Howard A, Constantine E, et al. Evidence into practice: pediatric orthopaedic surgeon use of removable splints for common pediatric fractures. *J Pediatr Orthop*. 2015;35(1):18–23.
6. Drendel AL, Gorelick MH, Weisman SJ, et al. A randomized clinical trial of ibuprofen versus acetaminophen with codeine for acute pediatric arm fracture pain. *Ann Emerg Med*. 2009;54(4):553–560.
7. Koller DM, Myers AB, Lorenz D, et al. Effectiveness of oxycodone, ibuprofen, or the combination in the initial management of orthopedic injury-related pain in children. *Pediatr Emerg Care*. 2007;23(9):627–633.
8. Ting BL, Kalish LA, Waters PM, et al. Reducing cost and radiation exposure during the treatment of pediatric greenstick fractures of the forearm. *J Pediatr Orthop*. 2016;36(8):816–820.

ADDITIONAL READING

- Flynn JM, Skaggs DL, Waters PM, eds. *Rockwood and Wilkins' Fractures in Children*. 8th ed. Philadelphia, PA: Lippincott Williams & Wilkins; 2015.
- Mencio GA, Swiontkowski MF, eds. *Green's Skeletal Trauma in Children*. 5th ed. Philadelphia, PA: Saunders; 2015.
- Wenger DR, Pring ME, Pennock AT, et al, eds. *Rang's Children's Fractures*. 4th ed. Philadelphia, PA: Lippincott Williams & Wilkins; 2018.

CLINICAL PEARLS

- Examine surrounding bones/joints closely for accompanying injuries such as a both-bone forearm fracture or a Monteggia-variant fracture/dislocation.
- Incomplete fractures, like the greenstick, may require completing the fracture for adequate reduction.
- Reduce radial greenstick fractures by rotating the forearm so that the palm is pointing toward the apex of the fracture.
- Forearm fractures have tremendous potential for remodeling, but greenstick fractures require monitoring after reduction to ensure reduction is maintained.
- Beware of the long-term risk for a valgus deformity following greenstick fractures of the tibia.

HAGLUND DEFORMITY (PUMP BUMP)

Shaun P. Garff, DO • Brent S.E. Rich, MD, ATC

BASICS

DESCRIPTION

- Haglund deformity is an abnormal prominence of the posterosuperior surface of the calcaneus. It can give rise to Haglund disease, which consists of retrocalcaneal bursitis, insertional Achilles tendinitis, and pre-Achilles (superficial) bursitis. These occur due to compression of the distal Achilles tendon and the surrounding soft tissues.
- Named after the Swedish orthopedic surgeon Patrick Haglund in 1928 (1)
- Often chronic process but can present with acute exacerbation of pain
- Synonyms(s): Haglund disease; Haglund syndrome; pump bump

EPIDEMIOLOGY

Haglund deformity occurs in both sexes and is seen in all active age groups.

ALERT

More common in females, ages 20 to 30 yr, who wear high heels and shoes with restrictive heel counters (2)

- Also seen in individuals/athletes wearing shoes with rigid heel counters (e.g., pumps, ice skates, work boots) or experience an increase in training (e.g., increase in miles, running on hard surfaces)

RISK FACTORS

- Heel varus
- Pes cavus
- Rigid plantarly flexed 1st ray
- Rigid or poorly shaped heel counters
- Tight Achilles tendon

GENERAL PREVENTION

- Appropriate shoe wear (avoiding high heels and shoes with rigid heel counters)
- Heel lift/pad
- Stretching Achilles tendon
- Avoiding running on hard surfaces or uphill

DIAGNOSIS

HISTORY

- Posterior heel pain with palpable bump
- Increase in training program, specifically number of miles run or changing running surface
- Change in shoe wear (shoes with rigid heel counters can irritate the subcutaneous tissues and can inflame the underlying bursae)
- May be an incidental finding on imaging without any symptoms (3)

PHYSICAL EXAM

- Dull, achy, exertional posterior heel pain
- Tenderness and thickening of the overlying skin at the Achilles tendon attachment
- Palpable swelling anterior or posterior to the Achilles tendon
- Pain is intensified with active or passive dorsiflexion of the ankle.
- Prominent-appearing posterosuperior portion of the calcaneus
- Careful, discreet palpation to differentiate between swelling in the Achilles tendon and swelling in the retrocalcaneal bursa
- Assessment for gastrocnemius/soleus tightness is imperative.

DIFFERENTIAL DIAGNOSIS

- Pre-Achilles bursitis
- Achilles tendinitis/tendinosis
- Retrocalcaneal bursitis
- Calcaneal stress fracture
- Ankle impingement
- Tibiotalar degenerative joint disease

DIAGNOSTIC TESTS & INTERPRETATION

- Weight-bearing radiographs of both feet and/or ankles can assist in determining enthesopathic spurring and thus concern for state of the Achilles tendon degradation (1).
- Lateral radiographs may show a 2- to 3-mm bony extrusion on the posterosuperior angle of the calcaneus.
- Calcaneal body index assesses the shape of the calcaneus, and the calcaneal inclination angle assesses the orientation of the calcaneus; good predictors of posterior heel pain

- Calcaneal pitch lines and Fowler lines have been used in the past for diagnosis but in recent studies have been found to have no statistically significant relationship to posterior heel pain (4).
- Consider ordering magnetic resonance imaging (MRI) or musculoskeletal ultrasound (US) to evaluate the integrity of the Achilles tendon and the retrocalcaneal bursa.

TREATMENT

GENERAL MEASURES

- Shoe modification (5)[C]
- Achilles stretching program
- U-shaped pad
- Heel pad/heel lift (2)
- Soft tissue modalities (i.e., ice, US, iontophoresis, Astym, Graston Technique)
- Decrease in mileage and hill running
- Minimization of hard-surface running
- Nonsteroidal anti-inflammatory drugs (NSAIDs) (topical and/or oral)
- Immobilization with a short leg cast or walking boot

ALERT
Corticosteroid injections are generally avoided to prevent injury or damage to Achilles tendon (5)[C].

ADDITIONAL THERAPIES

Dry needling of the gastrocnemius/soleus

SURGERY/OTHER PROCEDURES

- Partial (posterosuperior) calcaneal osteotomy (open or endoscopic) with excision of Haglund prominence; may include complete resection of the bursal projection or Achilles tendon débridement
- Systematic reviews have shown better results with endoscopic versus open approach (1).
- Postoperative course: immobilization in short leg cast or walking boot for 2 to 6 wk, followed by 2 wk partial weight-bearing, then full weight-bearing over succeeding 6 wk; course shortened with endoscopic procedure
- Results of open surgery have generally shown good results, although failure rates have occurred in up to 25–30% (1).
- Rehabilitation program consisting of conditioning exercises and functional retraining

ONGOING CARE

FOLLOW-UP RECOMMENDATIONS

Return to clinic in 4 to 6 wk for reevaluation and discussion of management options after initial conservative interventions

COMPLICATIONS

- Achilles tendon rupture
- Postoperatively: infection, hematoma, recurrent exostosis, persistent pain, hypoesthesia (1)
- Chronic heel pain
- Sural nerve injury

REFERENCES

1. Syed TA, Perera A. A proposed staging classification for minimally invasive management of Haglund's syndrome with percutaneous and endoscopic surgery. *Foot Ankle Clin*. 2016;21(3):641–664.
2. Vaishya R, Agarwal AK, Azizi AT, et al. Haglund's syndrome: a commonly seen mysterious condition. *Cureus*. 2016;8(10):e820.
3. Aronow MS. Posterior heel pain (retrocalcaneal bursitis, insertional and noninsertional Achilles tendinopathy). *Clin Podiatr Med Surg*. 2005;22(1):19–43.
4. Bulstra GH, van Rheenen TA. Can we measure the heel bump? Radiographic evaluation of Haglund's deformity. *J Foot Ankle Surg*. 2015;54(3):338–340.
5. Thomas JL, Christensen JC, Kravitz SR, et al. The diagnosis and treatment of heel pain: a clinical practice guideline-revision 2010. *J Foot Ankle Surg*. 2010;49(Suppl 3):S1–S19.

ADDITIONAL READING

Almaawi A, Boszczyk AM, Daniels TR. Exostosis (osteochondrosis, apophysites, and Haglund's deformity). In: Valderrabano V, Easley M, eds. *Foot and Ankle Sports Orthopaedics*. Cham, Switzerland: Springer; 2017:209–218.

CLINICAL PEARLS

- Posterior heel pain consistent with Haglund deformity needs bilateral foot/ankle x-rays.
- Not all radiographic evidence of a Haglund deformity produce symptoms.
- Initial treatment with conservative measures can be very successful.
- Return to play is dependent on the severity and number of associated conditions involved. Return to play after conservative treatment ranges from 2 to 8 wk, whereas surgery and postoperative course limit and prevent strenuous activity for 4 to 6 mo. Athletes may return to strenuous activity when local symptoms have resolved.

HALLUX VALGUS (BUNIONS)

Alan Shahtaji, DO, CAQSM • Sonya S. Ahmed, MD

BASICS

DESCRIPTION

- Hallux valgus (HV) refers to a subluxation of the 1st metatarsophalangeal (MTP) joint with lateral or valgus deviation of the great toe and medial or varus deviation of the 1st metatarsal, leading to a bony prominence at the medial aspect of the joint (medial eminence or bunion).
- Bunion comes from the Latin word *bunio*, which means turnip.
- Synonym(s): bunion; hallux abductovalgus (HAV); metatarsus primus varus

EPIDEMIOLOGY

- More common in females; female:male = 10:1
- Familial tendency
- Almost exclusively seen in shoe-wearing societies
- Prevalence is highest in women in their 4th through 6th decades of life; potential worsening with aging
- Subset of juvenile/adolescent onset

ETIOLOGY AND PATHOPHYSIOLOGY

- The dorsal, plantar, medial, and lateral structures attach to proximal phalanx and maintain alignment of MTP articulation. There are no attachments on the distal metatarsal, so deviation of proximal phalanx dictates deformity.
- As HV deformity develops, the abductor hallucis tendon is displaced in a plantar direction, and the joint loses most of its medial support.
- The adductor hallucis then pulls the proximal 1st phalanx laterally and exerts a rotational force, resulting in pronation of the 1st phalanx.
- With worsening of the HV deformity, the extensor hallucis longus shifts into the 1st metatarsal interspace and becomes a lateral force on the great toe.
- The sesamoid complex plantarward may shift laterally if the 1st metatarsal continues to deviate medially.
- Pes planus and forefoot pronation likely accelerate the progression when HV is present. These conditions increase pressure on the medial aspect of the great toe and attenuation of the medial capsular structures at the 1st MTP joint.

RISK FACTORS

- Hereditary influences
- Constrictive footwear, mostly with narrow toe box; conflicting literature regarding high-heeled shoes; neuromuscular disorders and collagen-deficient disorders
- A rounded MTP articulation and longer 1st metatarsal
- Metatarsus primus varus and an increased 1st and 2nd intermetatarsal angle (IMA) are often implicated in juvenile or adolescent HV.
- Possible associations:
  - Tight gastrocsoleus complex and Achilles tendon
  - Hypermobility of the 1st tarsometatarsal joint
  - Pes planus/planovalgus and forefoot pronation

GENERAL PREVENTION

Avoid tight-fitting shoes with narrow toe box.

COMMONLY ASSOCIATED CONDITIONS

- Lesser toe abnormalities, including hammertoes, crossover toes, and claw toes; ingrown toenails in the great toe or the 2nd toe
- Metatarsalgia (lateral)
- Plantar keratosis beneath the 2nd metatarsal head
- Bursitis with pressure erythema over deformed areas

DIAGNOSIS

HISTORY

- Pain over the medial MTP eminence aggravated by tight or rigid footwear is the most common complaint.
- Pain under the 2nd metatarsal head with a plantar keratosis is also common.
- Blisters, swelling, callus formation, or bursitis over the medial eminence may occur with athletic activities.
- Patients may describe forefoot widening or difficulty wearing shoes comfortably. Concern about foot appearance and footwear exists (1)[B]. Numbness or tingling of the medial aspect of the great toe may occur from compression of medial cutaneous nerve.
- May have weight shift and gait compensation to lateral foot resulting in metatarsalgia

ALERT

Lateral metatarsalgia may be presenting complaint (2)[B].

PHYSICAL EXAM

- Note the severity of HV and rotational deformity of the great toe in both the standing and non–weight-bearing positions.
- Assess for alignment of arch and hindfoot.
- Check active and passive range of motion (ROM) at the 1st MTP joint (normal extension is ~70 degrees) and tarsometatarsal joint.
- Evaluate sensation of the great toe.
- Assess for pain and location of great toe sesamoids.
- Evaluate for tightness of the gastrocsoleus complex.

DIFFERENTIAL DIAGNOSIS

- Hallux rigidus (degenerative arthritis of the great toe MTP joint with dorsal bunion)
- Trauma with torn medial capsule
- HV interphalangeus (valgus at the interphalangeal joint, not the MTP joint)
- Gout and other inflammatory conditions
- Osteoarthritis of the 1st MTP joint

DIAGNOSTIC TESTS & INTERPRETATION

Weight-bearing anteroposterior (AP) and lateral foot radiographs along with sesamoid views may be helpful.

ALERT

- Using the AP radiographs, the HV angle (HVA) can be measured. HVA is calculated using the bisection of the longitudinal axes from the proximal phalanx and the 1st metatarsal. HV is >15 degrees with wider angles associated with increased severity.
- The 1st to 2nd IMA is formed by the intersection of the longitudinal axis of the 1st and 2nd metatarsals; normal IMA <9 degrees
- Radiographs can assess MTP joint congruity and presence of arthritis. Subluxation of the MTP, position of the sesamoids, and shape of the metatarsal head are also evaluated (3)[B].

TREATMENT

GENERAL MEASURES

- Initial treatment consists of footwear modification and patient education.
- Wider toe box footwear will help decrease pressure and friction on the medial eminence.
- Shoes with flexible and nonconstricting stitching over the medial eminence are recommended (shoes can be professionally stretched to provide additional room).
- Medial longitudinal arch support may decrease pressure on the 1st metatarsal, especially in patients with pes planus. Custom-fabricated orthotics improve foot pain (4)[A] but do not change radiographic progression (5).
- Activity modification in joggers and runners (substituting bicycling or other nonimpact activities) may significantly decrease symptoms and stress on the forefoot.
- Bunion splints, spacers, and slings/guards may help alleviate symptoms but do not slow progression nor permanently "fix" HV.

MEDICATION

Topical and occasional use of oral nonsteroidal anti-inflammatory drugs (NSAIDs) may be beneficial in decreasing pain and inflammation.

ADDITIONAL THERAPIES

- Felt pads to protect the medial eminence
- Metatarsal pads to help unload the joint
- Treatment of an athlete with HV should be nonoperative until pain and symptoms are significantly affecting athletic performance.

SURGERY/OTHER PROCEDURES

- Surgery should be considered after conservative treatment has failed and is not solely indicated for cosmesis.
- Numerous surgical procedures have been developed to correct HV.
- Operative procedures include various osteotomies and soft tissue releases. MTP fusions are considered in severe HV, arthritic, inflammatory, and/or neuromuscular conditions.
- A distal chevron osteotomy may be beneficial in alleviating pain in mild and moderate HV (4)[A], whereas proximal crescentic osteotomy and distal soft-tissue repair has been used with moderate to severe cases (2)[A].

ONGOING CARE

FOLLOW-UP RECOMMENDATIONS

Patients should be referred for surgical consideration when nonoperative treatments, including footwear and activity modification, have not adequately relieved symptoms.

COMPLICATIONS

- Increased risk of falls secondary to pain and postoperative footwear, especially in the elderly
- Lesser toe deformities and local skin breakdown and ulceration
- Considerations: Stiffness, decreased ROM, and reduced function of the MTP joint are potential risks of surgery and may hamper athletic performance (especially in sprinters and dancers who require MTP motion for strength in toe push off).
- It is important that patients understand that bunion may still be present and not all patients will be able to wear desired shoes.

REFERENCES

1. Nix S, Vicenzino B, Collins N, et al. Characteristics of foot structure and footwear associated with hallux valgus: a systematic review. *Osteoarthritis Cartilage*. 2012;20(10):1059–1074.
2. Coughlin MJ, Jones CP. Hallux valgus and first ray mobility. A prospective study. *J Bone Joint Surg Am*. 2007;89(9):1887–1898.
3. Nix SE, Vicenzino BT, Smith MD. Foot pain and functional limitation in healthy adults with hallux valgus: a cross-sectional study. *BMC Musculoskelet Disord*. 2012;13:197.
4. Torkki M, Malmivaara A, Seitsalo S, et al. Surgery vs orthosis vs watchful waiting for hallux valgus: a randomized controlled trial. *JAMA*. 2001;285(19):2474–2480.
5. Reina M, Lafuente G, Munuera P. Effect of custom-made foot orthoses in female hallux valgus after one-year follow up. *Prosthet Orthot Int*. 2012;37(2):113–119.

ADDITIONAL READING

- Coughlin MJ, Jones CP. Hallux valgus: demographics, etiology, and radiographic assessment. *Foot Ankle Int*. 2007;28(7):759–777.
- Hawke F, Burns J, Radford JA, et al. Custom-made foot orthoses for the treatment of foot pain. *Cochrane Database Syst Rev*. 2008;(3):CD006801.

CLINICAL PEARLS

- HV deformities mostly occur in females with a hereditary predisposition in shod cultures.
- Activity modification, proper footwear, and selective use of orthotic arch supports may be used to control symptoms.
- Refractory symptoms are surgical indication, but the bunion may remain and loss of ROM postoperatively is significant for some athletes.
- Do not confuse with traumatic entity of medial capsule injury.

HAMMER/CLAW/MALLET TOE

Antonio Howard, MBBS, MSc, FAAPMR, CAQSM • Robert D. Martin, MD

BASICS

DESCRIPTION

- Toe joint deformities result from an imbalance between flexor and extensor forces about the interphalangeal (IP) and metatarsophalangeal (MTP) joints. Pain often results from abnormal distribution of pressure and increased friction against other toes or footwear:
  - Mallet toe is a flexion deformity at the distal interphalangeal (DIP) joint.
  - Hammer toe is a flexion deformity affecting the proximal interphalangeal (PIP) joint. Concomitant extension at the MTP joint may be present.
  - Claw toe is a flexion deformity affecting the PIP and DIP joints. Concomitant extension at the MTP joint is always present.
- Acute deformities are usually flexible/reducible. Chronic deformities may become rigid/fixed.

EPIDEMIOLOGY

- Incidence increases with age.
- Female preponderance, especially after age 70 yr
- Claw toe deformity may be present in up to 46% of patients within the first year after a severe stroke.
- Hammer toe deformity is the most common lesser toe deformity. The second toe is most commonly affected.

ETIOLOGY AND PATHOPHYSIOLOGY

Imbalance between flexor and extensor forces about the IP and MTP joints, secondary to:

- Toe crowding in ill-fitting footwear leading to chronic shortening of the flexor tendons and eventual flexion contracture
- Traumatic injury to the:
  - Terminal extensor tendon of the extensor expansion resulting in reduction of extensor forces and predominance of flexor tone at the DIP joint, or
  - Metatarsal/plantar plate resulting in dorsal subluxation of the MTP joint and predominant flexor tone at the IP joints
- Chronic synovitis leading to injury of the terminal extensor tendon, sagittal bands, and/or metatarsal/plantar plate
- Neurologic disease, such as:
  - Peripheral neuropathy and associated intrinsic foot muscle weakness. The foot intrinsic muscles are responsible for flexion at the MTP joint and extension at the IP joints. Weakness of the foot intrinsic muscles with preservation of the long flexor tone leads to the predominance of MTP extension and IP flexion forces that result in claw toe.
  - Spasticity leading to increased tone in the extrinsic muscles of the foot—the long flexors/extensors which overpower the small intrinsic muscles of the foot and have the combined effect of extension at the MTP joint and flexion at the IP joints
- Long flexor tendon contracture as a complication of posterior leg compartment syndrome

RISK FACTORS

- Constricting footwear—high heels, narrow and shallow toe box
- Abnormally long metatarsal and/or toe, relative to adjacent ray
- Neuromuscular disorders (more commonly associated with claw toe deformity), such as:
  - Peripheral neuropathy (e.g., secondary to diabetes mellitus and Charcot-Marie-Tooth disease)
  - Muscular dystrophies
  - Equinovarus associated with spasticity and/or dystonia (e.g., with stroke, cerebral palsy)
- Inflammatory joint disease
- Older age
- High body mass index
- Acute trauma

GENERAL PREVENTION

Avoidance of constrictive footwear

DIAGNOSIS

HISTORY

- Trauma
- Personal or family history of neuromuscular disorder
- Risk factors for peripheral neuropathy: diabetes mellitus, alcohol abuse, renal failure

PHYSICAL EXAM

- Inspect for:
  - Toe deformity and position of the MTP, PIP, and DIP joints. Observations should be made in the weight-bearing and non–weight-bearing position.
  - Signs of abnormal pressure: callous formation (usually dorsal IP joints, at the tip of the toe or at the metatarsal heads on the plantar surface), skin ulcers, injury to nails.
  - Other associated foot/toe deformities: equinovarus, pes planus/cavus, hallux valgus, under-riding or over-riding toes.
  - Gait evaluation: Observe for antalgic gait. Often times, spasticity is more pronounced during ambulation.
  - Palpate to assess for
    - The point of maximal tenderness to guide the need for pressure relief.
    - The presence or absence of synovitis.
    - Joint range of motion.
    - Flexible versus fixed deformity. This may be assessed by passively ranging the MTP and/or IP joints or by moving the ankle into plantar flexion and observing for resolution of hammer or claw toe deformities. Alternatively, dorsally directed pressure on the plantar surface of the involved metatarsal may reduce a flexible hammer toe deformity (push up test).
    - Heel cord tightness using the Silfverskiold test.
    - Neurovascular integrity and muscular tone.
- Examination considerations:
  - Patients should be examined in weight-bearing and non–weight-bearing positions because MTP extension may be more manifest during weight-bearing.
  - Similarly, hammer and claw toe deformities may be less apparent with ankle plantar flexion. Ankle equinus should be manually corrected and the toes reexamined for deformity in this position.
  - It is important to distinguish between flexible versus fixed deformity. If a deformity is completely correctable with manipulation, it is typically considered a "flexible" deformity. Flexible deformities are more likely to respond to nonoperative measures. Fixed deformities are more likely to require surgery.

DIAGNOSTIC TESTS & INTERPRETATION

Initial Tests (lab, imaging)

- Imaging is typically not necessary to make a diagnosis. When obtained, weight-bearing x-rays of the feet—anteroposterior (AP), lateral, and oblique—should
  - Confirm the presence of IP joint deformity and
  - Identify other associated foot abnormalities (e.g., MTP joint subluxation).
- Consider rheumatologic workup as guided by the clinical index of suspicion: erythrocyte sedimentation rate (ESR), C-reactive protein (CRP), complete blood count (CBC), rheumatoid factor (RF), and antinuclear antibody (ANA).
- Advanced imaging—bone scan or magnetic resonance imaging (MRI)—may be indicated in cases of ulceration with suspected underlying osteomyelitis.

Diagnostic Procedures/Other

- Nerve conduction study and electromyography (NCS/EMG) may be useful in the workup for neuromuscular causes.
- Motor nerve blocks with local anesthetic may be helpful in distinguishing between spasticity and contracture.

TREATMENT

GENERAL MEASURES

- Patient education about shoe selection/modification—flat/low heel, wider, and taller toe-box and adequate length (1)[C]. A good rule of thumb is, there should be a circumference of 1 cm around the foot and at the distal tip of the toes when standing on the insole.
- Orthotics/measures to reduce flexible deformities (e.g., Budin splint, figure of 8 taping) (1,2)[C]
- Other pressure relief measures:
  - Toe sleeves, typically with foam padding to relieve pressure over the dorsal toe
  - Toe crests relieve pressure at the tip of the toes.
  - Metatarsal pads relieve pressure under the metatarsal heads.
  - Rocker bottom sole can help reduce forefoot pressure during gait (3)[C].
- Attention to nail care and callous trimming, as necessary

MEDICATION

- Oral analgesics for pain—acetaminophen, nonsteroidal anti-inflammatory drugs (NSAIDs)
- Chemodenervation/neurolysis:
  - Alcohol or phenol neurolysis (e.g., tibial nerve motor branch block to treat equinus)
  - Botulinum toxin injection at muscle motor points in the flexor digitorum longus (FDL) and flexor hallucis longus and brevis (FHL and FHB) muscles (4)[B]
- Medication considerations:
  - Exercise the usual precautions in cases of known liver, renal, gastrointestinal, pulmonary, or cardiac disease.

ISSUES FOR REFERRAL

- Surgery *may* be indicated when nonoperative treatment is unsuccessful in relieving symptoms.
- The acute onset of toe deformity or pain, particularly in the athlete or in the presence of associated trauma, should lead to more prompt and urgent evaluation by a surgeon.

ADDITIONAL THERAPIES

Consider prescribing exercises for heel cord stretching (in subtalar neutral) and foot core strengthening as clinically indicated.

SURGERY/OTHER PROCEDURES

- Differentiation between flexible and rigid deformity must be incorporated into surgical planning:
  - Flexible hammer/claw toes may be repaired with flexor and extensor percutaneous tenotomies (1)[C].
  - Flexible mallet toes may be treated with percutaneous release of the FDL tendon (1)[C].
  - Transfer of the FDL tendon to the extensor mechanism is an option in some flexible deformities (1,5)[C].
  - Rigid deformities often require a capsulotomy or treatment with arthroplasty (joint resection) or arthrodesis (joint fusion) (5)[C].
- Involvement of the MTP joint may require additional soft tissue (i.e., capsulotomy, collateral ligament release, plantar plate repair) and/or bony (i.e., shortening osteotomy) procedures.

ONGOING CARE

FOLLOW-UP RECOMMENDATIONS

In the absence of any pressing surgical indication (e.g., acute trauma or competitive athlete), conservative treatment may be a long-term option given that the patient's expectations are being met, and symptoms do not create significant interruption in activities of daily living (ADLs).

PROGNOSIS

- Surgery may be unnecessary if conservative treatment is started early.
- Postoperative recovery time varies depending on the complexity and invasiveness of the procedure.
- Most patients are allowed to bear weight through the heel immediately following surgical intervention.
- Return to activity is highly dependent on the type of procedure performed. For example, after plantar plate repair, return to play may be delayed for 3 mo following surgery.

COMPLICATIONS

- Fixed toe deformity
- Toenail injury
- Callous formation
- Ulceration with the potential for osteomyelitis
- If surgery is performed:
  - Excessive shortening of the toe may lead to poor motor control of the affected digit.
  - Excessive shortening of the metatarsal may lead to a floating toe in addition to causing transfer metatarsalgia (adjacent metatarsal pain).
  - Persistent numbness of the toe and surrounding areas may occur as a result of nerve injury.
  - FDL tendon transfer results in the inability to actively flex the affected toe.

REFERENCES

1. Frey-Ollivier S, Catena F, Hélix-Giordanino M, et al. Treatment of flexible lesser toe deformities. *Foot Ankle Clin*. 2018;23(1):69–90.
2. Federer AE, Tainter DM, Adams SB, et al. Conservative management of metatarsalgia and lesser toe deformities. *Foot Ankle Clin*. 2018;23(1):9–20.
3. Malhotra K, Davda K, Singh D. The pathology and management of lesser toe deformities. *EFORT Open Rev*. 2017;1(11):409–419.
4. Lim EC, Ong BK, Seet RC. Botulinum toxin-A injections for spastic toe clawing. *Parkinsonism Relat Disord*. 2006;12(1):43–47.
5. Shirzad K, Kiesau CD, DeOrio JK, et al. Lesser toe deformities. *J Am Acad Orthop Surg*. 2011;19(8):505–514.

ADDITIONAL READING

- Hagedorn TJ, Dufour AB, Riskowski JL, et al. Foot disorders, foot posture, and foot function: the Framingham foot study. *PLoS One*. 2013;8(9):e74364.
- Hannan MT, Menz HB, Jordan JM, et al. High heritability of hallux valgus and lesser toe deformities in adult men and women. *Arthritis Care Res (Hoboken)*. 2013;65(9):1515–1521.
- Laurent G, Valentini F, Loiseau K, et al. Claw toes in hemiplegic patients after stroke. *Ann Phys Rehabil Med*. 2010;53(2):77–85.

CLINICAL PEARLS

- Remember: The joint will deform or pull to the strong (intact) side.
- Injecting botulinum toxin to both the long and the short flexors of the toes is well tolerated and efficacious in the treatment of toe clawing from spasticity, allowing for lower dosages to be used than injecting the long flexors alone.
- Surgery for cosmesis alone should be strongly discouraged.

HAMSTRING STRAIN

Alan Shahtaji, DO, CAQSM

BASICS

DESCRIPTION

- Hamstring injuries are among the most common reported muscle injuries in sports medicine.
- The musculotendinous unit (biceps femoris [BF], semitendinosus [ST], and semimembranosus [SM]) can be injured at multiple sites, including the proximal bony attachment, the proximal free tendon, the musculotendinous junction, the intramuscular tendon, the central muscle belly, and the distal tendon.
- The injury often occurs due to an excessive load during an eccentric contraction, such as with running or jumping.
- Time lost to this injury is significant, and rate of recurrence is high among athletes.
- Proximal hamstring tendinopathy is often a chronic process seen in runners.

EPIDEMIOLOGY

The BF is the most commonly injured muscle, with the myotendinous junction being most often affected.

Prevalence

- Research has focused on male athletes, but no gender predisposition exists.
- Incidence has been reported in high-level soccer clubs to be 22% over the course of a season.
- Prevalence rates vary but have been reported up to 29%.
- Reinjury is common and is reported at rates of 12–31%.

ETIOLOGY AND PATHOPHYSIOLOGY

- Strains are classified by severity of muscle fiber injury:
  - Mild strain (1st degree): stretch type injury with few muscle fibers injured, causing only minor swelling/pain and minimal loss of strength/motion
  - Moderate strain (2nd degree): partial tear with strength loss and functional limitations due to more extensive muscle injury
  - Severe strain (3rd degree): extensive or complete tear across whole muscle with disabling loss of muscle function
  - Magnetic resonance imaging (MRI) classifications vary and are either based on extent of edema and signal change versus location of injury.
  - The healing process in muscle injury includes initial muscle fiber insult with immediate hemorrhage followed by inflammatory cell introduction to the damaged tissue, production of connective scar tissue, and regeneration of damaged muscle fibers.
- The hamstring musculotendinous unit (BF, ST, and SM) is susceptible to injury for many reasons:
  - The hamstrings cross two joints, which can be moving in opposing directions.
  - The short head of the BF has a long, inconstant origin along the femur.
  - The hamstrings (specifically the biceps) have dual innervation, which causes forceful, uncoordinated contractions (the hamstrings, including the long head of the biceps, are innervated by the tibial branch of the sciatic nerve, with the exception being the short head of the biceps, which alone is innervated by the peroneal branch of the sciatic nerve).
  - During the gait cycle, the hamstrings have differing activity (the SM has increased eccentric activity to slow hip flexion during the swing phase, whereas the biceps are most active during takeoff).
- The usual mechanism of injury occurs in the later part of the swing phase as the hamstrings rapidly change from eccentrically working to decelerate knee extension to concentrically becoming an extensor of the hip.

RISK FACTORS

Strength imbalances, flexibility, core strength, lumbopelvic position, and fatigue have been quoted as risk factors.

ALERT

The only consistent finding is that previous history of hamstring injury increases risk of reinjury by 2 to 6 times. A proposed multifactorial model for hamstring injury includes poor flexibility, strength imbalances, inadequate warm-up, and muscle fatigue.

GENERAL PREVENTION

Primary prevention of acute hamstring injuries has been proven highly effective with use of Nordic hamstring exercises. Adherence and compliance are key factors (1)[A].

COMMONLY ASSOCIATED CONDITIONS

Pediatric Considerations

Apophyseal injury, such as traction apophysitis (found in children when the ischial apophysis appears at ages 13 to 15 yr and up to ages 20 to 25 yr when it fuses with the pelvis):

- Proximal avulsion injuries at the ischial tuberosity can occur with eccentric contraction during knee extension with hip flexion (i.e., hurdling in track with lead leg).
- Complete tendon rupture, with or without avulsion fracture (found mostly in adults, more commonly proximal at the ischium vs. distal, which is rare)

DIAGNOSIS

Most hamstring strain injuries occur in an acute setting with sudden onset of posterior thigh pain that often limits participation. The diagnosis can be made with history and physical exam.

HISTORY

- Hamstring strain is most commonly seen in kicking or speed athletes.
- In cases of avulsion injury, other activities are often reported, such as water skiing, dance, weight lifting, and ice skating.
- Acute or chronic:
  - Some hamstring strain injuries are more chronic in nature with recurring "tightness" or muscle "pull" complaints.
  - Treatment protocol is different for acute versus chronic injury as well as for initial versus recurrent injury.
- Severity: Discontinuation of activity, inability to ambulate following the injury, and/or describing an audible pop at the time of injury can point toward a more severe strain or an avulsion injury.
- Location of pain (distal, mid, or proximal posterior thigh)

PHYSICAL EXAM

- A "stiff-legged" gait may occur as patient tries to avoid hip flexion with knee extension.
- Position patient prone and inspect for swelling and/or ecchymosis.
- Palpate the entire length of each hamstring muscle going from common origin on ischial tuberosity moving distally until insertion on fibular head (BF), medial femur (SM), and medial tibia (ST).
- Note location of pain and also if any defect appreciated; active range of motion, strength, flexibility, and neurovascular testing of bilateral lower extremities
- Note severity of injury using maximal tolerance of passive straight leg raise/knee extension.

DIFFERENTIAL DIAGNOSIS

In addition to the associated injuries listed above, consider these in the differential diagnosis (2)[C]:

- Direct hamstring injury, including muscle laceration or contusion (common direct mechanism for injury as opposed to indirect strain mechanism)
- Posterior lateral corner knee injury, meniscal injury, or popliteal cyst formation or rupture
- Pelvic or proximal femoral stress fracture
- Piriformis syndrome, gluteus medius injury, or adductor strain
- Pain radiating from the lumbar back, sacroiliac joint, or hip

DIAGNOSTIC TESTS & INTERPRETATION

- Further examination beyond the physical exam is not typically necessary, but, if needed, radiographs, MRI, and sonography may be useful.
- Radiographs: Anteroposterior pelvis can be helpful acutely if an avulsion is suspected.

- Ultrasound (US) and MRI can help determine more accurate location and extent of injury (2)[C]:
  - US is as useful as MRI for acute hamstring injury and has added benefit of low cost.
  - MRI images of an acute injury appear as high signal in or around the muscle on T2-weighted images.
  - There is no significant change in MRI appearance over the first 7 days after acute hamstring injury.
  - MRI findings do not reliably predict time for return to play (RTP) (3)[A].
  - There is debate in the literature regarding the significance of injury to intramuscular tendon.

TREATMENT

- The treatment protocol is different for acute versus chronic injury as well as for initial versus recurrent injury. Location and type of injury also dictate treatment considerations (1,4)[A],(2)[C].
- The protocol should be individualized for the patient and have a criteria-based progression (5)[C].
- Acute:
  - Goals: control pain, swelling, hemorrhage, and muscle fiber adhesion; work toward restoration of normal gait (5)[C]
  - Treatment:
    - Protection, rest, ice, compression, and elevation (PRICE):
      - Avoid nonsteroidal anti-inflammatory drugs (NSAIDs) because no proven benefit and may disrupt natural healing process; also, risk of side effects (4)[A],(5)[C]
      - Platelet-rich plasma (PRP) has not been shown to be effective for reducing time to RTP (5)[C],(6)[A].
- Subacute/rehab and functional (days to weeks/months):
  - Goals: advance activity as tolerated and work toward regaining strength, flexibility, and psychological readiness (5)[C]
  - Treatment:
    - Several different protocols exist, and hamstring rehabilitation could be an entire chapter unto itself. Criteria-based programs are being employed at most sports medicine institutions.
    - There is variability but attention to core strength, neuromuscular influences, and lumbar stability (4)[A],(5)[C].
    - Gradual movement away from traditional sequential progression of isometric > concentric > eccentric hamstring exercises; may be able to incorporate eccentric load early in rehab based on patient tolerance (1)[A],(5)[C]:
      - Eccentric or lengthening programs tend to have better outcomes when compared to concentric-based rehab (1)[A],(5)[C].
      - Nordic hamstring exercises are effective in preventing recurrent hamstring injuries (1)[A].
- RTP:
  - Goals: safe and timely RTP with best possible functionality and least risk of repeat injury
  - MRI imaging at time of injury or at RTP is not necessary and not predictive in majority of cases (3,6)[A].
  - In nonprofessional athletes with grade 1 or grade 2 injuries, prognostic factors may include patient's predicted time to RTP and passive straight leg raise deficit (3)[A].
  - Treatment:
    - May RTP when able to perform pain-free sport-specific activity along with a normal physical examination and psychological readiness (3)[A],(5)[C]
    - Use sports medicine RTP models nonspecific to hamstring injuries that incorporate biopsychosocial influences.

SURGERY/OTHER PROCEDURES

- Surgical referral should be considered in proximal injuries with bony avulsions that are >2 cm displaced, two tendons that are retracted ≥2cm, or three tendon avulsions (2)[C].
- Distal tendon avulsions are less common but deserve special attention and may need primary surgical intervention, especially in high-level athletes (2)[C].
- Patients with proximal injuries that do not recover may develop hamstring syndrome, and surgical options exist for symptom relief (2)[C].

ONGOING CARE

FOLLOW-UP RECOMMENDATIONS

- Recovery time after hamstring strain injury can be as short as 2 wk and as long as several months, depending on the severity and chronicity of the injury.
- Although reinjury is common, proper functional rehab and appropriate RTP can minimize the risk.
- Maintenance and prevention protocols should focus on eccentric-based exercises and modifiable risk factors.

REFERENCES

1. Goode AP, Reiman MP, Harris L, et al. Eccentric training for prevention of hamstring injuries may depend on intervention compliance: a systematic review and meta-analysis. *Br J Sports Med*. 2015;49(6):349–356.
2. Ahmad C, Redler L, Ciccotti M, et al. Evaluation and management of hamstring injuries. *Am J Sports Med*. 2013;41(12):2933–2947.
3. Moen MH, Reurink G, Weir A, et al. Predicting return to play after hamstring injuries. *Br J Sports Med*. 2014;48:1358–1363.
4. Reurink G, Goudswaard G, Tol J, et al. Therapeutic interventions for acute hamstring injuries: a systematic review. *Br J Sports Med*. 2012;46(2):103–109.
5. Valle X, L Tol J, Hamilton B, et al. Hamstring muscle injuries, a rehabilitation protocol purpose. *Asian J Sports Med*. 2015;6(4):e25411.
6. Reurink G, Goudswaard GJ, Moen MH, et al. Platelet-rich plasma injections in acute muscle injury. *N Engl J Med*. 2014;370(26):2546–2547.

ADDITIONAL READING

- A Hamid MS, Mohamed Ali MR, Yusof A, et al. Platelet-rich plasma injections for the treatment of hamstring injuries: a randomized controlled trial. *Am J Sports Med*. 2014;42(10):2410–2418.
- Askling CM, Tengvar M, Thorstensson A. Acute hamstring injuries in Swedish elite football: a prospective randomised controlled clinical trial comparing two rehabilitation protocols. *Br J Sports Med*. 2013;47(15):953–959.
- Brukner P, Connell D. 'Serious thigh muscle strains': beware the intramuscular tendon which plays an important role in difficult hamstring and quadriceps muscle strains. *Br J Sports Med*. 2016;50(4):205–208.
- Reurink G. Managing acute hamstring injuries in athletes. *Br J Sports Med*. 2016;51(7):1–2.
- van der Horst N, Backx F, Goedhart EA, et al. Return to play after hamstring injuries in football (soccer): a worldwide Delphi procedure regarding definition, medical criteria and decision-making. *Br J Sports Med*. 2017;51(22):1583–1591.
- van der Made AD, Almusa E, Whiteley R, et al. Intramuscular tendon involvement on MRI has limited value for predicting time to return to play following acute hamstring injury. *Br J Sports Med*. 2018;52(2):83–88.
- Wangensteen A, Bahr R, Van Linschoten R, et al. MRI appearance does not change in the first 7 days after acute hamstring injury—a prospective study. *Br J Sports Med*. 2017;51(14):1087–1092.

CLINICAL PEARLS

- Previous history of hamstring injury is a significant risk factor for hamstring strain injury.
- Compliance with Nordic hamstring protocols is essential for prevention of hamstring injuries.
- Functional rehab with criteria-based progression and incorporation of eccentric strengthening is effective for acute hamstring injuries.
- There is no evidence to support PRP for RTP.
- The utility of MRI is questionable and does not seem to predict RTP in amateur athletes.
- Severe proximal and distal injuries may require surgery.

HEEL PAIN: HEEL FAT PAD SYNDROME, LATERAL PLANTAR NERVE ENTRAPMENT

Reno Ravindran, MD, CAQSM • Richard E. Rodenberg, MD, FAAP, CAQSM • Thomas L. Pommering, DO, FAAFP

BASICS

DESCRIPTION

- Heel fat pad syndrome:
  - The heel pad is composed of columns of adipose tissue (globules) separated by fibrous septae extending from the skin to the calcaneal periosteum.
  - The fibroelastic septae are arranged in a honeycombed structure, which runs vertically, diagonally, and transversely.
  - The encapsulated fat acts in a hydraulic fashion to absorb shock by resisting compressive loads.
  - The heel pad is located directly below the calcaneus and acts as a shock-absorbing layer allowing the heel to tolerate repetitive high load bearing, allowing for pain-free ambulation (1,2).
- Lateral plantar nerve (LPN) entrapment:
  - LPN and the first branch of the LPN (FBLPN) are branches of the tibial nerve, which supplies autonomic, sensory, and motor fibers to the plantar foot. The LPN is the most common cause of plantar heel pain of neural origin (3).
- Synonym(s): calcaneodynia; heel pain syndrome; heel pad atrophy; calcaneal neuritis; policeman's heel; runner's heel; tennis heel; stone bruise; tuber calcanei pain; subcalcaneobursitis

EPIDEMIOLOGY

- 1 in 10 people develop heel pain in their lifetime.
- Peak age 40 to 60 yr (2)
- More common with increasing age, obesity, and diabetes
- LPN: relationship with long-distance running and sports that require repetitive hyperdorsiflexion (4)
- More common with prolonged standing or walking on hard surfaces (2)

ETIOLOGY AND PATHOPHYSIOLOGY

- Heel fat pad syndrome:
  - With aging, the heel pad becomes less elastic, making the patient more prone to atrophy of the pad which results in less shock absorption.
  - Trauma and inflammation may also lead to degeneration of the heel pad or rupture of the fibrous tissue septa, leading to decreased compressibility and heel pad atrophy.
  - The cause is often multifactorial leading to heel pad atrophy and pain (1,2).
- LPN entrapment can occur at different sites:
  - Where the nerve passes at the sharp edge of the deep fascia of the abductor hallucis
  - Distal to the medial edge of the calcaneus
  - Between the abductor hallucis and the medial head of quadratus plantae muscle (3,4)
  - Predisposing factors include abductor hallucis, muscle hypertrophy, local trauma, local venous engorgement, or calcaneal enthesophytes.

RISK FACTORS

- Elderly, advancing age
- Obesity
- Prolonged standing, walking, and running on hard surfaces
- Overuse in recreational and athletic activities
- Poorly constructed shoes
- Repetitive steroid injection due to potential for heel pad atrophy (2)
- Possible associated altered biomechanics, including hyperpronation, decreased ankle dorsiflexion, decreased metatarsophalangeal joint extension, pes cavus, and pes planus
- Presence and absence of heel spurs do not correlate with heel pain.

DIAGNOSIS

HISTORY

- Gradual onset of plantar heel pain, which may be unilateral or bilateral
- May have a history of local trauma
- Pain may radiate into the arch or proximally to the medial heel area.
- If pain is severe enough, a patient may walk on the ball or lateral aspect of the foot.
- Heel fat pad syndrome:
  - Pain primarily with weight-bearing and relieved with rest
  - Symptoms can be exacerbated by walking barefoot or on hard surfaces.
  - Pain described as deep and nonradiating involving the central weight-bearing portion of the calcaneal tuberosity and commonly misdiagnosed as plantar fasciitis.
  - Pain does not tend to radiate or increase with dorsiflexion (1,2)[C].
- LPN entrapment:
  - Burning, sharp, shooting, shock-like pain; localized to the medial inferior aspect of the heel and proximally into the medial ankle region. Pain may radiate across the plantar aspect of the heel to the lateral aspect of the foot.
  - Pain worse during or after weight-bearing activities and improves with rest
  - Pain at night may be due to nerve compression as a result of venostasis and venous engorgement.
  - Poststatic dyskinesia: plantar heel pain when patient first stands after periods of rest; can be typical in patients with heel pain of neural origin, but this can also occur in plantar fasciitis
  - Sensory deficit may not be common but occasionally, can cause tingling and/or numbness in the heel or foot (3)[C].

PHYSICAL EXAM

- Heel fat pad syndrome:
  - Thorough examination of the lower extremity, including neurovascular exam, is recommended.
  - Exam is facilitated by having the patient lie prone.
  - Observe for any signs of fat pad atrophy.
  - Observe gait for signs of pes planus, pes cavus, hindfoot deformity, hyperpronation, as well as look for indications of posterior tibial tendon dysfunction.
  - Observe ankle range of motion (ROM) and pain is not reproducible with passive motion of the ankles or toes.
  - Tenderness directly over the central weight-bearing portion of the calcaneal tuberosity rather than on the distal tuberosity
  - Typically, negative calcaneal squeeze test
  - In prolonged cases, the underlying bone can be felt underneath the skin due to significant fat pad atrophy (1,2).
- LPN entrapment:
  - Palpation over the FBLPN deep to the abductor hallucis muscle or medial calcaneal tuberosity with reproduction of pain/symptoms proximally and distally; should have minimal tenderness over the plantar fascia origin
  - Dorsiflexion with eversion of the ankle can reproduce symptoms; although not specific, can help with diagnosis
  - Plantar flexion-inversion may reproduce symptoms, although not specific (5)[C].
  - Positive Tinel test (4)[C]

DIFFERENTIAL DIAGNOSIS

- Calcaneal fracture or stress fracture
- Plantar fasciitis/fasciopathy
- Plantar aponeurosis rupture
- Local inflammatory conditions (subcalcaneal bursitis, osteomyelitis, tendonitis/tenosynovitis)
- Systemic inflammatory conditions (enthesitis, ankylosing spondylitis, Reiter syndrome, psoriatic arthritis, rheumatoid arthritis, inflammatory bowel–induced inflammation, gout, and pseudogout)
- Entrapment neuropathy (tarsal tunnel syndrome, medial calcaneal nerve, LPN/Baxter nerve)
- Infectious (osteomyelitis, tuberculosis)
- Benign neoplasm: (glomus tumor of heel pad, osteoid osteoma, intraosseous lipoma, giant cell tumor)
- Malignant neoplasm: (osteogenic sarcoma, chondrosarcoma, Ewing sarcoma, metastatic tumor)
- Neuropathy (diabetes mellitus, alcoholism, reflex sympathetic dystrophy)
- Metabolic (osteomalacia, Paget disease)
- Calcaneal apophysitis
- Referred pain from the low back (S1 radiculopathy) (2)

DIAGNOSTIC TESTS & INTERPRETATION

Initial Tests (lab, imaging)

- Radiographic studies are typically not needed to diagnose heel fat pad syndrome or LPN but can be used to rule in or out other diagnoses in the differential (2)[C].
- Anteroposterior, lateral, and oblique plain radiographs. Radiographs may reveal calcaneal spurs or calcifications, fractures, tumors, arthrosis, or other unusual causes of heel pain.
- High-resolution ultrasound (US) or magnetic resonance imaging (MRI) to look for benign tumors or neuromas entrapping a nerve
- MRI may reveal edema in abductor hallucis or quadratus plantae muscle or surrounding fascia (5)[C].
- Lumbar spine radiographs and MRI to rule out causes of lumbar radiculopathy
- Consider bone scan or MRI to rule out suspected stress fracture.

Diagnostic Procedures/Other

LPN:

- Electromyography and nerve conduction studies can reveal abnormalities in LPN (6)[C].
- Quantitative sensory testing, also known as the pressure-specified sensory device, determines pain mechanisms by assessing function of large and small sensory nerve fibers.
- If nerve entrapment is suggested by history and exam, a diagnostic injection with local anesthetic providing complete pain relief can help with diagnosis (4)[C].

TREATMENT

- The earlier treatment is started generally lends to improvement in most patients.
- Nonsteroidal anti-inflammatory drug (NSAID) of choice
- Rest, modified weight-bearing activities
- Injections of local anesthetics/steroids at site of nerve entrapment for LPN. Caution should be exercised with repeated injections of steroid or improper technique due to the risk of irreversible damage to the heel pad by mechanical disruption of the heel septae and by steroid-induced fat necrosis (4,5)[C].
- Immobilization rarely necessary, symptom directed
- Orthotics, heel cups
- Treatment of other associated conditions (e.g., night splints in plantar fasciitis)

ADDITIONAL THERAPIES

Various methods for altering the biomechanical forces on the heel have been advocated but little evidence-based proof is available:

- Low-quality evidence for shock wave therapy (6)[A]
- Low-quality evidence that orthoses were effective in the reduction of heel pain. A well-fitted heel cup cushions the heel and prevents the heel pad from splaying, thereby improving the intrinsic cushioning of the calcaneus. There is no consensus as to which type of orthosis is best. Regardless of whether over-the-counter heel cups/orthoses versus custom orthoses are used; consistent features should be support of the arch, presence of adequate cushioning material, recess for area of pain beneath the heel, and slight medial elevation (6)[A].
- Moderate quality evidence that low-level laser therapy, dry-needling of lower leg and foot muscle trigger points, and calcaneal taping were effective in the reduction of persistent heel pain. Taping of the heel in fat pad syndrome can provide support and limit movement of the heel's fat pad (6)[A].
- High-quality evidence that ultrasound-guided pulsed radiofrequency (USGPRF) achieved heel pain reduction (6)[A].
- Weight control
- Shoes with softer midsoles, which provide more cushioning of the fat pad
- Raising the heel may thereby transfer the weight-bearing anteriorly with heel strike and in midstance.
- Medial heel wedge to relieve the pressure on the medial tuberosity, causing more lateral pressure
- Physical therapy to focus on Achilles tendon and plantar fascia flexibility and strengthening of foot intrinsics and the ankle (5)[C]

SURGERY/OTHER PROCEDURES

- Heel fat pad syndrome:
  - Surgery is reserved for patients when conservative treatment fails to provide adequate pain relief and should be considered a last resort. There are no proven techniques that can recreate or replace the normal anatomy of the heel pad (1)[C].
  - Surgical options are directed toward the cause of heel pain and include spur resection, wide release of plantar fascia, drilling decompression, and neurolysis.
  - It is important to have an exact diagnosis of the pain before surgical intervention due to the multifactorial and often recurrent nature of plantar heel pain.
- LPN entrapment:
  - Considered after failure of conservative treatment for 6 to 12 mo (5)[C]
  - Surgical nerve decompression of the first branch of LPN or fascial release provides good to excellent results in >85% of surgically treated patients (4)[C].

ONGOING CARE

FOLLOW-UP RECOMMENDATIONS

- Heel fat pad syndrome responds very well to conservative treatment and is usually self-limited.
- LPN: Approximately 90% of patients improve with nonoperative management.
- 52% of patients required at least 6 mo to reach maximum improvement (5)[C].

REFERENCES

1. Lareau C, Sawyer G, Wang JH, et al. Plantar and medial heel pain: diagnosis and management. *J Am Acad Orthop Surg*. 2014;22(6):372–380.
2. Hossain M, Makwana N. "Not plantar fasciitis": the differential diagnosis and management of heel pain syndrome. *Orthop Trauma*. 2011;25(3):198–206.
3. Alshami AM, Souvlis T, Coppieters MW. A review of plantar heel pain of neural origin: differential diagnosis and management. *Man Ther*. 2008;13(2):103–111.
4. Ferkel E, Davis WH, Ellington JK. Entrapment neuropathies of the foot and ankle. *Clin Sports Med*. 2015;34(4):791–801.
5. Meadows JR, Finnoff JT. Lower extremity nerve entrapment in athletes. *Curr Sports Med Rep*. 2014;13(5):299–306.
6. Salvioli S, Guidi M, Marcotulli G. The effectiveness of conservative, non-pharmacological treatment, of plantar heel pain: a systematic review with meta-analysis. *Foot (Edinb)*. 2017;33:57–67.

ADDITIONAL READING

- Aldridge T. Diagnosing heel pain in adults. *Am Fam Physician*. 2004;70(2):332–338.
- Alvarez-Nemegyei J, Canoso JJ. Heel pain: diagnosis and treatment, step by step. *Cleve Clin J Med*. 2006;73(5):465–471.
- Bateman JE. *Disorders of the Foot and Ankle, Medical and Surgical Management*. Philadelphia, PA: WB Saunders; 1991.
- Franson J, Baravarian B. Tarsal tunnel syndrome: a compression neuropathy involving four distinct tunnels. *Clin Podiatr Med Surg*. 2006;23(3):597–609.
- Toomey EP. Plantar heel pain. *Foot Ankle Clin*. 2009;14(2):229–245.

CLINICAL PEARLS

- Both soft heel cups and more rigid ones have been used with some success. The hard cups are intended to encompass the heel pad beneath the calcaneus, helping to restore some of its compressibility. The softer cups are designed primarily to cushion the fat pad. Athletes who run a lot in their sport often prefer softer heel cups or orthotics.
- To prevent heel fat pad syndrome, training errors should be identified and corrected. The athlete should wear proper shoes with an energy-absorbing heel cushion, avoiding excessive wear of the shoes. Mileage should be increased gradually, and running on steep hills should be avoided. Training on safe and shock-absorbing surfaces is essential (e.g., running on an all-weather track or on a surface softer than concrete or asphalt).

HEMATOMAS, EPIDURAL AND SUBDURAL

Greg Nakamoto, MD, FACP

BASICS

DESCRIPTION

- Both epidural hematoma (EDH) and subdural hematoma (SDH) are structural brain injuries that can result from traumatic brain injury (TBI). However, they can follow different courses and have different prognoses.
- In EDH, blood is confined to the space between the inner table of the calvaria (inner surface of the skull and the dura mater).
- In SDH, localized bleeding occurs below the dura mater, directly adjacent to brain parenchyma.
- SDH can be acute or chronic (this topic focuses on acute SDH, commonly defined as an SDH diagnosed within 72 hr of TBI).
- Successful treatment of EDH and acute SDH involves treatment principles of TBI as well as considerations specific to EDH and SDH.
- Synonyms:
  - EDH: epidural hemorrhage, extradural hematoma, extradural hemorrhage
  - SDH: subdural hemorrhage
  - EDH and SDH: intracranial hematoma, intracranial hemorrhage, extra-axial hematoma, extra-axial hemorrhage

ALERT

EDH and acute SDH are neurosurgical emergencies. With prompt appropriate treatment, a patient with an EDH can often achieve complete neurologic recovery, whereas a missed diagnosis may result in death within hours. Mortality for patients with acute SDH is much higher (36–79%) due to greater associated underlying injury to the brain tissue itself.

EPIDEMIOLOGY

- EDH: Incidence is reported between 2.7% and 4% of TBI admissions (1):
  - Peak incidence is in the 2nd decade.
  - More frequently located in temporoparietal and temporal regions of the skull, with a slight right-sided predominance; bilateral in 2–5% of patients
  - Typically attributed to bleeding from the middle meningeal artery due to a temporal skull fracture. Other sources of EDH blood include the middle meningeal vein, the diploic veins, or the venous sinuses.
- Acute SDH: Incidence is reported between 12% and 29% of TBI admissions (2):
  - Mean age reported to be between 31 and 47 yr, with the vast majority being male
  - Most SDH are caused by motor vehicle accidents (MVAs), falls, and assaults; predominant mechanism varies by age.
  - Acute SDH occurs either secondary to a parenchymal laceration (which implies a severe underlying brain tissue injury) or due to disruption of a surface or bridging vessel (in which case underlying brain injury may be less severe).
  - SDH is the most common athletic injury resulting in death.

RISK FACTORS

- EDH and SDH: high-energy head trauma
- SDH: Bridging veins can be torn during acceleration-deceleration injuries without actual head impact.

COMMONLY ASSOCIATED CONDITIONS

- EDH: associated temporal or other skull fracture
- SDH: underlying brain parenchymal injury
- EDH and SDH:
  - Sequelae of increased intracranial pressure (ICP), including obtundation, Cushing reflex, respiratory distress, and death
  - Due to high-energy mechanisms of injury, cervical spine and other orthopedic trauma are often seen.

DIAGNOSIS

Prehospital:

- EDH: <50% of the patients have the classically described "lucid interval" that is commonly associated with EDH (1):
  - Patient suffers TBI, which is often followed by an initial period of altered consciousness.
  - The patient subsequently improves, exhibiting for a period of the appearance of recovery.
  - The period of improvement, however, ends with secondary deterioration of the patient's mental status, ending the so-called "lucid interval."
- SDH: Lucid interval has been described in between 12–38% of patients with SDH (2):
  - Between 37% and 80% of patients with acute SDH present with initial Glasgow Coma Scale (GCS) scores of 8 or less, thus meeting criteria for severe head injury (2).

HISTORY

- Mechanism: Higher energy trauma resulting in skull fracture is a risk factor for EDH. Acute SDH due to high-energy trauma implies more underlying brain tissue damage. Also, mechanism of injury can guide the search for associated traumas in the poorly responsive patient.
- Lucid interval: more common with EDH
- Deterioration in mental status: Regardless of mechanism or level of recovery after initial injury, any patient with a deterioration of mental status after TBI should be evaluated for a possible neurosurgical emergency.

PHYSICAL EXAM

- Trauma assessment as necessitated by search for coexisting injuries
- Complete neurologic exam initially, followed by serial exams to assess for herniation (ipsilateral pupillary dilatation, contralateral hemiparesis) and signs of increased ICP (obtundation, hypertension, bradycardia, respiratory depression)
- Calculation of GCS, which helps guide treatment (mild TBI: GCS ≥13; moderate TBI: GCS 9 to 12; severe TBI: GCS ≤8)
- EDH: skull exam to look for fracture

DIFFERENTIAL DIAGNOSIS

- Concussion
- Uncomplicated skull fracture
- Intracerebral hemorrhage/cerebrovascular accident
- Subarachnoid hemorrhage
- Second-impact syndrome

DIAGNOSTIC TESTS & INTERPRETATION

- Perform appropriate laboratories for any associated trauma and coagulation studies for neurosurgical planning.
- In infants, EDH in an expansile cranium with open sutures can result in significant blood loss and resultant hemodynamic instability. Therefore, in infants with EDH, careful monitoring of the hematocrit is also warranted.
- Computed tomography (CT) is the study of choice in EDH and SDH (1,2)[A]:
  - EDH: Lesion is hyperdense (acute blood), biconvex, sharply demarcated, and adjacent to the skull; mass effect is common.
  - SDH: Lesion can be slightly less dense than in EDH (from mixing with cerebrospinal fluid (CSF)), concave, and conforming to the underlying brain; accompanying parenchymal injury and edema may be seen; may become isodense with brain parenchyma as early as 4 days

TREATMENT

In addition to the primary structural injury caused by TBI, neurotrauma also results in an inflammatory response that causes secondary brain injury. Targeting elements that are believed to contribute to secondary injury and minimizing ICP are the goals of presurgical neuroresuscitation (3,4).

GENERAL MEASURES

- Prehospital:
  - As would be expected for any trauma patient:
    - Stabilize vital signs, achieve airway control, support blood pressure (BP), and address acute life-threatening injuries.
    - Establish intravenous (IV) access.
    - Cervical spine precautions as indicated
- Emergency room (ER) treatment:
  - Complete prehospital care steps not already addressed as per *Advanced Trauma Life Support* guidelines
  - If intubation is indicated, consider esmolol at 1.5 mg/kg IV to blunt the hemodynamic response to intubation (use only if hypotension not a concern) (3)[C]. Preferred induction agents include ketamine and etomidate (for their hemodynamic sparing properties) or fentanyl (for neuroprotective effects although can lead to hypotension) (3)[C].
  - Once spine is cleared, **elevate the head of the bed** to 30 degrees to reduce ICP and increase venous drainage (3)[C].
  - Maintain **systolic BP** >100 mm Hg (>110 mm Hg if >70 yr of age) or mean arterial pressure (MAP) >70 to 80 mm Hg (3,5)[B].
  - Maintain goal **temperature** between 36°C and 38°C (3)[C]. Moderate hypothermia (goal temperature of 32–34°C) may be used as a short-term intervention (2 to 3 days) to decrease refractory elevated ICP (3)[C].
  - Consider phenytoin to reduce early posttraumatic (within 7 days of injury) **seizures** (3,5)[C].
  - Once the patient is stabilized and any suspected ICP elevation is controlled, **head CT** is the preferred imaging modality in TBI (1,2)[A].
  - **If clinical signs of increased ICP despite the above**, then consider osmotic agents (mannitol or hypertonic saline), followed by propofol or pentobarbital coma and hyperventilation:
    - Mannitol 0.25 to 1.0 g/kg IV bolus; avoid in hypotensive patients due to diuretic effects (3,5)[C].
    - **Hypertonic saline** 3% 150 to 250 mL IV boluses, with goal serum sodium >145 mEq/L (maximum 155 to 160 mEq/L) (3)[C]
    - Propofol 1 to 3 mg/kg IV bolus to reduce ICP, followed by infusion of 200 μg/kg/min (3)[B]; although indicated to reduce ICP, has not been shown to improve mortality or 6-mo outcomes (5)

- Pentobarbital coma to control ICP not responsive to maximum standard measures (5)[B]: bolus of 10 mg/kg IV over 30 min, followed by 5 mg/kg/hr IV for 3 hr and maintenance of 1 to 4 mg/kg/hr; may be continued for 24 to 96 hr (3)[C]
- **Hyperventilation** targeting $Paco_2$ to 30 to 35 mm Hg may be considered; avoid during first 24 hr when cerebral blood flow is often reduced; should be viewed as a short-term intervention for patients with life-threatening elevated ICP (5)[B]

– Reversal of coagulopathy and platelet inhibition:
  - Coagulopathy can be due to patient medications, resuscitation-related hemodilution, or the release of tissue factor from damaged brain tissue (3,4).
  - Correction of coagulopathy in TBI (including in patients taking anticoagulants for medical reasons) is necessary for patients undergoing cranial surgery, requiring ICP monitor placement, and suffering from intracranial hemorrhage (including EDH and SDH) (4)[C].
  - Patients on warfarin can be given vitamin K 10 mg IV push and either prothrombin complex concentrate or fresh frozen plasma (3)[C].
  - Patients on **novel oral anticoagulants** can be given prothrombin complex concentrate or medication-specific antidotes (3)[C].
  - **Platelet inhibitors** should be discontinued. Platelet transfusion is usually limited to surgical patients only to maintain a level >75,000. Despite lack of evidence, some guidelines recommend a single dose of desmopressin (DDAVP; 0.4 μg/kg IV) in patients with intracranial hemorrhage on platelet inhibitors (6)[C].

– **ICP monitoring:**
  - Patients with a GCS ≤8, any acute abnormality on CT (hematomas, contusions, swelling, herniation, or compressed basal cisterns), or a systolic BP <90 mm Hg should undergo placement of an ICP monitor (3,5)[B].
  - Treatment of ICP >22 mm Hg is recommended because values above this level are associated with increased mortality in patients with TBI (5)[B].

– Rapid **neurosurgical consultation** for any symptomatic EDH or SDH or for any asymptomatic EDH or SDH meeting the CT criteria listed under "Surgery/Other Procedures"

– Medical interventions to control elevated ICP should not delay definitive neurosurgical treatment.

ALERT

Corticosteroids have been shown to **increase mortality** when used acutely in patients with head injury (5)[A].

ADDITIONAL THERAPIES

- If there is a high index of suspicion of EDH or SDH but a negative CT scan, such patients should be admitted for observation because EDH and SDH can evolve slowly. If headache or other symptoms persist, or the patient otherwise simply fails to improve, repeat CT in 6 to 12 hr before considering discharge (7)[C]:
  – Delayed EDH (hematoma not present on initial CT but found on follow-up scan) comprises up to 10% of cases in most series. A high index of suspicion is necessary to make the diagnosis.
- Drilling **burr holes (trephination)**:
  – Reserved for patients with raised and deteriorating ICP refractory to medical management when neurosurgical intervention is not available (3)[C]
  – Contraindications to drilling burr holes include GCS >8, no imaging obtained, and neurosurgical intervention is available (3)[C].
  – Burr hole procedure:
    - Drill hole adjacent to, but not over, skull fracture in the area located by CT scan
    - In the absence of CT scan (such as in a wilderness situation), place burr hole on the side of the dilated pupil, 2 fingerwidths anterior to tragus of ear and 3 fingerwidths above.

SURGERY/OTHER PROCEDURES

Acute neurosurgical referral is merited for any patient who is found to have either an EDH or acute SDH:

- **CT guidelines for surgical management of EDH (1,3)[A]:**
  – GCS <9 with anisocoria
  – Size >30 cm^3
  – In patients initially being treated nonoperatively, the first follow-up CT scan should be obtained within 6 to 8 hr after TBI (1)[C]:
    - Enlargement of an EDH is common, resulting in the need for follow-up CT scans in patients initially being treated nonoperatively.
    - Mean time to enlargement in one study was 8 hr after TBI, with no enlargement after 36 hr.
- **CT guidelines for surgical management of SDH (2,3)[A]:**
  – Thickness >10 mm or midline shift >5 mm regardless GCS
  – GCS decline by >2
  – Fixed and dilated or asymmetric pupils
  – ICP >20 mm Hg
  – Patients who present with coma (GCS <9) but with an SDH with a thickness <10 mm and a midline shift (MLS) <5 mm can be treated nonoperatively, provided they undergo ICP monitoring, are neurologically stable since the injury, have no pupillary abnormalities, and have no intracranial hypertension (no ICP >20 mm Hg) (2)[B].
- Any patient with known EDH or SDH who is initially stable but later develops new symptoms suggestive of mass effect, herniation, or increased ICP is a candidate for emergent neurosurgical intervention.

ONGOING CARE

FOLLOW-UP RECOMMENDATIONS

- EDH: In the case of nonsurgical EDH, the consulting neurosurgeon may consider discharge if the patient is neurologically stable after some period of observation. For patients treated both surgically and nonsurgically, follow-up CT scan in 1 to 2 wk is commonly pursued in even asymptomatic patients to monitor for signs of progression or recurrence (5)[C], although the preferred timing of follow-up CT scans is not established in the literature and largely institution dependent.
- SDH: Due to its association with underlying brain injury (2), period of observation required before determination of clinical stability in SDH may be longer than for EDH. Furthermore, patients with an underlying brain injury may be more likely to need rehabilitation or temporary/permanent skilled nursing care.

PROGNOSIS

- EDH: mortality about 10% (range 7–12%) for EDH, as low as 5% if treated optimally within a few hours. The mortality rate is twice as high if there was no lucid interval, presumably because of associated brain parenchyma injury (1).
- SDH: Mortality in SDH is more varied but generally worse than for EDH; ranges from 40% to 60% in those requiring surgery and up to 68% in surgical cases presenting to the hospital in coma (2)

COMPLICATIONS

- Complications seen in patients with TBI include:
  – Neurologic deficits associated with parenchymal brain injury, which is more commonly seen in acute SDH than EDH.
  – Neurologic deficits associated with increased ICP and subsequent herniation.
  – Posttraumatic seizures, which can occur early or late after TBI.
- Postoperative complications include:
  – Recurrent or residual hematoma, which may require repeat operations.
  – Wound infection, meningitis, or cerebral abscess after craniotomy.
  – CSF leak.

REFERENCES

1. Bullock MR, Chesnut R, Ghajar J, et al. Surgical management of acute epidural hematomas. *Neurosurgery*. 2006;58(Suppl 3):S7–S15.
2. Bullock MR, Chesnut R, Ghajar J, et al. Surgical management of acute subdural hematomas. *Neurosurgery*. 2006;58(Suppl 3):S16–S24.
3. Long B, Koyfman A. Secondary gains: advances in neurotrauma management. *Emerg Med Clin North Am*. 2018;36(1):107–133.
4. Davanzo JR, Sieg EP, Timmons SD. Management of traumatic brain injury. *Surg Clin North Am*. 2017;97(6):1237–1253.
5. Carney N, Totten AM, O'Reilly C, et al. Guidelines for the management of severe traumatic brain injury, fourth edition. *Neurosurgery*. 2017;80(1):6–15.
6. Al-Mufti F, Mayer SA. Neurocritical care of acute subdural hemorrhage. *Neurosurg Clin N Am*. 2017;28(2):267–278.
7. DeCuypere M, Klimo P Jr. Spectrum of traumatic brain injury from mild to severe. *Surg Clin North Am*. 2012;92(4):939–957.

ADDITIONAL READING

Servadei F, Compagnone C, Sahuquillo J. The role of surgery in traumatic brain injury. *Curr Opin Crit Care*. 2007;13(2):163–168.

CLINICAL PEARLS

- EDH and acute SDH are neurosurgical emergencies that merit rapid neurosurgical evaluation.
- CT is the study of choice in evaluating intracranial lesions in a patient with head injury (1,2)[A].
- In patients who need operative treatment, delay in time to surgery is associated with poorer outcomes.

HEMATURIA IN SPORTS

Charles W. Webb, DO, FAAFP, CAQSM • Cody Franzen, MD, CAQSM

BASICS

Exercise-induced hematuria (EIH):

- Occurs with or without trauma in males and females; resolves with rest in 2 to 3 days (1,2)
- Although a benign condition, it is a diagnosis of exclusion.
- Directly correlated with exercise intensity, duration, core temperature, acidosis, oxidative stress (3)
- **Traumatic mechanisms:**
  - Direct urologic trauma
  - Foot strike and bladder trauma (3)
- **Atraumatic mechanisms:**
  - Physiologic decreased renal blood flow during exercise causing hypoxic damage to the nephron and leading to increased permeability for red blood cells (RBCs) and proteins
  - Increased glomerular filtration pressure favoring excretion of RBCs and protein
  - Hydration and a partially full bladder during exercise may help to prevent or minimize this condition (3).
- Persistent recurrent, symptomatic, or traumatic hematuria warrants further evaluation (1,3,4).

DESCRIPTION

- **Microscopic hematuria**: ≥3 RBCs per high-powered field (HPF) in 2 of 3 properly collected urine samples:
  - A urine dipstick of 1+ blood corresponds to ~1 to 5 RBCs/HPF.
  - Can also be caused by free hemoglobin, myoglobin, or other substances (see "Diagnosis")
  - Urine dipstick is **not** diagnostic of hematuria.
  - Prompt microscopic analysis is important for detection.
- **Gross hematuria**: red-brown urine with numerous RBCs seen on microscopy:
  - *Note*: 1 mL of blood per liter of urine can produce a visible color change.
- **EIH**: transient, usually microscopic hematuria following physical exertion
- **Symptomatic hematuria**: gross or microscopic hematuria in the presence of any lower or upper urinary tract symptoms (e.g., flank pain, renal colic, dysuria, urgency, etc.)
- **Asymptomatic hematuria**: either gross or microscopic hematuria in the absence of any urinary tract symptoms

EPIDEMIOLOGY

- **EIH**: idiopathic
- **All other causes:**
  - Age <40 yr: usually infection
  - Age >40 yr: increasing incidence of tumor
  - Males >60 yr: usually prostatic obstruction, calculi, or tumor
  - Females >60 yr: usually malignancy (1,3)

Prevalence

- Prevalence of hematuria in the general population ranges from 2.5% to 20% (3).
- Prevalence increases to 18–80% following athletic competition and usually resolves in 48 hr (1,4).

RISK FACTORS

- Previous or chronic urinary tract infection (UTI)
- Anticoagulation
- Strenuous exercise
- History of calculi, prostatitis, trauma, malignancy, coagulopathy, or sexually transmitted illness
- Travel to Africa, India, or the Middle East (1,3)

GENERAL PREVENTION

Routine screening of adults for microscopic hematuria with urinalysis (UA) is not indicated.

DIAGNOSIS

- Hematuria is rarely a medical emergency but may be a sign of underlying pathology.
- History and exam will help to guide which patients need further workup.
- Benign asymptomatic microscopic hematuria can be achieved with urine microscopy on ≥2 separate urine samples.
- >50 RBCs/HPF is generally considered significant hematuria and may warrant *immediate* further investigation.
- Symptomatic/gross hematuria warrants further workup.
- **Causes:**
  - Unexplained/idiopathic: 87% of all cases of microhematuria and 72% of gross hematuria seen at a referral clinic
  - Spurious:
    - Menstruation
    - Sexual intercourse
  - Pseudohematuria (a.k.a. dipstick hematuria)
  - Rhabdomyolysis
  - Foods (beets, rhubarb, blackberries)
  - Drugs (doxorubicin, chloroquine, rifampin)
  - UTI: acute cystitis or pyelonephritis:
    - If UTI is suspected, obtain urine culture, treat infection, and repeat test in 6 wk before further workup.
  - Prostatitis or urethritis
  - Urinary tract calculi
  - Exercise induced
  - Trauma to flank or abdomen (renal fracture)
  - Cancer: renal, bladder, prostate, ureter:
    - Present in 19–25% of gross hematuria but <1.5% of microhematuria in the general population:
      - Exceedingly rare at age <40 yr
    - Transient/intermittent hematuria is common.
    - Benign prostatic hyperplasia (BPH)
    - Glomerular disease
    - Sickle cell disease
- **Rare causes:**
  - Polycystic kidney disease (PCKD)
  - *Schistosoma haematobium*
  - Radiation cystitis
  - Urethral strictures
  - Tuberculosis
  - Medullary sponge kidney
  - Cyclophosphamide-induced cystitis
  - Arteriovenous malformation
  - Renal artery thrombosis
  - Papillary necrosis of any cause
  - Loin pain hematuria syndrome
- **EIH** (5,6):
  - Not fully understood; thought to be multifactorial
  - Diagnosis of exclusion
  - Can make the diagnosis without further workup in athletes <40 yr old who have hematuria within 12 hr of vigorous activity that resolves completely within 48 to 72 hr
  - More common with increased intensity of exercise
  - Bladder trauma in runners; can be alleviated by keeping a small amount of urine in bladder
  - Cyclist can experience direct trauma to the prostate and urethra (4).
  - Hemoglobinuria can be caused by RBC lysis for a number of reasons.
  - Dehydration and increased blood viscosity
  - Increased body temperature
  - Oxidative damage myoglobinuria
  - March, or foot-strike, hematuria is thought to occur from trauma to the foot capillaries.
- Traumatic hematuria:
  - More likely to present as gross hematuria
  - Children are more likely to have renal injury following trauma owing to lack of perinephric fat and less protection by the ribs.
  - There is a lower threshold for imaging of children.
  - In children, additional criteria for imaging include >50 RBCs/HPF and abdominal/flank pain or ecchymosis.
  - Serious renal injury is much more likely to occur after a fall, bike, or motor vehicle accident (high-velocity accidents and/or collisions) than with athletic participation.
  - Football was the most common sport causing traumatic renal injury.

HISTORY

- Recent physical activity: type, intensity, and duration; EIH can occur up to 12 hr after activity (2).
- Trauma
- Urinary tract symptoms: flank pain, renal colic, dysuria, weak stream, and so forth.
- Medication use, including herbals and over-the-counter drugs: Anticoagulants do not increase the risk of hematuria and should not influence the workup.
- Family history of sickle cell disease/trait or hematuria.
- Red flags for malignancy or tuberculosis such as fevers, night sweats, and weight loss
- Assess risk factors for significant urologic disease:
  - Abuse of analgesic drugs (nonsteroidal anti-inflammatory drugs [NSAIDs])
  - Age >40 yr increases likelihood of cancer.
  - Exposure to pelvic radiation
  - Irritative voiding symptoms
  - Occupation exposure to chemicals or dyes
  - Smoking
  - Recent sore throat could suggest poststreptococcal glomerulonephritis or immunoglobulin A (IgA) nephropathy.
  - Travel to developing nations
  - Unilateral flank pain suggests calculi or pyelonephritis.

PHYSICAL EXAM

- Many patients will not have any signs or symptoms. Nearly all patients with EIH will be asymptomatic. The symptoms listed below suggest something *other than* benign EIH:
  - Fever
  - Urethral discharge
  - Flank pain or ecchymosis
  - Painless red or brown urine
  - Dysuria
  - Frequency
  - Hesitancy
  - Suprapubic pain
- Physical examination:
  - Vitals
  - Abdominal and flank exam
  - Genitourinary exam

- **Stepwise approach to the patient:**
  - Step 1: history and physical as above:
    - If patient <40 yr of age, observe and repeat UA after 48 to 72 hr.
    - If UA is normal, no further studies are warranted. Observe the patient for recurrence.
    - If hematuria persists or exam suggests cause other than EIH, proceed to step 2.
  - Step 2: Obtain the following laboratory tests:
    - Urine culture and serum creatinine, blood urea nitrogen (BUN), complete blood count (CBC), prothrombin time (PT), partial thromboplastin time (PTT), sickle-cell preparation
    - Consider serum creatine kinase.
    - If serum creatinine is normal, obtain intravenous pyelogram (IVP) to evaluate for obstruction, mass, and kidney function.
    - If results of these tests are normal, proceed to step 3.
  - Step 3: cystoscopy. If normal, proceed to step 4.
  - Step 4: ultrasound (US) or computed tomography (CT) scan:
    - Include bladder, especially if patient >40 yr of age.
    - If normal, proceed to step 5.
  - Step 5: Consider renal arteriogram:
    - Evaluate for vasculitis, atriovenous (AV) malformation, and renal infarction/thrombosis.
    - If normal, proceed to step 6.
  - Step 6: Consider renal biopsy:
    - If at any time concurrent proteinuria, dysmorphic RBCs, or casts are present, obtain 24-hr urine for protein, creatinine, calcium, citrate, and uric acid.
    - Consider antistreptolysin O (ASO) titer, Venereal Disease Research Laboratory (VDRL), antineutrophil cytoplasmic antibodies (ANCA), compliment levels, antiglomerular basement membrane antibody levels, and hepatitis serology.

DIFFERENTIAL DIAGNOSIS

- **Painless:**
  - EIH
  - Malignancies
  - Glomerulonephropathy, especially in children
  - PCKD
  - Sickle cell trait or disease
  - Coagulation defect (clotting factor deficiency, thrombocytopenia, polycythemia)
  - Vasculitis (lupus, Goodpasture syndrome)
  - Infection (endocarditis, tuberculosis, syphilis)
  - Iatrogenic: anticoagulation, catheterization, NSAIDs
  - Early calculi formation: hypercalciuria, hyperuricosuria, hypocitruria (Citrate helps to prevent stone formation.)
  - Myoglobinuria—rhabdomyolysis (no RBCs on microscopy)
  - Hemolysis—"march hematuria" (no RBCs on microscopy)
  - Medications: phenothiazine, phenolphthalein laxatives, rifampin, phenazopyridine, phenytoin, quinine
  - Porphyria
  - Vegetable dyes (beets, rhubarb)
  - Vaginal blood contamination (4)
- **Painful:**
  - Pyelonephritis
  - Prostatitis
  - Cystitis
  - Urethritis
  - Calculi
  - Trauma
  - Bladder or renal tumor
  - Renal artery aneurysm
  - Renal vein thrombosis

DIAGNOSTIC TESTS & INTERPRETATION

- **Initial testing**: UA with microscopy; further testing indicated if UA not clear in 48 to 72 hr (1):
  - Must include cell count
  - RBCs alone suggest prostatic disease, pelvic or ureteral calculi, trauma, heavy exercise, or malignancy.
  - Dysmorphic RBCs can be seen in EIH as well as intrinsic renal disease.
  - White blood cells (WBCs) + RBCs suggests infection.
  - RBCs + protein/casts/dysmorphic RBCs or absence of clots suggests glomerular disease.
  - RBC casts are virtually diagnostic of glomerulonephritis or vasculitis.
  - RBC clots usually indicate extraglomerular bleeding.
  - Proteinuria suggests renal disease.
- Urine culture
- 24-hr urine protein, creatinine, calcium, uric acid, and citrate
- Spot urine protein:creatine ratio usually sufficient
- CBC, PT, and PTT
- Serum creatinine/BUN/electrolytes
- Urine cytology is rarely helpful.
- Imaging is needed only if hematuria does not clear on UA after 48 to 72 hr of rest (4).
- Imaging is rarely needed, unless there is a traumatic incident or suspected nephrolithiasis or tumor.
- Non–contrast-enhanced CT scan is the preferred modality for evaluating calculi with a sensitivity of 98–100% and a specificity of 92–100%. Many institutions have a renal stone CT scan protocol to minimize radiation exposure.
- CT urography is preferred test to evaluate urologic malignancy or obstruction.
- The combination of CT urography and cystoscopy generally is considered sufficient to rule out serious urinary tract pathology.
- US can be used safely in children and pregnant women but low sensitivity for calculi or tumors <3 cm.
- Retrograde pyelography also can be used to visualize the bladder and collecting system.
- Voiding cystourethrogram (VCUG) is used to detect vesicoureteral reflux.
- Magnetic resonance (MR) urography can be used in place of CT scan.
- Arteriography detects renovascular hypertension, polyarteritis nodosa, thromboemboli, mass, and aneurysm (5).

TREATMENT

- **General:**
  - Treatment targeted to the underlying condition
  - Antibiotics for infection
  - Pain control, if applicable; avoid NSAIDs until renal injury and nephritis are ruled out.
  - Pyridium can be given for cystitis.
- **EIH:**
  - Rest and reassurance
  - Emphasize hydration during exercise and avoidance of urination within 15 to 20 min of onset of exercise to minimize bladder trauma.
- **Traumatic hematuria:**
  - Assess life-threatening and coexisting injuries.
  - Immediate surgical consultation for signs of shock or severe trauma
  - Evaluate need for imaging.
- **Management of asymptomatic microscopic hematuria:**
  - Confirm in 2/3 properly collected specimens.
  - No further workup needed if present in only one sample or no RBCs seen on microscopic analysis
  - Consider further workup if >50 RBCs/HPF in single sample.
  - Rule out transient or spurious causes; treat if present.
  - If age ≥40 yr, refer for urologic evaluation with imaging and cystoscopy.
  - If age <40 yr, assess for:
    - Glomerular filtration rate (GFR) <60 mL/min.
    - Proteinuria (albumin:creatinine ratio ≥30 or protein:creatine ratio ≥50).
    - Hypertension (BP ≥140/90 mm Hg).
  - If any of the above are abnormal, refer to nephrology.
  - If no diagnosis is found, monitor GFR, proteinuria, and hypertension yearly.
- **Management of symptomatic microscopic hematuria:**
  - Rule out transient and spurious causes.
  - Consider immediate referral to urology.
  - May follow the same algorithm as for anti-müllerian hormone (AMH)
- **Management of gross hematuria:**
  - Consider referral to urology.
  - Evaluate and treat transient causes.
  - Assess renal function, and consider imaging before referral (1,5).

ONGOING CARE

Referral to urology or nephrology useful when other etiologies cannot be found and the hematuria persists

PROGNOSIS

- Based on underlying diagnosis, if known
- Unexplained hematuria is relatively common in the general population and carries a favorable prognosis as long as an appropriate diagnostic workup has been done (3,5).

REFERENCES

1. Rao PK, Jones JS. How to evaluate 'dipstick hematuria': what to do before you refer. *Cleve Clin J Med*. 2008;75(3):227–233.
2. Varma PP, Sengupta P, Nair RK. Post exertional hematuria. *Ren Fail*. 2014;36(5):701–703.
3. Shephard RJ. Exercise proteinuria and hematuria: current knowledge and future directions. *J Sports Med Phys Fitness*. 2016;56(9):1060–1076.
4. Alhazmi HH. Microscopic hematuria in athletes: a review of the literature. *Saudi J Sports Med*. 2015;15(2):131–136.
5. Bernard J. Renal trauma: evaluation, management, and return to play. *Curr Sports Med Rep*. 2009; 8(2):98–103.
6. Kelly JD, Fawcett DP, Goldberg LC. Assessment and management of non-visible haematuria in primary care. *BMJ*. 2009;338:a3021.

CLINICAL PEARLS

- Return to play is acceptable if hematuria resolves after 48 to 72 hr of rest; otherwise, counsel patients on an individual basis depending on the diagnosis.
- Transient hematuria is usually benign but should be worked up further in people ≥40 yr of age.
- Persistent hematuria always should be evaluated further.
- Painless gross hematuria should be considered bladder cancer until proven otherwise.

H

HEMOGLOBINOPATHIES IN SPORT: THALASSEMIA, SICKLE CELL TRAIT

Bernadette Pendergraph, MD • Evan S. Bass, MD, FAAFP, CAQSM

BASICS

DESCRIPTION

Thalassemia and sickle cell trait are genetic disorders of hemoglobin production. Thalassemias are a mixed collection of quantitative abnormal production, leading to either absent or decreased production of normal α or β subunits. Sickle cell trait produces an abnormal β subunit in normal amounts.

EPIDEMIOLOGY

Incidence

- Thalassemia: 1 in 1,000 people has thalassemia in the United States.
- Sickle cell trait: United States–screened newborns—73 cases per 1,000 African Americans, 7 per 1,000 Hispanics, and 3 per 1,000 whites; 1 in 3 persons in West Africa and 1 in 5 persons in the eastern province of Saudi Arabia have sickle cell trait (1).

Prevalence

Thalassemia is the most common single genetic disorder known. In the thalassemia belt (Mediterranean, Turkey, Iran, India, Thailand, Cambodia, and southern China), the prevalence is 2.5–15%; 2.5 million people in the United States and 300 million people worldwide have sickle cell trait (2).

ETIOLOGY AND PATHOPHYSIOLOGY

- Thalassemia occurs when there is an abnormal gene on chromosome 16 or 11 that impairs the production of α or β subunits of hemoglobin, respectively. Abnormalities include point mutations, total deletions, or the rearrangement of gene loci. Thalassemia minor occurs when a single abnormal gene is inherited, resulting in normal or low-normal hemoglobin measurement with significant microcytosis. More severe forms of β thalassemia impair erythropoietin production, cause hemolytic anemia, and reduce oxygen capacity (2).
- Sickle cell trait occurs from the inheritance of one normal hemoglobin gene (HbA) and one abnormal B1 globin gene (HbS). In this carrier state, hemoglobin A1 and hemoglobin S is produced in a 60:40 ratio. The B1 gene is found on the short arm of chromosome 11. Red blood cells (RBCs) will sickle and polymerize under certain conditions, such as severe tissue hypoxia, acidosis, dehydration, increased viscosity, and hypothermia (1).

Genetics

Both conditions are caused by the inheritance of an autosomal-recessive gene.

GENERAL PREVENTION

Genetic screening and preconception counseling

COMMONLY ASSOCIATED CONDITIONS

- Sickle cell trait: increased incidence of hyposthenuria, microhematuria, renal papillary necrosis, exertional rhabdomyolysis, exercise-related sudden death, and renal medullary carcinoma; 2-fold increase in venous thrombosis; splenic infarcts reported at high altitude (>7,000 feet) (1)
- Thalassemia minor is usually asymptomatic. Other forms of thalassemia are associated with erythroid hyperplasia (extramedullary erythropoietic tissue development in face, chest, abdomen, and pelvis), resulting in frontal bossing, coarse facies, and splenomegaly. Heart failure occurs secondary to hemolytic anemia. Other bone abnormalities include shortened upper extremities, pathologic fractures of long bones and vertebral bodies, notching, and osteolytic lesions of the ribs because of marrow masses. Growth retardation, delayed pubertal development, insulin resistance, hypothyroidism, and hypoparathyroidism are also possible complications.

DIAGNOSIS

Prehospital:

- Thalassemia minor: usually asymptomatic
- Sickle cell trait: usually asymptomatic; may present with cramping or sudden collapse, usually within the first 30 min of intense practice and initial conditioning with normal core temperature (3)

HISTORY

- Thalassemia: symptoms of anemia—dizziness, fatigue, light-headedness, weakness
- Sickle cell trait: usually asymptomatic; may present with gradual deterioration over minutes with symptoms of muscle cramping/pain, dyspnea, severe weakness, fatigue provoked by multiple bursts of vigorous exertion often combined with ambient temperatures ≥80°C or high altitude (4)

PHYSICAL EXAM

- Thalassemia: no findings or signs of anemia—pallor, elevated heart rate, low blood pressure, cool extremities, brittle nails
- Sickle cell trait: Muscles are soft and nontender to palpation; no visible contractions

DIFFERENTIAL DIAGNOSIS

- α-Thalassemia (5):
  - One-gene deletion
  - Asymptomatic; normal hematologically
- α-Thalassemia:
  - Two-gene deletion
  - Microcytosis and mild anemia, not reversed with iron
- β-Thalassemia minor:
  - One normal gene and one abnormal
  - Microcytosis and mild anemia not reversed with iron
- Sickle cell trait combined with β-thalassemia minor or α-thalassemia:
  - Usually symptomatic
- Sickle cell trait combined with hemoglobin C
- Iron deficiency anemia:
  - Microcytosis, decreased iron stores; improves with iron repletion
- Dilutional pseudoanemia:
  - Increased volume expansion related to exercise; normal RBC indices and iron stores

DIAGNOSTIC TESTS & INTERPRETATION

- Sickle solubility test: initial screening test that detects HgS. It cannot differentiate between sickle cell disease or trait; needs confirmation by hemoglobin electrophoresis, high-performance liquid chromatography (HPLC), or isoelectric focusing (IEF). HPLC and IEF identify α-thalassemias (1)[C].
- Hemoglobin electrophoresis: Sickle cell trait shows hemoglobin AS (hemoglobin A1, 55–60%, and hemoglobin S, 40–45%) (2)[C].
- Complete blood count (CBC): Both sickle cell trait and thalassemia lead to microcytosis and hypochromia.

- Reticulocyte count: normal in sickle cell trait but increased when combined with α- or β-thalassemia
- Indirect bilirubin: normal in sickle cell trait but increased when combined with α- or β-thalassemia
- DNA analysis: identifies α-thalassemias

TREATMENT

- No treatment for asymptomatic sickle cell trait; focus is on prevention of exertional rhabdomyolysis and exertional collapse.
- Collapse in sickle cell athlete:
  - Occurs from sickling of RBCs in exerting limbs, with resultant rhabdomyolysis from continued exertion in the face of ischemia
  - Severe lactic acidosis from anaerobic metabolism of ischemic muscles can develop, leading to eventual shock.
  - Rapid diagnosis and treatment are necessary to prevent acute renal failure from the rhabdomyolysis, subsequent hyperkalemia, eventual ventricular fibrillation, and death.
- Prehospital:
  - Thalassemia: fluid resuscitation if abnormal vital signs
  - Sickle cell trait: If with cramping or collapse, check vital signs, administer high-flow oxygen, cool athlete if necessary, and activate emergency medical services (if patient is obtunded or vital signs are unstable).
- Emergency department (ED) treatment:
  - Continued support: oxygen, intravenous (IV) fluids
  - Evaluation for rhabdomyolysis: CBC, electrolytes, blood urea nitrogen (BUN), creatinine, liver function tests, coagulation panel
  - Correction of hyperkalemia

ISSUES FOR REFERRAL

Hematology referral: patients with symptomatic sickle cell trait, concern for misdiagnosis and need for more advanced testing, thalassemias requiring transfusions

ADDITIONAL THERAPIES

- Thalassemia: in severe cases, transfusions to keep the hemoglobin 9 to 10.5 g/L; chelation therapy in those receiving transfusions with deferasirox, deferoxamine, or deferiprone (2)[C]:
  - Deferasirox: 20 to 30 mg/kg/day orally; associated with nausea, abdominal pain, diarrhea, rash, or liver/kidney dysfunction
  - Deferoxamine: 20 to 40 mg/kg/day subcutaneous (SC) infusion; minimal side effects
  - Deferiprone: 25 to 33 mg/kg TID orally; associated with neutropenia and agranulocytosis
- Stem cell transplant: curative (2)[C]
- Sickle cell trait:
  - Education of the athlete on importance of conditioning and identification of cramping as a sign of sickling
  - All athletes with the sickle cell trait should be counseled on preseason strength and conditioning programs, gradual progression during session training, and stopping activity if cramping, difficulty catching breath, weakness, or pain (3)[C].
  - When performing repetitive sprints/interval training, longer periods should be allowed for athlete to recover in between exertional activities.
  - Exertion should be limited when conditions exist that may precipitate sickling: illness, high ambient temperature, dehydration, asthma, and altitude (3)[C].

ONGOING CARE

PATIENT EDUCATION

- Sickle Cell Disease Association of America: http://www.sicklecelldisease.org/about/sickle-cell-101/
- American Society of Hematology: http://www.hematology.org/about/history/50-years/1534.aspx
- Thalassemia International Federation: http://www.thalassemia.org.cy/education/

PROGNOSIS

Excellent, if prevention measures are instituted

REFERENCES

1. Naik RP, Haywood C. Sickle cell trait diagnosis: clinical and social implications. *Hematology Am Soc Hematol Educ Program*. 2015;2015:160–167.
2. Fibach E, Rachmilewitz EA. Pathophysiology and treatment of patients with beta-thalassemia—an update. *F1000Res*. 2017;6:2156.
3. Asplund CA, O'Connor FG. Challenging return to play decisions: heat stroke, exertional rhabdomyolysis, and exertional collapse associated with sickle cell trait. *Sports Health*. 2016;8(2):117–125.
4. Maron BJ, Harris KM, Thompson PD, et al. Eligibility and disqualification recommendations for competitive athletes with cardiovascular abnormalities: Task Force 14: sickle cell trait: a scientific statement from the American Heart Association and American College of Cardiology. *J Am Coll Cardiol*. 2015;66(21):2444–2446.
5. Taher A, Vichinsky E, Musallam K, et al. *Guidelines for the Management of Non Transfusion Dependent Thalassaemia*. 2nd ed. Nicosia, Cyprus: Thalassemia International Federation; 2013.

ADDITIONAL READING

Quattrone RD, Eichner ER, Beutler A, et al. Exercise collapse associated with sickle cell trait (ECAST): case report and literature review. *Curr Sports Med Rep*. 2015;14(2):110–116.

CLINICAL PEARLS

- Use preventive strategies to minimize the risk of an event in an athlete known to have sickle cell trait.
- Recognize thalassemia as a cause of microcytic anemia, and avoid iron supplementation unless athlete is truly iron deficient.
- Additional testing beyond hemoglobin electrophoresis is necessary to identify α-thalassemias.

HERPES GLADIATORUM

Stephen Shaheen, MD, CAQSM

BASICS

DESCRIPTION

Variant of cutaneous herpes disease caused by herpes simplex virus type 1 (HSV-1) or type 2 (HSV-2) occurring among wrestlers and transmitted by direct skin-to-skin contact

EPIDEMIOLOGY

Affects 2.6% of high school wrestlers and 7.6% of collegiate wrestlers. Current estimates from the National Collegiate Athletic Association (NCAA) indicate possible increased incidence rates of 20–40% in collegiate wrestlers (1).

RISK FACTORS

- Abrasions or physical trauma increase the likelihood of acquiring infection.
- Physical and mental stressors (i.e., weight loss, sleep deprivation, competition, school responsibilities) may increase likelihood of recurrence.

GENERAL PREVENTION

- Isolate infected wrestler to prevent skin contact with other wrestlers (control outbreaks among previously infected wrestlers).
- Regular wrestling matt cleaning and general hygiene (e.g., avoid sharing towels, soap, razors)
- Consider using prophylactic antiviral medications during the season or before competition (2).
- Acyclovir 200 mg BID
- Valacyclovir 500 mg or 1 g daily
- Famciclovir 250 mg BID
- Teach skin hygiene (e.g., showering after activity), and protect other skin abrasions from secondary contact.
- Educate athletes on how to identify lesions/recurrence, and seek early treatment.

DIAGNOSIS

HISTORY

- Initial versus recurrent eruption
- Similar location as previous infection
- Previous treatment and length of infection
- History of recent stressors (e.g., school, sleep, weight loss, emotional)

PHYSICAL EXAM

- Incubation period for primary infection is 2 to 14 days.
- Prodrome of burning, stinging pain, or itching at the infected site, followed by clusters of vesicles on an erythematous base
- Common locations include head, neck, and upper body.
- Erythema and grouped vesicles, ulcers, or crusts on head, face, neck, or upper extremities most common but may occur anywhere on the body
- Symptoms of fever, localized lymphadenopathy, malaise, myalgia, or pharyngitis may accompany infection, especially with initial episode.
- Repeated outbreaks usually are less severe and involve a smaller area.
- Infections around the eye increase the risk of corneal or retinal involvement, such as keratoconjunctivitis or retinal necrosis.
- Think herpes if infection fails to improve after 3 to 4 days of oral antibiotic therapy and if lesions cross the midline and involve the face and scalp.

DIFFERENTIAL DIAGNOSIS

- Impetigo
- Herpes zoster
- Folliculitis
- Allergic or contact dermatitis
- Tinea gladiatorum
- Cellulitis

- Diagnosis can be made by viral culture or Tzanck smear of vesicle fluid, although neither is as sensitive as polymerase chain reaction (PCR).
- PCR testing is a sensitive but costly method to determine viral presence and is considered the gold standard for detecting HSV-1 or HSV-2 in individuals with a rash suggestive of a herpes infection.

TREATMENT

- Initial infection:
  - Started early in the clinical course, during vesicle formation, oral antiviral medications can arrest viral replication and shorten the duration of infection (2).
  - Acyclovir 200 mg 5 times a day or 400 mg TID for 10 days
  - Valacyclovir 1 g BID for 10 days
  - During the ulcer stage, benzoyl peroxide and use of a hair dryer can help dry crusts more rapidly and minimize secondary bacterial infections.
- Recurrent infection:
  - Antiviral medications begun during the prodromal phase can effectively shorten the duration of recurrent infections (2).
  - According to a recent study, treatment with 1 g valacyclovir daily reduced herpes gladiatorum (HG) outbreaks by 92% in individuals with a $<$2-yr history of recurrent HG, and treatment with 300 mg valacyclovir daily reduced HG outbreaks in 88% of those with a $<$2-yr history of recurrent infection (2).
  - Valacyclovir 1 g PO daily or 500 mg BID for 3 to 7 days
  - Valacyclovir 2 g $\times$ 1 dose; repeat in 12 hr.
  - Acyclovir 800 mg BID for 5 days or 400 mg TID for 5 days
  - Famciclovir 125 mg BID for 5 days or 1 g PO BID for 1 day

- Treatments and levels of evidence:
  - Level 1 (strong, good quality, patient-oriented evidence): treatment with systemic oral antivirals in initial and recurrent infections (1,2,3)
  - Level 2 (limited-quality patient-oriented evidence): prevention of outbreak via season-long antiviral prophylaxis for players with history of HG outbreak (1)
  - Level 3 (limited, case-oriented, disease-oriented evidence): isolating players with weeping lesions, educating players on importance of not returning to play with active lesions, covered or not (3)

REFERENCES

1. Wilson EK, deWeber K, Berry JW, et al. Cutaneous infections in wrestlers. *Sports Health*. 2013;5(5):423–437.
2. Anderson BJ, McGuire DP, Reed M, et al. Prophylactic valacyclovir to prevent outbreaks of primary herpes gladiatorum at a 28-day wrestling camp: a 10-year review. *Clin J Sport Med*. 2016;26(4):272–278.
3. Shah N, Cain G, Naji O, et al. Skin infections in athletes: treating the patient, protecting the team. *J Fam Pract*. 2013;62(6):284–291.

ADDITIONAL READING

- Anderson BJ. The effectiveness of valacyclovir in preventing reactivation of herpes gladiatorum in wrestlers. *Clin J Sport Med*. 1999;9(2):86–90.
- Anderson BJ. The epidemiology and clinical analysis of several outbreaks of herpes gladiatorum. *Med Sci Sports Exerc*. 2003;35(11):1809–1814.
- Anderson BJ. Valacyclovir to expedite the clearance of recurrent herpes gladiatorum. *Clin J Sport Med*. 2005;15(5):364–366.
- Annunziato PW, Gershon A. Herpes simplex virus infections. *Pediatr Rev*. 1996;17(12):415–424.
- Johnson R. Herpes gladiatorum and other skin diseases. *Clin Sports Med*. 2004;23(3):473–484, x.
- Stacey A, Atkins B. Infectious diseases in rugby players: incidence, treatment and prevention. *Sports Med*. 2000;29(3):211–220.

CLINICAL PEARLS

- Return to play: National Federation of State High School Associations Sports Medicine Advisory Committee guidelines:
  - Herpetic lesions (simplex, fever blisters/cold sores, zoster, gladiatorum): To be considered "noncontagious," all lesions must be scabbed over with no oozing or discharge, and no new lesions should have occurred in the preceding 48 hr, with no lymph node swelling near affected area. For primary (first episode of HG), wrestlers should be treated and not allowed to compete for a minimum of 10 days. If general body signs and symptoms like fever and swollen lymph nodes are present, that minimum period of treatment should be extended to 14 days. Recurrent outbreaks require a minimum of 120 hr or 5 full days of oral antiviral treatment, again so long as no new lesions have developed and all lesions are scabbed over. Herpesvirus may spread prior to vesicle formation; therefore, anyone in contact with the infected individual during the 3 days prior to the outbreak must be isolated from any contact activity for 8 days and be examined daily for suspicious skin lesions.
- NCAA guidelines on herpes simplex:
  - Primary infection: (i) Wrestler must be free of systemic symptoms of viral infection (fever, malaise, etc.). (ii) Wrestler must have developed no new blisters for 72 hr before the examination. (iii) Wrestler must have no moist lesions; all lesions must be dried and surmounted by a *firm adherent crust* with no evidence of secondary bacterial infection. (iv) Wrestler must have been on appropriate dosage of systemic antiviral therapy for at least 120 hr before and at the time of the meet or tournament. (v) Active herpetic infections shall not be covered to allow participation. See above criteria when making decisions for participation status.
  - Recurrent infection: (i) Blisters must be completely dry and covered by a *firm adherent crust* at time of competition, or wrestler shall not participate. (ii) Wrestler must have been on appropriate dosage of systemic antiviral therapy for at least 120 hr before and at the time of the meet or tournament. (iii) Active herpetic infections shall not be covered to allow participation. See above criteria when making decisions for participation status.
  - Questionable cases:
    - Tzanck preparation and/or HSV antigen assay (if available)
    - Wrestler's status deferred until Tzanck preparation and/or HSV assay results complete
    - Wrestlers with a history of recurrent herpes labialis or HG could be considered for season-long prophylaxis. This decision should be made after consultation with the team physician.

HIGH ANKLE SPRAIN

Brandon Eck, DO • Delmas Bolin, MD, PhD, FACSM

BASICS

- A syndesmosis is defined as a fibrous joint in which two adjacent bones (in this case, tibia and fibula) are linked by a strong membrane or ligaments.
- Involves disruption of ligaments supporting the integrity of the ankle mortise joint
- Associated with prolonged symptoms of pain and dysfunction
- Relevant injured structures can include anterior tibiofibular, posterior tibiofibular and transverse tibiofibular ligaments, interosseous membrane, and interosseous ligament, which serve to prevent lateral displacement of distal fibula during weight-bearing.
- Synonym(s): Syndesmodial injury of the lower leg

DESCRIPTION

- Mechanism of injury involves sudden, forced external rotation and hyperdorsiflexion of the ankle.
- The talus is pressed against the fibula, opening the distal tibiofibular articulation and rupturing the tibiofibular syndesmosis and tibiofibular ligaments.

EPIDEMIOLOGY

- 1–10% of all ankle sprains (Underdiagnosis may be common.)
- Higher percentage (as high as 35%) involve the syndesmosis when occurring in collision sports such as football, rugby, and lacrosse.

RISK FACTORS

- Collision sports are at higher risk:
  - Football
  - Rugby
  - Lacrosse
- Sports that immobilize the foot in a high ankle shoe or boot:
  - Hockey
  - Slalom skiing; catching inner ski on gate
  - Wrestling
- Sports played on turf (e.g., soccer)

COMMONLY ASSOCIATED CONDITIONS

- Deltoid ligament tear
- Fibular or medial malleolar fracture
- Pronation-external rotation (PER) and supination-external rotational (SER) fractures
- Proximal fibular fractures (Maisonneuve injuries)
- Heterotopic ossification or synchondrosis of the syndesmosis in 25–100% of cases
- Tibiofibular synostosis resulting in prolonged pain and chronic disability
- Longer healing time and more missed practices
- Occult talar dome fracture

DIAGNOSIS

HISTORY

- Patient is often unable to adequately or completely describe mechanism; patients commonly report an inversion mechanism.
- The clinician should delineate any prior ankle injuries.
- Focus history on mechanism of injury and direct location of pain; raise index of suspicion with history of forceful external rotation, hyperdorsiflexion, or hyperplantar flexion.
- Examples of common mechanisms include soccer (player tackling ball), football (player prone, has foot stepped on, leading to forceful external rotation), and skiing (slalom skiers, catch ski on gate).
- Pain is usually between anterior distal tibia and fibula and also posteromedially at ankle joint.
- Pain can be persistent on weight-bearing or an unusually long period of recovery after the initial injury.
- Pain is also worse with pushing off or with external rotation.

PHYSICAL EXAM

- Less swelling than anticipated with severe lateral ankle sprain
- Palpation of the tibia and fibula helpful to rule out fracture:
  - Anterior joint line and anterior syndesmosis are often tender.
- Squeeze test: Compression above midcalf produces distal pain in the anterior ankle joint (syndesmosis).
- External rotation test: Distal lower leg is stabilized with ankle in neutral position while mediolateral force/external rotation of the foot is performed; positive test noted by pain and/or increased rotation relative to unaffected side
- Push-off test: Push off/heel raise on affected side may be weak or absent.
- Fibular translation (drawer) test: pain or increased translation of fibula from anterior to posterior or loss of firm end point relative to uninjured side
- Stabilization test: Distal syndesmosis is stabilized with athletic tape and assess if symptoms are decreased with running and jumping.
- Cotton test: increased translation or pain with translation of talus from medial to lateral (may indicate deltoid ligament tear)
- Crossed-leg test: pain at syndesmosis with gentle pressure exerted on the medial side of the knee while resting the midtibia of affected leg on uninjured knee
- Evaluate distal neurovascular status with any lower leg injury to rule out acute compartment syndrome (1)[B].

DIFFERENTIAL DIAGNOSIS

- PER ankle fracture (Weber C)
- SER ankle fracture (Weber B)
- Fracture of the proximal fibula (Maisonneuve)
- Ossification of the syndesmosis
- Calcification of the syndesmosis
- Deltoid ligament tear
- Talar dome fracture
- Tibiofibular synostosis resulting in prolonged pain and chronic disability

DIAGNOSTIC TESTS & INTERPRETATION

ALERT

- X-rays: Initial studies are static films. 50% of syndesmotic injuries have avulsion fractures associated:
  - Weight-bearing anteroposterior view:
    - Tibiofibular clear space is among most sensitive indicators of syndesmotic injuries. Measured 1 cm proximal to ankle joint; widening demonstrated by >6 mm between medial border of fibula and medial cortical density of tibia
    - Tibiofibular overlap; measured 1 cm proximal to joint; normal is >6 mm overlap between medial border of fibula and lateral border of tibia.
    - Medial clear space should be <4 mm; >4 mm termed *diastasis*
  - Standing mortise view to evaluate talocrural angle; the angle of a line drawn across tips of malleoli intersecting with a line perpendicular to a line drawn across the superior aspect of tibial plafond. Variation from contralateral side of >5 degrees is significant.
  - Lateral
- Dynamic radiographs:
  - Cotton test: Grasp distal fibula and pull laterally; modified cotton test: Push or pull fibula in sagittal plane. Comparison to contralateral side is frequently required.
  - Varus and valgus ankle stress views are essential to assess instability.
  - External rotation stress views not considered reliable indicators of syndesmotic injury
- Magnetic resonance imaging (MRI) can clarify diagnosis and extent of soft tissue injury:
  - Compared with ankle arthroscopy, had sensitivity 100%/100% and specificity 93%/100% for anterior inferior/posterior inferior tibiofibular ligament disruption, respectively
  - Although sensitive and specific for syndesmotic injuries, MRI is not predictive for instability because it is a static test.
- Computed tomography (CT) helpful for bony detail of suspected talar dome injuries (2)[B]
- Ultrasound (US) imaging can be used to diagnose ligament ruptures of the lower leg (3)[B].

TREATMENT

- High ankle sprains/Syndesmosis injuries without fracture (1)[B]: Consensus is three- to four-phase rehabilitation protocol. If no frank diastasis, most injuries result in inability to bear weight without symptoms:
  - Phase I is to limit inflammatory response and protect the joint, usually with nonsteroidal anti-inflammatory drugs (NSAIDs) and short-term (10 days to 2 wk) non–weight-bearing protection in a cast, boot, or brace with crutches. Include protection, rest, ice, compression, and elevation and modalities to minimize edema.
  - Phase II is typically restoration of range of motion and normalization of gait pattern. In this phase, high ankle braces (DonJoy Velocity and others) may facilitate rehabilitation.
  - Phase III progression once patient can ambulate and hop without dysfunction. Progress to agility drills, plyometrics, sports-specific tasks, and strengthening.
  - Return to play is challenging and is typically based on a functional testing evaluation and physical examination; usually 6 to 8 wk
  - Patient may return to play with demonstration of tasks such as backward pedaling, vertical hopping, or running in figure-8 pattern.
- Syndesmosis injuries with fracture or diastasis noted on radiographs:
  - Referral to orthopedic surgeon indicated if frank diastasis is noted on stress radiographs or if fracture is present
- Screw fixation followed by non–weight-bearing cast immobilization for 6 wk, followed by appropriate rehabilitation (1)[B]
- Suture-button fixation followed by non–weight-bearing cast immobilization for 6–8 wk, followed by appropriate rehabilitation
- Platelet-rich plasma injections under US guidance have been used in elite athletes for faster return to play (3).

REFERENCES

1. Fort NM, Aiyer AA, Kaplan JR, et al. Management of acute injuries of the tibiofibular syndesmosis. *Eur J Orthop Surg Traumatol*. 2017;27(4):449–459.
2. Herscovici D Jr, Anglen JO, Archdeacon M, et al. Avoiding complications in the treatment of pronation-external rotation ankle fractures, syndesmotic injuries, and talar neck fractures. *J Bone Joint Surg Am*. 2008;90(4):898–908.
3. Laver L, Carmont MR, McConkey MO, et al. Plasma rich in growth factors (PRGF) as a treatment for high ankle sprain in elite athletes: a randomized control trial. *Knee Surg Sports Traumatol Arthrosc*. 2015;23(11):3383–3392.

ADDITIONAL READING

- Amendola A, Williams G, Foster D. Evidence-based approach to treatment of acute traumatic syndesmosis (high ankle) sprains. *Sports Med Arthrosc Rev*. 2006;14(4):232–236.
- Hopkinson WJ, St Pierre P, Ryan JB, et al. Syndesmosis sprains of the ankle. *Foot Ankle*. 1990;10(6):325–330.
- Kellett JJ. The clinical features of ankle syndesmosis injuries: a general review. *Clin J Sport Med*. 2011;21(6):524–529.
- Sman AD, Hiller CE, Rae K, et al. Prognosis of ankle syndesmosis injury. *Med Sci Sports Exerc*. 2014;46(4):671–677.
- Switaj P, Mendoza M, Kadakia A, et al. Acute and chronic injuries to the syndesmosis. *Clin Sports Med*. 2015;34(4):643–677.

CLINICAL PEARLS

- A high ankle sprain involves ligaments that stabilize the ankle mortise joint. It is not a "routine ankle sprain" and must be treated differently.
- High ankle sprains should be immobilized as soon as the diagnosis is made for a variable period ranging from a few days in elite professional and collegiate athletes to 2 wk for high school athletes. Suspect a high ankle sprain in a "regular ankle sprain" that is not improving as you expect.
- Although anecdotal, some find high ankle stirrup braces helpful in the subacute setting for stabilizing the mortise joint, limiting rotational stress at the ankle, and permitting a more vigorous rehabilitation.

HIGH-ALTITUDE ILLNESS

Joseph E. Allen, MD, MS, FAAFP, CAQSM

BASICS

- Altitude sickness was described and documented by missionaries to South America in the late 16th century.
- High-altitude illness (HAI) is primarily caused by hypobaric hypoxemia. Rapid ascent to elevation in excess of 2,000 m, without adequate physiologic acclimation, can result in a spectrum of HAI, ranging from a mild acute mountain sickness (AMS) to more severe and potentially fatal forms of high-altitude pulmonary edema (HAPE) and high-altitude cerebral edema (HACE).
- High-altitude environment:
  - Intermediate: 1,520 to 2,440 m (5K to 8K feet)
  - High: 2,440 to 4,270 m (8K to 14K feet)
  - Very high: 4,270 to 5,500 m (14K to 18K feet)
  - Extreme altitude: above 5,500 m (>18K feet)
- Optimal prevention of HAI involves slow, graded ascent to altitude. Certain medications and portable oxygen or hypobaric chamber may mitigate and alleviate symptoms.

ALERT

Once symptoms are recognized, the definitive solution to HAI is descent to lower altitude.

DESCRIPTION

- The atmospheric percentage of oxygen is a constant 21%. However, the partial pressure of oxygen decreases with increase in altitude. Hypobaric hypoxia forms the physiologic basis for the HAIs, AMS, HAPE, and HACE.
- Initial AMS symptoms are typically mild and self-limited, progressing to more severe HACE if not adequately recognized and treated.
- HAPE or HACE can present independently and progress rapidly, with or without initial warning of AMS symptoms.
- Untreated, HAPE or HACE can be fatal.

EPIDEMIOLOGY

- Incidence and severity of HAI increase with higher altitude and speed of ascent.
- At high altitude, AMS may affect 25% of unacclimated individuals, increasing to 50–85% afflicted at very high altitude (>4,000 m).
- HAPE and HACE are rarely seen <4,000 m, accounting for an estimated 0.1–0.4% of all cases.

GENERAL PREVENTION

ALERT

- Graded ascent is the best way to prevent HAIs.
- Never ascend to a higher sleeping altitude with HAI symptoms.
- If travel is planned from sea level to above 2,500 m, spend one night at an intermediate elevation.
- Above 2,500 m, do not ascend >500 m sleeping altitude per day.
- Spend an extra night of acclimatization for every 1,500 m altitude gained.
- Pharmaceutical agents: Acetazolamide and dexamethasone may be used for prevention of AMS/HACE and sustained-release; nifedipine for individuals prone to HAPE

ETIOLOGY AND PATHOPHYSIOLOGY

- Hypobaric hypoxia:
  - With ascent to high altitude comes decreased partial pressure of oxygen. Decreased atmospheric PaO_2 affects absorption into the circulation at the alveolar level. Hypoxemia at the cellular level causes a myriad of physiologic stress responses.
  - Decreased partial pressure of oxygen triggers the carotid body to signal the respiratory centers in the medulla to increase ventilation. The extent of compensatory hypoxic ventilatory response (HVR) is thought to be determined at the genetic level. Increased ventilatory rate causes hypocapnia and respiratory alkalosis, which results in an increase in renal excretion of bicarbonate.
- **AMS:**
  - Hypoxic stress induces the trigeminovascular system (TVS), leading to increased cerebral blood flow and resultant nausea, headache, and malaise.
  - The central respiratory center responds to HVR-induced respiratory alkalosis with periods of apnea causing disturbed sleep.
- **HACE:**
  - Vasogenic cerebral edema, caused by a myriad of responses to hypobaric hypoxia, including TVS induction, endothelial activation, and sympathetic activity
- **HAPE:**
  - Acute pulmonary edema induced by hypoxic pulmonary hypertension increases capillary hydrostatic pressure causing extravasation of fluid across the vascular endothelium and into the alveolar space.
  - Impaired reabsorption of alveolar fluid and amplified inflammatory mediator response then accelerate and exacerbates the process.

RISK FACTORS

- Rapid ascent
- Sleeping at altitude >2,000 m; exceeding >500 m/day sleeping altitude above 2,500 m
- Lack of acclimatization
- Young age
- Strenuous exertion at high altitude
- Previous history and/or individual susceptibility to altitude illness
- Obesity
- Chronic obstructive pulmonary disease, sickle cell disease, uncompensated congestive heart failure, or pulmonary hypertension
- Well-controlled hypertension and asthma are not considered risk factors.
- Physical fitness does not predict or prevent altitude illness.

DIAGNOSIS

- AMS:
  - Nausea
  - Light-headedness
  - Headache
  - Insomnia
  - Anorexia
  - Malaise
  - Fatigue
  - Weakness
  - Impaired memory
  - Inability to focus or concentrate
- HAPE: Symptoms of AMS may present initially and then progress 2 to 5 days after ascent to dyspnea on exertion and/or dyspnea at rest:
  - Persistent cough, progressing to pink, foamy sputum
  - Chest tightness
  - Fatigue
  - Muscle weakness
- HACE: Ataxia and confusion are hallmark symptoms heralding progression from AMS to HACE:
  - Headache
  - Vomiting
  - Incoordination
  - Disorientation
  - Irrational behavior
  - Auditory or visual hallucination
  - Lethargy
  - Altered level of consciousness
  - Unconsciousness or coma within 24 hr after the onset of ataxia

HISTORY

- Rapid ascent to high altitude
- AMS:
  - Onset of symptoms typically 12 to 24 hr and self-limited (as early as 2 hr after arrival but rarely after 36 hr)
- HAPE:
  - Symptoms usually begin 2 to 5 days after arrival to high altitude and classically the second night sleeping at high altitude.
  - May have a sudden onset (e.g., gondola or helicopter ascent), especially in sedentary individuals at altitude
  - Decreased exercise performance and increased recovery time, cough, dyspnea on exertion, and progressive worsening of symptoms, especially at night. Pink, frothy sputum is usually a late finding.
- HACE:
  - AMS symptomatology with progressive worsening of neurologic symptoms, including ataxia, extreme lassitude, mental status changes, and coma
  - Commonly associated with HAPE
  - AMS progression to HACE at altitude may be within 12 hr but more commonly 1 to 3 days.
  - HACE generally occurs above 3,000 m but has been described at altitude as low as 2,100 m.

PHYSICAL EXAM

- **AMS:**
  - Specific physical findings are uncommon in mild AMS.
  - Tachycardia or bradycardia
  - Normotensive
- **HAPE:**
  - Breathlessness at rest
  - Cyanosis
  - Crackles in right middle lobe are typical but can be anywhere in the lung field.
  - Tachycardia
  - Tachypnea
  - Low-grade fever
  - Orthopnea

- **HACE:**
  - Inability to perform activities such as dressing or eating
  - Truncal ataxia demonstrated by poor heel-toe walking
  - Mental status changes
  - Occasionally focal neurologic deficits
  - Funduscopic examination can demonstrate papilledema and retinal hemorrhages (not diagnostic).

DIFFERENTIAL DIAGNOSIS

- **AMS:**
  - Dehydration
  - Exhaustion
  - Viral syndrome
  - Gastroenteritis
  - Hangover
  - Hypothermia
  - Carbon monoxide exposure
  - Hyponatremia
  - Seizures or focal neurologic deficits are uncommon.
- **HAPE:**
  - Pneumonia
  - Asthma
  - Pulmonary embolism
  - Congestive heart failure
  - Myocardial infarction
  - Fever >101°F, chills, or mucopurulent sputum are typically absent.
- **HACE:**
  - In addition to AMS differential:
    - Cerebrovascular accident
    - Alcohol intoxication
    - Brain tumor
    - Central nervous system (CNS) infection (e.g., meningitis)
    - Acute psychosis/delirium

DIAGNOSTIC TESTS & INTERPRETATION

Initial Tests (lab, imaging)

- **HAPE:**
  - Chest x-rays demonstrate normal heart size with patchy infiltrates.
- **HACE:**
  - Brain magnetic resonance imaging (MRI) T2-weighted images show increased signal in the white matter, particularly the splenium of the corpus callosum, consistent with vasogenic edema and microhemorrhage.

TREATMENT

ALERT

- Descent to a lower altitude is the mainstay of treatment for any HAI.
- Low-intensity descent of at least 500 m is recommended.
- Avoid further ascent until symptoms resolve.
- Supplemental oxygen 2 to 4 L/min if available
- Preventative/treatment options

MEDICATION

- Oral acetaminophen 650 to 1,000 mg or ibuprofen 600 mg for pain or headache; ondansetron orally disintegrating tablet (ODT) 4 mg PO q4–6h for nausea and vomiting
- Acetazolamide 125 to 250 mg PO BID, starting 8 to 24 hr prior to ascent (1)[A]
- Ibuprofen 600 mg PO TID for AMS prevention and symptomatic relief of headache (2)[B]
- Dexamethasone 2 mg PO q6h, or 4 mg PO q12h, can be used as alternative for AMS prevention if sulfa/acetazolamide allergic. Start the day of ascent, continuing for first 2 days at altitude, or for rapid increase in altitude (1,3)[A].
- For treatment of HAPE, dexamethasone 4 mg PO/intramuscular (IM)/intravenous (IV) q6h
- For treatment of HACE, dexamethasone 8 mg loading dose, followed by 4 mg PO/IM/IV q6h

ALERT

Rebound symptoms of AMS have been described after discontinuation of dexamethasone and continued ascent should be avoided.

- Budesonide 200 μg inhaled BID starting 3 days prior to ascent has been shown effective in preventing AMS (4)[B].
- Nifedipine 30 mg extended-release PO BID to treat HAPE if oxygen unavailable and rapid descent is delayed (5)[C].
- Tadalafil 10 mg PO BID, as an alternative to nifedipine (due to potential hypotension with concomitant use), has been described for treatment of HAPE in case reports (2)[C].
- When extreme weather or additional factors preclude rapid descent, medical treatment has been shown to be a viable option up to 4,240 m (6)[B].
- If available, a portable hypobaric chamber, or Gamow bag, manually inflated to 2 psi, may be effectively used to simulate a descent of 1,000 to 3,000 m.
- Upon return to low altitude, transition to inpatient hospital care as soon as possible.

COMPLEMENTARY & ALTERNATIVE MEDICINE

Limited research on Ginkgo biloba for AMS prophylaxis has produced conflicting results but may be a viable alternative for those seeking natural sources. Coca preparations have shown potential for increasing blood oxygenation and decreasing AMS symptoms in some studies (7)[B].

ONGOING CARE

- General measures:
  - Minimize heavy exertion for 2 to 3 days upon arrival to high altitude.
  - Maintain adequate hydration.
  - Eat frequent, small, high-carbohydrate meals.
  - Avoid alcohol or other sedative/hypnotic medications which could suppress respiratory drive.
  - Smoking worsens hypoxia and should be avoided.
- In critically ill patients:
  - Monitor vital signs periodically because hypotension may lead to cerebral hypoperfusion.
  - Intravenous fluid (IVF) is not contraindicated in HAPE. Administer if available to treat dehydration and maintain cardiac perfusion.
  - Gradually decompress portable hypobaric chambers to minimize potential barotrauma to the middle ear.
  - HACE progressing to coma warrants advanced airway management and bladder decompression if possible. Hyperventilation may lead to further cerebral ischemia and should be avoided.

REFERENCES

1. Kitsteiner J, Whitworth JD, Nashelsky J. FPIN's clinical inquiries. Preventing acute mountain sickness. *Am Fam Physician*. 2011;84(4):398–400.
2. Lipman GS, Kanaan NC, Holck PS, et al. Ibuprofen prevents altitude illness: a randomized controlled trial for prevention of altitude illness with nonsteroidal anti-inflammatories. *Ann Emerg Med*. 2012;59(6):484–490.
3. Eide RP III, Asplund CA. Altitude illness: update on prevention and treatment. *Curr Sports Med Rep*. 2012;11(3):124–130.
4. Chen GZ, Zheng CR, Qin J, et al. Inhaled budesonide prevents acute mountain sickness in young Chinese men. *J Emerg Med*. 2015;48(2):197–206.
5. Davis C, Hackett P. Advances in the prevention and treatment of high altitude illness. *Emerg Med Clin North Am*. 2017;35(2):241–260.
6. Fagenholz PJ, Gutman JA, Murray AF, et al. Treatment of high altitude pulmonary edema at 4240 m in Nepal. *High Alt Med Biol*. 2007;8(2):139–146.
7. Biondich AS, Joslin JD. Coca: high altitude remedy of the ancient Incas. *Wilderness Environ Med*. 2015;26(4):567–571.

ADDITIONAL READING

- Centers for Disease Control and Prevention. https://wwwnc.cdc.gov/travel/yellowbook/2018.
- Flaherty G, O'Connor R, Johnston N. Altitude training for elite endurance athletes: a review for the travel medicine practitioner. *Travel Med Infect Dis*. 2016;14(3):200–211.
- Shackleton M, Tondora CM, Whiting S. The effect of homeopathic coca on high altitude mountain sickness: Mt. Everest base camp. *J Evid Based Integr Med*. 2000;6:44–55.
- Sutton JR, Coates G, Houston CS, eds. The Lake Louise consensus on the definition and quantification of altitude illness. In: *Hypoxia and Mountain Medicine*. Burlington, VT: Queen City Press; 1992:272–274.
- Wilderness Medical Society. http://m.wms.org/

CLINICAL PEARLS

- Proper acclimatization (i.e., graded ascent) is the best method for preventing HAI.
- Never ascend to a higher sleeping altitude if symptoms of HAI are present.
- Acetazolamide 125 to 250 mg PO BID remains a safe and effective means to prevent and treat AMS.
- Dexamethasone is effective for treating significant AMS as well as HACE.
- Early recognition and treatment of HAPE/HACE are critical.
- Once the symptoms of HAI are recognized, supplemental oxygen (if available), and/or controlled descent to a lower altitude are the mainstay of treatment.

HIP APOPHYSITIS

Anthony J. Saglimbeni, MD, Board Certified Internal Medicine, CAQSM • Anthony Kwon, MS

BASICS

DESCRIPTION

- Hip apophysitis is a chronic inflammatory injury seen only in child, adolescent, and skeletally immature athletes.
- Repetitive overload of hip muscles applies excessive forces to pelvic apophyses resulting in hip pain and inflammation.

EPIDEMIOLOGY

Incidence

- Hip apophysitis is common among young athletes.
- Hip apophyses appear and fuse later than growth plates in long bones, placing adolescents at increased risks for apophysitis, especially during periods of growth spurts (boys 13 to 14, girls 11 to 12 yr old).
- Apophysitis of the hip occurs more commonly in male athletes compared to females.

ETIOLOGY AND PATHOPHYSIOLOGY

- The apophyses serve as the origination and insertion site for muscles and tendons with bones.
- In the growing child, the apophysis is a weak point in the muscle-tendon-bone connection.
- Overuse and repetitive exercise of the larger pelvic muscles exerts excessive force on hip apophyses causing microtrauma and inflammation.

RISK FACTORS

- Skeletal immaturity
- Limited flexibility
- Rapid bone growth
- Early sport specialization
- Excessive sport participation

GENERAL PREVENTION

- Strength and flexibility program to improve hip range of motion and symmetrical balance between hip muscles
- Caution should be taken to avoid repetition and overuse.

COMMONLY ASSOCIATED CONDITIONS

Increased stress on an injured apophysis or rapid eccentric loading of the attached muscle can cause a hip avulsion fracture.

DIAGNOSIS

HISTORY

- Increase in physical activity duration, frequency, and intensity
- Recent growth spurt
- Gradually increasing pain, exacerbated by physical activity (i.e., running or jumping) (1)[A]
- Limited range of motion (1)[A]
- Biomechanical and gait changes (2)[A]

PHYSICAL EXAM

- Localized tenderness and swelling near the affected apophysis (Commonly affected apophyses include anterior superior iliac spine [ASIS], anterior inferior iliac spine [AIIS], and ischial tuberosity.) (2)[A]
- Swelling or tenderness near tendon-bone junction (2)[A]
- Pain with resistance testing (1)[A]
- Diminished range of motion (1)[A]

DIFFERENTIAL DIAGNOSIS

Avulsion fracture

DIAGNOSTIC TESTS & INTERPRETATION

Initial Tests (lab, imaging)

- Anteroposterior radiographs of the hip and pelvis may show open apophysis (1)[A].
- Affected apophysis may or may not show minimal widening (1)[A].
- Magnetic resonance imaging (MRI) may sometimes show bone marrow and soft tissue edema, indicative of apophysitis and inflammation (1)[A].
- Ultrasound findings may include regional hypoechogenicity, widening of the hypoechoic physis, or hyperemia (1)[A].

TREATMENT

GENERAL MEASURES

- Dependent on degree of pain and instability
- Rest from physical activity (1)[A]
- Ice
- Modified activity (1)[A]
- Protected weight-bearing
- Physical therapy (1)[A]
- Gentle stretching, avoid vigorous stretching (2)[A]

ISSUES FOR REFERRAL

Physical therapy for hip and abdominal strengthening and flexibility

ADDITIONAL THERAPIES

Neoprene shorts for warmth and compression (2)[A]

SURGERY/OTHER PROCEDURES

Surgery consult may be necessary in cases of severe avulsion fracture (1,2)[A].

ONGOING CARE

FOLLOW-UP RECOMMENDATIONS

Follow up weekly or as needed intervals on a case by case basis.

PROGNOSIS

- Dependent on severity of pain and disability
- Crutches can be used to avoid weight-bearing if necessary.
- Rest from physical activity
- Progress to improving strength and flexibility of the hip and abdominal muscles
- Once athlete achieves full range of motion without pain, gradual return to sport may begin ideally under the supervision of an athletic trainer or physical therapist.

REFERENCES

1. Belair JA, Hegazi TM, Roedl J, et al. Core injuries remote from the pubic symphysis. *Radiol Clin North Am*. 2016;54(5):893–911.
2. Weiss JE, Stinson JN. Pediatric pain syndromes and noninflammatory musculoskeletal pain. *Pediatr Clin North Am*. 2018;65(4):801–826.

ADDITIONAL READING

- Arnaiz J, Piedra T, de Lucas EM, et al. Imaging findings of lower limb apophysitis. *AJR Am J Roentgenol*. 2011;196(3):316–325.
- Houghton KM. Review for the generalist: evaluation of pediatric hip pain. *Pediatr Rheumatol Online J*. 2009;7:10.
- Paluska SA. An overview of hip injuries in running. *Sports Med*. 2005;35(11):991–1014.

CLINICAL PEARLS

- Hip strength and flexibility are key to reducing the risk of hip apophysitis.
- Ensure that athletes recover to full pain-free range of motion before returning to sport.
- Hip apophysitis can recur in the growing athlete; be cautious to avoid overtraining.

HIP POINTER

Brent S.E. Rich, MD, ATC

BASICS

DESCRIPTION
- Iliac crest contusion (1)
- Avulsion fracture of the iliac crest
- Iliac crest apophysitis
- Synonym(s): bruised hip or contusion

EPIDEMIOLOGY
- Most common in contact/collision sports such as football, wrestling, soccer, and lacrosse
- Occasionally, caused by violent contraction of the abdominal musculature (2)

RISK FACTORS
- Collision sports
- Inadequate iliac crest protection

DIAGNOSIS

HISTORY
Usually caused by direct blow to the iliac crest

PHYSICAL EXAM
- Signs and symptoms:
  - Acute, severe pain at the site of contusion (3)
  - Athlete usually not able to continue activity
  - Posture often flexed to side of injury
- Physical examination:
  - Inspect for swelling, deformity, or ecchymosis.
  - Tenderness to palpation over iliac crest
  - Abdominal exam may reveal muscle spasm but should not be tender to palpation.
  - Weakness and pain with active abdominal contraction, trunk rotation, side bending, resisted hip abduction, and/or hip flexor contraction

DIFFERENTIAL DIAGNOSIS
- Compression fracture to iliac crest
- Avulsion fracture of anterosuperior iliac spine
- Intra-abdominal injury
- Cutaneous nerve injury (superior cluneal nerves)
- Avulsion of internal/external oblique, latissimus dorsi, and/or paraspinal musculature

DIAGNOSTIC TESTS & INTERPRETATION
- Plain anteroposterior (AP) pelvis radiographs to rule out fracture
- Oblique views or comparison side radiographs may be helpful.
- Often, radiographs are normal.
- Often, iliac crest ossifications centers will be open. Closure is usually between 14 to 16 yr of age.
- Musculoskeletal ultrasound may be used for evaluation of the extent of a hematoma.

TREATMENT

GENERAL MEASURES
- Analgesia:
  - Minimize bleeding and swelling with compression and ice.
  - Consideration of narcotics may be appropriate for first 48 to 72 hr if there is severe, debilitating pain.
  - Nonsteroidal anti-inflammatory drugs (NSAIDs) are indicated at onset until resolution.
  - Some clinicians prefer to give corticosteroid burst to decrease symptoms.

- Physical therapy:
  - Modalities per certified athletic trainer or physical therapist in acute phase
  - Hip spica wrap with ace bandage or commercial neoprene wrap may be helpful for compression and comfort.

ADDITIONAL THERAPIES

- Most cases resolve with 4 to 6 wk of conservative management (4).
- Crutches for partial or non–weight-bearing may be necessary for first few days of treatment.
- Some clinicians prefer to inject with local anesthetic and corticosteroid to decrease symptoms and speed recovery; increases risk of infection and bleeding
- Musculoskeletal ultrasound may be useful to aspirate or inject an iliac crest hematoma.
- Rehabilitation:
  - Gentle abdominal and hip stretching when tolerated
  - Gradual abdominal and hip strengthening
  - Progressive functional activity
  - Protection with padding on return to play

ONGOING CARE

FOLLOW-UP RECOMMENDATIONS

In cases of intra-abdominal trauma (consider surgical evaluation) or displaced iliac crest fracture

COMPLICATIONS

Recurrent or recalcitrant injury or hematoma if athlete is returned to sport before resolution of symptoms

REFERENCES

1. Hall M, Anderson J. Hip pointers. *Clin Sports Med*. 2013;32(2):325–330.
2. Anderson K, Strickland SM, Warren R. Hip and groin injuries in athletes. *Am J Sports Med*. 2001;29(4):521–533.
3. Wilson JJ, Furukawa M. Evaluation of the patient with hip pain. *Am Fam Physician*. 2014;89(1): 27–34.
4. Bolia I, Utsunomiya H, Locks R, et al. Twenty-year systematic review of the hip pathology, risk factors, treatment, and clinical outcomes in artistic athletes-dancers, figure skaters, and gymnasts. *Clin J Sport Med*. 2018;28(1):82–90.

CLINICAL PEARLS

Return to play can take place when there is minimal to no tenderness at the contusion site, near-normal or normal abdominal and hip muscle strength, full range of motion to hip flexion, trunk rotation, and side bending. Athlete then should be given adequate protection/padding.

HYPERMOBILITY SYNDROME

Adrian Tabares, MD, CAQSM

BASICS

DESCRIPTION

- Joint hypermobility syndrome, once viewed as a distinct clinical entity comprising of joint laxity and skin fragility, currently falls under the classification for Ehlers-Danlos syndrome hypermobility type (1).
- It is a diagnosis of exclusion that requires the absence of other features of Ehlers-Danlos syndrome subtypes, in addition to other connective tissue disorders. Although there is still ongoing debate on how the clinical diagnosis is made, it is currently based on a combination of clinical history and physical exam findings (1,2).
- There is no confirmatory genetic test, and the phenotype is variable.
- Manifestations in individuals can range from asymptomatic to chronic widespread pain (2).
- Many affected individuals pursue athletics that require a large degree of flexibility, such as yoga, dance, and gymnastics.

EPIDEMIOLOGY

Incidence

Actual incidence is unknown.

Prevalence

The prevalence of joint hypermobility syndrome is estimated to be between 1:5,000 and 1:15,000 (1).

ETIOLOGY AND PATHOPHYSIOLOGY

- The pathophysiology of joint hypermobility syndrome is poorly understood because there are no observable structural abnormalities on examination of collagen fibers or other associated molecules or the genes encoding for them in the majority of patients.
- This is in contrast to other disorders such as Ehlers-Danlos and Marfan syndrome, which can be distinguished, based on genetic markers (1).

Genetics

- No genetic marker identified to date
- Believed to be inherited through an autosomal dominant pattern
- Incomplete penetrance and variable phenotype (1)

RISK FACTORS

More commonly seen in childhood, adolescence, female gender, and people of Asian and West African descent (1,2)

GENERAL PREVENTION

Unknown

COMMONLY ASSOCIATED CONDITIONS

- Recurrent joint subluxation and dislocation
- Pes planus
- Chronic pain
- Anxiety and depression
- Gastroesophageal reflux disease (GERD)
- Irritable bowel syndrome (IBS)
- Syncope
- Orthostatic hypotension (1,2)

DIAGNOSIS

HISTORY

The diagnosis of joint hypermobility syndrome relies on appropriate history taking and the exclusion of other types of connective tissue disorders, joint arthritides, and myopathy. A family history should be elicited to determine if genetic testing for other conditions is warranted (1,2)[B].

PHYSICAL EXAM

- The Beighton score has been developed to assess joint hypermobility and consists of a nine-point scoring system. One point is given for each positive test: (i) if the patient is able to demonstrate apposition of the thumb to the forearm, (ii) extension of the 5th finger beyond 90 degrees, (iii) extension of the elbow beyond 10 degrees, (iv) extension of the knee beyond 10 degrees,(v) and being able to place both palms flat on the floor with forward flexion of the trunk while keeping the legs straight (1,2).
- The sum of all positive tests is then calculated with a maximum score of 9/9.
- Major criteria for the diagnosis of hypermobility syndrome include a score of 4/9 or greater, or arthralgia for over 3 mo among four or more joints.
- Minor criteria for hypermobility syndrome include the following:
  - A Beighton score of 1 to 3/9 (0 to 3 if age 50 yr or older)
  - Arthralgia over 3 months in one to three joints, or back pain for over 3 months
  - Dislocation/subluxation in more than one joint or on more than one occasion
  - Soft tissue rheumatism with more than three lesions
  - Marfanoid habitus (tall, thin, wingspan to height ratio >1.03, upper to lower body ratio <0.89, arachnodactyly (positive Steinberg wrist sign)
  - Abnormal skin: striae, hyperextensibility, thin skin, papyraceous scars
  - Drooping eyelids, myopia, or "antimongoloid slant"
  - Varicose veins, hernia or rectal/uterine prolapse
- The diagnosis of joint hypermobility is made if any of the following are met: (i) two major criteria, or (ii) one major and two minor criteria, or (iii) four minor criteria, or (iv) two minor criteria and an affected first-degree relative (1,2)[B].
- If joint hypermobility is suspected but the individual does not meet Beighton score criteria, a five-point questionnaire may be used to assess for historical joint hypermobility. This consists of the following questions:
  - Could you ever place your hands flat on the floor without bending your knees?
  - Could you ever bend your thumb to touch your forearm?
  - As a child, did you amuse your friends by contorting your body into strange shapes OR could you do the splits?
  - As a child or teenager, did your shoulder or kneecap dislocate on more than one occasion?
  - As a child or teenager, did you consider yourself "double-jointed?"
- A positive answer to two or more questions increases the suspicion of joint hypermobility (1)[B].

DIFFERENTIAL DIAGNOSIS

- Ehlers-Danlos syndrome classic type
- Marfan syndrome
- Loeys-Dietz syndrome
- Ankylosing spondylitis
- Rheumatoid arthritis
- Fibromyalgia
- Multiple sclerosis
- Amyotrophic lateral sclerosis
- Autonomic polyneuropathies
- Myopathy
- Chronic fatigue syndrome
- Osteogenesis imperfecta
- Arterial tortuosity syndrome
- Lateral meningocele syndrome

DIAGNOSTIC TESTS & INTERPRETATION

Initial Tests (lab, imaging)

There are no diagnostic labs or imaging to confirm joint hypermobility syndrome, and the diagnosis relies on history and physical exam findings (1).

Follow-Up Tests & Special Considerations

Additional testing may be performed to rule out other conditions or to evaluate for other pathology and may include:

- X-ray, diagnostic ultrasound, computed tomography (CT), or magnetic resonance imaging (MRI) of involved joints.
- Inflammatory markers, uric acid levels, autoimmune markers, evaluation for endocrine or hematologic conditions, muscle biopsy.
- Echocardiography if Ehlers-Danlos or Marfan syndromes are suspected.
- Bone mineral density testing for osteogenesis imperfecta (1)[C].

Pediatric Considerations
In pediatric patients, a second evaluation in adult age is recommended or laboratory testing to exclude other disorders before the diagnosis is made (1)[C].

Diagnostic Procedures/Other
Arthrocentesis may be considered if joint infection or other arthritides such as gout or pseudogout are suspected.

Test Interpretation
Tissue pathology does not play a role in diagnosis.

TREATMENT

GENERAL MEASURES
- Although there are no treatment options that lead to the resolution of joint hypermobility syndrome, treatment should be individualized and focus on symptom management (2,3).
- Physical and occupational therapy: There is limited evidence to suggest therapy can be effective in pain reduction, improved proprioception, strength, balance, and improvement of quality of life. However, joint-specific exercise has not been found to be more effective than exercise in general (3)[A].
- Splints and orthotics may provide additional support but high-quality evidence is lacking (3)[C].
- Pain management using a team approach, including behavioral therapy, pharmacologic and nonpharmacologic methods can provide an adjunct to overall symptom control (2)[C].

MEDICATION
Medication has not been found to be effective for the long-term treatment of hypermobility syndrome. However, analgesics, such as acetaminophen; nonsteroidal anti-inflammatories; muscle relaxants; antidepressants, such as selective serotonin reuptake inhibitors (SSRIs) and tricyclics; and antiseizure medications, such as gabapentin, may prove helpful in reducing acute and chronic pain (2)[C].

ISSUES FOR REFERRAL
- A referral to a rheumatologist or clinical geneticist may be considered for additional testing if the diagnosis remains uncertain.
- Cardiology, endocrinology, gastroenterology, neurology, ophthalmology, orthopedic surgery, and podiatry referrals may be considered for additional evaluation.
- Psychiatry, clinical psychology, and pain management referrals may be indicated for assistance in management (1)[C].

ADDITIONAL THERAPIES
N/A

SURGERY/OTHER PROCEDURES
Surgery may be recommended for recurrent joint dislocations and instability on an individualized basis.

COMPLEMENTARY & ALTERNATIVE MEDICINE
- A number of supplements have been proposed to treat joint hypermobility syndrome including calcium, carnitine, coenzyme Q10, glucosamine, magnesium, methylsulfonylmethane, pycnogenol, silica, vitamin C, and vitamin K.
- However, large-scale, randomized controlled trials demonstrating efficacy are lacking (4)[C].

ADMISSION, INPATIENT, AND NURSING CONSIDERATIONS
N/A

ONGOING CARE

FOLLOW-UP RECOMMENDATIONS

Patient Monitoring
Follow-up is recommended at the clinicians discretion based on the specific needs of the individual.

DIET
N/A

PATIENT EDUCATION
- The goal of education is to help individuals understand the nature of the condition and recommended treatment options.
- Education may help reduce rates of joint dislocations and other associated injuries.
- Self-help groups such as the Hypermobility Syndromes Association (HMSA) located in the United Kingdom may provide further support (2).

PROGNOSIS
- Joint hypermobility syndrome is a lifelong condition that in many individuals may manifest as recurrent episodes of joint pain. However, the majority of those affected are asymptomatic.
- Some individuals experience reduction in symptoms along with reduced flexibility that occurs with age.
- Longitudinal studies examining the progression of the condition are currently unavailable (1,2).

COMPLICATIONS
- Although recurrent joint subluxation, dislocation and pes planus are commonly associated conditions, exact rates of these complications remain unknown (2).
- Physical therapy including a strengthening protocol is thought to reduce the rates of these complications, but high-quality studies that provide measurement of these outcomes are lacking (2,3).

REFERENCES

1. Colombi M, Dordoni C, Chiarelli N, et al. Differential diagnosis and diagnostic flow chart of joint hypermobility syndrome/Ehlers-Danlos syndrome hypermobility type compared to other heritable connective tissue disorders. *Am J Med Genet C Semin Med Genet*. 2015;169C(1):6–22.
2. Pacey V, Tofts L, Wesley A, et al. Joint hypermobility syndrome: a review for clinicians. *J Paediatr Child Health*. 2015;51(4):373–380.
3. Palmer S, Bailey S, Barker L, et al. The effectiveness of therapeutic exercise for joint hypermobility syndrome: a systematic review. *Physiotherapy*. 2014;100(3):220–227.
4. Mantle D, Wilkins RM, Preedy V. A novel therapeutic strategy for Ehlers-Danlos syndrome based on nutritional supplements. *Med Hypotheses*. 2005;64(2):279–283.

ADDITIONAL READING

- Grahame R, Bird HA, Child A. The revised (Brighton 1998) criteria for the diagnosis of benign joint hypermobility syndrome (BJHS). *J Rheumatol*. 2000;27(7):1777–1779.
- Hakim AJ, Grahame R. A simple questionnaire to detect hypermobility: an adjunct to the assessment of patients with diffuse musculoskeletal pain. *Int J Clin Pract*. 2003;57(3):163–166.

SEE ALSO

Connective Tissue Disorders; Ehlers-Danlos Syndrome Hypermobility Type; Joint Hypermobility Syndrome

CLINICAL PEARLS
- Joint hypermobility syndrome is a chronic condition and a diagnosis of exclusion that includes joint laxity and skin fragility.
- The diagnosis is based on history and physical exam and relies on the exclusion of other connective tissue disorders such as Marfan and Ehlers-Danlos syndromes.
- Treatment should be tailored to address symptoms and include physical therapy to improve strength, balance, proprioception, and quality of life.

HYPERTHERMIA: HEAT STROKE, EXHAUSTION, AND CRAMPS

Christopher C. Trigger, MD, FACEP, CAQSM

BASICS

DESCRIPTION

- Heat illness is the result of increased heat production and impaired heat dissipation.
- Exertional heat illness is a continuum but based on signs and symptoms can be divided into the following groups:
  - Heat cramps
  - Heat exhaustion
  - Heat stroke

EPIDEMIOLOGY

Incidence

- ~400 deaths per year can be attributed to all types of heat illness in the United States.
- Exertional heat stroke is the third leading cause of death in athletes (1,2).

Prevalence

- Football has been identified as the sport with the greatest number of heat-related fatalities.
- From 2005 to 2009, 49 deaths were reported in high school, collegiate, and professional football due to heat stroke (2).

ETIOLOGY AND PATHOPHYSIOLOGY

Heat dissipation occurs via four processes (1,2):

- Radiation is the direct release of heat from the body to the environment.
- Conduction occurs with direct transfer of heat during contact with a cooler object.
- Convection is when cooler air passes over the warmer exposed skin, lifting the heat away.
- Evaporation through perspiration is the body's most effective way of eliminating heat, although limited when humidity is high.

RISK FACTORS

- Hot, humid weather
- Dehydration
- Sickle trait
- Age (<15 yr or >65 yr)
- Poorly trained and/or overweight athletes
- Cumulative heat load from previous days' exposures
- Improper attire (plastic suits)
- Equipment (football pads/helmet)
- Poor acclimatization
- Medications:
  - Dietary supplements (i.e., ephedra, diet pills)
  - Antihypertensives (i.e., diuretics, β-blockers, calcium channel blockers)
  - Tricyclic antidepressants
  - Monoamine oxidase inhibitors
  - Antihistamines
  - Amphetamines
  - Illicit drugs (i.e., cocaine, heroin, phencyclidine)
- Concurrent illness (viral illness, skin disorders, cardiac disease)

GENERAL PREVENTION

- Pre/posthydration
- Modify time; intensity; and exposure in hot, humid weather:
  - Exercise in the early morning or evening.
  - Limit sun exposure if possible.
  - Remove unnecessary equipment and/or clothing.
- Heat acclimatization (usually takes 10 to 14 days) (3)[C]
- Increase electrolyte intake, mainly sodium (Na), using sports drinks.

DIAGNOSIS

HISTORY

- Heat cramps:
  - Painful involuntary contractions of muscles, most commonly the calf, quadriceps, and abdomen
  - Heat cramps are more commonly thought of as an electrolyte problem than a heat issue.
- Heat exhaustion:
  - Fatigue
  - Shortness of breath
  - Dizziness or syncope
  - Nausea and vomiting
  - Normal mental status
- Heat stroke:
  - Central nervous system (CNS) symptoms with the correct environmental conditions (hot and humid)
  - Previous history of heat exhaustion

PHYSICAL EXAM

- Heat cramps:
  - Normal temperature and vital signs
  - Tense, tender, involuntary contraction of the muscle belly
- Heat exhaustion:
  - Normal or elevated core temperature but <40°C (104°F)
  - Vital signs usually normal but can be variable depending on severity
  - Normal mental status
  - Flushed skin
  - Profuse sweating
  - Cold, clammy skin
- Heat stroke:
  - Core (rectal) temperature >40°C (104°F) (3,4)
  - CNS disturbances (confusion, ataxia, irritability, coma)
  - Tachycardic, tachypneic, and hypotensive
  - Hot skin with or without sweating
  - End-organ damage/failure

DIFFERENTIAL DIAGNOSIS

- Dehydration
- Electrolyte abnormality
- Cardiovascular disease
- Exercise-associated collapse
- CNS lesion
- Thyroid dysfunction
- Infection

DIAGNOSTIC TESTS & INTERPRETATION

Initial Tests (lab, imaging)

Routine lab work typically unnecessary for minor heat illness, but depending on the clinical picture, you may need to check the following:

- Complete blood count (CBC)
- Basic metabolic panel
- Urinalysis to detect myoglobin
- Serum creatine kinase to evaluate for rhabdomyolysis
- Toxicology screen
- Cardiac enzymes
- Liver function tests
- Coagulation studies to evaluate disseminated intravascular coagulation

Diagnostic Procedures/Other

Electrocardiography (ECG): Consider in heat stroke to look for cardiac damage/dysfunction.

TREATMENT

- Acute treatment:
  - Use basic or advanced cardiac life support for all unstable patients and transfer them to the nearest medical facility.
  - Common theme in treating all heat illnesses is to lower the core temp to an acceptable (38°C) level as quickly as possible.
- Heat cramps (2,5):
  - Rest
  - Oral replacement of fluids and electrolytes (Na) using sports drinks (1)
  - Intravenous (IV) fluids if unable to tolerate by mouth
  - Passive stretching and/or ice massage of the affected muscles
- Heat exhaustion (2,3):
  - More aggressive cooling techniques:
    - Move to cool environment.
    - Rest and remove excess clothing.
    - Apply ice bags to neck, axilla, and groin (3)[C].
  - Place in supine position and elevate legs.
  - Replacement of fluids and electrolytes
  - IV fluids if unable to tolerate oral rehydration
- Heat stroke (2,3,5):
  - Support airway, breathing, and circulation.
  - Rapid cooling of the patient is first line:
    - Cold/ice water immersion most rapid form of cooling (3,4)[A]
    - If immersion unavailable, place wet towels/sheets and ice bags to neck, axilla, and groin (2,3,5)[C]
  - IV fluids
  - If doctor of medicine/doctor of osteopathic medicine (MD/DO) onsite and cooling occurs immediately and patient is asymptomatic 1 hr postcooling, transport to emergency department (ED) may be unnecessary (4)[B].
- ED treatment:
  - Any person exhibiting signs of worsening heat illness, specifically those with mental status changes and a temperature >40°C, should be immediately cooled and transferred for improved monitoring and management.
  - Once in the ED, the patient should undergo similar cooling techniques as noted above.

ONGOING CARE

FOLLOW-UP RECOMMENDATIONS

Return to play recommendations (2,3):

- Heat cramps (3)[C]:
  - May return immediately after symptoms resolve with rest and fluid replacement
  - Depending on severity, may require 24 hr of relative rest
- Heat exhaustion (3)[C]:
  - Immediate return not recommended
  - Generally, can return to activity within 24 to 48 hr
  - Gradually increase intensity and volume of training
- Heat stroke (4)[B]:
  - Consider at least 7 days of rest or until asymptomatic and lab values have normalized.
  - Consider follow-up no later than 1 wk after event or even sooner based on severity of symptoms and lab abnormalities.
  - When cleared, begin training in cool environment and acclimate to heat over a 2-wk period.
  - Clear the athlete for full competition if heat tolerance exists after 2 to 4 wk of training.
  - If athlete does not tolerate return to play progression or has recurrent heat illnesses, consider laboratory exercise-heat tolerance test.

PATIENT EDUCATION

- Avoid risks listed above.
- "Salty sweaters" may be at higher risk for heat cramps due to loss of Na; encourage increased salt intake with meals and hydration with electrolytes.

COMPLICATIONS

- Death
- End-organ failure
- Seizures
- Cardiovascular collapse
- Acute respiratory distress syndrome
- Liver failure
- Acute renal failure
- Rhabdomyolysis
- Disseminated intravascular coagulation

Danger Category	Apparent Temperature (°F)	Heat Syndrome
IV. Extreme danger	130°F or higher	Heat stroke highly likely with continued exposure
III. Danger	105–130°F	Heat cramps or heat exhaustion likely and heat stroke possible with prolonged exposure and/or physical activity
II. Extreme caution	90–105°F	Heat stroke, heat cramps, and heat exhaustion possible with prolonged exposure and/or physical activity
I. Caution	80–90°F	Fatigue possible with prolonged exposure and/or physical activity

REFERENCES

1. Casa DJ, DeMartini JK, Bergeron MF, et al. National Athletic Trainers' Association position statement: exertional heat illnesses. *J Athl Train*. 2015;50(9):986–1000.
2. Howe AS, Boden BP. Heat-related illness in athletes. *Am J Sports Med*. 2007;35(8):1384–1395.
3. Armstrong LE, Casa DJ, Millard-Stafford M, et al; and American College of Sports Medicine. American College of Sports Medicine position stand. Exertional heat illness during training and competition. *Med Sci Sports Exerc*. 2007;39(3):556–572.
4. Casa DJ, Armstrong LE, Kenny GP, et al. Exertional heat stroke: new concepts regarding cause and care. *Curr Sports Med Rep*. 2012;11(3):115–123.
5. Pryor RR, Bennett BL, O'Connor FG, et al. Medical evaluation for exposure extremes: heat. *Clin J Sport Med*. 2015;25(5):437–442.

CLINICAL PEARLS

- Remember the principle "cool first, transport second."
- General Heat Stress Index (2,5) (see Table)

HYPERTROPHIC CARDIOMYOPATHY

Anne M. Garrison, DO, CAQSM • Lisa Falotico, DO, CAQSM

BASICS

DESCRIPTION

- Asymmetric nondilated left ventricular hypertrophy (LVH), with or without outflow obstruction
- Mostly inherited autosomal dominant disease, but many cases are sporadic
- Primary cause (35%) of sudden atraumatic death in athletes aged <35 yr
- Death results from ventricular tachycardia either due to, or in the absence of, LV outflow obstruction (some patients have arrhythmogenic foci).

EPIDEMIOLOGY

- Incidence of hypertrophic cardiomyopathy (HCM) is 0.2% or 1:500 in the general population, meaning there are about 600,000 patients in the United States.
- Incidence of sudden cardiac death (SCD) in athletes <35 yr, mostly due to HCM, is 1:250,000.
- Many patients remain undiagnosed.

RISK FACTORS

- Family history of unexplained or early (<40 yr) cardiac death
- Age from 12 to 30 yr old
- Prior history of syncope
- Abnormal blood pressure (BP) response to exercise

DIAGNOSIS

HISTORY

- History is negative for most patients.
- Direct and specific questions are important, and parents should be questioned as well.
- Providers should also inquire about prescription medications and drugs of abuse.

PHYSICAL EXAM

- Most common initial presentation is syncope or SCD with exertion.
- Palpitations
- Exertional chest pain
- Most patients with HCM have a completely normal physical examination.
- Murmur: In rare cases where murmur is detected, it is usually midsystolic and heard at the midleft sternal border:
  - Murmur is ominous if it increases with maneuvers to decrease LV end-diastolic (LVED) filling. These maneuvers cause dynamic obstruction in the LV outflow tract.
  - Maneuvers include rising from squatting to standing, moving from supine to vertical position, and performing the Valsalva maneuver.
  - Murmur decreases when LVED filling increases while moving from standing to squatting (LV free wall moves away from the septum with increased filling).
  - Benign murmurs usually become louder while squatting and decrease on rising.
  - Benign murmurs are common with improved fitness from training, as described with the athletic heart syndrome (AHS).
  - Athletes with significant outflow obstruction eventually may have pansystolic blowing murmur of mitral regurgitation radiating to the axilla.
- Any diastolic murmur indicates other cardiac pathology requiring workup.
- Screening electrocardiogram (ECG) as part of the preparticipation exam can help detect cardiac disorders with the potential to cause SCD (such as HCM), but they also create false positives (1)[C].

DIFFERENTIAL DIAGNOSIS

- AHS
- Myocarditis/pericarditis
- Coronary artery anomalies
- Aortic stenosis
- Prolonged QT syndrome
- Marfan syndrome
- Wolff-Parkinson-White syndrome
- Arrhythmogenic right ventricular dysplasia
- Exercise-induced asthma
- Costochondritis
- Gastroesophageal reflux

DIAGNOSTIC TESTS & INTERPRETATION

Initial Tests (lab, imaging)

- Genetic family screening is available and may help identify first-degree family members at risk for developing HCM (2)[B].
- Clinicians may be increasingly faced with the dilemma of making recommendations regarding sports participation for subjects who have only preclinical evidence of HCM (genotype positive-phenotype negative).
- Patients with pathologic mutations who do not express HCM phenotype are recommended to have ECG, echocardiogram, and clinical assessments (every 12 to 18 mo in children and adolescents, and every 5 yr in adults) (2)[B].
- ECG (2)[C]:
  - LVH findings
  - Increased voltage
  - Repolarization abnormalities
  - Prominent deep Q waves in left precordial leads, ischemic ST changes in 90% of cases
  - ECG findings do not correlate with severity or pattern of hypertrophy noted on imaging.
- 24-hr Holter monitor (2)[B]:
  - Not commonly used for screening (but recommended in initial HCM evaluation), may reveal paroxysmal atrial fibrillation and ventricular tachycardia, which frequently are symptomatic
- Echocardiogram:
  - Echocardiogram usually shows LV wall thickening measured on the free wall as >15 mm in adults or >2 standard deviations above the mean for children (2)[B].
  - The wall thickness is characteristically asymmetric, with the interventricular septum and anterolateral thicker than the posterior wall.
  - Has the advantage of using provocative maneuvers
  - Unlike patients with HCM, athletes with AHS (fit, young adults who also have murmurs) have right ventricular hypertrophy and increased LV volumes or total LV diameter. These findings represent physiologic adaptations to increased plasma volume rather than pathologic.
- Cardiac magnetic resonance imaging (2)[B]:
  - Superior for identifying atypical hypertrophy locations and apical aneurysms
  - Indicated when echo is inconclusive

Diagnostic Procedures/Other

Exercise stress testing is useful for evaluation and management of symptomatic patients, but its value in screening asymptomatic subjects is controversial (2)[B].

TREATMENT

- Acute treatment/emergency action plan:
  - Cardiopulmonary resuscitation (CPR) for syncope or arrest and defibrillation with automated external defibrillator (AED) as soon as possible if indicated
- Long-term treatment (for symptomatic patients):
  - Implantable cardiac defibrillator (ICD) for primary or secondary prevention of SCD (2)[B]
  - Medication (typically β blockers) (2)[B]
  - Myomectomy or ablation (2)[B]
  - Activity restrictions (2)[C]
  - Treatment is individualized based on degree/location of LV thickening, symptoms, and concomitant cardiac pathology.

ONGOING CARE

The 36th Bethesda Conference recommendations for activity for individuals with HCM:

- Athletes with a probable or unequivocal clinical diagnosis of HCM should be excluded from most competitive sports, except possibly low-intensity sports. This recommendation includes athletes with and without symptoms or LV outflow obstruction.
- Given that the risk of SCD may be reduced in older individuals (>40 yr) with HCM, an alternative of individual judgment may be used in selected older athletes only when each of the following clinical features is absent:
  - Ventricular tachycardia (sustained or nonsustained) on ambulatory ECG
  - Family history of SCD due to HCM, particularly if <40 yr old
  - History of syncope or other clinically relevant episodes of impaired consciousness
  - Severe hemodynamic abnormalities, including dynamic LV outflow tract gradient >50 mm Hg
  - Exercise-induced hypotension
  - Moderate-to-severe mitral regurgitation, enlarged left atrium (>50 mm), or paroxysmal atrial fibrillation
  - Presence of abnormal myocardial perfusion
  - These recommendations are not altered if medical or surgical treatment is undertaken in a given athlete.
- Competitive athletic participation is reasonable in asymptomatic genotype positive/phenotype negative (no LV hypertrophy noted on echo or cardiovascular magnetic resonance imaging [CMRI]); HCM patients—especially if there is no family history of SCD (3)[C]

REFERENCES

1. Drezner JA, O'Connor FG, Harmon KG, et al. AMSSM position statement on cardiovascular preparticipation screening in athletes: current evidence, knowledge gaps, recommendations, and future directions. *Clin J Sport Med*. 2016;26(5):347–361.
2. Gersh BJ, Maro BJ, Bonow RO, et al. 2011 ACCF/AHA guideline for the diagnosis and treatment of hypertrophic cardiomyopathy: a report of the American College of Cardiology Foundation/American Heart Association Task Force on Practice Guidelines. *J Am Coll Cardiol*. 2011;58(25):e214–e260.
3. Maron BJ, Udelson JE, Bonow RO, et al. Eligibility and disqualification recommendations for competitive athletes with cardiovascular abnormalities: task force 3: hypertrophic cardiomyopathy, arrhythmogenic right ventricular cardiomyopathy and other cardiomyopathies, and myocarditis: a scientific statement from the American Heart Association and American College of Cardiology. *Circulation*. 2015;132(22):e273–e280.

ADDITIONAL READING

- Houston BA, Stevens GR. Hypertrophic cardiomyopathy: a review. *Clin Med Insights Cardiol*. 2014;8(Suppl 1):53–65.
- Maron BJ, Ommen SR, Semsarian C, et al. Hypertrophic cardiomyopathy: present and future, with translation into contemporary cardiovascular medicine. *J Am Coll Cardiol*. 2014;64(1):83–99.

CLINICAL PEARLS

- Patients should avoid physical activities that require exertion while awaiting diagnosis as this may exacerbate a potentially deadly condition.
- HCM is a rare genetic disease that can cause abnormal beating of the heart, especially with exercise. It is difficult to control, and even those who are treated probably should avoid all strenuous exercise, unless HCM is proven not to be the diagnosis.
- Genotype positive/phenotype negative patients may spontaneously convert to LV hypertrophy, often without cardiac symptoms, at any age, but appears to occur most often between ages 12 and 20 yr.
- There is a significant risk of death in people who have true HCM. Exercise increases this risk in some athletes. Certain exercises may be permitted after the true diagnosis and extent of the problem are clear.
- Only very low-intensity exercises (class IA sports) are considered possibly acceptable, including golf, billiards, bowling, cricket, curling, and riflery.

HYPHEMA

Jennifer J. Mitchell, MD, FAAFP, CAQSM • Kelly T. Mitchell, MD

BASICS

DESCRIPTION

- Blood in the anterior chamber of the eye
- Traumatic hyphema grading:
  - Microhyphema:
    - Circulating red blood cells (RBCs) usually seen by slit lamp exam only
  - Grade I:
    - <1/3 anterior chamber with layered blood
  - Grade II:
    - 1/3 to 1/2 of anterior chamber filled with blood
  - Grade III:
    - >1/2 anterior chamber filled with blood
  - Grade IV:
    - 100% anterior chamber filling (blackball or 8-ball hyphema) (1)

EPIDEMIOLOGY

Incidence

- Annual incidence of traumatic hyphema:
  - 17/100,000 <18 yr
  - 20.7/100,000 <20 yr (1)
- Males:females 3:1 (2)

ETIOLOGY AND PATHOPHYSIOLOGY

- Trauma:
  - Blunt trauma 2/3
  - Lacerating injury 1/3 (2)
- Spontaneously: association with certain medical conditions
- Postocular procedure (laser, surgery)

RISK FACTORS

- Traumatic hyphema:
  - High-risk sports causing blunt injury to eye with projectile or body part:
    - Hockey, lacrosse, racquetball, basketball
- Spontaneous hyphema:
  - Neovascularization; diabetes mellitus
  - Blood dyscrasias/hemoglobinopathies
  - Uveitis
  - Ocular tumors

GENERAL PREVENTION

- Protective eyewear during sports involving contact or use of a ball
- One-eyed athletes should wear impact resistant eye protection at all times.

COMMONLY ASSOCIATED CONDITIONS

- Corneal abrasion
- Corneal scleral laceration
- Perforation
- Intraocular foreign body
- Subconjunctival hemorrhage/hemorrhagic chemosis
- Orbital fracture
- Iridodialysis

DIAGNOSIS

HISTORY

- Mechanism of injury to determine whether associated injuries such as open globe or orbital fracture may be present (2)[B].
- Presence of sickle cell disease or blood dyscrasias, which changes prognosis and management (2)[B]. Sickle-shaped RBCs clog trabecular meshwork and cause more severe type of glaucoma.
- Predisposing medical conditions and medications related to increased risk of spontaneous hyphema
- If mechanism does not match degree of injury, evaluate for child abuse, diabetes mellitus, clotting disorder, or tumors (1)[A],(2)[B].

PHYSICAL EXAM

Acute systematic exam (3,4)[C]:

- Sports-related ocular trauma evaluated on site
- Mechanism of injury if not personally witnessed
- Best corrected visual acuity, pocket Snellen chart or smart phone app
- Confrontation visual fields
- Pupil exam with penlight, including evaluation for afferent pupillary defect
- Penlight exam of the anterior chamber looking for haziness with red tinge (microhyphema) or boat-shaped layering of blood inferiorly
- Ocular motility
- External exam looking for conjunctiva, corneal, or orbital injury
- Funduscopic exam, if possible, but not likely to provide much useful information
- Topical anesthetic may be used to facilitate exam.
- Intraocular pressure evaluation should be deferred to ophthalmology.
- If concern for ruptured globe, place protection (shield or sturdy sunglasses) over affected eye, make nothing by mouth (NPO), refer emergently; defer further ocular exam or manipulation to ophthalmologist.

DIFFERENTIAL DIAGNOSIS

- Iris tear, traumatic mydriasis
- Orbital fracture
- Retrobulbar hematoma
- Ruptured globe:
  - Anterior corneal scleral rupture
  - Occult posterior scleral rupture
- Traumatic cataract
- Traumatic subconjunctival hemorrhage/hemorrhagic chemosis
- Vitreous hemorrhage

DIAGNOSTIC TESTS & INTERPRETATION

Initial Tests (lab, imaging)

- Sickle cell rapid preparation in high-risk populations (African American, Afro-Caribbean, Hispanic); hemoglobin electrophoresis, if positive (2)[B]
- Spontaneous hyphema: complete blood count (CBC), prothrombin time, partial thromboplastin time, international normalized ratio, liver function to screen for bleeding dyscrasias
- Plain film x-ray for ocular or orbital injury has a high false-negative rate and is not useful to plan therapeutic intervention.
- Orbital computed tomography (CT) scan if concern for globe rupture, intraocular foreign body, orbital fracture
- CT: thin-sliced helical CT with coronal reconstructions; if helical CT not available, CT scan with slices of 3 mm or less in axial and coronal planes
- Magnetic resonance imaging (MRI) is contraindicated in cases of possible metallic foreign body.
- Ultrasound evaluation in primary evaluation is controversial due to concern for presence of ruptured globe.
- Ultrasound in acute evaluation has questionable diagnostic yield and carries risk of further injury from inadvertent compression of the injured eye.
- Use of ultrasound in this setting should be deferred to the consulting ophthalmologist.

Diagnostic Procedures/Other

- A gonioscopy exam, to assess for glaucoma, puts pressure on the eye and is contraindicated with an acute hyphema.
- Once the blood is completely resolved, no earlier than 4 wk, the managing ophthalmologist will perform gonioscopy to check for angle recession (trauma to the angle) to determine whether there is increased risk for glaucoma. Gonioscopy can precipitate rebleeding if done too early, before the hyphema has resolved.

TREATMENT

GENERAL MEASURES

- Prehospital:
  - Place rigid eye shield to protect the eye.
  - Minimize mobility of the patient.
  - Head of transport bed elevated 30 to 45 degrees so blood will tend to settle inferiorly.
  - Do not give any nonsteroidal anti-inflammatory drugs (NSAIDs) or aspirin.
  - Keep NPO in case surgery is required.
- Emergency department treatment:
  - Assess and treat life-threatening injuries.
  - To facilitate further exam, provide additional pain control with topical anesthetic: proparacaine or tetracaine ophthalmic.
  - Fluorescein dye can be used to detect a corneal abrasion.
  - Assess carefully for ocular perforation (open globe).
  - Treat emesis and pain to prevent sudden intraocular hypertension and extrusion of ocular contents.
  - Do not give NSAIDs or aspirin due to the platelet-inhibiting properties.
  - Evaluate for underlying hemoglobinopathy or bleeding dyscrasias if indicated. When not being examined, keep eye protected with shield and head of bed elevated to 30 to 45 degrees.
  - Arrange for urgent ophthalmology assessment.

MEDICATION

- Medication management should be directed by ophthalmology.
- Anticoagulant medications risk: Hyphema persistence or rebleed so risk of continuation versus benefit for underlying medical conditions are made on a case by case basis (1)[A].
- Mydriatics and cycloplegics permit visualization of the posterior pole, provide comfort from iritis, facilitate clot resolution, and decrease the risk of posterior synechiae related to scarring of the iris to the lens:
  - Cyclopentolate ophthalmic drops 1 gtt BID
  - Atropine ophthalmic drops 1 gtt QD to BID (1)[A]

- Ophthalmic topical steroids help decrease intraocular inflammation, minimize long-term iris scarring, and may facilitate clot stabilization to minimize rebleeding, which is a priority early in the course of hyphema (1)[A].
- Oral steroids may have a role to decrease inflammation and minimize rebleeding risk.
- Antifibrinolytic agents lower the rate of rebleeding but may delay clot resorption. Their use is controversial for a variety of reasons. They do not offer any major advantage in preventing most complications related to hyphema (1,5)[A]:
  - Aminocaproic acid:
    - 50 mg/kg by mouth (PO) q4h × 5 days, adult dosing
    - 30% gel q6h × 5 days, adult dosing
    - Side effects: nausea, vomiting, hypotension; more likely with oral versus topical
    - Contraindicated in pregnancy, renal disease, hemophilia, thromboembolic disease
  - Tranexamic acid:
    - 75 mg/kg divided TID × 5 days, adult dosing
    - 5% solution 1 gtt q6h × 5 days, adult dosing
  - *Not U.S. Food and Drug Administration (FDA) approved*

ISSUES FOR REFERRAL

Any hyphema warrants urgent early ophthalmologic referral to categorize the severity of the ocular injury and of the hyphema, which is critical in management decisions.

ADDITIONAL THERAPIES

- Eye protection with hard plastic eye shield at all times, including sleep, until hyphema is resolved
- Strict bed rest for severe hyphema, sickle cell trait/disease, children, bleeding predisposition and noncompliant patients. This may require hospitalization.
- Bed rest with quiet activity at home otherwise
- Consulting ophthalmologist will guide the care regarding continued use of medications and management of intraocular pressure.
- Traumatic hyphema and intraocular hypertension require medication to decrease intraocular pressure:
  - Topical medications used: β-adrenergic blocker eye drops (timolol), α-agonist eye drops (brimonidine—avoid in children <3 yr due to risk of apnea), prostaglandin analogs (latanoprost), and topical carbonic anhydrase inhibitors (CAIs), if sickle cell hemoglobinopathy has been ruled out
- In sickle cell, CAIs may cause increased sickling in anterior chamber due to decreasing the pH.
- After complete resolution of the hyphema, and usually at the 2- to 4-wk follow-up appointment, the ophthalmologist will:
  - Perform gonioscopy to evaluate for permanent angle injury (angle recession) that may predispose the patient to chronic, posttraumatic glaucoma.
  - Perform dilated retinal exam to assess for any occult breaks or tear.
- If vision is still blurrier than expected, an optical coherence tomography (OCT) or fluorescein angiography may be performed to assess for occult, posttraumatic injury to the macula or retinal vessels.

SURGERY/OTHER PROCEDURES

- 5–7% require surgery (1)[A].
- Indications for surgical intervention after hyphema:
  - Corneal blood staining
  - Intraocular pressure >24 mm Hg for >24 hr in patient with sickle cell disease
  - Intraocular pressure >60 mm Hg for >2 days
  - Intraocular pressure ≥50 mm Hg for 5 days
  - 50% or greater hyphema unresolved for 7 days (1)[A]
- Other surgeries considered by ophthalmologist to optimize vision:
  - Trabeculectomy glaucoma surgery to treat persistently elevated intraocular pressure even after clot evacuation
  - Corneal transplant if blood staining has occurred, impacting visual axis; can cause amblyopia in children
  - Cataract surgery for associated posttraumatic cataract

ADMISSION, INPATIENT, AND NURSING CONSIDERATIONS

Inpatient management is recommended for:

- Other ocular or facial injuries requiring hospital care.
- Bleeding dyscrasias or sickle hemoglobinopathy.
- Active young children or unstable home.
- Large hyphemas (grade III or IV) with early signs of elevated intraocular pressure.
- Suspected child abuse.
- Evidence of secondary rebleeding on follow-up examination.

ONGOING CARE

PATIENT EDUCATION

- Patient must understand need for strict compliance with all activity restrictions and medication dosing and follow-up appointments.
- Review symptoms of rebleeding or elevated intraocular pressure (sudden decreased vision and pain).
- Provide medications and medication schedule prior to discharge to improve adherence.

PROGNOSIS

- Final visual acuity depends on size of hyphema and related complications.
- Secondary hemorrhages usually result in hyphemas that are larger than the initial injury. When this complication occurs, the patients usually have a poorer outcome due to the higher occurrence of severe glaucoma and blood staining of the cornea.
- A final vision of 20/50 or worse is seen in 10% of patients with grade I and in 50–75% with grade III or IV. The poorer visual outcome is usually due to more severe optic atrophy secondary to the initial trauma or secondary glaucoma or visually significant blood staining.
- 14% of hyphema patients have poor visual outcomes as a result of associated sequelae (vitreous hemorrhage, retinal detachment, ocular rupture).
- Blunt eye injury and hyphema increase risk of late developing traumatic glaucoma.
- Anticipate return to normal activities within a week, but no athletic participation for up to a month.

COMPLICATIONS

- Rebleeding
- Glaucoma: early/late developing
- Corneal blood staining
- Traumatic cataract: early/late developing
- Potential for significant vision loss

REFERENCES

1. Bansal S, Gunasekeran DV, Ang B, et al. Controversies in the pathophysiology and management of hyphema. *Surv Ophthalmol*. 2016;61(3):297–308.
2. Trief D, Adebona OT, Turalba AV, et al. The pediatric traumatic hyphema. *Int Ophthalmol Clin*. 2013;53(4):43–57.
3. Micieli JA, Easterbrook M. Eye and orbital injuries in sports. *Clin Sports Med*. 2017;36(2):299–314.
4. Cass SP. Ocular injuries in sports. *Curr Sport Med Rep*. 2012;11(1):11–15.
5. Gharaibeh A, Savage HI, Scherer RW, et al. Medical interventions for traumatic hyphema. *Cochrane Database Syst Rev*. 2013;(12):CD005431.

ADDITIONAL READING

- American Academy of Ophthalmology. *Protective Eyewear for Young Athletes*. https://www.aao.org/clinical-statement/protective-eyewear-young-athletes. Accessed June 3, 2018.
- Bizrah M, Verma S. Nerf gun eye injuries: traumatic hyphema [published online ahead of print September 18, 2017]. *BMJ Case Rep*. doi:10.1136/bcr-2017-220967.
- Black AM, Eliason PH, Patton DA, et al. Epidemiology of facial injuries in sport. *Clin Sports Med*. 2017;36(2):237–255.
- Romaniuk VM. Ocular trauma and other catastrophes. *Emerg Med Clin North Am*. 2013;31(2):399–411.
- Walton W, Von Hagen S, Grigorian R, et al. Management of traumatic hyphema. *Surv Ophthalmol*. 2002;47(4):297–334.

CLINICAL PEARLS

- Appropriate protective eyewear is needed for all athletic events involving a ball, projectile, or physical contact:
  - The American Society for Testing and Materials has established performance standards for selected eyewear that are most appropriate for sports with a risk of ocular injury.
  - The American Academy of Ophthalmology has helpful guidelines online.
- Concern for hyphema requires prompt evaluation and emergent referral to an ophthalmologist.
- Detailed education of the patient for adherence to activity restrictions is essential.
- Return to athletic competition may be prolonged.

HYPOTHENAR HAMMER SYNDROME

Holly J. Benjamin, MD, FAAP, FACSM • Tarek S. Hadla, MD, CAQSM

BASICS

DESCRIPTION

Lesion of the superficial palmar arch of the ulnar artery in the hand caused mainly by repetitive compression or blunt trauma or even a single severe trauma over the hook of the hamate-hypothenar eminence as a result of occupational or sport activities usually (1,2,3,4)[A]

EPIDEMIOLOGY

- Rare: traditionally regarded as a rare condition, although may be underdiagnosed
- Male:female ratio is 9:1.
- Age bracket is 40 to 50 yr.

ETIOLOGY AND PATHOPHYSIOLOGY

- Etiology (1,2)[B]:
  - *Trauma*: by frequent use of the hand as "hammer"
  - *Vascular pathology*: thrombosis, abnormal anatomy, or aneurysm of the ulnar artery, prothrombotic factors. Unilateral symptoms with hypothenar hammer syndrome (HHS) are suspected to occur when persons with preexisting palmar ulnar artery fibrodysplasia experience repetitive palmar trauma. This revised theory for the etiology of HHS explains why HHS does not develop in most patients with repetitive palmar trauma (1)[C].
  - *Work related*: auto mechanics, metal workers, Lathe operators, miners, machinists, butchers, bakers, carpenters, and brick layers
  - *Sport related*: golf, baseball catchers, heavy weight lifting, martial arts, mountain biking
- Pathophysiology:
  - Hypothenar relates to the muscles of the 5th finger.
  - Unilateral, dominant ring finger +/− small finger
  - Less commonly, index and middle fingers
  - Thumb is spared.
  - Mnemonic AFO:
    - A-bductor digiti minimi
    - F-lexor digiti minimi
    - O-pponens digiti minimi
  - The hand obtains its arterial supply through the ulnar and radial arteries. The ulnar artery and nerve pass through Guyon canal next to the hamate bone before dividing into the superficial and deep palmar branches. Just distal to the canal, a short segment of the superficial branch that forms the origin of the superficial palmar arch is unprotected between the skin and the bone in the hypothenar area. Over distal 2 cm, the artery is directly anterior to the hook of the hamate, covered by palmaris brevis, subcutaneous tissue, and skin. Chronic trauma to this area can lead to pathology of the ulnar artery.
  - Types of HHS:
    - *Type 1*: stenosis of superficial palmar arch around the hook of the hamate
    - *Type 2a*: occlusion of the superficial palmar arch around the hook of the hamate
    - *Type 2b*: occlusion of superficial and deep palmar arches around the hook of the hamate
    - *Type 3a*: occlusion of the ulnar artery at the proximal part of the wrist
    - *Type 3b*: occlusion of the ulnar artery near the wrist

DIAGNOSIS

Early diagnosis allows more effective therapeutic strategies and is important to prevent long-term negative medical sequelae (5)[B].

HISTORY

Symptoms (2):

- Paresthesia in fingers; pins and needles sensation
- Pain in fingers caused by cold or repetitive movements
- Raynaud-like phenomenon that spares the thumb

PHYSICAL EXAM

- A hypothenar mass or callus; pulsatile mass if aneurysm is present
- Tenderness over the hypothenar eminence
- Raynaud phenomenon–like symptoms in the fingers and on the ulnar side of the hand (6,7)
- Positive Allen test (see below)
- Dependent rubor
- Finger tips ulceration, blanching, mottling, cyanosis, pallor, gangrene (rare)
- *Allen tests*: Allen test is often used before cannulating the radial artery or in assessment of the hand trauma. The technique is as follows:
  - Patient elevates the hand and makes a fist for 20 sec.
  - Firm pressure is held against both the radial and ulnar arteries.
  - The patient opens the hand and it should blanche (changes color to white).
  - The examiner releases compression of the ulnar but not radial artery.
  - A normal hand flushes within 5 to 7 sec.
  - If the hand remains white, then there is an abnormal circulation—positive Allen test.

DIFFERENTIAL DIAGNOSIS

- Hand–arm vibration syndrome (6)
- Raynaud phenomena (RP) (2)[A]: RP involves the thumb, whereas HHS does not.

DIAGNOSTIC TESTS & INTERPRETATION

- Complete blood count (CBC) and international normalization ratio (INR) if thrombosis is suspected
- Doppler ultrasound (US)—first line. Measure digital brachial index: <0.7 necessitates reconstruction (2)[B].
- Arteriography (gold standard)
- Magnetic resonance (MR) angiography
- Computed tomography (CT) angiography
- *Finding*: tortuous "corkscrew" ulnar artery

TREATMENT

Optimal therapy for HHS has not been determined.

- Nonsurgical:
  - Lifestyle modification: Avoid further trauma, smoke cessation, alteration of sport activity.
  - Urokinase has been used to clear obstruction, as has prostaglandin E1 with heparin. Because the etiology of acute hand ischemia is not always obvious at the time of presentation, a trial of Urokinase infusion is warranted because it is relatively safe and its use may obviate the need for complex microsurgical reconstruction.
  - Calcium channel blockers, vasodilators, and platelet inhibitors have been also used (7)[C].
  - Treat underlying atherosclerosis and prothrombotic factors (e.g., smoking and hyperlipidemia).
- Surgical:
  - Surgical reconstruction (end-to-end anastomosis of the ulnar artery): This requires microsurgical techniques. Arteries may be transplanted from other sites or a venous graft may be used (3)[B].
  - Sympathectomy appears to give poor results.

ONGOING CARE

- *Complications*: gangrene of the fingers in severe cases, which may require surgery
- *Prognosis*: Many patients improve with non-surgical treatments as mentioned above (about 80% success). Results of reconstructive surgery were variable, and recurrence was fairly common (2)[B].
- *Prevention*: education focusing at improving work practices, sports modification, hand protection, and avoiding use of the palm of the hand as a hammer to pound, push, or twist objects (2,5)[A]

REFERENCES

1. Ferris BL, Taylor LM Jr, Oyama K, et al. Hypothenar hammer syndrome: proposed etiology. *J Vasc Surg*. 2000;31(1, Pt 1):104–113.
2. Jagenburg A, Goyen M, Hirschelmann R, et al. Hypothenar hammer syndrome: causes, sequelae and diagnostic aspects [in German]. *Rofo*. 2000;172(3):295–300.
3. Brodmann M, Stark G, Aschauer M, et al. Hypothenar hammer syndrome caused by post-traumatic aneurysm of the ulnar artery. *Wien Klin Wochenschr*. 2001;113(17–18):698–700.
4. Swofford BP, Swofford DP. Management of hypothenar hammer syndrome a case report. *Am J Case Rep*. 2018;19:150–152.
5. Schröttle A, Czihal M, Lottspeich C, et al. Hypothenar hammer syndrome. *Vasa*. 2015;44(3): 179–185.
6. Cooke RA. Hypothenar hammer syndrome: a discrete syndrome to be distinguished from hand-arm vibration syndrome. *Occup Med (Lond)*. 2003;53(5):320–324.
7. Conn J Jr, Bergan JJ, Bell JL. Hypothenar hammer syndrome: posttraumatic digital ischemia. *Surgery*. 1970;68(6):1122–1128.

CLINICAL PEARLS

- Avoid using hand as a *hammer*.
- Rare condition, but needs high suspicion in certain groups
- Doppler US—first line
- CT angiography—gold standard
- Prevention is the best management modality.
- Surgery if no improvement to avoid complication

HYPOTHERMIA AND FROSTBITE

Rania L. Dempsey, MD, MS • Craig C. Young, MD

BASICS

DESCRIPTION

- Frostbite:
  - Severe, local cold-related injury, resulting in freezing of soft tissue:
    - Superficial: partial or complete freeze of skin
    - Deep: involvement of skin and underlying tissue (may include muscles, vessels, nerves, fat, and bone)
- Hypothermia:
  - Systemic cold injury, classified as:
    - Mild: core body temperature 32–35°C (90–95°F)
    - Moderate: 30–32°C (86–90°F)
    - Severe: <30°C (86°F)

EPIDEMIOLOGY

Incidence

- True incidence of hypothermia and frostbite is unknown in athletes:
  - Mild cases of both are likely common in cold environments.
  - Hypothermia reported in up to 69% of athletes in cold water swimming events (1)
- Annual incidence of hypothermia-related deaths 4 per 1,000,000 general population in the United States:
  - More common in men (68% of cold-related deaths)
  - Aged ≥45 yr account for 78% of cold-related deaths.

ETIOLOGY AND PATHOPHYSIOLOGY

- Frostbite:
  - Fluids in body tissues and cellular spaces freeze and crystallize.
  - Cyclic vasodilation and vasoconstriction contribute to hypoxia/ischemia of affected tissue.
  - Severe or prolonged exposure can lead to irreversible tissue damage.
- Hypothermia:
  - Body heat is lost to the environment at a rate that overwhelms normal temperature homeostasis, resulting in decreased core body temperature.
  - With decreasing temperature, heart rate, cardiac output, and cerebral blood flow decrease:
    - May lead to cardiac rhythm disturbance and death

RISK FACTORS

- Hypothermia:
  - Environmental factors: cold temperature, wind chill, prolonged exposure, high altitude
  - Wet clothing (increases heat loss 2 to 5 times) or immersion (increases heat loss 10 to 25 times)
  - Fatigue
  - Low body fat
  - Alcohol use (inhibits shivering, enhances heat loss through peripheral vasodilation, and may lead to false sense of warmth)
  - Extremes of age (very young or old)
  - Underlying medical disease (e.g., sickle cell anemia, peripheral vascular disease, diabetes, seizure disorder, hypothyroidism)
  - Use of neuroleptic drugs
- Frostbite:
  - Environmental factors:
    - Cold temperature, wind chill, prolonged exposure, high altitude:
      - Risk of frostbite is <5% with temperatures >5°F (−15°C), but significant risk of frostbite increases with wind chill temperature ≤−18°F (−27°C) (2).
  - Wet clothing (increases heat loss 2 to 5 times) or immersion (increases heat loss 10 to 25 times)
  - Prior cold injury
  - Petroleum or oil lubricants
  - Constrictive clothing or shoes
  - Smoking
  - Vasospastic disorders (i.e., Raynaud syndrome)

GENERAL PREVENTION

Best treatment for hypothermia and frostbite is prevention:

- Event planning based on the potential temperature ranges
- Proper clothing, including hats, mittens, and multiple layers, as necessary
- Avoid alcohol and other mood-altering drugs.
- Recognize the signs and symptoms of hypothermia that indicate a need to seek shelter (shivering, slurred speech, somnolence).

DIAGNOSIS

- Frostbite:
  - Skin may appear erythematous and swollen, or waxy, white, yellow, or blue-purple.
  - Vesicles/blisters may be present.
  - Patients with superficial frostbite complain of numbness and pain in affected area, but in severe/deep frostbite, pain may be absent.
  - Technetium 99 bone scanning (1)[B] or magnetic resonance imaging may be useful in establishing disease severity and prognosis.
- Hypothermia:
  - Mild: Patient displays shivering and mild mental status changes, including confusion, amnesia, dysarthria, and ataxia.
  - Moderate: As core temperature declines, patient may develop severely impaired judgment or stupor, loss of deep tendon reflexes, loss of shivering with muscle rigidity, and cardiac arrhythmias.
  - Severe: Patient may have dilated pupils and appear comatose, with nearly undetectable blood pressure (BP) and respiration.

HISTORY

- Duration and severity of cold exposure (Prolonged exposure to very cold temperatures increases risk of severe frostbite or hypothermia.)
- Recent alcohol or drug use (impairs judgment and increases susceptibility to cold injury)
- History of cold water immersion (Wet clothing and skin significantly increase continued heat loss.)
- Underlying medical conditions (increases risk of severe frostbite or hypothermia)
- Pain in affected area suggests superficial versus deep frostbite.

PHYSICAL EXAM

- Measure core body temperature with a thermometer capable of measuring hypothermic temperatures:
  - To avoid further cold exposure, rectal temperature is not advisable until the patient is in a warm environment (3)[C].
  - Oral temperature is inadequate for diagnosis but can rule out hypothermia (3)[C].
  - Esophageal temperature has greatest accuracy but should be used only when patient's airway is secured (3)[C].
  - Epitympanic thermometer (not to be confused with the widely available much less accurate infrared tympanic thermometer) may be used if airway is not secured (3)[C].
- Assess pulse and cardiac rhythm:
  - Tachycardia may be seen with mild hypothermia.
  - May progress to bradycardia, atrial fibrillation, or ventricular fibrillation with more severe hypothermia
  - In severe hypothermia, may be difficult to manually palpate pulse
- Assess mental status:
  - Degree of mental status alteration correlates with severity of hypothermia.
- Perform complete neurologic examination:
  - Intact sensation to pinprick indicates a better prognosis for patients with frostbite.
  - Decreased muscle coordination, delayed deep tendon reflexes, and slowed pupillary reflexes suggest more severe hypothermia.
  - Focal neurologic deficit suggests etiology of mental status changes other than hypothermia.
- Inspect appearance of skin:
  - Cold, yellow-white, or purple skin suggests frostbite.
  - Tissue pliability suggests superficial frostbite; hard tissue without pliability suggests deep frostbite.
- Electrocardiogram (ECG): may see tachycardia; bradycardia; atrial fibrillation; ventricular fibrillation; prolonged PR, QRS, and QT intervals; and J waves (positive deflection occurring at junction of QRS complex and ST segment)
- Electrolytes and basic chemistries: Hypothermic patients are at high risk for acid–base disturbances.

DIFFERENTIAL DIAGNOSIS

- Frostbite:
  - Frostnip: freezing injury to superficial skin layers
  - Trench foot: swelling, cyanosis, and erythema of extremity without freezing of tissue
  - Chilblains: local cold-related erythematous skin lesions
  - Raynaud phenomenon: cold-induced vasospasm resulting in sequential pallor, cyanosis, and erythema of digits
- Hypothermia:
  - Altered mental status from metabolic abnormalities, alcohol/toxic ingestion, or closed head injury

TREATMENT

- Prehospital:
  - Frostbite:
    - Avoid thawing until no further risk of refreezing.
    - Immerse affected part in 37–39°C (98.6–102°F) (2)[C].
    - Remove wet clothing and protect from further cold injury.
    - Ensure adequate hydration with warmed oral or intravenous (IV) fluids.
    - Avoid rubbing or massaging skin, which may compound tissue damage (4)[C].
    - Monitor and treat for concurrent hypothermia. Moderate and severe hypothermia should be treated before treating frostbite injury (5)[C].
    - Arrange transport to medical facility for moderate or severe frostbite.
  - Hypothermia:
    - Mild:
      - Passive external rewarming: Prevent further heat loss with blankets, dry clothing, shared body heat, and moving patient to shelter (3)[C].
      - Active external rewarming: direct application of heat sources (heating pad, hot water bottle, warm water immersion, electric blanket) applied to trunk and used cautiously. Application of heat sources to extremities can result in rapid reversal of cold-induced peripheral vasoconstriction, leading to hypotension (rewarming shock) and further decreases in core temperature ("afterdrop").
      - Hot drinks for patients with normal gag reflex.
    - Moderate/severe: in addition to the above measures:
      - Active emergency medical system. Perform a primary survey and institute cardiopulmonary resuscitation (CPR) if needed.
      - Attempts at field rewarming should not delay transport to emergency facility for patients with moderate or severe hypothermia.
      - Avoid agitation or jarring due to high risk of arrhythmias.
- Emergency department (ED) treatment:
  - Frostbite:
    - After rewarming, débride white blisters and apply topical aloe vera. For hemorrhagic blisters, apply aloe vera without débridement (5)[C].
  - Hypothermia (moderate or severe):
    - Continuous cardiac monitoring (6)[C]
    - Active external rewarming with forced-air rewarming blanket (6)[C]
    - Active internal rewarming with heated (43°C [109°F]) IV fluid or heated humidified air or oxygen (6)[C]:
      - Peritoneal, gastric, pleural, or bladder lavage with heated (40°C [104°F]) fluids may be used.
      - For severe cases, cardiopulmonary bypass may improve survival in young, otherwise healthy individuals (6)[C].
    - Monitor electrolytes; rewarming usually corrects electrolyte and acid–base disturbances.
    - Conventional wisdom has held that hypothermia with cardiac arrest requires a modified Advanced Cardiac Life Support (ACLS) protocol; however, evidence to support this is insufficient, and the recommendation of administering or withholding medications is not clear (6)[C]:
      - In the case of hypothermia with cardiac arrest, establish airway and start CPR. It may be reasonable to consider administration of a vasopressor according to the standard ACLS algorithm concurrent with rewarming strategies (6)[C].

MEDICATION

- Frostbite:
  - Administer tetanus prophylaxis if indicated according to standard tetanus guidelines (4)[C].
  - Administer analgesics/nonsteroidal anti-inflammatory medications unless contraindicated.
  - Administration of penicillin G (500,000 IU every 6 hr for 48 to 72 hr) prophylactically is controversial and not shown to reduce amputation rate (5)[C].
  - Administration of intra-arterial tissue plasminogen activator within 6 to 24 hr of rewarming may decrease amputation rate (2)[C].
  - IV iloprost administered up to 48 hr after rewarming may decrease amputation rate. IV iloprost is not currently available in the United States (2)[C].
- Hypothermia:
  - No evidence to support routine use of antibiotics, steroids, or barbiturates

ADDITIONAL THERAPIES

Range of motion and strengthening exercises may benefit frostbite-affected limbs.

SURGERY/OTHER PROCEDURES

Surgical débridement or amputation may be indicated for late treatment of necrotic or gangrenous tissue due to frostbite.

ONGOING CARE

PROGNOSIS

- Mild to moderate cases of both hypothermia and frostbite generally recover fully without complication.
- Severe cases may lead to significant disability and death.

COMPLICATIONS

- Frostbite:
  - Limb and digit loss
  - Premature closure of the epiphysis (younger athletes)
  - Autonomic dysfunction of affected extremity
  - Permanent cold sensitivity and susceptibility to cold injury
- Hypothermia:
  - Cardiac arrhythmias
  - Electrolyte and acid–base disorders
  - Inefficient clotting leading to disseminated intravascular coagulation

REFERENCES

1. Cauchy E, Marsigny B, Allamel G, et al. The value of technetium 99 scintigraphy in the prognosis of amputation in severe frostbite injuries of the extremities: a retrospective study of 92 severe frostbite injuries. *J Hand Surg Am*. 2000;25(5):969–978.
2. Cauchy E, Davis CB, Pasquier M, et al. A new proposal for management of severe frostbite in the austere environment. *Wilderness Environ Med*. 2016;27(1):92–99.
3. Zafren K, Giesbrecht GG, Danzl DF, et al. Wilderness Medical Society practice guidelines for the out-of-hospital evaluation and treatment of accidental hypothermia: 2014 update. *Wilderness Environ Med*. 2014;25(Suppl 4):S66–S85.
4. Handford C, Thomas O, Imray CHE. Frostbite. *Emerg Med Clin North Am*. 2017;35(2):281–299.
5. McIntosh SE, Opacic M, Freer L, et al. Wilderness Medical Society practice guidelines for the prevention and treatment of frostbite: 2014 update. *Wilderness Environ Med*. 2014;25(Suppl 4):S43–S54.
6. Vanden Hoek TL, Morrison LJ, Shuster M, et al. Part 12: cardiac arrest in special situations: 2010 American Heart Association Guidelines for Cardiopulmonary Resuscitation and Emergency Cardiovascular Care. *Circulation*. 2010;122(18, Suppl 3):S829–S861.

ADDITIONAL READING

- Cappaert TA, Stone JA, Castellani JW, et al. National Athletic Trainers' Association position statement: environmental cold injuries. *J Athl Train*. 2008;43(6):640–658.
- Castellani JW, Young AJ, Ducharme MB, et al. American College of Sports Medicine position stand: prevention of cold injuries during exercise. *Med Sci Sports Exerc*. 2006;38(11):2012–2029.

CLINICAL PEARLS

- Hypothermia can occur even at moderate temperatures (50–65°F [10–18°C]) if wind, rain, sweat, or wet clothing lead to heat loss that is greater than metabolic heat production.
- Prolonged exposure to cold temperatures, wet clothing, drug or alcohol use, and underlying medical conditions increase risk of hypothermia and frostbite.
- Avoid freeze-thaw-freeze cycles which worsen tissue damage.
- Prevention is the best treatment for hypothermia and frostbite.

ILIOPSOAS INJURY

Kevin E. Burroughs, MD, CAQSM

BASICS

- The iliopsoas is the most powerful hip flexor with a major role in posture, walking, and running (1).
- Pathology can include iliopsoas bursitis, tendonitis, impingement, and snapping hip (coxa saltans).
- Aching pain; can be in groin or over the anterior thigh
- Occasionally, onset of pain is acute or subacute, with sharp lancinating or burning pain; more common with tendon tears
- More often, it is insidious in onset, with pain exacerbated by running, climbing stairs, getting in/out of bed, or rising from a seated position.
- Inflammatory or degenerative hip diseases may be complicated by iliopsoas bursitis (2).

DESCRIPTION

- Bursitis is inflammation and secondary pain in a bursal structure.
- Two types of bursae have been described constant and adventitial. Constant bursae are formed in embryogenesis and are endothelial-lined saclike structures (e.g., iliopsoas and trochanteric). Adventitial bursae form later in life through myxomatous degeneration of fibrous tissues at sites of friction (e.g., a bunion).
- The iliopsoas bursa is the largest synovial bursa in the body and is present in >95% of adults. It averages 3 cm (width) × 6 cm (length) in size. There is often communication with the hip joint capsule (~14% of adults).
- Synonym(s): snapping hip syndrome
- Snapping hip syndrome is usually broken down into intra-articular and extra-articular.
- Extra-articular is subclassified into medial (internal), which is associated with iliopsoas pathology, and lateral (external), which is associated with iliotibial band and greater trochanteric pathology.
- Avulsion fractures/apophyseal separation of the lesser trochanter can occur in younger patients, although these injuries occur in <1% of hip injuries in an orthopedic practice (3).

EPIDEMIOLOGY

- Iliopsoas disorders are the primary cause of chronic groin pain in 12–36% of athletes and in 25–30% of athletes with acute groin injury (2).
- Bursitis is reported to account for 0.4% of all visits to primary care, but in runners, the incidence may be as high as 10%.
- In a 6-yr study of ballet dancers, 21 of 73 hip problems reported were attributed to iliopsoas bursitis/tendonitis (4).
- Reported in patients of all ages, but average age is 25 yr, with a range of 12 to 56 yr
- Snapping hip syndrome more common in females than males

ETIOLOGY AND PATHOPHYSIOLOGY

- The psoas and iliacus muscles originate from the lumbar spine and the internal aspect of the pelvic brim, respectively. They converge to form the iliopsoas muscle-tendon complex and insert distally on the lesser trochanter. It is a hip flexor and external rotator.
- The muscle-tendon complex crosses over the anterior pelvic brim and hip capsule. The iliopsoas bursa lies between the tendon and the bony pelvic brim.
- Frictional compression of the bursa between these structures leads to an inflammatory reaction.

RISK FACTORS

- Rheumatoid arthritis, osteoarthritis (OA), acute trauma, overuse, or mechanical factors (tightened hip flexors)
- Common sports associated: competitive track and field, strength training, rowing, uphill running, dancing, aerobics
- Running, jumping, and overextension are typical mechanisms for avulsion injuries at the lesser trochanter and for distal tendon tears (3).

COMMONLY ASSOCIATED CONDITIONS

- OA
- Rheumatoid arthritis (5)
- Pigmented villonodular synovitis
- Synovial chondromatosis
- Infection
- Trauma
- Status post total hip arthroplasty
- Avascular necrosis of the femoral head
- Leg-length discrepancy

DIAGNOSIS

- Pain can be present ± snapping.
- If pain is the predominant feature, it will be in the groin or anterior thigh.
- Irritation of the femoral nerve can be a cause of anterior thigh pain.
- If there is remarkable bursal swelling, a pelvic or inguinal mass may be palpated.
- Stride may be abbreviated during gait to avoid extension.

HISTORY

- Pain is typically achy but may be sharp and located in the groin or anterior thigh. One must differentiate from L1 disk disease (uncommon).
- Hip flexion and/or extension may cause pain. Stride length of gait may be shortened.

PHYSICAL EXAM

- Local tenderness to pressure beneath the midpoint of the inguinal ligament may be present.
- In significant cases, the hip may be passively held in flexion, and the gait may be shortened to avoid hip extension.
- Pain is present in the inguinal region with resisted hip flexion supine and external rotation in a seated position. Pain also should be in same location with passive hip extension or internal rotation, but there should not be a fixed limitation of motion.
- Positive Thomas test

DIFFERENTIAL DIAGNOSIS

- Inguinal mass present: lymphadenopathy, malignant tumor, hernia, vascular malformation, hematoma
- Pain or paresthesia present: L1 disk disease, meralgia paresthetica, hip arthritis, stress fracture of the hip, acetabular labral tear, proximal rectus femoris avulsion fracture at the anteroinferior iliac spine in an adolescent
- Acute trauma leading to muscle/tendon tear or avulsion fracture of the lesser trochanter (2)

DIAGNOSTIC TESTS & INTERPRETATION

Initial Tests (lab, imaging)

- X-rays: Anteroposterior (AP) view of the pelvis and lateral (Dunn) view of the affected hip may show OA (associated cause in older patients) or other bony pathology (i.e., femoro-acetabular impingement [FAI]) to be considered in the differential diagnosis.
- Ultrasound (US): Musculoskeletal US (MSKUS) is a noninvasive, cost-effective diagnostic modality that can demonstrate the fluid nature of an enlarged bursa. Dynamic US can demonstrate abnormal snapping or movement of the tendon over the anterior pelvic brim. MSKUS also can be used to guide aspiration/injection of the bursa (1).

- Joint effusions were present in ~50% of OA patients with iliopsoas bursitis (5).
- Contrast bursography: not often used. It will not show communication with hip joint if present, and it is difficult to interpret.
- Arthrography: clearly shows if there is communication of bursa with hip joint
- Computed tomography (CT) scan: seldom used; can demonstrate abnormal bony pathology causing friction at the pelvic brim or a malpositioned lesser trochanter
- Magnetic resonance imaging (MRI)/MR arthrogram: MRI is a more sensitive and specific means of identifying lesions other than bursa as the source of hip pain. MR arthrography may be required to increase the sensitivity of detecting an acetabular labral tear (1).

TREATMENT

- In mild cases of tendonitis/bursitis, relative rest, nonsteroidal anti-inflammatory drugs (NSAIDs), and heat or other physical therapy modalities (6)
- If there is a palpable mass or remarkable enlargement of the bursa by imaging or CT scan, US-guided aspiration and instillation of a steroid preparation may be indicated.

GENERAL MEASURES

- Two basic premises: reduce pain and inflammation and rehabilitation and prevention of reinjury
- Treatment depends on the severity and nature of the underlying cause.
- Acute tendon injuries and avulsions should undergo conservative treatment unless the avulsion fragment is separated >2 cm (3)[C].

ADDITIONAL THERAPIES

- Stretching of the hip flexors, including iliopsoas and quadriceps
- Strengthening of same and of hip rotators (internal and external)
- An eccentric hip and core loading protocol has been outlined by Rauseo (7)[C].
- Modification of any underlying mechanical abnormality (i.e., correcting leg-length discrepancy)

SURGERY/OTHER PROCEDURES

- Typically, only as a last resort after several attempts at directed conservative measures (typically at least 3 mo)
- May be necessary if bony pathology causes the bursal irritation
- Partial surgical release or lengthening of the distal tendinous portion has demonstrated good outcomes but can have residual atrophy (25% volume loss) and weakness (19% reduction in seated hip flexion strength) (8)[B]
- Mild hip weakness and loss of sensation in the lateral femoral cutaneous nerve distribution have occurred following surgical release.

ONGOING CARE

PATIENT EDUCATION

- A study by Johnston and colleagues showed that a home-based exercise program leads to the majority of individuals being pain free or essentially pain free (9)[B].
- The program included:
  - Exercises performed in a seated position with an elastic resistance strap. Three sets of 20 repetitions of both internal and external rotation of the hip were performed. These were performed daily for 2 wk.
  - The patient continued these exercises but with the hip in less flexion and now only 2 to 3 days per week. The patient added a side-lying abduction/external rotation with the hip at 45 degrees of flexion. These again were performed daily for 2 wk.
  - At 1 mo, an additional exercise of a one-legged mini squat on the affected side was added; three sets of 20 repetitions, 2 to 3 times per week
  - Daily stretching targeting the hip flexor, quadriceps, and lateral hip/piriformis and hamstring muscles was performed.

PROGNOSIS

Good prognosis with reduction of inflammation, appropriate rehabilitation, and proper attention to alteration of mechanical issues

REFERENCES

1. Chopra A, Robinson P. Imaging athletic groin pain. *Radiol Clin North Am*. 2016;54(5):865–873.
2. Anderson CN. Iliopsoas: pathology, diagnosis, and treatment. *Clin Sports Med*. 2016;35(3):419–433.
3. Homma Y, Baba T, Ishii S, et al. Avulsion fracture of the lesser trochanter in a skeletally immature freestyle footballer. *J Pediatr Orthop B*. 2015;24(4):304–307.
4. Johnston CA, Wiley JP, Lindsay DM, et al. Iliopsoas bursitis and tendinitis. A review. *Sports Med*. 1998;25(4):271–283.
5. Tormenta S, Sconfienza LM, Iannessi F, et al. Prevalence study of iliopsoas bursitis in a cohort of 860 patients affected by symptomatic hip osteoarthritis. *Ultrasound Med Biol*. 2012;38(8): 1352–1356.
6. Di Sante L, Paoloni M, De Benedittis S, et al. Groin pain and iliopsoas bursitis: always a cause-effect relationship? *J Back Musculoskelet Rehabil*. 2014;27(1):103–106.
7. Rauseo C. The rehabilitation of a runner with iliopsoas tendinopathy using an eccentric-biased exercise—a case report. *Int J Sports Phys Ther*. 2017;12(7):1150–1162.
8. Brandenburg JB, Kapron AL, Wylie JD, et al. The functional and structural outcomes of arthroscopic iliopsoas release. *Am J Sports Med*. 2016;44(5): 1286–1291.
9. Johnston CA, Lindsay DM, Wiley JP. Treatment of iliopsoas syndrome with a hip rotation strengthening program: a retrospective case series. *J Orthop Sports Phys Ther*. 1999;29(4):218–224.

ADDITIONAL READING

- Adler RS, Buly R, Ambrose R, et al. Diagnostic and therapeutic use of sonography-guided iliopsoas peritendinous injections. *AJR Am J Roentgenol*. 2005;185(4):940–943.
- Lachiewicz PF, Kauk JR. Anterior iliopsoas impingement and tendinitis after total hip arthroplasty. *J Am Acad Orthop Surg*. 2009;17(6):337–344.
- Pelsser V, Cardinal E, Hobden R, et al. Extraarticular snapping hip: sonographic findings. *AJR Am J Roentgenol*. 2001;176(1):67–73.
- Schon L, Zuckerman JD. Hip pain in the elderly: evaluation and diagnosis. *Geriatrics*. 1988;43(1):48–62.
- Toohey AK, LaSalle TL, Martinez S, et al. Iliopsoas bursitis: clinical features, radiographic findings, and disease associations. *Semin Arthritis Rheum*. 1990;20(1):41–47.

CLINICAL PEARLS

- The iliopsoas bursa is the largest synovial bursa in the body and is present in >95% of adults and communicates with the hip joint in 14%.
- Pain involving the iliopsoas can come from tendon overuse or injury, or inflammation of the bursa from activity or intra-articular pathology.
- Diagnostic US or MRI is best means of imaging.
- Aspiration or injection of inflamed bursa improved with US guidance.
- Rehab focused on improving flexibility.

ILIOTIBIAL BAND FRICTION SYNDROME

Kyle Meyer, DO • Rahul Kapur, MD, CAQSM

BASICS

DESCRIPTION

- Iliotibial band friction syndrome (ITBS or ITBFS) is an overuse tendinopathy that occurs from compression of the iliotibial band (ITB) against the lateral femoral epicondyle.
- Pain is especially sharp after foot strike in the gait cycle, usually at ~30 degrees of knee flexion.
- Synonym(s): ITB tendinopathy

EPIDEMIOLOGY

- Incidence as high as 12% of all running-related overuse injuries
- Second to patellofemoral syndrome as the most common running injury

ETIOLOGY AND PATHOPHYSIOLOGY

- The ITB is composed of dense fibrous connective tissue that originates off the iliac crest. Its course runs inferiorly, passing over the lateral femoral epicondyle prior to insertion distally on the tibia at Gerdy tubercle.
- The ITB is compressed against the lateral femoral epicondyle with knee flexion, with the greatest compression at 30 degrees of knee flexion.
- Etiology is unclear, but it appears that the repetitive compression leads to inflammation of the band as well as inflammation of the connective tissue and fat pad between the band and the epicondyle (1).

RISK FACTORS

- Training factors: higher weekly mileage, downhill running, disproportionate running on a track in the same direction
- Increased peak hip adduction (possibly owing to significant weakness of the hip abductors of one limb as compared with the other) and increased knee internal rotation during stance phase, with running (2)

DIAGNOSIS

HISTORY

- Lateral knee sharp pain or burning
- Pain is not present when the patient starts exercising but begins at a predictable time or distance within the workout.
- Symptoms that subside shortly after the workout but return with the next workout
- Pain worse with downhill running, stride lengthening, or sitting for long periods of time with a flexed knee
- Involvement in sports that require continuous running or repetitive knee flexion (i.e., bicycling)

PHYSICAL EXAM

- Lateral knee pain made worse with running (3)[C]
- Pain with ascending and descending stairs
- Stiff-legged walking in advanced cases
- Extensive musculoskeletal exam with particular attention to the lower extremities: With a patient with ITBS, the clinician may notice local tenderness and swelling as well as crepitation, snapping, or pitting edema over the distal ITB where it passes over the lateral femoral epicondyle, and there may be pain or paresthesia along the length of the band (3)[C].
- Perform Ober test: Position the patient on the unaffected side with the involved knee in 90 degrees of flexion. The leg is abducted at the hip, and the examiner then grasps the ankle and extends leg, allowing the knee to return to an adducted position. A person with ITB tightness will remain abducted (4).
- Perform Noble compression test: With the patient on his or her side with the affected knee up and flexed at 90 degrees, apply pressure on the ITB at the lateral femoral epicondyle and extend the knee. A positive test occurs when pain occurs as the knee approaches 30 degrees of flexion (4).
- Evaluate for excessive ankle pronation and causes of it, including evaluation for tight gastrocnemius or soleus muscles, pes planus, or femoral or tibial torsion. Excessive ankle pronation increases knee flexion.
- Evaluate for muscle imbalances, especially pelvic and core musculature.
- Exclude lumbar spine and intra-articular hip pathology.
- Feet and footwear should be evaluated closely. Footwear can give clues to the pronation pattern.
- Evaluate iliac crests and leg length. Discrepancies of leg length can cause tightening of the ITB.

DIFFERENTIAL DIAGNOSIS

- Patellofemoral syndrome
- Degenerative joint disease
- Lateral meniscal damage or pathology
- Lateral collateral ligament sprain
- Superior tibiofibular joint sprain
- Popliteal or biceps femoris tendinopathy
- Peroneal nerve injury
- Gout and other metabolic arthropathy
- Referred pain

DIAGNOSTIC TESTS & INTERPRETATION

- Generally not needed except to rule out other disease processes
- Consider a standing anteroposterior (AP) view of pelvis (in adult) to assess leg-length discrepancy if clinically indicated.

TREATMENT

GENERAL MEASURES

- Initially, patient should rest and avoid offending activities, such as running and biking (3,5)[C].
- Control inflammation and pain with ice and nonsteroidal anti-inflammatory drugs (NSAIDs) (3,4)[C].
- Physical therapy should focus on hip and core strengthening, stretching, and soft tissue release with a foam roller (5).
- Gait training should focus on increasing gait width, reducing hip adduction changing from heel strike to forefoot landing, and avoiding excess pronation (4,5).
- Relative rest is important, but no forms of immobilization are used.

ADDITIONAL THERAPIES

- Corticosteroid injections have been shown to be more effective than placebo in controlling pain related to ITBS (4)[B]. However, cases of ITB rupture after steroid injection has been documented.
- There is currently no conclusive data regarding the effectiveness of platelet-rich plasma (PRP), prolotherapy, or stem cell therapy in treating this condition.

SURGERY/OTHER PROCEDURES

- Only after exhaustive nonoperative therapy
- Techniques include ITB release, open partial excision, or lengthening. Bursectomy and synovial recess excision have also been reported (4).

ONGOING CARE

FOLLOW-UP RECOMMENDATIONS

If no improvement is seen after extensive therapy and training modification, then referral to an orthopedic surgeon is warranted.

REFERENCES

1. Fairclough J, Hayashi K, Toumi H, et al. The functional anatomy of the iliotibial band during flexion and extension of the knee: implications for understanding iliotibial band syndrome. *J Anat*. 2006;208(3):309–316.
2. Noehren B, Davis I, Hamill J. ASB clinical biomechanics award winner 2006 prospective study of the biomechanical factors associated with iliotibial band syndrome. *Clin Biomech (Bristol, Avon)*. 2007;22(9):951–956.
3. Fredericson M, Wolf C. Iliotibial band syndrome in runners: innovations in treatment. *Sports Med*. 2005;35(5):451–459.
4. Strauss EJ, Kim S, Calcei JG, et al. Iliotibial band syndrome: evaluation and management. *J Am Acad Orthop Surg*. 2011;19(12):728–736.
5. Barton CJ, Bonanno DR, Carr J, et al. Running retraining to treat lower limb injuries: a mixed-methods study of current evidence synthesised with expert opinion. *Br J Sports Med*. 2016;50(9):513–526.

CLINICAL PEARLS

- An attempt to return too early with pain can result in significant delay. Activity can be resumed when symptoms have improved nearly 100% or have resolved. Earlier return can be accomplished using non–weight-bearing activities such as swimming or running in the deep end of a pool. Return should be gradual with gentle buildup on level ground progressing in distance/resistance and elevation.
- Most patients recover in about 6 wk and are able to resume full activity at that time.
- To prevent ITBFS, maintain flexibility with adequate warm-up periods and stretching before and after exercise.

I

IMPETIGO

Arturo J. Aguilar, MD, CAQSM

BASICS

DESCRIPTION

- Superficial skin infection of the epidermis with *Staphylococcus aureus* or group A β-hemolytic streptococcus or a combination of the two, classically characterized as well-defined erythematous papules and pustules with honey-colored crust (1)
- Divided into bullous and nonbullous types (1)
- Bullous (2,3):
  - Caused by epidermolytic toxin from *S. aureus*
  - Favors intertriginous areas
  - Is a localized form of scalded skin syndrome
  - Starts as a vesicular eruption that develops into bullae and then may rupture to form honey crusts
- Nonbullous (more contagious) (2,3):
  - Caused by *S. aureus* and group A β-hemolytic streptococcus (GAS)
  - Starts as macules or papules and progresses to vesicular eruption, which rupture to form erosions with honey crusts
- Impetiginous (or common) impetigo is a nonbullous subtype that is a complication of systemic diseases such as diabetes mellitus or HIV. It may also develop as a secondary infection of a cut, scrape, or insect bite (1).
- May be transmitted person to person or person to athletic equipment by direct contact (1,4)
- Can also be spread by autoinoculation from skin excoriations in contact with other parts of the body (1,4)
- Synonym(s): scrum strep (1)

EPIDEMIOLOGY

- Most common bacterial skin infection in children (2)
- Third most common skin infection overall (2)
- Most common in areas of skin-to-skin contact between athletes (1,4)
- Most common on face and upper extremities (1)
- Incidence is greatest in the summer months (1).
- 14.2% of skin infections in men's wrestling practices (4)

ETIOLOGY AND PATHOPHYSIOLOGY

- Bullous (2,3):
  - Epidermolytic toxin from *S. aureus*
- Nonbullous (2,3):
  - *S. aureus* and/or GAS

RISK FACTORS

- Abrasions or open cuts allow passage of bacteria through the epidermis (1).
- Sweat- and water-soaked clothes allow easy passage of bacteria through the first protective layer of the epidermis (stratum corneum) (1).
- Poor hygiene (1,4)

GENERAL PREVENTION

Techniques (1,4):

- Avoid sharing equipment, towels, tape, and ointments.
- Avoid dispensing ointments from common containers.
- Clean equipment and clothes daily.
- Shower immediately after sports activity with antibacterial soap.
- Avoid communal hot tubs.
- Wear moisture-wicking, synthetic clothing.
- Discourage body shaving in contact sports.
- Frequent skin checks by athletic trainers and athletes in contact sports
- Frequent handwashing by athletic trainers and affected athletes
- Cover any injured skin immediately.
- Use topical triple antibiotic for skin wounds.

DIAGNOSIS

HISTORY

- Mild itching and soreness (1,3)
- May be an infection of a minor skin injury or occur on unimpaired skin (1)
- May have accompanying pharyngitis (2)
- Bullous (1,2,3):
  - Starts with superficial vesicles, which progress to flaccid bullae without surrounding erythema
  - When the bullae rupture, they ooze and create honey-colored crusts.
  - Self-limited and may spontaneously resolve in weeks if left untreated
- Nonbullous (more contagious) (1,2,3):
  - Starts as a single macule or papule that develops into a vesicle
  - Vesicle may rupture and form an erosion, and the contents become honey-colored crusts that are often pruritic.
  - May spontaneously resolve without scarring if left untreated for weeks

PHYSICAL EXAM

Findings (1,2,3):

- Clear vesicles in the early stages
- Some may progress to pustules and/or bullae.
- When vesicles or pustules/bullae break, they will have a honey-colored crust with erythematous papules or erosions.
- Lesions may range from millimeters up to several centimeters in diameter.
- Mainly located on face and upper extremities
- Regional lymphadenopathy
- Diagnosis is based on history and clinical appearance (1).
- Cultures can be done if history or epidemic of methicillin-resistant *S. aureus* (MRSA).

DIFFERENTIAL DIAGNOSIS

- Acne vulgaris (1)
- Folliculitis (2)
- Poison ivy (2)
- Atopic dermatitis (2)
- Herpes gladiatorum (1)
- Tinea corporis gladiatorum (1)

DIAGNOSTIC TESTS & INTERPRETATION

- Wound culture to confirm or rule out MRSA if recent epidemic on the athletic team (1)
- Throat culture if symptoms of pharyngitis for GAS (2)

TREATMENT

Methods (1)[C]:

- Soak affected skin in warm water for 5 to 10 min 3 times daily until cleared.
- Gently remove honey-colored crusts to improve antibiotic penetration.

MEDICATION

First Line

- Mild (1,3,5)[A]:
  - Topical 2% mupirocin 2 times a day for 5 days
  - Topical fusidic acid (not available in the United States)
  - Topical 1% retapamulin 2 times a day for 5 days
- Moderate or widespread (adult dosing) (1,3,5)[A]:
  - Topical therapy in combination with oral antibiotic coverage
  - Amoxicillin/clavulanate 250 to 500 mg 2 times a day for 7 days
  - Dicloxacillin 250 to 500 mg 3 to 4 times a day for 7 days
- Cephalexin 250 to 500 mg 3 to 4 times a day for 7 days (5)[A]
- Penicillin-allergic oral therapy (3,5)[A]:
  - Erythromycin
  - Clindamycin
- MRSA-positive lesions (1,5)[A]:
  - Trimethoprim/sulfamethoxazole or clindamycin for at least 7 days

ADDITIONAL THERAPIES

- Clean clothes in bleach and water at a temperature of at least 71°C (1)[C].
- Clean equipment with diluted bleach solution (1)[B].

ONGOING CARE

Return-to-play guidelines (4)[C]:

- College:
  - National Collegiate Athletic Association wrestling rules for competition:
    - Oral antibiotics for at least 72 hr prior to competition
    - No new lesions for 48 hr before a meet or tournament
    - No moist, exudative, or purulent lesions at the meet or tournament time
    - Active purulent lesions shall not be covered to allow participation.
    - Noninfectious lesions may be covered with a nonpermeable dressing that will not dislodge.
- High school:
  - Each state's high school association has varying guidelines for competition.

FOLLOW-UP RECOMMENDATIONS

Patient Monitoring

Recurrent infection should be considered for evaluation and possible treatment for *S. aureus* carrier state (2).

PATIENT EDUCATION

Educate athletes and athletic staff regarding the importance of good hygiene (4).

PROGNOSIS

Untreated, may last several weeks to months but ultimately self-limiting (1,3)

COMPLICATIONS

Secondary (1,2,3):

- Poststreptococcal glomerulonephritis up to 3 wk after skin infection:
  - Occurs in 20% of nonbullous-type impetigo
  - Risk not decreased with antibiotic treatment
- Hyperpigmented area after healed lesions mostly in dark-skinned athletes
- Cellulitis
- Lymphangitis
- Guttate psoriasis
- Toxic shock syndrome
- Staphylococcal scalded skin syndrome
- Sepsis
- Osteomyelitis
- Pneumonia

REFERENCES

1. Adams BB, ed. Bacterial skin infections. In: *Sports Dermatology*. New York, NY: Springer; 2006:3–8.
2. Habif PT, ed. Bacterial infections. In: *Clinical Dermatology*. New York, NY: Mosby; 2004:267–272.
3. Hartman-Adams H, Banvard C, Juckett G. Impetigo: diagnosis and treatment. *Am Fam Physician*. 2014;90(4):229–235.
4. National Collegiate Athletic Association. Skin infections. In: *2014–15 NCAA Sports Medicine Handbook*. Indianapolis, IN: National Collegiate Athletic Association; 2014:65–70.
5. Stevens DL, Bisno AL, Chambers HF. Practice guidelines for the diagnosis and management of skin and soft tissue infections: 2014 update by the Infectious Diseases Society of America. *Clin Infect Dis*. 2014;59(2):e10–e52.

CLINICAL PEARLS

- Impetigo is a superficial skin infection caused by *Staphylococcus* or *Streptococcus*.
- Signs include vesicles, with/without bullae, erythematous papules, and honey-colored crusts.
- Treat mild or localized infection with mupirocin 2%, retapamulin 1%, or fusidic acid.
- Treat moderate or widespread infection with topical treatment above plus oral antibiotics such as Augmentin, dicloxacillin, or cephalexin.
- Treat MRSA-positive infection with trimethoprim/sulfamethoxazole or clindamycin orally:
  - NCAA wrestling guidelines require 72 hr of oral treatment and no new lesions for 48 hr before competition.

IMPINGEMENT, SUBACROMIAL BURSITIS AND ROTATOR CUFF TENDINITIS

Andrew Cheung, DO • Mark E. Lavallee, MD, CSCS, FACSM

BASICS

DESCRIPTION

- Repetitive shoulder activity causes breakdown in the rotator cuff muscles from tensile overload and results in tendinopathy.
- Weakness in the rotator cuff muscles (supraspinatus, infraspinatus, teres minor, or subscapularis) results in loss of effective dynamic glenohumeral movement.
- This causes impingement of the cuff muscles under the acromion, enhancing the pain and inflammation.
- Synonym(s): subacromial bursitis; shoulder impingement syndrome

EPIDEMIOLOGY

- Very common in athletes, especially in those with repetitive motion of the arms (i.e., throwing, racquet sports, swimming, weight lifting)
- In individuals <25 yr of age, impingement is usually related to laxity caused by instability.
- In those 25 to 40 yr of age, impingement is usually due to overuse of the rotator cuff.
- In those >40 yr of age, impingement is caused by use of the cuff muscles over threshold. This may result in partial- or full-thickness tears in addition to impingement.

RISK FACTORS

- Weight lifting (Olympic style) and CrossFit
- Throwing or racquet sports
- "Industrial" athletics (repetitive, overhead motion)
- Shoulder instability
- Previous shoulder surgery or trauma (to ipsilateral or contralateral shoulder)
- Individuals with more "hooked" acromial morphology (type III > type II > type I)
- Smoking
- Diabetes

COMMONLY ASSOCIATED CONDITIONS

- Rotator cuff tear (partial or full)
- Adhesive capsulitis
- Thoracic outlet syndrome
- Brachial plexus injury
- Axillary nerve entrapment
- Pancoast tumor
- Suprascapular nerve palsy

DIAGNOSIS

HISTORY

- Rule out cervical spine disease, neck pain.
- Symptoms: weakness, crepitation, numbness, "slipped out," night pain, dead arm
- Exacerbation: Pain presents more at rest or with activity.
- Duration: chronic (overuse) versus acute (traumatic)
- Activation: right or left handed, type of job, sports, hobby
- History of previous trauma or surgery

PHYSICAL EXAM

- Shoulder pain with overhead activity
- Weakness in the shoulder musculature
- Crepitus
- Numbness/paresthesias (usually between the lateral neck to the elbow)
- Night pain
- Pain at rest (usually in more severe cases)
- Medial upper scapular border or medial upper trapezius pain
- Observation:
  - How the athlete carries arm/shoulder (e.g., recent dislocation, guarding, obvious asymmetry)
  - Deltoid atrophy (i.e., C5 plexus injury)
  - Scapular winging (i.e., long thoracic nerve palsy, cranial nerve XI palsy)
  - Infraspinatus fossa scalloping (inferior branch of the suprascapular nerve)
- Palpation:
  - Cervical spinous process: Rule out cervical neck pathology as cause of shoulder pain.
  - Subacromial bursa: distal to acromion
  - Biceps tendon (long head)/bicipital groove
  - Insertion of the deltoid on the humerus: pain at site but no pain with palpation; axillary nerve pain referral site
  - Coracoid process: pain referral site for impingement
- Range of motion (ROM):
  - Abduction (0 to 180 degrees)
  - Adduction (0 to 50 degrees)
  - Flexion: forward (0 to 180 degrees) and horizontal (0 to 130 degrees)
  - Extension (0 to 90 degrees)
  - Internal rotation (0 to 100 degrees) (adduction and internal rotation: "bra strap")
  - External rotation (0 to 60 degrees) (abduction and external rotation: "shampoo hair")
- Manual muscle testing:
  - Deltoid: full abduction, resist at 90 degrees
  - Supraspinatus: abduction to 90 degrees forward flexion to 30 degrees, resist downward pressure (empty can/Jobe test)
  - Infraspinatus and teres minor: arm at side, 90 degrees at elbow, resist external rotation (i.e., "opening the door")
  - Subscapularis: hand on lower back, push against resistance; Gerber lift-off test
- Special tests:
  - Hawkins test: 90 degrees of forward flexion at the shoulder and elbow, support elbow, pain with internal rotation of arm
  - Arc test: Shoulder abduction gets "stuck" or painful at 60 to 120 degrees.
  - Infraspinatus test: 90 degrees of flexion at the elbow; elbow held against body while patient attempts to externally rotate arm against examiner's resistance, pain in shoulder with external rotation
  - Neer test: arm straight, thumb down, passive forward flexion (pain at 60 to 120 degrees)
  - Impingement test: Inject subacromial bursa with lidocaine; helps to differentiate between impingement and tear; after injection, pain, ROM, and strength should improve if impingement and not a tear.
  - Drop arm test: Patient cannot hold arm at 90 degrees of abduction; indicates cuff tear
  - Speed test: arm straight, forward flexion to 90 degrees, palm up, resisted downward pressure; palpate the bicipital tendon at groove; pain indicates bicipital tendonitis.

DIFFERENTIAL DIAGNOSIS

- Rotator cuff tear (partial or full thickness)
- Adhesive capsulitis
- Acromioclavicular sprain/injury
- Labral tear
- Bicipital tendonitis
- Thoracic outlet syndrome
- Brachial plexus injury
- Fracture: clavicle, humerus, scapula
- Subluxation of glenohumeral joint
- Axillary nerve entrapment
- Pancoast tumor
- Bankart lesion (avulsion fracture of glenoid labrum)
- Hill-Sachs lesion (impact fracture of humeral head)
- Septic arthritis
- Glenohumeral arthritis
- Thrombosis of subclavian or brachial artery

DIAGNOSTIC TESTS & INTERPRETATION

- Imaging is often not needed in light of good history and physical exam and a straightforward case.
- Radiography (1,2):
  - Anteroposterior (AP) view and axillary (transscapular) views bare minimum to order; radiographs helpful for acute injuries to rule out fractures, dislocations; with impingement, may be helpful to get additional views
  - Internal and external AP rotational views help to visualize humerus (i.e., Hill-Sachs lesions).
  - Stryker notch view helps to visualize posterolateral humeral head deformity (i.e., Hill-Sachs lesions).
  - West Point (modified axillary) view allows visualization of the anterior/inferior glenoid (i.e., Bankart lesions).
  - Outlet or Alexander view allows for visualization of subacromial space; helpful in elderly patients with severe impingement
  - Calcification on the tendon is associated with bicipital tendonitis or severe impingement.
- Ultrasound (US) (3):
  - Dependent on skill and comfort of practitioner, can be cost-effective in-office imaging choice for static and dynamic view of soft tissue structures of the shoulder (i.e., rotator cuff muscles, biceps tendons, subacromial bursa, calcification in tendons)
  - Also, can be used to guide injections into biceps tendon sheath, subacromial bursa, or intra-articular area
- Magnetic resonance imaging (MRI):
  - In severe or confusing cases, MRI is helpful in diagnosis of rotator cuff tears, labrum tears, biceps tendon rupture as well as assessing volume and capsule thickening in adhesive capsulitis (1).
  - An MRI arthrogram is often useful to further displace a torn labrum, thus improving visualization of the anatomy.
- Electromyography/nerve conduction study: helpful if there is weakness in addition to an altered neurologic exam (sensation, reflexes); has the highest sensitivity when symptoms have persisted >3 wk

TREATMENT

MEDICATION

- Oral analgesia: nonsteroidal anti-inflammatory drugs (NSAIDs), acetaminophen, tramadol; in severe cases, short-term pain relief with narcotics. Prednisone: short course of 40 mg daily for 5 days
- Dermal: topical cream or transdermal patches (NSAID or lidocaine based)
- Injectable: subacromial bursa injection (5 to 10 mL 2:2:1 mixture of lidocaine/bupivacaine, corticosteroid; use a 22- to 25-gauge, 1.5-inch-long needle)

ADDITIONAL THERAPIES

- Management of acute phase (4):
  - Relative rest: Decrease use of affected shoulder.
  - Home exercise program (HEP): exercise done daily, three sets per exercise
  - ROM: dangling arm circles, finger wall-walking, broom-handle exercises
  - Strengthening: sword-from-sheath exercises, posterior dumbbell raises, proprioceptive neuromuscular facilitation (PNF), augmented soft tissue mobilization (ASTM), scapular stabilizing exercises using light weights or flexible elastic cords
- Rehabilitation for long-term treatment:
  - Formal physical therapy: pain relief via contrast baths, hydrocollator, ice, mobilization/manipulation, modalities (e.g., electrostimulation, US therapy)
  - ROM strengthening: deltoid, rotator cuff musculature, scapular stabilizers, biceps
  - ROM flexibility: biceps, triceps, glenohumeral joint
  - Transmembrane corticosteroid (i.e., phonophoresis, iontophoresis)
  - Return to normal function.
  - Sports-specific retraining
- In the younger athlete, impingement is often due to another underlying problem (i.e., instability, scapular dyskinesis [5], muscular imbalance).
- Certain athletes (i.e., mentally challenged, unmotivated, etc.) may need assistance of formal physical therapy without a trial of HEP.

SURGERY/OTHER PROCEDURES

- Anterior acromioplasty: The acromion is "shaved" to allow more space for the rotator cuff. It is used only if conservative measures fail. There is a less favorable outcome in younger (50% success rate) than older athletes.
- Surgical débridement/repair of rotator cuff: often accompanies an anterior acromioplasty
- Surgical débridement/repair of labrum

COMPLEMENTARY & ALTERNATIVE MEDICINE

Mentioned in literature for recalcitrant cases: prolotherapy, platelet-rich plasma (PRP) injections, acupuncture, dry needling, autologous stem cell therapy, and topical nitrates

ONGOING CARE

FOLLOW-UP RECOMMENDATIONS

- Presence of a fever and a tense joint capsule (i.e., a potentially septic joint, orthopedic surgical emergency)
- Severe disease that is refractory to physical therapy, modalities, and steroid injections
- Rotator cuff tear, full or partial thickness, nonresponsive to conservative care
- Cervical rib, causing shoulder symptoms
- superior labrum anterior and posterior (SLAP)
- Gross instability of shoulder not improved with physical therapy

REFERENCES

1. Corpus KT, Camp CL, Dines DM, et al. Evaluation and treatment of internal impingement of the shoulder in overhead athletes. *World J Orthop*. 2016;7(12):776–784.
2. Parker B, Zlatkin M, Newman J, et al. Imaging of shoulder injuries in sports medicine: current protocols and concepts. *Clin Sports Med*. 2008;27(4):579–606.
3. Iannotti JP, Ciccone J, Buss DD, et al. Accuracy of office-based ultrasonography of the shoulder for the diagnosis of rotator cuff tears. *J Bone Joint Surg Am*. 2005;87(6):1305–1311.
4. Steuri R, Sattelmayer M, Elsig S, et al. Effectiveness of conservative interventions including exercise, manual therapy and medical management in adults with shoulder impingement: a systematic review and meta-analysis of RCTs. *Br J Sports Med*. 2017;51(18):1340–1347.
5. Burn MB, McCulloch PC, Lintner DM, et al. Prevalence of scapular dyskinesis in overhead and nonoverhead athletes: a systematic review. *Orthop J Sports Med*. 2016;4(2):2325967115627608.

ADDITIONAL READING

Monica J, Vredenburgh Z, Korsh J, et al. Acute shoulder injuries in adults. *Am Fam Physician*. 2016;94(2):119–127.

CLINICAL PEARLS

- If caught early with no other shoulder pathology and treated with aggressive conservative therapy, many athletes are able to return to their prior level of competition.
- With subacromial injections, often pain relief is immediate, due to the analgesia (i.e., lidocaine/bupivacaine). This will wear off. Corticosteroid injections may have a delay in onset of up to 3 days.
- If no other shoulder pathology is present, and the injury is treated with aggressive conservative therapy, most athletes respond well and are able to avoid surgery.

INGROWN TOENAIL

Rodney S. Gonzalez, MD, FAAFP

BASICS

DESCRIPTION

- Onychocryptosis is commonly called ingrown toenail and most commonly affects the great toe.
- Puncturing of the periungual skin by the nail plate; this leads to a foreign body (the nail plate), inflammatory, and (possibly) infectious processes (1).
- Alteration in the proper fit of the nail plate into the lateral or medial nail groove
- Improper fit leads to callous formation, edema, and perforation in the nail groove as a result of the rubbing of the nail plate against the nail groove.
- Three stages (2):
  - Stage 1 (mild): erythema, slight edema, and pain when pressure is applied to the lateral nail groove
  - Stage 2 (moderate): increased stage 1 symptoms, drainage, and infection
  - Stage 3 (severe): worsening stage 1 symptoms, presence of granulation tissue, and lateral wall hypertrophy
- Recurrence is not uncommon.
- Synonym(s): unguis incarnatus; in-fleshed toenail; embedded toenail

EPIDEMIOLOGY

- Most commonly affects the great toe
- Lateral nail edge more common than medial nail edge
- 26% of pathologic nail conditions
- Most cases occur in males in their 2nd and 3rd decades.
- Predominant gender: male > female (2:1 <30 yr of age, 1:1 >30 yr of age)

ETIOLOGY AND PATHOPHYSIOLOGY

- Nail spicules form on the medial or lateral nail plate owing to trauma, disease processes, or improper hygiene.
- Nail plate punctures the periungual skin, causing a foreign-body and inflammatory reaction.
- Biologic agents (e.g., bacteria and fungi) may cause an infection of the periungual skin.

RISK FACTORS

- Shoes with tight-fitting toe box
- Improperly fitting cleats
- Poor stance and gait
- Improper nail-trimming techniques (including tearing of nails)
- Senior athletes
- Onychomycosis
- Diabetes
- Hyperhidrosis
- Obesity
- Subungual neoplasms
- Arthritis
- Immune deficiency
- Trauma, acute and repetitive
- Skeletal abnormalities
- Family history of incurvated nails
- Congenital and acquired nail disorders

GENERAL PREVENTION

- Properly fitting footwear
- Proper nail trimming

COMMONLY ASSOCIATED CONDITIONS

- Paronychia
- Cellulitis
- Osteomyelitis

DIAGNOSIS

HISTORY

- Ask about tight-fitting shoes: Small toe boxes predispose to onychocryptosis.
- Signs of infection: erythema, edema, and pain
- Ask about recurrence and previous treatment: may affect treatment choice
- History of immune deficiency or abnormal wound healing: increased chance for severe infection and possibly requires the use of antibiotics

PHYSICAL EXAM

- Signs and symptoms:
  - Pain, swelling, and limitation of activities
  - Cardinal signs of inflammation (redness, warmth, and drainage)
  - Incurvated nail margin
- Physical examination:
  - Tenderness, erythema, edema, drainage
  - Inspect for foreign bodies.
  - Cardinal signs of ascending infection (redness traveling up the foot); this is more common in individuals with poor circulation or diabetes.
  - Presence of excess medial or lateral wall tissue

DIFFERENTIAL DIAGNOSIS

- Osteomyelitis
- Cellulitis
- Felon
- Paronychia
- Foreign body
- Tumor

DIAGNOSTIC TESTS & INTERPRETATION

- Labs usually not necessary
- Consider complete blood count (CBC), erythrocyte sedimentation rate (ESR), and C-reactive protein (CRP) ± blood cultures if there is concern for a more severe infection (e.g., osteomyelitis).
- Plain films and/or bone scan may be required for a severely infected toe if osteomyelitis is suspected.

TREATMENT

- Long-term treatment
- Acute treatment
- Analgesia (1)[C]:
  - Depends on planned treatment option and patient discomfort level
  - Recommend performing local anesthesia or a digital block with 1–2% lidocaine without epinephrine before manipulation.
  - Ibuprofen or acetaminophen for postoperative pain control

- Immobilization (1)[C]:
  - Patients may be full weight-bearing after nonsurgical treatment.
  - Partial weight-bearing for 24 to 48 hr after surgery may be needed, but generally, weight-bearing is well tolerated.
- Nonsurgical treatment (1,2)[C]:
  - There are no trials that compare the cost-benefit of nonsurgical versus surgical treatment options.
  - Patients should be instructed in maintenance of proper foot hygiene, avoidance of shoes with a tight-fitting toe box, soaking the feet, properly trimming nails (cutting the nail straight across), and avoidance of repetitive trauma.
  - Conservative treatment options (1,2)[C]:
    - Foot soaking: 10 to 20 min in warm, soapy water, followed by application of topical antibiotic ointment for a few days until resolution
    - Cotton wisps: Place cotton under the ingrown nail edge (also may be done with dental floss).
    - Gutter splint: using plastic tubing (e.g., intravenous [IV] infusion tubing) with a vertical slit and placing this over the ingrown nail edge
    - Small metal brace placement (such as KD device) around both edges of nail to relieve nail pressure (3)[C]
    - Cure rates can be as high as 75% with good patient compliance for stage 1 lesions.
    - If infection is suspected, it is important to remove the source of the infection. Antibiotics are usually not required when doing surgical treatment; when using antibiotics, they should be directed against gram-positive bacteria (e.g., *Staphylococcus aureus* and *Streptococcus* spp.).

SURGERY/OTHER PROCEDURES

- Surgery may be recommended for recurrent stage 1 lesions as below for stage 2 lesions:
  - Stage 2: Remove with a wedge excision the distal outer nail edge without matrixectomy.
  - Stage 2 or 3: partial removal of the medial or lateral nail with matricectomy (medial/lateral nail avulsion) ± electrosurgical or phenol cauterization
  - Stage 3: in addition to the preceding, ablation of medial or lateral wall tissue to promote normalization of the medial/lateral nail fold
- Major contraindications include disorders causing digital ischemia (e.g., diabetes, peripheral vascular disease, and collagen diseases).
- Studies show that antibiotics before or after surgery do not affect healing time and should be withheld in most cases. One study showed increased risk of infection after nail matrixectomies compared to clean foot and ankle surgery. They suggest providers should consider this a clean-contaminated surgery and may provide indication for antibiotic prophylaxis (4)[C].
- Partial nail removal with phenolization decreases the risk of recurrence; however, there may be a slight increase in postoperative infections (1,5)[C].
- Matricectomy with electrocautery and radiofrequency and carbon dioxide laser is also effective; the high cost of these procedures may be prohibitive, however (2)[C].

ONGOING CARE

FOLLOW-UP RECOMMENDATIONS

Immunocompromised individuals with a severe infection may require hospitalization for administration of IV antibiotics.

PATIENT EDUCATION

- Properly fitting footwear
- Proper nail trimming (and foot hygiene)
- Online patient handouts:
  - https://familydoctor.org/condition/ingrown-toenails
  - www.aafp.org/afp/20090215/311ph.html

COMPLICATIONS

- Osteomyelitis
- Narrowing of nail (when matrix ablation performed)
- Recurrence

REFERENCES

1. Heidelbaugh JJ, Lee H. Management of the ingrown toenail. *Am Fam Physician*. 2009;79(4):303–308.
2. Park DH, Singh D. The management of ingrowing toenails. *BMJ*. 2012;344:e2089.
3. Arik HO, Arican M, Gunes V, et al. Treatment of ingrown toenail with a shape memory alloy device. *J Am Podiatr Med Assoc*. 2016;106(4):252–256.
4. Rusmir A, Salerno A. Postoperative infection after excisional toenail matrixectomy: a retrospective clinical audit. *J Am Podiatr Med Assoc*. 2011;101(4):316–322.
5. DeBrule MB. Operative treatment of ingrown toenail by nail fold resection without matricectomy. *J Am Podiatr Med Assoc*. 2015;105(4):295–301.

CLINICAL PEARLS

- Antibiotics have not been shown to change the healing from ingrown toenails when using surgical treatment options.
- Impact activities should be avoided until the patient is pain free and clear of infection.
- The frequencies of symptomatic nail regrowth following distal nail wedge resection is 70%, nail avulsion in 50–80%, phenol cauterization is 4–25%, and electrosurgical cauterization is <5%.

INNER EAR INJURIES (TYMPANIC MEMBRANE PERFORATION)

Rochelle M. Nolte, MD, FAAFP, CAQSM • John W. Hariadi, MD, FAAFP

BASICS

DESCRIPTION

Disruption of the tympanic membrane, exposing the middle ear to the external auditory canal

EPIDEMIOLOGY

Incidence

The incidence of tympanic membrane perforation in the general population has not been studied.

ETIOLOGY AND PATHOPHYSIOLOGY

- Blunt trauma (slap to the ear)
- Penetrating trauma (Q-tip)
- Rapid pressure change (diving, flying)
- Extreme noise (blast)
- Lightning
- Spontaneous perforation of acute otitis media
- Acute necrotic myringitis

DIAGNOSIS

HISTORY

- Ear pain (mild)
- Decreased hearing (partial)
- Severe pain or complete hearing loss in the affected ear suggests additional injuries.
- Purulent or bloody discharge from ear canal
- Tinnitus
- Vertigo
- Otorrhea

PHYSICAL EXAM

- Direct visualization of tympanic membrane with otoscope
- Test hearing in both ears with audiogram or finger rub:
  - Weber test (tuning fork on midline bone):
    - Sound should be equal or louder in the injured ear, consistent with decreased conduction.
    - Sound localizing to the opposite side of injury indicates possible otic nerve injury.
  - Rinne test: usually normal (air conduction detected after bone conduction fades) or shows a small conductive loss
- Note any nystagmus with changes of position or pressure on the tragus occluding the canal (fistula sign).
- Insufflation via pneumatic otoscope:
  - Will not cause the perforated tympanic membrane to move normally
  - Holding pressure for 15 sec (the fistula test) may cause nystagmus or vertigo if the pressure is transmitted through the middle ear and into a labyrinthine fistula.

DIFFERENTIAL DIAGNOSIS

- Temporal bone fracture
- Serous otitis media
- Suppurative otitis media
- Otitis externa
- Cerumen impaction
- Barotrauma
- Acoustic trauma
- Foreign body
- Child abuse

DIAGNOSTIC TESTS & INTERPRETATION

- Radiography and magnetic resonance imaging (MRI) are of no value unless the clinical picture suggests ossicular destruction and/or cholesteatoma.
- Asymptomatic perforations, especially if hearing is near normal, require no imaging studies.

TREATMENT

GENERAL MEASURES

- Medical treatment for perforations is directed at controlling otorrhea.
- Clean debris from the ear canal.
- Prescribe antibiotics if there is evidence of infection.
- Acute otitis media with tympanic membrane perforation should be treated with an oral antibiotic (1)[A].
- Oral antibiotic choices (administered for 7 to 10 days):
  - Amoxicillin
  - Trimethoprim-sulfamethoxazole
  - Augmentin
- Prophylactic antibiotics are not indicated.
- Use topical antibiotics with low acidity/ototoxicity, such as ofloxacin or ciprofloxacin otic, in combination with oral systemic antibiotics.
- Topical quinolones (± steroids) are the best treatment for chronic suppurative otitis media (1)[A].
- Analgesics if needed for pain

ALERT

Do not prescribe topical ototoxic eardrops such as gentamicin, neomycin sulfate, or tobramycin.

MEDICATION

- Amoxicillin: 250 to 500 mg (children: 20 to 40 mg/kg/24 hr) PO TID
- Trimethoprim-sulfamethoxazole (Bactrim DS): 1 tablet (children: 6 to 12 mg/kg/24 hr) PO BID
- Augmentin: 250 to 500 mg (children: 20 to 40 mg/kg/24 hr) PO TID
- Ofloxacin otic topical 0.3%: 10 drops in affected ear BID × 7 days
- Ciprofloxacin 0.3% and dexamethasone 0.1% otic suspension (Ciprodex): 4 drops in affected ear BID × 7 days (1)

ISSUES FOR REFERRAL

Arrange ear, nose, throat (ENT) specialist follow-up:

- After detailed examination and formal audiometric tests, most otolaryngologists follow the perforation with monthly examinations.
- Operative repair is reserved for the 10–20% that do not heal spontaneously.

SURGERY/OTHER PROCEDURES

- Office procedures such as paper patch method (up to 90% success) (2)
- Surgical tympanoplasty under local or general anesthesia (87–94% success) (3)

ADMISSION, INPATIENT, AND NURSING CONSIDERATIONS

Admission criteria:

- Associated injuries requiring admission
- Severe vertigo impairing ambulation

ONGOING CARE

PATIENT EDUCATION

- Provide detailed discharge instructions.
- Occlude the ear canal with cotton coated in petroleum jelly or antibiotic ointment when showering to prevent entry of water into the middle ear, which can be painful.
- Swim only with fitted earplugs.
- Avoid forceful blowing of the nose.
- Patients may return to play when all clinical symptoms are improved, including inner ear symptoms and hearing, and the tympanic membrane is intact.

PROGNOSIS

ALERT

Most perforations heal spontaneously over a few months (76% within 1 mo, 97% within 3 mo) (4).

- A few require operative repair using a fat graft or a temporalis fascia graft (3).
- Perforations caused by molten metal or electrical burns are less likely to heal spontaneously.

ALERT

Forceful entry of water, as in a water skiing accident, is more likely to lead to infection.

COMPLICATIONS

- Infection
- Dislocation of ossicles
- Perilymph leak
- Cholesteatoma

REFERENCES

1. Wright D, Safranek S. Treatment of otitis media with perforated tympanic membrane. *Am Fam Physician*. 2009;79(8):650, 654.
2. Simsek G, Akin I. Early paper patching versus observation in patients with traumatic eardrum perforations: comparisons of anatomical and functional outcomes. *J Craniofac Surg*. 2014;25(6):2030–2032.
3. Gün T, Boztepe OF, Atan D, et al. Comparison of hyaluronic acid fat graft myringoplasty, fat graft myringoplasty and temporal fascia techniques for the closure of different sizes and sites of tympanic membrane perforations. *J Int Adv Otol*. 2016;12(2):137–141.
4. Jellinge M, Kristensen S, Larsen K. Spontaneous closure of traumatic tympanic membrane perforations: observational study. *J Laryngol Otol*. 2015;129(10):950–954.

ADDITIONAL READING

Golz A, Goldenberg D, Netzer A, et al. Paper patching for chronic tympanic membrane perforations. *Otolaryngol Head Neck Surg*. 2003;128(4):565–570.

CLINICAL PEARLS

- Infections are responsible from more tympanic membrane perforations than sports-related trauma.
- No imaging is needed for uncomplicated tympanic membrane perforations.
- Avoid ototoxic eardrops/solutions in the setting of tympanic membrane perforations.

INTERMETATARSAL (MORTON'S) NEUROMA

Amy Kakimoto, MD, DAAFP, CAQSM

BASICS

DESCRIPTION

- An inflammatory fibrosing process of the interdigital nerve of the foot, characterized by pain on the plantar surface of the foot
- Most commonly occurs between the heads of the 3rd and 4th metatarsals, although may also involve the 2nd or 4th intermetatarsal spaces
- Occurs just before the nerve bifurcates at the metatarsal area to innervate sides of two adjacent toes
- Usually unilateral symptoms

EPIDEMIOLOGY

- Occurs more often in women than men
- Athletes most at risk include kickboxers, ballet dancers, and runners.

ETIOLOGY AND PATHOPHYSIOLOGY

- Caused by nerve thickening from repetitive dorsiflexion of the toes, causing microtrauma to the nerve as it is compressed either under the transverse metatarsal ligament or by an inflamed intermetatarsal bursa (1)
- The repetitive trauma causes swelling of the plantar digital nerve that pathologically resembles other nerve entrapment syndromes.

GENERAL PREVENTION

- Avoidance of tight footwear
- Limit overpronation.

DIAGNOSIS

HISTORY

- Intermittent, episodic pain, usually on the plantar surface of the foot between the 3rd and 4th metatarsals
- Forefoot pain radiating to the affected interspace and toes (1)[C]
- Numbness or paresthesias in the toes and interdigital space are common (1)[C].
- Pain on weight-bearing, exacerbated with exercise, and relieved with rest

PHYSICAL EXAM

- Tenderness to palpation on the plantar surface of the foot, usually between the 3rd and 4th metatarsals
- Mulder click: palpable click after compressing the metatarsal heads while palpating the digital interspace on plantar aspect of foot
- No weakness noted on strength testing of the foot
- Primarily a clinical diagnosis without need for imaging typically (2)[A]

DIFFERENTIAL DIAGNOSIS

- Metatarsalgia
- Metatarsal stress fracture
- Ganglion cyst
- Neuropathies (diabetic, alcoholic, toxic, nutritional)
- Intermetatarsal bursitis
- Freiberg disease (metatarsal avascular necrosis)

DIAGNOSTIC TESTS & INTERPRETATION

- Imaging usually not needed (2)[A]
- X-ray imaging can be used to exclude other causes of foot pain.
- Electromyography and nerve conduction studies are not helpful.
- Ultrasound may identify neuromas with higher sensitivity than magnetic resonance imaging (MRI), depending on the skill of the interpreter (3)[A].
- MRI may show neuroma and edema surrounding the interdigital nerve but is not routinely recommend because many in the population may have features on MRI suggestive of asymptomatic neuromas.

TREATMENT

GENERAL MEASURES

- Conservative treatment is almost always indicated initially.
- Decrease pressure on metatarsal heads.
- Wide toe box shoes or open footwear
- Avoid repetitive toe dorsiflexion activities.
- Metatarsal pad proximal to the affected interspace may be helpful (1)[B].
- Strengthening exercises for intrinsic foot muscles
- Women should avoid wearing high heels.

MEDICATION

- Nonsteroidal anti-inflammatory drugs (NSAIDs) for pain
- If conservative measures are unsuccessful or unhelpful, injection of the intermetatarsal bursa with corticosteroid, following a dorsal approach, may help (4)[B].

ISSUES FOR REFERRAL

Referral for surgical evaluation for failure to improve with conservative treatment

SURGERY/OTHER PROCEDURES

- If nonpharmacologic and acute treatments do not give sufficient relief, surgical treatment has been shown to be successful (5)[A].
- Surgical excision of the neuroma has variable success rates (6).

REFERENCES

1. McKean KA. Neurologic running injuries. *Neurol Clin*. 2008;26(1):281–296.
2. Pastides P, El-Sallakh S, Charalambides C. Morton's neuroma: a clinical versus radiological diagnosis. *Foot Ankle Surg*. 2012;18(1):22–24.
3. Fazal MA, Khan I, Thomas C. Ultrasonography and magnetic resonance imaging in the diagnosis of Morton's neuroma. *J Am Podiatr Med Assoc*. 2012;102(3):184–186.
4. Shapiro BE, Preston DC. Entrapment and compressive neuropathies. *Med Clin North Am*. 2009;93(2):285–315.
5. Akermark C, Saartok T, Zuber Z. A prospective 2-year follow-up study of plantar incisions in the treatment of primary intermetatarsal neuromas (Morton's neuroma). *Foot Ankle Surg*. 2008;14(2):67–73.
6. Monacelli G, Cascioli I, Prezzemolo G, et al. Surgical treatment of Morton's neuroma: our experience and literature review. *Clin Ter*. 2008;159(3):165–167.

ADDITIONAL READING

Kang JH, Chen MD, Chen SC, et al. Correlations between subjective treatment responses and plantar pressure parameters of metatarsal pad treatment in metatarsalgia patients: a prospective study. *BMC Musculoskelet Disord*. 2006;7:95.

CLINICAL PEARLS

- Morton neuroma usually causes pain in the 3rd intermetatarsal space.
- Numbness or paresthesias are common.
- Morton neuroma is a clinical diagnosis without need for routine imaging.
- Treat first with conservative measures.

I

INTERPHALANGEAL COLLATERAL LIGAMENT SPRAIN

Lindsay A. Lafferty, MD • Shawn Phillips, MD, MSPT • Matthew L. Silvis, MD

BASICS

DESCRIPTION

- Injury to a collateral ligament at the interphalangeal (IP) joint of the finger, usually the proximal interphalangeal (PIP) joint:
  - 1st degree: pain but no laxity
  - 2nd degree: pain and laxity but firm end point when ligament is stressed
  - 3rd degree: pain and loss of firm end point when ligament is stressed
- Mechanisms: axial loading with radial or ulnar stress applied to the finger, usually while extended
- Synonym(s): jammed finger

EPIDEMIOLOGY

Incidence

- 1st- and 2nd-degree sprain more common than 3rd-degree sprain
- Index finger most often affected
- Combined injury to both collateral ligaments is more common than isolated radial collateral ligament (RCL) or ulnar collateral ligament (UCL) injury.

RISK FACTORS

- Ball handling, collision, and contact sports: football, basketball, volleyball, wrestling
- Prior injury or dislocation of the PIP joint

DIAGNOSIS

HISTORY

- Finger struck by player or ball during play
- Axial trauma causing forced ulnar or radial deviation
- Usually presents acutely but may become chronic

PHYSICAL EXAM

- Pain and swelling over radial or ulnar aspects of PIP joint
- Decreased range of motion (ROM) secondary to pain and edema
- Confirm neurovascular integrity, especially with on-field assessment.
- Ensure that maximum tenderness is over lateral aspects and not dorsal or volar.
- Dorsal pain may suggest central slip injury.
- Collateral ligament stability is best evaluated with the metacarpophalangeal (MCP) joint in 90 degrees of flexion and the IP joint stressed in extension and in 30 degrees of flexion (1)[C].
- Hyperextension is concerning for a volar plate injury.
- Compare with uninjured fingers.
- Instability with lateral stress (opening beyond 10 degrees or lack of firm end point) suggests loss of integrity (1)[C].
- Assess function of flexor and extensor tendons by isolating MCP, PIP, and distal interphalangeal (DIP) joints separately to rule out tendon injury.
- Loss of active ROM may be due to either pain or volar plate/central slip injury, so digital block may be necessary to test ROM (2)[C].

DIFFERENTIAL DIAGNOSIS

- Phalangeal fracture
- IP dislocation
- Central slip injury
- Volar plate injury
- Often associated with one or more of above

DIAGNOSTIC TESTS & INTERPRETATION

- Plain radiographs are generally not required for 1st-degree injuries but may be considered for 2nd- or 3rd-degree injuries or to rule out associated fracture.
- Posteroanterior, true lateral, and oblique radiographs of involved fingers (1)[C]
- Avulsion fracture may be seen at ligamentous insertion.
- Look for dorsal subluxation to suggest instability.
- Ultrasound (US) may be used to evaluate finger ligament integrity (1)[C].

TREATMENT

GENERAL MEASURES

- Immobilization:
  - Guided by level of activity, degree of pain, and disability
  - Mild injures may be "buddy taped," and patient may consider immediate return to play depending on function and sport requirements (1)[C].
  - 1st and 2nd degree: protected motion with "buddy tape" continuously for up to 3 wk (3)[B]. Consider taping during physical activity for an additional 2 to 4 wk (2)[C].
  - 3rd degree: Treat as severe 2nd degree. Surgery may be warranted if "unstressed instability," tissue interposition limiting joint motion, or lack of joint congruity is observed on radiographs (1,4)[C].

– In general, "buddy tape" to adjacent finger; for example, long finger to index and ring to small finger to prevent additional trauma to the index or small finger (3)[B]
– Continuous immobilization for >3 wk may lead to permanent stiffness (4)[C].
- Rehabilitation: Depending on severity, begin passive ROM exercises in 1st wk and active ROM after 1 to 2 wk, later for more severe injuries (2)[C].

ADDITIONAL THERAPIES

- Displaced intra-articular and large avulsion fractures with displacement may require open reduction and internal fixation (ORIF) (1)[C].
- Hyperextension and/or dorsal dislocation injuries and central tenderness over the volar aspect should raise concern for volar plate injuries requiring different treatment.
- Central tenderness over the dorsal PIP joint suggests central slip injury, which can lead to a chronic boutonnière deformity and requires a different management approach.

Pediatric Considerations

Collateral ligament injury in children should raise concern for growth plate involvement, and there should be a low threshold for referral to a hand specialist (5)[C].

SURGERY/OTHER PROCEDURES

- Generally necessary if instability with active ROM, tissue interposition limiting joint motion, or lack of joint congruity is observed on radiographs (1,4)[C]
- Routine surgical repair for complete tears is controversial. Most complete tears heal well with conservative treatment, and operative trauma may limit joint motion (1)[C].

ONGOING CARE

FOLLOW-UP RECOMMENDATIONS

- Follow up in 1 to 2 wk for reevaluation of laxity.
- Refer significant fractures for possible ORIF (4)[C].
- If uncertain of possible central slip/volar plate injury, refer to surgeon or follow up in 7 to 10 days for reevaluation (5)[C].
- Chronic symptoms may respond to extended splinting and "buddy taping" with protected ROM exercises for several weeks to months (5)[C].
- Surgical repair may be indicated if disability and instability persist after a sufficient trial of conservative treatment (5)[C].

PATIENT EDUCATION

Advise patients that some persistent deformity may be noted after injury has healed.

REFERENCES

1. Carruthers KH, Skie M, Jain M. Jam Injuries of the finger: diagnosis and management of injuries to the interphalangeal joints across multiple sports and levels of experience. *Sports Health*. 2016;8(5):469–478.
2. Freiberg A, Pollard BA, Macdonald MR, et al. Management of proximal interphalangeal joint injuries. *Hand Clin*. 2006;22(3):235–242.
3. Roh YH, Koh YD, Go JY, et al. Factors influencing functional outcome of proximal interphalangeal joint collateral ligament injury when treated with buddy strapping and exercise. *J Hand Ther*. 2018;31(3):295–300.
4. Khouri JS, Bloom JM, Hammert WC. Current trends in the management of proximal interphalangeal joint injuries of the hand. *Plast Reconstr Surg*. 2013;132(5):1192–2014.
5. Leggit JC, Meko CJ. Acute finger injuries: part I. Tendons and ligaments. *Am Fam Physician*. 2006;73(5):810–816.

ADDITIONAL READING

- Alexy C, De Carlo M. Rehabilitation and use of protective devices in hand and wrist injuries. *Clin Sports Med*. 1998;17(3):635–655.
- Palmer RE. Joint injuries of the hand in athletes. *Clin Sports Med*. 1998;17(3):513–531.

CLINICAL PEARLS

- Ensure active ROM in all affected and surrounding joints to rule out more significant ligamentous injuries.
- Return to play depends on severity and demands of sport, but frequently, immediate return to play can be accomplished with "buddy taping."
- Most injuries can be managed with protected motion through "buddy taping" for up to 3 wk and early ROM to prevent stiffness.
- Some residual soreness can be expected for months and sometimes up to a year.
- The joint affected may appear permanently enlarged owing to scarring during the healing process.

INTERSECTION SYNDROME

Jennifer Scott Koontz, MD, MPH, FAAFP, CAQSM

BASICS

DESCRIPTION

- Intersection syndrome is an inflammatory condition located in the distal radial forearm where the tendons of the 1st extensor compartment cross over the tendons of the 2nd compartment.
- Patient usually presents with pain, crepitus, and squeaky sensation in the dorsal distal forearm; may have localized swelling
- Pain usually occurs about 4 cm (range of 4 to 8 cm) proximal to the radial styloid.
- Synonym(s): Oarsman wrist; crossover syndrome; squeaker wrist; peritendinitis crepitans

EPIDEMIOLOGY

- Most common in rowers and weight lifters
- Skiers, other athletes, or workers who do repetitive forceful wrist flexion and extension activities are also at risk.

ETIOLOGY AND PATHOPHYSIOLOGY

- The abductor pollicis longus (APL) and extensor pollicis brevis (EPB) tendons comprise the 1st compartment.
- The extensor carpi radialis longus (ECRL) and brevis (ECRB) tendons comprise the 2nd compartment.
- Friction occurs at the intersection where the APL and EPB of the 1st compartment cross over the tendon sheath of the ECRL and ECRB in the 2nd compartment (1).
- This results in a tenosynovitis of the 2nd compartment.

RISK FACTORS

Sports with increased risk include:

- Rowing.
- Weight lifting.
- Skiing.
- Racquetball.
- Tennis.
- Any activity with repetitive forceful flexion and extension of the wrist.

GENERAL PREVENTION

Avoid or modify activity involving repetitive forceful flexion and extension of the wrist.

DIAGNOSIS

HISTORY

- Commonly misdiagnosed as de Quervain tenosynovitis
- History of increase in activity that requires repetitive wrist flexion/extension
- Athletes will report pain in the distal forearm or radial side of wrist, typically 4 cm (range of 4 to 8 cm) proximal to the radial styloid; may complain of localized swelling and a squeaking sensation

PHYSICAL EXAM

- Localized swelling 4 to 8 cm proximal to the radial styloid may be present.
- Crepitus on palpation is classic for intersection syndrome.
- Pain exacerbated by ulnar deviation of the hand
- Movement of wrist typically causes more pain than movement of thumb, as seen in de Quervain.
- Bony palpation is typically nontender, and neurovascular status should be intact.

DIFFERENTIAL DIAGNOSIS

- De Quervain tenosynovitis
- Extensor pollicis longus tendinitis (drummer boy palsy)
- Wartenberg syndrome (neuritis of superficial radial nerve)
- Degenerative joint disease of carpometacarpal joint
- Radial styloid fracture
- Scaphoid fracture
- Forearm stress fracture

DIAGNOSTIC TESTS & INTERPRETATION

Initial Tests (lab, imaging)

- Radiographs should be taken to evaluate for any underlying abnormalities. Anteroposterior, lateral, and oblique views of the wrist and distal forearm are the images of choice.
- If diagnostic ultrasound is available, this can be helpful for differentiating intersection syndrome from other disorders (2)[C].
- Magnetic resonance imaging (MRI) would not be indicated in the initial evaluation of this syndrome. If diagnosis is not clear or pain is persistent, MRI could be considered to evaluate for soft tissue masses or bony abnormalities. The MRI should include the forearm in addition to the wrist (3)[B].

Follow-Up Tests & Special Considerations

If symptoms persist and diagnosis is not clear, electromyography (EMG)/nerve conduction testing (NCT) may be helpful to evaluate for nerve entrapment.

TREATMENT

GENERAL MEASURES

Initial treatment (for 2 to 3 wk) (4)[C]:

- Rest
- Ice
- Nonsteroidal anti-inflammatory drugs (NSAIDs)
- Thumb spica splint in 15 to 20 degrees of extension

ADDITIONAL THERAPIES

- All treatment requires subsequent activity modification to prevent recurrence.
- Occupational therapy may be helpful for stretching program, local swelling reduction, and to help with activity modification. Manual therapy may be used in chronic cases to reduce scar tissue or tendinopathy.
- Injection is usually reserved after no improvement with 2 to 3 wk of splinting and activity modification.
- 2 to 3 mL of a local anesthetic and steroid combination may be injected into the area of maximal swelling or guided into intersection of 1st and 2nd compartment under ultrasound guidance.
- Saline hydrodissection under ultrasound guidance is an additional treatment option (5)[C].

SURGERY/OTHER PROCEDURES

- Surgery is reserved for recalcitrant cases.
- Surgery may include tenosynovectomy or bursectomy.

ONGOING CARE

FOLLOW-UP RECOMMENDATIONS

- If no improvement after adequate course of conservative therapy, surgical referral is warranted.
- Surgery may be needed if fibrosis of the tendon sheath has occurred (6)[C].

PROGNOSIS

- Recovery is achieved in majority of patients after initial treatment of activity modification, splinting, and NSAIDs for 2 to 3 wk.
- If surgery is necessary, postoperative rehabilitation typically lasts 4 to 6 wk.
- Return to play may occur once symptoms have resolved.

REFERENCES

1. Adams JE, Habbu R. Tendinopathies of the hand and wrist. *J Am Acad Orthop Surg*. 2015;23(12):741–750.
2. De Maeseneer M, Marcelis S, Jager T, et al. Spectrum of normal and pathologic findings in the region of the first extensor compartment of the wrist: sonographic findings and correlations with dissections. *J Ultrasound Med*. 2009;28(6):779–786.
3. Lee RP, Hatem SF, Recht MP. Extended MRI findings of intersection syndrome. *Skeletal Radiol*. 2009;38(2):157–163.
4. Chatterjee R, Vyas J. Diagnosis and management of intersection syndrome as a cause of overuse wrist pain [published online ahead of print September 28, 2016]. *BMJ Case Rep*. doi:10.1136/bcr-2016-216988.
5. Skinner TM. Intersection syndrome: the subtle squeak of an overused wrist. *J Am Board Fam Med*. 2017;30(4):547–551.
6. Fulcher SM, Kiefhaber TR, Stern PJ. Upper-extremity tendinitis and overuse syndromes in the athlete. *Clin Sports Med*. 1998;17(3):433–448.

ADDITIONAL READING

- Grundberg AB, Reagan DS. Pathologic anatomy of the forearm: intersection syndrome. *J Hand Surg Am*. 1985;10(2):299–302.
- Rettig AC. Wrist and hand overuse syndromes. *Clin Sports Med*. 2001;20(3):591–611.
- Rumball JS, Lebrun CM, Di Ciacca SR, et al. Rowing injuries. *Sports Med*. 2005;35(6):537–555.

CLINICAL PEARLS

- Intersection syndrome is an overuse syndrome.
- Pain is located 4 to 8 cm proximal to radial styloid.
- Athletes will often report a squeaking sensation in their wrist.
- Be able to consider both intersection syndrome and de Quervain tenosynovitis in the differential of distal forearm pain.
- The mainstay of treatment is conservative, utilizing activity modification and a short course of NSAIDs and possibly thumb spica splinting.

INTRAOCULAR FOREIGN BODIES

Kevin Waninger, MD, MS, FAAFP, FACEP, FACSM, CAQSM

BASICS

EPIDEMIOLOGY

- *Adults*: often the result of work accidents (high-risk mechanisms include hammering, chiseling, or grinding, especially metal on metal contact; machine-yard work such as lawn mowing; exposure to explosives or blast injuries; high-speed machines like drills, saws; windy environments)
- *Children*: often with explosives, weapons (toys that shoot projectiles), sports, windy weather.
- Similar to most other traumatic injuries, patients with IOFBs are mostly male, with the peak incidence in middle age (25 to 40 yr) (1,2).
- Although most IOFBs are related to accidental work-related injuries, an increasing number are related to sports activities.

GENERAL PREVENTION

- Protective eyewear of appropriate quality (3 mm of polycarbonate) prevents virtually all injuries from IOFBs. Patients should be instructed to wear appropriate protective eyewear in any situation that may lead to a higher risk of particles or objects getting into the eyes (sports; play activities with toys that shoot projectiles, like BB guns and air rifles; construction; workshops; explosives, industries; machine-yard work).
- The eyes should not be rubbed while working with wood or metal pieces. If a foreign body (FB) should enter the eye, no attempt should be made by the patient to remove the FB if perforation of the eye is suspected. If perforation is not suspected, eye irrigation may be attempted to wash out any potential foreign materials.

DIAGNOSIS

- Superficial FBs that are removed after the injury typically leave no permanent sequelae. However, corneal scarring, cataracts, and infection may occur, and the longer the time interval between the eye injury and treatment, the greater the likelihood that complications may occur.
- Morbidity increases if the FB penetrates into the anterior or posterior chambers of the eye, as damage to the iris, lens, and retina can occur and severely affect visual acuity. Any IOFB may lead to infection and endophthalmitis if not managed appropriately, which can threaten loss of the eye.
- Prehospital:
  - If an IOFB is suspected, place a hard shield over the injured eye to protect the eye from further damage until emergency department (ED) and/or ophthalmologic evaluation. Make sure to cover both eyes if IOFB with globe perforation is suspected.
  - Instruct the patient not to squeeze the affected eye.
  - Position the patient sitting upright to decrease intraocular pressure.

HISTORY

- The activities of the patient and their surroundings at the time of the injury are important and should lead to a high index of suspicion for IOFB.
- Patients frequently feel something entering their eye with no obvious external changes; hence, the incident is often dismissed quickly. Sometimes, patients may not complain of vision loss or severe pain.
- Past medical history should be obtained, including prior surgeries, medications, allergies, tetanus status, last meal (if surgery is a possibility).
- Does patient wear contacts (daily or extended wear) or glasses? Document if wearing at time of accident.
- Inquire whether the patient was wearing eye protection at the time of injury and whether the eyewear was still intact.
- The usual IOFB is a very small (<2 mm), sharp-edged object that enters the eye at high speed (2). Explosives often cause binocular changes with multiple FBs:
  - *Organic* (high incidence of infection): wood, soil, plants, insect parts
  - *Inorganic*: oxidizing metals (e.g., iron, copper). Iron can cause long-term toxicity as siderosis bulbi; copper FBs are very irritating and can cause a marked inflammatory response.
  - *Inert material*: paint, glass, plastic, gold, fiberglass, nonoxidizing metals, sand. Inert materials can be left in the eye for longer periods of time because they usually do not cause an immediate inflammatory response.

PHYSICAL EXAM

- Note that IOFBs can be deceptively subtle on initial presentation. The symptoms of an ocular FB may range from irritation to intense, excruciating pain. This is dependent on the size, location, material, and injury pattern.
- Note that high-speed projectiles may not produce pain or visual acuity problems initially because the FB may be located below the epithelial or conjunctival surface.
- In 20–40% of cases, IOFBs are located in the anterior chamber, allowing identification with slit-lamp exam alone. However, most IOFBs are located in the posterior chamber of the eye and will require a fully dilated pupil examination to identify accurately (2).
- Eye pain and FB sensation may be relieved significantly by topical anesthesia.
- Eye redness and tearing are common complaints, and light sensitivity (photophobia) may be present during your examination.
- Although patients may present with blurred/decreased vision, vision problems are not a reliable indicator of an IOFB because visual acuity might remain excellent as long as the visual axis is not involved.
- Look for any site of ocular penetration with visualization using a slit lamp.
- Always remember to look at the eyelids for signs of skin penetration; however, most IOFBs enter through or near the cornea.
- A complete examination of both eyes should be documented, including visual acuity and visual field examination, with lid eversion to check for retained FB. Pupil size, shape, and reactivity should be documented; any pupillary irregularities like a peaked pupil shape should alert the investigator of the possibility of a corneal perforation. Carefully access the pupillary direct reflex and look for an abnormal afferent pupillary defect on examination.
- Note the wound location and size, if visible, depth of the anterior chamber (compared to other side), iris and lens condition, blood in the anterior chamber (hyphema), or vitreous humor leakage. Document any cataracts, conjunctiva chemosis, or hemorrhage.
- Slit lamp, fluorescein, and funduscopic examinations should all be performed as soon as possible. Perform intraocular pressures if there is no suspicion or evidence of perforation.
- Minimize manipulation of the globe and exercise caution during examination if perforation is suspected to prevent prolapse of ocular contents.
- Note normal or decreased visual acuity, any conjunctival injection, ciliary injection (especially if an "anterior chamber reaction" occurs), any visible FB, any rust ring (especially if a metallic FB has been embedded for at least several hours), any epithelial defect that stains with fluorescein, any corneal edema, or any anterior chamber floating cells and flare noted.
- If a corneal infiltrate is present, an infectious cause needs to be considered.
- The Seidel sign is used to look for globe penetration that is not obvious on initial examination. In the case of a positive Seidel sign, the oozing aqueous humor at the site of the penetration through the cornea appears under ultraviolet or blue light as a "dark waterfall," clearing away excess fluorescein as it flows over the cornea.
- History, physical, and imaging studies should be used to access number, size, shape, location, composition, visibility, trajectory, and accessibility of any identified IOFBs.

DIFFERENTIAL DIAGNOSIS

- Corneal abrasion
- Conjunctival and corneal FBs
- Corneal perforation
- Ruptured globe
- Other trauma without retained IOFB
- Corneal ulcer
- Keratitis, bacterial and/or fungal

DIAGNOSTIC TESTS & INTERPRETATION

- Unless an infectious corneal infiltrate, corneal ulcer, or IOFB is suspected, no laboratory work is indicated.
- Infectious corneal infiltrates and corneal ulcers generally require scrapings for smears and cultures.
- Imaging is required whenever a patient is believed to have a retained IOFB.
- Plain radiographs, with Caldwell or Water projections, may demonstrate the presence of metallic or glass (lead content), but radiographs have low sensitivity for small and nonmetallic objects (like wood or plant material). The Sweet localization techniques utilizing frontal and lateral projections can be used if necessary to help localize IOFB locations when computed tomography (CT) scanning is not available.
- Orbital CT scanning with 0.5-mm cuts in both the axial and coronal planes allows the most precise and accurate identification and localization of IOFBs (2,3).
- Ocular ultrasound is also excellent for identifying and localizing IOFBs, but it must be performed with caution to avoid placing too much pressure on the globe and causing vitreous prolapse (2).
- Magnetic resonance imaging (MRI) is initially contraindicated due to the risk of magnetized IOFBs but may be used to localize small nonmetallic IOFBs after metallic IOFBs have been ruled out by CT scanning.

TREATMENT

- No topical medications or ointments should be administered if globe perforation is suspected.
- Topical anesthetics (proparacaine/tetracaine) may be used to assist with the examination and decrease discomfort unless globe perforation is suspected.
- Try to minimize patient nausea and vomiting to prevent the resultant increase in intraocular pressure.
- Pediatric patients may require sedation to facilitate examination and FB removal.

- If an IOFB is suspected, place a hard shield over the injured eye to protect the eye and avoid any pressure on the globe. Both eyes should be shielded to prevent contralateral eye movement/tracking if IOFB with globe perforation is suspected. Instruct the patient not to squeeze the affected eye. Position the patient sitting upright to decrease intraocular pressure.
- Topical antibiotics may be started to prevent infection until any epithelial defect heals. If perforation is suspected, systemic antibiotics may be started prior to surgical intervention. Endophthalmitis rates have been shown to decrease with early antibiotic administration.
- Topical corticosteroids may be used to decrease inflammation but such intervention should only be started after consultation with an ophthalmologist and a slit-lamp exam to rule out herpetic infection.
- Topical cycloplegic agents may be initiated to relieve pain and photophobia.
- Tetanus should be updated if indicated.
- Liberal use of opioid and other pain medications should be given because these injuries are extremely painful.
- Corneal patching is no longer recommended (4)[A].
- ED treatment:
  - For deep penetrating FBs, immediate referral to an ophthalmologist is recommended because endophthalmitis and permanent scarring may occur. Delayed surgical removal of IOFBs has been associated with significantly worse outcomes.
  - For superficial FBs, those who are trained in the technique can remove these manually. Anesthesia (topical anesthetic ophthalmic solution) is necessary prior to the FB removal procedure to facilitate the examination and removal process. The procedure risks, benefits, and complications must be discussed with the patient, and an informed consent must be signed. If a globe perforation is suspected, this procedure should not be attempted, and the patient should be referred.
  - If the FB is superficial, the eye should be irrigated to moisten the cornea. Removal of the FB should be attempted by using a gentle rolling motion with a wet cotton-tipped applicator. Pressure should not be applied, as this may push the FB deeper into the cornea or even create a corneal abrasion. An attempt to wash the FB off the cornea may be attempted by directing a stream of sterile normal saline at an oblique angle off the cornea.
  - An embedded FB should not be removed with irrigation or a cotton-tipped applicator. An embedded FB should be removed by using a gentle flicking motion with an eye spud, if available, or with a 25-gauge or 27-gauge sterile needle. Using a slit lamp to immobilize the patient's head and visualize the FB, the hub of the needle may be placed on a 3-mL syringe for easier control. The cornea should be approached from the side with the needle in a plane tangent to the cornea and the bevel away from the corneal surface to minimize the chance of corneal perforation. Good anesthesia of the corneal surface is important to the safety and success of this technique. Once dislodged from its embedded position in the cornea, remaining FB debris can be removed with a wet cotton-tipped applicator.
  - Within 3 hr, iron-containing FBs oxidize, leaving a rust ring/stain on adjacent epithelial cells, which can delay healing and act as an irritant focus. Removal of a rust ring at the time of FB removal may be attempted with a small-gauge needle or a pothook burr, but a rust ring often seems to be easier to remove 24 hr after the FB was initially removed, when the cells around the ring have loosened and can be readily lifted off and removed with a small burr instrument (5,6)[B].
  - Documenting a negative Seidel sign after removal of a corneal FB is good practice, especially after using sharp instruments in the FB removal process. This will confirm that no iatrogenic penetration of the corneal occurred during the procedure.

MEDICATION

- Prophylactic antibiotics are recommended to reduce infection and decrease endophthalmitis rates. Systemic penicillins, vancomycin, cephalosporins, and fluoroquinolones are commonly administered orally or intravenously. The fluoroquinolones have been shown to have excellent intraocular penetration after administration (2).
- Topical anesthetics may prolong epithelial healing and are not routinely prescribed for home pain relief.
- Ophthalmic nonsteroidal medications appear to be useful for decreasing pain in patients with corneal injury (7)[A].

ISSUES FOR REFERRAL

- Patients who present to the ED with emergent conditions should be discussed and/or referred to an ophthalmologist on the day of presentation. Patients with urgent conditions can be seen the following day.
- Emergent conditions:
  - Hyphema (blood in the anterior chamber) associated with a suspected IOFB
  - Diffuse corneal defect or opacity
  - Laceration of the cornea or sclera
  - Single dilated pupil or an abnormally shaped pupil
  - A deep or shallow anterior chamber (when compared to the other eye)
  - Suspected penetration of the globe
  - Positive Seidel sign
  - Multiple eye FBs
  - Extremely uncooperative patient (e.g., young child, intoxicated individual, patient with mental disability)
- Urgent conditions:
  - Significant lid edema
  - Large corneal abrasion
  - Corneal ulceration

ADMISSION, INPATIENT, AND NURSING CONSIDERATIONS

- Patients who have a history of assault, gunshot wound, explosive injury, or an inability to communicate an effective history need a systemic examination with vital signs and occasionally a general ED referral (1).
- If the examination in the office or the ED is not sufficient to rule out a FB or ocular perforation, then an examination under anesthesia should be considered. This is especially true for children, where there should be a low threshold to examine the child in the operating room.
- FBs that present any potential for intraocular penetration must be explored in the operating room. These injuries should be explored within 24 hr of initial examination.
- All corneal FBs, corneal ulcers, and corneal abrasions should follow up in 24 to 48 hr for reexamination. If rust rings are not completely removed, follow-up should be made within 24 hr for rust ring removal.

ONGOING CARE

FOLLOW-UP RECOMMENDATIONS

Patient Monitoring

- Follow-up every 1 to 2 days until all epithelial defects are well healed and all corneal infiltrates have resolved
- No activity or positioning restrictions are necessary once the wound heals.
- Gonioscopy should be performed by opthalmology after resolution and improvement. Annual follow-up care for intra-ocular pressure should be planned if the severity of trauma raises a suspicion of angle recession glaucoma in later life.
- A dilated fundus examination should be performed on a routine basis after any injury severe enough to potentially damage the retina.

PATIENT EDUCATION

Eye protection when taking part in risky activities (e.g., hammering, mowing the lawn) is strongly recommended.

PROGNOSIS

Prognosis is good unless a rust ring or scarring involves the visual axis. If infection develops, prognosis is more guarded. Globe-penetrating injuries and IOFB have much worse prognoses, but reading vision is usually retained/regained, if properly treated.

COMPLICATIONS

Endophthalmitis, corneal scarring, elevated intraocular pressure, cataract, retinal detachment, proliferative vitreoretinopathy, and metallosis (e.g., chalcosis, siderosis) are possible complications.

REFERENCES

1. Karth PA, Kamjoo S, Shah VA. Intraocular foreign bodies (IOFB). EyeWiki. http://eyewiki.aao.org/Intraocular_Foreign_Bodies (IOFB). Updated December 7, 2017. Accessed July 2, 2018.
2. Parke DW III, Flynn HW Jr, Fisher YL. Management of intraocular foreign bodies: a clinical flight plan. *Can J Ophthalmol*. 2013;48(1):8–12.
3. Dass AB, Ferrone PJ, Chu YR, et al. Sensitivity of spiral computed tomography scanning for detecting intraocular foreign bodies. *Ophthalmology*. 2001;108(12):2326–2328.
4. Turner A, Rabiu M. Patching for corneal abrasion. *Cochrane Database Syst Rev*. 2006;(2):CD004764.
5. Weichel ED, Yeh S. Techniques of intraocular foreign body removal. *Tech Ophthalmology*. 2009;7:45–52.
6. Yeh S, Colyer MH, Weichel ED. Current trends in the management of intraocular foreign bodies. *Curr Opin Ophthalmol*. 2008;19(3):225–233.
7. Weaver CS, Terrell KM. Evidence-based emergency medicine. Update: do ophthalmic nonsteroidal anti-inflammatory drugs reduce the pain associated with simple corneal abrasion without delaying healing? *Ann Emerg Med*. 2003;41(1):134–140.

CLINICAL PEARLS

- Accurate history taking that involves attention to the mechanism of ocular injury should be obtained.
- Remember that the clinical presentation of IOFB can be subtle on initial presentation.
- Make sure you have adequate pain relief for your patient so that you can get an adequate examination. You need an adequate examination to rule out significant ocular injury.
- Do not limit your clinical focus to the eye injury and forget to do a complete examination on your patient to rule out other systemic injury beyond that of the presentation of an ocular injury.
- Discuss any ocular pathology with an ophthalmologist and plan adequate referral.
- Protective eyewear of appropriate quality prevents virtually all injuries from IOFB.

I

KLIPPEL-FIEL SYNDROME: FUSION OF CERVICAL VERTEBRAE

Tracy Zaslow, MD, FAAP, CAQSM

BASICS

- A malformation sequence
- Clinical triad of short neck, low hairline, and fusion of multiple cervical vertebrae resulting in decreased range of motion (ROM)

DESCRIPTION

- First described independently by Maurice Klippel and Andre Feil in 1912. They described patients who had the triad of short, webbed neck; decreased ROM in the cervical spine; and a low hairline.
- Original classification by Gunderson et al (1):
  – Type I: massive fusion of cervical spine
  – Type II: fusion of one or two cervical interspaces
  – Type III: thoracic or lumbar vertebrae involved
- A newer classification system by Samartzis (2,3) modifies the classification system as: Type I patients have a single-level fusion; type II patients have multiple, noncontiguous fused segments; and type III patients have multiple, contiguous fused segments.

EPIDEMIOLOGY

- Occurrence is sporadic.
- However, cases with autosomal dominant and autosomal recessive inheritance with variable expression have been reported.

Incidence

- The true incidence of Klippel-Feil syndrome is unknown.
- Estimated as 1:40,000 to 42,000; recent computed tomography (CT) study of asymptomatic patients demonstrated a prevalence of 1 in 172 (4).

ETIOLOGY AND PATHOPHYSIOLOGY

- Etiology of Klippel-Feil syndrome and its associated conditions are unknown.
- The sequence may be a part of a serious neural tube development caused by a failure in the normal segmentation or division of the cervical vertebrae during the early weeks (3rd and 8th wk) of fetal development.
- Other possible etiologies include vascular disruption and global fetal insult.
- Recent molecular studies have suggested genetic mutations (MEOXI gene, GDF6, GDF3, PAX1, RIPPLY2) may be involved in the pathogenesis (5,6,7,8).

GENERAL PREVENTION

- Prevention of complications can be done by initial broad evaluation of systems commonly affected by Klippel-Feil and regular evaluation of associated features.
- Motion at each intervertebral space should be evaluated annually by lateral flexion–extension radiographs of the cervical spine.

COMMONLY ASSOCIATED CONDITIONS

- Klippel-Feil triad is associated with congenital abnormalities of the genitourinary (GU) tract, musculoskeletal system, spinal cord/neurologic system, cardiovascular system, and auditory system.
- GU tract:
  – GU tract structure abnormalities occur in 30–40% of patients with Klippel-Feil; double collecting systems, renal aplasia, horseshoe kidney, and recurrent pyelonephritis are common; however, absence of a kidney is the most common finding.
  – The extent of cervical abnormality does not correlate with severity of GU abnormalities; thus, thorough GU evaluation is indicated in all patients.
- Musculoskeletal:
  – Short stature
  – Atlantoaxial instability
  – Scoliosis is present in 60% of patients with Klippel-Feil syndrome.
  – Scoliosis may be due to fusion in the thoracic or lumbar spine, or a developmental compensation for the cervical/cervicothoracic scoliosis.
  – Cervical spinal stenosis can also occur in association with Klippel-Feil syndrome; although uncommon, when present, cervical stenosis can increase risk of neurologic involvement.
  – Sprengel anomaly (congenital elevation of the scapula) occurs in 20–30% of those with Klippel-Feil. A higher than expected incidence of scoliosis occurs in those with Sprengel anomaly.
  – Upper extremity abnormalities, including syndactyly, hypoplastic thumb, supernumerary digits, and hypoplasia of the upper extremity
- Cardiovascular:
  – Septal defects
  – Situs inversus
  – Coarctation of the aorta
- Pulmonary:
  – Lobar agenesis
- Neurologic:
  – Chiari I malformation
  – Syringomyelia
  – Diastematomyelia
  – Sleep-disordered breathing
  – Dermoid cyst in the posterior fossa
  – Hereditary neuropathies
- Auditory system:
  – Hearing impairment: occurs in >1/3 of Klippel-Feil patients
- Other:
  – Ptosis of the eye
  – Duane eye contracture
  – Lateral rectus palsy
  – Facial nerve palsy
  – Cleft palate
  – Synkinesia or mirror movement
  – Facial asymmetry
  – Craniosynostosis

DIAGNOSIS

- Clinical presentation is variable due to the presence/absence of different associated anomalies.
- Often Klippel-Feil syndrome is discovered incidentally on physical examination.
- The complete triad is present in <50% of cases.

HISTORY

- Often asymptomatic
- Neck/back pain +/− neurologic symptoms, including numbness, tingling, weakness
- Decreased hearing

PHYSICAL EXAM

- Low hairline
- Short neck
- Decreased cervical ROM; rotational loss is usually more pronounced than loss of flexion and extension.
- Torticollis
- Facial asymmetry
- Heart examination to evaluate for heart position and murmurs
- Chest examination to evaluate for rib fusion and other chest wall anomalies
- Back examination for Sprengel deformity and scoliosis

DIFFERENTIAL DIAGNOSIS

- Congenital muscular torticollis
- Acquired spinal fusion (postinfection, spine inflammatory disorders)
- Wildervanck (cervicooculoacoustic) syndrome
- Mayer-Rokitansky-Küster syndrome
- Cervical spina bifida
- Congenital scoliosis
- Brachial plexus injury
- Central nervous system (CNS) lesion (brain tumor)
- Iniencephaly
- Dyssegmental dysplasia

DIAGNOSTIC TESTS & INTERPRETATION

Initial Tests (lab, imaging)

- Plain radiography (anteroposterior/lateral of the cervical spine) is the basis for the diagnosis of Klippel-Feil syndrome.
- Flexion–extension radiographs are indicated if instability is suspected at the craniocervical junction or if two fused segments are separated by an open segment.
- Plain radiographs of the entire spine must be obtained to detect other spinal anomalies.
- Rib series radiography to evaluate for possible rib anomalies, such as multiple rib fusions, also is necessary.
- CT scanning may be done in patients being evaluated for surgery but is not required for diagnosis.

- Magnetic resonance imaging (MRI) is indicated in patients with neurologic deficits to most accurately assess subluxation, cord compression, spinal stenosis, and additional CNS anomalies.
- Ultrasound (US) of the kidneys: indicated to screen for renal anomalies. Intravenous (IV) pyelography should be performed if further definition of a kidney abnormality is required.

Diagnostic Procedures/Other

Full age–appropriate hearing screening: due to the high incidence of hearing loss

TREATMENT

GENERAL MEASURES

- No known treatment for underlying etiology
- Treatment is symptomatic, which includes modification of activities, bracing, and, for subluxation, traction. Response to traction may also predict the success of surgery.
- Surgical interventions should be delayed as long as possible. Indications for surgery include progressive symptomatic segmental instability and neurologic compromise.
- Physical therapy may help to maximize ROM and minimize functional limitations.
- General activity limitations, even without presence of symptoms or instability:
  - Avoid contact sports.
  - Avoid occupations and recreational activities with risk of head and neck trauma.
- Sports participation limitations:
  - All types: Avoid contact sports and activities with risk of head and neck trauma.
  - Type I: absolute contraindication to participation in contact sports
  - Type II:
    - Fusion of one or two interspaces at C2 or above with limited cervical ROM, occipitocervical anomalies, involvement of C2, instability, disk disease, or degenerative changes → absolute contraindication
    - Fusion of one or two interspaces at C3 or below with full cervical ROM AND no occipitocervical anomalies, no involvement of C2, no instability, no disk disease, and no degenerative changes → no additional contraindications; may participate in contact sports

SURGERY/OTHER PROCEDURES

- Referral to otolaryngology for airway issues and evaluation for hearing loss (9)
- Surgical interventions should be delayed as long as possible.
- Indications for surgery include progressive symptomatic segmental instability, neurologic compromise, and/or severe scoliosis.
- Surgical techniques involve occipitocervical arthrodesis, halo immobilization, and atlantoaxial arthrodesis.

ONGOING CARE

FOLLOW-UP RECOMMENDATIONS

Patient Monitoring

- Annual cervical spine radiographs to evaluate for instability
- Additional follow-up studies based on individual system involvement

PATIENT EDUCATION

If hypermobility is noted in the upper cervical segment, there is increased risk of developing neurologic impairment and patients should not be cleared for activities that increase risk of neck injury (i.e., gymnastics, cheerleading, contact sports).

PROGNOSIS

- Prognosis is good if features of the disorder are treated early and appropriately.
- If hypermobility is noted in the upper cervical segment, there is increased risk of developing neurologic impairment and patients should not be cleared for activities that increase risk of neck injury (i.e., gymnastics, cheerleading, contact sports).
- If hypermobility is noted in the lower cervical segment, there is increased risk for degenerative disk disease and patients should be treated symptomatically and held from sports based on symptoms.

REFERENCES

1. Gunderson CH, Greenspan RH, Glaser GH, et al. The Klippel-Feil syndrome: genetic and clinical reevaluation of cervical fusion. *Medicine (Baltimore)*. 1967;46(6):491–512.
2. Samartzis D, Herman J, Lubicky JP, et al. Sprengel's deformity in Klippel-Feil syndrome. *Spine (Phila Pa 1976)*. 2007;32(18):E512–E516.
3. Samartzis DD, Herman J, Lubicky JP, et al. Classification of congenitally fused cervical patterns in Klippel-Feil patients: epidemiology and role in the development of cervical spine-related symptoms. *Spine (Phila Pa 1976)*. 2006;31(21):E798–E804.
4. Gruber J, Saleh A, Bakhsh W, et al. The prevalence of Klippel-Feil syndrome: a computed tomography-based analysis of 2,917 patients. *Spine Deform*. 2018;6(4):448–453.
5. Mohamed JY, Faqeih E, Alsiddiky A, et al. Mutations in MEOX1, encoding mesenchyme homeobox 1, cause Klippel-Feil anomaly. *Am J Hum Genet*. 2013;92(1):157–161.
6. David KM, Thorogood PV, Stevens JM, et al. The dysmorphic cervical spine in Klippel-Feil syndrome: interpretations from developmental biology. *Neurosurg Focus*. 1999;6(6):e1.
7. Karaca E, Yuregir OO, Bozdogan ST, et al. Rare variants in the notch signaling pathway describe a novel type of autosomal recessive Klippel–Feil syndrome. *Am J Med Genet A*. 2015;167A(11):2795–2799.
8. McGaughran JM, Oates A, Donnai D, et al. Mutations in PAX1 may be associated with Klippel–Feil syndrome. *Eur J Hum Genet*. 2003;11(6):468–474.
9. Kenna MA, Irace AL, Strychowsky JE, et al. Otolaryngologic manifestations of Klippel-Feil syndrome in children. *JAMA Otolaryngol Head Neck Surg*. 2018;144(3):238–243.

ADDITIONAL READING

- Brown MW, Templeton AW, Hodges FJ III. The incidence of acquired and congenital fusions in the cervical spine. *Am J Roentgenol Radium Ther Nucl Med*. 1964;92:1255–1259.
- Driscoll DJ, Rigamonti D, Gailloud P. Klippel-Feil syndrome. In: National Organization for Rare Disorders. *NORD Guide to Rare Disorders*. Philadelphia, PA: Lippincott Williams and Wilkins; 2003:720.
- Gjorup PA, Gjorup L. Klippel-Feil's syndrome. *Dan Med Bull*. 1964;11:50–53.
- Hensinger RN, Lang JE, MacEwen GD. Klippel-Feil syndrome; a constellation of associated anomalies. *J Bone Joint Surg Am*. 1974;56(6):1246–1253.
- Klippel-Feil sequence. In: Jones KL, Jones MC, del Campo, Miguel. *Smith's Recognizable Patterns of Human Malformation*. 7th ed. Philadelphia, PA: W.B. Saunders; 2013:810–811.
- Klippel-Feil syndrome In: Behrman RE, Kliegman RM, Jenson HB. *Nelson Textbook of Pediatrics*. 16th ed. Philadelphia, PA: W.B Saunders; 2000:2090.
- McGaughran JM, Kuna P, Das V. Audiological abnormalities in the Klippel-Feil syndrome. *Arch Dis Child*. 1998;79(4):352–355.
- Thomsen MN, Schneider U, Weber M, et al. Scoliosis and congenital anomalies associated with Klippel-Feil syndrome types I–III. *Spine (Phila Pa 1976)*. 1997;22(4):396–401.
- Tracy MR, Dormans JP, Kusumi K. Klippel-Feil syndrome: clinical features and current understanding of etiology. *Clin Orthop Relat Res*. 2004;(424):183–190.
- Wheeless CR. Klippel-Feil syndrome. In: *Wheeless' Textbook of Orthopaedics*. Brooklandville, MD: Data Trace Internet; 1995–2009.

CLINICAL PEARLS

- When examining the back, always look at the scapula for Sprengel deformity.
- If Sprengel deformity is observed, consider cervical spine x-rays to rule out fusion associated with Klippel-Feil syndrome.

KNEE DISLOCATION

Timothy Tiu, MD, FAAPMR, CAQSM

BASICS

- The true incidence of knee dislocations is unknown, owing to frequent spontaneous reduction (1,2,3,4). Missed spontaneous reductions may cause detrimental neurovascular damage. It is unnecessary to have complete dislocation for injury to occur at the intimal wall of the popliteal artery (PA) (1,2,3,5).
- Traumatic knee dislocation is defined as complete disruption of the integrity of the tibiofemoral articulation (2,3).
- A multiligamentous knee injury is defined as a grossly unstable knee with disruption of at least two of the four major ligamentous structures (2,3).
- Knee dislocation is a rare but potentially devastating injury. It may lead to amputation or inability to return to full function.
- High-velocity injuries involving a sudden violent force, such as a motor vehicle accident (MVA), falls from skiing, and injuries from gymnastics and extreme sports, are usually associated with an increased risk for neurovascular damage, owing to more extensive disruption to the joint capsule.
- Low-velocity injuries are usually due to sports, such as football or rugby, and usually have less soft tissue damage with better prognosis.
- Ultra low–velocity injuries are due to falls and occur more commonly in obese females (6).
- There are six structures within the knee that are at risk of injury with knee dislocation: anterior cruciate ligament (ACL), posterior cruciate ligament (PCL), medial cruciate ligament (MCL), lateral cruciate ligament (LCL), medial meniscus, and lateral meniscus. *Cautions*:
  - Documentation of pulses and motor response (ankle dorsiflexion) is essential.
  - Splint in slight flexion to prevent traction or compression of the PA (2,5)[C].

DESCRIPTION

- Categorized by the position of the tibia in relationship to the distal femur
- Anterior dislocation (40%):
  - Hyperextension of the knee of at least 30 degrees
  - Rupture of the posterior capsule followed by the PCL
- Posterior dislocation (33%):
  - Direct blow to the anterior tibia with the knee flexed at 90 degrees ("dashboard" injury or falling onto flexed knee)
  - ACL is usually spared.
- Medial dislocation (4%):
  - Varus stress causing tear to ACL, PCL, and LCL; highest risk of posterolateral corner (PLC) damage and thus the highest risk of irreducible dislocation
  - Associated with tibial plateau fracture
- Lateral dislocation (18%):
  - Valgus stress causing tear to ACL, PCL, and MCL
  - Associated with tibial plateau fracture
- Rotatory dislocation:
  - Twisting mechanism (planted foot and body twisting in opposite direction) that can be further divided into anteromedial, anterolateral, posterolateral
  - Posterolateral dislocations are nearly impossible to be reduced by closed method.
- PA injury:
  - Reported in as high as 64% of dislocations. Recent large-scale study reports frequency of 3.3% (7).
  - Artery is fixed proximally at the fibrous insertion of the adductor magnus onto the medial femoral epicondyle and distally tethered by the tendinous arch of the soleus (1,7).
  - The PA sits within the popliteal fossa with branches to the collateral artery supply. The geniculate collateral arteries cannot compensate for a ruptured PA.
  - If vascular injury is not reversed within 6 to 8 hr, amputation rate approaches 90% (1,3,7).
  - Anterior dislocations place traction on the PA and cause contusion or intimal injury, which may result in delayed thrombosis.
  - Posterior dislocations (most common) cause direct intimal fracture or transection of the artery with immediate thrombosis.
- Fibular nerve injury:
  - The fibular nerve wraps around the fibular head.
  - May occur in up to 50% of dislocations.
  - Characterized by hypesthesia of anterolateral leg and dorsum of foot, weakness of ankle dorsiflexion
  - Poor prognosis for recovery
  - Medial dislocations cause injury by traction to the nerve.
  - Rotatory injuries have a high incidence of traction and transection.

EPIDEMIOLOGY

- The most common mechanism of injury is an MVA.
- Most commonly anterior (40%), followed by posterior (33%); most common types associated with PA damage (1)
- PA injury rate previously reported up to 64%; newer data reports 3.3% (7).
- Full recovery of the fibular nerve is unlikely.

Prevalence

- MVAs (50–60%)
- Sports (30–50%)
- Falls (1–17%)

ETIOLOGY AND PATHOPHYSIOLOGY

- High-energy injuries such as MVAs, auto versus pedestrian accidents, and athletic injuries
- Football is the most common source of athletic injuries.
- Ground-level falls in obese patients

RISK FACTORS

- Morbid obesity is a potential risk factor for posterior dislocations.
- Contact or high-velocity sports

DIAGNOSIS

HISTORY

- Patient will usually hear a pop at time of injury.
- Have patient describe mechanism of injury, if possible.

PHYSICAL EXAM

- The initial physical exam may be difficult, owing to excessive swelling and pain.
- Subjective pain, instability, and swelling
- Grossly deformed knee/asymmetry
- Grossly unstable knee in anterior/posterior plane or on varus/valgus stress:
  - ACL and PCL, collateral ligament injuries
  - Suspect a relocated knee dislocation if the patient had a high-impact injury with multiple ligamentous laxity.
- Lateral/posterolateral (irreducible) dislocation:
  - Grossly deformed
  - Dimple sign: dimple of the medial skin and soft tissues
  - Pucker sign: Puckering of skin results from its attachment to the invaginated capsule (3).
- Evaluate vasculature:
  - By palpation, Doppler, ankle-brachial pressure indexes, and distal perfusion (5)[C]
  - Dorsalis pedia, posterior tibialis, popliteal
  - Popliteal thrill or expanding pulsatile hematoma
  - Signs of distal ischemia: pallor, paresthesias, pain, paralysis, unequal temperature
  - If peripheral pulses are normal initially, it is essential to do serial, frequent exams with documentation of pulses (2,3,4,5)[C].
  - Estimated 5–15% of knee dislocations may have a strong distal pulse initially with delayed expansion of intimal tear (5)[B].
- Neurologic examination:
  - Sensory: anterolateral lag, dorsum of foot, first web space
  - Motor: ankle dorsiflexion, eversion

DIFFERENTIAL DIAGNOSIS

- Tibial plateau fracture
- Supracondylar femoral fracture
- Isolated fibular nerve injury
- ACL injury/rupture

DIAGNOSTIC TESTS & INTERPRETATION

Initial Tests (lab, imaging)

- Complete blood count (CBC)
- Basic metabolic protein with blood urea nitrogen/creatinine (BUN/Cr)
- International normalized ratio (INR)/coagulation studies

- Knee x-rays: fractures common (periarticular, avulsion fracture, tibial plateau)
- Ankle brachial index (ABI): systolic blood pressure (BP) from all four extremities with Doppler probe and BP cuff; ABI: highest pressure from dorsal pedal pulse or posterior tibial pulse/highest brachial BP (5):
  - Prospective study: ABI >0.90 had 100% negative predictive value for arterial injury requiring surgical repair (2,3,4).
  - Patients with asymmetric pulses, normal reperfusion, and ABI <0.90 should undergo arteriography (2)[C].
- Angiography remains the "gold standard," but there is evidence to support the use of selective angiography or computed tomography (CT) angiography (1,2,3,4)[C].
- Duplex Doppler
- Magnetic resonance imaging (MRI)

TREATMENT

- Prehospital:
  - If covering a game or event with potential high-impact injuries, initially assess for life-threatening injuries.
  - Basic life support: circulation, airway, breathing (CAB); assess for head and neck injury.
  - If knee dislocation is suspected, immediate neurovascular assessment becomes the focus of evaluation. If safe, remove shoes and socks for better neurovascular exam.
  - Splint knee in 20 degrees flexion in order to prevent spontaneous posterior tibia translation and preserve safety of the popliteal neurovascular structures (2,5)[C].
  - Plan for reduction in emergency room (ER)
- ER treatment:
  - Reduction to reduce pressure on both the neurovascular structures and the skin. Successful under conscious sedation in most cases. Intraoperative closed and, rarely, open reduction may be necessary (3).
  - If a "pucker sign" or "dimple sign" is evident, suspicion of an irreducible posterolateral knee dislocation should be raised and an emergency open reduction in the operating room is to be undertaken (2).
  - Intravenous (IV) analgesia for patient comfort
  - Vascular and orthopedic surgical consultation for open injury, evidence of PA injury, or unable to reduce dislocation

SURGERY/OTHER PROCEDURES

- All vascular injuries will need a vascular surgeon consult.
- Orthopedic consult
- Patients with hard signs of vascular injury should undergo immediate surgical exploration with or without intraoperative arteriography (2)[C].
- Ligamentous repair/reconstruction versus conservative treatment with splinting alone depends on activity level of patient.
- Goal of repair is to provide a functional, stable joint:
  - Nonoperative care is reserved only for sedentary patients or if unable to undergo surgery (1,4)[C].
- Physical therapy will be essential for conservative and postoperative treatment.
- Rehabilitation depends on specific ligaments torn.
- Goal of 90 degrees knee flexion 6 wk postoperatively and 120 degrees at 12 wk (4)[C].
- No return to full activity or sports before 9 mo (4)[C]

ADMISSION, INPATIENT, AND NURSING CONSIDERATIONS

- All patients with knee dislocation require admission for either arterial injury repair or observation of limb perfusion.
- Patients with normal pulses and ABI >0.90 should undergo 24 to 48 hr of serial examinations (2,3,4,5)[C].

ONGOING CARE

PROGNOSIS

- Prognosis depends on neurovascular damage, which depends on velocity of injury.
- Fibular nerve damage portends a worse prognosis. Full recovery is unlikely, but younger patients may have better nerve recovery (8).
- Complications include joint stiffness, joint contractures, ongoing knee instability, joint pain, and swelling (3,4).
- Recovery to good function of the knee for daily activities of living is likely, but return to demanding sports is not predictable (1,9).

COMPLICATIONS

- Amputation
- Compartment syndrome
- Neurovascular deficit
- Chronic pain
- Stiffness
- Instability

REFERENCES

1. McKee L, Ibrahim MS, Lawrence T, et al. Current concepts in acute knee dislocation: the missed diagnosis? *Open Orthop J*. 2014;8:162–167.
2. Maslaris A, Brinkmann O, Bungartz M, et al. Management of knee dislocation prior to ligament reconstruction: what is the current evidence? Update of a universal treatment algorithm. *Eur J Orthop Surg Traumatol*. 2018;28(6):1001–1015.
3. Walker RE, McDougall D, Patel S, et al. Radiologic review of knee dislocation: from diagnosis to repair. *AJR Am J Roentgenol*. 2013;201(3): 483–495.
4. Skendzel JG, Sekiya JK, Wojtys EM. Diagnosis and management of the multiligament-injured knee. *J Orthop Sports Phys Ther*. 2012;42(3):234–242.
5. Nicandri GT, Chamberlain AM, Wahl CJ. Practical management of knee dislocations: a selective angiography protocol to detect limb-threatening vascular injuries. *Clin J Sport Med*. 2009;19(2): 125–129.
6. Werner BC, Gwathmey FW Jr, Higgins ST, et al. Ultra-low velocity knee dislocations: patient characteristics, complications, and outcomes. *Am J Sports Med*. 2014;42(2):358–363.
7. Natsuhara KM, Yeranosian MG, Cohen JR, et al. What is the frequency of vascular injury after knee dislocation? *Clin Orthop Relat Res*. 2014;472(9): 2615–2620.
8. Peskun CJ, Chahal J, Steinfeld ZY, et al. Risk factors for peroneal nerve injury and recovery in knee dislocation. *Clin Orthop Relat Res*. 2012;470(3): 774–778.
9. Ibrahim SA, Ahmad FH, Salah M, et al. Surgical management of traumatic knee dislocation. *Arthroscopy*. 2008;24(2):178–187.

ADDITIONAL READING

Cush GJ, Maloney PJ, Irgit K. Drop foot after knee dislocation: evaluation and treatment. In: Fanelli G, ed. *The Multiple Ligament Injured Knee*. New York, NY: Springer; 2013:343–353.

CLINICAL PEARLS

- Knee dislocations often reduce spontaneously. If it is a high-impact injury with knee deformity or multiple ligamentous laxity, suspect a knee dislocation (1,2,3,4).
- Anterior dislocations are the most common (1).
- PA injury incidence may be much lower than previously reported (7).
- Normal pulse does not necessarily indicate normal PA. Angiography remains the "gold standard," but there is evidence to support the use of selective angiography or CT angiography (1,2,3,4)[C].
- Neurologic deficit indicates worse injury and prognosis.
- Splint knee in 20 degrees flexion to protect neurovascular structures (2,5)[C].
- PA damage that is not surgically repaired within 8 hr is likely to result in above-knee amputation (1,3,7). Ultra low–velocity injuries are more common in obese females and due to falls (6).

KÖHLER DISEASE (ASEPTIC NECROSIS OF THE TARSAL NAVICULAR)

Kevin E. Burroughs, MD, CAQSM

BASICS

DESCRIPTION

- Pediatric osteochondrosis of the tarsal navicular, first described by Alban Köhler in 1908 (1)
- Osteochondrosis is a disease process that causes necrosis of the ossification center of a developing bone and is followed by regeneration.

EPIDEMIOLOGY

ALERT

- Predominant age: occurs in children 2 to 7 yr of age (average age 5 yr and 10 mo) (2)
- Predominant gender: males > females (4 to 6:1)
- Usually occurs unilaterally; bilateral in only ~15–20% of cases
- Appears to be no relation between weight and incidence

Consideration:

- Adult onset navicular osteonecrosis is known as Mueller-Weiss disease (also known as Brailsford disease).

ETIOLOGY AND PATHOPHYSIOLOGY

- Navicular development:
  - The navicular becomes evident on radiographs between 18 and 24 mo in girls and between 30 and 36 mo in boys.
  - A more irregular and dense navicular is often present in children whose navicular ossifies at later times than these, and these findings are similar to those in Köhler disease.
  - The navicular ossifies from a single center in 2/3 of children and from multiple centers in the remainder. Those ossifying later than normal tend to be from multiple centers.
  - A dense perichondral network of blood vessels has been described on the nonarticular surfaces, with numerous penetrating arteries.
- Theories of etiology:
  - Questionably a normal variant but does not explain why some individuals are asymptomatic
  - Some believe that it is avascular necrosis; however, this wouldn't explain acute onset of pain, lack of correlation with radiographic changes in that short amount of time, and no matter the treatment, a normal navicular is the end result (true necrosis should cause deformity).
  - Most likely a syndrome or continuum of disease because radiographic changes can be seen in asymptomatic individuals. Perhaps those who are symptomatic have experienced a stress injury to the ossifying bone. This would explain radiographic changes, with remodeling to a normal-appearing bone.

RISK FACTORS

- May be caused by repetitive microtrauma to the maturing navicular ossification center (the last tarsal bone to ossify) (3)
- Compression of the bony nucleus at a critical phase of growth may occlude the penetrating blood vessels and produce ischemia and aseptic necrosis of the bone.
- Delayed ossification leading to irregular ossification centers may predispose to this condition.
- Occurrence is not related to acute macrotrauma, age at first walking, foot type, or family history.

DIAGNOSIS

Although variations in morphology of the navicular have been described, the diagnosis of Köhler disease is made on the basis of both clinical and radiographic findings.

HISTORY

- It is often difficult for young children to localize pain, but it should be over the midfoot area.
- Repetitive microtrauma may be a risk factor in sports.
- A history of macrotrauma should lead the practitioner to consider other causes of foot pain.

PHYSICAL EXAM

ALERT

Signs and symptoms:

- Insidious onset of foot pain and limp aggravated by activity
- Time to presentation varies from days to months after onset of pain.

Physical examination:

- Look for localized edema and warmth in the area of the tarsal navicular.
- Palpate the entire foot and ankle; tenderness should be localized to the medial midfoot.
- Check the range of motion of the ankle and subtalar joints, which should be normal.
- Examine the knee and hip, which can be the source of referred pain and limp.

DIFFERENTIAL DIAGNOSIS

- Normal variants: Variations of size and shape of the navicular ossification center may be indistinguishable from Köhler disease except for the absence of symptoms.
- Osteochondritis dissecans
- Localized involvement on the articular surface
- Well demarcated from the normal bone by a crescent-shaped area of radiolucency

DIAGNOSTIC TESTS & INTERPRETATION

ALERT

Radiographs:

- Standard anteroposterior, lateral, and oblique radiographs of the foot should be obtained.

- Findings (4):
  - Varying degrees of navicular sclerosis
  - Diminished size or flattening of the navicular ("Alka-Seltzer-on-end" appearance)
  - Occasional loss of trabecular pattern and fragmentation

- A person with an asymptomatic foot with abnormal radiographic features found incidentally does not have Köhler disease.
- Bone scintigraphy (4)[C]:
  - If diagnosis not evident, bone scan can show decreased uptake in the navicular, indicating decreased or interrupted blood supply early when radiographs still normal.
  - In the later phases, can show increased uptake indicating revascularization
- Pathologic findings:
  - Patchy areas of bone destruction and dead trabeculae with interference of normal ossification

TREATMENT

GENERAL MEASURES

- Acute treatment:
  - Apply ice to midfoot.
  - Nonsteroidal anti-inflammatory drugs (NSAIDs) or acetaminophen can be used for analgesic effect.
  - Immobilization to affect relief of symptoms, although the type and duration of treatment do not influence long-term outcomes

ALERT

Despite not altering the long-term outcome, immobilization has been shown to decrease the duration of symptoms (4)[C].

- Immobilization:
  - Patients with cast immobilization are typically pain free at 3 mo, whereas those treated without casting were symptomatic until 15 mo on average.
  - Those casted for a minimum of 2 mo were asymptomatic in the shortest time.
  - Weight-bearing status does not appear to affect outcome.

ADDITIONAL THERAPIES

- Orthoses have not been found to be effective.
- Rehabilitation: usually not indicated

SURGERY/OTHER PROCEDURES

Rarely required

ONGOING CARE

FOLLOW-UP RECOMMENDATIONS

Orthopedic referral is indicated if symptoms do not resolve with conservative management.

Patient Monitoring

- In a study of 12 cases, complete restoration of normal bone structure occurred in 8 mo (minimum 6 mo and maximum of 13 mo) (5)[C].
- At 30-yr follow-up, no patient showed degenerative changes at the tarsonavicular joint, and no radiographic differences were seen with the unaffected foot (5)[C].

PROGNOSIS

- Complete resolution of symptoms with reconstitution of the navicular can be expected in all patients.
- No evidence of cartilage degeneration in long-term follow-up studies

REFERENCES

1. Köhler A. A frequent disease of individual bones in children. *Munch Med Wochenschr*. 1908;55:1923–1925.
2. Santos L, Estanqueiro P, Matos G, et al. Köhler disease: an infrequent or underdiagnosed cause of a child's limping? *Acta Reumatol Port*. 2015;40(3):304–305.
3. Alhamdani M, Kelly C. Kohler's disease presenting as acute foot injury. *Am J Emerg Med*. 2017;35(11):1787.e5–1787.e6.
4. Khoury J, Jerushalmi J, Loberant N, et al. Kohler disease: diagnoses and assessment by bone scintigraphy. *Clin Nucl Med*. 2007;32(3):179–181.
5. Ippolito E, Ricciardi Pollini PT, Falez' F. Köhler's disease of the tarsal navicular: long-term follow-up of 12 cases. *J Pediatr Orthop*. 1984;4(4):416–417.

ADDITIONAL READING

- Borges JL, Guille JT, Bowen JR. Köhler's bone disease of the tarsal navicular. *J Pediatr Orthop*. 1995;15(5):596–598.
- Gips S, Ruchman RB, Groshar D. Bone imaging in Kohler's disease. *Clin Nucl Med*. 1997;22(9):636–637.
- Manusov EG, Lillegard WA, Raspa RF, et al. Evaluation of pediatric foot problems: part I. The forefoot and the midfoot. *Am Fam Physician*. 1996;54(2):592–606.
- Sharp RJ, Calder JD, Saxby TS. Osteochondritis of the navicular: a case report. *Foot Ankle Int*. 2003;24(6):509–513.
- Stanton BK, Karlin JM, Scurran BL. Köhler's disease. *J Am Podiatr Med Assoc*. 1992;82(12):625–629.
- Williams GA, Cowell HR. Köhler's disease of the tarsal navicular. *Clin Orthop Relat Res*. 1981;(158):53–58.

CLINICAL PEARLS

- Although all patients eventually will have complete resolution of symptoms, immobilization with a cast for at least 8 wk shortens the duration of symptoms by ~1 yr.
- Sports may be resumed once symptoms have resolved.
- Long-term follow-up studies have found no increase in the rate of arthritis or other chronic foot problems in adults who had Köhler disease during childhood.

K

KYPHOSIS

Joseph Medellin, MD, MPH, MBA • Mark E. Lavallee, MD, CSCS, FACSM

BASICS

DESCRIPTION

- Kyphosis is a fixed exaggerated anteroposterior (AP) curvature of the thoracic spine.
- Scoliosis is a fixed lateral curvature of the spine (>10 degrees by Cobb angle) and vertebral rotation.
- Lordosis is a fixed concave exaggerated AP curvature of the lumbar spine.
- Kyphoscoliosis is a combination of lateral and AP curvatures of the spine.
- Scheuermann juvenile kyphosis is osteochondrosis of the secondary ossification center of a vertebrae causing thoracic kyphosis.
- Synonym(s): curvature of the spine; hunchback; dowager's hump; postural round back

EPIDEMIOLOGY

- Most commonly seen in postmenopausal women who have osteoporosis
- Rare occurrence in skeletally maturing patients; occasionally seen in adolescents as they transition through their secondary growth spurt
- Females > males
- Kyphosis has an incidence of 1 in 1,000, whereas scoliosis is about 2 in 100.
- Scheuermann juvenile kyphosis has been reported to be between 0.4% and 10% between ages 13 and 17 yr.

ETIOLOGY AND PATHOPHYSIOLOGY

Genetics

In 2007, CHD7 was identified as the first gene with polymorphisms associated with susceptibility to scoliosis. No consistent genetic loci have been associated purely with kyphosis (1).

RISK FACTORS

- Female gender and remaining growth potential
- Family history is the primary risk. Inheritance patterns are still being actively elucidated.
- Myelodysplasia, Marfan syndrome, Ehlers-Danlos syndrome, osteogenesis imperfecta type 2, and achondroplasia have all been associated with kyphosis and/or scoliosis.

COMMONLY ASSOCIATED CONDITIONS

- Osteoporosis
- Vertebral fracture
- Scoliosis
- Scheuermann juvenile kyphosis
- Marfan syndrome
- Ehlers-Danlos syndrome
- Osteogenesis imperfecta type 2
- Neurofibromatosis

DIAGNOSIS

HISTORY

- Upper back curvature, often painless
- Often noticed by an observer, such as a parent, partner, or spouse
- Cases of nonpainful, nontraumatic kyphosis are often discovered in school-based screenings, preparticipation examinations, or general wellness exams.
- A family history of kyphosis, scoliosis, connective tissue disorder, or neurologic disorder should be sought.

PHYSICAL EXAM

- Subtle findings, such as noticeable "hump" on back and/or hyperlordosis in lumbar spine (a.k.a. "swayback")
- Pain is not often a feature for idiopathic kyphosis, but if present, other causes of kyphosis need to be ruled out.
- Check posture, leg-length discrepancy, muscle tone, and abdominal reflexes.
- A complete neuro-orthopedic exam (i.e., cavus feet seen in Charcot-Marie-Tooth syndrome)
- Assess patient's ability to "correct" deformity with attempted thoracic hyperextension. Postural round back will improve, whereas true kyphosis will have minimal improvement.
- Marfanoid body habitus, hypermobile joints, or hyperextensible skin (i.e., Marfan or Ehlers-Danlos syndrome)
- Café-au-lait spots (i.e., neurofibromatosis)
- Adam forward bending test (to look for associated scoliosis): Patient stands with legs locked, bends at the waist, and arms toward feet. Examiner stands behind patient, lowers head, and views across patient's back, looking for elevated and rotated vertebral segments.
- A scoliometer may also be used to assess if patient has scoliosis. Measure the angle of trunk rotation (ATR). An ATR of 7 degrees or greater correlates (83% sensitivity, 86% specificity) to a clinically significant curve. The ATR multiplied by three estimates the curvature (Cobb angle).

DIFFERENTIAL DIAGNOSIS

- Congenital kyphosis: anomalies of vertebral segmentation and/or formation (Klippel-Feil syndrome, VACTERL [vertebral defects, anal atresia, cardiac defects, tracheo-esophageal fistula, renal anomalies, and limb abnormalities] syndrome)
- Neuromuscular scoliosis: upper motor neuron (Friedreich ataxia, cerebral palsy, Charcot-Marie-Tooth syndrome, syringomyelia, muscular dystrophy) or lower motor neuron (poliomyelitis, spina bifida), spinal dysraphism (myelomeningocele)
- Scheuermann juvenile kyphosis: pathognomonic Schmorl nodes on at least two consecutive levels
- Kyphosis secondary to bone demineralization (osteoporosis)
- Vertebral fractures/trauma
- Benign or malignant tumors (i.e., Paget disease of bone)
- Parkinson disease: "stooping posture"
- Spinal tuberculosis
- Rickets
- Marfan syndrome
- Osteogenesis imperfecta type 2
- Achondroplasia
- Ehlers-Danlos syndrome, especially kyphoscoliotic type
- Ankylosing spondylitis

DIAGNOSTIC TESTS & INTERPRETATION

- Kyphosis: AP/lateral chest x-ray is usually the first imaging test. Able to assess for degenerative joint disease, fractures, Schmorl nodes, angle of kyphosis. Secondary or more complete view is a lateral standing radiograph of entire spine. Look for Schmorl nodes (protrusions of intervertebral disc cartilage through vertebral body end plate of adjacent vertebra that are pathognomonic for Scheuermann).
- If scoliosis is associated with kyphosis: standing posteroanterior and lateral radiographs of the entire spine. Pelvis is analyzed to determine Risser score.
- In children and adolescents, make sure with radiographs to image the iliac crests, including the iliac epiphyses to help with the Risser scoring.
- Indications for magnetic resonance imaging (MRI):
  - Age <10 yr
  - Rapid progression of a curve
  - Abnormal neurologic examination
  - Atypical pain with inconclusive radiograph

TREATMENT

- Management options include observation, bracing, physical therapy, oral medicine (osteoporosis), and surgical invention (in rare cases).
- Idiopathic kyphosis in adolescence and Scheuermann kyphosis rarely need surgical intervention.
- Treatment of painful kyphosis is first to determine cause.
- <50 degrees in young adolescents without evidence of progression may be observed. Strengthening and stretching of abdominals, hamstrings, and paraspinal muscles are recommended to prevent excessive lordosis and hamstring contractures.
- Painful curves between 50 and 70 degrees or progressive deformity >65 degrees may be braced (many associated with Scheuermann) with a Rigo-Cheneau de rotational brace, thoracic lumbar sacral orthosis (TLSO) zero-degree brace, or a Milwaukee brace.
- Literature supports surgical correction indicated at >75 degrees with Scheuermann kyphosis and 60 degrees for congenital kyphosis.
- Observation:
  - Juveniles/adolescents with moderate curves of <60 degrees: Manage by following with serial radiographs every 4 to 6 mo, depending on skeletal maturity (Risser score; see "Scoliosis" chapter).
  - Skeletally mature with curves <40 degrees: Follow with history, physical exam, and occasional radiograph.

- Check bone densitometry (dual energy x-ray absorptiometry) on patient with nontraumatic vertebral fracture and those with osteoporosis. Treatment of osteoporosis with bisphosphonates has been shown to improve kyphosis-related back pain. *Do not use bisphosphonates in women of reproductive age due to potential long-term teratogenic effects.*
  - Standing lateral radiographs of whole spine every 6 mo
- Brace:
  - Immature with curve >60 degrees or in those who progresses >10 degrees during observation to a curve >40 degrees
  - Bracing options include:
    - Milwaukee brace (for curves above T7).
    - TLSO with an underarm rigid brace (if curve is below T7).
    - Wood-Cheneau-Rigo de rotational brace.
  - Once the curve is supported, the patient should wear the brace 20 hr/day. The brace use may be tapered to nighttime use once the progression of the curve is controlled.
  - Goal is to delay/prevent curve progression until skeletally mature.
  - Contraindication to bracing: curves >80 degrees, extreme thoracic hypokyphosis, high thoracic or cervical curves
  - Standing radiograph images every 6 mo (or 4 mo if progressing and skeletally immature)
- Surgery:
  - Wedge osteotomies of the posterior aspect of the vertebrae have been done to correct those with severe kyphosis in skeletally mature patients without osteoporosis.
  - Vertebroplasty and balloon kyphoplasty are procedures available to patients who develop kyphosis related to osteoporosis or trauma-related collapse of thoracic vertebral body.
  - Once a curve reaches 80 degrees, it is assumed it is not controlled by bracing; operative correction with posterior instrumentation/fusion is recommended.
  - Upper thoracic kyphosis with curves >100 degrees causes significant restrictive lung disease.
- Some clinicians advocate following juvenile patients with exaggerated kyphotic curves of >40 degrees at 4- to 6-mo intervals until iliac crest growth plates close (2).

ADDITIONAL THERAPIES

- Postural "round back," not true kyphosis, has been shown to improve with physical therapy focused on postural control and core/shoulder girdle strengthening.
- Bracing in juvenile/adolescent patients should be continued as long as there is no progression of curvature and vertical growth is still occurring. In young women, this means a Risser stage of at least 3, whereas in young men, a Risser stage of 4.

ONGOING CARE

FOLLOW-UP RECOMMENDATIONS

- Refer to orthopedic/spine specialist when there is a:
  - Nonbraceable curve of the thoracic spine (apex of curve higher than T6).
  - Worsening curvature despite bracing.
  - Curvature in the newborn and infant and any children <10 yr old.
  - Curvature associated with severe trauma/vertebral fracture.
  - Curvature-associated malignancy.
- Juvenile/adolescent kyphosis is often diagnosed or progresses during a sensitive time of life. Studies have demonstrated a negative effect on body image, self-esteem, and attitude with treatment. This may affect compliance. Treatment is time-consuming, confining, and can be uncomfortable. The adolescent is faced with many lifestyle changes. Providers should be aware of the possible psychological impact from new demands on the patient and family. Discussions about patient's thoughts/feelings on treatment as well as support groups should be considered (3,4).

REFERENCES

1. Palazzo C, Sailhan F, Revel M. Scheuermann's disease: an update. *Joint Bone Spine*. 2014;81(3):209–214.
2. Weinstein SL, Dolan LA, Wright JG, et al. Effects of bracing in adolescents with idiopathic scoliosis. *N Engl J Med*. 2013;369(16):1512–1521.
3. Bezalel T, Kalichman L. Improvement of clinical and radiographical presentation of Scheuermann disease after Schroth therapy treatment. *J Bodyw Mov Ther*. 2015;19(2):232–237.
4. Reichel D, Schanz J. Developmental psychological aspects of scoliosis treatment. *Pediatr Rehabil*. 2003;6(3–4):221–225.

ADDITIONAL READING

- Dobbs MB, Weinstein SL. Infantile and juvenile scoliosis. *Orthop Clin North Am*. 1999;30(3):331–341.
- Dolan LA, Haggerty KA, Weinstein SL, et al. Evaluation of TLSOS in the bracing in adolescent idiopathic scoliosis trial (BrAIST). *Scoliosis*. 2013;8(Suppl 1):O48.
- Ferrell MC. The spine in swimming. *Clin Sports Med*. 1999;18(2):389–393.
- Grossman DC, Curry SJ, Owens DK, et al; for US Preventive Services Task Force. Screening for adolescent idiopathic scoliosis: US Preventive Services Task Force recommendation statement. *JAMA*. 2018;319(2):165–172.
- Gao X, Gordon D, Zhang D, et al. CHD7 gene polymorphisms are associated with susceptibility to idiopathic scoliosis. *Am J Hum Genet*. 2007;80(5):957–965.
- Hawes MC. The use of exercises in the treatment of scoliosis: an evidence-based critical review of the literature. *Pediatr Rehabil*. 2003;6(3–4):171–182.
- Hresko MT, Talwalkar VR, Schwend RM. Position statement—screening for the early detection for idiopathic scoliosis in adolescents: SRS/POSNA/AAOS/AAP position statement. https://www.srs.org/about-srs/news-and-announcements/position-statement–screening-for-the-early-detection-for-idiopathic-scoliosis-in-adolescents. Published September 2, 2015. Accessed March 19, 2018.
- Jarvis J, Garbedian S, Swamy G. Juvenile idiopathic scoliosis: the effectiveness of part-time bracing. *Spine (Phila Pa 1976)*. 2008;33(10):1074–1078.
- Marks DS, Qaimkhani SA. The natural history of congenital scoliosis and kyphosis. *Spine (Phila Pa 1976)*. 2009;34(17):1751–1755.
- Miller NH. Cause and natural history of adolescent idiopathic scoliosis. *Orthop Clin North Am*. 1999;30(3):343–352.
- Negrini S, Fusco C, Minozzi S, et al. Exercises reduce the progression rate of adolescent idiopathic scoliosis: results of a comprehensive systematic review of the literature. *Disabil Rehabil*. 2008;30(10):772–785.
- Roach JW. Adolescent idiopathic scoliosis. *Orthop Clin North Am*. 1999;30(3):353–365.
- Schiller JR, Eberson CP. Spinal deformity and athletics. *Sports Med Arthrosc Rev*. 2008;16(1):26–31.
- Staheli LT. *Fundamentals of Pediatric Orthopedics*. 5th ed. Philadelphia, PA: Lippincott Williams & Wilkins; 2016.
- Staheli LT, Song K. Spine and Pelvis. In: *Practice of Pediatric Orthopedics*. 2nd ed. Philadelphia, PA: Lippincott Williams & Wilkins; 2006:220–224.
- Wood KB. Spinal deformity in the adolescent athlete. *Clin Sports Med*. 2002;21(1):77–92.

CLINICAL PEARLS

- Sports and athletic activity are allowed and encouraged for all patients with nonpainful kyphosis in nonoperative treatment.
- Postoperative patients' return to play is at the discretion of the surgeon.
- Braces are used to prevent progression and are not intended to correct the curve. Compliance is essential to treatment success.
- Most studies support results with brace wear of 18 to 20 hr/day. Night-only braces have also been shown to have success.
- Braces for juvenile/adolescent patients should be worn until the Risser score is 4 (closed growth plates).
- Manipulation therapy has not been proven to help correct curvature of the spine.

LACERATIONS AND SOFT TISSUE INJURIES IN ATHLETES

Ross Osborn, MD, FAAFP, CAQSM

BASICS

DESCRIPTION

- Lacerations, contusions, hematomas, and abrasions are disruptions to the skin resulting from trauma.
- Soft tissue injuries include:
  - Friction blisters—pressure and shear forces causing delamination of the stratum spinosum.
  - Chafing —repetitive friction of the skin without separation of dermis from epidermis.
  - Hematomas—blunt trauma to the skin and underlying structures, causing extravasation of blood into surrounding soft tissue.
  - Abrasions—superficial skin wounds caused by tangential friction, involving stripping of the epidermis from the underlying dermis.
  - Lacerations—full-thickness skin wounds involving the epidermis and dermis and may occur with injury to connective tissue, cutaneous nerves, and vasculature.
  - Seromas—a collection of clear serous fluid that develops after surgery.
- Soft tissue injuries can occur on any part of the body:
  - Blisters generally occur at sites where the skin encounters repetitive friction.
  - Chafing most commonly occurs in areas of skin-to-skin contact (i.e., groin, axilla) or where clothes rub (i.e., "jogger's nipple").
  - Abrasions most commonly occur on the knees and elbows.
  - Lacerations most often occur on the head and neck (50%) or upper extremities (35%).

EPIDEMIOLOGY

11 million lacerations are treated in emergency departments, but this number doesn't include those injuries treated in an office or on the sideline.

ETIOLOGY AND PATHOPHYSIOLOGY

- Hematomas, lacerations, and abrasions are most commonly caused by blunt trauma.
- Lacerations caused by sharp objects are common and usually involve the equipment used for the sport (i.e., shoe spikes, sticks, skates).

Pediatric Considerations

Any nonaccidental trauma in a child should raise the suspicion for abuse.

RISK FACTORS

- Most common preventable cause of skin trauma is improper equipment use or lack of use.
- Risk factors for friction blisters include moisture, temperature, external load, activity duration, characteristics of footwear, and adaptation and/or conditioning (1).

COMMONLY ASSOCIATED CONDITIONS

Associated symptoms can include:

- Bleeding.
- Foreign body.
- Paresthesia.
- Loss of motor function.
- Diminished vascularization.

DIAGNOSIS

- First and foremost, observe standard universal precautions; assess airway, breathing, and circulation (ABCs); and control bleeding as initial steps.
- Determine the time, mechanism, and circumstances of injury.
- Obtain history to determine the potential for foreign body presence.
- Evaluate nerve and motor function as well as possibility of underlying fracture.
- Assess presence of devitalized tissue.
- Obtain medical history for comorbid conditions that may impede wound healing.

HISTORY

- Estimate the amount of blood loss.
- Assess tendon, muscle, or nerve injury:
  - Complaints of weakness, numbness, or tingling
  - Local sensory nerve/peripheral nerve function should be assessed by two-point discrimination prior to administration of anesthetic.
- Medication history:
  - Aspirin, nonsteroidal anti-inflammatory drugs (NSAIDs), clopidogrel, Coumadin (warfarin), or other blood-thinning medications and/or supplements
- Allergies:
  - Latex, lidocaine, iodine, or pain medications
- Immunization status:
  - Assess if tetanus status is up-to-date.
- In minors, parental consent should be obtained prior to procedure if possible.
- Have a consent form in sideline bag.

PHYSICAL EXAM

- Vitals:
  - Blood pressure (BP) and pulse should be assessed for hemodynamic stability.
- General:
  - Pallorous, ashen, or faint (hemodynamic vs. vagal)
- Cardiovascular:
  - Peripheral pulses distal to the site of injury:
    - Decreased or absent pulses should initiate prompt referral.
  - Capillary refill
- Pulmonary:
  - Assess ease of respiration after chest wall trauma.
  - Adequate and equal breath sounds:
    - Unequal breath sounds necessitate further evaluation for pneumothorax.
- Head/eyes/ears/nose/throat:
  - Cranial nerve assessment in cases of trauma to the head
  - Assess for concussion.
- Musculoskeletal:
  - Deformities or concerns for fracture under an open wound should prompt referral.
- Neurologic:
  - Sensory exam distal to site of injury to evaluate underlying nerve damage
- Skin:
  - Patients with thin skin may require adapting the repair modality.
- Psychological:
  - Psychomotor agitation may make following universal precautions more challenging.
  - May also signify underlying head trauma

DIFFERENTIAL DIAGNOSIS

- Skin avulsion
- Contusion
- Abrasion
- Laceration
- Hematoma
- Seroma
- Rash/dermatitis

DIAGNOSTIC TESTS & INTERPRETATION

- Radiographs:
  - For concerns of underlying fracture
  - Plain radiography may help to identify some foreign bodies.
- Ultrasound (US) is emerging as a useful tool in the imaging of suspected foreign bodies:
  - A few small clinical studies show increasing reliability in the detection of foreign bodies (2).
  - The portable US units make them a readily available imaging modality.
  - US is useful to identify foreign bodies with the same density as soft tissue (e.g., splinters).

TREATMENT

- Initial stabilization:
  - Manage ABCs.
  - Ensure hemostasis prior to further evaluation, treatment, or repair.
- Initial examination:
  - Explore wound for foreign body.
  - Remove devitalized tissue.
  - Assess injury to underlying structures.
- Irrigation and preparation:
  - Clean surrounding skin with soap and water if superficial or copious irrigation.
  - Employ appropriate universal precautions.
  - Remove foreign bodies or contaminants in wound:
    - A fine-pore sponge may be used in cases of contamination or fine particulate matter.
    - Indications for removal of a foreign body include potential or actual injury to tendons, nerves, and vasculature; toxic substance or reactive agent; and source of pain.
    - Retained foreign bodies in abrasions may result in "tattooing" of the skin.
  - Irrigate wound with clean tap water:
    - This has been found to be superior for irrigation (3)[A].
    - A "rule of thumb" is to use 50 to 100 mL of irrigant per centimeter of laceration (3).
  - Débride devitalized tissue and revise wound edges if necessary to achieve a good closure.
  - Clip hair near the wound, but avoid shaving because it may introduce bacteria into the wound.
  - Friction blisters:
    - Larger blisters can be drained to prevent expansion or epidermal "roof" intact to act as a biologic dressing (4).
    - Blisters <1 cm can be left intact and covered with a protective dressing (4).
- Time to treatment:
  - Blisters, chafing, and abrasions can be treated immediately, and the athlete can return to play:
    - Blister treatment with fixation dressings is inferior to adhesive tape for treatment (5).
  - Lacerations may heal by primary closure, delayed primary closure, or secondary intention:
    - Close all "clean" wounds primarily, except puncture wounds not able to be adequately irrigated.
    - Wounds presenting for treatment after a delay, contaminated wounds, and noncosmetic animal bites should be irrigated, débrided, and have bleeding controlled.
    - Can perform delayed primary closure after 3 to 5 days to allow the patient's immune system to decrease the bacterial load. The lowest load occurs 96 hr after the initial injury (5).
    - Secondary closure is allowing a wound to heal by granulation. This is appropriate for partial-thickness avulsions, contaminated small wounds, and infected wounds (5).

- Analgesia:
  - Topical anesthesia:
    - Can be useful to treat abrasions, chafing, and blisters as well as to further evaluate skin lacerations (6)
    - Options include 1% or 2% lidocaine jelly, LET (4% lidocaine, 0.1225% epinephrine, and 0.5% tetracaine), EMLA (eutectic mixture of local anesthetics: 2.5% lidocaine and 2.5% prilocaine), or LMX (formerly known as ELA-Max-liposomal lidocaine) (5).
  - Local or regional anesthesia:
    - Preferred type of anesthesia for lacerations: Amide agents (lidocaine and bupivacaine) and ester agents (procaine) are the two basic types.
    - Allergy to one group is not associated with allergy to anesthetic from the other group.
    - Most allergies are caused by the preservatives used in the anesthetic, so a pure agent, such as cardiac lidocaine, could be used as an alternative.
    - Intradermal diphenhydramine can be used for those patients allergic to the above anesthetics (3).
    - Epinephrine will improve the duration of injected anesthetics (4) and will promote vasoconstriction:
      - Local anesthetic with epinephrine (up to 1:100,000) is safe for repair of the digits, including digital block (3)[B].
    - Patient comfort can be increased by using a smaller gauge needle to inject, injecting subcutaneously through the open wound, using a slower injection rate, and with the addition of sodium bicarbonate to the anesthetic (1:10 of total volume injected) (5).
- Sterility:
  - Using clean, nonsterile versus sterile exam gloves does not increase the risk of infection (3)[B].
- Modalities for closure:
  - Laceration location determines the type of material used for closure due to differences in skin tension.
  - Materials include surgical tapes, skin adhesives, staples, and sutures:
    - Surgical tape: Advantages: rapid application, patient comfort, lower infection rates, least tissue reactivity, and low cost. Disadvantages: can't apply to areas with hair, must remain dry, highest dehiscence rates, and low tensile strength. Application: Use benzoin tincture, apply only to dry skin edges, and ensure adequate approximation of skin edges.
    - Skin adhesives: Advantages: rapid application, resists bacterial growth, no need for removal, no anesthesia needed, good cosmetic results, and excellent for children. Disadvantages: not adequate for moderate or heavy tension areas of the skin. Application: Apply on to dry skin edges, approximate skin edges.
    - Staples: Advantages: rapid application, low tissue reactivity, low cost, and can be used in areas with a lot of hair. Disadvantages: inability to provide a meticulous closure, interference with imaging (computed tomography [CT] or magnetic resonance imaging [MRI]), and removal required. Application: Sterilize area, anesthesia, and roughly approximate edges.
    - Sutures: Advantages: meticulous closure, most tensile strength, and lowest dehiscence rate. Disadvantages: anesthesia required, slow application, most tissue reaction, and removal required. Application: Determine single or multiple layer closure, remove foreign material or devitalized tissue, and create sterile field.
- Skin closure:
  - Suture choice:
    - Use the smallest suture that provides adequate strength for reapproximation.
    - There is no significant difference in cosmetic outcome, infection rate, or wound dehiscence between absorbable and nonabsorbable suture (3).
    - There is no advantage to braided over monofilament sutures with regard to cosmesis, infection rate, or dehiscence (3):
      - Single versus multiple layer closure:
        - Single layer—performed with staples, adhesives, surgical tape, or sutures depending on location of laceration
        - Multiple layer closure—closes deep tissue dead space; lessens tension at the epidermal level, improving the cosmetic result; absorbable suture should be used to close subcutaneous (SC) tissue.
- Wound dressing:
  - Blisters: should be covered with protective membrane or dressing, or a semipermeable membrane, or hydrocolloidal dressing if draining:
    - Treatment with adhesive tape is superior to fixation dressing with regard to healing time, pain scores, infection rates, and need for additional medical treatment (5).
  - Abrasions can be covered by a nonstick dressing, such as Telfa or Adaptic, then covered by an absorbent gauze dressing:
    - Alternative dressings include Tegaderm, zinc oxide–impregnated gauze, and occlusive hydrocolloidal dressings such as DuoDERM.
  - Hematomas can be covered by a pad or padded dressing for comfort if the athlete is able to return to play.

- Lacerations should be covered with a sterile gauze or nonadherent pad until the stitches or staples are removed:
  - Uncovering wounds for routine bathing within the first 12 hr does not increase risk of infection (5).
  - Occlusive and semiocclusive dressing lead to faster wound healing, decreased wound contamination, decreased infection rates, and increased comfort compared to dry gauze dressings (5).

MEDICATION

- Antibiotics:
  - Uncomplicated lacerations, abrasions, blisters, and chafing do not require systemic antibiotics:
    - A meta-analysis did not show benefit to prophylactic oral antibiotics for reducing wound infection in simple, nonbite wounds (5).
  - Open fractures, exposed tendon injuries, or exposed joint injuries typically require systemic antibiotics:
    - Ointments containing neomycin and bacitracin have shown to have lower rates of infection (3).
- Tetanus prophylaxis guidelines should be followed (4).

ADMISSION, INPATIENT, AND NURSING CONSIDERATIONS

Admission criteria (6):

- Soft tissue injuries require hospitalization for:
  - Grossly contaminated wounds or wounds requiring extensive débridement.
  - Open fractures.
  - Hemodynamically unstable patient.
  - Neurovascular compromise.
  - Comorbid conditions such as a head injury or abdominal trauma.
  - Wounds requiring ongoing intravenous (IV) antibiotics.
- Eyelid lacerations should prompt a referral to an ophthalmologist.

ONGOING CARE

FOLLOW-UP RECOMMENDATIONS

Suture removal (3)

Wound Location	Timing (Days)
Face	3–5
Scalp	7–10
Arms	7–10
Trunk	10–14
Legs	10–14
Hands or feet	10–14
Palms or soles	14–21

REFERENCES

1. Worthing RM, Percy RL, Joslin JD. Prevention of friction blisters in outdoor pursuits: a systematic review. *Wilderness Environ Med*. 2017;28(2):139–149.
2. Blankenship RB, Baker T. Imaging modalities in wounds and superficial skin infections. *Emerg Med Clin North Am*. 2007;25(1):223–234.
3. Forsch RT, Little SH, Williams C. Laceration repair: a practical approach. *Am Fam Physician*. 2017;95(10):628–636.
4. Honsik KA, Romeo MW, Hawley CJ, et al. Sideline skin and wound care for acute injuries. *Curr Sports Med Rep*. 2007;6(3):147–154.
5. Janssen L, Allard NAE, Ten Haaf DSM, et al. First-aid treatment for friction blisters: "walking into the right direction?" *Clin J Sport Med*. 2018;28(1):37–42.
6. Cordoro KM, Ganz JE. Training room management of medical conditions: sports dermatology. *Clin Sports Med*. 2005;24(3):565–598.

CLINICAL PEARLS

- Traumatic skin lesions are commonly seen in the athletic arena, and their proper management can facilitate a safe and rapid return to play.
- Proper assessment and preparation will allow the best possible outcome for skin injuries.
- Materials for treatment should be based on the location and type of injury as well as the experience of the treating provider.
- Return-to-play decisions should be based on the ability to treat the injury and dress the wound to limit the exposure of bodily fluids.

LATERAL COLLATERAL LIGAMENT TEAR

David Milo Hirschi III, MD • Brent S.E. Rich, MD, ATC

BASICS

DESCRIPTION

- Partial or complete sprain of the lateral collateral ligament (LCL) owing to an acute force, usually from a medial direction
- Consists of a cordlike fiber bundle that runs from the lateral femoral condyle to the anterolateral aspect of the fibular head about 1 cm anterior to the apex: discrete extracapsular structure
- Primary restraint to varus stress with the knee in extension
- Isometric between 0 and 70 degrees of flexion, followed by slackening trend with deeper flexion (1)

EPIDEMIOLOGY

- Least commonly injured knee ligament; isolated injuries are rare.
- Infrequent site of overuse injury or rupture
- Wrestling is the most likely associated sport.
- May be associated with injury to other ligaments (anterior cruciate ligament [ACL] or posterior cruciate ligament [PCL]) or structures of the posterolateral corner (popliteus tendon, biceps femoris, iliotibial band, popliteofibular ligament) and peroneal nerve injuries (2)

RISK FACTORS

- Unclear if previous LCL injuries predispose to recurrent injury
- Varus knee, otherwise normal, does not seem to be predisposed to LCL injury.
- PCL deficiency may increase risk of LCL injury.

DIAGNOSIS

HISTORY

- Contact or noncontact varus stress to partially flexed knee in internal tibial rotation from direct force or, more rarely, distal indirect stress (e.g., stepping into a hole) with fixed foot
- Acute lateral knee pain
- Many hear/feel an associated "pop."
- LCL is extra-articular; mild to moderate swelling is associated with isolated injury.
- Mild disability with low-grade injury; difficult weight-bearing with high-grade injury/associated injuries owing to pain and instability
- Instability with high-grade or moderate injury
- Check for possible peroneal nerve symptoms.

PHYSICAL EXAM

- Signs and symptoms:
  - Acute lateral knee pain associated with a mechanism of varus stress with knee in flexion of 25 to 30 degrees
  - Patient may feel or hear a "pop" at time of injury.
  - Swelling variable, effusion not common with low-grade injuries; associated ligamentous injuries may cause significant effusion.
  - Instability symptoms in high-grade injury or with associated underlying varus knee
  - Possible peroneal nerve symptoms
- Physical examination:
  - Local swelling over ligament
  - Tender to palpation over ligament
  - Readily palpated in "figure-of-4 position": normally, a pencil-like structure but less distinct with partial tears (grade II) or complete tears (grade III)
  - Varus stress testing: grade I sprain, no increased laxity; grade II sprain, increase in laxity with semifirm endpoint at 25 to 30 degrees of flexion isolates the LCL; grade III sprain, increase in laxity with soft or no endpoint compared with the uninjured knee indicates injury.
  - Special tests:
    - Careful assessment of ACL (Lachman test) and PCL (posterior drawer test), posterolateral structures (external rotation recurvatum test, external rotation roll-out test at 90 and 30 degrees, posterolateral drawer sign), and pivot shift if possible. Grade I injuries may be confused with lateral meniscal tears (3).
  - Peroneal nerve sensory and motor function should be checked as well.

DIFFERENTIAL DIAGNOSIS

- Proximal fibula avulsion fracture
- Biceps femoris strain
- Iliotibial band strain
- Popliteus strain/tear/tendinopathy
- Associated anterior or posterior cruciate injury
- Lateral meniscus tear
- Lateral compartment chondral/osteochondral injury
- Tibial plateau fracture
- Proximal tibiofibular syndesmosis injury
- Associated loose body
- Peroneal nerve injury (4)

DIAGNOSTIC TESTS & INTERPRETATION

- Plain films to rule out occult fracture of tibial plateau, lateral femoral condyle, or fibular head on all patients
- Magnetic resonance imaging (MRI) to better assess integrity of LCL and associated knee structures (ACL, PCL, lateral meniscus, popliteus tendon, posterolateral corner) (3)

TREATMENT

- Acute treatment (3)
- Analgesia:
  - Ice and compression in acute setting
  - Nonsteroidal anti-inflammatory drugs (NSAIDs) until acute pain subsides
  - Narcotics appropriate for 24 to 72 hr for grade II or III injuries or combined ligamentous injuries
- Immobilization:
  - Grade I injury: crutches PRN for pain; hinged bracing (stabilization while allowing range of motion [ROM]), 4 to 5 wk during weight-bearing activities
  - Grade II: crutches and knee immobilizer × 1 to 2 wk for pain control and then progress from non–weight-bearing to partial–weight-bearing weeks 2 to 3. A hinged brace may be used once the patient is partial–weight-bearing, usually at 2 to 3 wks.
  - Grade III: immobilization, non–weight-bearing with crutches, and consultation with an orthopedic surgeon. Immobilization will likely be maintained until surgery is performed, preferably within 2 wk of injury.

ADDITIONAL THERAPIES

- May consider more prolonged immobilization and bracing in varus knee, which is thought to increase stress on the injured ligament. This is somewhat controversial (3,5).
- Functional rehabilitation:
  - In the acute setting, start isometric quadriceps exercises and straight-leg lifts.
  - Electrical stimulation/biofeedback to vastus medialis oblique (VMO) quads
  - Gentle hamstring and calf strengthening in protective ROM
  - ROM exercises with progression to full ROM over 4 to 8 wk to allow ligament to heal without too much stress
  - Stair stepper or similar for cardiovascular (CV) conditioning can be added, limiting knee flexion to 45 to 60 degrees when tolerated.
  - Stationary bike later in rehabilitation when able to flex knee to 115 degrees without pain or residual swelling afterwards
  - When gait is normal, begin jogging and enhanced resistance exercises.
  - Progress to half sprints, full sprints, and cutting maneuvers once ligament fully healed

SURGERY/OTHER PROCEDURES

Surgery is considered for grade III and combined ligamentous injuries.

ONGOING CARE

FOLLOW-UP RECOMMENDATIONS

- Referral to orthopedic surgery for any fracture, associated ligament injury, complex meniscal tear, or grade III injury that is not amenable to the initial 2 to 4 wk of rehabilitation
- Associated neurovascular injuries should be considered emergent, and appropriate surgical/radiographic consultations should be initiated and performed on the same day.

REFERENCES

1. Wilson WT, Deakin AH, Payne AP, et al. Comparative analysis of the structural properties of the collateral ligaments of the human knee. *J Orthop Sports Phys Ther*. 2012;42(4):345–351.
2. Swenson DM, Collins CL, Best TM, et al. Epidemiology of knee injuries among U.S. high school athletes, 2005/2006–2010/2011. *Med Sci Sports Exerc*. 2013;45(3):462–469.
3. Levy BA, Stuart MJ, Whelan DB. Posterolateral instability of the knee: evaluation, treatment, results. *Sports Med Arthrosc Rev*. 2010;18(4):254–262.
4. Kozanek M, Fu EC, Van de Velde SK, et al. Posterolateral structures of the knee in posterior cruciate ligament deficiency. *Am J Sports Med*. 2009;37(3):534–541.
5. Victor J, Wong P, Witvrouw E, et al. How isometric are the medial patellofemoral, superficial medial collateral, and lateral collateral ligaments of the knee? *Am J Sports Med*. 2009;37(10):2028–2036.

ADDITIONAL READING

Duke University. *Wheeless' Textbook of Orthopaedics*. Durham, NC: Duke University; 2012. http://www.wheelessonline.com/ortho/lateral/collateral/ligament.

CLINICAL PEARLS

- Average return to play for grade I injury approximately 4 wk; grade II approximately 10 wk. Return to play is greatly dependent on the type of activity.
- Once healed, there are no data to suggest that the ligament is more predisposed to recurrent injury.

LATERAL EPICONDYLITIS

Bryant Walrod, MD, CAQSM • Craig C. Young, MD

BASICS

DESCRIPTION

- Lateral epicondylitis, or lateral elbow tendinosis, is an overuse injury of the forearm and wrist extensor muscles, which causes pain at the lateral elbow.
- Synonym(s): tennis elbow, common extensor tendinopathy, epicondylalgia

EPIDEMIOLOGY

- Prevalence: 1.3% of general population
- Represents 20% of tennis injuries
- Accounts for ~90% of elbow epicondylitis
- Precipitated by tennis and other activities that require repetitive wrist extension, radial deviation, and forearm supination
- Occurs in dominant arm 75% of the time

RISK FACTORS

- Age 40 to 60 yr
- Smoking, obesity
- Improper equipment (e.g., inappropriate grip size, overstrung racquet, inappropriate-weight racquet)
- Poor technique (e.g., backhand with excessive wrist extension)
- Recreational tennis player
- Playing tennis for >2 hr daily
- Repetitive movement of >2 hr a day

COMMONLY ASSOCIATED CONDITIONS

Posterior interosseous nerve entrapment (radial tunnel syndrome)

DIAGNOSIS

HISTORY

- Pain pattern: Patients typically report an insidious onset, but they will often relate a history of overuse without specific trauma. Pain can vary from mild (e.g., present only with aggravating activities like tennis or the repeated use of a hand tool), or it can be severe (e.g., holding a coffee cup will act as a trigger for the pain).
- Numbness or tingling: Radicular symptoms suggest nerve entrapment or radiculopathy.
- Backhand hitting style: Lateral epicondylitis is much more common in players who hit with a one-handed backhand.
- Improper technique: hitting late in the backhand, improper positioning when striking the ball or insufficient follow-through
- Equipment used, location, and frequency of play: Many cases of lateral epicondylitis are associated with improper equipment, old or wet tennis balls, racquets that are strung too tightly or too heavy, and fast surfaces. Shock-absorbing rubber vibration dampeners have not been shown to reduce risk.
- Poor conditioning: Poor general conditioning leads to fatigue of the core and shoulder muscles, which puts an overemphasis on the extensor muscles of the forearm.
- Scapular dyskinesis and poor rotator cuff control can lead to the development of lateral elbow pain.

PHYSICAL EXAM

- Pain at lateral elbow
- Pain with wrist and forearm movements
- Pain with gripping objects ("coffee cup sign") and shaking hands ("politician's sign")
- Localized tenderness over lateral epicondyle; also pain just distal and anterior to lateral epicondyle ~1 to 2 cm distal to the origin of the extensor carpi radialis brevis
- Tenderness with resisted wrist extension with wrist pronated and radially deviated
- Tenderness with resisted middle finger extension
- Tenderness with resisted supination
- Decreased internal rotation of ipsilateral shoulder causing compensatory excessive wrist flexion
- Scapular dyskinesia

DIFFERENTIAL DIAGNOSIS

- Posterior interosseous nerve entrapment
- Radial tunnel syndrome
- Osteoarthritis
- C7 radiculopathy
- Musculocutaneous nerve entrapment
- Chronic compartment syndrome of anconeus muscle
- Radiocapitellum osteochondritis dissecans (OCD) lesion
- Lateral collateral ligament strain
- Stress fracture
- Humeral fracture

DIAGNOSTIC TESTS & INTERPRETATION

Initial Tests (lab, imaging)

- Not usually needed for initial treatment
- Standard elbow radiography series (anteroposterior and lateral) should be obtained if other potential injuries are suspected (e.g., fracture, tumor, degenerative joint disease) or if injury is not responding to appropriate treatment.
- Up to 25% of cases have associated calcification in extensor aponeurosis; however, presence of these deposits does not affect initial treatment.
- Musculoskeletal (MSK) ultrasound (US) may reveal tendon thickening, calcifications, hypoechoic changes and vascular ingrowth in the tendons.
- Magnetic resonance imaging (MRI) may reveal partial intrasubstance tears and tendinosis; MRI may assist with evaluation of other potential causes of lateral elbow pain like OCD lesions and stress fractures.

Diagnostic Procedures/Other

- A local anesthetic block may lead to symptom resolution and confirmation of the diagnosis.
- Pathologic findings:
  - Microscopic evaluation of the tendons does not show signs of inflammation but rather angiofibroblastic degeneration and collagen disarray.
  - Light microscopy reveals both an excess of fibroblasts and blood vessels that are consistent with neovessels or angiogenesis.
  - The tendons are relatively hypovascular near the tendon insertion. This hypovascularity may predispose the tendon to hypoxic tendon degeneration and has been implicated in the etiology of tendinopathies.
  - These findings support a failed healing response rather than a true inflammatory process.

TREATMENT

- Acute treatment:
  - Ice after activity
  - Relative rest: Limit activities that cause pain.
  - Anti-inflammatory medications: Consider nonsteroidal anti-inflammatory drugs (NSAIDs), either topical or by mouth.
  - Counterforce bracing: can be effective in treating acute symptoms (1)[B]
  - Wrist splints (2)[B]:
    - Use at night may decrease morning symptoms.
  - Taping during activities may be useful (3)[B].
  - Corticosteroid injections have proven effectiveness for short-term relief of symptoms but may not be effective for long-term management of chronic tendinopathies (4,5)[A].
  - Modalities: Consider the use of US, phonophoresis, or iontophoresis. Some studies have shown them to be useful in returning an athlete to activity sooner, but they show no long-term benefit.

- Long-term treatment:
  - Watchful waiting: 83% of patients symptom-free at 1 yr
  - Autologous blood, platelet-rich plasma, prolotherapy, topical nitrates, botulinum toxin have demonstrated effectiveness in small studies (5)[A].
  - Extracorporeal shock wave therapy may provide short-term relief of symptoms but may not be effective for long-term management of chronic tendinopathies (6)[B].
  - Newer interventions include hyaluronic acid, bone marrow aspiration, and direct tenocyte injections (5)[A].
  - US-guided percutaneous tenotomy procedure has been shown to be effective for chronic symptoms.
  - Surgical intervention has been shown to be useful in recalcitrant cases.
  - Physical therapy consisting of forearm stretching and strengthening program with progression to eccentric muscle strengthening of the common extensor tendon

ISSUES FOR REFERRAL

Consider referral for surgical intervention for individuals whose symptoms do not respond to a high-quality nonoperative treatment program for >6 mo.

ADDITIONAL THERAPIES

- Technique modification: lessons from a professional instructor or coach about proper serve and backhand techniques
- Improve ergonomics in the work environment.
- Equipment: Ensure athlete is using properly sized, weighted, and strung racquet.
- Stretching and strengthening: Ensure athlete is on an appropriate conditioning program, preactivity warm-up, and postactivity cool-down programs.
- Evaluate and treat biomechanical risk factors such as scapular dyskinesis and rotator cuff weakness.

REFERENCES

1. Nishizuka T, Iwatsuki K, Kurimoto S, et al. Efficacy of a forearm band in addition to exercises compared with exercises alone for lateral epicondylitis: a multicenter, randomized, controlled trial. *J Orthop Sci*. 2017;22(2):289–294.
2. Najafi M, Arazpour M, Aminian G, et al. Effect of a new hand-forearm splint on grip strength, pain, and function in patients with tennis elbow. *Prosthet Orthot Int*. 2016;40(3):363–368.
3. Dilek B, Batmaz I, Sariyildiz MA, et al. Kinesio taping in patients with lateral epicondylitis. *J Back Musculoskelet Rehabil*. 2016;29(4):853–858.
4. Arirachakaran A, Sukthuayat A, Sisayanarane T, et al. Platelet-rich plasma versus autologous blood versus steroid injection in lateral epicondylitis: systematic review and network meta-analysis. *J Orthop Traumatol*. 2016;17(2):101–112.
5. Krogh TP, Bartels EM, Ellingsen T, et al. Comparative effectiveness of injection therapies in lateral epicondylitis: a systematic review and network meta-analysis of randomized controlled trials. *Am J Sports Med*. 2013;41(6):1435–1446.
6. Yang TH, Huang YC, Lau YC, et al. Efficacy of radial extracorporeal shock wave therapy on lateral epicondylosis, and changes in the common extensor tendon stiffness with pretherapy and posttherapy in real-time sonoelastography: a randomized controlled study. *Am J Phys Med Rehabil*. 2017;96(2):93–100.

ADDITIONAL READING

- Bisset L, Paungmali A, Vicenzino B, et al. A systematic review and meta-analysis of clinical trials on physical interventions for lateral epicondylalgia. *Br J Sports Med*. 2005;39(7):411–422.
- Branson R, Naidu K, du Toit C, et al. Comparison of corticosteroid, autologous blood or sclerosant injections for chronic tennis elbow. *J Sci Med Sport*. 2017;20(6):528–533.
- Chou LC, Liou TH, Kuan YC, et al. Autologous blood injection for treatment of lateral epicondylosis: a meta-analysis of randomized controlled trials. *Phys Ther Sport*. 2016;18:68–73.
- Claessen FMAP, Heesters BA, Chan JJ, et al. A meta-analysis of the effect of corticosteroid injection for enthesopathy of the extensor carpi radialis brevis origin. *J Hand Surg Am*. 2016;41(10):988.e2–998.e2.
- Grewal R, MacDermid JC, Shah P, et al. Functional outcome of arthroscopic extensor carpi radialis brevis tendon release in chronic lateral epicondylitis. *J Hand Surg Am*. 2009;34(5):849–857.
- Mi B, Liu G, Zhou W, et al. Platelet rich plasma versus steroid on lateral epicondylitis: meta-analysis of randomized clinical trials. *Phys Sportsmed*. 2017;45(2):97–104.
- Pattanittum P, Turner T, Green S, et al. Non-steroidal anti-inflammatory drugs (NSAIDs) for treating lateral elbow pain in adults. *Cochrane Database Syst Rev*. 2013;(5):CD003686.
- Petrella RJ, Cogliano A, Decaria J, et al. Management of tennis elbow with sodium hyaluronate periarticular injections. *Sports Med Arthrosc Rehabil Ther Technol*. 2010;2:4.
- Placzek R, Drescher W, Deuretzbacher G, et al. Treatment of chronic radial epicondylitis with botulinum toxin A. A double-blind, placebo-controlled, randomized multicenter study. *J Bone Joint Surg Am*. 2007;89(2):255–260.
- Sims S, Miller K, Elfar J, et al. Non-surgical treatment of lateral epicondylitis: a systematic review of randomized controlled trials. *Hand (N Y)*. 2014;9(4):419–446.
- Sirico F, Ricca F, Di Meglio F, et al. Local corticosteroid versus autologous blood injections in lateral epicondylitis: meta-analysis of randomized controlled trials. *Eur J Phys Rehabil Med*. 2017;53(3):483–491.
- Smidt N, van der Windt DA, Assendelft WJ, et al. Corticosteroid injections, physiotherapy, or a wait-and-see policy for lateral epicondylitis: a randomised controlled trial. *Lancet*. 2002;359(9307):657–662.
- Tarpada S, Morris M, Lian J, et al. Current advances in the treatment of medial and lateral epicondylitis. *J Orthop*. 2018;15(1):107–110.
- Vellilappilly DV, Rai HR, Varghese J, et al. Counterforce orthosis in the management of lateral epicondylitis. *J Ayub Med Coll Abbottabad*. 2017;29(2):328–334.

CLINICAL PEARLS

- The lateral elbow serves as the origin of the forearm supination and wrist extensor muscles, and thus, elbow pain may result from repetitive use.
- Histologic biopsies of chronic lateral epicondylitis reveal no inflammation but rather signs of poor and disordered healing, a term called *angiofibroblastic degeneration*. Chronic lateral epicondylosis is not an inflammatory condition. Consider other treatments such as physical therapy and proinflammatory modalities in this case.
- Equipment modifications: appropriate racquet grip size; decrease racquet string tension; use only new, dry tennis balls; play on grass court if available.

LEGG-CALVÉ-PERTHES DISEASE

Christopher McGrew, MD, FACSM, CAQSM

BASICS

DESCRIPTION

- Juvenile idiopathic avascular necrosis of the capital femoral epiphysis of the femoral head
- Synonym(s): Perthes disease; aseptic necrosis of the femoral head; osteochondritis deformans juvenilis; osteonecrosis of capital femoral epiphysis of the femoral head

EPIDEMIOLOGY

- Incidence in general population 1/1,200 to 1/12,000
- Prevalence 75/100,000 person-years
- Predominant age: affects children 3 to 12 yr of age but is most common between the ages of 4 and 9 yr; median age 7 yr
- Predominant gender: male > female (4 to 5:1)
- Most prevalent among whites and Chinese; rare in blacks and Native Americans
- Bilateral hip involvement in 15–20% of patients

ETIOLOGY AND PATHOPHYSIOLOGY

Etiology of Legg-Calvé-Perthes disease (LCPD) is unclear, but the following has been proposed as a theoretical sequence of events (1):

- Blood supply to the capital femoral epiphysis is interrupted.
- Bone infarction occurs, especially in the subchondral cortical bone, whereas the articular cartilage continues to grow (articular cartilage receives its nutrients from synovial fluid).
- Revascularization occurs, and new bone ossification starts. At this point, a percentage of patients develop LCPD, whereas others have normal bone growth and development.
- LCPD is present when a subchondral fracture occurs. This is the result of normal physical activity, not direct trauma to the area.
- Changes to the epiphyseal growth plate occur secondary to the subchondral fracture.

RISK FACTORS

- Low birth weight
- Short stature
- Delayed bone maturation
- Involved family member (after index sibling, incidence 1/35)
- Familial thrombophilia and hypofibrinolysis (controversial)
- Lower socioeconomic status

DIAGNOSIS

HISTORY

Symptoms of LCPD usually have been present for weeks because the child often does not complain:

- Limp worsened by activity, usually most pronounced at end of day (may be painless)
- Hip or groin pain, which may be referred to the thigh
- Mild or intermittent pain in anterior thigh or knee
- Usually no history of trauma
- Inflammatory synovitis can mimic LCPD but usually resolves in 10 to 14 days.

PHYSICAL EXAM

- Examine the musculoskeletal system with a focus on the pelvis and lower extremities.
- Include range of motion (ROM) testing to evaluate for limited abduction and internal rotation and the presence or absence of hip flexion contracture.
- Evaluate for muscle atrophy of the thigh, calf, and buttocks, which may be seen in long-standing cases.
- Measure for possible leg-length discrepancy, which indicates advanced involvement of the femoral head.
- Evaluate gait. Trendelenburg gait is observed with abductor weakness.
- Perform log roll test of extended leg on examining table; painful and reduced ROM is observed compared with the opposite side.
- Short stature: Children with LCPD often have delayed bone age.

DIFFERENTIAL DIAGNOSIS

- Inflammatory: septic arthritis, osteomyelitis, transient synovitis
- Trauma: fracture
- Neoplasm
- Congenital: limb abnormality
- Developmental: hip dysplasia, slipped capital femoral epiphysis
- Sickle cell anemia, other hemolytic anemias, and hemophilia: osteonecrosis secondary to vascular infarcts
- Gaucher disease: osteonecrosis secondary to cerebroside and infarcts
- Certain genetic mutations (trisomy 21 and Klinefelter syndrome)

DIAGNOSTIC TESTS & INTERPRETATION

- Anteroposterior and frog-leg lateral views of pelvis; can appear normal early in course
- Femoral head appears smaller then opposite head with a widened articular cartilage space.
- With disease progression, a crescent-shaped radiolucent line may be seen in the central portion of the femoral head, especially on the lateral view.
- Fracture, fragmentation, and resorption
- Extent of femoral head involvement determines severity of disease. Radiographic changes can be divided into five distinct stages representing a continuum of the disease process, as follows:
  - Stage 1—cessation of femoral epiphyseal growth
  - Stage 2—subchondral fracture
  - Stage 3—resorption
  - Stage 4—reossification
  - Stage 5—healed or residual stage
- Bone scan and magnetic resonance imaging (MRI) can be used to evaluate and diagnose LCPD before radiographic changes are apparent.
- MRI may also be used to evaluate disease progression and/or resolution over time if radiographs provide inadequate detail.
- Ultrasonography is useful to evaluate the presence of synovitis or effusion.

TREATMENT

GENERAL MEASURES

- The healing process involves revascularization of the femoral head, removal of necrotic bone, and replacement with viable bone. It is a biologic process that requires many months. No current interventions accelerate this process.
- Treatment is controversial; goal is to prevent a prearthrotic deformity and subsequent arthritis.
- Requires individual adaptations and close follow-up
- Treatment courses vary widely among patients.
- Nonsurgical treatment:
  - Treatment may involve simple observation, especially in children <6 yr of age.
  - Analgesia: nonsteroidal anti-inflammatory drugs (NSAIDs) or acetaminophen
  - Activity restriction, crutches or wheelchair for non–weight-bearing, and abduction stretching exercises and occasionally bed rest. Abduction bracing/casting can be used for symptom relief and to hold the femoral head in the acetabulum.
  - Casting/bracing may be discontinued when there is radiographic evidence of subchondral reossification, usually after 12 to 18 mo.

ADDITIONAL THERAPIES

- Both surgical and nonsurgical treatments are aimed at symptom reduction, prevention of capital femoral epiphysis destruction, and attainment of a spherical femoral head at healing.
- Rehabilitation:
  - Formal therapy program is recommended during and after bracing owing to extensive atrophy, contracture, and loss of motion.
  - A home stretching program is encouraged to maintain ROM.

SURGERY/OTHER PROCEDURES

- Goal is containment of femoral head to maintain or restore joint congruence during the period of biologic plasticity, leading to the restoration of a round femoral head.
- Results of surgical containment appear to be better than those of nonsurgical containment (orthosis). Surgical management typically involves either femoral osteotomy to redirect the involved portion within the acetabulum or innominate osteotomy. The two procedures yield equivalent results, but femoral osteotomy may cause shortening of the limb, leading to a chronic limp (2).
- Techniques vary depending on age of child and severity of femoral head involvement.
- Advantages include less time required in a brace and earlier return to activity.
- Disadvantages include necessity of two operations.

ONGOING CARE

FOLLOW-UP RECOMMENDATIONS

All patients with suspected LCPD should be referred to a pediatric orthopedic surgeon promptly.

PROGNOSIS

- The younger the age of onset of LCPD, the better is the prognosis.
- Children >10 yr of age have a very high risk of developing osteoarthritis (3).
- Most patients have a favorable outcome.
- Prognosis is proportional to the degree of radiologic involvement as well as later age of onset, obesity, severely limited ROM, and female sex.

COMPLICATIONS

- Femoral head deformity (i.e., irregular contouring, flattening, or mushrooming of the head and shortening and broadening of the neck) along with flattening of the vertical wall of the acetabulum
- Degenerative joint disease (onset of severe arthritis varies from adolescence to more commonly in geriatric years)

REFERENCES

1. Berthaume MA, Perry DC, Dobson CA, et al. Skeletal immaturity, rostral sparing, and disparate hip morphologies as biomechanical causes for Legg-Calvé-Perthes' disease. *Clin Anat*. 2016;29(6):759–772.
2. Wiig O, Terjesen T, Svenningsen S. Prognostic factors and outcome of treatment in Perthes' disease: a prospective study of 368 patients with five-year follow-up. *J Bone Joint Surg Br*. 2008;90(10):1364–1371.
3. Heesakkers N, van Kempen R, Feith R, et al. The long-term prognosis of Legg-Calvé-Perthes disease: a historical prospective study with a median follow-up of forty one years. *Int Orthop*. 2015;39(5):859–863.

ADDITIONAL READING

- Ibrahim T, Little DG. The pathogenesis and treatment of Legg-Calvé-Perthes disease. *JBJS Rev*. 2016;4(7). doi:10.2106/JBJS.RVW.15.00063.
- Johansson T, Lindblad M, Bladh M, et al. Incidence of Perthes' disease in children born between 1973 and 1993. *Acta Orthop*. 2017;88(1):96–100.
- Leroux J, Abu Amara S, Lechevallier J. Legg-Calvé-Perthes disease. *Orthop Traumatol Surg Res*. 2018;104(Suppl 1):S107–S112.

CLINICAL PEARLS

- Etiology of LCPD is unclear.
- Treatment courses vary widely among patients, and close follow-up is essential.
- Both surgical and nonsurgical treatments are aimed at symptom reduction, prevention of capital femoral epiphysis destruction, and attainment of a spherical femoral head at healing.
- Results of surgical containment appear to be better than those of nonsurgical containment (orthosis) in more advanced cases.

L

LITTLE LEAGUE SHOULDER

Mike LaGrange, MD, FAAFP, CAQSM • Tracy Ray, MD, FACSM, CAQSM

BASICS

DESCRIPTION

- Also known as thrower's shoulder
- Remodeling and deformation of the proximal humeral physis
- Overuse injury from recurrent, excessive torque placed on the growth plate
- Typically seen in overhead athletes, especially adolescent baseball pitchers; results from recurrent, excessive overhead activity
- First described in 1966 as osteochondrosis of the proximal humeral epiphysis and then reported again in 1974 as proximal humeral epiphysiolysis in adolescent baseball players

EPIDEMIOLOGY

- Uncertain exact prevalence due to underreporting of pain with throwing
- Most common in male baseball players between ages of 11 and 16 yr
- Has also been reported in swimming, volleyball, and cricket
- Can occur in any adolescent athlete involved in repetitive overhead rotational activities

ETIOLOGY AND PATHOPHYSIOLOGY

- Unknown exact etiology
- Biomechanical studies have revealed shear stress arising from high torque during late cocking phase is large enough to lead to deformation of the proximal humeral growth plate.

Genetics

No known genetic disposition

RISK FACTORS

The following risk factors are based on expert opinion because no studies have evaluated this to the author's knowledge:

- Year-round pitching without 3 mo of rest from throwing during the course of the year
- Playing in multiple leagues at the same time
- Going over recommended age-specific pitch count for game, season, or year (1)[C]
- Inadequate rest between pitching outings
- Improper throwing mechanics
- Throwing with a fatigued shoulder

GENERAL PREVENTION

Prevented by avoiding excessive, repetitive overhead activities; having adequate rest between outings; and not throwing with shoulder fatigue or pain

DIAGNOSIS

Diagnosis based on history, physical, and classic radiographic findings

HISTORY

- Patients typically complain of pain while throwing or with overhead activity.
- Pain with throwing is typically constant throughout throwing cycle.
- Most commonly presents with pain laterally over the proximal humeral physis but can present with diffuse pain all over shoulder or referred pain to upper arm
- Insidious onset of pain
- Patients may report recent increase in number of pitches thrown or recent change to playing on a larger field.

PHYSICAL EXAM

- Typical physical exam finding is tenderness to palpation over the proximal humeral physis without erythema, increased warmth, or soft tissue swelling.
- Can present with painful range of motion, including pain with abduction or forward flexion >150 degrees
- Can present with decreased strength of the rotator cuff musculature secondary to pain. Most common is reduced strength and pain with resisted external rotation.
- Can have reduced internal rotation of the shoulder due to posterior capsular tightness, but this finding can also be normal in an adolescent overhead athlete and is not pathognomonic for injury

DIFFERENTIAL DIAGNOSIS

- Rotator cuff tendonitis/impingement
- Multidirectional instability
- Labral tear (usually superior labrum anterior posterior [SLAP] tear)
- Salter-Harris type I fracture of the proximal humeral physis
- Biceps tendonitis
- Osteochondral fragment of the glenoid

DIAGNOSTIC TESTS & INTERPRETATION

- Standard x-rays are the diagnostic gold standard.
- Ultrasound can be helpful and can help to document tenderness at the physis.
- Anteroposterior of the affected shoulder in external rotation and internal with comparison films of the unaffected side are standard.
- Typical findings are widening of the affected growth plate, especially on the lateral side of the growth plate.
- May also see osteolysis and cortical irregularity of the bone surrounding the physis
- Although not required for diagnosis, magnetic resonance imaging (MRI) will also show widening of the growth plate on the T1-weighted images with possible extension of signal into the metaphysis on T1 and gradient echo images.

TREATMENT

GENERAL MEASURES

- Treatment consists of rest from throwing and limited use of over-the-counter (OTC) pain medications such as acetaminophen or nonsteroidal anti-inflammatory drugs (NSAIDs) as needed for pain (2)[C].
- Recommend rest from throwing for 3 to 12 mo (3)[C].
- Physical therapy during rest period should focus on rotator cuff strengthening, core muscle strengthening, and improved range of motion at the shoulder.
- Recommended to complete an interval throwing program after finishing physical therapy or 3-mo rest before returning to full activity

MEDICATION

Age-appropriate dose of any NSAID or acetaminophen can be used as needed for pain during initial period of rest.

SURGERY/OTHER PROCEDURES

No surgical correction required

ONGOING CARE

FOLLOW-UP RECOMMENDATIONS

- After 3- to 12-mo rest/physical therapy to reassess exam and give guidance on starting an interval throwing program
- Repeat x-rays are not necessary because it can take up to a year for growth plate to return to normal.

PATIENT EDUCATION

- Patients, parents, and coaches should be educated on age-appropriate pitching recommendations, including pitch counts and age restrictions on throwing specialty pitches.
- Should also stress importance of not throwing with a fatigued arm or painful shoulder because this can lead to future injury

PROGNOSIS

Patients treated with appropriate rest have an excellent long-term prognosis.

COMPLICATIONS

Alteration of throwing mechanics from throwing with pain may lead to other injuries, such as labral tears or injuries to the elbow of the same arm.

REFERENCES

1. Little League. Regular season pitching rules—baseball and softball. https://www.littleleague.org/playing-rules/pitch-count/. Accessed October 17, 2018.
2. Shanley E, Thigpen C. Throwing injuries in the adolescent athlete. *Int J Sports Phys Ther*. 2013;8(5):630–640.
3. Arnold A, Thigpen C, Beattie PF, et al. Overuse physeal injuries in youth athletes. *Sports Health*. 2017;9(2):139–147.

ADDITIONAL READING

DiFiori JP, Benjamin HJ, Brenner JS, et al. Overuse injuries and burnout in youth sports: a position statement from the American Medical Society for Sports Medicine. *Br J Sports Med*. 2014;48(4):287–288.

CLINICAL PEARLS

- An adolescent should never throw with shoulder pain or fatigue.
- Loss of velocity or pitch control during an outing are signs of shoulder fatigue.
- Pain with external rotation and pain along physis can indicate thrower's shoulder.

L

LITTLE LEAGUER'S ELBOW (MEDIAL APOPHYSITIS)

Robert Hosey, MD, FACSM, CAQSM • Andrew Schleihauf, DO, CAQSM

BASICS

DESCRIPTION

- Classic definition: valgus stress lesion of the medial epicondylar physis
- On a continuum with avulsion fracture of the medial epicondyle
- Now, Little League elbow (LLE) used as a catch-all phrase for elbow pain in a young athlete:
  - Medial epicondylar fragmentation and avulsion
  - Lateral pain from osteochondrosis (Panner disease) and osteochondritis dissecans of the capitellum
  - Delayed or accelerated apophyseal growth of the medial epicondyle
  - Delayed closure of the medial epicondylar growth plate
  - Deformation and osteochondritis of the radial head
  - Hypertrophy of the ulna
  - Olecranon apophysitis

EPIDEMIOLOGY

- It has been estimated that 20–40% of 9 to 12 yr baseball players suffer from elbow pain.
- Of the symptomatic elbows, about 67% have pain in the medial elbow.
- Roughly 5% of youth pitchers sustain an elbow or shoulder injury that requires surgery or forces them to leave baseball.

ETIOLOGY AND PATHOPHYSIOLOGY

- There are six distinct secondary centers of ossification in the elbow: capitellum, radius, medial epicondyle, trochlea, olecranon, and lateral epicondyle (CRMTOL).
- The medial epicondyle may arise from more than one ossific nucleus and is commonly the last epiphyseal center to fuse with the humeral shaft. In the normal child, it may fuse as late as 17 yr of age.
- The medial epicondyle is the site of attachment for the flexor muscle origins and the ulnar collateral ligament (UCL).
- LLE is caused by valgus stress forces placed on the elbow during cocking and acceleration phases of throwing.

RISK FACTORS

- Position: shows magnitude of stress (pitcher > catcher > infielder > outfielder)
- Activity level: types of pitches, number of pitches, innings pitched, typical pitching rotation
- Longitudinal study found a 35% increase in elbow pain in players aged 9 to 12 yr who threw >75 pitches a game and a similar increase in pitchers who threw >600 pitches in a season.
- Fatigue: Pitchers who ignore fatigue and continue to pitch are at a >10 times risk of injury.
- Lack of physical conditioning has been associated with LLE.
- Family history of osteochondrosis
- Glenohumeral internal rotation deficit (GIRD) >25 degrees shown to increase shoulder and elbow pathology.

GENERAL PREVENTION

- All pitchers should be taught to incorporate proper form and mechanics.
- Core strengthening and stretching exercises should be implemented, including yearlong general conditioning and proper warm-up.
- The most important factor is monitoring number of competitive pitches in practice and games.
- Current recommendations for 8 to 14 yr olds include a maximum of 50 to 95 pitches per game, 75 to 125 per week, and 1,000 pitches for an entire season.
- The USA Baseball Medical & Safety Advisory Committee recommends pitchers <13 yr old only throw fastballs and changeups.

COMMONLY ASSOCIATED CONDITIONS

- Flexion contracture
- If avulsion fragment is incarcerated in the joint, it can severely damage the articular surface.

DIAGNOSIS

HISTORY

- Age: important because of the different ages at which each growth center appears and/or closes
- Location: Most commonly, pain is located at medial epicondyle; however, sometimes pain presents laterally or posteriorly.
- Duration (pain characteristics): The length of time that the athlete has had pain is usually an indirect measure of the severity of the problem. If the pain occurs during and after throwing as well as when the athlete is throwing, it is an ominous sign.
- Radiation: If pain or numbness radiates into the last two fingers, consider ulnar nerve involvement (neuritis).
- Mechanism (acute vs. chronic): Acute pain in the young athlete in the medial elbow is more consistent with avulsion fracture of the medial epicondyle. In chronic pain, athletes may complain of pulling, popping, giving out, or decreased velocity during throwing; pain accentuated during early and late cocking of throwing motion

PHYSICAL EXAM

- Pain in the medial elbow
- Bilateral comparison of elbow appearance
- Inspection: Note presence of swelling, muscle atrophy/hypertrophy, symmetry, and carrying angle (normal 5 to 10 degrees in males, 10 to 15 degrees in females); ecchymosis is indicative of an avulsion.
- Palpation: medial/lateral epicondyles (point tenderness along medial epicondyle consistent with avulsion fracture), olecranon process, radial head collateral ligaments, ulnar nerve
- Range of motion: flexion/extension (flexion contracture >15 degrees consistent with avulsion fracture); supination/pronation usually normal; assess for UCL stability with valgus stress at 20 to 30 degrees of flexion (1)[C].
- Evaluation of the shoulder to assess for scapular dyskinesia, GIRD, and rotator cuff strength
- Neurologic: Check sensation along the ulnar nerve distribution; check Tinel sign at the cubital tunnel; check interosseous muscle strength in the hand.

DIFFERENTIAL DIAGNOSIS

- Medial epicondylitis
- Avulsion fracture
- UCL sprain/tear
- Osteochondritis dissecans
- Avascular necrosis of the capitellum (may have lateral pain)
- Neoplasms
- Referred pain: neck, shoulder, wrist

DIAGNOSTIC TESTS & INTERPRETATION

- Radiology is indicated if there is decreased range of motion or there is a suspicion of an avulsion fracture. X-ray films are found to be normal up to 85% of the time.
- Anteroposterior/lateral views of elbow
- Appearance of growth centers: CRMTOL:
  - Capitellum: appears at 1 to 2 yr of age
  - Radial epiphysis (3 to 4 yr)
  - Medial epicondyle (medial, 5 to 6 yr)
  - Trochlea (9 to 10 yr)
  - Lateral epicondyle (lateral, >10 yr)
  - Obtain bilateral elbow views if needed for comparison.
- Assess for presence of anterior and especially posterior fat pads.
- Bilateral elbow images to compare medial epicondylar ossification centers
- Assess for displacement of epicondylar fragment (2)[C].
- Magnetic resonance imaging (MRI), computed tomography (CT), or bone scan rarely indicated but may be helpful if athlete fails to show signs of improvement

TREATMENT

- Long-term treatment (3)[C]:
  - Pitch-count guidelines:
    - Most recent guidelines 2016
    - Ages <8 yr (50 pitches per game), 9 to 10 yr (75 pitches), 11 to 12 yr (85 pitches), 13 to 14 yr (95 pitches)
- Acute treatment:
  - Typically 4 to 6 wk of rest:
    - Athletes should work on general conditioning, endurance, and core strengthening exercises.
    - Range of motion exercises, stretches, and strengthening with bands or light dumbbells can be beneficial.
  - Followed by progression of noncompetitive throwing program
  - Ice and nonsteroidal anti-inflammatory drugs (NSAIDs) as needed

ADDITIONAL THERAPIES

- Treatment depends on the amount of displacement of the medial epicondylar physis (4)[C].
- If fragment is minimally displaced (2 to 5 mm):
  - Apply posterior splint until acute symptoms resolve (2 to 3 wk).
  - Gradual active motion
  - Radiologic healing by ~6 wk; at this time, start aggressive active motion.
  - When bony union achieved, allow patient to throw if pain free.
  - Allow return to competitive play when there is normal range of motion/strength/endurance while throwing and having completed throwing program.
- If fragment is displaced >5 mm:
  - Open reduction and internal fixation
  - Two cancellous screws to prevent rotation
  - Allow early gradual active motion.
  - After 6 wk, aggressive rehabilitation program

ONGOING CARE

Closed reduction is associated with pseudoarthrosis, causing pain and instability as well as formation of double epicondylar epiphyses.

REFERENCES

1. Marsh D. Little League elbow: risk factors and prevention strategies. *Strength Cond J*. 2010;32(6):22–37.
2. Wu M, Fallon R, Heyworth BE. Overuse injuries in the pediatric population. *Sports Med Arthrosc Rev*. 2016;24(4):150–158.
3. Leahy I, Schorpion M, Ganley T. Common medial elbow injuries in the adolescent athlete. *J Hand Ther*. 2015;28(2):201–211.
4. Zellner B, May MM. Elbow injuries in the young athlete—an orthopedic perspective. *Pediatr Radiol*. 2013;43(Suppl 1):S129–S134.

ADDITIONAL READING

- Benjamin HJ, Briner WW Jr. Little League elbow. *Clin J Sport Med*. 2005;15(1):37–40.
- Klingele KE, Kocher MS. Little League elbow: valgus overload injury in the paediatric athlete. *Sports Med*. 2002;32(15):1005–1015.
- Osbahr DC, Chalmers PN, Frank JS, et al. Acute, avulsion fractures of the medial epicondyle while throwing in youth baseball players: a variant of Little League elbow. *J Shoulder Elbow Surg*. 2010;19(7):951–957.

CLINICAL PEARLS

- LLE or medial epicondylar apophysitis is the most common elbow injury in childhood and the most common cause of medial elbow pain in young baseball pitchers.
- At present, baseball youth leagues have rules that limit the number of innings per week and length of time between pitching appearances. In addition, specific pitch count recommendations have been published and adopted by the Little League in conjunction with the Major League Baseball (MLB) in a program called Pitch Smart (http://m.mlb.com/pitchsmart/).
- Best prevention is to follow established pitching guidelines set forth by the Little League. An off-season conditioning program, including core and upper body strengthening along with a throwing program, may also be helpful. It is generally recommended to take 4 mo off (at least 2 to 3 consecutive mo) of throwing per year in adolescent athletes. If pain does begin to occur, the player should stop throwing and see a physician.
- The initial rest period is 4 to 6 wk and should include pain-free stretching and range of motion exercises along with core and upper body strengthening. A gradual return to full throwing activity >4 to 6 wk is typical making average return to full competition 8 to 12 wk.

LOW BACK PAIN AND LUMBAR STRAINS

John Kiel, DO, MPH • M. Kyle Smoot, MD

BASICS

DESCRIPTION

- Acute low back pain is pain of <3 mo duration localized below the costal margin but above the inferior gluteal folds with or without leg pain.
- Synonym(s): lumbar strain; lumbar sprain; lumbago; low back syndrome
- Acute pain is felt in the low lumbar, lumbosacral, or sacroiliac region. It may be accompanied by sciatica, pain radiating down the distribution of the sciatic nerve.
- Chronic low back pain is the same unremitting pain that has been present for >3 mo.

EPIDEMIOLOGY

- The total costs of low back pain in the United States exceed $100 billion per year from direct and indirect costs.
- It is the most common musculoskeletal reason for office visits to primary care providers.
- Most common between the ages of 35 and 55 yr
- ~1% of the U.S. population is chronically disabled because of back problems, and another 1% is temporarily disabled.

Incidence

- 90% of people experience low back pain in their lifetime; 5–10% will develop chronic back pain.
- Approximately 9.8% will develop sciatic nerve or radicular back pain.
- Various authors have reported incidences of 16–22% in populations 8 to 14 yr of age.

Prevalence

- Annual prevalence in the U.S. population is 15–20%.
- Increases with age, peaking during the 6th decade of life

RISK FACTORS

- Age
- Activity
- Occupation
- Obesity
- Smoking
- Sedentary lifestyle
- Psychosocial factors
- Poor posture
- Chronic flexion injuries

GENERAL PREVENTION

- Exercise programs, posture training, body mechanics training, and weight loss have been advised.
- U.S. Preventive Services Task Force has concluded that current evidence is not adequate to recommend for or against the routine use of interventions to prevent low back pain in adults.

DIAGNOSIS

HISTORY

- Initial history should focus on the patient's age and pain characteristics (onset, duration, severity, quality, radiation, aggravating factors, alleviating factors).
- Question patient about mechanism of injury and occupation.
- Determine if serious underlying conditions (red flags) are responsible for the back pain: fracture (steroid use, trauma, menopausal status); infection (fever, intravenous [IV] drug use, adenopathy, immunosuppression); cancer (weight loss, adenopathy, previous cancer); cauda equina syndrome (bowel or bladder incontinence, saddle anesthesia, major limb motor weakness).
- Assess psychological and socioeconomic problems.
- The patient should be assessed for the following red flags:
  - Is patient <20 or >55 yr with no prior history of back pain?
  - Known or previous cancer? Assume bone metastasis until otherwise proven.
  - IV drug abuse? Assume spinal abscess if tender.
  - Is pain increased or unrelieved by rest? Is low back pain relieved by bed rest?
  - Is pain associated with fever, chills, or weight loss? Look for infection or tumor.
  - Loss of bowel or bladder control and/or caudal anesthesia? Look for cauda equina syndrome.

PHYSICAL EXAM

- Pain located below the costal margin but above the inferior gluteal folds
- Possible radiation of pain to buttocks and lower extremity
- Pain aggravated by movement and alleviated by rest
- Limited range of motion of the lumbar spine
- Paraspinal muscular spasm is common.
- Assess severity of pain by observing the patient's gait, posture, and demeanor.
- Prior to examining the back, check the temperature, weight, skin, abdomen, pelvis, groin, peripheral pulses, and lymph nodes for pathology that may mimic spinal disease. A rectal exam should be performed to assess sphincter tone.
- With the patient standing, assess stance, spinal curvature, range of motion, heel-walk, toe-walk, and squat. Locate area of maximal pain.
- With patient sitting, assess patellar and Achilles deep tendon reflexes.
- With the patient supine, assess the straight-leg raise and contralateral straight-leg raise, ankle and great toe dorsiflexion, hip range of motion, sacroiliac joint stability, muscle strength testing, and sensory testing.
- With the patient in the prone position, assess buttock symmetry and perform femoral stretch test.
- Pain in low back is exacerbated by movement and is often accompanied by focal muscle spasm in the lumbar extensors.
- Patients prefer to stand in a semiflexed position and move slowly rather than sit motionless on the exam table.
- Walk on heels (L4–L5) and then toes (S1–S2).
- Assess back muscles for uncoordination or guarding (signs for spasm).
- Straight-leg raising and crossed straight-leg raising (can suggest radicular etiology such as acute disc herniation)

DIFFERENTIAL DIAGNOSIS

- Herniated disc
- Musculoskeletal sprains and strains
- Degenerative joint disease
- Posterior facet syndrome
- Spondylolisthesis
- Spinal stenosis
- Osteoporosis
- Ankylosing spondylitis
- Referred pain
- Tumor
- Infection
- Fracture
- Genitourinary
- Gynecologic
- Psychogenic
- 85% mechanical back pain (MBP)
- 5% symptomatic herniated disc
- 4% compression fracture
- 4% spondylolysis/spondylolisthesis
- 2% tumor, infection, rheumatologic disease, or referred pain

DIAGNOSTIC TESTS & INTERPRETATION

- In the absence of red flag symptoms, imaging can usually be delayed until 30 days after the initial assessment. This approach allows 90% of patients to recover spontaneously and avoids unneeded testing and procedures.
- If symptoms persist >30 days, consider plain radiographs, computed tomography (CT) scan, magnetic resonance imaging (MRI), and bone scan.
- If no red flags are identified in the history, then no imaging tests or laboratory tests are indicated.
- If a red flag is identified, then proceed with diagnostic testing as indicated.

TREATMENT

- Natural history of MBP, regardless of treatment: 33% resolve within 1 wk, 70% resolve within 1 mo, and 90–95% resolve within 3 mo.
- Analgesia:
  - Acetaminophen for 2 wk (as effective as nonsteroidal anti-inflammatory drugs [NSAIDs] if given on schedule)
  - NSAIDs provide pain relief and allow early ambulation (caution for renal insufficiency, pregnancy, hypertension [HTN], gastrointestinal [GI] intolerance, history of gastric ulcers or bleeding).
  - Short-term tramadol on a schedule basis (50 mg TID)
  - Opioids have low-to-moderate evidence of short-term efficacy in chronic low back pain. The efficacy and safety of long-term use remains unproven (1). Caution should be taken before initiating opioids for chronic back pain given risk of dependence and abuse.
  - Muscle relaxants are effective in the management of nonspecific low back pain, but due to adverse effects, they should be used with caution.
- Manipulative medicine:
  - Massage therapy may be effective for treatment of chronic back pain (2).
  - Passive therapies, such as spinal manipulation therapy, muscle energy, and traction have no proven benefit.
  - Physical therapy modalities including muscle energy, low-level laser therapy, and ultrasound have no evidence to support their use.
  - Exercise therapy appears to be slightly effective at decreasing pain and increasing function in adults with chronic low back pain (3).
  - The McKenzie method results in a decrease in and disability, but not pain, for acute low back pain (4).
  - There is evidence that yoga results in small to moderate improvements in back related function at 3 and 6 mo; it may be slightly more effective for pain (5).
  - Motor control exercise has low-to-moderate quality evidence that helps in chronic low back pain (6).
  - Combined chiropractic interventions slightly improved pain and disability for acute and subacute lower back pain (7).
  - Aquatic exercise appears to be beneficial in patients suffering from chronic back pain and pregnancy-related low back pain (8).

- Systemic corticosteroids: no proven benefit and significant potential harm (avascular necrosis of the hip) (9)
- Antidepressants: There is no evidence that antidepressants are more effect than placebo in the management of nonspecific low back pain (10). There is some evidence that tricyclic antidepressants may be similar in effectiveness to gabapentinoids (11).
- Antiepileptic medications: Gabapentin and pregabalin use has shown nonsignificant improvement in pain compared to placebo (12). Topiramate is also slightly better than placebo for nonradicular back pain.
- Behavioral therapy: There is moderate quality evidence that behavioral therapy can help individuals with chronic low back pain (13).
- Herbal medicine: Low-to-moderate quality evidence shows that four topical herbal medicines may reduce pain in acute and chronic low back pain compared to placebo: cayenne, harpagoside, willow bark, and comfrey.
- Injection therapy: There is conflicting evidence regarding the efficacy of prolotherapy. When used alone, it is not an effective treatment; however, when combined with other modalities, it may improve chronic low back pain (14). There is insufficient evidence to support any specific drug for injection (NSAIDS, corticosteroids, etc.) or location (disc, muscles, etc.).
- Radiofrequency denervation: There is low-quality evidence supporting the use of radiofrequency denervation in patients with chronic low back pain (15).
- Transcutaneous electrical nerve stimulation (TENS): There is no evidence from the small number of placebo-controlled trials to support the use of TENS (16).
- Acupuncture: may have a favorable effect on self-reported pain and functional limitations in nonspecific chronic low back pain (17)
- Insoles: There is strong evidence that insoles are ineffective for prevention of chronic back pain (18).
- Lumbar support: There is moderate evidence that lumbar support is not more effective than no intervention in preventing low back pain (3).
- Long term:
  - Systematic review of the literature of chronic low back pain concluded that individualized exercise therapy programs that incorporated stretching or strengthening and supervision may improve pain and function in chronic nonspecific low back pain (19).
  - Cochrane review of the literature added that there is evidence that a graded activity program improves absentee outcomes in subacute low back pain. In acute low back pain, exercise therapy is as effective as either no treatment or other conservative treatments (20).

ISSUES FOR REFERRAL

Rapidly progressive neurologic deficits, symptoms of cauda equina syndrome or cord compression, acute vertebral collapse, suspicion of infection

ADDITIONAL THERAPIES

- Bed rest for 2 to 4 days may be required in patients with severe initial symptoms of sciatica. Prolonged bed rest (>4 days) should be avoided.
- Patients should be advised to stay active because this speeds recovery and reduces time away from work. It takes twice as long to regain conditioning as it does to lose it.
- Begin with low-stress aerobic activity such as walking, riding a bicycle, swimming, and eventually jogging.
- After ~2 wk of general activity, specific conditioning exercises for trunk muscles may be helpful.
- Physical therapy may be helpful during the 1st mo of symptoms. Goal of therapy is increasing function, not absence of pain.

SURGERY/OTHER PROCEDURES

- Considered only when serious spinal pathology or nerve root dysfunction due to a herniated lumbar disc is detected
- Patients with acute low back pain alone, without findings of serious conditions or significant nerve root compression, rarely benefit from surgery.
- Surgery has not been proven to help back pain without radiculopathy (21).

ONGOING CARE

FOLLOW-UP RECOMMENDATIONS

- Begin walking as soon as possible.
- Early osteopathic or chiropractic referral is often beneficial.
- Early orthopedic or physical therapy referral is rarely indicated.

REFERENCES

1. Chaparro LE, Furlan AD, Deshpande A, et al. Opioids compared with placebo or other treatments for chronic low back pain: an update of the Cochrane review. *Spine (Phila Pa 1976)*. 2014;39(7):556–563.
2. Kumar S, Beaton K, Hughes T. The effectiveness of massage therapy for the treatment of nonspecific low back pain: a systematic review of systematic reviews. *Int J Gen Med*. 2013;6:733–741.
3. van Middelkoop M, Rubinstein SM, Verhagen AP, et al. Exercise therapy for chronic nonspecific low-back pain. *Best Pract Res Clin Rheumatol*. 2010;24(2):193–204.
4. Garcia AN, Costa Lda C, da Silva TM, et al. Effectiveness of back school versus McKenzie exercises in patients with chronic nonspecific low back pain: a randomized controlled trial. *Phys Ther*. 2013;93(6):729–747.
5. Cramer H, Lauche R, Haller H, et al. A systematic review and meta-analysis of yoga for low back pain. *Clin J Pain*. 2013;29(5):450–460.
6. Byström MG, Rasmussen-Barr E, Grooten WJ. Motor control exercises reduces pain and disability in chronic and recurrent low back pain: a meta-analysis. *Spine (Phila Pa 1976)*. 2013;38(6):E350–E358.
7. Cherkin DC, Sherman K, Kahn J, et al. A comparison of the effects of 2 types of massage and usual care on chronic low back pain. *Ann Intern Med*. 2011;155(1):1–9.
8. Baena-Beato PÁ, Artero EG, Arroyo-Morales M, et al. Aquatic therapy improves pain, disability, quality of life, body composition and fitness in sedentary adults with chronic low back pain. A controlled clinical trial. *Clin Rehabil*. 2014;28(4):350–360.
9. Chou R, Deyo R, Friedly J, et al. Systemic pharmacologic therapies for low back pain: a systematic review for an American College of Physicians clinical practice guideline. *Ann Intern Med*. 2017;166(7):480–492.
10. Kuijpers T, van Middelkoop M, Rubinstein SM, et al. A systematic review on the effectiveness of pharmacological interventions for chronic non-specific low-back pain. *Eur Spine J*. 2011;20(1):40–50.
11. Dharmshaktu P, Tayal V, Kalra BS. Efficacy of antidepressants as analgesics: a review. *J Clin Pharmacol*. 2012;52(1):6–17.
12. Atkinson JH, Slater MA, Capparelli EV, et al. A randomized controlled trial of gabapentin for chronic low back pain with and without a radiating component. *Pain*. 2016;157(7):1499–1507.
13. Cherkin DC, Sherman KJ, Balderson BH, et al. Effect of mindfulness-based stress reduction vs cognitive behavioral therapy or usual care on back pain and functional limitations in adults with chronic low back pain: a randomized clinical trial. *JAMA*. 2016;315(12):1240–1249.
14. Enke O, New HA, New CH, et al. Anticonvulsants in the treatment of low back pain and lumbar radicular pain: a systematic review and meta-analysis. *CMAJ*. 2018;190(26):E786–E793.
15. Leggett LE, Soril LJ, Lorenzetti DL, et al. Radiofrequency ablation for chronic low back pain: a systematic review of randomized controlled trials. *Pain Res Manag*. 2014;19(5):e146–e153.
16. Buchmuller A, Navez M, Milletre-Bernardin M, et al. Value of TENS for relief of chronic low back pain with or without radicular pain. *Eur J Pain*. 2012;16(5):656–665.
17. Lam M, Galvin R, Curry P. Effectiveness of acupuncture for nonspecific chronic low back pain: a systematic review and meta-analysis. *Spine (Phila Pa 1976)*. 2013;38(24):2124–2138.
18. Chuter V, Spink M, Searle A, et al. The effectiveness of shoe insoles for the prevention and treatment of low back pain: a systematic review and meta-analysis of randomised controlled trials. *BMC Musculoskelet Disord*. 2014;15:140.
19. Searle A, Spink M, Ho A, et al. Exercise interventions for the treatment of chronic low back pain: a systematic review and meta-analysis of randomized controlled trials. *Clin Rehabil*. 2015;29(12):1155–1167.
20. Macedo LG, Smeets RJ, Maher CG, et al. Graded activity and graded exposure for persistent nonspecific low back pain: a systematic review. *Phys Ther*. 2010;90(6):860–879.
21. Chou R, Baisden J, Carragee EJ, et al. Surgery for low back pain: a review of the evidence for an American Pain Society clinical practice guideline. *Spine (Phila Pa 1976)*. 2009;34(10):1094–1109.

ADDITIONAL READING

Vijan S, Manaker S, Qaseem A. Noninvasive treatments for acute, subacute, and chronic low back pain. *Ann Intern Med*. 2017;167(11):835–836.

CLINICAL PEARLS

- Acute low back pain is the most common musculoskeletal complaint seen by primary care providers associated with a significant morbidity, health care cost, and missed work.
- In the absence of red flags, imaging is generally not necessary on initial evaluation, and most patients will improve within 1 mo.
- Initial conservative management includes minimal bed rest, nonopioid analgesia, muscle relaxants, and physical therapy.
- Alternative, evidence-based treatments include exercise therapy, yoga, chiropractic interventions, aquatic exercise therapy, behavioral therapy, and herbal medicine.
- There is no evidence supporting the use of corticosteroids, with increased risk of adverse events.

LUMBAR DISC DISEASE

Jin Choi, DO

BASICS

DESCRIPTION

- Any disease process that alters the normal anatomy of the discs between the vertebral bodies, causing various musculoskeletal and/or neurologic symptoms (low back pain, radiculopathy, urinary/bowel incontinence, etc.)
- It represents a broad spectrum of pathology, including disc herniations, disc space narrowing, disc desiccation, discogenic pain, and sclerosis of the end plates as well as many other lumbar spine abnormalities with various etiologies.
- Most commonly, the term refers to lumbar disc herniation, and this topic most specifically addresses lumbar disc herniation.
- Lumbar disc herniations are the most common cause of sciatica, although not the only cause (1).
- Per North American Spine Society, disc herniation is defined as a localized displacement of disc material beyond the normal margins of the intervertebral disc space resulting in pain, weakness or numbness in myotomal, or dermatomal distribution (2).

EPIDEMIOLOGY

Incidence

- Approximately 3:1 male to female ratio
- Peak incidence is between the 4th and 6th decades of life (ages 30s to 50s).

ETIOLOGY AND PATHOPHYSIOLOGY

- Compromise in the integrity of the annulus fibrosus may allow herniation of the nucleus pulposus (3,4).
- Herniation of the nucleus pulposus of the disc may compress and irritate the adjacent nerve root.
- The disc herniates when the pressure within the nucleus pulposus increases from a torsional strain or compression, and it pushes against the outside ring of the annulus fibrosis and overcomes its tensile strength (3,4).
- Most common location of herniation is paracentral (posterior longitudinal ligament is the weakest at this location), followed by foraminal (lateral), and then central.
- Different stages of herniation include protrusion, extrusion, and sequestration.
- Due to vertical anatomy of lumbar nerve roots, paracentral and foraminal disc herniation will affect different nerve roots.
- Most common site of herniation is L5–S1, affecting the S1 nerve root with a paracentral herniation and the L5 nerve root with a foraminal herniation (4).
- Second most common site of herniation is L4–L5, affecting the L5 nerve root with a paracentral herniation and the L4 nerve root with a foraminal herniation (4).
- Central herniation may present with back pain only, but the clinician should take caution for other possible red flags, such as cauda equina syndrome (see below).

RISK FACTORS

- Lifestyle risks, such as sedentary occupations, physical inactivity, and smoking
- Family history of acquired spinal disorders, such as ankylosing spondylitis and degenerative arthritis
- Prior low back injuries or surgeries
- Increased height and weight

DIAGNOSIS

HISTORY

- Often presents with history of multiple episodes of back pain that vary in severity and duration:
  - This accumulated recurrent back pain can lead to disc herniation.
  - May present following an acute lifting or twisting injury
  - Often worsened by coughing, sneezing, and Valsalva maneuver
- May present with sciatic pain, which is pain originating in the low back and radiating to the buttock and down the posterior or lateral thigh to the ankle or foot:
  - Patients may have a difficult time finding a position of comfort.
- Sciatica has a high sensitivity for lumbar disc herniation but low specificity (1):
  - More specific for disc herniation if the pain is greater in the leg than in the back or if the pain is worse with Valsalva maneuver
- Can present with back pain that does not radiate, but patient may note motor or sensory deficits
- Red flag symptoms that may indicate an alternative diagnosis, including cauda equina syndrome, infection, or neoplasm:
  - Fecal incontinence
  - Loss of motor function
  - Perianal numbness
  - Radicular symptoms lasting >6 wk
  - Saddle anesthesia
  - Urinary retention or incontinence
  - Unexplained fever
  - Unintentional weight loss
  - No improvement with >6 wk of conservative management

PHYSICAL EXAM

- A full physical exam of the back, pelvis, and lower extremities should be done, including a detailed neurologic exam:
  - Visual exam of the lower back and lower extremities and gait exam
  - Palpation of lower back, sacrum, and hips
  - Range of motion of lower back and lower extremities
  - Lower extremity strength, sensation, and reflex
- Provocative tests should include a straight-leg raise (SLR) test, the most sensitive test for lumbar disc herniation (1):
  - SLR: can be done seated or supine, although for lumbar disc herniation supine test has higher sensitivity (1)
  - Crossed SLR: highly specific for lumbar nerve root entrapment, including that caused by lumbar disc herniation (1)
  - Lasègue sign, which is SLR aggravated by forced ankle dorsiflexion, is also helpful to increase sensitivity and specificity.
- Other less commonly used provocative tests:
  - Bowstring sign: SLR aggravated by compression on popliteal fossa
  - Kernig test: pain reproduced with neck flexion, hip flexion, and leg extension
  - Naffziger test: pain reproduced by coughing, which is instigated by lying patient supine and applying pressure on the neck veins
  - Milgram test: pain reproduced with straight-leg elevation for 30 sec in the supine position
- Other findings may include:
  - Decreased or loss of sensation:
    - Medial lower leg and foot, including plantar aspect of 1st toe (L3–L4 involvement)
    - Anterior lower leg, dorsum of the foot, and 1st dorsal web space (L4–L5 involvement)
    - Lateral foot and posterior heel (S1–S2 involvement)
  - Tendon reflex changes:
    - Diminished or lost patellar tendon reflex (L4 involvement)
    - Diminished or lost Achilles tendon reflex (S1 involvement)
    - No L1, L2, L3, or L5 tendon reflexes
  - Motor finding (often late findings):
    - Weak knee extension or hip flexion (L3–L4 involvement)
    - Weak ankle dorsiflexion (L4 involvement)
    - Weak 1st toe extension (extensor hallucis longus [EHL]) or hip abduction (L5 involvement)
    - Weak ankle plantarflexion (S1 involvement)
- Waddell signs: to assess for possible nonorganic cause of back pain (psychological, socioeconomic, secondary gain, etc.):
  - Tenderness:
    - Superficial tenderness with light palpation or tenderness on deep palpation but nonanatomic over a large area
  - Simulated tests:
    - Axial loading causes low back pain, or rotation of the hips and shoulders together causes low back pain.
  - Distraction:
    - Formal straight-leg raise is positive but when distracted, straight-leg raise does not produce pain.
  - Regional sensory or motor changes:
    - Glove and stocking sensation loss or nonanatomic muscular weakness (various muscles innervated by different nerve roots)
  - Overreaction:
    - Exaggerated response or emotions

DIFFERENTIAL DIAGNOSIS

- Cauda equina syndrome
- Hip arthritis
- Knee arthritis
- Meralgia paresthetica
- Piriformis syndrome
- Sacroiliitis
- Spinal neoplasms
- Spinal stenosis

- Trochanteric bursitis
- Vascular insufficiency
- Vertebral fracture
- Spondylolisthesis
- Spondylolysis
- Infection/abscess

DIAGNOSTIC TESTS & INTERPRETATION

- Magnetic resonance imaging (MRI) is the preferred imaging modality; however, in the absence of red flag symptoms, MRI should be delayed for a 6-wk trial of conservative treatment. If symptoms persist beyond 6 wk, MRI may then be considered (1)[A]:
  - Important to note that imaging evidence of degenerative disc disease in asymptomatic individuals is very common and its prevalence increases with age (5).
- Emergent imaging may be considered for red flag symptoms such as urinary retention, fecal incontinence, saddle anesthesia, progressive neurologic changes, and intractable pain.
- Plain radiographs may be beneficial to rule out osseous abnormalities (such as metastatic disease or fractures); in addition, they may demonstrate age-related degenerative changes.
- Computed tomography (CT) is also useful in evaluating osseous abnormalities and for those whom an MRI is contraindicated.
- CT-myelogram can be useful for patient with contraindications for MRI or with history of prior back surgeries (instrumentation can cause artifacts on MRI) (5).

TREATMENT

GENERAL MEASURES

- Clinicians should advise patients that most acute low back pain with or without sciatic symptoms resolves within the 1st month, and it generally has a very favorable prognosis.
- Given that most patients with acute or subacute low back pain improve over time regardless of treatment, clinicians and patients should select nonpharmacologic treatment with superficial heat (moderate-quality evidence), massage, acupuncture, or spinal manipulation (low-quality evidence) (grade: strong recommendation per American College of Physicians [ACP] grading system) (6).
- If pharmacologic treatment is desired, clinicians and patients should select nonsteroidal anti-inflammatory drugs (NSAIDs) or skeletal muscle relaxants (moderate-quality evidence) (grade: strong recommendation per ACP grading system) (6).

MEDICATION

First Line

- NSAIDs, acetaminophen, and muscle relaxants may be effective for nonspecific low back pain, but studies for lumbar disc herniation are limited (1)[B].
- In the treatment of pain associated with lumbar disc herniation, systemic steroids are no better than placebo (1)[A].
- Opioid medications and opioid agonists, such as tramadol, are often included as a standard component in the conservative treatment of patients with severe pain, although their use has not been extensively studied.

Second Line

Epidural steroid injections can improve pain in the short term (2 to 4 wk) but do not provide long-term relief (1,2)[A].

SURGERY/OTHER PROCEDURES

- Common surgical techniques include:
  - Open discectomy.
  - Microdiscectomy.
- Immediate indications for surgery include:
  - Cauda equina syndrome.
  - Acute myelopathy.
  - Severe motor deficits.
  - Intractable pain.
- In addition, surgery may be considered with the failure of conservative therapy to provide relief within 6 to 12 wk (1)[A].
- Discectomy is suggested to provide more effective symptom relief than medical/interventional care for patients with lumbar disc herniation with radiculopathy whose symptoms warrant surgical intervention. In patients with less severe symptoms, surgery or medical/interventional care appear to be effective for both short- and long-term relief (2)[B].
- In comparison to conservative management, surgical discectomy has been shown to provide quicker and better relief of pain associated with lumbar disc herniation in the first 4 yr:
  - The performance of surgical decompression is suggested to provide better medium-term (1 to 4 yr) symptom relief as compared with medical/interventional management of patients with radiculopathy from lumbar disc herniation whose symptoms are severe enough to warrant surgery, but there is inconsistent evidence for long-term (>4 yr) symptom relief (2)[B].

COMPLEMENTARY & ALTERNATIVE MEDICINE

- Physical therapy is often incorporated as a component of conservative therapy; however, there is insufficient data to make recommendation for or against the use of physical therapy or structured exercise regimen as stand-alone treatment for lumbar disc disease (2)[C].
- Modalities such as ultrasound and transcutaneous electrical nerve stimulation (TENS) do not have enough quality evidence to clearly assess their effectiveness (2)[C], although they may provide some short-term benefit.
- Traction produces conflicting evidence, and systemic reviews indicate that the results are inconsistent (2)[C].
- Aerobic conditioning and trunk muscle strengthening are important for good outcomes and preventing future injuries.

REFERENCES

1. Gregory DS, Seto CK, Wortley GC, et al. Acute lumbar disk pain: navigating evaluation and treatment choices. *Am Fam Physician*. 2008;78(7):835–842.
2. Kreiner DS, Hwang SW, Easa JE, et al. An evidence-based clinical guideline for the diagnosis and treatment of lumbar disc herniation with radiculopathy. *Spine J*. 2014;14(1):180–191.
3. Amin RM, Andrade NS, Neuman BJ, et al. Lumbar disc herniation. *Curr Rev Musculoskelet Med*. 2017;10(4):507–516.
4. Humphreys SC, Eck JC. Clinical evaluation and treatment options for herniated lumbar disc. *Am Fam Physician*. 1999;59(3):575–582, 587–588.
5. Hoeffner EG, Mukherji SK, Srinivasan A, et al. Neuroradiology back to the future: spine imaging. *AJNR Am J Neuroradiol*. 2012;33(6):999–1006.
6. Qaseem A, Wilt TJ, McLean RM, et al. Noninvasive treatments for acute, subacute, and chronic low back pain: a clinical practice guideline from the American College of Physicians. *Ann Intern Med*. 2017;166(7):514–530.

ADDITIONAL READING

- Brinjikji W, Luetmer PH, Comstock B, et al. Systematic literature review of imaging features of spinal degeneration in asymptomatic populations. *AJNR Am J Neuroradiol*. 2015;36(4):811–816.
- Greer S, Chambliss L, Mackler L, et al. Clinical inquiries. What physical exam techniques are useful to detect malingering? *J Fam Pract*. 2005;54(8):719–722.
- Jarvik JG, Deyo RA. Diagnostic evaluation of low back pain with emphasis on imaging. *Ann Intern Med*. 2002;137(7):586–597.
- Kerr RS, Cadoux-Hudson TA, Adams CB. The value of accurate clinical assessment in the surgical management of the lumbar disc protrusion. *J Neurol Neurosurg Psychiatry*. 1988;51(2):169–173.
- Peul WC, van Houwelingen HC, van den Hout WB, et al. Surgery versus prolonged conservative treatment for sciatica. *N Engl J Med*. 2007;356(22):2245–2256.
- Weinstein JN, Lurie JD, Tosteson TD, et al. Surgical vs nonoperative treatment for lumbar disk herniation: the Spine Patient Outcomes Research Trial (SPORT) observational cohort. *JAMA*. 2006;296(20):2451–2459.

CLINICAL PEARLS

- Obtaining detailed and careful history and physical exam is the key for making proper diagnosis and treatment plan for any lumbar disc disease etiology.
- Although the specificity is low, the straight-leg raise test in supine position is the most sensitive physical exam test for lumbar disc herniation.
- In the absence of red flag symptoms, conservative management may be attempted for 6 wk prior to obtaining diagnostic imaging such as MRI.
- Conservative management may include NSAIDs, acetaminophen, muscle relaxants, and opioid analgesics for severe pain:
  - Oral steroids have not been shown to be beneficial compared to placebo.
- There is insufficient data to make recommendation for or against the use of physical therapy or structured exercise regimen for symptoms associated with lumbar disc herniation.
- Epidural steroids may provide short-term relief but have not been shown to provide long-term relief.
- Although surgery offers better improvement of pain in the first 4 yr compared to conservative management, there is no difference in outcome beyond 4 yr.

LUNATE DISSOCIATION

Aleem Bakhtiar, MS, MD • Kory Gill, DO, FAAFP, CAQSM

BASICS

DESCRIPTION

- Dissociation, or *dislocation*, is classified by the pattern of carpal collapse, either dorsal or volar in nature, after wrist trauma or injury.
- The carpal bones in the wrist are stabilized by multiple extrinsic and intrinsic ligaments. The scaphoid, lunate, and triquetrum have no tendon insertions and are described as an intercalated segment (motion depends on mechanical signals from ligamentously intact neighboring articulations) (1).
- The dorsal component of the scapholunate interosseous ligament (SLIL) is the primary stabilizer of the lunate. Important secondary stabilizers include the short radiolunate ligament (SRL), which maintains the position of the lunate adjacent to the radius, and the dorsal intercarpal (DIC) ligament. Several other extrinsic ligaments serve as secondary restraints (1,2).
- Injury typically occurs when an extended wrist undergoes a forced axial load, such as in a fall on outstretched hand (FOOSH) with the hand in ulnar deviation or when pushing a heavy object.
- Isolated carpal dislocations are rare. Most information on them comes from case reports and surgical technique papers (2).
- A number of injury patterns can occur with this mechanism, depending on several factors: position of the extremity at impact, quality of the bone, ligamentous strength, and direction of the force (2).
- Secondary stabilizers include the scaphotrapezial ligamentous complex, palmar radial extrinsic ligaments, and palmar ulnar extrinsic ligaments. The scapho-trapezio-trapezoid ligament complex plays a major role in preventing flexion of the scaphoid (3).
- Another important secondary stabilizer is the DIC ligament, which, if injured, can lead to increase in the scapholunate angle and dorsal intercalated segment instability (DISI) deformity when injured inconjunction with a primary stabilizer (3).
- The terms *lunate dissociation*, *scapholunate dissociation (SLD)*, and *perilunate dissociation* and *dislocation* have overlapping features. Similarly, injury patterns to the lunate and adjacent structures have overlapping characteristics and nomenclatures.
- Perilunate injuries are disruptions of the carpal anatomy defined by dislocation of the capitate head from the concavity of the distal lunate. Injuries to the scapholunate ligament can have concomitant perilunate injuries such as dislocation involving the greater or lesser arcs (3).
- Mayfield initially described four stages of perilunate instability in 1980 that have since been modified (2):
  - Stage 1: disruption of scapholunate articulation
  - Stage 2: lunocapitate dislocation
  - Stage 3: lunotriquetral disruption
  - Stage 4: volar lunate dislocation
- A four-stage classification system is used commonly to describe SLD (4):
  - Stage 1: Predynamic instability consists of the mildest form of scapholunate injury and results from a stretched or partially torn SLIL. This may cause abnormal motion, synovitis, and wrist pain. Plain and stress radiographs are normal; arthroscopy may show attenuation of the SLIL or hemorrhage within the scapholunate joint. Untreated, secondary stabilizers may become attenuated and progress to dynamic or static instability.
  - Stage 2: Dynamic instability is characterized by ligamentous tear of the palmar or dorsal aspect of the SLIL. Portions of the ligament may be still intact. Plain radiographs will be normal, but stress views show widening of the scapholunate interval. An arthrogram may show abnormalities within the ligament.
  - Stage 3: Static instability occurs with complete tear to the SLIL *and* attenuation or attrition of the supporting wrist ligaments. Radiographic changes become evident on plain radiography (gap of 3 mm or greater between the lunate and scaphoid or a scapholunate angle >60 degrees on lateral views). DISI is often present.
  - Stage 4: Scapholunate advanced collapse (SLAC) refers to longstanding carpal misalignment; this will result in cartilage damage and eventual arthritis. Changes begin at the radial styloid joint and can progress to the radioscaphoid fossa and eventually to the midcarpal joint.
- Synonym(s): wrist sprain; perilunate dissociation; SLD; scapholunate instability
- Dislocation is often used interchangeably with dissociation; a dislocated bone is always dissociated, but a dissociated bone is not always dislocated.

EPIDEMIOLOGY

- Perilunate dislocations (PLDs) are the most common carpal dislocation (2).
- More common in men in the 2nd and 3rd decades of life; less common in the elderly (distal radius fails/fractures before ligamentous injury occurs) and children (Radial physis is weaker, resulting in Salter-Harris fractures.) (2)
- SLD is more common in football than in any other sport.
- Wrist injuries account for an estimated 3–9% of all athletic-related injuries.
- A 10-yr study done at the Cleveland Clinic revealed that 14.8% of athletic participants aged <16 yr sustained upper extremity injuries, and of these, 9% involved the wrist.
- The incidence of lunate dissociation is uncommon, but failure to identify the injury results in long-term disability.

RISK FACTORS

- Any injury involving excessive wrist extension and ulnar deviation with intracarpal supination, typically a FOOSH injury
- Chronic crutch-walkers, gymnasts, American football players, collision sports
- Increased ulnar negative variance

GENERAL PREVENTION

- Controversy exists as to whether braces or wrist guards effectively prevent wrist injuries.
- One cadaveric model showed decreased carpal fractures, ligament, and capsular tears with bracing.
- In-line skating-type guards have not been shown to prevent wrist fractures.
- European studies of snowboarders show a significant decrease in the incidence of wrist fractures and injuries with wrist guards.
- Some are concerned that bracing/guards simply alter the area of force transmission.

COMMONLY ASSOCIATED CONDITIONS

- Scaphoid fractures occur with a similar mechanism of injury (FOOSH) and therefore must be ruled out.
- Failure to diagnose and treat lunate dissociation increases the risk of arthritic degeneration and development of SLAC wrist.

DIAGNOSIS

HISTORY

- Determine duration of pain: Most patients present acutely, but some report a history of painful clicking, reduced grip strength, and giving way with activities.
- Obtain detailed mechanism of injury to determine if SLD is a possible injury (typically a FOOSH with ulnar deviated wrist).
- Rule out any distracting injuries (elbow, forearm, etc.).

PHYSICAL EXAM

- Signs and symptoms:
  - 100% of patients have dorsal wrist pain, 91% have decreased grip strength, and 71% have decreased range of motion (ROM).
  - Clicking with wrist motion (nonspecific)
- Physical examination:
  - Inspect for swelling and deformity; compare with contralateral wrist.
  - Tenderness is typically on radial aspect of the wrist; palpate just distal to Lister tubercle, which is often tender as well.
  - Scaphoid tenderness (anatomic snuffbox) is a scaphoid fracture until proven otherwise.

- Document ROM of wrist and neurovascular status (pulses, sensation, particularly median nerve distribution because it can be diminished in severe dissociations owing to mechanical forces).
- Finger extension test: Hold wrist in flexion, and test active finger extension against resistance; causes pain over lunate
- Watson scaphoid test may be positive. The examiner places the thumb on the scaphoid tubercle, and the four fingers wrap around the distal radius. While the wrist is in ulnar deviation, pressure is directed dorsally with the thumb at the volar scaphoid. The wrist is then radially deviated. Pain is the hallmark of a positive test result, although a dramatic "clunk" may be felt or heard.
- Kleinman shear stress test for lunotriquetral instability: Wrist in neutral position, examiner's contralateral thumb is placed over dorsal lunate while ipsilateral thumb loads the pisotriquetral joint with a dorsally directed force. Pain is a positive test.
- The Reagan shuck test and Linscheid compression test are other maneuvers to determine lunotriquetral instability.

DIFFERENTIAL DIAGNOSIS

- Scaphoid fracture
- Colles fracture
- Scaphoid impaction syndrome
- Dorsal wrist ganglion cyst
- Other carpal bone injury

DIAGNOSTIC TESTS & INTERPRETATION

Initial Tests (lab, imaging)

- Radiographs: posteroanterior (PA), lateral, and oblique views of the wrist, clenched-fist view:
  - Gap of 3 mm on PA films ("Terry Thomas" or "Dave Letterman" sign, in reference to their gapped teeth) is classically used. However, Cautilli obtained PA radiographs on 100 normal wrists and found the mean gap in males was 4.0 mm and in females it was 3.6 mm. Zhu performed a similar study and found the mean gap to be 3.14 mm. Both studies revealed that gaps up to 5 mm were not necessarily indicative of carpal instability. Consequently, contralateral wrist films should be obtained for comparison.
  - Lateral views: Dorsal extension of the lunate is referred to as DISI and is highly suggestive of injury to the SLIL and at least one secondary stabilizer.
  - Scapholunate angle is normally 30 to 60 degrees on lateral view; an angle >70 degrees is diagnostic (5); clenched-fist view accentuates injury.

Follow-Up Tests & Special Considerations:

- Recent evidence shows that multidetector computed tomography (CT) arthrogram is superior to magnetic resonance angiography (MRA) in detecting partial ligament injuries (6).
- Magnetic resonance imaging (MRI) (1,5):
  - Complete SLIL tears are characterized by distinct area of discontinuity within the ligament, outlined by fluid-like T2 hyperintensity, or by complete absence of the ligament. Fluid signal at attachments also can be seen.
  - Detection of lunotriquetral interosseous ligament (LTIL) tears is more difficult, with a decreased sensitivity and specificity given the smaller size of this structure.
- MRI arthrography appears to have greater sensitivity at detecting partial tears of the SLIL than does MRI or traditional arthrograms. Extravasation of contrast material indicates a full-thickness ligamentous defect.
- MRI arthrography has a sensitivity of 83–92% and a specificity of 46–100%.

Diagnostic Procedures/Other

Arthroscopic evaluation is the "gold standard" for identifying and grading scapholunate injuries (3).

TREATMENT

- Acute treatment
- Analgesia; nonsteroidal anti-inflammatory drugs (NSAIDs), narcotics
- Reduction techniques:
  - Only for least severe injury (e.g., dynamic instability; see above)
  - Recommended for experienced providers only
- Immobilization:
  - Partial tears of SLIL can be treated conservatively with splinting. Immobilize with splint in correct anatomic position. Symptoms guide management.
  - Patients with suspected ligamentous injury should be referred promptly to an orthopedist, preferably a hand specialist, because misdiagnoses can have significant consequences.

ISSUES FOR REFERRAL

- Timely referral to hand surgeon if any question in the diagnosis
- Immediate referral to hand surgeon if abnormal neurovascular status

ADDITIONAL THERAPIES

- Long-term treatment
- Surgical referral:
  - Standard of care is operative repair.
  - Prolonged immobilization for weeks to months after surgery is necessary to maintain carpal bone alignment and to prevent SLAC wrist
- Rehabilitation: physical therapy after immobilization to improve ROM and strength
- Typically considered a season-ending injury

SURGERY/OTHER PROCEDURES

Standard of care typically involves open reduction, ligament repair, and internal fixation (2).

REFERENCES

1. Lau S, Swarna SS, Tamvakopoulos GS. Scapholunate dissociation: an overview of the clinical entity and current treatment options. *Eur J Orthop Surg Traummot*. 2009;19(6):377–385.
2. Grabow RJ, Catalano L III. Carpal dislocations. *Hand Clin*. 2006;22(4):485–500.
3. Chennagiri RJ, Lindau TR. Assessment of scapholunate instability and review of evidence for management in the absence of arthritis. *J Hand Surg Eur Vol*. 2013;38(7):727–738.
4. Chim H, Moran SL. Wrist essentials: the diagnosis and management of scapholunate ligament injuries. *Plast Reconstr Surg*. 2014;134(2):312e–322e.
5. Bencardino JT, Rosenberg ZS. Sports-related injuries of the wrist: an approach to MRI interpretation. *Clin Sports Med*. 2006;25(3):409–432.
6. Pappou IP, Basel J, Deal DN. Scapholunate ligament injuries: a review of current concepts. *Hand (N Y)*. 2013;8(2):146–156.

ADDITIONAL READING

- Cohen MS. Ligamentous injuries of the wrist in the athlete. *Clin Sports Med*. 1998;17(3):533–552.
- Manuel J, Moran SL. The diagnosis and treatment of scapholunate instability. *Orthop Clin North Am*. 2007;38(2):261–277.
- Mastey RD, Weiss AP, Akelman E. Primary care of hand and wrist athletic injuries. *Clin Sports Med*. 1997;16(4):705–724.
- Nguyen DT, McCue FC III, Urch SE. Evaluation of the injured wrist on the field and in the office. *Clin Sports Med*. 1998;17(3):421–432.
- Rettig AC. Epidemiology of hand and wrist injuries in sports. *Clin Sports Med*. 1998;17(3):401–406.
- Ritchie JV, Munter DW. Emergency department evaluation and treatment of wrist injuries. *Emerg Med Clin North Am*. 1999;17(4):823–842.
- Sauder DJ, Athwal GS, Faber KJ, et al. Perilunate injuries. *Orthop Clin North Am*. 2007;38(2):279–288.
- Slade JF III, Milewski MD. Management of carpal instability in athletes. *Hand Clin*. 2009;25(3):395–408.
- Young D, Papp S, Giachino A. Physical examination of the wrist. *Orthop Clin North Am*. 2007;38(2):149–165.

CLINICAL PEARLS

- Surgery results in ∼35% loss of flexion and extension. This should still allow an athlete to return to activity in most cases.
- The ligament in the wrist has torn in this injury, and the bones have shifted, so they cannot heal correctly without surgery.

MALLET FINGER

Rachel A. Coel, MD, PhD, FAAP, CAQSM • Quynh Hoang, MD, FAAP, CAQSM

BASICS

DESCRIPTION

- Mallet finger is defined as a stretching or tearing of the extensor tendon or a complete avulsion of the tendon insertion from the dorsal base of the distal phalanx with or without bony avulsion.
- The injury results in the inability to actively extend the distal interphalangeal (DIP) joint.
- It is most commonly caused by sudden forced flexion of the fingertip while the DIP joint is actively extended.
- Less commonly, it can occur when the DIP joint is forcefully hyperextended with a resulting fracture at the dorsal base of the distal phalanx.
- Chronic mallet finger is defined as a mallet injury presenting >4 wk after injury.

EPIDEMIOLOGY

- Usually occurs during sports participation when an extended finger is struck on the tip by a ball
- Also occurs in the work environment or with minor household trauma
- The most commonly injured digit is the 3rd (middle) finger of the dominant hand, although any digit, including the thumb, can be involved.

RISK FACTORS

Sports, especially those involving ball contact and hand-to-hand contact

DIAGNOSIS

HISTORY

- Patient reports axial loading and/or hyperflexion of the DIP joint while the finger is held in extension. Classically, the extended finger is struck on the tip by a ball.
- Patient complains of pain, swelling, and deformity at the DIP joint of the affected finger as well as tenderness especially at the dorsal aspect, with inability to actively extend the DIP joint.

PHYSICAL EXAM

- There is tenderness to palpation over the dorsum of the DIP joint.
- Patient is unable to actively extend the DIP joint, although passive extension is possible.
- To effectively establish the diagnosis, hold the proximal interphalangeal (PIP) joint in a fixed position, and then have the patient extend at the DIP joint.
- An extensor lag at the DIP joint generally is present immediately after injury, but the deformity may be delayed by hours and even days or weeks.
- In general, also evaluate for open skin lesions, collateral stability, and digit rotation or angulation.
- There are three classification systems used to describe the type of mallet injury: Doyle, Wehbe and Schneider, and Burton classification (used for chronic mallet finger) (1)[C].
- Using the Doyle classification scheme, mallet finger injuries can be divided into four types:
  - Type I: closed injury ± small dorsal avulsion fracture
  - Type II: open injury with tendon laceration
  - Type III: open injury with deep abrasion, causing loss of skin, subcutaneous tissue, and tendon substance
  - Type IV: mallet fracture:
    - Transepiphyseal injury fracture in children
    - Hyperflexion injury with fracture involving 20–50% of articular surface
    - Hyperextension injury with fracture involving >50% of articular surface

DIFFERENTIAL DIAGNOSIS

- Tuft or distal phalanx fracture with deformity
- In the pediatric age group, injury to the epiphysis at the base of the distal phalanx may mimic a mallet finger.
- In the pediatric age group, consider Seymour fracture—an open physeal fracture involving the nail bed and germinal matrix.

DIAGNOSTIC TESTS & INTERPRETATION

- Radiographs are recommended in all cases to evaluate for accompanying fracture or joint subluxation.
- Three views of the affected finger: posteroanterior, lateral, and oblique
- Three patterns: no avulsion fracture, small avulsion fracture (<30% articular surface), large avulsion fracture (>30% articular surface)
- Consider obtaining repeat radiographs at conclusion of continuous splinting to evaluate fracture healing.

TREATMENT

GENERAL MEASURES

- There is general consensus in current literature that nonoperative treatment is indicated in almost all mallet finger injuries in the absence of large articular disruption or distal phalanx (1,2)[C],(3,4)[A].
- The involved finger should be splinted in full extension or slight hyperextension at the DIP joint.
- No flexion should occur at any time until treatment is complete.
- Splint continuously for at least 6 to 8 wk and with additional weeks of immobilization in cases of persistent lag (1,2)[C],(4)[A].
- If bone avulsion fracture, extension splint should be applied for 6 wk.
- If tendon injury without bone involvement, splint in extension for at least 8 wk
- Although most recommend additional 2 to 4 wk of nighttime splinting, the effectiveness of night splinting after initial treatment of mallet finger is unknown.
- A recent prospective randomized controlled trial comparing night splinting with no splinting after treatment of mallet finger found that supplemental night splinting does not improve outcome of mallet finger (5)[A].
- Compliance should be assessed at 2-wk intervals until healing has occurred.
- Monitor skin for signs of ulceration, maceration, or local allergic reactions.
- Controversy still exists regarding the optimal nonoperative treatment of each type of mallet finger with respect to the type of splint used and the length of immobilization.
- Regardless of the type of material the splint is or whether it is applied dorsally or volarly over the finger, any type of splint maintaining DIP joint in extension is effective (2)[C].
- The most commonly used is the Stack splint (plastic or custom-made thermoplastic), whereas AlumaFoam splints and Abouna metal splints are also often used.
- A Cochrane Review (2009) concluded that there is insufficient evidence from existing studies to establish the relative effectiveness of different types of finger splints used versus the standard Stack splint. Additionally, there is insufficient evidence to determine when surgery is indicated (5)[A].

ADDITIONAL THERAPIES

- DIP joint often is stiff after prolonged immobilization.
- After 6 to 8 wk of continuous splinting, start DIP joint gentle active and passive range of motion (ROM) exercises.
- At the end of continuous immobilization, if a mallet deformity of >20 degrees recurs, continue splinting for an additional 1 to 2 mo.
- Consider extension splinting during athletic activities for an additional 2 mo after continuous splinting has been completed.
- For chronic mallet finger injury, treatment includes initial trial of prolonged splinting (10 wk). Surgery is considered if there is extensor lag of 40 degrees or if there is functional deficit (2)[C].

SURGERY/OTHER PROCEDURES

ALERT

Although operative treatment is generally recommended for mallet fractures involving >30% of the articular surface or if there is volar subluxation of the distal phalanx, indications for surgical intervention remain controversial.

A 2009 Cochrane Review concluded that there is insufficient evidence to determine when surgery is specifically indicated (6)[A].

ONGOING CARE

FOLLOW-UP RECOMMENDATIONS

- Regular physician assessment and diligent patient compliance are critical for successful nonoperative treatment.
- Assess compliance with continuous splinting at follow-up visits at 2-wk intervals.
- Consider repeat radiographs at the conclusion of continuous splinting to assess for bone healing.

PATIENT EDUCATION

- This injury requires careful patient compliance.
- The patient must understand the necessity of keeping the finger in extension for the entire duration of treatment, including during splint changes and skin care.
- The patient must monitor dorsal skin for signs of vascular compromise from continuous extension splinting.

COMPLICATIONS

ALERT

Patients may develop a slight extensor lag (5 to 10 degrees) with a mild loss of total motion, but it should not result in a functional deficit.

- Complications tend to be related to splinting and typically are short term, such as skin ulcerations, splint-related pain, and tape allergies.
- Other complications include permanent DIP joint stiffness, persistent flexion deformity, recurrence of mallet deformity, and, in cases of open injuries, osteomyelitis.
- Swan neck deformity at the level of the PIP joint can occur if mallet finger injury is left untreated or if there is poor patient compliance with splinting.
- Surgery may need to be considered in patients with chronic mallet deformities after failing a trial of splinting.
- Surgical complications may be long term, including pain, deformity, and treatment failure.

Pediatric Considerations

- Physeal and epiphyseal involvement at the base of the distal phalanx is common in pediatric mallet finger injuries.
- Children <12 yr are more likely to have a Salter-Harris type I or II fracture rather than a true mallet injury.
- In the pediatric age group, nondisplaced mallet finger injury may be treated with continuous splinting of the DIP joint in extension or slight hyperextension for 4 to 6 wk. Effectiveness of additional nighttime splinting after that remains unknown.
- Extension splints should also be worn for sports activities for an additional 4 wk.
- Reduction is necessary for displaced fractures. If closed reduction is unsuccessful, then referral for surgical repair is indicated.
- Extra attention should be paid to open fractures in pediatric patients, specifically Seymour fractures. A Seymour fracture is an open physeal fracture of the distal phalanx with associated injury to the nail bed of the finger. Evaluate the injured finger for nail bed laceration with possible germinal matrix interposition. Seymour fractures require surgery to reduce the entrapped germinal matrix at the fracture site. Complications include growth deformity of the nail or phalanx, flexion deformity, and osteomyelitis (2)[A].

REFERENCES

1. Bachoura A, Ferikes AJ, Lubahn JD. A review of mallet finger and jersey finger injuries in the athlete. *Curr Rev Musculoskelet Med*. 2017;10(1):1–9.
2. Lamaris G, Matthew M. The diagnosis and management of mallet finger injuries. *Hand (N Y)*. 2017;12(3):223–238.
3. Lin JS, Samora JB. Surgical and nonsurgical management of mallet finger: a systematic review. *J Hand Surg Am*. 2018;43(2):146.e2–163.e2.
4. Valdes K, Naughton N, Algar L. Conservative treatment of mallet finger: a systematic review. *J Hand Ther*. 2015;28(3):237–246.
5. Gruber J, Bot A, Ring D. A prospective randomized controlled trial comparing night splinting with no splinting after treatment of mallet finger. *Hand (N Y)*. 2014;9(2):145–150.
6. Handoll H, Vaghela M. Interventions for treating mallet finger injuries. *Cochrane Database of Syst Rev*. 2004;(3):CD004574.

ADDITIONAL READING

Alla S, Deal N, Dempsey I. Current concepts: mallet finger. *Hand (N Y)*. 2014;9(2):138–144.

CLINICAL PEARLS

- The typical mechanism of injury is a "jamming" or axial load to the fingertip, resulting in the inability to actively extend the DIP joint.
- Without treatment, mallet finger may result in hyperextension (swan neck) deformity at the PIP joint or osteoarthritis at the DIP joint.
- Controversy exists regarding optimal treatment of each type of mallet finger with respect to the type of splint used, the length of immobilization, and the surgical technique used when operative repair is indicated.
- However, there is general consensus that nonoperative management with splinting is the treatment of choice and is effective for most mallet finger injuries involving less than a third of the articular surface or without DIP joint subluxation.

M

MARFAN SYNDROME

Rebecca L. Carl, MD, MSCI

BASICS

DESCRIPTION

- An autosomal dominant genetic disorder of connective tissue
- System(s) affected: musculoskeletal, cardiovascular, ocular, skin/integument, endocrine/metabolic, pulmonary
- Genetics: autosomal dominant with high penetrance; 15–25% spontaneous mutation
- Incidence/prevalence in United States: 1/5,000 to 1/15,000
- Predominant age: genetic condition. Generally, clinical manifestations become apparent during late childhood or adolescence. There is a more severe early-onset form of this condition; affected individuals are generally diagnosed in the newborn period.
- Predominant gender: no gender, ethnic, or racial predilection

ETIOLOGY AND PATHOPHYSIOLOGY

Genetic: ~75% of affected individuals have an affected parent; the remainder has a spontaneous mutation in the fibrillin-1 (*FBN-1*) gene.

RISK FACTORS

Advanced paternal age gives rise to a slightly increased risk only in cases that are not clearly familial.

GENERAL PREVENTION

Primary prevention: In families where a *FBN-1* gene mutation has been identified, preimplantation genetic diagnosis can be used to identify embryos without the mutation.

DIAGNOSIS

- Genetic testing, looking for mutations in the *FBN-1* gene, is available. Mutations can be identified in ~90% of affected individuals (1)[A].
- The mainstay of diagnosis is clinical evaluation and application of established diagnostic criteria. These criteria, now known as the *Ghent nosology*, were revised most recently in 2010 (2)[C].
- The criteria for diagnosis in individuals with no family history include any of the following:
  - Pathologic *FBN-1* mutation and either ectopia lentis or aortic root dilatation (*Z*-score ≥2 points)
  - Ectopia lentis and aortic root dilatation (*Z*-score ≥2 points)
  - Aortic root dilatation (*Z*-score ≥2 points) and other systemic features (≥7 points)
- The criteria for diagnosis in individuals who have a first-degree relative with Marfan syndrome include any of the following:
  - Ectopia lentis
  - Systemic features (≥7 points)
  - Aortic root dilatation (*Z*-score ≥2 points or *Z*-score ≥3 points for individuals <20 yr of age)
- Echocardiography, spine radiographs, and slit-lamp exam may be important in making the diagnosis.

PHYSICAL EXAM

- Features listed below with diagnostics points in parentheses (where applicable)
- Musculoskeletal:
  - Pectus carinatum (2 points)
  - Pectus excavatum (1 point)
  - Reduced upper segment to lower segment ration with increased arm span: height ratio (>1.05) in the absence of scoliosis (1 point)
  - Positive thumb sign (thumb can protrude from ulnar side of a clenched fist) and/or wrist sign (thumb and 5th finger can encircle wrist and overlap) (3 points if both present, 1 point if one is present)
  - Decreased elbow extension (1 point)
  - Pes planovalgus (1 point, 2 points with medial displacement of the medial malleolus)
  - Protrusio acetabuli on radiographs (2 points)
  - Scoliosis of >20 degrees or thoracolumbar kyphosis (1 point)
  - High-arched palate with crowding of teeth
  - Three out of five characteristic facial features (1 point)
- Cardiovascular:
  - Mitral valve prolapse (1 point)
  - Dilatation of the main pulmonary aorta (age <40 yr)
  - Calcification of the mitral valve annulus (age <40 yr)
  - Dilatation or dissection of the descending or abdominal aorta (age <50 yr)
- Ocular:
  - Myopia >3 diopters (1 point)
  - Flat cornea
  - Decreased miosis owing to hypoplastic iris or ciliary muscles
- Pulmonary (minor criteria only):
  - Spontaneous pneumothorax (2 points)
  - Apical blebs
- Skin/integument (minor criteria only):
  - Striae (1 point)
  - Recurrent hernia or hernia at an incision site
- Dura: lumbosacral dural ectasia (2 points)

DIFFERENTIAL DIAGNOSIS

- Loeys-Dietz syndrome
- Homocystinuria
- Marfanoid habitus
- Marfanoid skeletal and skin features (MASS) phenotype
- Ehlers-Danlos syndrome
- Beal syndrome (congenital contractural arachnodactyly)

DIAGNOSTIC TESTS & INTERPRETATION

- Targeted-gene genetic testing to look for *FBN-1* mutation (1)[A]
- Genomic sequencing may be indicated when clinical picture is less convincing for Marfan syndrome.
- Drugs that may alter lab results: N/A
- Disorders that may alter lab results: N/A
- Plain radiographs of the spine are useful prior to skeletal maturity to detect and quantify scoliosis.
- Initial diagnostic echocardiogram, followed by serial screening echocardiograms, is recommended beginning in adolescence to look for dilatation of the aorta and valvular changes.
- Pathologic findings:
  - Cystic medial necrosis of the aorta
  - Myxomatous degeneration of the cardiac valves

TREATMENT

- Long-term treatment
- Acute treatment: outpatient

MEDICATION

First Line

- No specific medical therapy is available. Medications may be used to treat manifestations of Marfan syndrome.
- β-Blockers have been used to slow progression of aortic root dilatation.
- Angiotensin-converting-enzyme (ACE) inhibitors and calcium channel blockers have been used in patients who don't tolerate or fail to respond to β-blockers.
- Angiotensin II receptor blockers do not appear to be effective as adjunctive therapy in slowing aortic root dilatation (3,4)[A].
- Contraindications for β-blockers: asthma, depression, Raynaud phenomenon
- Precautions: Refer to the manufacturer's profile for each drug.
- Significant possible interactions: Refer to the manufacturer's profile for each drug.

ISSUES FOR REFERRAL

- In addition to health supervision visits with primary care physicians, individuals with Marfan syndrome should have regular follow-up with cardiology and ophthalmology (5)[C].
- Geneticists generally are involved in making the initial diagnosis.
- Orthopedic consultation is often helpful.
- Affected individuals should have echocardiograms every 6 to 12 mo to screen for the presence of aortic root dilatation and worsening valvular insufficiency.
- Skeletally immature patients should be offered the opportunity to meet with an endocrinologist if they would like to consider hormonal therapy to limit growth (5)[C].

ADDITIONAL THERAPIES

- Antibiotic prophylaxis for endocarditis prior to medical and dental procedures is not uniformly recommended for Marfan patients with mitral valve prolapse (6)[C].
- Individuals with significant valvular regurgitation/insufficiency should consult their cardiologists about the necessity of infective endocarditis prophylaxis for their specific conditions (6)[C].
- Antibiotic prophylaxis should be given to individuals with a prior history of infective endocarditis or a history of valve replacement or repair of the aorta using graft material (6)[C].

SURGERY/OTHER PROCEDURES

Cardiac surgery is often required for people with Marfan syndrome who have aortic root diameter >5 cm, rapid rate of aortic root dilatation, or significant aortic valve regurgitation (6)[C].

ONGOING CARE

FOLLOW-UP RECOMMENDATIONS

- Athletes with Marfan syndrome can participate in low to moderate static/low-dynamic sports as long as they do not have moderate or severe mitral regurgitation, left ventricular dysfunction, aortic root dilatation, and have no family history of aortic root >50 mm, aortic dissection, or sudden death owing to Marfan syndrome (6)[C].
- Individuals with Marfan syndrome should not participate in contact sports or weight lifting (6)[C].

Patient Monitoring

- Routine health maintenance visits with a primary care physician
- Regular follow-up with cardiology; athletes should have screening echocardiograms every 6 to 12 mo.
- Yearly ophthalmology follow-up owing to high rate of retinal detachment. Patients also have higher rates of myopia and glaucoma.

DIET

No special diet

PATIENT EDUCATION

Information is available from the National Marfan Foundation, 382 Main St., Port Washington, NY 11959; 800–8MARFAN, www.marfan.org.

PROGNOSIS

Life-threatening complications are cardiovascular. With the advancement of techniques to replace the aortic root, individuals with Marfan have a near-normal life span.

COMPLICATIONS

- Aortic dissection or aortic rupture
- Aortic valvular insufficiency owing to aortic root dilatation
- Mitral valve insufficiency, often associated with myxomatous change
- Bacterial endocarditis
- Spontaneous pneumothorax
- Retinal detachment

Pediatric Considerations

Early medical or surgical intervention may reduce the degree of scoliosis.

Pregnancy Considerations

Pregnant women with the Marfan syndrome need to be managed as high-risk patients, preferably with involvement of a cardiologist. The outcome is usually excellent.

REFERENCES

1. Faivre L, Masurel-Paulet A, Collod-Béroud G, et al. Clinical and molecular study of 320 children with Marfan syndrome and related type I fibrillinopathies in a series of 1009 probands with pathogenic FBN1 mutations. *Pediatrics*. 2009;123(1):391–398.
2. Loeys BL, Dietz HC, Braverman AC, et al. The revised Ghent nosology for the Marfan syndrome. *J Med Genet*. 2010;47(7):476–485.
3. Milleron O, Arnoult F, Ropers J, et al. Marfan Sartan: a randomized, double-blind, placebo-controlled trial. *Eur Heart J*. 2015;36(32):2160–2166.
4. Muiño-Mosquera L, De Nobele S, Devos D, et al. Efficacy of losartan as add-on therapy to prevent aortic growth and ventricular dysfunction in patients with Marfan syndrome: a randomized, double-blind clinical trial. *Acta Cardiol*. 2017;72(6):616–624.
5. Tinkle BT, Saal HM; for Committee on Genetics. Health supervision for children with Marfan syndrome. *Pediatrics*. 2013;132(4):e1059–e1072.
6. Braverman AC, Harris KM, Kovacs RJ, et al. Eligibility and disqualification recommendations for competitive athletes with cardiovascular abnormalities: Task Force 7: aortic diseases, including Marfan syndrome: a scientific statement from the American Heart Association and American College of Cardiology. *Circulation*. 2015;132(22):e303–e309.

CLINICAL PEARLS

- Clinicians should be on the lookout for the musculoskeletal manifestations of Marfan syndrome when performing preparticipation screening.
- Physicians should carefully evaluate individuals with increased arm span: height ratio (>1.05), characteristic facial features, and other stigmata of Marfan syndrome and consider referral to genetics, cardiology, and/or ophthalmology when appropriate.

MCP (METACARPOPHALANGEAL) COLLATERAL LIGAMENT SPRAIN

Jason L. Zaremski, MD, CAQSM, FAAPMR, FACSM

BASICS

DESCRIPTION

- Injury to the collateral ligaments of the metacarpophalangeal (MCP) joints; most commonly the MCP joint of the thumb
- An injury to the MCP ligament may result in a simple sprain to a complete tear of both proper and accessory ligaments.

EPIDEMIOLOGY

- Isolated injuries to collateral ligaments of the MCP joints are uncommon, except for those of the MCP joint of the thumb, which is the focus of this chapter.
- Ulnar collateral ligament (UCL) injuries of the MCP joint of the thumb (gamekeeper's thumb or skier's thumb) occur more often than radial collateral ligament (RCL) injuries (1).
- UCL sprain is the second most common injury encountered by skiers and most common ligamentous injury to the thumb.
- UCL injury incidence is ~50/100,000 (1).
- The ligamentous injury can occur either at the proximal or more commonly the distal attachment of the ligament.
- ~50% of these injuries will have an associated base of the proximal phalanx fracture.
- Acute UCL injury is seen frequently in athletes including ball-handling athletes and other contact sports participants.

COMMONLY ASSOCIATED CONDITIONS

- Complete rupture of the collateral ligament (proper and accessory) and volar plate (1,2)
- Stener lesion: The adductor pollicis aponeurosis is interposed between the torn end of the UCL (thumb) and its insertion into the base of the proximal phalanx, inhibiting healing (not seen in RCL complete tears) (2,3).
- Three types of avulsion fractures: small fragment at the base of the proximal phalanx; a large, intra-articular fracture that involves at least 25% of the articular surface of the base of the proximal phalanx; and an avulsion fracture involving the volar plate (2)
- Dislocation of the thumb MCP joint

DIAGNOSIS

HISTORY

- MCP collateral ligament sprain is most commonly an acute injury related to trauma.
- Mechanism of injury to the UCL of the MCP joint of the thumb is sudden, forced, radial deviation (abduction) and extension resulting in partial or complete tear of the ligament.
- Mechanism of injury to the RCL of the MCP joint of the thumb is force adduction or twisting of the flexed joint.
- Prompt diagnosis is the key to a good outcome.
- Chronic MCP collateral ligament sprain is usually secondary to a missed diagnosis from an earlier acute injury.

PHYSICAL EXAM

- Hallmark symptom of acute UCL injury is pain and swelling localized to the ulnar aspect of the MCP joint along the UCL.
- Acute injury: ecchymosis and pain over the ligament
- Chronic injuries may not be painful.
- A palpable mass may be present.
- Weakness of thumb; weakness with pinch noted with UCL injury (1)
- RCL injuries have pain and swelling localized to the radial aspect of the metacarpal head, and activities such as twisting open a jar lid can exacerbate the symptoms.
- A careful physical exam differentiates a sprain from a complete tear (1,2).
- Always compare with asymptomatic thumb (1).
- Examine the joint for swelling, ecchymosis, and areas of tenderness.
- Anteroposterior (AP) and lateral radiographs should be obtained prior to stressing the joint because a nondisplaced fracture can be displaced as a result of the stress.
- If radiographs are negative, the stability of the ligament should be tested.
- Test the ligaments by applying radial stress (UCL) or ulnar stress (RCL) to the MCP joint in full extension and in 30 degrees of flexion.
- A collateral ligament injury should be suspected if during stress testing, a firm end point is lacking.
- Valgus stress of the flexed MCP joint with opening of ≥30 degrees or 15 degrees greater than the contralateral thumb indicates collateral ligament proper complete rupture; <30 degrees of laxity assume a partial tear (1).
- Valgus stress of the extended MCP joint with opening of ≥30 degrees suggests an accessory collateral ligament tear or volar plate tear (1).

ALERT

If unable to make a clear distinction on clinical exam, stress ultrasound or magnetic resonance imaging (MRI) is indicated.

DIFFERENTIAL DIAGNOSIS

- Grade 1 sprain = pain but no instability
- Grade 2 sprain = partial tear with laxity but firm end point with valgus testing
- Complete tear of collateral ligament (grade 3)
- Dislocation of the thumb MCP joint
- Fracture

DIAGNOSTIC TESTS & INTERPRETATION

- AP and lateral radiographs of the thumb to evaluate for a fracture (1,2)
- Stress radiographs are controversial because there is concern for displacement of nondisplaced ligaments or fractures (1,3).
- Additional radiographic signs that indicate a complete rupture are volar subluxation of the proximal phalanx seen on lateral view and radial deviation of the proximal phalanx seen on AP view ("Sag Sign").

ALERT
Stress films are contraindicated in children because of risk of Salter-Harris fractures.

- MRI and ultrasound (US) may be used to evaluate for a ligament injury and Stener lesion (4).

TREATMENT

GENERAL MEASURES

- Analgesia: nonsteroidal anti-inflammatory drugs (NSAIDs), ice
- Non–thumb-related collateral ligament sprains, depending on severity, can be splinted immobilized or "buddy taped" (2)[C].
- No detectable instability: immobilization (thumb spica splint) for 2 to 4 wk dependent on severity (1)[C]
- Partial tear with stable joint: thumb spica splint or cast for 4 to 6 wk depending on severity of the injury (2)[C]; thumb is immobilized in slight flexion in the spica cast; the interphalangeal joint is not immobilized to allow active motion and prevent scarring of the extension mechanism.
- Complete tear: Repair surgically (5)[A].
- Avulsion fracture: small avulsions that are not intra-articular can be treated nonoperatively; nondisplaced fractures, thumb spica cast (application as above) for 4 to 6 wk (5)[B]
- Avulsion fracture: Rotated, displaced, or large intra-articular fragments require surgical repair (5)[A].
- Surgical repair is necessary for Stener lesion; failure to recognize this injury or inadequate treatment can result in chronic instability (5)[A].

ISSUES FOR REFERRAL

Prompt referral to an orthopedist or hand surgeon is indicated for all but uncomplicated injuries.

ADDITIONAL THERAPIES

- When the cast is removed, range of motion (ROM) exercises are performed several times a day; a removable splint is worn for an additional time dependent on severity of injury.
- Sports participation: Protect the thumb for ~3 mo with splinting (6).
- Return to sport and play in a splint is dependent on sport-specific needs of the athlete (6).

SURGERY/OTHER PROCEDURES

ALERT

- Surgical treatment is recommended for fractures that are displaced, rotated, or have significant articular involvement.
- Surgical repair is necessary for complete ligament tears and Stener lesions.
- The goal of surgery is restoration of anatomy and joint stability.

ONGOING CARE

COMPLICATIONS

Inadequate treatment of UCL thumb injuries may result in chronic painful instability, weakness of pinch, and arthritis (6).

REFERENCES

1. Avery DM III, Inkellis ER, Carlson MG. Thumb collateral ligament injuries in the athlete. *Curr Rev Musculoskelet Med*. 2017;10(1):28–37.
2. Carlsen BT, Moran SL. Thumb trauma: Bennett fractures, Rolando fractures, and ulnar collateral ligament injuries. *J Hand Surg Am*. 2009;34(5):945–952.
3. McKeon KE, Gelberman RH, Calfee RP. Ulnar collateral ligament injuries of the thumb: phalangeal translation during valgus stress in human cadavera. *J Bone Joint Surg Am*. 2013;95(10):881–887.
4. Arend CF, da Silva TR. The role of US in the evaluation of clinically suspected ulnar collateral ligament injuries of the thumb: spectrum of findings and differential diagnosis. *Acta Radiol*. 2014;55(7):814–823.
5. Samora JB, Harris JD, Griesser MJ, et al. Outcomes after injury to the thumb ulnar collateral ligament—a systematic review. *Clin J Sport Med*. 2013;23(4):247–254.
6. Goldfarb CA, Puri SK, Carlson MG. Diagnosis, treatment, and return to play for four common sports injuries of the hand and wrist. *J Am Acad Orthop Surg*. 2016;24(12):853–862.

CLINICAL PEARLS

- Acute (thumb) UCL injuries are common injuries in all athletes.
- The MOI is a sudden, forced, radial deviation (abduction).
- Timely diagnosis is important to determine the severity of the injury and immobilization timeframe.
- If a displaced avulsion and/or Stener lesion is present, prompt referral to an orthopedist or hand surgeon is recommended.

MCP (METACARPOPHALANGEAL) DISLOCATION

Jessica Stumbo, MD, CAQSM • Steven T. Brown, MD

BASICS

- The metacarpophalangeal (MCP) joints are relatively stable joints, especially in flexion.
- Stability is provided by collateral ligaments on either side of the joint or the volar plate. The collateral ligaments are lax in extension and taut in flexion. The volar plate has a firm distal attachment to the proximal phalanx and a less stable proximal attachment to the metacarpal. It is the proximal attachment that is disrupted in a dislocation (1,2,3).
- The index finger, thumb, and 5th finger are most vulnerable to dislocations.

DESCRIPTION

- An MCP joint dislocation involves dislocation of the proximal phalanx in relation to the distal metacarpal.
- Requires disruption of stabilizing structures
- Dislocations may occur dorsally (most common), laterally (uncommon), or volarly (rare).
- The typical mechanism for a dorsal dislocation is hyperextension at the MCP joint:
  - With hyperextension, there is rupture of the volar plate from its proximal attachment, and due to the anatomy of the joint, there is also proximal dorsal translocation of the base of the proximal phalanx over the distal metacarpal (4).
- The neurovascular bundle is located anterior to the lumbrical muscle and metacarpal head, placing it at risk for injury during traumatic dislocation (1).

ALERT

Classification of dislocations (4):

- Simple dorsal: Articular surfaces are in partial contact, and there is no soft tissue interposed in the joint.
- Complex dorsal: The volar plate or other tissue is interposed between articular surfaces and is, by definition, an irreducible dislocation.
- Lateral: Results from an injury to the collateral ligament, either ulnar collateral ligament (UCL) or radial collateral ligament (RCL). The collateral ligaments of the thumb are more commonly injured than the collateral ligaments of the fingers (5).
- Volar: rare, but may result from severe or repetitive blows to knuckle, leading to rupture of dorsal capsule with subsequent volar displacement of the proximal phalanx

EPIDEMIOLOGY

- MCP dislocations are much less common than proximal interphalangeal (IP) dislocations because of support from surrounding structures and protected position (2).
- Usually occurs in index finger, thumb, or 5th finger
- Nearly always, a single digit but multiple digits may be involved.

RISK FACTORS

- Contact and ball-handling sports
- Prior history of injury or dislocation

DIAGNOSIS

HISTORY

- Will complain of pain, loss of function, and usually an obvious deformity
- Dorsal dislocation generally results from forced hyperextension of digit, as in striking the heel of an opponent while diving to make a tackle, or a fall on an outstretched hand (1,2)[C].
- Lateral dislocation is caused by an ulnar or radially directed blow to the MCP joint, usually while in a flexed position (2)[C].
- Volar dislocation may be seen with punching in boxing and martial arts.

PHYSICAL EXAM

- Evaluate and document neurovascular status before and after reduction attempts.
- With dorsal dislocations, the metacarpal head is volarly displaced and will be easily palpable in the palm (1)[C].
- Simple dorsal: There is obvious deformity, with the phalanx resting at 60 to 90 degrees of hyperextension over the head of the metacarpal (4)[C].
- Complex dorsal: much more subtle deformity, with only slight hyperextension (10 to 15 degrees) of the phalanx; may find dimpling or puckering of the palmar aspect of the finger where the volar plate is caught between the ends of the bones (proximal phalanx and head of metacarpal). This is pathognomonic for a complex dislocation; slight ulnar deviation of the involved digit also may be noted (1,4)[C].
- Lateral: swelling and tenderness along the ulnar or radial side of the MCP joint; assess for injury and laxity of the collateral ligaments by stressing the ligament with the MCP joint in flexion (5)[C].
- Volar: obvious deformity, with the phalanx positioned palmar to metacarpal

DIFFERENTIAL DIAGNOSIS

- Fracture of phalanx or metacarpal
- Tendon rupture
- Disruption of volar plate

DIAGNOSTIC TESTS & INTERPRETATION

- Anteroposterior (AP), lateral, and oblique views of involved digit (not the entire hand) generally show deformity, joint space widening, and any accompanying fracture.
- Brewerton view (MCP joint flexed to 65 degrees, with the dorsum of the proximal phalanx flat against the film cassette and the beam angled 15 degrees ulnar to radial) helpful in identifying collateral ligament avulsion fractures and fractures of the metacarpal head (2,5)[C]

ALERT

- Presence of a sesamoid in the widened joint space of the involved digit is pathognomonic for a complex dorsal dislocation (because sesamoids are embedded in the volar plate) (1)[C].
- In skeletally immature patients, it is important to image the contralateral side to adequately evaluate for growth plate injuries.
- In skeletally mature patients, stress radiographs are sometimes used. Stress x-rays should only be done after static x-rays to prevent nondisplaced fractures from becoming displaced fractures. In the thumb, MCP joint laxity >30 to 35 degrees on stress x-rays is usually associated with a complete collateral ligament tear. Stress x-rays are not typically used in the skeletally immature patient because those patients are more likely to have a growth plate injury.
- Postreduction views: AP, lateral, and oblique to evaluate for joint congruity and/or fracture

ALERT

Up to 50% of MCP joint dislocations may have a concomitant fracture of the proximal phalanx base and/or the metacarpal head.

TREATMENT

- Anesthesia:
  - Various methods of anesthesia can be used for reduction, including local intra-articular, regional block, or intravenous (IV) sedation. Typically for intra-articular injections, a short-acting local anesthetic such as 1% lidocaine without epinephrine is used, although a longer acting agent such as bupivacaine may also be used. It is important to document neurovascular status prior to the administration of the anesthetic agent.
  - Usually not necessary for simple dislocations but intra-articular anesthesia or wrist block may facilitate reduction and prevent false conclusion that dislocation is complex if patient prevents reduction due to pain.
  - For complex dislocations, digital block or general anesthesia in the operating room may be necessary if closed reduction is to be attempted.
  - Evaluate and document neurovascular status before and after reduction.

ALERT

- In general, reduction of dorsal MCP dislocations differs from most other dislocations in that distal traction should be avoided. By using traction, a simple dislocation can be converted to a complex one because the volar plate gets displaced and locked within the joint space (1,2)[C].
- Simple dorsal: First, relax flexors by placing wrist and IP joints into flexion; next, accentuate dislocation slightly by hyperextending proximal phalanx to 90 degrees (controversial), and then push base of proximal phalanx distally over the articular surface of the metacarpal into flexion while maintaining contact with metacarpal head to prevent entrapment of the volar plate (thus converting a simple dislocation into a complex one) (2)[C].

- Reduction:
  - Complex dorsal: Attempt at closed reduction is warranted but usually not successful; reduction technique is similar to that of a simple dislocation (2)[C].
  - Lateral: Closed reduction is usually accomplished with gentle longitudinal traction, taking care not to interpose any soft tissue.
  - Volar: Generally, reduction is performed open because of concomitant dorsal hood injury needs repair.
  - Reasons for failed closed reductions: Volar plate is interposed in the joint space or metacarpal head has buttonholed through the palmar structures (1)[C].
  - Evaluate tendon and ligament function. With thumb MCP dislocations, it is very important to assess the integrity and stability of the collateral ligaments, particularly the UCL.
  - Postreduction imaging: AP, lateral, and oblique radiographs of the involved digit to evaluate for joint congruity and/or fracture
  - Simple dorsal: Dorsal blocking splint to prevent extension beyond neutral with the MCP joint in 50 to 70 degrees of flexion for 7 to 10 days if no evidence of significant instability; buddy taping also may be implemented. Active flexion exercises are permitted. With thumb MCP dislocations, a thumb spica splint is used for immobilization (1)[C].
  - Complex dorsal: Postoperative immobilization is at the prerogative of the surgeon (ranges from buddy taping for 4 to 6 wk to immobilization in 60 degrees of flexion).
  - Lateral: Majority of complete ligamentous injuries are splinted in 30 to 50 degrees of MCP flexion for 2 to 4 wk followed by buddy taping; with significant instability especially of the border digits, primary surgical repair of the collateral ligament may be considered. Incomplete MCP collateral ligament injuries and complete tears in nonborder digits are usually treated with buddy taping and early range of motion (ROM) exercises (5)[C].
  - Volar: Postoperative management varies and is at the prerogative of the surgeon.

MEDICATION

- Nonsteroidal anti-inflammatory drugs (NSAIDs) for pain relief
- If surgery is planned, may consider acetaminophen to avoid potential bleeding risks

ADDITIONAL THERAPIES

- PRICE: protection, rest, ice, compression, elevation
- In dislocations of the thumb, assessment of the UCL is essential. With a hyperextension/hyperabduction injury, a Stener lesion can result. A Stener lesion occurs when the adductor aponeurosis becomes interposed between the torn end of the UCL and its bony attachment on the proximal phalanx. Spontaneous healing cannot occur, because the ligament is no longer in contact with its bony attachment (3).
- Occupational therapy may be indicated in more severe injuries.
- Dorsal dislocations that are stable postreduction need to be placed in a dorsal extension blocking splint to prevent extension beyond neutral and hyperextension. This position allows the volar plate to heal. Time frame is variable but typically 2 to 3 wk. While in the extension blocking splint, active ROM is encouraged to prevent joint stiffness.
- Thumb MCP dislocations require immobilization in a forearm-based thumb spica splint or cast for 4 to 6 wk.
- Initial therapy will focus on control of pain and swelling. General progression through rehab includes regaining full active ROM, followed by strengthening, and then function (activities of daily living and work-/sport-specific functions).
- If the injury can be properly protected in a splint or cast, an athlete may be able to return to activities immediately. Otherwise, after the injury has healed (3 to 6 wk), an athlete can return to play with buddy taping for 1 to 3 more wk for additional protection.

SURGERY/OTHER PROCEDURES

Surgery is often necessary for reduction, specifically for the complex dorsal and volar dislocations, as discussed above, and may be indicated for repair of severely damaged structures in other forms of dislocation (i.e., complete tear of UCL or RCL in lateral MCP joint dislocation) (6)[B].

ONGOING CARE

FOLLOW-UP RECOMMENDATIONS

After successful closed reduction, most MCP dislocations should be followed up with an orthopedic surgeon or hand surgeon within a week.

PATIENT EDUCATION

Warn patients that finger and hand swelling can take months to resolve.

PROGNOSIS

Prognosis of most MCP dislocations is good if identified early and managed appropriately.

COMPLICATIONS

- Joint stiffness and/or flexion contracture
- Degenerative/posttraumatic arthritis
- Avascular necrosis
- Osteochondral fracture
- Tendon adhesions/stiffness
- Ligamentous laxity
- Damage to the neurovascular bundle during open reduction, especially when using a volar approach
- Premature closure of the physeal plate (rare) (1,2,6)

REFERENCES

1. Dinh P, Franklin A, Hutchinson B, et al. Metacarpophalangeal joint dislocation. *J Am Acad Orthop Surg*. 2009;17(5):318–324.
2. Hubbard LF. Metacarpophalangeal dislocations. *Hand Clin*. 1988;4(1):39–44.
3. Owings FP, Calandruccio JH, Mauck BM. Thumb ligament injuries in the athlete. *Orthop Clin North Am*. 2016;47(4):799–807.
4. Schupp CM, Rand SE, Hanson TW, et al. Sideline management of joint dislocations. *Curr Sports Med Rep*. 2016;15(3):140–153.
5. Lourie GM, Gaston RG, Freeland AE. Collateral ligament injuries of the metacarpophalangeal joints of the fingers. *Hand Clin*. 2006;22(3):357–364.
6. Rubin G, Orbach H, Rinott M, et al. Complex dorsal metacarpophalangeal dislocation: long-term follow-up. *J Hand Surg Am*. 2016;41(8):e229–e233.

ADDITIONAL READING

- Ashkenaze DM, Ruby LK. Metacarpal fractures and dislocations. *Orthop Clin North Am*. 1992;23(1):19–33.
- Lee SJ, Montgomery K. Athletic hand injuries. *Orthop Clin North Am*. 2002;33(3):547–554.
- Palmer RE. Joint injuries of the hand in athletes. *Clin Sports Med*. 1998;17(3):513–531.
- Rettig AC. Athletic injuries of the wrist and hand: part II: overuse injuries of the wrist and traumatic injuries to the hand. *Am J Sports Med*. 2004;32(1):262–273.
- Shah SS, Techy F, Mejia A, et al. Ligamentous and capsular injuries to the metacarpophalangeal joints of the hand. *J Surg Orthop Adv*. 2012;21(3):141–146.

SEE ALSO

MCP (Metacarpophalangeal) Collateral Ligament Sprain; Thumb Ulnar Collateral Ligament Sprain (Skier's Thumb)

CLINICAL PEARLS

- Dorsal dislocations are the most common type of MCP joint dislocations.
- When attempting to reduce a dorsal MCP joint dislocation, do not use distal traction; risk converting simple dislocation to a complex one
- In general, complex dorsal and volar MCP joint dislocations require surgery.

MEDIAL COLLATERAL LIGAMENT TEAR

Claudia Dal Molin, DO • Delmas Bolin, MD, PhD, FACSM

BASICS

ANATOMY:

- The medial collateral ligament (MCL) has a single origin on the femur but two separate insertions on the tibia (1).
- The distal attachment of the superficial MCL is just >6 cm distal to the joint line (1).
- The superficial component is the primary restraint to valgus stress (1).
- The deep portion has a direct connection to medial meniscus (1):
  - It connects with the posteromedial corner (PMC) structures and is a secondary stabilizer in resisting external rotation and anterior-posterior translation of the knee (1).

DESCRIPTION

- Tension injury to the MCL occurs most commonly with a valgus stress (i.e., a blow to the lateral knee).
- Grade of injury classified by symptoms and physical exam by degree of joint opening with applied valgus stress at 0 degree and 30 degrees of flexion (1)
- I—minimal fiber tearing, localized tenderness, no instability (0 to 5 mm of laxity)
- II—greater degree of ligamentous tearing, slight to moderate abnormal motion (6 to 10 mm of laxity)
- III—complete tear, demonstrable instability (>10 mm of laxity)

EPIDEMIOLOGY

- MCL is the most frequently injured ligament of the knee (2).
- The most injurious sports are contact sports (e.g., wrestling, hockey, martial arts) (2).
- Intercollegiate athletes are at greater risk than intramural athletes (2).

COMMONLY ASSOCIATED CONDITIONS

- Medial meniscal tear
- Anterior cruciate ligament (ACL) tear
- Posterior oblique ligament (POL)/PMC injury
- Dislocation of the knee (rare)
- Patellar dislocation

DIAGNOSIS

HISTORY

- Mechanisms of injury:
  - Closed chain injury:
    - In contact/collision sports, an acute blow to the lateral aspect of the knee when the foot is planted results in valgus stress.
  - Open chain injury:
    - In kicking sports, the injury may be seen in players who are struck on the instep while passing the ball.
    - Skiers can injure the MCL by a noncontact valgus external rotation injury.
    - Overuse injuries to the MCL have been reported in breaststroke swimmers.
- History of a "pop" is concerning for an associated meniscal or ACL injury.
- Because the MCL is an extra-articular structure, the presence of an effusion is concerning for an associated intra-articular injury.
- Ask if the knee feels "loose" or if it is "moving in ways it wasn't intended to."

PHYSICAL EXAM

- INSPECTION: Note any antalgic gait, ecchymosis, swelling, effusion, presence of deformity. In pediatric patients, ecchymosis and swelling are concerning for a physeal injury.
- PALPATION: Check for tenderness to palpation over the entire medial joint line and along the MCL from the adductor tubercle to its insertion on the anteromedial proximal tibia. Evaluate the entire knee to avoid missing concomitant injuries.
- RANGE OF MOTION (ROM): Assess for any deficit of extension or flexion. ROM deficits or a locked knee can be a sign of a more serious concomitant injury (e.g., bucket handle meniscal tear).
- LIGAMENTOUS EXAM:
  - Valgus stress at 0 degree and at 20 degrees. Laxity at 20 degrees alone indicates an isolated MCL injury. Laxity at both 0 degree and 20 degrees indicates an injury to the MCL and POL, knee capsule, and/or ACL (1).
  - Compare to the unaffected side.
  - Clinical grading: 1st degree = pain without laxity; 2nd degree = pain and laxity but firm endpoint; 3rd degree = no endpoint is present (1).
  - Estimate joint line opening—if >10 mm, coexisting intra-articular pathology (torn ACL or meniscus) will be present 80% of the time (1).
  - Assess for POL injury, which can lead to anteromedial rotatory instability (AMRI) and posterior horn meniscal tears. Estimate the amount of anteromedial tibial rotation by performing the anterior drawer test with the foot in both neutral and in 15 degrees of external rotation (1).
  - Evaluate all other ligamentous structures (Lachman test, posterior drawer test, varus stress).
- SPECIAL TESTS: In addition to the above, a McMurray exam should be used to evaluate for meniscal injury.
- NEUROVASCULAR EXAM: Popliteal nerve and artery injuries can occur with multiligament injuries and should not be missed.

DIFFERENTIAL DIAGNOSIS

- Medial meniscal tear
- Medial knee contusion (soft tissue or bony)
- Patellar instability (subluxation or dislocation)
- Fracture of the distal femoral or proximal tibial physis
- Tibial plateau fracture

DIAGNOSTIC TESTS & INTERPRETATION

- RADIOGRAPHY—standard weight-bearing knee series (anteroposterior [AP], notch, lateral, and sunrise views) are typically normal but can identify avulsions or osteochondral injuries. A Pellegrini-Stieda lesion is a calcification of the proximal MCL that can be seen in chronic injuries.
- Magnetic resonance imaging (MRI)—T2-weighted imaging is the gold standard for viewing edema and fiber continuity. Associated bone contusions (45% of MCL injuries) and concomitant injuries can also be seen.

TREATMENT

GENERAL MEASURES

- GRADE I and II INJURIES:
  - PRICE (protection, rest, ice, compression, elevation) and nonsteroidal anti-inflammatory drugs (NSAIDs) are first line.
  - Weight-bearing as tolerated, with or without assistive devices based on comfort (1,3)[C]
  - The clinical utility of bracing is unclear but may help with comfort. A hinged knee brace is often used for comfort and support. An extension block of 15 to 20 degrees in the first 1 to 2 wk can potentially encourage healing in an anatomically shortened position. The brace can then be unlocked and weaned as tolerated if this mode of bracing is used. Braces can typically be discontinued in 3 to 12 wk depending on the severity of the injury and clinical course (1,3)[C].

- Active ROM is started immediately (1,3)[C].
- Strengthening exercises are started immediately, progressing from static to dynamic as tolerated. Both open and closed chain exercises are used.
- Proprioception, agility, and sport-specific training can begin when full ROM and functional strength are regained (1,3)[C].
- Athletes typically return to play in 1 to 4 wk. Criteria include resolution of tenderness, full and pain free ROM and strength, and successful progression of sport-specific drills (1,3)[C].

- GRADE III INJURIES:
  - Isolated acute grade III injuries to the medial knee are often successfully treated nonoperatively. Operative treatment can be considered in specific situations involving complete ligament disruption, including intra-articular entrapment of the end of the ligament, a large bony avulsion injury, a tibial plateau fracture, a complete tibial side avulsion in athletes, or when AMRI is present (1,3)[C].
  - Nonoperative management follows the same management principles outlined above in grade I and II injuries (1,3)[C]:
    - A period of non–weight-bearing is used initially (1 to 3 wk).
    - Early bracing may be preferred in order to reapproximate disrupted fibers and facilitate healing. Some providers lock the knee in extension, whereas others limit parts of ROM (90 degrees flexion block vs. terminal extension block at 20 degrees).
    - Avoid valgus and external rotation forces during the acute phase of healing (typically the first 3 to 4 wk).
    - Strengthening exercises can begin once painless and full ROM is achieved. Progression to proprioceptive, agility, and sport-specific drills occurs similarly to grade I and II injuries.
    - Athletes typically return to play in 5 to 7 wk.
- There are a subset of patients who do not clinically improve with conservative measures. It is possible that these patients have a PMC injury with a component of AMRI. These patients can benefit from reconstruction (4)[A].
- EXPERIMENTAL OPTIONS:
  - Platelet-rich plasma (PRP) injections can be considered in injuries refractory to conservative management as long as continued instability and AMRI don't appear to be present (typically grades I and II with persistent pain) (5)[C].
  - Evidence for PRP injections in MCL injuries is limited to case studies and studies using animal models.
- COMBINED MCL/ACL INJURIES:
  - Early referral to orthopedics
  - MRI is helpful.
  - Surgical approach remains controversial, but most authors recommend ACL reconstruction after a period of rehabilitation to allow the MCL to heal. This approach has been shown to minimize postoperative arthrofibrosis. Initial rehab mirrors that of grade III MCL injuries for the first 5 to 7 wk while ACL reconstruction is typically delayed. Time is given for swelling to improve and for full ROM to be regained.
  - ACL/MCL reconstruction may be recommended for excessive valgus laxity. These patients typically require a more substantial initial period of non–weight-bearing.

MEDICATION

Short-term use of NSAIDs can help decrease pain and swelling. There is evidence that NSAID therapy can impair bone fracture healing and tendon-to-bone (enthesis) healing. The effects of specific NSAIDs on ligament healing are variable, with most data originating from animal model studies (6)[C].

ONGOING CARE

COMPLICATIONS

The Pellegrini-Stieda lesion can be seen on radiographs. It represents calcification of the previously injured MCL.

REFERENCES

1. Stannard JP. Evaluation and treatment of medial instability of the knee. *Sports Med Arthrosc Rev*. 2015;23(2):91–95.
2. Roach CJ, Haley CA, Cameron KL, et al. The epidemiology of medial collateral ligament sprains in young athletes. *Am J Sports Med*. 2014;42(5):1103–1109.
3. Weber AE, Kopydlowski NJ, Sekiya JK. Nonsurgical management and postoperative rehabilitation of medial instability of the knee. *Sports Med Athrosc Rev*. 2015;23(2):104–109.
4. Varelas AN, Erickson BJ, Cvetanovich GL, et al. Medial collateral ligament reconstruction in patients with medial knee instability: a systematic review. *Orthop J Sports Med*. 2017;5(5):2325967117703920.
5. Yoshida M, Marumo K. An autologous leukocyte-reduced platelet-rich plasma therapy for chronic jury of the medial collateral ligament in the knee: a report of 3 successful cases [published online ahead of print November 29, 2017]. *Clin J Sport Med*. doi:10.1097/JSM.0000000000000515.
6. Su B, O'Connor JP. NSAID therapy effects on healing of bone, tendon, and the enthesis. *J Appl Physiol (1985)*. 2013;115(6):892–899.

ADDITIONAL READING

- Roth J, Taylor DC. Management of acute isolated medial and posteromedial instability of the knee. *Sports Med Arthrosc Rev*. 2015;23(2):71–76.
- Westermann RW, Spindler KP, Hettrich CM, et al. Outcomes following ACL and grade III MCL injuries: is there a role for MCL repair? *Orthop J Sports Med*. 2017;5(3 Suppl 3):2325967117S00126.

CLINICAL PEARLS

Common questions and answers:

- Q: How long until I can play again?
- A: For most sports, athletes with grade I injuries return in an average of 10 days. Those with grade II sprains may return in as little as 2 to 3 wk. Grade III injuries can take 5 to 7 wk for full recovery. Sport can influence speed of return: Soccer players may require more time because of the use of the instep to kick and pass the ball. Operative treatment of combined injuries can take 6 to 12 mo.
- Q: Should I wear a brace?
- A: Bracing is typically used for all grades of MCL injuries. Grade III injuries can require a full year of bracing depending on the athlete and injury. Prophylactic bracing is controversial. Use hasn't demonstrated a clinically significant trend to MCL injury prevention.
- Q: Will I get early arthritis?
- A: A 10-yr follow-up on isolated MCL injuries suggests that most patients have excellent function and no major radiographic evidence of arthritis.
- Q: Will it always bother me?
- A: After rehabilitation, most patients note only minor symptoms, if any at all. 10-yr studies show most perform well with only minor decreases in physical ability.

MEDIAL EPICONDYLITIS

Emily B. Porter, MD, ATC • Craig C. Young, MD

BASICS

DESCRIPTION

Medial epicondylitis is clinically defined as pain at the medial epicondyle due to repetitive flexion and pronation at the elbow. A more accurate term may be *medial epicondylosis* or *epicondylalgia*. It is usually an overuse injury that can affect both athletes and nonathletes. *Golfer's elbow* is a common term used for medial epicondylitis.

EPIDEMIOLOGY

- Diagnosed less often than lateral epicondylitis, a similar condition affecting the origin of the common extensor tendon on the lateral epicondyle
- Overall prevalence of <1% in general population but may be as high as 3.8–8.2% in occupational settings (1)[C]
- Diagnosis is often made in the 4th and 5th decades, although the condition has been seen in patients ranging from 12 to 80 yr of age.
- Men and women are affected equally.
- The dominant hand is most often affected.

ETIOLOGY AND PATHOPHYSIOLOGY

- Initially thought to be an inflammatory process, but histologic studies do not show inflammatory cells in chronic epicondylitis.
- Inflammation may play a role in the initial acute injury when microtearing of the tendon occurs.
- Histologic studies of chronic epicondylitis have shown abnormal collagen architecture due to a fibroblastic and immature vascular response, which causes incomplete tendon repair.
- Degenerative changes often seen in the pronator teres and flexor carpi radialis muscles and their tendons:
  - Palmaris longus, flexor digitorum superficialis, and flexor carpi ulnaris may also be involved.
- Common causes:
  - Activities that involve forceful and/or continuous wrist flexion and/or forearm pronation or a large amount of stabilization—especially with forearm supinated (2)[B], such as racquet sports, swimming, swinging a golf club, throwing, playing tennis, waterskiing, using a computer keyboard, or playing piano
  - Certain occupations (carpenters, plumbers, meat cutters, etc.) may be more at risk.

DIAGNOSIS

HISTORY

- Pain and tenderness along the medial elbow, extending into the forearm, which worsen with resisted forearm pronation or wrist flexion at 90 degrees of elbow flexion and/or full elbow extension
- Difficulty gripping without pain
- Decreased wrist strength
- Tightness/stiffness when stretching elbow and wrist

PHYSICAL EXAM

- Tenderness to palpation over the medial epicondyle, pronator teres, and flexor carpi radialis
- Local swelling and warmth may be present.
- Active and resisted range of motion may be full or limited depending on the severity of the injury.

DIFFERENTIAL DIAGNOSIS

- Entrapment neuropathy (i.e., cubital tunnel syndrome, carpal tunnel syndrome)
- Ulnar neuritis
- Ulnar collateral ligament (UCL) insufficiency
- Medial elbow apophysitis (i.e., "Little Leaguer's elbow")
- Inflammatory arthritis
- Cervical radiculopathy
- Thoracic outlet syndrome
- Myofascial pain

DIAGNOSTIC TESTS & INTERPRETATION

- Generally not needed for initial evaluation
- In cases that are refractory to treatment or where the diagnosis is in question, basic elbow x-rays followed by ultrasound (US) or magnetic resonance imaging (MRI) may be considered.

TREATMENT

- More studies are needed specifically on medial epicondylitis; most studies focus on treatment of lateral epicondylitis. Many of these treatments are used for medial epicondylitis as well.
- Initial treatment includes relative rest, ice, and acetaminophen or over-the-counter (OTC) nonsteroidal anti-inflammatory drugs (NSAIDs) as needed.
- The mainstay of treatment involves stretching and strengthening with progression to eccentric training exercise with or without formal physical therapy (3)[A].
- Bracing may be helpful.
- If no improvement in 6 wk, consider obtaining x-rays and initiating formal physical therapy.
- If still symptomatic, consider injection. Various techniques have been proposed, including dry needling of tendon, corticosteroid injection, or use of newer techniques, including prolotherapy or injection of platelet-rich plasma or autologous blood (4)[A].
- Other treatments to consider include nitric oxide via topical nitroglycerin, extracorporeal shock wave therapy, or percutaneous ultrasonic tenotomy performed under local anesthesia (4,5)[A],(6)[B].
- If symptoms persist, consider advanced imaging with US or MRI to confirm diagnosis.
- Rarely, recalcitrant symptoms >6 mo in duration may require surgical intervention.

ONGOING CARE

Home exercise program as follows:

- Strengthening:
  - Stay below the level of pain.
  - Perform two to three sets of 10 to 15 repetitions 2 to 4 times a week. Once three sets of 15 repetitions can be performed easily, increase the weight, reduce the repetitions to 10, and build back up to 15.
  - Wrist extension curls: With the forearm supported on a firm surface and the palm facing downward, lift and lower the weight.
  - Wrist flexion curls: With the forearm supported on a firm surface and the palm facing upward, lift and lower the weight.
  - Forearm pronation/supination: With the forearm supported on a firm surface, turn the palm up and then down while holding onto a weight.
  - Gripping: Gently grip a rubber ball, a towel, or putty and then advance to items with more resistance. Perform 10 to 30 repetitions, increasing in intensity once 30 repetitions can be performed.
  - Finger extension: Wrap a rubber band around the outside of all the fingers and thumb, gently extend the hand by opening the fingers, and then close the fingers. Perform 10 to 30 repetitions.
- Stretching:
  - Keep the stretch to a comfortable level.
  - Hold each stretch for ~30 sec.
  - Repeat each stretch 3 to 6 times.
  - Wrist flexion stretch: Bend the involved wrist down gently by grasping it with the other hand until a pulling sensation is felt. Keep the elbow straight.
  - Wrist flexion stretch (advanced): same as for the wrist flexion stretch but with the addition of wrist movement toward the side of the little finger
  - Wrist extension stretch: Bend the involved wrist up gently by grasping it with the opposite hand until a pulling sensation is felt. Keep the elbow straight.

REFERENCES

1. Amin NH, Kumar NS, Schickendantz MS. Medial epicondylitis: evaluation and management. *J Am Acad Orthop Surg*. 2015;23(6):348–355.
2. Rosa D, Di Donato SL, Balato G, et al. Supinated forearm is correlated with the onset of medial epicondylitis in professional slalom water-skiers. *Muscles Ligaments Tendons J*. 2016;6(1):140–146.
3. Hoogvliet P, Randsdorp MS, Dingemanse R, et al. Does effectiveness of exercise therapy and mobilisation techniques offer guidance for the treatment of lateral and medial epicondylitis? A systematic review. *Br J Sports Med*. 2013;47(17):1112–1119.
4. Hussain N, Johal H, Bhandari M. An evidence-based evaluation on the use of platelet rich plasma in orthopedics—a review of the literature. *SICOT J*. 2017;3:57.
5. Gambito ED, Gonzalez-Suarez CB, Oquiñena TI, et al. Evidence on the effectiveness of topical nitroglycerin in the treatment of tendinopathies: a systematic review and meta-analysis. *Arch Phys Med Rehabil*. 2010;91(8):1291–1305.
6. Barnes DE, Beckley JM, Smith J. Percutaneous ultrasonic tenotomy for chronic elbow tendinosis: a prospective study. *J Shoulder Elbow Surg*. 2015;24(1):67–73.

ADDITIONAL READING

- Gündüz R, Malas FÜ, Borman P, et al. Physical therapy, corticosteroid injection, and extracorporeal shock wave treatment in lateral epicondylitis. Clinical and ultrasonographical comparison. *Clin Rheumatol*. 2012;31(5):807–812.
- Han SH, Lee JK, Kim HJ, et al. The result of surgical treatment of medial epicondylitis: analysis with more than a 5-year follow-up. *J Shoulder Elbow Surg*. 2016;25(10):1704–1709.
- Paoloni JA, Appleyard RC, Nelson J, et al. Topical nitric oxide application in the treatment of chronic extensor tendinosis at the elbow: a randomized, double-blinded, placebo-controlled clinical trial. *Am J Sports Med*. 2003;31(6):915–920.
- Stasinopoulos D, Stasinopoulos I. Comparison of effects of eccentric training, eccentric-concentric training, and eccentric-concentric training combined with isometric contraction in the treatment of lateral elbow tendinopathy. *J Hand Ther*. 2017;30(1):13–19.
- Suresh SP, Ali KE, Jones H, et al. Medial epicondylitis: is ultrasound guided autologous blood injection an effective treatment? *Br J Sports Med*. 2006;40(11):935–939.
- Thiese MS, Hegmann KT, Kapellusch J, et al. Psychosocial factors related to lateral and medial epicondylitis: results from pooled study analyses. *J Occup Environ Med*. 2016;58(6):588–593.

CLINICAL PEARLS

- Wrist splints are often more helpful than counterforce bracing if the patient has significant pain upon awakening. However, counterforce braces are often better tolerated during the day.
- The cost of nitroglycerin patches can be decreased by cutting them in half or quarters.

MEDIAL GASTROCNEMIUS INJURY, TENNIS LEG

Daniel C. Herman, MD, PhD, FAAPMR, FACSM, CAQSM • Glenn H. Sapp II, MD

BASICS

DESCRIPTION

Musculotendinous disruption of varying degrees in the medial head of the gastrocnemius muscle, resulting from sudden dorsiflexion of the foot during an eccentric loading (Athlete is actively plantarflexing as an outside force causes a sudden stretch/dorsiflexion moment.)

RISK FACTORS

- Male
- 4th to 6th decades of life (1)
- Participation in sports involving quick accelerations, including racquet sports (tennis, squash), hill running, and track events involving jumping activities but may also involve relatively low stress activities such as ascending stairs (1,2)
- Muscles that have not been properly warmed up may be greater at risk.
- Participation during prolonged activities as fatigued muscles with impaired coordination increases the risk of injury.
- Recurrent calf strains

DIAGNOSIS

- Audible pop or tearing sensation when injury to the medial calf occurs
- Pain in the area of the calf with radiation to the knee or the ankle
- Pain with range of motion (ROM) of the ankle, particularly dorsiflexion
- Swelling or bruising of the posterior calf

HISTORY

Athlete reports audible pop or experiencing tearing sensation at time of injury to the medial calf. The patient may complain of feeling like a stick struck their calf.

PHYSICAL EXAM

- Asymmetric calf swelling and increased circumference that can be serially measured. Swelling may be noted all the way to the ankle.
- Calf ecchymosis
- A visible or palpable defect may be present in the medial gastrocnemius muscle.
- Tenderness on palpation of the medial gastrocnemius muscle (more painful at the medial musculotendinous junction)
- Peripheral pulses should be normal.
- Pain with passive ankle dorsiflexion
- Pain with active resistance to ankle plantar flexion
- Palpation of the Achilles tendon demonstrates an intact tendon.
- Thompson test is negative: Thompson test should always be performed in the clinical setting of atraumatic, acute-onset pain in the posterior lower leg associated with an audible "pop."

DIFFERENTIAL DIAGNOSIS

- Baker cyst rupture
- Deep vein thrombosis (DVT)
- Plantaris tendon rupture
- Achilles tendon rupture
- Acute compartment syndrome after rupture of the medial head of the gastrocnemius (3)
- Chronic exertional compartment syndrome (posterior)
- Posterior tibial tendon rupture or tendonitis
- Popliteal artery entrapment syndrome
- Anomalous gastrocnemius muscle rupture

DIAGNOSTIC TESTS & INTERPRETATION

- X-ray films of the tibia/fibula may be ordered to rule out an avulsion fracture or calcific tendinosis.
- Magnetic resonance imaging (MRI): the most sensitive and specific imaging method to show the area of disrupted soft tissue and surrounding structures (4)
- Ultrasound (US): will aid in ruling out a DVT or Achilles tendon rupture. The calf can also be serially imaged to assess the extent of injury and healing (4).
- Advanced imaging (MRI, US) is usually not necessary because the diagnosis is commonly made on clinical findings.

TREATMENT

GENERAL MEASURES

- Prevention/reduction of swelling: elevation, compression dressing/sleeve, and ice for 20 min 3 to 4 times a day (1)[C]
- Early weight-bearing (may need crutches and/or bilateral heel lifts for normal gait)
- Ankle/foot bracing to keep the ankle in maximally tolerable dorsiflexion: In the early stages of treatment, using the splint at night may be helpful (5)[C].

MEDICATION

Nonsteroidal anti-inflammatory drugs (NSAIDs): Clinicians must carefully consider pain therapy in the initial 48 hr because decreased platelet activity may result in increased bleeding and larger hematoma formation with resultant effects on healing:

- Ibuprofen: adult: 600 mg PO q8h; children: 10 mg/kg PO q8h
- Naproxen: adult: 250 to 500 mg PO BID
- Ketorolac: adult: 30 mg intravenous (IV)/intramuscular (IM) q6h or 10 mg PO q4–6h

ADDITIONAL THERAPIES

- Ice therapy for control of pain and swelling
- Active resistance dorsiflexion exercises until the athlete is pain free (2)[B]
- Apply compression dressing from the metatarsal heads to the gastrocnemius for the first 2 wk (6)[B].
- Partial weight-bearing ambulation as soon as tolerable to maximize the contact of the sole of the foot to the ground (1,2)[C]
- Stationary cycling, leg presses, and heel raises
- Proprioception and balance training

ONGOING CARE

PROGNOSIS

- Prognosis is excellent for the tennis leg sufferer to return to sports endeavors.
- Noncompliance can prevent players from returning to sports for 3 to 4 mo.
- Early and aggressive rehabilitation allows most patients to recover within a few weeks.

REFERENCES

1. Fields KB, Rigby MD. Muscular calf injuries in runners. *Curr Sports Med Rep.* 2016;15(5):320–324.
2. Millar AP. Strains of the posterior calf musculature ("tennis leg"). *Am J Sports Med.* 1979;7(3):172–174.
3. Tao L, Jun H, Muliang D, et al. Acute compartment syndrome after gastrocnemius rupture (tennis leg) in a nonathlete without trauma. *J Foot Ankle Surg.* 2016;55(2):303–305.
4. Delgado GJ, Chung CB, Lektrakul N, et al. Tennis leg: clinical US study of 141 patients and anatomic investigation of four cadavers with MR imaging and US. *Radiology.* 2002;224(1):112–119.
5. Ryu DJ, Kim JM, Kim BS. Concomitant contracture of the knee and ankle joint after gastrocnemius muscle rupture: a case report. *J Foot Ankle Surg.* 2017;56(1):87–91.
6. Kwak HS, Lee KB, Han YM. Ruptures of the medial head of the gastrocnemius ("tennis leg"): clinical outcome and compression effect. *Clin Imaging.* 2006;30(1):48–53.

ADDITIONAL READING

Delgado GJ, Chung CB, Lektrakul N, et al. Tennis leg: clinical US study of 141 patients and anatomic investigation of four cadavers with MR imaging and US. *Radiology.* 2002;224(1):112–119.

CLINICAL PEARLS

- Although the mechanism of injury is often during athletic events with quick or explosive motions, this injury may also occur during relatively minor activities.
- In light of the occasionally severe pain experienced at the time of the injury and subacutely, the patient should be counseled and reassured regarding the excellent prognosis of this injury.
- Weight-bearing and splints for maximizing tolerable ankle dorsiflexion early in the course of treatment is key to functional progression and prevention of contractures and prolonged return to activities.
- Thompson test must be performed to rule out Achilles tendon rupture.

MEDIAL SYMPTOMATIC PLICA

Laura J. Murphy, DO • David E.J. Bazzo, MD, FAAFP, CAQSM

BASICS

DESCRIPTION

- Plica is a Latin term meaning fold.
- Medial plica syndrome is inflammation of the synovial lining forming an intra-articular band located over the medial aspect of the knee, resulting in fibrosis and persistent pain.

EPIDEMIOLOGY

Incidence

Estimates range from 8% to 45% of children, adolescents, and young adults presenting with acute knee pain.

Prevalence

- Unknown, likely from underdiagnosis due to lack of strict diagnostic criteria
- Females more often than males
- Usually occurs during 1st through 3rd decade

ETIOLOGY AND PATHOPHYSIOLOGY

Repetitive injury and inflammation of the medial synovium from the femur or from the femur and the patella pinching tissue with subsequent fibrosis, thickening, and loss of elasticity of the plica caused by:

- Repetitive knee flexion/extension (e.g., running, squatting)
- Direct trauma
- Underlying intra-articular abnormalities (e.g., foreign bodies, osteochondritis dissecans, or inflammatory arthritis)

Genetics

There is some evidence to suggest a genetic component due to the embryologic etiology of plica development, although this has not yet been established.

RISK FACTORS

- Congenital presence of plica
- Multiple injuries or surgeries over medial aspect of knee
- Poor structural mechanics, including weak quadriceps, tight hamstrings, and increased Q angle

GENERAL PREVENTION

Proper knee extension alignment and mechanics

COMMONLY ASSOCIATED CONDITIONS

- Knee valgus
- Heel valgus and midfoot pronation

DIAGNOSIS

HISTORY

- Complaint of anterior and medial knee pain just proximal to medial joint line
- Pain is often unilateral.
- Often exacerbated by activity, including running, squatting, and ascending or descending stairs
- Patients commonly report popping, snapping, and catching with knee flexion.

PHYSICAL EXAM

- Palpable fibrotic cord located between medial border of the patella and medial femoral condyle
- Cord is painful with full knee extension or flexion (nonspecific).
- May have soft tissue swelling medial to patellar border
- Medial patellar plica (MPP) test: With patient supine, examiner applies pressure with thumb over inferior and medial aspect of the patellofemoral joint while passively flexing the knee from 0 to 90 degrees; positive test if pain in extension is relieved at 90 degrees of flexion

DIFFERENTIAL DIAGNOSIS

- Medial collateral ligament strain
- Patellofemoral pain syndrome
- Patellar subluxation
- Osteochondritis dissecans
- Osteoarthritis
- Pes anserinus pain syndrome
- Medial meniscus tear

DIAGNOSTIC TESTS & INTERPRETATION

Initial Tests (lab, imaging)

- Dynamic ultrasound (US) in office/training room may help establish diagnosis.
- X-rays are often normal, but certain views (standing anteroposterior [AP], lateral, and sunrise views) may be useful in identifying bony abnormalities that may irritate the plica (e.g., osteoarthritis, osteochondritis dissecans, fractures) and also in excluding other diagnoses (1)[C].

Follow-Up Tests & Special Considerations

Additional imaging may be useful in identifying alternative etiologies (2)[C].

Diagnostic Procedures/Other

- Intra-articular 1% lidocaine injection
- Arthroscopy provides definitive diagnosis but only indicated when conservative therapy fails.

TREATMENT

GENERAL MEASURES

- Acute phase:
  - Rest to reduce repetitive flexion/extension of the knee.
  - Ice
  - Compression knee sleeves or braces may be helpful to reduce swelling.
  - Elevating the knee above the level of the heart may help reduce swelling.
- Recovery phase:
  - Physical therapy (PT) or home exercise program (HEP) focusing on strengthening quadriceps, stretching of hamstring/quadriceps/gastrocnemius/abductors for 6 to 8 wk after diagnosis (1)[C]
  - Intra-articular corticosteroid injection if no improvement with PT or those with significantly irritated plicas in which PT may not be directly beneficial

MEDICATION

Oral or topical nonsteroidal anti-inflammatory drugs (NSAIDs)

ISSUES FOR REFERRAL

Referral to orthopedic surgeon may be warranted if no improvement with conservative therapy.

ADDITIONAL THERAPIES

Orthotics to correct heel valgus if present

SURGERY/OTHER PROCEDURES

- Arthroscopic resection may be considered if conservative therapy fails after 6 mo and has a generally high success rate with the majority of patients able to resume to their previous level of activity (3,4)[A].
- Surgery is more successful in adolescents.
- Surgery is considered with caution because it may cause development of scar tissue that is more painful than the fibrotic plica itself.

ONGOING CARE

FOLLOW-UP RECOMMENDATIONS

Consider follow-up once monthly while patient is in recovery phase to evaluate for progress.

PROGNOSIS

The majority of patients respond to conservative therapy and rehabilitation.

COMPLICATIONS

Erosion of the articular cartilage may develop in patients where the plica is acting as a shelf catching over the medial femoral condyle.

REFERENCES

1. Griffith CJ, LaPrade RF. Medial plica irritation: diagnosis and treatment. *Curr Rev Musculoskelet Med*. 2008;1(1):53–60.
2. Patel DR, Villalobos A. Evaluation and management of knee pain in young athletes: overuse injuries of the knee. *Transl Pediatr*. 2017;6(3):190–198.
3. Lee PYF, Nixion A, Chandratreya A, et al. Synovial plica syndrome of the knee: a commonly overlooked cause of anterior knee pain. *Surg J (N Y)*. 2017;3(1):e9–e16.
4. Al-Hadithy N, Gikas P, Mahapatra AM, et al. Review article: plica syndrome of the knee. *J Orthop Surg (Hong Kong)*. 2011;19(3):354–358.

CLINICAL PEARLS

- Medial plica syndrome is suspected by the history of anterior knee pain after blunt trauma, twisting injury, or repetitive flexion/extension injury.
- Diagnosis is clinical and only made when alternative pathologies are ruled out (usually by imaging).
- Treatment is primarily rehabilitation and avoiding exacerbating activities.
- Corticosteroid injections are generally not recommended but may be helpful when the conservative therapeutic measures have not provided relief within 2 to 4 wk.
- Surgical intervention through complete arthroscopic excision of the fibrotic plica should only be considered after at least 6 mo when conservative therapy has failed and has a good reported success rate.

MEDIAL TIBIAL STRESS SYNDROME

Alecia Gende, DO • Britt Marcussen, MD, FAAFP, CAQSM

BASICS

DESCRIPTION

- Typically an overuse injury, with exercise-induced pain over the posteromedial border of the middle to distal 2/3 of the tibia
- Exact pathophysiology is unknown, thought due to traction on periosteum and repetitive loading across tibia (1).
- May be on a continuum with stress fracture
- Synonym(s):
  - "Shin splints"
  - Tibialis posterior myofasciitis
  - Soleus syndrome

EPIDEMIOLOGY

- 13.6–20% incidence in runners (1)
- 5.7% incidence and second most common musculoskeletal injury in military recruits (2)

RISK FACTORS

Risks for development of lower extremity overuse syndromes are a point of interest in literature.
First 4 higher risk (1,3,4):

- Female sex
- Higher body weight
- Navicular drop (an indicator of excessive pronation)
- Prior running injury
- Limited external/internal rotation of hip
- Limited ankle range of motion (ROM)
- Higher body mass index (BMI)
- Overall poor conditioning
- Limited core strength

GENERAL PREVENTION

- Prevention methods often encouraged (5,6)[C]:
  - Shock-absorbing insoles: most promising in studies (5,6)
  - Pronation control insoles if navicular drop
  - Replacing running shoes after 300 to 600 miles
  - Gradually increasing running programs
- Systematic review shows no statistical benefit from any prevention strategy (6).

DIAGNOSIS

HISTORY

- Often insidious and progressive
- Temporally related to sudden increase in intensity/duration of activity, or change in playing/running surface from a softer surface to a harder surface such as concrete
- Early in course: Pain occurs during activity rather than at onset:
  - Sometimes relieved as activity continues
  - Often worse with toe-off
  - Often aches after rest which is in contrast to chronic exertional compartment syndrome where pain is relieved quickly by rest
- Late in course: pain through full duration of activity:
  - Pain and aching continue after cessation of inciting activity.

PHYSICAL EXAM

- Tenderness to palpation along the middle to distal 2/3 of the tibia, along the posteromedial border
- Diffuse posteromedial pain with palpation is most sensitive finding (5).
- Lower extremity kinetic chain examination may reveal excessive pronation, navicular drop, or other alignment abnormalities, core weakness, and instability
- Chronic cases: induration, soft tissue swelling, or nodularity
- Shoe examination reveals overpronation wear pattern, excessive age of shoes

DIFFERENTIAL DIAGNOSIS

- Stress fracture
- Compartment syndrome
- Muscular strain
- Nerve entrapment
- Fascial defects
- Popliteal artery entrapment syndrome
- Effort-induced venous thrombosis

DIAGNOSTIC TESTS & INTERPRETATION

ALERT

- Overall a clinical diagnosis, but imaging needed to evaluate for other etiologies such as stress fracture
- Plain films of anteroposterior and lateral tibia are often normal.
- Bone scan: Diffuse uptake along the posteromedial border of the tibia, often seen better on delayed images, involves radiation, shows whole body (if concern for bilateral or other associated areas of bony tenderness as in multiple stress fractures); sensitivity 74–84% (5)
- Computed tomography (CT): Posteromedial cortical osteopenia, sensitivity 42–100%, specificity 82–100% in various studies, like bone scan involves radiation. May be useful in unclear clinical diagnosis; magnetic resonance imaging (MRI) typically preferred over CT (5)
- MRI: Bone marrow edema and periosteal signal may be seen, similar sensitivity and specificity to bone scan, no radiation (5).

TREATMENT

Acute treatment (6)[C]:

- Nonsteroidal anti-inflammatory drugs (NSAIDs) and ice most beneficial in acute stages
- Complete rest if possible
- Otherwise, graded running program, gradual increase in inciting activities
- Cross-training with nonimpact activities: swimming, water running, bicycling
- Low-energy extracorporeal shock wave therapy (ESWT) may provide some benefit.
- No benefit to immobilization
- Surgery rarely indicated

ADDITIONAL THERAPIES

- Special considerations (5)[C]:
  - Special taping techniques by athletic trainers may improve symptoms.
  - For very flat feet (pes planus), consider more supportive shoes or supportive inserts.
  - For very high-arched feet (pes cavus), consider increased cushioning in shoes or shock-absorbing inserts.
- Rehabilitation (5)[C]:
  - Target-specific stretching and strengthening exercises
  - Core strengthening
  - Towel calf stretches
  - Tracing alphabet with toes
  - Alternate heel/toe walking

SURGERY/OTHER PROCEDURES

- Generally limited success to fully return to level of presymptoms activity but more success with relief of pain
- Surgical procedures for recalcitrant cases:
  - Surgical release of the investing fascia around the soleus insertion on the posteromedial aspect of the tibia. Medial tibial stress syndrome is not a compartment syndrome, but releasing this fascia has helped with pain.
  - Surgical division of the insertion of the soleus on the periosteum can relieve associated periostitis.
  - Cauterization of the periosteum over the posteromedial tibia allows scarring and reattachment of the periosteum.

ONGOING CARE

- Changes in training techniques:
  - Increase rest days.
  - Add in cross-training days with non–weight-bearing activity such as swimming and biking.
  - Slow increase in training intensity/duration, with no more than a 10% increase per week
- Correct shoe type for foot type:
  - Some people may benefit from orthotics.

PATIENT EDUCATION

- Much education required
- Prolonged recovery course
- Gradual increase of training intensity (5,6)[C]
- Rest sufficiently to overcome symptoms.
- Return slowly to avoid recurrence.
- New shoes every 3 to 6 mo, 200 to 300 miles of wear (6)[C]

REFERENCES

1. Winkelmann ZK, Anderson D, Games KE, et al. Risk factors for medial tibial stress syndrome in active individuals: an evidence-based review. *J Athl Train*. 2016;51(12):1049–1052.
2. Sharma J, Greeves JP, Byers M, et al. Musculoskeletal injuries in British Army recruits: a prospective study of diagnosis-specific incidence and rehabilitation times. *BMC Musculoskelet Disord*. 2015;16:106.
3. Reinking MF, Austin TM, Richter RR, et al. Medial tibial stress syndrome in active individuals: a systematic review and meta-analysis of risk factors. *Sports Health*. 2017;9(3):252–261.
4. Hamstra-Wright KL, Bliven KC, Bay C. Risk factors for medial tibial stress syndrome in physically active individuals such as runners and military personnel: a systematic review and meta-analysis. *Br J Sports Med*. 2015;49(6):362–369.
5. Reshef N, Guelich DR. Medial tibial stress syndrome. *Clin Sports Med*. 2012;31(2):273–290.
6. Craig DI. Medial tibial stress syndrome: evidence-based prevention. *J Athl Train*. 2008;43(3):316–318.

ADDITIONAL READING

- Korakakis V, Whiteley R, Tzavara A, et al. The effectiveness of extracorporeal shockwave therapy in common lower limb conditions: a systematic review including quantification of patient-rated pain reduction. *Br J Sports Med*. 2018;52(6):387–407.
- Lopes AD, Hespanhol LC Jr, Yeung SS, et al. What are the main running-related musculoskeletal injuries? A systematic review. *Sports Med*. 2012;42(10):891–905.
- Winters M, Eskes M, Weir A, et al. Treatment of medial tibial stress syndrome: a systematic review. *Sports Med*. 2013;43(12):1315–1333.

CLINICAL PEARLS

- Activity should be avoided until pain and tenderness resolve, followed by a slow, structured return to prior level of activity.
- There is no good evidence that special taping or an ACE bandage will shorten recovery, but it may help to improve symptoms.
- If time cannot be taken off from training, relative rest, with a 20–50% decrease in training intensity/duration. Work in cross-training days, with non–weight-bearing activity.
- Rehabilitation exercises should aim at stretching and strengthening involved musculotendinous units.
- Use a towel to pull your foot toward you and stretch your calf. Trace the alphabet with your feet. Alternate walking on toes and heels; "toe raises" to strengthen lower leg while standing on stairs or steps

MENISCAL TEARS

Saif Usman, MD, FAAFP, CAQSM

BASICS

DESCRIPTION

- Menisci are cartilaginous structures whose functions include distribution of joint fluid, shock absorption, deepening of the joint, nutrient distribution, load or weight-bearing, and joint stabilization especially in rotation.
- The peripheral 1/3 zone (red-red) has good vascular supply, central third zone (red-white) has limited vascular supply, whereas inner third zone (white) is avascular.
- The most common tear patterns are longitudinal, radial, horizontal, displaced, root, complex, and bucket-handle tears.
- Meniscal tears can disrupt knee biomechanics, causing varying degrees of symptoms and predisposing the knee to other short- and long-term sequelae, including quadriceps or hamstring inhibition, patellofemoral pain syndrome, altered gait, and osteoarthritis.
- Synonym(s): cartilage tear (common usage by patients for a meniscal tear)

EPIDEMIOLOGY

- One of the most common knee problems; annual incidence is 66/100,000 persons per year (1).
- Traumatic tears typically occur in 13- to 40-yr-old individuals with sports-related injuries.
- Degenerative tears typically develop in patients >40 yr.
- Posterior horn of medial meniscus is most commonly affected location.
- More common in males than females, with ratio between 2.5:1 and 4:1 (1)
- In athletic population, >1/3 are associated with anterior cruciate ligament (ACL) tears.

ETIOLOGY AND PATHOPHYSIOLOGY

- A meniscal tear may occur following twisting, shearing, or compressive forces from contact or noncontact mechanisms.
- Injury mechanism is typically a twisting moment through the knee in the flexed, weight-bearing position.

RISK FACTORS

- Male gender
- Abnormal mechanical axis
- Playing soccer or rugby (2)[A]
- Ligament deficiency
- Degenerative joint disease
- Discoid meniscus
- Poor quadriceps control
- Waiting >12 mo between ACL tear and reconstruction surgery is a risk factor for medial meniscus tear (2)[A].

COMMONLY ASSOCIATED CONDITIONS

- ~1/3 of traumatic meniscal tears associated with ACL injury in athletes
- Tibial plateau and femoral shaft fractures

DIAGNOSIS

HISTORY

- The diagnosis can be accurately made in 69% of cases by a skilled musculoskeletal examiner by history alone (3)[C].
- Traumatic tears in the younger, athletic population are most frequently associated with a significant cutting/twisting injury, whereas degenerative tears in older patients usually lack identifiable trauma.
- Pain along joint line
- Pain with weight-bearing and twisting/turning of knee or squatting
- Degree of pain is variable, and patient may or may not be able to ambulate after acute injury.
- May be associated with slow onset of effusion over several hours
- Catching, locking, or clicking sensation
- Episodes of giving way
- Symptoms may wane but typically recur with resumption of activities.
- Subsequent intermittent effusions not uncommon

PHYSICAL EXAM

Exam findings suggestive of meniscal tear:

- Effusion/hemarthrosis may be a sign of meniscal, ligament, or osteochondral injury.
- Locked knee is suggestive of bucket-handle meniscal tear, ligament tear, or loose body.
- Valgus/varus instability suggestive of medial collateral ligament (MCL)/lateral collateral ligament sprain, which may have associated meniscal injury
- Positive anterior/posterior drawer or Lachman test indicates cruciate ligament injury, which may have associated meniscal injury.
- An effusion combined with joint line tenderness is one of the most sensitive and reliable signs of a meniscal tear (4)[C].
- Positive McMurray test: palpable click and pain over joint line produced when meniscal fragment catches during test (diagnostic accuracy up to 63% when performed by skilled examiner) (3)[C]
- Positive Apley test: pain over the respective joint line with the patient prone and the knee flexed to 90 degrees, whereas the leg is internally and externally rotated under an axial load (diagnostic accuracy up to 58% when performed by skilled examiner) (3)[C]
- Positive Thessaly test: pain over the respective joint line with the patient standing on the affected leg at 5 and 20 degrees of knee flexion, followed by internal and external rotation of the leg and torso (diagnostic accuracy up to 59% when performed by skilled examiner) (3)[C]
- Atrophic quadriceps suggestive of chronic inhibition by pain or effusion
- May have decreased range of motion secondary to pain or effusion

DIFFERENTIAL DIAGNOSIS

- Synovitis
- Intra-articular loose body
- Articular cartilage defect (osteochondritis dissecans [OCD])
- Ligamentous injury, particularly ACL and/or MCL
- Patellar subluxation/dislocation
- Degenerative joint disease
- Chondromalacia patellae
- Tibial plateau fracture

DIAGNOSTIC TESTS & INTERPRETATION

- Standard weight-bearing anteroposterior/lateral/tunnel/patellar (sunrise, merchant) views to rule out other conditions such as loose body, arthritis, osteochondral defect, loose body, OCD, or fracture
- Magnetic resonance imaging (MRI) useful to evaluate for concomitant structural damage when the diagnosis is in question or for operative planning

- Should be performed quickly for locking symptoms or suspicion for substantial injury; otherwise, is typically reserved for symptoms persisting >4 to 8 wk in the otherwise healthy knee
- MRI findings of meniscal tear include meniscal cleavage signal, which extends to the meniscal surface.

TREATMENT

GENERAL MEASURES

- Initial treatment is RICE—rest, ice (20 min several times per day), compression, elevation—and nonsteroidal anti-inflammatory drugs (NSAIDs).
- Immobilization is not recommended unless evaluating for fracture or major ligamentous injury; however, a hinged knee brace may offer support, protection, and symptom relief.
- Although infrequently required, crutches with partial weight-bearing may provide acute relief.
- Sports activity should be restricted until symptoms resolve or (if indicated) MRI is performed.
- Further management decisions are based on patient's age, symptomatology, type of tear, and coexisting knee conditions.
- Younger patients with traumatic tears should be thoroughly evaluated and more aggressively treated.

ISSUES FOR REFERRAL

- Expedited surgical referrals should be made for:
  - Locked knee.
  - Younger patients with vertical longitudinal tears in periphery of meniscus (5)[C].
  - Locking symptoms, flap tears, and bucket-handle tears.
  - Associated cruciate ligament injury, osteochondral defect, loose bodies, or fracture.
  - Nonurgent referrals include tears treated nonoperatively but that continue to cause pain or disability.
- Individuals with degenerative joint disease will likely have meniscal tears, and the presence of one is not necessarily a cause for a surgical referral.

ADDITIONAL THERAPIES

- For discomfort persisting several weeks, intra-articular corticosteroid injections often provide significant relief.
- Stationary bicycle riding or a home exercise program/physical therapy addressing balance, quadriceps, and hamstring strength can reduce pain, increase range of motion, and help protect the knee from further injuries.
- Although surgery is not contraindicated, nonoperative interventions (including NSAIDs and corticosteroid injections) are appropriate initial treatment for:
  - Smaller central tears.
  - Complex/degenerative tears.
  - Tears in setting of degenerative joint disease.

SURGERY/OTHER PROCEDURES

- Both partial meniscectomy and meniscal repair are outpatient-based procedures.
- Partial meniscectomy is frequently performed for flap and bucket-handle tears or for tears failing nonoperative treatment.
- Horizontal tears are typically degenerative tears and have a minimal chance of healing. Because they may progress to flap tears, they may be excised.
- Meniscal repair is indicated for vertical longitudinal tears in the outer 25–30% of the meniscus, corresponding to the "red-red" zone (5)[C].
- Occasionally, bucket-handle tears are amenable to repair.

ONGOING CARE

PROGNOSIS

- In the carefully chosen patient, meniscal repair is successful in up to 95% (5)[C].
- Successful repair compared to meniscectomy has a lower incidence of degenerative change and better functional scores at 10 yr follow-up (6)[C].
- Total meniscectomy in previously normal knees results in significant arthrosis in 2/3 of patients by 15 yr from surgery (6)[C].

COMPLICATIONS

- Injury to peroneal nerve possible with lateral meniscus repair
- Injury to infrapatellar branch of saphenous nerve possible with medial meniscus repair
- Repair could fail, resulting in repeat arthroscopy.
- Infection

REFERENCES

1. Morelli V, Braxton TM Jr. Meniscal, plica, patellar, and patellofemoral injuries of the knee: updates, controversies and advancements. *Prim Care*. 2013;40(2):357–382.
2. Snoeker BA, Bakker EW, Kegel CA, et al. Risk factors for meniscal tears: a systematic review including meta-analysis. *J Orthop Sports Phys Ther*. 2013;43(6):352–367.
3. Blyth M, Anthony I, Francq B, et al. Diagnostic accuracy of the Thessaly test, standardised clinical history and other clinical examination tests (Apley's, McMurray's and joint line tenderness) for meniscal tears in comparison with magnetic resonance imaging diagnosis. *Health Technol Assess*. 2015;19(62):1–62.
4. Bronstein RD, Schaffer JC. Physical examination of the knee: meniscus, cartilage, and patellofemoral conditions. *J Am Acad Orthop Surg*. 2017;25(5):365–374.
5. Jarit GJ, Bosco JA III. Meniscal repair and reconstruction. *Bull NYU Hosp Jt Dis*. 2010;68(2):84–90.
6. Lutz C, Dalmay F, Ehkirch FP, et al. Meniscectomy versus meniscal repair: 10 years radiological and clinical results in vertical lesions in stable knee. *Orthop Traumatol Surg Res*. 2015;101(8 Suppl):S327–S331.

ADDITIONAL READING

- Brelin Am, Rue JP. Return to play following meniscus surgery. *Clin Sports Med*. 2016;35(4):669–678.
- Nguyen JC, De Smet AA, Graf BK, et al. MR imaging-based diagnosis and classification of meniscal tears. *Radiographics*. 2014;34(4):981–999.
- Persson F, Turkiewicz A, Bergkvist D, et al. The risk of symptomatic knee osteoarthritis after arthroscopic meniscus repair vs partial meniscectomy vs the general population. *Osteoarthritis Cartilage*. 2018;26(2):195–201.

CLINICAL PEARLS

- Not all meniscus tears require surgery.
- Posterior horn of medial meniscus is most commonly affected.
- Younger patients with traumatic tears should be treated more aggressively.
- Patients with degenerative joint disease will likely have meniscal tears, and the presence of one is not necessarily a cause for a surgical referral.
- MRI is a good imaging modality for identifying tears when diagnosis in question and to evaluate for concomitant structural damage.

MENSTRUAL DISORDERS IN THE ATHLETE

Kayla Daniel, MD • Anastasia Fischer, MD, FAAFP, FACSM

BASICS

DESCRIPTION

- Menstrual dysfunction: a lack of regular menstrual periods (every 22 to 35 days) 1 to 2 yr after menarche (1):
  - Primary amenorrhea is the lack of spontaneous uterine bleeding:
    - By the age of 14 yr without development of secondary sexual characteristics or
    - By the age of 15 yr with otherwise normal development.
  - Secondary amenorrhea is absence of menstruation for 3 consecutive months with previously regular menses (or <9 per year) *or* absence of menstruation for 6 to 12 mo if previously oligomenorrheic.
  - Oligomenorrhea is when menstrual cycles occur >35 days apart.
- Related conditions of menstrual dysfunction (2,3):
  - Female athlete triad refers to the interrelationships among energy availability (EA), menstrual function, and bone mineral density (BMD).
  - Relative energy deficiency in sport (RED-S) describes a syndrome of impairment in physiologic function, health, and athletic performance secondary to imbalance of dietary energy intake and energy expenditure:
    - Impairments in metabolic rate, menstrual function, bone health, immunity, protein synthesis, and cardiovascular health

EPIDEMIOLOGY

Prevalence

Prevalence of menstrual dysfunction (4):

- High school 19–54%
- College 25–36%
- Professional 44–69%

ETIOLOGY AND PATHOPHYSIOLOGY

Functional hypothalamic amenorrhea is a low estrogen state, resulting from suppression of the hypothalamic-pituitary-ovarian axis due to energy deficit (1).

RISK FACTORS

- EA is defined as energy intake minus exercise energy expenditure divided by kilograms lean body mass (LBM) (2).
- In adult women, menstrual dysfunction presents when EA is <30 kcal/kg LBM per day.

COMMONLY ASSOCIATED CONDITIONS

- Altered BMD
- Nutritional deficiencies
- Decreased EA
- Disordered eating or eating disorders
- Psychiatric conditions (depression)

DIAGNOSIS

HISTORY

- Menstrual history:
  - Age of menarche, family history of menarche
  - Last menstrual period
  - Frequency and duration of menses
  - Longest time between menses
  - Changes in menstrual cycle with exercise
  - Previous or current use of hormonal therapy
- Diet history
- Exercise history:
  - Overtraining, history of sport-specific training
- Sexual history
- Changes in weight
- Psychosocial stressors
- History of stress fractures or sports-related injuries
- Medication use (including hormonal medications such as oral contraceptives)
- Symptoms of androgen excess, abnormal thyroid function, autoimmune and pituitary disorders:
  - Hair growth, acne
  - Temperature intolerance, palpitations, diarrhea, constipation, tremor, mood changes, dry skin
  - Headaches, visual changes, galactorrhea

PHYSICAL EXAM

- Vital signs and general appearance:
  - Height, weight, body mass index (BMI)
  - Heart rate, blood pressure, body temperature
  - Dysmorphic features such as webbed neck, short stature, low hairline
- Thyroid palpation
- Tanner stage
- Skin findings: acne, lanugo, hirsutism
- Exertional genitalia exam:
  - Virilization, outflow tract obstruction, anomalies
- Pelvic examination:
  - Evidence of clitoromegaly, outflow tract obstruction, thin vaginal mucosa

DIFFERENTIAL DIAGNOSIS

- Hypothalamic dysfunction:
  - Functional hypothalamic amenorrhea:
    - Energy deficiency–related amenorrhea secondary to excessive exercise, weight loss, disordered eating
  - Primary gonadotropin-releasing hormone (GnRH) deficiency:
    - Congenital disorders such as Kallmann syndrome
  - Secondary/acquired GnRH deficiency:
    - Traumatic brain injury, brain tumor
- Physiologic:
  - Pregnancy
  - Hormonal contraception
  - Menopause
- Pituitary dysfunction:
  - Hyperprolactinemia
  - Prolactinoma
  - Cushing syndrome
  - Empty sella syndrome
  - Sheehan syndrome
  - Autoimmune disease
  - Medications
- Anatomic abnormality/outflow tract obstruction:
  - Congenital: müllerian agenesis, imperforate hymen, transverse vaginal septum, androgen insensitivity
  - Acquired: Asherman syndrome
- Primary ovarian insufficiency:
  - Congenital: gonadal dysgenesis, Turner syndrome
  - Acquired: ovarian neoplasm, ovarian destruction secondary to medications, radiation, autoimmune disorder
- Other endocrine gland dysfunction:
  - Thyroid dysfunction
  - Polycystic ovary syndrome (PCOS)
  - Adrenal dysfunction

DIAGNOSTIC TESTS & INTERPRETATION

- Initial labs:
  - Pregnancy test (human chorionic gonadotropin [HCG]), prolactin, thyroid-stimulating hormone (TSH)
- If normal, consider:
  - Progesterone challenge test:
    - If the patient has no menses following progesterone, confirm estrogen deficiency with estrogen challenge test.
  - Luteinizing hormone (LH), follicle-stimulating hormone (FSH) to evaluate for ovarian failure
- If evidence of hyperandrogenism and concern for PCOS, check estradiol, testosterone (total and free), dehydroepiandrosterone sulfate (DHEA-S), and early morning salivary 17-hydroxyprogesterone.
- Pelvic ultrasound to rule out suspected anatomic abnormalities or polycystic ovaries
- Head magnetic resonance imaging (MRI) to look for pituitary abnormalities or space-occupying lesions
- Electrocardiogram (ECG) to evaluate for arrhythmia
- Electrolytes to evaluate for abnormalities from disordered eating
- Dual energy x-ray absorptiometry (DEXA) scan:
  - Indications:
    - One or more "high risk" triad factors
    - History of *Diagnostic and Statistical Manual of Mental Disorders, fifth edition (DSM-5)* diagnosed eating disorder
    - BMI:
      - Adults: BMI ≤17.5 kg/m^2, <85% estimated weight, *or* recent weight loss of 10% or more in 1 mo
      - Adolescents: BMI <5% for age
    - Menarche at 16 yr of age or older
    - Current or history of <6 menses >12 mo
    - Two prior stress reactions/fractures, one high-risk stress reaction/fracture, or a low-energy nontraumatic fracture
    - Prior *Z*-score of <−2.0 (after at least 1 yr from baseline DEXA)
  - Two or more "moderate risk" triad factors:
    - Current or history of disordered eating for 6 mo or greater
    - BMI between 17.5 and 18.5, <90% estimated weight, *or* recent weight loss of 5–10% in 1 mo
    - Menarche between ages 15 and 16 yr
    - Current or history of 6 to 8 menses >12 mo
    - One prior stress reaction/fracture
    - Prior *Z*-score between −1.0 and −2.0 (after at least 1-yr interval from baseline DEXA) (5)[C]

TREATMENT

GENERAL MEASURES

Functional hypothalamic amenorrhea:

- Primary goal of treatment (+/− female athlete triad) is weight restoration or normalization of body weight through nutritional rehabilitation and exercise modifications with the goal of increasing EA (1,5)[C].
- The expert panel on treatment and return to play of the female athlete concluded there is no evidence at this time to unequivocally recommend pharmacologic therapy in athletes with the female athlete triad disorders due to lack of evidence-based research in this population (5)[C].
- Combined oral or nonoral routes of contraceptive therapy create an exogenous ovarian steroid environment inducing withdrawal bleeding but do not restore spontaneous menses (5)[C].
- Combined oral contraceptive therapy is not associated with improved BMD in amenorrheic athletes (1,5)[C].
- Consider pharmacologic therapy if there is a lack of response to nonpharmacologic management >1 yr period and there is occurrence of a new clinically significant fracture during nonpharmacologic management (5)[C].
- Optimal calcium intake is between 1,000 and 1,300 mg/day and daily intake of 1,000 IU vitamin D for children <18 yr and 600 to 2,000 IU for adults up to age 70 yr; recommended that vitamin D levels be maintained between 32 and 50 ng/mL (5)[C]
- If a definitive cause of menstrual dysfunction is found, treatment targeting the disease is recommended (1)[C].

ADMISSION, INPATIENT, AND NURSING CONSIDERATIONS

Admission criteria specifically with suspected anorexia or bulimia:

- Bradycardia: heart rate <50 bpm in daytime or <45 bpm at night
- Tachycardia: >110 bpm
- Hypotension: systolic blood pressure (SBP) <90 mm Hg
- Postural tachycardia: >20 bpm differential
- Postural hypotension: >10 mm Hg differential
- Syncope
- Potassium <3.2 mmol/L
- Chloride <88 mmol/L
- QTc >430 ms or evidence of arrhythmia
- Weight loss or failure to gain weight, which renders the patient at <75% of ideal body weight
- Refusal to eat or drink
- Intractable vomiting or hematemesis
- Suicide risk

REFERENCES

1. Klein DA, Poth MA. Amenorrhea: an approach to diagnosis and management. *Am Fam Physician*. 2013;87(11):781–788.
2. Nattiv A, Loucks AB, Manore MM, et al. American College of Sports Medicine position stand. The female athlete triad. *Med Sci Sports Exerc*. 2007;39(10):1867–1882.
3. Mountjoy M, Sundgot-Borgen J, Burke L, et al. The IOC consensus statement: beyond the female athlete triad—relative energy deficiency in sport (RED-S). *Br J Sports Med*. 2014;48(7):491–497.
4. Rauh MJ, Nichols JF, Barrack MT. Relationships among injury and disordered eating, menstrual dysfunction, and low bone mineral density in high school athletes: a prospective study. *J Athl Train*. 2010;45(3):243–252.
5. DeSouza MJ, Nattiv A, Joy E, et al. 2014 Female Athlete Triad Coalition consensus statement on treatment and return to play of the female athlete triad: 1st International Conference held in San Francisco, California, May 2012 and 2nd International Conference held in Indianapolis, Indiana, May 2013. *Br J Sports Med*. 2014;48(4):289.

CLINICAL PEARLS

- There is a correlation between BMD decline and number of missed menstrual cycles; loss of BMD is not fully reversible.
- Relative risk for stress fracture is 2 to 4 times greater in amenorrheic than eumenorrheic athletes.
- Indications for ordering a DEXA scan for BMD testing in a female athlete should follow the triad risk stratification guidelines.
- Treatment for menstrual dysfunction in the setting of functional hypothalamic amenorrhea should be focused on optimizing EA from a multidisciplinary team approach.

MERALGIA PARESTHETICA (MP)

Amanda Babcock, MD, CAQSM

BASICS

DESCRIPTION

- Entrapment or compression of the lateral femoral cutaneous nerve (LFCN) (at inguinal ligament) causes anterolateral thigh pain and paresthesia.
- The LFCN is completely sensory, thus there are no motor complaints.

EPIDEMIOLOGY

Incidence

- 4.3 cases per 10,000 patient-years in general population (1)
- 247 cases per 100,000 patient-years in those with diabetes mellitus (DM) (2)
- Males affected more commonly than females

ETIOLOGY AND PATHOPHYSIOLOGY

- Mechanical, metabolic, and iatrogenic causes
- Mechanical-tight garments, belts, body armor, direct trauma, iliacus hematoma
- Iatrogenic postoperatively after anterior approach for total hip arthroplasty or after lumbar spine surgery

Genetics

Possible autosomal dominant trait as shown in one case series in four-generation family (1)

RISK FACTORS

- Tight garments
- Weight gain

COMMONLY ASSOCIATED CONDITIONS

- DM
- Obesity
- Pregnancy

Pediatric Considerations

Children treated for osteoid osteoma of the hip may develop meralgia paresthetica (MP) (1). MP has also been described with anterior superior iliac spine (ASIS) avulsion (1).

Pregnancy Considerations

Associated with pregnancy

DIAGNOSIS

HISTORY

- Burning, tingling, numbness in anterolateral thigh
- May worsen with prolonged standing and walking and improve with sitting

PHYSICAL EXAM

- Diagnosis is often clinical.
- Overall, there is a paucity of clinically validated tests.
- Pelvic compression test—side lying with symptomatic side up. Examiner places downward pressure on pelvis for 45 sec, considered positive if symptoms alleviated (2,3)[B]; small study with 20 patients confirmed by neurodiagnostic testing, sensitivity of 95% and a specificity of 93.3%
- Neurodynamic testing—patient side lying with symptomatic side up, extend and adduct hip (2)[C]
- Tinel sign—tapping over lateral inguinal ligament causes symptoms; no diagnostic studies (2)[C]

DIFFERENTIAL DIAGNOSIS

- Lumbar radiculopathy
- Lumbar stenosis
- Trochanteric bursitis

DIAGNOSTIC TESTS & INTERPRETATION

Initial Tests (lab, imaging)

- Consider pelvic x-ray to evaluate for bony tumor (1).
- Nerve conduction studies may be used but are limited by body habitus because adipose can make exam difficult (1). Somatosensory evoked potentials have 81.3% sensitivity, and sensory nerve conduction has 65.2% sensitivity (2)[B].

Follow-Up Tests & Special Considerations

- Magnetic resonance neurography (1)
- Consider appropriate imaging to evaluate for lumbar pathology.

Diagnostic Procedures/Other

- Diagnostic nerve block by landmarks: injection of 1% lidocaine 1 cm medial and 1 cm inferior to ASIS or at point of maximum tenderness; considered positive if immediate relief that lasts 30 min (2)[B]
- Diagnostic injection by ultrasound guidance is preferred because landmark-guided injection failure rate is as high as 60%. LFCN appears hypoechoic and swollen (4)[C]. Large anatomical variation of the LFCN. Majority exit as single nerve, 1.9 cm medial to ASIS and inferior to inguinal ligament (5).

TREATMENT

GENERAL MEASURES

- Objective evidence for treatment is weak.
- Weight loss
- Protect area.
- Avoid compression activities or clothing.
- Physical therapy such as stretching exercises for the hip and abdominal core exercises

MEDICATION

First Line

Nonsteroidal anti-inflammatory drugs (NSAIDs) (2)[C]

Second Line

Topical lidocaine and capsaicin (1)

ADDITIONAL THERAPIES

- Pulsed radiofrequency ablation (1,2)[C]
- Nerve block (1,2)[C]—small prospective study of 20 patients. 16 had relief after one injection, 4 patients had relief after two injections; however, follow-up was only for 3 mo.

SURGERY/OTHER PROCEDURES

- Neurolysis—may have reoccurrence
- Nerve resection—much symptom relief but likely to have permanent numbness (2)[C]

COMPLEMENTARY & ALTERNATIVE MEDICINE

- Active release techniques (ART), mobilization of the pelvis, myofascial therapy for the abdominal musculature
- Acupuncture (2)[C]

ONGOING CARE

PROGNOSIS

According to a Cochrane Data review, there are no randomized control trials (RCTs) to guide treatment or prognosis; however, some high-quality observational studies showed (6):

- 69% (20 of 29) of patients resolved spontaneously.
- 83% (130 of 157) of patients improved or resolved after perineural steroid injection.
- 88% (264 of 300) improved after surgical decompression and 94% (44 of 48) improved with neurectomy.
- 97% (99 of 102) of iatrogenic cases completely recovered.

REFERENCES

1. Harney D, Patijn J. Meralgia paresthetica: diagnosis and management strategies. *Pain Med*. 2007;8(8):669–677.
2. Cheatham SW, Kolber MJ, Salamh PA. Meralgia paresthetica: a review of the literature. *Int J Sports Phys Ther*. 2013;8(6):883–893.
3. Nouraei SA, Anand B, Spink G, et al. A novel approach to the diagnosis and management of meralgia paresthetica. *Neurosurgery*. 2007;60(4):696–700.
4. Onat SS, Ata AM, Ozcakar L. Ultrasound-guided diagnosis and treatment of meralgia paresthetica. *Pain Physician*. 2016;19(4):E667–E669.
5. Tomaszewski KA, Popieluszko P, Henry BM, et al. The surgical anatomy of the lateral femoral cutaneous nerve in the inguinal region: a meta-analysis. *Hernia*. 2016;20(5):649–657.
6. Khalil N, Nicotra A, Rakowicz W. Treatment for meralgia paraesthetica. *Cochrane Database Syst Rev*. 2012;(12):CD004159.

ADDITIONAL READING

Tagliafico A, Serafini G, Lacelli F, et al. Ultrasound-guided treatment of meralgia paresthetica (lateral femoral cutaneous neuropathy): technical description and results of treatment in 20 consecutive patients. *J Ultrasound Med*. 2011;30(10):1341–1346.

CLINICAL PEARLS

- LFCN impingement leads to sensory symptoms or paresthesias in the anterolateral thigh.
- Diagnosis is often clinical and based on history, but there is no strong evidence for current clinical examination maneuvers.
- There is great variability in nerve anatomy and therefore ultrasound-guided injections, rather than palpation-guided, are preferred.
- Based on a most recent Cochrane review in 2012, prognosis is good, including for those treated conservatively.

M

MOLLUSCUM CONTAGIOSUM

Steven K. Poon, MD, CAQSM • Kimberly G. Harmon, MD

BASICS

DESCRIPTION
Superficial pox virus skin infection

EPIDEMIOLOGY
- Prevalence 5.1–11.5% in pediatric age group
- Coinfection rate of 5–18% in HIV-positive patients (1)

ETIOLOGY AND PATHOPHYSIOLOGY
- Caused by the *Molluscipoxvirus* strain of the Poxviridae family
- Four major subtypes with molluscum contagiosum virus (MCV)-1 as the most common strain

RISK FACTORS
- Skin-to-skin contact
- Contact sports (i.e., wrestling)
- Sexual contact
- Autoinoculation
- Contaminated fomites (i.e., dirty towels) and community swimming pools

GENERAL PREVENTION
Avoid sharing used towels and sponges.

DIAGNOSIS

- Characteristic rash that is usually asymptomatic but can become pruritic
- Located most frequently at the trunk, extremities, and face; can be in the perineum if sexually transmitted
- Typically, small (1 to 5 mm), smooth, pearly, flesh-colored papules with umbilication
- Can be larger in immunocompromised patients
- No associated prodrome, fever, or illness

HISTORY
- How long has it been there?
- Does it itch?
- Any blisters (usually more associated with herpetic lesions)?
- Do new lesions keep appearing?
- Sexually active or previous sexually transmitted disease (STD)?
- Contact sports participation?

PHYSICAL EXAM
Small, raised, 1- to 2-mm, flesh-colored umbilicated lesions containing white core substance

DIFFERENTIAL DIAGNOSIS
- Acne/ectopic sebaceous glands
- Warts
- Ingrown hairs
- Chicken pox
- Superficial or subepidermal cyst
- Benign skin tumor (i.e., acantholytic acanthoma)

DIAGNOSTIC TESTS & INTERPRETATION
- Diagnosis is almost always clinical.
- Polymerase chain reaction (PCR) and excision biopsy with histopathologic staining can be used for difficult diagnosis.

TREATMENT

GENERAL MEASURES

- Keep lesions covered.
- Avoid skin-to-skin contact with other individuals with lesions.
- Always use clean linens and towels.
- Acute treatment:
  - Watchful waiting for self-limited resolution with mean duration 6 to 13 mo but can persist for longer
  - Mechanical removal (2,3,4)[C]:
    - Cryotherapy
    - Curettage and deroofing
    - Pulsed dye laser therapy (less common)
  - Chemical therapy (2,3,4)[C]:
    - Cantharidin
    - Salicylic acid gel or in combination products
    - Potassium hydroxide 5–10%
    - Podophyllotoxin
    - Retinoids
  - Immunomodulatory methods (2,3,4)[C]:
    - Topical imiquimod
    - Oral cimetidine
    - Interferon-α for severely immunocompromised patients

ONGOING CARE

PROGNOSIS

Most lesions are self-limiting and not associated with complications but can persist for months to years. Coexisting atopic dermatitis and immunodeficiency can lead to persistent lesions.

REFERENCES

1. Dohil MA, Lin P, Lee J, et al. The epidemiology of molluscum contagiosum in children. *J Am Acad Dermatol*. 2006;54(1):47–54.
2. Leung AKC, Barankin B, Hon KLE. Molluscum contagiosum: an update. *Recent Pat Inflamm Allergy Drug Discov*. 2017;11(1):22–31.
3. Forbat E, Al-Niaimi F, Ali FR. Molluscum contagiosum: review and update on management. *Pediatr Dermatol*. 2017;34(5):504–515.
4. Sterling J. Treatment of warts and molluscum: what does the evidence show? *Curr Opin Pediatr*. 2016;28(4):490–499.

ADDITIONAL READING

- National Collegiate Athletic Association. Appendix C: skin infections in wrestling. In: *2017-18 and 2018-19 NCAA Wrestling Rules*. Indianapolis, IN: National Collegiate Athletic Association; 2017:96–99.
- Zinder SM, Basler RS, Foley J, et al. National athletic trainers' association position statement: skin diseases. *J Athl Train*. 2010;45(4):411–428.

CLINICAL PEARLS

- Molluscum contagiosum can be contracted from another athlete via close contact, such as football or wrestling.
- Molluscum contagiosum is contagious, and it is spread by physical or sexual contact. Should keep them covered when participating; ideally, athletes should wait to resume contact sports for 24 to 48 hr after lesions are gone.
- Some regulatory bodies, such as the National Collegiate Athletic Association (NCAA), require that molluscum lesions are eradicated prior to any participation in contact/combat sports.

MONONUCLEOSIS

Brandon Hockenberry, MD • Christopher McGrew, MD, FACSM, CAQSM

BASICS

DESCRIPTION

- Acute viral syndrome classically resulting from infection with the Epstein-Barr virus (EBV)
- EBV is a lymphotropic γ-herpesvirus that replicates in epithelial cells and B lymphocytes.
- Characterized by classic triad of fever, pharyngitis, and lymphadenopathy
- Synonym(s): "mono"; glandular fever

EPIDEMIOLOGY

- Peak incidence in the United States is between the ages of 15 and 19 yr.
- Estimated prevalence 1–3% of adolescent/young adult population. U.S. incidence is 45:100,000.
- Evidence of infection via EBV antibody seroconversion occurs earlier in lower socioeconomic groups.
- In all populations, >90% seroconversion by the end of the 3rd decade of life, although many are not aware of having the disease
- No evidence to suggest that infectious mononucleosis (IM) is more or less prevalent in student athletes than among the general student population

ETIOLOGY AND PATHOPHYSIOLOGY

IM is caused by the EBV, which is a lymphotrophic γ-herpesvirus that replicates in epithelial cells and B lymphocytes (1).

RISK FACTORS

- Transmission via passage of infected mucous membrane secretions, most commonly saliva ("the kissing disease"); incubation period typically 30 to 50 days (2)
- EBV also felt to be passed via respiratory tract secretions, blood, rectal, and potentially genital secretions, raising the possibility of sexual transmission. No aerosol transmission has been found.
- Lack of mononucleosis epidemics supports concept of low-level contagiousness.
- Relative risk of contracting EBV increased by factors negatively affecting the overall status of the immune system: baseline fatigue, overtraining, poor nutritional status

GENERAL PREVENTION

- General hand washing/hygiene measures
- Avoidance of sharing of water bottles, food, other utensils
- Proper rest/avoid overtraining
- Good nutrition
- Vaccines have been developed and tested, but none are currently approved.

COMMONLY ASSOCIATED CONDITIONS

Group A β-hemolytic streptococcal pharyngeal/tonsillar infection coexistent in up to 30% of cases

DIAGNOSIS

- IM remains a clinical diagnosis based on history, physical, and selected laboratory testing.
- Hoagland criteria are frequently cited for establishing diagnosis.
- Complete blood count (CBC) shows at least 50% lymphocytes, of which 10% are atypical (1)[C].
- Presence of fever, pharyngitis, and adenopathy
- Serologic confirmation
- Only 50% of patients with suggestive symptoms and serologic confirmation meet all of Hoagland criteria.

HISTORY

- Prodrome of malaise/fatigue followed by development of the classic triad of fever, sore throat, and enlarged lymph nodes
- Headache in many cases
- Patient often does not have known history of EBV exposure.
- Athlete may complain of poor exercise performance.
- Fatigue is often disabling, even for activities of daily living.

PHYSICAL EXAM

- Classic triad: fever, pharyngitis, and cervical lymphadenopathy (anterior and posterior)
- Many patients manifest a prodrome of disabling fatigue/malaise.
- Pharyngitis characterized by yellow-gray tonsillar exudate and palatal edema
- Fevers of 39–40°C with evening peaks, typically for 10 to 14 days
- Abdominal pain
- Notable decline in exercise tolerance
- Fever often demonstrable
- Patient may appear fatigued and mildly to moderately ill but generally nontoxic.
- Exudative pharyngitis
- Palatal petechiae
- Periorbital edema
- Prominent anterior and posterior cervical lymphadenopathy (Lymphadenopathy may also involve axillary and inguinal regions.)
- Although splenomegaly is probably present in nearly all patients, peaking in the 2nd and 3rd wk, physical exam for splenomegaly has poor sensitivity and specificity, and interexaminer reliability is poor.
- Overzealous abdominal exam may precipitate splenic injury in rare cases.
- With splenic rupture, may develop Kehr sign (patient supine, raise left leg, intra-abdominal blood tracks up to diaphragm, creates referred pain to left shoulder)
- Maculopapular, urticarial or petechial rash (Petechial rashes should raise suspicion for potential aplastic anemia, thrombocytopenia, or disseminated intravascular coagulation [DIC].)
- Maculopapular rash may often develop after antimicrobial administration: most commonly ampicillin or amoxicillin but has also been reported with the use of azithromycin, levofloxacin, and cephalexin.

DIFFERENTIAL DIAGNOSIS

- Primarily must be differentiated from nonspecific viral syndromes, lymphoma, leukemia, and *Streptococcus* pharyngitis.
- Concomitant *Streptococcus* infection is not uncommon.
- Many infectious agents may cause mononucleosis-like syndromes: cytomegalovirus, adenovirus, hepatitis A, human herpesvirus 6, HIV, rubella, toxoplasmosis.
- Medications causing mononucleosis-like syndromes: phenytoin, sulfa drugs

DIAGNOSTIC TESTS & INTERPRETATION

- Primary means of laboratory testing via nonspecific heterophile antibody studies (i.e., monospot qualitative agglutination slide test)
- Heterophile antibody (+) 60–70% at 1 wk, 80–90% by 3 to 4 wk (1)
- Definitive diagnosis: EBV viral capsid antigen (VCA) immunoglobulin M (+) for acute infections, (−) for recent or past infections (1)
- EBV VCA immunoglobulin G confirms past infection and generation of protective antibody.
- May use more specific EBV-associated antigens if necessary to determine exact phase of illness
- Classic hematologic findings include >10% atypical lymphocytes (Downey cell-activated cytotoxic suppressor [CD8] T lymphocytes), relative leukocytosis (up to 20,000), followed by mild neutropenia during week 2 of illness, mild hemolytic anemia, and mild thrombocytopenia (100,000 to 140,000/mm^3)
- Mild hepatitis (2- to 3-fold increase in liver function tests) may be seen in week 2 to 3 of illness.
- No routine imaging used for diagnosis or management of mononucleosis
- One-time imaging of the spleen for assessment of splenomegaly at the time of illness is not recommended because of the wide variability encountered in normal values (2,3)[B].
- Serial imaging may be useful (2)
- Contrasted abdominal computed tomography (CT) for concerns about splenic rupture (incidence of 1 to 2 per 1,000 cases of mononucleosis, often spontaneous)

TREATMENT

GENERAL MEASURES

- Care is primarily supportive/symptomatic.
- No effective treatment presently is available.
- Care should be taken to avoid splenic trauma; avoid exercise and activities with jarring movements; use stool softeners to avoid increasing intra-abdominal pressure.
- Avoid alcohol and other liver toxins.

ISSUES FOR REFERRAL

Splenic rupture

ADDITIONAL THERAPIES

- Acyclovir/valacyclovir have been shown to decrease viral shedding but have no effect on the natural course of the illness, and no clinical benefit has been demonstrated (1)[B].
- Corticosteroids may be clinically indicated in cases with airway compromise, severe dysphagia, massive/painful spleen enlargement, myocarditis, or hemolytic anemia (4)[C].
- A Cochrane review evaluating the use of corticosteroids for symptom control in IM concluded that although symptoms were decreased for the first 12 hr, these benefits were lost at 2 to 4 days. Because there was no clear evidence on the effectiveness of steroids and, given the potential for adverse effects from the use of steroids, the Cochrane review recommended that corticosteroid use be avoided in uncomplicated cases (4)[A].

SURGERY/OTHER PROCEDURES

- Splenic rupture may be treated with either splenectomy or observation in selected situations (5)[A].
- Earlier return to play with splenectomy but must be weighed against risks of asplenia.
- If splenectomy chosen, *Haemophilus influenzae*, pneumococcal, and meningococcal vaccination should be provided prior to splenectomy (1)[C].

COMPLEMENTARY & ALTERNATIVE MEDICINE

None

ONGOING CARE

DIET

No special recommendations other than balanced diet with adequate fluids and fiber to avoid constipation; avoid alcohol.

PROGNOSIS

- Most patients who contract IM have an uneventful clinical course with an unremarkable recovery.
- Athletes often kept out of noncontact activities for 2.5 to 3 wk and contact activities for 3 to 4 wk, although return to activity decision is individualized (2)[C].
- Some athletes may take as long as 3 mo to return to their preillness levels of activity (6).
- Adult form of mononucleosis is different from the disease in children and adolescents:
  - Most adults: pharyngitis or lymphadenopathy
  - Fever is often more prolonged.
  - Abnormal liver function more frequent
  - Lymphocytosis/presence of atypical lymphocytes less common

COMPLICATIONS

- A wide variety of complications can occur, involving virtually all organ systems:
  - Edema of Waldeyer ring, resulting in airway compromise and/or severe dysphagia
  - Splenomegaly: nearly universal in IM, so not truly a complication
  - Splenic rupture: reported in 0.1–2% of cases; most cases occur in first 3 to 4 wk of illness; in one study, 50% nontraumatic. Splenic rupture can occur up to 8 wk after onset of illness (5).
  - Guillain-Barré syndrome
  - Cranial nerve palsies
  - Aseptic meningitis
  - Meningoencephalitis
  - Aplastic anemia
  - Hemolytic uremic syndrome
  - DIC
  - Jaundice
  - Acute acalculous cholecystitis
  - Myocarditis
- Conjecture that chronic fatigue syndrome may be associated with chronic EBV infection is not well supported in the literature.
- Immunocompromised (e.g., HIV, transplant patients, etc.): Lymphoma and other lymphoproliferative disorders are potential severe complications.

REFERENCES

1. Dunmire S, Verghese P, Balfour H Jr. Primary Epstein-Barr virus infection. *J Clin Virol*. 2018;102:84–92.
2. Putukian M, O'Connor FG, Stricker P, et al. Mononucleosis and athletic participation: an evidence-based subject review. *Clin J Sport Med*. 2008;18(4):309–315.
3. Hosey RG, Mattacola CG, Kriss V, et al. Ultrasound assessment of spleen size in collegiate athletes. *Br J Sports Med*. 2006;40(3):251–254.
4. Candy B, Hotopf M. Steroids for symptom control in infectious mononucleosis. *Cochrane Database Syst Rev*. 2006;(3):CD004402.
5. Bartlett A, Williams R, Hilton M. Splenic rupture in infectious mononucleosis: a systematic review of published case reports. *Injury*. 2016;47(3):531–538.
6. Becker J, Smith J. Return to play after infectious mononucleosis. *Sports Health*. 2014;6(3):232–238.

ADDITIONAL READING

Shephard R. Exercise and the athlete with infectious mononucleosis. *Clin J Sport Med*. 2017;27(2):168–178.

CLINICAL PEARLS

- In most cases, athletes will not feel well enough to participate in activity for several weeks. In addition, although the risk for splenic rupture is extremely low, given that most of these occur within the first 3 wk of illness, independent of spleen size, it is generally felt that it is safe to resume light activity 3 wk from the onset of symptoms, as long as the athlete is afebrile, has a good energy level, and does not have any significant associated abnormalities. The risk of splenic rupture likely diminishes as more time progresses; therefore, delaying return to play should be considered if clinical features, lack of athlete readiness, and/or associated complications are present. Treatment must, therefore, be individualized to account for all of these issues (6)[C].
- The appropriate time for safe return to contact play is unclear, although, given the risk for splenic rupture, a time frame of at least 3 wk commonly is recommended. Return can occur only after the athlete has no remaining clinical symptoms, is afebrile, and has a normal energy level. The risk for splenic rupture likely decreases as more time passes, allowing for individualized return-to-play decisions, depending on the athlete, sport, and other factors (6)[C].
- It is unclear what role exercise has on the natural history of IM disease. Although many athletes can self-regulate on return to ad lib activity if afebrile, it would appear that premature return to heavy exertion might prolong the duration of symptoms, most notably fatigue, and also be associated with a decrease in performance (2)[C].
- Fortunately, because of the nature of transmission, epidemics of mononucleosis are uncommon. Care should be taken to avoid shared water bottles, utensils, and so forth. Teams that travel extensively together have greater potential contacts for transmission. As the incubation period is lengthy, identifying index cases is difficult. It is not practical or necessary to exclude infected teammates if appropriate measures are taken to avoid spread of the virus. Appropriate rest, proper nutrition, and avoiding overtraining may reduce susceptibility to IM.

MYOFASCIAL PAIN SYNDROME AND TRIGGER POINTS

Navid Mahooti, MD, MPH, CAQSM

BASICS

DESCRIPTION

- Descriptions of painful muscle and "thickenings" or "knots" dates back to at least the 16th century. In the mid-1900s, Kellgren injected hypertonic saline into various anatomical structures such as fascia, tendon, and muscle in healthy volunteers and was able to chart zones of referred pain in neighboring and distant tissue called "target zones" (TZs). Kellgren's work influenced the U.S. physician Janet Travell, who, with David Simons, published the two-volume "Red Books" on *Myofascial Pain and Dysfunction*, arguably the most comprehensive works on myofascial pain syndrome (MPS).
- Travell classically defined a myofascial trigger point (MTP) as "a hyperirritable spot in skeletal muscle that is associated with a hypersensitive palpable nodule in a taut band. The spot is painful on compression and can give rise to characteristic referred pain, referred tenderness, motor dysfunction, and autonomic phenomena."
- ***Active*** MTPs cause spontaneous pain to the adjacent soft tissues and often to TZs.
- ***Latent*** MTPs (LMTPs) do not cause spontaneous pain but are tender and may exhibit features of active MTPs but only when palpated. Decision to treat LMTPs is debatable.
- MTPs are associated with muscle dysfunction, muscle weakness, limited range of motion, and autonomic phenomena.
- MPS implies the presence of more than one MTP. The definition and pathogenesis of MPS is still not fully understood, and disagreement persists about whether MPS is a disease or process, rather than a syndrome.
- Several authors have questioned the theory of MPS caused by MTPs, pointing out the lack of standardized diagnostic criteria as well as the many unanswered questions and knowledge gaps.

EPIDEMIOLOGY

Prevalence

Epidemiologic data are wide-ranging from 30% to 100% prevalence, likely because of the relatively high prevalence of musculoskeletal (MSK) pain in general, poor understanding of MPS, lack of widely accepted objective diagnostic criteria, and diagnostic misattribution to conditions that mimic MPS (see "Differential Diagnosis").

ETIOLOGY AND PATHOPHYSIOLOGY

- Lack of objective diagnostic techniques makes theories of MPS pathogenesis and pathophysiology speculative.
- Various hypotheses incorporating central nervous system (dorsal root ganglia and dorsal horn neurons), peripheral nervous system (motor endplate [MEP]), or both, have been described.
- It is generally accepted that the nodule of an MTP is comprised of multiple "contraction knots," described as perpetually contracted sarcomeres that have not (or will not) relax as a result of dysfunctionally overactive MEPs. In addition, metabolic alterations of the local soft tissue milieu cause cellular stress and release of myokines, inflammatory cytokines, and neurotransmitters. Neurogenic inflammation, sensitization, and limbic system dysfunction also may all play a role in MPS initiation, amplification, and perpetuation.

RISK FACTORS

Associated factors: overuse, repetitive motions, acute strain, posttraumatic, poor posture, poor ergonomics, poor mechanics, deconditioned muscle, fatigue, poor sleep hygiene, inactivity, prolonged sitting, infections, metabolic problems, and nutritional deficiencies

GENERAL PREVENTION

Recommendations are expert opinion: posture, core strength, ergonomics, correct biomechanics, adequate warm-up and cool down, foam-rolling (preexercise, and especially postexercise), massage, stretching, optimal hydration and nutrition, adequate sleep.

COMMONLY ASSOCIATED CONDITIONS

- *Fibromyalgia syndrome* (FMS) is distinct from MPS. Both conditions are associated with mood, health-related quality of life, sleep disturbance, disability, and dysfunction. However, FMS pain is typically widespread and symmetrically distributed, and exam reveals doughy muscles. MPS is usually local or regional, and exam reveals firm/ropey muscles.
- *Patients with FMS may develop MTPs, but most patients with MPS do not have FMS*. Successful treatment of MTPs in FMS has been reported to improve quality of life.
- MPS may be more common in patients with certain nutritional deficiencies (e.g., iron, vitamin D and vitamin B_{12}, Mg, selenium, zinc); gluten sensitivity; metabolic, visceral, endocrine (hypothyroid), infectious (parasitic infestation, recurrent vaginal yeast infections), and psychological conditions.

DIAGNOSIS

HISTORY

- Patients often report vague, persistent, or intermittent symptoms in a region of the body that do not fit a more classic MSK diagnosis, or resemble a common orthopedic/medical problem; typical examination and diagnostic tests are negative or equivocal, and traditional treatments are not effective (*see "Differential Diagnosis" for conditions mimicked by MPS*).
- Symptoms are more often unilateral but may be bilateral and can perplex the clinician and patient alike ("the pain moves around").
- MTPs can develop suddenly, hours to days after a particular activity or idiopathically.
- Pain severity ranges from mild and intermittent to excruciatingly debilitating and persistent.
- MTPs often present with weakness of regional muscles and nerve-like pain, and hence misdiagnosed as a radiculopathy or myelopathy. Advanced imaging findings (or lack thereof) that do not correlate with clinical presentation should raise suspicion for MTP (or other) etiology.
- Patients often report that massage, foam rolling, and stretching provide temporary pain relief.
- It is not uncommon for patients to see multiple physicians and allied health professionals and pursue numerous diagnostic tests and treatments, with no firm diagnosis and a generic treatment plan. Some patients with undiagnosed (or properly diagnosed but ineffectively treated) MPS may be labeled with psychiatric diagnoses, fibromyalgia, or chronic pain syndrome.

PHYSICAL EXAM

- Diagnosis is clinical and dependent on a clinician's thorough, meticulous palpation of regional muscles and soft tissues in search of the pain-generating central MTPs, which are arguably the hallmark of diagnosis.
- Familiarity and recognition of the remarkable referral patterns of MTPs to TZs is essential for the accurate diagnosis and treatment of MPS.
- Satisfaction of the following three criteria (which are inherently subjective, examiner-dependent, and lack robust sensitivity and specificity data) are currently considered the gold standard of diagnosis: (i) palpation of a taut band, (ii) identification of an exquisitely tender nodule in the taut band, and (iii) reproduction of the patient's index pain with sustained pressure on the MTP. Satisfaction of all three criteria is most specific and probably pathognomonic for a trigger point.
- Clinicians with a good understanding of the referral patterns and TZs often develop a skill at identifying the culprit trigger points and may choose to treat empirically (often with needling)—even in cases when just one or two of the aforementioned criteria are met.
- The presence of an MTP can also be confirmed by strumming or snapping the taut band in a direction perpendicular to the muscle fibers, which almost always produces a characteristic "local twitch response" (LTR), which is thought to be a quick contraction and then relaxation of the muscle fibers. The mechanism of the LTR is not fully understood.
- Diagnosis is complicated by the understanding that MTPs are prevalent across a wide range of MSK disorders and associated conditions.

DIFFERENTIAL DIAGNOSIS

- No body part is exempt from the painful effects of MPS; it should be on the differential diagnosis of every pain presentation. The following commonly occurring diagnoses (painful areas in bold) often have pain contributions, or turn out to be exclusively due to regional MTPs ("→" points to culprit muscles) (1,2,3)[B].
- **Cervical radiculopathy** → pectoralis minor, scalenes, cervical/shoulder girdle
- **Shoulder pain** → deltoid, long head biceps, pectorals, cuff muscles, latissimus dorsi, trapezius
- **Lateral epicondylosis** → common extensors, supinator, brachioradialis
- **Medial epicondylosis** → common flexors
- **Carpal tunnel syndrome** → volar forearm

- **Ulnar neuropathy/neuritis** → forearm
- **Triangular fibrocartilage complex (TFCC)** → extensor carpi ulnaris
- **Basilar thumb pain** → thenars, scalenes, supinator, brachialis, brachioradialis
- **Costochondritis** → pectoralis
- **Abdominal/flank** → intercostals, abdominal
- **Low back** → quadratus lumborum (QL), paraspinals, lower trapezius
- **Buttocks (piriformis syndrome, "sciatica," sacroiliac dysfunction)** → gluteals, piriformis/deep hip abductors, tensor fascia lata (TFL)
- **Greater trochanteric pain syndrome** → gluteals, piriformis, vastus lateralis (VL), QL
- **Hip osteoarthritis**: hip flexors, quadriceps
- **Meralgia paresthetica** → sartorius, VL, TFL
- **Knee pain** (*all causes*) → rectus femoris (RF), VL, vastus medialis obliquus (VMO), adductors, gastrocsoleus (GS), hamstrings, and others
- **Calf strain, shin splints, restless leg syndrome** → GS/calf muscles
- **Plantar heel/arch pain** → GS, calf muscles
- **Achilles tendon** → GS, tibialis posterior
- **Sesamoiditis** → Flexor hallucis brevis

DIAGNOSTIC TESTS & INTERPRETATION

- Diagnosis is clinical. Currently, there are no widely accepted objective criteria. Lack of consistent nomenclature, universally accepted diagnostic criteria, objective assessments (e.g., biomarkers, electrodiagnostics, or images), and conclusive biopsy findings has led to controversy and generally, poor understanding and acceptance by mainstream medicine (4)[B].
- Emerging imaging modalities: magnetic resonance elastography, ultrasound vibration elastography, infrared thermography (1)[B]

TREATMENT

GENERAL MEASURES

- There are numerous treatments described in the literature for MSK pain in general. It is unclear how often MPS is misdiagnosed as a condition that (i) presents similarly and (ii) responds to traditional treatments (e.g., subacromial impingement syndrome vs. deltoid trigger point).
- Availability of experienced practitioner to perform first-line treatments may affect outcomes.

First Line

- Identify and address causative biomechanical factors (e.g., postural, ergonomics, overuse, core weakness, etc.) (4,5,6,7)[B].
- Needling techniques (dry needling [DN], trigger point injection [TPI], acupuncture; heterogeneously described in the literature) emerging as treatment of choice for MPS. Popularized by Travell who wrote extensively on its effectiveness. Highly practitioner dependent. No universally accepted "best practice" regarding technique variables (needle length, bore, filiform vs. hypodermic, wet vs. dry). Mechanism of action not entirely clear (anatomical/mechanical, physiologic/biochemical, improved local blood flow and oxygenation, clearance of nociceptive substances all likely involved). Needling typically elicits LTRs (anywhere from 1 to >100) and results in immediate pain relief (even if LTR not elicited). Postprocedural discomfort for a few days is typical ("worse before it gets better") and associated with number of needle passes and LTRs. Several needling sessions over weeks to months may be necessary (4)[B],(6)[B],(7)[B],(8)[A].
- Physical therapy and manual techniques by practitioners experienced in MPS (often performed in conjunction with needling) (4,6,7)[B]. Therapists often employ various modalities and manual therapies, spray, and stretch.
- Exercise, stress reduction (7)[C]

Second Line

- Ultrasound (therapeutic): insufficient evidence to recommend
- Amitriptyline helpful for some MPS presentations
- Botulinum toxin effectively denervates the MEP, shown to provide pain relief, but study results are mixed, and it is unclear whether it is more effective than TPI or DN (7)[B].
- Topical nonsteroidal anti-inflammatories
- Oral nonsteroidal anti-inflammatories (benefit unknown for MPS)
- Kinesio-taping: temporary relief of cervical MPS
- Benzodiazepines/muscle relaxants may be effective for orofacial/temporomandibular joint (TMJ), MPS; may have side-effects
- Lidocaine patch (temporary relief)
- Serotonin and norepinephrine reuptake inhibitors may be beneficial in MPS especially if concomitant mood disorder.

ONGOING CARE

PATIENT EDUCATION

- *Trigger Point Therapy Workbook* by Clair Davies
- National Association of Myofascial Physical Therapists (https://www.myofascialtherapy.org/)
- https://www.painscience.com/tutorials/trigger-points.php (e-book)

PROGNOSIS

Most cases improve with consistent first-line treatments. If not responsive: Seek opinion of different physical/manual therapist, improve needling techniques, consider second-line treatment options, and broaden differential diagnosis and workup.

COMPLICATIONS

- Needling techniques are widely practiced and generally safe, but do carry risk. Vasovagal symptoms, postprocedural pain and bruising are not uncommon. Pneumothorax, cardiac tamponade, spinal epidural hematoma, abdominal visceral injury, as well as radial, median, peroneal, and other nerve injuries have been reported. Practitioners should be familiar with anatomy of treatment area.
- Ultrasound guidance may be helpful but not considered standard of care.

REFERENCES

1. Gerwin RD. Diagnosis of myofascial pain syndrome. *Phys Med Rehabil Clin N Am*. 2014;25(2):341–355.
2. Dor A, Kalichman L. A myofascial component of pain in knee osteoarthritis. *J Bodyw Mov Ther*. 2017;21(3):642–647.
3. Sergienko S, Kalichman L. Myofascial origin of shoulder pain: a literature review. *J Bodyw Mov Ther*. 2015;19(1):91–101.
4. Shah JP, Thaker N, Heimur J, et al. Myofascial trigger points then and now: a historical and scientific perspective. *PM R*. 2015;7(7):746–761.
5. Jafri MS. Mechanisms of myofascial pain. *Int Sch Res Notices*. 2014;2014:523924.
6. Desai MJ, Saini V, Saini S. Myofascial pain syndrome: a treatment review. *Pain Ther*. 2013;2(1):21–36.
7. Borg-Stein J, Iaccarino MA. Myofascial pain syndrome treatments. *Phys Med Rehabil Clin N Am*. 2014;25(2):357–374.
8. Kietrys DM, Palombaro KM, Azzaretto E, et al. Effectiveness of dry needling for upper-quarter myofascial pain: a systematic review and meta-analysis. *J Orthop Sports Phys Ther*. 2013;43(9):620–634.

ADDITIONAL READING

- Simons DG, Travell JG, Simons LS. *Travell & Simmon's Myofascial Pain and Dysfunction: The Trigger Point Manual. Upper Half of Body*. Vol 1. 2nd ed. Baltimore, MD: Williams & Wilkins; 1999.
- Travell J, Simons DG. *Myofascial Pain and Dysfunction: The Trigger Point Manual. The Lower Extremities*. Vol 2. 1st ed. Baltimore, MD: Williams & Wilkins; 1993.

CLINICAL PEARLS

- Pathophysiology not fully understood
- Commonly overlooked cause of numerous pain presentations; include MPS in the differential diagnosis of every pain presentation.
- Diagnosis is clinical, requires careful palpation along with suggestive history.
- Understanding the principle of referred pain and "TZs" is essential to avoid misattribution and provide proper treatment.
- Needling techniques are growing in favor and largely considered first-line gold standard. Study quality is improving, but many questions remain, and further research is needed.
- Consistent, concomitant incorporation of all "first-line" treatments is often necessary.

MYOSITIS OSSIFICANS

Shawn Skarpnes, MD, CAQSM

BASICS

DESCRIPTION

- A localized, nonneoplastic, heterotopic ossification that develops in muscle from physical trauma
- Anterior muscle groups of the thigh and arm are most frequently affected but may occur at any site.
- Occurs more commonly from muscle contusion than from muscle strain
- Osteoblasts proliferate inappropriately in a healing muscle hematoma and lay down bone over a period of weeks to months.
- Bone maturation usually takes 6 to 12 mo to complete.
- Once ossification takes place, little can be done to accelerate the resorptive process, which may take months to years.
- Average duration of symptoms related to myositis ossificans (MO) is 1.1 yr.
- Synonym(s): MO traumatica (MOT), MO circumscripta

EPIDEMIOLOGY

- MOT is an acquired condition after injury and represents 60–75% of all MO.
- MO progressiva is a rare autosomal dominant genetic disorder that leads to an irreversible severe generalized form. Neurogenic MO is nontraumatic and associated with severe burns, hemophilia, and neuromuscular disorders.
- MOT most frequently occurs in adolescent and young adult men from a sport-related injury.
- Occurs in 9–14% of muscle contusions overall
- Highest prevalence following a quadriceps muscle contusion
- Incidence increases with severity of injury.

ETIOLOGY AND PATHOPHYSIOLOGY

- No clear pathogenesis established
- It is postulated that after a muscle is crushed or torn, an inflammatory cascade recruits an influx of macrophages into the necrotic tissue. A prolonged macrophage invasion may lead to inappropriate differentiation and stimulation of mesenchymal cells into osteoblastic stem cells under anoxic conditions.
- A lesion matures over 3 to 6 mo and forms an eggshell-like calcification on imaging.

RISK FACTORS

- Contact sports
- Application of heat or massage to injury site
- Premature return to activity
- Reduced range of motion of injured muscle
- Previous muscle injury
- Delay in treatment >3 days
- Adjacent joint effusion

GENERAL PREVENTION

- Immobilize the muscle in slight tension immediately after injury for 24 hr: for example, knee placed in 120 degrees of flexion for quadriceps injury.
- Minimize hemorrhage within the first 48 hr with rest, ice, compression, and elevation.
- Avoid soft tissue therapy within the first 48 hr of injury.
- Avoid forceful stretching and active range of motion.
- Nonsteroidal anti-inflammatory drugs (NSAIDs) like indomethacin, if used within the 5 days postinjury, may prevent heterotopic bone formation.

COMMONLY ASSOCIATED CONDITIONS

MO is a complication seen in 1 of 5 total hip arthroplasties and may occur in the joint capsule, adjacent tendon, ligament, or fascia.

DIAGNOSIS

HISTORY

- Muscle contusion or strain becomes unresponsive to conservative therapy within the first 2 wk.
- Symptoms intensify 2 to 3 wk after trauma.
- Injured muscle becomes indurated and range of motion progressively declines.
- Night pain is often present.

PHYSICAL EXAM

- Initially, may palpate a doughy mass at 1 to 2 wk that gradually becomes indurated
- Persistent tenderness to palpation with local edema that fails to resolve
- Reduced range of motion that worsens 2 to 3 wk after injury

DIFFERENTIAL DIAGNOSIS

- Muscle contusion
- Muscle or tendon tear
- Fracture
- Malignant neoplasm: osteosarcoma, lymphoma, or rhabdomyosarcoma
- Compartment syndrome
- Abscess
- Rhabdomyolysis

DIAGNOSTIC TESTS & INTERPRETATION

Initial Tests (lab, imaging)

- Ultrasound: detects calcifications within 2 wk of injury but may be difficult to differentiate from malignancy (1)[B]
- X-ray: detects calcifications within 3 to 4 wk of injury, initially with periosteal bone reaction at the periphery (1)[B]

- Computed tomography (CT): often not required but is the best modality to demonstrate characteristic zoning pattern of MO with ossification at the periphery versus central zoning seen with osteosarcoma
- Magnetic resonance imaging (MRI): order if clinical picture uncertain or no history of trauma to rule out malignant soft tissue mass
- Once bone maturation is complete, imaging often reveals a well-circumscribed, peripherally calcified mass, with a radiolucent center that has an eggshell-like appearance.
- Radiographic evidence of calcifications persists long after clinical resolution.
- Erythrocyte sedimentation rate (ESR), C-reactive protein (CRP), and alkaline phosphatase may be elevated but are nonspecific.

Follow-Up Tests & Special Considerations

Bone scan can determine if lesion is fully developed. A mature lesion is positive only on the delayed phase whereas developing bone is positive on pool, flow, and delayed phases.

TREATMENT

GENERAL MEASURES

- Rest, ice, compression, and elevation are universally recommended in the acute phase (2)[A],(3,4)[B].
- Perform nonpainful passive stretching and strengthening (2)[A],(4)[B].
- MO is often a self-limiting condition, in which clinical and radiologic follow-up will suffice without pharmacologic or surgical intervention (3,4)[B].
- Corticosteroid injections are contraindicated (2)[A].

MEDICATION

- Most low-grade MO does not require NSAIDs.
- High-risk cases: Indomethacin at 75 to 100 mg/day, if initiated within 24 to 48 hr of injury and continued 7 to 14 days, is indicated to reduce new bone formation (3)[B].

ADDITIONAL THERAPIES

Once heterotopic ossification develops:

- Extracorporeal shockwave therapy may improve muscle function and pain but has not been shown to reduce ossification size.
- Local electrotherapy may reduce muscle spasms.
- Bisphosphonate therapy has been used in case reports but must be initiated early in disease course and continued for several months (5)[C]:
  - Should be avoided in women of childbearing age

SURGERY/OTHER PROCEDURES

- Surgical excision is rarely indicated and often not considered in the 1st yr.
- Surgery is contraindicated for immature lesions due to a high reoccurrence rate.
- Criteria for excision include lesion maturation complete, limited range of motion/function, neurovascular disturbance, and predisposition for further injury.
- Biopsy has a high false-positive rate and should be avoided, especially during the early or intermediate stages of the disease.

ONGOING CARE

PROGNOSIS

- 90% of athletes return to light physical activity within 3 mo and full sport activity within 6 mo (4)[C].
- Average duration of symptoms related to MO is 1.1 yr, but complete resorption of calcifications may take years or remain indefinitely.

REFERENCES

1. Koh ES, McNally EG. Ultrasound of skeletal muscle injury. *Semin Musculoskelet Radiol* 2007;11(2):162.
2. King JB. Post-traumatic ectopic calcification in the muscles of athletes: a review. *Br J Sports Med*. 1998;32(4):287–290.
3. Mehallo CJ, Drezner JA, Bytomski JR. Practical management: nonsteroidal antiinflammatory drug (NSAID) use in athletic injuries. *Clin J Sport Med*. 2006;16(2):170.
4. Simon T, Guillodo Y, Madouas G, et al. Myositis ossificans traumatica (circumscripta) and the return to sport: a retrospective series of 19 cases. *Joint Bone Spine*. 2016;83(4):416–420.
5. Mani-Babu S, Wolman R, Keen R. Quadriceps traumatic myositis ossificans in a football player: management with intravenous pamidronate. *Clin J Sport Med*. 2014;(5):e56–e58.

ADDITIONAL READING

Sferopoulos NK, Kotakidou R, Petropoulos AS. Myositis ossificans in children: a review. *Eur J Orthop Surg Traumatol*. 2017;27(4):491–502.

CLINICAL PEARLS

- MO can occur in the absence of trauma and may mimic other benign or malignant pathology during its early stage.
- Ultrasound is the most sensitive modality in early detection of MO.
- Reduced range of motion of the injured muscle is the most reliable predictor of MO formation.
- Most athletes with MO return to full sport activity within 6 mo but can be symptomatic for 1 yr or longer.

M

NASAL SEPTAL HEMATOMAS

Brandon M. Bockewitz, MD, CAQSM

BASICS

- Nasal bone fractures are the third most common fracture in the human skeleton, 90% of which involve septal injury.
- Nasal bone fractures are the most common facial bone fracture in sports injuries.
- Hematoma contained in the tight submucosal space can lead to pressure necrosis or abscess. Cartilage destruction, collapse of the nasal dorsum, or a saddle nose deformity may result.
- Dorsal nose deformity causes significant cosmetic and functional morbidity that usually is permanent.
- Once identified, nasal septal hematomas require urgent management.
- Although rare, monitor for the presence of septal hematoma in every case of nasal trauma and treat promptly when diagnosed.

DESCRIPTION

- Trauma causing bleeding between the septal cartilage and perichondrium resulting in hematoma collection which separates the cartilage from nutrient source
- Septal hematomas can occur bilaterally or unilaterally.

DIAGNOSIS

HISTORY

Trauma to the nose, most often an inferior blow, because the supportive structure of the lower 2/3 of the nose is composed entirely of cartilage

PHYSICAL EXAM

- Signs and symptoms:
  - Epistaxis, nasal deformity and swelling, ecchymosis, pain, and crepitant to palpation, usually from associated nasal fracture
  - Difficulty breathing through one or both sides of the nose
- Physical examination:
  - Septal hematoma will appear as a bluish red bulge from the septum into the nasal vestibule or as an asymmetric mucosal fold. Newly formed hematomas may lack the classic bluish red discoloration, making direct palpation a more reliable exam finding.
  - Control bleeding with direct pressure, topical decongestants, or cautery, as indicated for optimal visualization.
  - Septal hematomas do not shrink with use of decongestants.
  - Ensure the absence of cerebrospinal fluid (CSF) leak.
  - Patient positioning: Drainage of blood from the nose is best achieved with the patient in a supine position with the head elevated.
  - Visualize the anterior septum, preferably using a nasal speculum or otoscope with the tip inserted past the nasal vestibule. If necessary, a rigid nasal endoscope may be needed. Sufficient lighting and suction are helpful.
  - Direct palpation: Using a gloved finger or cotton tip applicator, gently palpate along the entire nasal septum, feeling for swelling, fluctuance, widening of the septum, or any other abnormalities.
  - Septal hematomas remain compressible with palpation via finger or cotton tip applicator:
    - Blood clots adjacent to the nasal septum can falsely represent a septal hematoma and should be evacuated before examining the nasal septum.
    - Masses located deep within the nasal cavity, out of the reach of a gloved finger, may require palpation by a cotton swab, again, feeling for a soft mass as opposed to the firm cartilaginous septum.

DIAGNOSTIC TESTS & INTERPRETATION

- Rarely necessary for routine cases
- Delayed presentation to health care providers or failed drainage can lead to nasal septal abscess.
- Purulent specimens should be sent for Gram stain and culture, both aerobic and anaerobic.
- Suspicion for CSF leak should be ruled out.

TREATMENT

Prompt intervention:

- Needle aspiration or sharp incision and drainage under local or general anesthesia followed by suction of the clot, if needed, and irrigation (1,2,3):
  - Mucosal incision should be made over the area of greatest fluctuance, with care taken not to damage the underlying cartilage.
  - Bilateral hematomas should be treated with staggered incisions to decrease risk of possible through-and-through perforation.
- Wick or drain placement is unnecessary unless suspicious for septal abscess (4)[C].
- If a drain was placed, it can be removed when drainage has stopped for 24 hr.
- Bilateral anterior nasal packing to approximate the perichondrium and prevent recurrence of the hematoma (3)[C]
- Continue nasal packing for 2 to 4 days (5).
- Systemic antibiotic coverage with clindamycin or amoxicillin-clavulanic acid provides appropriate coverage against the most common abscess pathogens (1,2,3)[C], including:
  - *Staphylococcus aureus*.
  - *Streptococcus pneumoniae*.
  - Group A β-hemolytic *Streptococcus*.
  - *Haemophilus influenzae*.

ONGOING CARE

FOLLOW-UP RECOMMENDATIONS

- Patients and parents should be instructed on signs and symptoms of nasal septal hematoma because formation may be delayed up to 14 days after the initial trauma (3).
- Close follow-up after diagnosis and drainage for evaluation of possible failed drainage or reaccumulation of blood after successful drainage
- After immediate management, continue nasal packing and follow up with otolaryngologist in 2 to 4 days (5).
- Children should be followed for 12 to 18 mo for cartilaginous changes and cosmetic defects (3).

COMPLICATIONS

- Reaccumulation of hematoma
- Nasal septal abscess
- Saddle nose deformity

REFERENCES

1. Menger DJ, Tabink I, Nolst Trenité GJ. Treatment of septal hematomas and abscesses in children. *Facial Plast Surg*. 2007;23(4):239–243.
2. Lopez MA, Liu JH, Hartley BE, et al. Septal hematoma and abscess after nasal trauma. *Clin Pediatr (Phila)*. 2000;39(10):609–610.
3. Savage RR, Valvich C. Hematoma of the nasal septum. *Pediatr Rev*. 2006;27(12):478–479.
4. Perkins SW, Dayan SH. Management of nasal trauma. *Aesthetic Plast Surg*. 2002;26(Suppl 1):S3.
5. Marston AP, O'Brien EK, Hamilton GS III. Nasal injuries in sports. *Clin Sports Med*. 2017;36(2):337–353.

ADDITIONAL READING

- Kaufman BR, Heckler FR. Sports-related facial injuries. *Clin Sports Med*. 1997;16(3):543–562.
- Puricelli MD, Zitsch RP III. Septal hematoma following nasal trauma. *J Emerg Med*. 2016;50(1):121–122.

SEE ALSO

Incision and Drainage of a Septal Hematoma or Abscess

CLINICAL PEARLS

- Special populations: children (4)[C]:
  - Increased incidence of septal hematoma secondary to highly cartilaginous nasal skeleton
  - Minor trauma can lead to hematoma formation, even without signs of external injury.
  - Any history of nasal trauma warrants intranasal examination.
- The nasal packing usually is left in for about 2 to 4 days so that the mucosa can heal and fill in the space where the hematoma formed.
- Return to play is not advised until the packing is removed owing to impaired breathing and the need to protect the septal mucosa while it heals.
- After removal of packing, return to play is based on consideration of the associated nasal fracture and whether or not an infection is present.

NEAR-DROWNING/DROWNING

Kevin Waninger, MD, MS, FAAFP, FACEP, FACSM, CAQSM

BASICS

- Drowning is the process of experiencing respiratory impairment from submersion (airway goes below the surface of the liquid)/immersion (water splashed over the face) in water (1,2).
- The terms "drowned" and "near-drowned" have been used to describe the outcomes dead or alive, respectively. The term "near-drowned" has also been used to describe patients who subsequently died from drowning. This usage has led to uncertainty about the meaning of the term. Therefore, the term "near-drowning" has lost favor. The term "drowned" will continue to refer to a person who died or suffered injury from drowning.
- Near-drowning, dry drowning, wet drowning, delayed drowning, and secondary drowning are all terms that are not medically accepted diagnosis. These terms should be abandoned in favor of understanding and communicating drowning as a process that is mild, moderate, and severe with fatal or nonfatal outcomes. Someone who drowns has three outcomes: (i) fatal, (ii) nonfatal with injury/illness, and (iii) nonfatal without injury/illness.

DESCRIPTION

- Drowning is a process resulting in primary respiratory impairment from submersion or immersion in a liquid medium. The pathophysiology is primarily related to abnormal gas exchange, with resultant hypoxia.
- Hypoxia may result from laryngospasm causing no pulmonary gas exchange or aspiration of fluids causing pulmonary injury and subsequent disruption of productive gas exchange.
- The drowning process is a continuum that begins when the victim's airway lies below the surface of a liquid, usually water, at which time the victim voluntarily holds their breath (submersion or immersion).
- Breath holding is usually followed by an involuntary period of laryngospasm secondary to the presence of liquid in the oropharynx or larynx, resulting in hypoxemia, hypercarbia, and acidosis.
- During this laryngospasm, there is no exchange of air, and the victim may swallow large quantities of water. As arterial oxygen tension drops further, laryngospasm abates, and the victim actively breathes liquid. The amount of liquid inhaled varies considerably from victim to victim.
- Changes occur in the lungs, body fluids, blood-gas tensions, acid–base balance, and electrolyte concentrations, which are dependent on the composition and volume of the liquid aspirated and the duration of submersion. Surfactant washout, pulmonary hypertension (HTN), and shunting also contribute to the development of hypoxemia.
- The clinical presentation and prognosis vary due to different water temperatures, different fluid properties (fresh water, seawater, Dead Sea water, water contaminated with chemicals and bacteria), and the variety of environments (from toilets to hurricane sea conditions) in which drowning occurs.
- The heart and brain are the organs at greatest risk for permanent, detrimental changes from relatively brief periods of hypoxia. Posthypoxic encephalopathy, with or without cerebral edema, is the most common cause of death in hospitalized drowning victims.
- Reinstitution of adequate ventilation and oxygenation before the occurrence of circulatory arrest and irreversible nervous system damage may result in complete and dramatic restoration of function (if aspiration does not occur).
- When aspiration occurs, due to ventilation/perfusion mismatch and shunting, prolonged hypoxemia and subsequent complications are more likely to occur (1,2,3).

EPIDEMIOLOGY

- Drowning incidents occur in swimming pools, lakes, rivers, streams, storm drains, hot tubs, bathtubs, and even toilets and buckets in toddlers.
- A swimming pool is 14 times more likely than a motor vehicle to be involved in the death of a child age ≤4 yr.
- 80% of drowning victims age >1 yr are males.
- Although drowning rates have slowly declined, fatal drowning remains the second leading cause of unintentional injury-related death for children ages 1 to 14 yr.
- 19% of drowning deaths involving children occur in public pools with certified lifeguards present. Of all preschoolers who drown, 70% are in the care of one or both parents at the time of the drowning, and 75% are missing from sight for <5 min.
- The majority of children who survive without sequelae are discovered within 2 min following submersion, and most children who die are found after 10 min (2,4).

Incidence

- From 2005 to 2014, fatal unintentional drownings in the United States averaged about 10 deaths per day (5).
- Among those 1 to 14 yr old, fatal drowning remains the second leading cause of unintentional injury-related death behind motor vehicle accidents (2,4).
- For every child who died from drowning, another five children received emergency department (ED) care for nonfatal submersion injuries.
- Children (<5 yr) and adolescents (ages 15 to 24 yr) have the highest drowning rates.

Prevalence

- Rates of fatal drowning are notably higher among African Americans (1.3 times) and American Indians and Alaskan Natives (1.8 times) compared to Caucasians (2,4).
- For children ages 5 to 14 yr, the fatal drowning rate of African American children (3.2 times) and American Indian and Alaskan Native children (2.4 times) is higher than for Caucasian children (5).

ETIOLOGY AND PATHOPHYSIOLOGY

- Unexpected submersion. Struggle does not always occur. Splashing, waving, and yelling rarely occur during actual drowning events. People in distress still have the ability to keep afloat and may signal for help, but drowning patients are suffocating and are in imminent danger of death within seconds.
- Aspiration of variable amounts of water. Grossly contaminated water poses a risk of pulmonary infection.
- Laryngospasm
- Hypoxia
- Metabolic acidosis
- Myocardial dysfunction
- Coagulation abnormalities
- Multisystem organ dysfunction with renal failure
- Central nervous system (CNS) dysfunction (posthypoxic encephalopathy)

RISK FACTORS

- Unattended children at water sites; inadequate adult supervision
- Alcohol and/or drug abuse (50% cases involving adolescents and adults)
- Limited swimming ability and exhaustion
- Trauma
- Risky behavior in the water; rough play
- Shallow water blackout is the deliberate prolonged submersion with intentional hyperventilation after breath-hold diving or swimming, with no warning felt prior to sudden loss of consciousness from hypoxia (4).
- Ascent "deep water" blackout caused by latent hypoxia during ascent from depth due to changes in lung partial pressure of oxygen
- Exacerbation of existing medical problems (seizure disorder, cardiac disease, diabetes, syncope, cerebrovascular accident)
- Cold-water immersion or hypothermia; cold shock response; young children more susceptible due to larger body surface-to-mass ratio; decreases the metabolic rate, survival to full recovery possible
- SCUBA: contamination of air supply with toxic gases (i.e., carbon monoxide), running out of air at depth
- Oxygen-induced seizures in divers using oxygen-enriched air mixtures
- Panic/anxiety
- Improper fencing of pools (at least 5 feet high with self-closing latches should be required) (1,4)

GENERAL PREVENTION

Drowning is preventable! Prevention is the key:

- Parental supervision of children around water; watch empty pails, buckets, and toddlers around toilets.
- Carefully watching children while they bathe
- Swimming lessons: Children 1 to 4 yr old who drowned were significantly less likely to have attended swimming classes than matched controls (6)[B].
- The American Academy of Pediatrics recommends that all children be taught to swim after age 5 yr but makes no recommendation for younger children (5,6)[C].
- Adequate pool fencing; wearing properly sized life jackets; improved pool design preventing children from being trapped when submerged
- Poor pool maintenance resulting in murky or cloudy water
- Instruction/supervision of lifeguards in methods of waterfront surveillance and resuscitation techniques
- Education of public in prudent consumption of alcoholic beverages; impose severe sanctions against boaters who are intoxicated.
- Encourage people to learn to swim, understand the limits of their swimming ability, and never swim alone.
- Restricted swimming areas; post proper signage in areas of dangerous underwater tow; pay attention to the weather, tides and water conditions, and especially currents. Currents are usually perceived from the outside as weaker than they actually are.
- Understand the water environment where you are swimming, diving, or boating.
- Instruct greater numbers of the public in basic life support (BLS) and proper cardiopulmonary resuscitation (CPR) techniques.
- Bring a cordless telephone to the pool so children are not left unsupervised while answering a phone call.

DIAGNOSIS

Pediatric Considerations

- Hypothermia may be protective, as the rate of cerebral oxygen consumption is reduced.
- Diving reflex in young children is triggered by submersion of face in cold water, with bradycardia and redistribution of blood flow to heart and brain.
- Family history of sudden death by drowning may suggest a genetic cause for syncope, such as prolonged QT syndrome (LQTt1) because swimming can trigger arrhythmias that cause unexplained drowning.

HISTORY

- See "Risk Factors."
- Information from witnesses or emergency medical services personnel at the scene

PHYSICAL EXAM

- Cardiac presentation depends on severity of exposure, ranging from sinus tachycardia to cardiac arrest and apnea. It is not uncommon for these patients to respond to prolonged CPR. Children who still require CPR at the time they arrive at the ED have a poor prognosis, with at least half of survivors suffering significant neurologic impairment.

- The process of drowning is characterized by a gradual decrease in arterial oxygen saturation with a simultaneous decrease in cardiac output. Cardiac arrest is, therefore, not sudden but is preceded by a brief period of tachycardia and HTN, followed by bradycardia with hypotension and electromechanical dissociation (pulseless electrical activity).
- Ventricular fibrillation is rare after submersion, unless resulting from acute hypothermia or triggered by mechanical irritation. The sequence of cardiac rhythm deterioration is usually tachycardia followed by bradycardia, pulseless electrical activity, and finally asystole. Drowning victims in cardiac arrest may not respond to defibrillation. The automated external defibrillator may not play a major role in improving the success of resuscitation after drowning (1,3)[A].
- Whether the drowning event occurs in fresh water or seawater, the end result is pulmonary edema, a decrease in pulmonary compliance, and an increase in the ventilation/perfusion mismatch.
- Patients with water aspiration may present with minimal symptoms, severe bloodstained pulmonary edema, or frank cardiopulmonary arrest. Cyanosis, dyspnea, and/or copious pulmonary secretions may be present.
- Cerebral edema/injury
- Look for evidence of trauma/cervical spine injury.
- Look for hypothermia; full vital signs with rectal temperature required

DIFFERENTIAL DIAGNOSIS

- Consider a potential underlying cause of submersion injury, such as alcohol or drug intoxication, myocardial infarction, syncope (prolonged QT syndrome), seizure (including O_2 induced), stroke, hypoglycemia, or trauma.
- Head or spinal cord injury/trauma (accidents involving diving, waterskiing, surfing, or watercraft)
- Venomous stings by aquatic animals
- Decompression sickness or arterial gas embolism, nitrogen narcosis from scuba diving
- Consider child abuse/neglect.

DIAGNOSTIC TESTS & INTERPRETATION

- Most drowning victims do not aspirate enough fluid to cause life-threatening changes in electrolytes or blood volume.
- Rarely is there a need for emergent treatment of electrolyte abnormalities unless very large volumes of water are aspirated or the drowning event occurs in a highly concentrated liquid medium such as the Dead Sea.
- Arterial blood gases should be obtained.
- Complete blood count (CBC); significant changes of hemoglobin and hematocrit are seldom seen in human drowning victims.
- Chemistry panels usually normal, but rule out hyperkalemia, hypernatremia, hyponatremia, or signs of renal failure
- Urinalysis
- Coagulation panel with prothrombin time (PT)/ international normalized ratio (INR)
- Alcohol and toxicology screen
- Chest x-rays may be normal initially or show infiltrates ranging from a patchy distribution to global pulmonary edema.
- Computed tomography (CT) scan of head may be needed to rule out acute or chronic intracranial process in unconscious patients.
- Obtain cervical spine films if you suspect head/neck trauma.

TREATMENT

- Prehospital:
  - Airway, breathing, and circulation (ABCs), remove wet clothing, initiate rewarming as soon as possible, intravenous (IV) with 0.9% normal saline (Watch fluids in patients with pulmonary edema.)
  - Initiate CPR as soon as possible if indicated; begin in the water if can be done without putting rescuer at risk; in-water resuscitation consists of ventilation alone because attempts at chest compression are futile as long as the rescuer and drowning patient are in deep water. Assessment of a pulse serves no purpose until the rescuer and patient are out of the water and on some solid space (2).
  - BLS, and sometimes rescue breathing alone, performed by laypersons, play a key role in the survival of the drowning victim (2,3)[A]. Drowning patients with only respiratory arrest may respond after a few rescue breaths.
  - CPR with chest compression only is not recommended in management of drowned patients (2)[C].
  - Endotracheal administration of drugs is not recommended in drowning patients (2)[C].
  - Although unusual, recovery with normal neurologic function has been reported even after prolonged cardiac arrest.
  - Avoid further aspiration; apply cricoid pressure during bag-valve-mask ventilation. Secure airway if needed, and protect against aspiration of stomach contents; intubation with 100% oxygen
  - Strict cervical spine precautions (1,2,3)[A]
  - The subdiaphragmatic thrust (Heimlich) maneuver to remove water from the abdomen is not recommended unless a foreign body is suspected of obstructing the airway (1,3)[A].
- ED treatment:
  - Correct hypoxia; titrate to oxygen saturation; intubation with positive end-expiratory pressure can be effective in reversing the abnormal V/Q relationships. In patients who are alert, nasal continuous positive airway pressure may be used for ventilation support.
  - The risk for aspiration from water and stomach contents is still present, so strict aspiration precautions with elevation of head of bed if possible are recommended.
  - If bronchospasm is present or suspected, give nebulized β_2-agonist treatments.
  - Evaluate and treat traumatic injuries.
  - If in cardiopulmonary arrest, initiate advanced cardiac life support measures; continue resuscitation until core temperature >32°C or until spontaneous pulse and respirations return.
  - Follow temperature and continue rewarming efforts if indicated.
  - Insert a nasogastric tube to decompress the stomach. The most frequent complication during a resuscitation attempt is regurgitation of stomach contents.

- Insert Foley catheter, if needed, to follow urine output.
- Check and correct severe electrolyte abnormalities, and monitor acid–base balance.
- Antibiotics needed only in those patients who become febrile, develop new pulmonary infiltrates, or have purulent secretions. Prophylactic antibiotics do not improve morbidity or mortality (3)[A].

- There is very little evidence to support the use of steroids for reducing pulmonary injury (2,3)[A].
- Management of patients with suspected hypoxic brain injury includes hyperventilation (maintain Pa_{CO_2} at 25 to 30 mm Hg), head elevation (if no C-spine injury is present), diuretics, and muscle relaxants.
- It appears that in the absence of hypothermia that may have occurred during the drowning process, aggressive brain resuscitation in the neurologically impaired drowning patient, using current techniques, is of limited benefit in returning patients to normal neurologic function.

ADMISSION, INPATIENT, AND NURSING CONSIDERATIONS

- Admission criteria:
  - Intensive care unit (ICU):
    - Patients who required CPR or artificial resuscitation
    - Abnormal chest x-ray
    - Arterial blood gas abnormalities
    - Glasgow Coma Scale (GCS) <13
  - Admit observation:
    - Submersion unknown or >1 min
    - History of cyanosis or apnea
    - Required brief assisted ventilation
    - GCS >13
    - Delayed pulmonary edema (up to 12 hr)
    - Delayed neurologic abnormalities
- Discharge criteria:
  - Questionable history of submersion, after observation in ED for 6 to 8 hr
  - Normal chest x-ray
  - No respiratory distress
  - No neurologic deterioration
  - Discharge to reliable home, with instructions to return for shortness of breath or mental status changes.
  - There has never been a case published in the medical literature of a patient who received a clinical assessment, was initially without symptoms, and who later deteriorated and died. People who have drowned and have minimal symptoms will usually either get better or get worse within 6 hr.

ONGOING CARE

PROGNOSIS

- Prognosis of resuscitated drowning victim is related to degree of damage secondary to the anoxic episode and the duration of immersion and pulmonary insult.
- Residual complications of near-drowning may include intellectual impairment, convulsive disorders, and pulmonary or cardiac complications.

REFERENCES

1. Bierens JJ, Lunetta P, Tipton M, et al. Physiology of drowning: a review. *Physiology (Bethesda)*. 2016;31(2):147–166.
2. Szpilman D, Bierens JJ, Handley AJ, et al. Drowning. *N Engl J Med*. 2012;366(22):2102–2010.
3. Layon AJ, Modell JH. Drowning: update 2009. *Anesthesiology*. 2009;110(6):1390–1401.
4. Boyd C, Levy A, McProud T, et al. Fatal and nonfatal drowning outcomes related to dangerous underwater breath-holding behaviors—New York State, 1988–2011. *MMWR Morb Mortal Wkly Rep*. 2015;64(19):518–521.
5. Centers for Disease Control and Prevention Childhood Injury Report. Unintentional drowning: get the facts. https://www.cdc.gov. Accessed April 22, 2018.
6. Brenner RA, Taneja GS, Haynie DL, et al. Association between swimming lessons and drowning in childhood: a case-control study. *Arch Pediatr Adolesc Med*. 2009;163(3):203–210.

ADDITIONAL READING

- Engel SC. Drowning episodes: prevention and resuscitation tips. *J Fam Pract*. 2015;64(2):E1–E6.
- Idris AH, Berg RA, Bierens J, et al. Recommended guidelines for uniform reporting of data from drowning: the "Utstein style." *Circulation*. 2003;108(20):2565–2574.
- Mott TF, Latimer KM. Prevention and treatment of drowning. *Am Fam Physician*. 2016;93(7):576–582.
- Papa L, Hoelle R, Idris A. Systematic review of definitions for drowning incidents. *Resuscitation*. 2005;65(3):255–264.

CLINICAL PEARLS

- Medical authorities traditionally made a great distinction between salt water and fresh water drowning. The theory was that because of its high salt content, seawater in the lungs would affect the body very differently from fresh water in a variety of ways. Although this is true in theory, very few survivors of near-drowning ingest enough water to make a difference, and this rarely becomes an issue in treating patients who arrive at the hospital. In practice, water temperature and the presence of any contaminants are much more important considerations.
- Hypoxia is the main threat in drowning victims, and resuscitation efforts should be directed toward restoration of optimal oxygenation.
- Key risk factors include male sex, age <14 yr, alcohol/drug use, low income, poor education, rural residency, aquatic exposure, risky behavior, and lack of supervision.
- Prevention is the key to saving lives.
- Sometimes respiratory symptoms and hypoxia are delayed for up to 6 hr after submersion or immersion.

NECK LACERATIONS AND PENETRATING INJURIES

Se Won Lee, MD

BASICS

- Unstawble patients with penetrating neck trauma should receive definitive care in the operating room.
- Stable patients should be transferred to a trauma center.
- Occlusive dressings that are soaked in petroleum jelly should be applied to lacerations over major veins to prevent air embolism. If possible, patients should also be placed in Trendelenburg position.
- Before attempting to secure the airway, be sure to have a surgical airway kit at the bedside.
- Do not be fooled by the seemingly stable patient. These patients can decompensate rapidly and without warning.
- Immediate surgical exploration is required in 15–20% of cases of penetrating neck injury (1).

Pediatric Considerations

Esophageal and venous injuries present with very subtle findings, and the diagnosis of injuries to these structures is often delayed

DESCRIPTION

- Penetrating neck trauma is defined as a wound that violates the platysma muscle.
- Anatomic consideration: The neck is divided into *three zones* based on superficial landmarks and are numbered from most caudal to cephalad:
  - Zone I extends from the top of the sternum to the sternal notch or cricoid cartilage:
    - Penetrating trauma in this zone carries the highest mortality due to injury to thoracic structures.
    - An isolated Horner syndrome may be the only presenting sign of injury to this zone.
  - Zone II extends from the cricoid cartilage to the angle of the mandible:
    - The majority of penetrating neck wounds occur in this zone.
    - However, because injured structures are more easily identified, treatment, both in the emergency department (ED) and the operating room, is more often successful. Therefore, mortality rates are the lowest in this zone.
  - Zone III extends cephalad from the angle of the mandible to the base of the skull:
    - Least commonly injured
    - Injuries to the distal carotid artery can mimic a stroke.

EPIDEMIOLOGY

- Penetrating neck injuries: 5–10% of all trauma cases
- Most common in young (a mean age around 30 yr), male (>80%) (2)
- Mortality: approximately 5%:
  - Exsanguination: 50% of mortality, most common cause of immediate death
- Concomitant injuries (3):
  - Aerodigestive tract injury (most common, ~10% per airway and digestive tract, respectively)
  - Vascular injury (9%): internal jugular and carotid artery
  - Spinal cord injury: ≤3%

ETIOLOGY AND PATHOPHYSIOLOGY

- Stab wounds from a violent assault (most common worldwide) followed by gunshot wounds
- Miscellaneous (self-harm, road traffic accidents, glass shards, metal fragments)
- Sports trauma (cleat spikes, hockey stick laceration, shattered baseball bat fragments, etc.)

DIAGNOSIS

- Careful examination of the wound to determine integrity of the platysma
- Wounds should never be blindly probed because this may result in uncontrolled hemorrhage.
- Lateral neck radiograph to evaluate soft tissue injury and detect foreign bodies
- Chest radiograph for suspected zone I injuries to detect hemopneumothorax, mediastinal air, or bleeding that extends into the upper mediastinum

PHYSICAL EXAM

- Signs and symptoms vary depending on the specific structures injured.
- Vascular injury:
  - Active hemorrhage or hematoma
  - Tracheal deviation
  - Loss of normal anatomic landmarks
  - Pulse deficits in upper extremities
  - Thrills or bruits in neck
  - An intact pulse does not rule out a vascular injury.
- Laryngotracheal injury:
  - Respiratory distress
  - Hoarseness, voice changes
  - Hemoptysis
  - Neck pain or tenderness
  - Crepitus/subcutaneous (SC) emphysema
- Pharyngoesophageal injury:
  - A high index of suspicion required as obvious clinical findings are frequently absent
  - Dysphagia
  - Odynophagia
  - Hematemesis
- Neurologic injury:
  - Central or peripheral nervous system deficits
  - Horner syndrome

DIFFERENTIAL DIAGNOSIS

- Vascular injury
- Pharyngoesophageal injury
- Laryngotracheal injury
- Peripheral or central nervous system injury
- Cervical spine injury
- Associated head or thoracic trauma

DIAGNOSTIC TESTS & INTERPRETATION

Can be divided by best tests to detect damage to a particular system; however, because there is no consensus on the best diagnostic approach, all decisions should be made in cooperation with the trauma service:

- Aerodigestive:
  - Multidetector helical computed tomography (MDCT) with esophageal studies (contrast swallow with endoscopy)
- Laryngotracheal injury:
  - MDCT in stable patients
- Vascular injuries:
  - Stable patients can undergo multidetector helical CT with angiography (MDCT-A). The sensitivity and specificity of this approaches traditional angiography, which was the former gold standard. However, MDCT-A is faster and more readily available (2)[B].
  - Ultrasonography with color flow Doppler combined with frequent, repeated physical exam is a fast, noninvasive therapeutic modality; however, this does not fully evaluate injuries to zone I or III, is operator dependent, and can miss subtle findings.
- Pharyngoesophageal injury:
  - Should always suspect esophageal injury in zone I injuries
  - MDCT is being used increasingly to evaluate esophageal injury.
  - The chest x-ray can demonstrate nonspecific findings but does not rule out esophageal injury.
  - 100% sensitivity is reached only with the combination of esophagography and flexible endoscopy (4)[B].
- Lab:
  - Type and crossmatch
  - Baseline complete blood panel and chemistry panel
  - Coagulation studies

TREATMENT

GENERAL MEASURES

- Esophageal and venous injuries are subtle and often missed.
- Initial stabilization: "C-ABCDE" approaches. "C" refers to circulation and hemorrhage control and "A" refers to airway management, "B" to breathing, "D" to disability or neurologic status, and "E" to exposure (undress) and environment (temperature control) (5)[C].

- Airway management:
  - Although penetrating neck trauma often does not involve the cervical spine, the cervical spine should be evaluated and cleared appropriately. Airway management should be done with the patient in cervical spine precautions until cleared.
  - Patients who are comatose or in respiratory distress require immediate intubation.
  - Stable patients without evidence of respiratory distress may be aggressively managed with prophylactic intubation or closely observed with airway equipment at the bedside.
  - Bag-valve-mask can force air through fascial planes and should be done carefully.
  - Orotracheal intubation with rapid sequence induction is the method of choice for securing the airway.
  - Nasotracheal intubation is contraindicated with apnea, severe facial injury, or airway distortion because of the risk of puncturing an expanding hematoma.
  - Fiberoptic intubation is contraindicated with active bleeding that may obscure the scope.
  - Percutaneous transtracheal ventilation may be useful when oral or nasotracheal intubation fails and should be used only as a temporizing measure until a more secure airway is obtained. Care should be taken to ensure proper placement:
    - Leaves the airway unprotected and is contraindicated in cases of upper airway obstruction because it may cause barotrauma
  - If the trachea is exposed due to a complete or partial transection, the caudal end should be directly intubated.
  - In all patients in whom intubation is attempted, there should be a surgical airway kit at the bedside. The physician must be prepared for a cricothyroidotomy or tracheostomy because these are required in cases of severe facial injury, laryngotracheal injury, and uncontrolled upper airway hemorrhage.
- Breathing:
  - Zone I injury can cause pneumothorax or subclavian vein injury and hemothorax, requiring needle decompression and tube thoracostomy.
- Circulation:
  - Two large-bore intravenous (IV) catheters should be placed contralateral to the side of the injury to avoid ipsilateral venous injury.
  - External hemorrhage should be controlled with direct pressure. Blind clamping of vessels is contraindicated due to the risk of further neurovascular injury.
  - If bleeding cannot be controlled, a Foley catheter can be inserted and inflated with saline to help tamponade the bleeding.
  - Patients with uncontrolled bleeding or hemodynamic instability must go directly to the operating room.
- Prehospital:
  - Impaled objects should not be removed.
  - Gently suction to clear the airway of blood, secretions, or vomitus.
  - Lateral decubitus or prone positioning may be required to prevent aspiration.
  - The airway must be vigilantly monitored because edema or expanding hematoma can progress to airway compromise.
  - Early oral intubation is indicated for clinical signs of respiratory distress, such as stridor, air hunger, or labored breathing, or if an expanding neck hematoma is present.
  - Cervical spine injury is uncommon in the context of low-velocity penetrating injury and immobilization is not routinely advocated unless clinically suspected (5)[C].
- ED treatment:
  - Alert and seemingly stable patients are known to rapidly decompensate; therefore, an airway setup should be at the bedside.
  - Nasogastric tube should not be placed due to risk of rupturing a pharyngeal hematoma.
  - Prophylactic antibiotics are recommended if a hollow viscous injury (such as pharyngoesophageal injuries) is suspected (3)[C]: cefoxitin, clindamycin, penicillin G plus metronidazole.
  - Surgical consult for all wounds that penetrate the platysma muscle:
    - Immediate surgical exploration: airway compromise, massive SC emphysema, air bubbling through a wound, profuse active bleeding, refractory shock/hemodynamic instability, evolving stroke or rapidly expanding hematoma (5)[C]
    - Selective approach in stable patients, especially in those with zone II injuries (2)[B]:
      - Surgical exploration for specific indications, including expanding or pulsatile hematoma, active bleeding, absence of peripheral pulses, hemoptysis, Horner syndrome, bruit, SC emphysema, respiratory distress, or air bubbling through a wound
  - Mandatory approach indicating surgical exploration in all cases of penetrating neck trauma is no longer widely practiced, tetanus prophylaxis.
  - Traumatic arrest in patients with penetrating neck injury is an indication for the ED thoracotomy.

MEDICATION

- Cefoxitin: adult: 2 g IV q8h; pediatrics: 80 to 160 mg/kg/day intramuscular (IM)/IV divided doses q6h *or*
- Clindamycin: adult: 600 to 900 mg IV q8h; pediatrics: 25 to 40 mg/kg/day IV divided doses q6–8h *or*
- Penicillin G: adult: 24 million IU/day divided doses q4–6h; pediatrics: 150,000 to 250,000 IU/kg/day divided doses q4–6h *plus*
- Metronidazole: adult: 1 g load and then 500 mg IV q6h; pediatrics: 30 mg/kg/day IV divided doses q12h

ADMISSION, INPATIENT, AND NURSING CONSIDERATIONS

- All patients with penetrating neck trauma should be admitted and observed for at least 24 hr.
- Observation must take place in a facility capable of providing definitive surgical care.
- Patients with possible airway or vascular injury must be admitted to the intensive care unit.
- Asymptomatic patients who have negative studies may be discharged after at least 24 hr of observation.

REFERENCES

1. Kendall JL, Anglin D, Demetriades D. Penetrating neck trauma. *Emerg Med Clin North Am*. 1998;16(1):85–105.
2. Biffl WL, Moore EE, Rehse DH, et al. Selective management of penetrating neck trauma based on cervical level of injury. *Am J Surg*. 1997;174(4):678–682.
3. McConnell DB, Trunkey DD. Management of penetrating trauma to the neck. *Adv Surg*. 1994;27:97–127.
4. Arantes V, Campolina C, Valerio SH, et al. Flexible esophagoscopy as a diagnostic tool for traumatic esophageal injuries. *J Trauma*. 2009;66(6):1677–1682.
5. Burgess CA, Dale OT, Almeyda R, et al. An evidence based review of the assessment and management of penetrating neck trauma. *Clin Otolaryngol*. 2012;37(1):44–52.

ADDITIONAL READING

- Inaba K, Munera F, McKenney M, et al. Prospective evaluation of screening multislice helical computed tomographic angiography in the initial evaluation of penetrating neck injuries. *J Trauma*. 2006;61(1):144–149.
- Thal ER, Meyer DM. Penetrating neck trauma. *Curr Probl Surg*. 1992;29(1):1–56.

CLINICAL PEARLS

- The majority of penetrating neck injuries occur at zone II between the cricoid cartilage to the mandibular angle.
- Exsanguination is the most common cause of immediate death, so hemorrhage control is prioritized in the advanced trauma life support approach.
- Cervical spine immobilization is not routinely recommended in low-energy injuries.
- Surgical consult should be obtained in all penetrating neck injuries.

NONSTEROIDAL ANTI-INFLAMMATORY DRUG POISONING

Kenneth P. Barnes, MD, MSc, CAQSM, FACSM • Shane Hudnall, MD, CAQSM

BASICS

- Primary effect is competitive inhibition of cyclooxygenase (COX) enzyme, thus inhibiting production of prostaglandins, thromboxanes, and prostacyclin from arachidonic acid.
- There are two COX isoforms: COX-1 and COX-2.
- COX-1 is expressed in most tissues.
- COX-2 is induced more in inflammation and pain.
- Most adverse effects are attributed to COX-1 inhibition.
- Most are metabolized through the liver with urinary excretion.
- Class of drugs works as antipyretics, analgesics, and anti-inflammatory agents
- Reduction of circulating prostacyclin and thromboxane results in platelet aggregation and vasodilation, respectively.
- Over-the-counter (OTC) nonsteroidal anti-inflammatory drugs (NSAIDs) include ibuprofen, naproxen, and aspirin.
- Classification:
  - Carboxylic acids:
    - Salicylates: aspirin, diflunisal
    - Propionic acids: ibuprofen, naproxen, ketoprofen
    - Acetic acids: indomethacin, etodolac, ketorolac, sulindac, diclofenac
    - Fenamates: meclofenamate, mefenamic acid
  - Enolic acids:
    - Oxicams: piroxicam, meloxicam
    - Pyrazolones: phenylbutazone
  - COX-2 inhibitors: celecoxib
- Meloxicam and etodolac have greater inhibition of COX-2 than COX-1 at low doses.

EPIDEMIOLOGY

Incidence

- >20 million Americans take NSAIDs on a regular basis.
- It is estimated that >30 billion OTC NSAID tablets are sold annually in the United States.
- ~70 million NSAID prescriptions are written each year in the United States.
- Acute NSAID poisoning is rare despite their extensive use.
- In most fatalities involving NSAIDs, patients ingested other pharmaceutical agents as well.
- Most poisonings are attributable to ibuprofen (>80,000 total yearly).

ETIOLOGY AND PATHOPHYSIOLOGY

- Toxicity:
  - Only a small percentage of overdoses (<0.5%) lead to serious harm (i.e., gastrointestinal [GI] bleeding, renal failure).
  - Most are asymptomatic or have nonspecific symptoms (nausea, vomiting, dizziness, somnolence).
  - Generally, doses >400 mg/kg of NSAID are needed to cause severe toxicity.
- GI:
  - Most common adverse effects are GI related (i.e., vomiting, abdominal pain, dyspepsia, diarrhea, constipation).
  - Gastric, duodenal, and large intestinal ulceration may occur (1–4% of users annually).
  - 3 to 10 times more likely to have serious hemorrhage with NSAIDs
  - COX-2 inhibitors have been shown to delay ulcer healing in animal studies, but this has not been elucidated in humans.
  - Celecoxib associated with fewer ulcers at 12 wk and 6 mo but no difference at 1 yr (presence of ulcer or complications) compared to ibuprofen and diclofenac (1)[A]
  - In patients requiring low-dose aspirin, celecoxib plus a proton-pump inhibitor (PPI) resulted in less recurrent bleeding and ulcers compared to naproxen plus a PPI (2)[A].
  - Celecoxib may be associated with decreased colon adenomas, duodenal polyps, and cancer from inhibiting COX-2 and tumor growth, especially in those with familial adenomatous polyposis.
- Renal:
  - Second most common adverse effects
  - Inhibition of prostaglandins interferes with renal blood flow and glomerular filtration rate.
  - Leads to vasoconstriction (from blocking prostaglandin synthesis) and possibly acute renal failure or acute interstitial nephritis
  - Retention of sodium, potassium, and water may lead to congestive heart failure (CHF) exacerbation.
  - COX-2 inhibitors: adversely affect function in patients with volume depletion, underlying renal disease, heart failure, and cirrhosis (3)[A]
- Central nervous system (CNS):
  - About 30% of patients with NSAID overdose experience CNS toxicity.
  - Elderly particularly at risk
  - Can cause headache, confusion, delirium, psychosis, hallucinations, nightmares, tremor, seizures, tinnitus, transient hearing loss, and aseptic meningitis
- Cardiovascular:
  - Can raise blood pressure (BP) and worsen control of hypertension (HTN)
  - Increased risk of cardiovascular events in both nonselective NSAIDs and COX-2 inhibitors
  - Risk of bleeding and cardiovascular events further increased in patients on antithrombotic drugs concomitantly taking NSAIDs (4)[B]
  - Lowest risk NSAID based on current research appears to be naproxen (5,6)[A].
  - All are associated with increased risk of CHF exacerbation in those with a history of CHF.
- Pulmonary:
  - Respiratory arrest is rare.
  - Asthmatics are at increased risk for bronchospasm owing to increased production of leukotrienes.
  - COX-2 inhibitors are much less likely to trigger bronchospasm.
  - Pulmonary infiltrates with eosinophilia are also possible.
  - Patients with clinical triad of asthma, nasal polyps, and allergic rhinitis are at increased risk of anaphylaxis to both salicylates and NSAIDs.
- Hepatic:
  - Possibility (although rare) of fulminant hepatic failure, hepatitis, elevated transaminases
  - Generally, this is reversible and only rarely fatal.
- Hematologic:
  - Aplastic anemia (now rare with decreased use of phenylbutazone and indomethacin), agranulocytosis, neutropenia, hemolytic anemia, thrombocytopenia possible
  - Decreased platelet aggregation may lead to increased GI bleeding.
  - COX-2 inhibitors have not been shown to decrease platelet function and are associated with a decreased risk of bleeding compared with nonselective NSAIDs.
- Skin: Toxic epidermal necrolysis and Stevens-Johnson syndrome are uncommon, but relative risk is increased slightly with NSAID use (including celecoxib) compared with placebo.
- Metabolic: may lead to anion-gap metabolic acidosis

- Drug interactions:
  - Increased risk of GI bleeding when used with anticoagulants
  - Digoxin, lithium, sulfonylurea, and aminoglycoside levels are all increased with use of NSAIDs.
  - NSAIDs reduce antihypertensive effects of diuretics, β-blockers, and angiotensin-converting enzyme (ACE) inhibitors.
  - Celecoxib contains a sulfa moiety and may have cross reactivity in those allergic to sulfa antibiotics.

RISK FACTORS

- Suicidal ideation
- Untreated pain
- Patients unclear of maximum allowed dosage of NSAIDs

DIAGNOSIS

HISTORY

- Although significant symptoms may occur after 5 to 10 times the maximum dose has been ingested, there is a poor correlation between the amount ingested and toxic poisoning.
- Timing of ingestion
- Past medical history (i.e., peptic ulcer disease, chronic renal insufficiency)

PHYSICAL EXAM

- Airway, breathing, and circulation (ABCs)
- Vital signs: Monitor BP, respiratory rate, and oxygen saturation.
- Thorough neurologic examination (especially monitoring mental status)
- Rectal examination for gross or occult blood

DIAGNOSTIC TESTS & INTERPRETATION

- Complete blood count (CBC), comprehensive metabolic panel (CMP) (attention to transaminases), prothrombin time/partial thromboplastin time (PT/PTT); coagulation studies, arterial blood gas (ABG) (if patient has anion gap on CMP or altered mental status), fingerstick glucose (rule out hypoglycemia), pregnancy test (if child-bearing female)
- Consider salicylate and acetaminophen levels, but do not check serum or urine levels of other NSAIDs. Just treat presumptively.
- Electrocardiogram (ECG) to look for prolongation of QRS or QTc
- Imaging generally not necessary unless concern for perforated ulcer is present

TREATMENT

- Acute treatment:
  - Supportive measures:
    - Call poison control.
    - Secure the ABCs.
    - There is no antidote for NSAID poisoning.
    - Close monitoring is warranted for almost all patients, and usually, this is the only treatment necessary.
    - Consider giving intravenous (IV) fluids if there is any volume deficit clinically.
    - Benzodiazepines IV if patient has seizures
  - Decontamination:
    - Gastric lavage if patient presents within 1 hr of ingestion or patient has massive overdose
    - Activated charcoal (1 g/kg adults, 0.5 to 1 g/kg in children) should be given to all patients with acute NSAID ingestion presenting within 2 hr unless contraindicated (i.e., bowel perforation).
    - Dialysis is unnecessary and ineffective.
- Long-term treatment: disposition:
  - Admit patient for any signs of toxicity (e.g., renal failure, vital sign changes, somnolence, electrolyte abnormalities).
  - Asymptomatic patients should be monitored for 4 to 6 hr to ensure that they do not have any signs of toxicity before discharging home (possibly longer for drugs such as naproxen that have longer half-lives).
  - Obtain psychiatric consultation for suicide attempts once medically stable.

REFERENCES

1. Silverstein FE, Faich G, Goldstein JL, et al. Gastrointestinal toxicity with celecoxib vs nonsteroidal anti-inflammatory drugs for osteoarthritis and rheumatoid arthritis: the CLASS study: a randomized controlled trial. Celecoxib Long-term Arthritis Safety Study. *JAMA*. 2000;284(10):1247–1255.
2. Chan FKL, Ching JYL, Tse YK, et al. Gastrointestinal safety of celecoxib versus naproxen in patients with cardiothrombotic diseases and arthritis after upper gastrointestinal bleeding (CONCERN): an industry-independent, double-blind, double-dummy, randomised trial. *Lancet*. 2017;389(10087):2375–2382.
3. Swan SK, Rudy DW, Lasseter KC, et al. Effect of cyclooxygenase-2 inhibition on renal function in elderly persons receiving a low-salt diet. A randomized, controlled trial. *Ann Intern Med*. 2000;133(1):1–9.
4. Schjerning Olsen AM, Gislason GH, McGettigan P, et al. Association of NSAID use with risk of bleeding and cardiovascular events in patients receiving antithrombotic therapy after myocardial infarction. *JAMA*. 2015;313(8):805–814.
5. Trelle S, Reichenbach S, Wandel S, et al. Cardiovascular safety of non-steroidal anti-inflammatory drugs: network meta-analysis. *BMJ*. 2011;342:c7086.
6. Nissen SE, Yeomans ND, Solomon DH, et al. Cardiovascular safety of celecoxib, naproxen, or ibuprofen for arthritis. *N Engl J Med*. 2016;375(26):2519–2529.

ADDITIONAL READING

- Hunter LJ, Wood DM, Dargan PI. The patterns of toxicity and management of acute nonsteroidal anti-inflammatory drug (NSAID) overdose. *Open Access Emerg Med*. 2011;3:39–48.
- Perazella MA, Tray K. Selective cyclooxygenase-2 inhibitors: a pattern of nephrotoxicity similar to traditional nonsteroidal anti-inflammatory drugs. *Am J Med*. 2001;111(1):64–67.
- Phillips RK, Wallace MH, Lynch PM, et al. A randomised, double blind, placebo controlled study of celecoxib, a selective cyclooxygenase 2 inhibitor, on duodenal polyposis in familial adenomatous polyposis. *Gut*. 2002;50(6):857–860.
- Tintinalli JE, Kelen GD, Stapczynski JS, eds. *Emergency Medicine: A Comprehensive Study Guide*. New York, NY: McGraw-Hill; 2000.

CLINICAL PEARLS

- There is no additional benefit to giving >1 dose of activated charcoal.
- Ipecac has fallen out of favor for most acute ingestions and is not recommended for NSAID toxicity.

NURSEMAID'S ELBOW

John Munyak, MD • Yaffa Ilyaguyeva • Amity Tung, MD

BASICS

DESCRIPTION

- Results from a traumatic subluxation of the radial head, which is produced by sudden forcible traction on the pronated hand or wrist with the relaxed elbow extended
- Subluxation of the radial head only occurs in pronation when the anteroposterior (AP) plane of the radial head diameter is narrowest.
- As the radial head subluxes, there is an interposition of the annular ligament in the radiocapitellar joint resulting in entrapment.
- Synonym(s): pulled elbow; radiocapitellar subluxation; subluxation of the head of the radius; subluxation of the radius by elongation; temper tantrum elbow; Malgaigne injury

EPIDEMIOLOGY

- One of the most common musculoskeletal injuries in children age 4 yr and under
- Uncommon in children >5 yr of age because the distal attachments of the orbicular ligament are sufficiently strong to prevent occurrence
- Peak incidence is from age of 1 to 3 yr old (1), with a predominance in females (2).

RISK FACTORS

- Frequently, the traction force occurs when the child suddenly attempts to pull away from a parent or drops to the ground.
- Pulling a child as he or she stumbles, lifting him or her up by the hand, or swinging the child by the hand(s) can also generate sufficient traction force.

DIAGNOSIS

- History alone is the basis for diagnosis in most cases.
- Consider prereduction radiographs if there is a history of trauma.
- Postreduction views are unnecessary.
- Consider x-rays if the child's arm does not return to normal function after performing appropriate reduction maneuvers.
- Consider additional imaging of the forearm, wrist, or humerus in young children.

HISTORY

- In >80% of cases, there is a history of sudden longitudinal traction to a pronated, extended forearm (3).
- May be a history of a "click" felt or heard by the person who pulled the child's arm
- May be a history of an incidental fall in which the arm, elbow, and forearm were impacted between the ground and the child's trunk (3)
- Immediately following the injury, the child is usually tearful due to the pain and refuses to use the affected arm.
- Pain, if vocalized, may be referred toward the wrist.
- The child holds the forearm by his or her side, always in a pronated and partially flexed position (nursemaid's position).
- Often, there is no history of trauma and the parents may notice the affected extremity not being used.

PHYSICAL EXAM

- Child refuses to use the affected limb.
- The forearm is always pronated, and the elbow is partially flexed.
- The child typically holds the affected limb by his or her side, sometimes supporting the forearm with the other hand.
- The child may be tearful during physical exam.
- The child also may appear content and playful but declines to move the affected arm.
- Gentle palpation can reveal local tenderness over the anterolateral aspect of the radial head.
- By carefully avoiding movements involving the elbow and forearm, one can note painless range of motion of the wrist, hand, and shoulder.
- Typically, no obvious swelling or deformity
- There is minimal restriction to flexion and extension of the elbow, but supination of the forearm is markedly limited and resisted.
- Often, the appearance is that of a wrist injury with the wrist flexed and pronated.
- It is imperative to examine the joints above and below the suspected injury, as well as the clavicle, to increase the likelihood of identifying the primary injury site.

DIFFERENTIAL DIAGNOSIS

- Posterior elbow dislocation
- Distal radial buckle fracture (torus) or other radial fracture
- Ulnar fracture
- Supracondylar fracture or other fracture of the humerus
- Avulsion of the medial or lateral epicondyle
- Septic joint
- Synovitis

TREATMENT

GENERAL MEASURES

- Analgesia:
  - Not typically necessary for reduction
  - Consider acetaminophen (15 mg/kg) or ibuprofen (5 to 10 mg/kg) as needed.
- Reduction techniques: flexion–supination and hyperpronation (4)

- *Flexion–supination:*
  - The thumb is placed in the region of the radial head for palpation and the exertion of mild pressure (anterior to posterior).
  - The child's forearm is gently but firmly rotated into full supination.
  - The elbow is then flexed to 90 degrees by holding the child's forearm above the wrist and stabilizing the humerus and elbow with the other hand to prevent rotation of the shoulder. If any resistance is met, one should continue flexing the elbow to the point of maximal flexion.
  - As reduction is achieved, a palpable and sometimes audible "click" can be felt in the region of the radial head.
  - This maneuver will typically achieve instantaneous reduction of the radial head and instant relief of pain.
- *Hyperpronation*:
  - Additional pressure is exerted to pronate the forearm further as the elbow is moved into full extension; if done correctly, may be more effective and less painful (5)
- Postreduction evaluation:
  - Observation is necessary until there is a return of full function and use of the affected arm (often occurs immediately postmaneuver).
  - If function has not normalized in 15 min, a repeated attempt at reduction is recommended or obtain radiographs.
  - In some studies, the delay until normal use of the arm is achieved is longer when there has been a delay in treatment from the time of injury; therefore, near normal function or significant improvement in function and postreduction may be sufficiently reassuring to continue observation at home with close follow-up within 24 hr.
  - If there is no evidence of recovery after several reduction attempts, the diagnosis must be reconsidered.
- Immobilization:
  - Immobilization is not necessary for the first occurrence of subluxation.
  - If reduction is delayed for >12 hr, consider immobilization in a sling and swathe or with a posterior mold for 10 days with the elbow in 90 degrees of flexion and the forearm in full supination. Compliance is difficult in this age range.
  - For cases of multiple recurrences of nursemaid's elbow, some clinicians recommend a trial of immobilization of the upper limb in an above elbow cast or postmold for 2 to 3 wk in conjunction with pediatric orthopedic consultation.

ADDITIONAL THERAPIES

- Special considerations:
  - In a child <6 mo of age, consider abuse from a caretaker while evaluating the child. However, subluxation can occur while simply rolling over in this age group.
  - Recurrence of subluxation as a result of subsequent pulls occurs in ~5–40% of cases.
- Rehabilitation:
  - Prevention is key. The parent should be advised to avoid longitudinal traction strains on the arm by not pulling on the hand or wrist, but pick the child up by the trunk.
  - For the child who recovers fully after one or two reduction maneuvers, further therapy or intervention is unnecessary.

SURGERY/OTHER PROCEDURES

- Very rarely, the subluxed radial head may be irreducible by manipulation, especially in recurrent cases, requiring surgical intervention.
- The need for open reduction is extremely rare.

ONGOING CARE

FOLLOW-UP RECOMMENDATIONS

- Even when multiple attempts at closed reduction fail, spontaneous reduction almost always occurs.
- Usually no long-term sequelae
- Consider an occult fracture or cartilaginous injury if the response to treatment is not typical.

REFERENCES

1. Vitello S, Dvorkin R, Sattler S, et al. Epidemiology of nursemaid's elbow. *West J Emerg Med.* 2014;15(4):554–557.
2. Wong K, Troncoso AB, Calello DP, et al. Radial head subluxation: factors associated with its recurrence and radiographic evaluation in a tertiary pediatric emergency department. *J Emerg Med.* 2016;51(6):621–627.
3. Welch R, Chounthirath T, Smith GA. Radial head subluxation among young children in the United States associated with consumer products and recreational activities. *Clin Pediatr (Phila).* 2017;56(8):707–715.
4. Krul M, van der Wouden JC, Kruithof EJ, et al. Manipulative interventions for reducing pulled elbow in young children. *Cochrane Database Syst Rev.* 2017;(7):CD007759.
5. Bexkens R, Washburn FJ, Eygendaal D, et al. Effectiveness of reduction maneuvers in the treatment of nursemaid's elbow: a systematic review and meta-analysis. *Am J Emerg Med.* 2017;35(1):159–163.

ADDITIONAL READING

Schunk JE. Radial head subluxation: epidemiology and treatment of 87 episodes. *Ann Emerg Med.* 1990;19(9):1019–1023.

CLINICAL PEARLS

- Commonly occurring traction injury age <4 yr
- Educating families to avoid pulling or putting traction on the child's arm for several days following injury significantly decreases the risk of recurrence.
- Long-term sequelae unlikely
- Evaluate returned usage of the elbow by making the child reach for a favorite object, parent's hand, or "eye candy."
- Consider fracture in the setting of antecedent trauma, significant swelling, deformity, or in cases of failed reduction attempts.

OBESITY AND WEIGHT MANAGEMENT

David Carfagno, DO, CAQSM • Timothy Perdue, DO

BASICS

DESCRIPTION

- World Health Organization (WHO) definitions:
  - Overweight = body mass index (BMI) >25
  - Obesity = BMI >30
- Waist circumference and risk of cardiometabolic disease:
  - >94 cm/37 inches (men), >80 cm/31.5 inches (women): at risk
  - >102 cm/40 inches (men), >88 cm/35 inches (women): increased risk
- Obesity is caused by a complex interplay between biology, behavior, and environment factors.
- Weight gain occurs when energy intake exceeds energy expenditure (i.e., positive energy balance).
- *1 lb of fat is equivalent to ~3,500 kcal of energy.*

EPIDEMIOLOGY

Prevalence

- Overweight (BMI ≥25) or obesity (BMI ≥30) now affects almost 2/3 of Americans (1).
- According to the WHO, in 2016, 39% of men and 40% of women in the United States are overweight or obese, with particularly high rates among non-Hispanic black Americans and Mexican Americans.
- Worldwide, 11% of men and 15% of women are obese.
- The problem of obesity is growing in many developing countries. Rates of obesity have tripled in the last 20 yr in the developing world, with 18% of the world's children currently overweight or obese. The Middle East, Pacific Islands, Southeast Asia, and China are facing the greatest challenges.
- The effect of obesity on mortality has shown that there is a 20–40% increase in mortality in both men and women who were overweight in midlife and a 2- to 3-fold increased risk of mortality among obese individuals. This is according to the National Institutes of Health-American Association of Retired Persons (NIH-AARP) cohort in 2006.
- Extremely obese people—those who are ≥80 lb over a normal weight—live 3 to 12 yr fewer than their normal-weight peers. ~6% of people are extremely obese—that is, they have a BMI ≥40.
- Nonsmokers who are overweight—~29 lb over a healthy weight—do not have shortened lives.
- Smoking takes a toll, too, and very heavy smokers are affected most. An 18-yr-old white male who has normal weight and does not smoke can expect to live to age 81 yr. If he's extremely obese and a smoker, his life expectancy is 60 yr, a difference of 21 yr.
- The effect of extreme obesity appears to be greater for men than women and for whites than blacks.

ETIOLOGY AND PATHOPHYSIOLOGY

- Hormones in the regulation of body weight:
  - Leptin: A hormone made in the hypothalamus is activated when there is a decrease in appetite and when insulin is secreted. It is also made when there is an increase in the metabolic rate. Obese individuals are known to have elevated levels of leptin and become leptin resistant.
  - Ghrelin: the key appetite hormone of the stomach. It is secreted at high levels by an empty stomach but is decreased with feeding.
  - Other hormones involved in the regulation of appetite and satiety include adiponectin, resistin, glucagon-like peptide-1, tumor necrosis factor, plasminogen activator inhibitor type 1, and peptide YY.
- Metabolic syndrome comprises obesity, carbohydrate intolerance or type 2 diabetes, hypertension (HTN), dyslipidemia, and a prothrombotic inflammatory vascular environment:
  - It is more prevalent in males over females worldwide. Male accumulation of body fat, predominantly in the trunk and visceral rather than the subcutaneous fat. It is the visceral fat that is the metabolically active fat, which produces adipokines, which increase insulin resistance.
  - Insulin resistance is closely related to the amount of visceral fat deposition and is poorly correlated with BMI.

Genetics

- Genetic linkage to obesity comes from the data on the FTO gene (fat mass and obesity associated) gene.
- A number of variant alleles of the FTO have been shown in several independent genome-wide association studies to be strongly and significantly associated with obesity-related traits.
- Individuals who are homozygous for the high-risk alleles weigh roughly 3 kg more than those individuals homozygous for the low-risk allele. Homozygosity appears to occur in roughly 16% of several populations that have been studied.
- Certain alleles of the apolipoprotein C-III (APOC3) gene were found to be a risk factor for obesity.

COMMONLY ASSOCIATED CONDITIONS

- Obesity contributes to excess mortality from HTN, type 2 diabetes, coronary artery diseases (CAD), stroke, gallbladder disease, sleep apnea, and osteoarthritis.
- Cancers occurring more commonly in these individuals include endometrial, breast, prostate, colon, esophageal, and liver.
- Centripetal obesity, in which the waist-to-hip ratio is high, indicates a subset of individuals at much higher risk of cardiovascular diseases.
- Relative risk of HTN among obese adults aged 20 to 45 yr is 5 to 6 times that of their nonobese counterparts.
- Relative risk of diabetes and of hypercholesterolemia is increased 2.9 and 1.5 times, respectively, in obese individuals.
- Several drugs are associated with weight change of varying degree: amitriptyline, mirtazapine, olanzapine, quetiapine, risperidone, gabapentin, tolbutamide, pioglitazone, glimepiride, gliclazide, glyburide, sitagliptin, and nateglinide (2).
- Secondary causes of obesity include a number of endocrinopathies and syndromes, which result in abnormalities of systems regulating feeding behavior and/or energy expenditure:
  - Hypothyroidism
  - Hypercortisolism
  - Hypothalamic dysfunction
  - Growth hormone deficiency
  - Prader-Labhart-Willi syndrome
  - Bardet-Biedl syndrome
  - Pseudohypoparathyroidism
  - Polycystic ovary syndrome (PCOS)
  - Hypogonadism
  - Insulinoma
  - Menopause

DIAGNOSIS

HISTORY

- Obtain weight history, diet history, eating patterns, activity history, and mental health history.
- Search for trigger factors (e.g., medications).

PHYSICAL EXAM

- Vital signs, including blood pressure (BP), heart rate, weight, height, waist circumference
- Appearance, including android (apple shaped/excess fat in abdomen) or gynoid (pear shaped/excessive fat in the thighs and buttock) fat deposition. Android has a higher predisposition to cardiovascular disease.
- BMI and waist-to-hip ratio. In the office, are the most reliable methods to determine body fat in the office. The gold standard test is the dual energy x-ray absorptiometry (DEXA) body composition.
- Eye exam: funduscopic exam to evaluate for arteriosclerosis; visual fields to screen for homonymous hemianopsia, presence of a pituitary tumor
- Oropharynx: tooth enamel evaluation for chronic gastric reflux disease. Craniofacial abnormalities seen in conditions like Prader-Willi syndrome. A small posterior pharynx due to hypertrophic fat may be a clue for obstructive sleep apnea.
- Neck: thyroid abnormalities, including asymmetrical or enlarged. Carotid bruits may indicate atherosclerosis.
- Chest: Heart examination may reveal findings such as an enlarged heart, displaced Point of maximal impulse, S3, and S4, all corresponding with cardiovascular disease and HTN. Atelectasis and bibasilar rales occur due to decreased lung compliance.
- Abdomen: appearance of subcutaneous and visceral fat deposition. Liver may be more prominent due to fatty liver.
- Pelvis, rectal, and genitalia: manually may be difficult to examine. Android obesity raises suspicion of testicular failure in men and Stein-Leventhal syndrome in women.
- Musculoskeletal: Joint arthritis may be prevalent in obese patients; careful to evaluate every joint, especially weight-bearing joints for effusion and range of motion abnormalities
- Skin: maceration of the intertriginous skin folds. Acanthosis nigricans can be seen in Cushing, PCOS, and diabetes.
- Breast: Gynecomastia in men must be differentiated from pseudogynecomastia, an increase in subareolar fat; careful inspection in women due to larger breasts and adipose tissue

DIAGNOSTIC TESTS & INTERPRETATION

Initial Tests (lab, imaging)

- Complete blood count (CBC); complete metabolic panel, including glucose, liver function tests, lipid panel, thyroid-stimulating hormone with T4, morning cortisol, urinalysis, HbA1c
- DEXA scan body fat composition; the gold standard test for determining body fat
- Other reliable tests include hydrostatic weighing, air displacement, skin calipers, and body impedance.
- Chest x-ray, mammogram, colonoscopy (per routine screening guidelines, age, and medically appropriate)

Diagnostic Procedures/Other

- Nocturnal pulse oximetry or formal sleep study
- Electrocardiogram, graded exercise treadmill Bruce American College of Sports Medicine (ACSM) protocol when indicated
- Exercise testing may be beneficial for obese patients. When performing standard exercise testing, the level of deconditioning typically observed in this population will necessitate a low initial workload (2 to 3 metabolic equivalents [METs]) and small workload increments per test stage (0.5 to 1.0 METs).

- Other comorbidities (e.g., HTN and other chronic diseases) or concerns (orthopedic limitations or elderly) may dictate modifications to the testing procedures.
- Use of leg or arm ergometry may enhance testing performance.
- Special attention to proper cuff size is necessary for accurate BP measurements.

TREATMENT

MEDICATION

- Pharmacologic therapy is appropriate for patients as an adjunct to lifestyle interventions to facilitate weight loss and prevent weight regain. Current criteria for the use of pharmacologic therapy for obesity are a BMI >30 or a BMI >27 in the presence of coexisting conditions.
- As of 2014, six drugs are approved for use in obesity. Only naltrexone/bupropion and liraglutide are not contraindicated in pregnancy and breastfeeding. However, it is recommended to avoid all weight loss medications in pregnancy or breastfeeding.
- Phentermine/diethylpropion—α agonist. Large side effect profile; contraindicated in CAD, HTN, anxiety, hyperthyroidism, and glaucoma
- Orlistat—pancreatic and gastric lipase inhibitor. Side effects include decreased absorption of fat-soluble vitamins, flatulence, and steatorrhea. Contraindicated in malnourishment or malabsorption syndromes; cholestasis; or in patients taking levothyroxine, warfarin, or antiepileptic drugs. Caution when taking cyclosporine (must take at least 2 hr apart). It is now available over the counter (OTC) and is recommended for use in patients with cardiovascular disease.
- Lorcaserin—$5HT_{2c}$ receptor agonist. Well tolerated, side effects include headache, nausea, dry mouth, dizziness, fatigue, and constipation. Only absolute contraindication is use in pregnancy or breastfeeding; caution in patients taking selective serotonin reuptake inhibitors (SSRIs), serotonin and norepinephrine reuptake inhibitors (SNRIs), monoamine oxidase inhibitors (MAOIs), or other drugs that increase serotonin levels due to risk of serotonin syndrome
- Phentermine/topiramate—α agonist/γ-aminobutyric acid (GABA) receptor modulator. Can cause insomnia, dry mouth, constipation, paresthesia, dizziness, dysgeusia; contraindicated in hyperthyroidism, glaucoma, MAOI use, sympathomimetic use
- Naltrexone/bupropion—opioid antagonist/dopamine and SNRI. Side effects include nausea, constipation, headache, vomiting, and dizziness; contraindicated in uncontrolled HTN, seizure disorder, anorexia/bulimia, drug or alcohol withdrawal, MAOI use
- Liraglutide—GLP-1 agonist. Can cause nausea, vomiting, acute pancreatitis; contraindicated in history of medullary thyroid cancer or multiple endocrine neoplasia type 2
- High level of caution when pharmacologically treating patients with chronic kidney disease. Only consider using orlistat or liraglutide (3)[C].

ISSUES FOR REFERRAL

Ancillary services may be needed for a multidisciplinary approach, including psychotherapists, registered dietitian, exercise physiologist, and physical therapy; referral at times necessary for morbidly obese to bariatric surgery consult

SURGERY/OTHER PROCEDURES

- Bariatric surgical treatments reduce calorie intake by restrictive or malabsorptive operations on the gastrointestinal (GI) tract.
- The two main procedures are the Roux-en-Y bypass and the laparoscopic adjustable gastric banding, with similar weight loss outcomes.
- The National Institutes of Health guidelines for adults recommended consideration of bariatric surgery with BMI at least 40 kg/m^2 or a BMI at least 35 kg/m^2 with significant obesity-related comorbidities.
- Bariatric surgery in adults improved diabetes (77% of patients), hyperlipidemia (83%), HTN (66%), and sleep apnea (88%), although more information is needed about the long-term durability of comorbidity benefit.
- Adverse effects include perioperative complications, dehydration, bowel obstruction, anastomotic leaks, ulcers, cholelithiasis, and vitamin deficiencies.
- 30-day mortality rates are reported as 0.14% for bypass, 0.03% for gastric banding, and 0.08% for sleeve gastrectomy.

ONGOING CARE

DIET

The U.S. Department of Agriculture puts out the *Dietary Guidelines for Americans 2015–2020* every 5 yr, last published in 2015. For long-term weight maintenance, individuals should follow these dietary guidelines:

- Consume a *healthy eating pattern* that includes a variety of vegetables from all subgroups, fruits, grains, low-fat dairy, and a variety of protein foods.
- >50% of grain products consumed should come from whole grains.
- Consume <10% of daily calories from added sugars.
- Consume <10% of daily calories from saturated fats.
- Consume <2,300 mg of sodium per day (4)[C].

PATIENT EDUCATION

- Exercise prescription is based on working on the model of frequency, intensity, and duration, with goal in mind to encourage greater overall energy expenditure within the program for the obese individual.
- Primary mode should be large muscle group aerobic activities.
- The initial exercise training intensity should be moderate (e.g., 40–60% VO_2R or heart rate reserve [HRR]) with more emphasis placed on increased duration and frequency. Eventual progression to higher exercise intensities (50–75% VO_2R or HRR) allows for further increases in VO_2 max, which in turn allows for a more efficient exercise session.
- Frequency of training: 5 to 7 days per week
- Duration of training session: 45 to 60 min
- Volume of training: Initial training volume should focus on attainment of 150 min of moderate intensity exercise weekly. However, the optimal maintenance dose of physical activity is >2,000 kcal/wk.
- Special considerations: Obese individuals are at an increased risk for orthopedic injury. Obese individuals are at an increased risk of hyperthermia during exercise. Equipment modifications may be needed (i.e., wide seats on cycle ergometers and rowers) (5)[C].
- The 2011 Centers for Disease Control and Prevention (CDC) guide to strategies to increase physical activity in the community:
  - Community-wide campaigns: large-scale, visible campaigns via television, radio, newspaper, and so forth
  - Point of decision prompts: signs in elevators to promote stair usage
  - Behavioral and social approaches: Teach behavioral skills to help incorporate physical activity into daily routines.
  - Enhanced school-based physical education (PE): increasing the number or duration of PE classes within the school schedule to encourage youth to engage in enjoyable moderate-to-vigorous physical activity; can also be applied in settings such as community/recreation centers and after-school programs
  - Environmental and policy approaches: social networks of exercise groups increased access to places for physical activity; improvement of urban areas to make them more amenable to physical activity
  - Organized programs to encourage active transport to school (i.e., walking, bicycling, skating)
- Future directions of obesity research lie in the field of genetics and of responsiveness to lifestyle and pharmacologic interventions.
- Since identification of the leptin gene, new hormones and metabolic pathways involved in the regulation of body weight have been discovered (e.g., ghrelin). This may lead to the development of new classes of drugs that can alter/modify energy balance (5)[C].

REFERENCES

1. Centers for Disease Control and Prevention. Division of nutrition, physical activity, and obesity. https://www.cdc.gov/nccdphp/dnpao/index.html. Accessed September 22, 2018.
2. Domecq JP, Prutsky G, Leppin A, et al. Clinical review: drugs commonly associated with weight change: a systematic review and meta-analysis. *J Clin Endocrinol Metab*. 2015;100(2):363–370.
3. Apovian CM, Aronne LJ, Bessesen DH, et al. Pharmacological management of obesity: an endocrine society clinical practice guideline. *J Clin Endocrinol Metab*. 2015;100(2):342–362.
4. U.S. Department of Health and Human Services. *Dietary Guidelines for Americans 2015–2020*. 8th ed. New York, NY: Skyhorse Publishing Company; 2017.
5. Centers for Disease Control and Prevention. *Strategies to Prevent Obesity and Other Chronic Diseases: The CDC Guide to Strategies to Increase Physical Activity in the Community*. Atlanta, GA: U.S. Department of Health and Human Services; 2011.

CLINICAL PEARLS

- Insulin resistance is most closely associated with visceral fat deposition and the release of adipokines and is poorly correlated with BMI.
- Obesity is not only associated with certain lifestyles but also has a genetic component. Certain alleles of the FTO gene have been strongly associated with obesity.
- Pharmacologic treatment is reserved for those with a BMI >30 or for those with a BMI >27 and comorbidities. Surgery is reserved for patients with BMI >40 or BMI >35 with comorbidities.
- Treatment plans should be individualized and multifaceted. Diet and exercise are mainstays of treatment, but additional treatment options may be appropriate for some patients.

OLECRANON BURSITIS

James M. Daniels, MD, MPH, RMSK, FAAFP, FACOEM, FACPM • Alexei DeCastro, MD, FAAFP, CAQSM • Dwaipayan Choudhury, MD

BASICS

DESCRIPTION

Common condition, a superficial bursal or synovial-lined sack sits over the olecranon process of the ulna that fills with fluid

EPIDEMIOLOGY

- Bursitis (from all sources) accounts for approximately 2/10,000 hospitalizations a year (1)[A].
- Annual incidence of 10/100,000 (1)[A]
- Most common in males 18 to 88 yr of age (1)[A]
- 75% are noninfectious.

ETIOLOGY AND PATHOPHYSIOLOGY

- Direct injury
- Prolonged pressure (elbow leaning on table)
- Overuse
- Crystal induced
- Rheumatoid arthritis (1)
- Infection

RISK FACTORS

Favor Septic Bursitis	Favor Nonseptic Bursitis
• Underlying immunocompromised • Diabetes • Systemic symptoms	• Trauma • History of rheumatoid arthritis or gout

Warning: Patients with gout and rheumatoid arthritis may also have secondary infection of the bursa.

- Septic bursitis (1)[A]:
  - Altered immune system
  - Diabetes
  - Skin irritation or interruption around the area
  - Hematoma
- Noninfectious (1)[A]:
  - Trauma
  - Overuse
  - Any occupation in which elbow is flexed on regular basis or traumatized

GENERAL PREVENTION

- Infectious:
  - Care of overlying skin to prevent abrasions, lacerations
  - Good control of underlying medical conditions
- Noninfectious:
  - Soft pads not effective, hard or supported elbow pads, that is, like those worn by skateboarders
  - Avoid overuse.

COMMONLY ASSOCIATED CONDITIONS

- Rheumatoid arthritis—rheumatoid nodules
- Gout, pseudogout
- Repetitive flexion of elbow:
  - Direct trauma

DIAGNOSIS

HISTORY

- History of repetitive flexion of elbow (2)[A]
- History of trauma (2)[A]
- History of abovementioned systemic disease (2)[A]
- History of systemic inflammatory response syndrome (SIRS) criteria (2)[A]
- High risk of not only infection but also systemic involvement (1)[A]:
  - Temperature >38°C
  - Heart rate (HR) >90/min
  - Respiratory rate (RR) >20/min
  - White blood cell (WBC) >12,000/mL

PHYSICAL EXAM

- Bursal swelling
- Should have normal range of motion (ROM) of elbow, if not, concern or joint involvement
- Skin lesions, concern for infections
- Acute, may just be tendon over olecranon:
  - It is very difficult to distinguish between a septic and nonseptic arthritis when a patient does not have systemic symptoms (1,3)[A].

DIFFERENTIAL DIAGNOSIS

ALERT

A number of meta-analysis studies have attempted to develop algorithms for evaluating and treating olecranon bursitis, especially trying to separate out differentiating between septic and nonseptic bursitis and have failed.

- There are some general guidelines that can be followed.
- Chronic bursitis (>2 wk) will produce a more "well formed" bursa and appear like "Popeye elbow"; some of these, especially those that have chronic drainage, require further investigation (i.e., imaging, aspiration, surgical removal of bursa) to rule out chronic atypical infections (i.e., fungus or cancer).

DIAGNOSTIC TESTS & INTERPRETATION

- Historically, the bursa was drained and the fluid was analyzed to rule out septic bursitis.
- Recent meta-analysis revealed that glucose level, protein, and WBC content were not accurate in distinguishing between septic and infectious bursitis (1,2,3)[A].
- Gram stain was helpful with sensitivity approaching ≥90%.

- Radiographs may be useful in chronic cases to rule out tophi, spurs, foreign bodies, and so forth.
- The use of point-of-care ultrasound can be very useful in detecting fluid pockets but cannot differentiate between inflammation and infection.
- The same can be said about magnetic resonance imaging (MRI).
- 75% of olecranon bursitis is noninfective.
- Of the other 25%, systemic symptoms are the most accurate way to determine if the joint is septic, that is, inability to flex elbow and SIRS criteria.
- Open skin lesions, diabetes, and immunocompromised patients are of particular concern:
  - Meta-analysis of multiple studies found that aspiration did little to affect the course of the problem and that aspiration was associated with an increase in complications (3)[A].

TREATMENT

- For nonseptic bursitis, protection of the bursa from microtrauma with a stiff or hard type of elbow guard or pad has been useful (1,3)[A].
- Change of repetitive job or elimination of microtrauma has been useful for nonseptic bursitis.

ALERT

- If the patient has no contraindication, nonsteroidal anti-inflammatory drugs (NSAIDs) can be used for pain. They do not decrease the amount of inflammation and should be used cautiously in patients with altered kidney function or who are on disease-modifying antirheumatic drugs (DMARDs) for rheumatoid arthritis (2)[A].
- Recent literature shows that cases of noninfectious acute bursitis (75% of all cases of bursitis) do best with little intervention, no corticosteroid injection, and no aspiration. Protect the bursa from continued microtrauma with a "hard" elbow protector and give medication for pain relief. Be aware that chronic bursitis could be a sign of other pathology in the elbow or could be associated with other chronic conditions.

- A small number of patients with acute bursitis are septic. This condition is a bit more difficult to diagnose and in these patients, aspiration of the bursa is preferred.
- *Staphylococcus aureus* is the most common pathogen from infected olecranon bursitis. Broad anterior treatment causing *S. aureus* is preferred. Intravenous (IV) antibiotic without systemic symptoms harbors no advantage from treating the patient with by mouth (PO) antibiotics (1,3)[A].
- Any patient suspected of septic bursitis should have the bursa aspirated either in office with a large gauge needle or in the operating room (OR) with bursectomy.
- Synovectomy is sometimes necessary to make the diagnosis or to treat the condition if nonsurgical treatment fails.
- Patients with chronic bursitis or chronic drainage should be referred to a surgeon for consideration of bursectomy (1)[A].

ONGOING CARE

PATIENT EDUCATION

- The care of patients with olecranon bursitis has changed over the years to a "hands off" approach.
- Unless septic bursitis is suspected, the bursa should not be aspirated.
- Literature no longer supports the use of corticosteroid injections.
- Chronic bursitis may do better being treated by referral to a surgeon for bursectomy.

REFERENCES

1. Baumbach SF, Lobo CM, Badyine I, et al. Prepatellar and olecranon bursitis: literature review and development of a treatment algorithm. *Arch Orthop Trauma Surg*. 2014;134(3):359–370.
2. Blackwell JR, Hay BA, Bolt AM, et al. Olecranon bursitis: a systematic overview. *Shoulder Elbow*. 2014;6(3):182–190.
3. Sayegh ET, Strauch RJ. Treatment of olecranon bursitis: a systematic review. *Arch Orthop Trauma Surg*. 2014;134(11):1517–1536.

CLINICAL PEARLS

- Current evidence favors treating nonseptic bursitis conservatively without drainage.
- Patients with an olecranon bursitis with any of the following are not only at higher risk of septic bursitis but also of systemic infection:
  - Fever
  - Immunocompromised
  - History of recent surgery
- Aspiration and the injection of corticosteroids into nonseptic olecranon bursa have been associated with an increased risk of complications (infection, chronic fistula, skin atrophy). Corticosteroid injection into the bursa is no longer recommended. Needle aspiration should no longer be done for symptomatic treatment. It should only be used to help rule out infectious bursitis. Care should be followed to not "seed" the bursa with bacteria from the skin or by passing the needle through area of cellulitis before entering the bursa. Care should be taken not to enter the joint with the needle.

ORAL LACERATIONS

Brent H. Messick, MD, MS, FAAFP, CAQSM • Kevin E. Burroughs, MD, CAQSM

BASICS

DESCRIPTION

- Soft tissue injury in the orofacial area
- Typically results from a direct blow to the mouth resulting from a fall or impact by an opponent or object
- Lacerations may be an indirect result of an individual biting the cheek or lip.

EPIDEMIOLOGY

- Most common in contact sports not requiring face protection (basketball, soccer, baseball, wrestling)
- Other at-risk sports include bicycling, in-line skating, and gymnastics.
- Children are most susceptible between the ages of 7 and 11 yr (1).

Incidence

As high as 1.06/100,000 athlete exposures (2)

Prevalence

1.4/10,000 athlete exposures in football and 18.3/10,000 in basketball; 58–75% of these injuries are soft tissue lacerations (3).

RISK FACTORS

- Participation in collision or contact sports
- *Not* using a mouth guard

COMMONLY ASSOCIATED CONDITIONS

- Fracture of the mandible, dental arch, palate
- Dental luxation or avulsion
- Tooth fracture
- Temporomandibular joint (TMJ) trauma
- Vessel injury
- Nerve transection
- Salivary gland duct injury

DIAGNOSIS

HISTORY

- Determine where and how the injury was sustained; common in sports but also seen as result of fighting, assault, and abuse
- Determine areas of numbness or loss of muscle control to evaluate for nerve injury.
- Determine last tetanus immunization because wounds are often contaminated from the environment as well as from the oral cavity.
- Sensitivity of teeth (Assess for occult dental trauma.)

PHYSICAL EXAM

- Significant hemorrhage due to the abundant blood supply in the face and maxillofacial areas
- Visible defects with "through and through" lacerations (lacerations involving all layers: mucosa, muscular, subcutaneous [SC], and skin)
- Patient distress
- Head and neck examination for signs of neural injury
- Palpate over TMJ to evaluate for subcondylar mandibular fracture.
- Test mobility of jaw.
- Evaluate laceration for length and depth as well as for affected structures, including nerves and vessels (transected nerves need to be referred for surgical repair).
- Buccal lacerations need to be evaluated for parotid salivary flow from the Stensen duct. Parotid orifice is located opposite the maxillary 1st molar. Saliva should flow from opening when parotid gland is palpated (disruptions of the duct should be referred for repair).
- Evaluate for normal occlusion of the teeth. Dental examination should be performed to check for fractured, loose, or avulsed teeth.

DIFFERENTIAL DIAGNOSIS

- Contusion
- Abrasion
- Dental trauma (luxation, avulsion, fracture)

DIAGNOSTIC TESTS & INTERPRETATION

- If there is a clinical suspicion of a fracture or foreign body such as a tooth fragment, appropriate studies should be ordered: panorex x-rays for teeth, plain radiographs for foreign bodies, or computed tomography (CT) for facial fractures, etc.
- Bone fixation/repair, if needed, should be performed before soft tissue closure.

TREATMENT

GENERAL MEASURES

- Most oral lacerations can be left to heal by secondary intention. Only those that are >1 cm, gapping at rest, or require hemostasis may need to be repaired (4).
- Copious irrigation of the wound to remove foreign debris and wound contaminants
- Clean with antiseptic scrub.
- Regional anesthesia via nerve block is preferred over local injection to minimize tissue distortion, making approximation easier (especially for the vermilion border).
- Infraorbital nerve block numbs the upper lip.
- Mental nerve block numbs the anterior lower lip and teeth.
- Maxillary nerve second division numbs the entire maxilla on the blocked side.
- Interrupted stitches using 3–0 chromic or similar absorbable suture material
- Inside-out and bottom-up technique; eliminating dead spaces helps prevent hematoma and subsequent infection.

- Muscular layer: 4–0 slow-absorbing suture; polyglactic suture breaks down more slowly than chromic suture, maintaining wound strength for ~30 days.
- Oral mucosa: 3–0 or 4–0 chromic or other absorbable suture material on a cutting needle
- Small intraoral lacerations may be left to heal by secondary intention.
- SC layer: 3–0 or 4–0 plain gut on a cutting needle
- Skin: 4–0 to 6–0 nylon
- Lip defects involving >33% usually require flap reconstruction (5).
- Suture orbicularis oris first (see above suture suggestions).
- Loosely approximate the vermilion border (very important for cosmetic appearance) with a suture at the junction with the skin.
- Proceed in layers as above.
- Superficial tongue lacerations <1 cm and not gaping at rest do not require sutures unless required for hemostasis.
- Lacerations involving the muscular layer or labial margin require sutures.
- Lacerations involving the tip may require sutures to prevent a "forked tongue." Most can be left alone. Anterior tongue lacerations are rare and are often self-inflicted. Small ones can close, but large ones will require sutures. If the tongue heals "forked," it can also be corrected later, if necessary.
- Repair in layers: 4–0 slow-resorbing polyglactic suture for the muscle and chromic suture for the mucosa
- Small lacerations can be allowed to close by secondary intention.
- Hemorrhage typically from disruption of the muscular layer may require a stitch to obtain hemostasis.
- Large gaping lacerations can be repaired with one or two vertical sutures.

ADDITIONAL THERAPIES

- Tetanus immunization status
- Prophylactic antibiotics for severe or grossly contaminated laceration (Coverage for the oral flora includes amoxicillin, penicillin, clindamycin, or erythromycin.)
- Prophylactic antibiotic coverage for less severe laceration can be considered due to an infection rate of 10% (6).
- If fracture is present, leave wound open until fixation is completed.

ADMISSION, INPATIENT, AND NURSING CONSIDERATIONS

Initial stabilization:

- Evaluate airway, breathing, and circulation (ABCs).
- Control hemorrhage.
- Protect the airway if compromised.

ONGOING CARE

FOLLOW-UP RECOMMENDATIONS

- Laceration associated with fracture or involving nerves or salivary ducts should be referred for definitive care as soon as possible.
- Refer dental trauma to a dentist or oral surgeon.
- Patients receiving antibiotics should be rechecked in 48 hr to ensure improvement and antibiotic susceptibility.

REFERENCES

1. Inouye J, McGrew C. Dental problems in athletes. *Curr Sports Med Rep*. 2015;14(1):27–33.
2. Labella CR, Smith BW, Sigurdsson A. Effect of mouthguards on dental injuries and concussions in college basketball. *Med Sci Sports Exerc*. 2002;34(1):41–44.
3. Flanders RA, Bhat M. The incidence of orofacial injuries in sports: a pilot study in Illinois. *J Am Dent Assoc*. 1995;126(4):491–496.
4. Soto F, Murphy A, Heaton H. Critical procedures in pediatric emergency medicine. *Emerg Med Clin North Am*. 2013;31(1):335–376.
5. Marks M, Polecritti D, Bergman R, et al. Emergent soft tissue repair in facial trauma. *Facial Plast Surg Clin North Am*. 2017;25(4):593–604.
6. Katsetos SL, Nagurka R, Caffrey J, et al. Antibiotic prophylaxis for oral lacerations: our emergency department's experience. *Int J Emerg Med*. 2016;9(1):24.

ADDITIONAL READING

- American Dental Association Council on Access, Prevention and Interprofessional Relations, Council on Scientific Affairs. Using mouthguards to reduce the incidence and severity of sports-related oral injuries. *J Am Dent Assoc*. 2006;137(12):1712–1720.
- Echlin P, McKeag DB. Maxillofacial injuries in sport. *Curr Sports Med Rep*. 2004;3(1):25–32.
- Echlin PS, Upshur RE, Peck DM, et al. Craniomaxillofacial injury in sport: a review of prevention research. *Br J Sports Med*. 2005;39(5):254–263.
- Ranalli DN, Demas PN. Orofacial injuries from sport: preventive measures for sports medicine. *Sports Med*. 2002;32(7):409–418.

CLINICAL PEARLS

- Stitches placed inside the mouth will dissolve on their own. Sutures in the skin should be removed in 4 to 5 days to prevent significant scarring.
- Return to play depends on the severity of the injury, chance of reinjury, and availability/feasibility of protection for the wound.

OSGOOD-SCHLATTER DISEASE

Ayo Adu, MD, CAQSM

BASICS

DESCRIPTION

- Traction apophysitis of the tibial tubercle at the insertion of the patellar tendon
- Overuse injury due to repetitive strain or microtrauma of the secondary ossification center of the tibial tubercle

EPIDEMIOLOGY

- One of the most common causes of knee pain in active adolescents
- More prevalent in male gender
- Age of onset coincides with growth spurts, males age 10 to 15 yr, females age 8 to 13 yr.

ETIOLOGY AND PATHOPHYSIOLOGY

- Chronic repetitive strain and microtrauma cause chronic avulsion of the secondary ossification center (1).
- The force is increased after periods of rapid growth.
- Chronic avulsion may cause separation of the patellar tendon insertion from the tibial tubercle, swelling, and enlargement.

RISK FACTORS

- Adolescents
- Male gender
- Sports that involve running and jumping
- Activities that involve direct contact with the knee (e.g., kneeling)
- Higher body weight
- Quadriceps muscle tightness (2)[B]

DIAGNOSIS

HISTORY

- Anterior knee pain and swelling
- Symptoms are bilateral in 20–30% of patients.
- Pain begins as a dull ache that gradually increases with continued activity.
- Pain is worsened by running, jumping, direct trauma, kneeling, and squatting.
- Pain is improved with rest.

PHYSICAL EXAM

- Enlarged prominent tibial tubercle
- Tenderness of the proximal tibial tubercle at the patellar tendon insertion
- Poor flexibility of the quadriceps and hamstrings
- Able to maintain full, symmetric knee extension with active straight-leg raise
- Inability to maintain symmetric knee extension with straight-leg raise, especially in event of acute onset of pain at tibial tubercle, is highly suggestive for tibial tubercle avulsion fracture.
- Pain is exacerbated by knee extension against resistance, active or passive knee flexion, or by direct trauma to the tibial tubercle.

DIFFERENTIAL DIAGNOSIS

- Patellar tendonitis
- Sinding-Larsen-Johansson syndrome
- Tibial tubercle avulsion fracture
- Tibial plateau fracture
- Patellar fracture
- Osteochondritis dissecans
- Patellofemoral syndrome
- Pes anserine bursitis
- Patellar tendon rupture
- Patellar subluxation
- Chondromalacia patellae
- Hoffa disease (infrapatellar fat pad impingement)
- Osteomyelitis
- Tumor

DIAGNOSTIC TESTS & INTERPRETATION

- Osgood-Schlatter disease is a clinical diagnosis, and radiographs are not required for diagnosis. However, they may be helpful in ruling out other conditions, such as acute tibial apophyseal fracture, osteomyelitis, and tumors (3)[A].
- X-ray:
  - Lateral view may show an elevated tibial tubercle with anterior soft tissue swelling, fragmentation of the tibial tubercle, or calcification and ossicle formation in the distal patellar tendon.

TREATMENT

GENERAL MEASURES

- Relative rest or activity modification is recommended.
- Activity as tolerated, including sports, is allowed as long as symptoms are tolerable and resolve within 24 hr.
- Pain control with nonsteroidal anti-inflammatory drugs (NSAIDs) or acetaminophen
- Protective pad may be worn over tibial tubercle to prevent direct trauma.
- Ice application especially after exercise
- If significant symptoms, consider physical therapy consult.

ADDITIONAL THERAPIES

- Osgood-Schlatter disease is usually a benign and self-limited condition that resolves once growth plate closes.
- Usual course is 6 to 18 mo.
- Symptoms may continue into adulthood despite conservative measures in 5–10% of patients.
- Recommended exercises include stretching of the quadriceps and hamstring and strengthening of the quadriceps.

SURGERY/OTHER PROCEDURES

Surgical excision of the enlarged tibial tubercle and free ossicles may be considered in skeletally mature patients if conservative treatment has failed.

REFERENCES

1. Gholve PA, Scher DM, Khakharia S, et al. Osgood Schlatter syndrome. *Curr Opin Pediatr*. 2007;19(1):44–50.
2. Nakase J, Goshima K, Numata H, et al. Precise risk factors for Osgood-Schlatter disease. *Arch Orthop Trauma Surg*. 2015;135(9):1277–1281.
3. Kabiri L, Tapley H, Tapley S. Evaluation and conservative treatment for Osgood-Schlatter disease: a critical review of the literature. *Int J Ther Rehabil*. 2014;21:91–96.

ADDITIONAL READING

Bloom OJ, Mackler L, Barbee J. Clinical inquiries. What is the best treatment for Osgood-Schlatter disease? *J Fam Pract*. 2004;53(2):153–156.

CLINICAL PEARLS

- Athletes may participate in athletic activity as tolerated. Pain level should generally be tolerable, without a decrease in performance, and resolve within 24 hr of activity. If performance is decreased, the athlete should discontinue activity.
- Athlete should not "play through the pain." Instead, pain should be used as a measure of when to stop activity.
- Pain will resolve when the growth plate closes.
- Future complications can include persistent enlargement of the tibial tubercle, pain with kneeling, and possibly some limitation of activities.
- Prognosis is excellent, provided the athlete demonstrates good compliance with the physician's recommendations.

OSTEITIS PUBIS

James M. Daniels, MD, MPH, RMSK, FAAFP, FACOEM, FACPM • William H. Dixon, MD • Michael Connolly, MD

BASICS

DESCRIPTION

- Inflammation of the pubic symphysis and surrounding tissue often brought on by overuse in the athletic population
- Should be considered when treating athletes with groin pain
- The condition is usually self-limited but may require a lengthy period of rest.
- Classifications:
  - Unilateral symptoms, pain in abductor muscle; worse after training session
  - Bilateral symptoms, inguinal pain, abductor pain; worse after training session
  - Bilateral symptoms, inguinal pain, pain with kicking; can't continue sport
  - Inguinal pain, pelvis, lumbar spine; worse with Valsalva, cannot perform activities of daily living (ADLs)

EPIDEMIOLOGY

- 0.5 to 6.2 of all athletes
- Increase incidence in males; soccer, football, hockey, rugby

ETIOLOGY AND PATHOPHYSIOLOGY

- Increased incidence in "cutting sports"
- Change or increased training
- Happens gradually as opposed to patients with osteomyelitis pubis (These patients experience sudden onset of pain.)
- Imbalance of pelvic and hip musculature has abrupt onset.
- Patient may have more than one problem (i.e., femoro-acetabular impingement [FAI] and osteitis pubis [OP]).

RISK FACTORS

- Increased risk in patients with rheumatoid arthritis (RA)
- Pregnancy, pelvic trauma, pelvic surgery

COMMONLY ASSOCIATED CONDITIONS

- FAI
- Patients with RA
- Pelvic trauma
- Pelvic surgery
- Sports hernia

DIAGNOSIS

HISTORY

- No evidence-based guideline for diagnosis or treatment exists (1)[C].
- Slow progressive symptoms after increased or different athletic activity (1)[C]
- More common in men (2)[C]
- Can occur with other problems (2)[C]
- Condition is theorized to be secondary to weak abdominal and hip muscles (2)[C].

PHYSICAL EXAM

- Clinical diagnosis—anterior medial groin pain
- Single adductor test (patient resistant adduction leg) (3)[C]
- Bilateral adduction test (patient resistant adduction both legs) (3)[C]
- Squeeze test (patient squeeze knees together with towel or exam hand between them)
- The more tests are positive, the higher rate of congruence with magnetic resonance imaging (MRI diagnosis).
- Should also try to rule out other conditions:
  - Inguinal hernia (standard exam for inguinal hernia) (4)[C]
  - Sports hernia (squeeze test but pain occurs more laterally) (4)[C]
  - FAI (circumduction of hip with most pain with patient's knee from 12 o'clock to 3 o'clock position) (4)[C]

DIFFERENTIAL DIAGNOSIS

- Adductor sprain—usually recovery is sooner (2)[C]
- Sports hernia—pain more lateral, superior (2)[C]
- Hip pathology—increased pain with circumduction of hip (1)[C]
- Referred back pain—pain when femoral nerve stretched (1)[C]
- Inflammatory problem—RA, inflammatory bowel, infection, and so forth (1)[C]
  - Positive lab tests: complete blood count (CBC), C-reactive protein (CRP), sedimentation rate

DIAGNOSTIC TESTS & INTERPRETATION

- Plain radiographs may show widening of the pubic symphysis, osteopenia.
- The "Flamingo test":
  - Have patient stand on one leg while anteroposterior (AP) view of pelvis is taken. If over 2 mm of vertical displacement of the pubis, it is considered a positive test by some authors (2)[C].
- MRI can distinguish between OP and osteomyelitis, the latter showing bone destruction (4)[C].
- CBC and erythrocyte sedimentation rate (ESR) can help differentiate OP from an infective or inflammatory process (4)[C].

TREATMENT

GENERAL MEASURES

- Conservative treatment is best.
- Relative rest, followed by abdominal and hip strengthening exercises allows almost all athletes to return to a normal life outside of sports (5)[C].
- The majority of these athletes do not return to their former level of play.
- The patients are usually rested 2 to 3 mo, but it is not unusual for it to take longer than this time to return to full play (5)[C].
- Ice, compression, and elevation (ICE); nonsteroidal anti-inflammatory drugs (NSAIDs); and physical therapy (PT) are the mainstay of treatment.

ADDITIONAL THERAPIES

- Some authors propose injection of glucocorticoid into the OP for recalcitrant cases (2)[B].
- In cases of bone destruction, some clinicians operate on these patients mostly by curettage (5)[B].

REFERENCES

1. Beatty T. Osteitis pubis in athletes. *Curr Sports Med Rep*. 2012;11(2):96–98.
2. Angoules AG. Osteitis pubis in elite athletes: diagnostic and therapeutic approach. *World J Orthop*. 2015;6(9):672–679.
3. Kelm J, Ludwig O, André J, et al. What do we know about osteitis pubis in athletes [in German]? [published ahead of print February 8, 2018]. *Sportsverletz Sportschaden*. doi:10.1055/s-0043-122763.
4. Gaudino F, Spira D, Bangert Y, et al. Osteitis pubis in professional football players: MRI findings and correlation with clinical outcome. *Eur J Radiol*. 2017;94(4):46–52.
5. Gomella P, Mufarrij P. Osteitis pubis: a rare cause of suprapubic pain. *Rev Urol*. 2017;19(3):156–163.

ADDITIONAL READING

Yax J, Cheng D. Osteomyelitis pubis: a rare and elusive diagnosis. *West J Emerg Med*. 2014;15(7):880–882.

CLINICAL PEARLS

- This diagnosis should be considered in any patient with groin pain.
- Many of these patients have more than one problem (i.e., OP and FAI).
- No evidence-based guideline for treatment of this condition exists, and the majority of these patients improve with rest.
- MRI can distinguish between OP and osteomyelitis.

OSTEOARTHRITIS

Kevin deWeber, MD, FAAFP, FACSM, RMSK

BASICS

DESCRIPTION

A predominantly noninflammatory, slowly progressing, degenerative condition of articular cartilage, sometimes known as "degenerative joint disease"

EPIDEMIOLOGY

Incidence

Exact incidence depends on the definition or technology used to identify. Knee or hip replacement for osteoarthritis (OA) is performed on ~1/3 of Americans.

Prevalence

- Radiographic prevalence exceeds symptomatic prevalence.
- Symptomatic prevalence significantly increases with age and varies with affected joint (1):
  - Knee: 7–17% of adults >45 yr
  - Hip: 10% of adults >45 yr
  - Hand: 13% of men and 26% of women >71 yr
  - Foot: 2.0% age 15 to 74 yr
  - Glenohumeral: <1%
  - Acromioclavicular: unknown (28% of x-rays)

ETIOLOGY AND PATHOPHYSIOLOGY

- OA is caused by an imbalance between breakdown and repair of joint tissue:
  - Cartilage matrix (collagen, water, proteoglycans) slowly degrades.
  - Chondrocytes slowly die off; those that remain are unable to maintain adequate repair.
  - Mechanical forces contribute to progressive cartilage loss.
- Early stages: cartilage fibrillation (fine fraying)
- Middle and late stages: formation of extra subchondral bone and cysts and osteophytes (usually at joint margins)
- Predominantly noninflammatory, but occasional mild inflammatory clinical flares

RISK FACTORS

ALERT

Systemic risk factors (1) contribute to development of OA by creating an environment where the joint is vulnerable:

- Age: strongest risk factor—10-fold increase between ages 30 and 65 yr
- Genetics: comprises 40–65% or risk; stronger for hand/hip than for knee
- Obesity: 29% of risk; linear increase in risk with rising body mass index (BMI); increases risk in hand, knee, and hip, so metabolic as well as biomechanical factors involved
- Gender: female sex with higher severity and prevalence
- Nutritional factors: no conclusive data on vitamins or minerals

Joint biomechanical risk factors (1) cause direct trauma to articular cartilage:

- Joint injury (fractures, dislocations, ligament and meniscal ruptures, articular surface damage)
- Occupations involving high physical demands: repetitive use of joints, heavy lifting, frequent squatting
- Sports: knee OA associated with elite-level impact sports; hip OA associated with elite-level impact sports, especially handball, soccer, and hockey. Competitive running is associated with more knee and hip OA compared to recreational running (2)[A].
- Abnormal joint biomechanics (dysplasia [hip OA], leg length inequality [knee OA], malalignment, instability, abnormal innervation). Cam-type femoroacetabular impingement predisposes to hip OA.

Genetics

OA has a genetic component, especially in women. Primary, generalized OA is polygenic and multifactorial; environmental factors play a significant role in gene expression.

GENERAL PREVENTION

- Avoidance of joint trauma or extremes of joint activity (immobilization or gross overuse)
- Weight reduction

COMMONLY ASSOCIATED CONDITIONS

- Degenerative meniscal tears in knee OA
- Labral tears in hip OA
- Association between OA and both type 2 diabetes mellitus and cardiovascular disease (CVD) and early death from CVD
- Calcium pyrophosphate deposition disease (CPPD)—unsure if causes OA or associated with it

DIAGNOSIS

- OA is diagnosed primarily through history and physical examination and confirmed by plain films. It can be classified as primary or secondary.
- Primary classification (idiopathic): related to systemic risk factors mentioned earlier; may be particular or generalized
- Secondary classification: Causes include previous trauma/internal derangement and inflammatory or deposition joint diseases (e.g., gout, rheumatoid arthritis [RA], CPPD).

- Most commonly affected joints include the distal interphalangeal (DIP) and proximal interphalangeal (PIP) joints of the hands; carpometacarpal (CMC) joint of the thumb; and the 1st metatarsophalangeal (MTP), hips, knees, cervical spine, and lumbar spine.

HISTORY

- Insidious onset over months to years is typical.
- Most common symptoms are pain (especially after excessive activity), crepitus or grinding, and noninflammatory joint swelling.
- There is typically short-lived (<30 min) stiffness after immobilization (i.e., on awakening), improving with mobilization.
- Some patients experience muscular weakness in the surrounding soft tissue and pseudoinstability.
- There may be a personal history of antecedent joint trauma or a family history of OA.

PHYSICAL EXAM

- Joint line tenderness is common in hands and knees.
- Joints may have crepitus, decreased range of motion (ROM), effusion, and atrophy of surrounding muscles.
- In knees, involved compartments can include medial (most common), patellofemoral, and/or lateral, so accurate palpation is important. Effusion and trace joint warmth are common in acute flares.
- In hands, may see nodules in the DIP and PIP joints, termed *Heberden* and *Bouchard nodes*, respectively
- In hips, decreased and painful internal rotation are early signs, and tenderness over the anterior joint line is a later finding.
- Severely affected joints may appear misshapen or deformed due to osteophytes or malalignment.

DIFFERENTIAL DIAGNOSIS

- RA
- Collagen vascular diseases
- Crystal deposition disease (gout, CPPD)
- Meniscal or labral tears

DIAGNOSTIC TESTS & INTERPRETATION

Initial Tests (lab, imaging)

- Laboratory assessment only used to rule out other disorders, if clinically suspected:
  - Markers of inflammation (erythrocyte sedimentation rate, C-reactive protein) usually are normal but may be slightly elevated during inflammatory flare-ups.
  - Rheumatoid factor and antinuclear antibody titers are negative.

ALERT

Plain films are the modality of choice for diagnosis, severity assessment, and monitoring progression (3):

- Hip: Weight-bearing anteroposterior (AP) films are most sensitive.
- Knee: Weight-bearing AP in 20 to 45 degrees of flexion (Rosenberg view) is most sensitive and accurate for the medial and lateral compartments. Supine lateral and sunrise or merchant views are best for patellofemoral compartment.
- Shoulder: true glenohumeral AP (Grashey) view most sensitive
- Thumb CMC joint: true AP (Robert) view of the thumb, wrist AP, and oblique
- Hands: AP and lateral

- X-ray characteristics include osteophytes, joint space narrowing, subchondral sclerosis, and cyst formation.
- Radiographic severity does not correlate with symptom severity.

ALERT

Radiographic severity is quantified using the Kellgren-Lawrence scale; OA is grade 2 or higher:

- Grade 0: no features of OA
- Grade 1: equivocal osteophytes
- Grade 2: definite osteophytes
- Grade 3: joint space narrowing
- Grade 4: bone-on-bone appearance

- Computed tomography (CT) and magnetic resonance imaging (MRI) do not play a significant role in diagnosis of OA but should be considered if other conditions are suspected. MRI is sensitive in detecting OA of the knee, but there is a high rate of false-positive findings that may not correlate with signs and symptoms. However, MRI can help with differentiation of other causes of pain (i.e., insufficiency fracture, interosseous pathology).

Diagnostic Procedures/Other

Arthrocentesis and joint fluid examination are not routinely necessary unless the diagnosis is in question; there is a possibility of septic arthritis/crystal deposition disease, or for treatment of tense effusion.

TREATMENT

GENERAL MEASURES

- The "core set" of treatments for all patients should include patient education, weight loss if overweight/obese, and an exercise program (4)[A].

ALERT

Patient education is important and effective (5,6,7)[A]:

- Set reasonable expectations on outcome (pain reduction, increased function, not cure).
- Modification of activities to minimize pain and risk of joint trauma
- Importance of nonpharmacologic therapies

- Weight reduction of 5% or more improves knee and hip pain (4,5,6,7)[A].
- Exercise and weight reduction of 11.4% is associated with no pain at 18 mo in 38% of patients. Exercise has an immediate beneficial effect.
- Aquatic and low-impact land-based aerobic exercise, strength training, and ROM exercise are all beneficial; programs involving all types may be most beneficial (4,5,6,7)[A].
- Walking aids for knee and hip OA (cane, crutch in contralateral hand; walkers for bilateral OA) (5,6,7)[A]
- Optimal management requires a combination of nonpharmacologic and pharmacologic modalities (7)[A].

ALERT

Surgical replacement is best reserved for patients with severe pain that affects quality of life or activities of daily living who have failed multiple conservative measures (7)[C].

MEDICATION

No disease-modifying agents are yet available.

First Line

- Oral glucosamine sulfate (not hydrochloride [HCl]) 1,500 mg/day and/or chondroitin sulfate 1,200 mg/day modestly reduce pain in hip/knee/hand OA (5,7)[A] but probably have no disease-modifying effect.
- Topical nonsteroidal anti-inflammatory drugs (NSAIDs) are effective; onset of pain reduction 1 to 2 wk and work as well as oral NSAIDs (4,5,6,7)[A]
- Older studies show that topical capsaicin is effective for knee OA; high incidence of local irritation (4,5,6,7)[A]

Second Line

- Oral NSAIDs effective but have higher risks; reserved for short-term therapy (4,5,6,7)[A]:
  - Cyclooxygenase-2 (COX-2) inhibitors are not more effective; less gastrointestinal (GI) toxicity but not without risks
  - Discourage chronic use of NSAIDs; if necessary, add gastroprotection with a proton pump inhibitor or misoprostol.
- Viscosupplementation with intra-articular injection of hyaluronate derivatives may be modestly effective in pain reduction (4,5,6,7)[A]:
  - 2 to 5 weekly injections
  - 2- to 5-wk delay in effects
  - 1- to 6-mo duration of effects
- Intra-articular injections with corticosteroids are effective for 2 to 4 wk (4,5,6,7)[A]:
  - Reserve for patients not responding to oral medications or for inflammatory flare-ups
  - Limit to 3 to 4 injections per year per joint.
  - No long-term adverse effect on diabetic control

Third Line

- Duloxetine (a pain-modulating serotonin and norepinephrine reuptake inhibitor [SNRI]) reduces chronic pain in knee or multijoint OA, especially in those who catastrophize (4,5)[A].
- Weak opioids (e.g., tramadol, codeine) can be considered for short-term refractory pain; those requiring long-term use may benefit from maximization of nonpharmacologic therapies and/or surgery (4,5,6,7)[A]. Long-term use and stronger opioids should be avoided because research now shows no improved pain scores at 1 yr compared to acetaminophen or NSAIDs and greater risks. Opioids if given within 2 yr of total knee arthroplasty (TKA) worsen long-term outcomes after surgery.
- Intra-articular injection of platelet-rich plasma (PRP) improves pain and function in knee OA up to 12 mo after single injection, with greater efficacy than hyaluronate (8)[A].
- Intra-articular stem cell injection may improve pain and function in knee OA for 24 to 48 mo and may have disease-modifying activity, but results are limited by high risk of bias (9)[B].

ISSUES FOR REFERRAL

- A multidisciplinary approach may help patients make the most of available therapies: physical therapy, personal exercise training, health care education, nutrition, complementary and alternative medicine, and so on.
- Surgical referral when cartilage has thinned to "bone-on-bone" status and pain/dysfunction are marked despite conservative therapies.

ADDITIONAL THERAPIES

- Valgus bracing for isolated medial knee OA with varus malalignment improves stability and reduces pain in some patients (4,5,6,7)[A]. Ideal patients are not obese and are younger and more physically active.
- Soft braces for knee OA can improve pain and function (4,5,6)[A].
- Wedge insoles for isolated medial or lateral knee OA may be effective; evidence is conflicting (4,5)[A].
- Thermal therapies (heat, cold) may be effective (5)[A].
- Transcutaneous electrical nerve stimulation (TENS) can provide only short-term relief for knee OA (4)[A].
- Walking aids (e.g., cane) reduce pain in hip/knee OA (4,5,6,7)[A].

COMPLEMENTARY & ALTERNATIVE MEDICINE

- Acupuncture reduces pain briefly and slightly in knee OA (7)[A].
- Massage therapy may improve pain and function (7)[A].
- Balneotherapy (spa, mineral baths; common in Europe) may improve pain and function in knee OA (6)[A].
- Traditional Chinese medications are likely effective in improving pain in knee OA (10)[A].
- Therapies with no proof of efficacy include static magnets and electrotherapy/neuromuscular electric stimulation.

SURGERY/OTHER PROCEDURES

- Indicated in patients with recalcitrant pain and interference with activities of daily living despite maximizing conservative management (5)[B]
- Arthroscopic débridement for mechanical symptoms (catching, giving out) *not* effective, even for partial meniscal tears (5)[A]
- Medial or compartment knee OA:
  - Wedge osteotomy may be effective (5)[B].
  - Unicompartmental arthroplasty (replacement) effective (5)[B]
  - Interposition arthroplasty (joint spacer insertion); no data on safety/efficacy
- TKA: very effective (4)[C]:
  - Hardware durable 10 to 15 yr
  - Try to delay TKA until after 55 yr by maximizing other treatments.
  - Rate of hardware failure $<$10 yr is 3 times in $<$55 versus $>$70 yr of age.
- Patellofemoral joint (PFJ) OA in isolation (rare):
  - Elevation of tibial tubercle may be effective.
  - PFJ arthroplasty sometimes used
- Total hip arthroplasty or joint resurfacing is effective in hip OA (5)[B].
- Glenohumeral OA: total shoulder replacement more effective/durable than humeral head replacement

- Cartilage replacement techniques for severe focal defects are gaining in popularity and evidence:
  - Autologous cartilage implantation: Arthroscopy harvests patient's cartilage, chondrocytes are replicated in culture, and second arthroscopy fills cartilage defect with cells.
  - Osteoarticular cartilage transplant: Cartilage from patient's non–weight-bearing surface in knee joint is placed into defect.
  - Cadaver cartilage allografts to fill large defects

ONGOING CARE

FOLLOW-UP RECOMMENDATIONS

- Follow-up to monitor efficacy of treatments and to try additional treatments if needed may improve outcomes by building a trusting patient-provider relationship.
- Reassessment of radiographic joint space worsening in patients not responding to conservative measures can be considered every 2 to 4 yr to assist in planning surgical referral.

DIET

- Supplements that may produce large, clinically important short-term pain reduction in OA include collagen hydrolysate, passion fruit peel extract, *Curcuma longa* extract, *Boswellia serrata* extract, curcumin, pycnogenol, and L-carnitine (11)[A].
- Supplements that may produce clinically important medium-term pain reduction are green-lipped mussel extract and undenatured type II collagen (11)[A].
- Supplements that may produce statistically significant pain reduction of unclear clinical importance include undenatured type II collagen, avocado soybean unsaponifiables, methylsulfonylmethane (MSM), and diacerein (11)[A].

PATIENT EDUCATION

See "Treatment"/"General Measures":

- Public education materials: https://www.webmd.com/osteoarthritis/default.htm

PROGNOSIS

OA is a progressive arthropathy with highly variable course.

REFERENCES

1. Neogi T, Zhang Y. Epidemiology of osteoarthritis. *Rheum Dis Clin North Am*. 2013;39(1):1–19.
2. Alentorn-Geli E, Samuelsson K, Musahl V, et al. The association of recreational and competitive running with hip and knee osteoarthritis: a systematic review and meta-analysis. *J Orthop Sports Phys Ther*. 2017;47(6):373–390.
3. American College of Radiology. ACR Appropriateness Criteria. See Nontraumatic Knee Pain, Chronic Hip Pain, Chronic Ankle Pain, Chronic Wrist Pain. https://acsearch.acr.org/list. Accessed August 29, 2018.
4. Bruyère O, Cooper C, Pelletier JP, et al. An algorithm recommendation for the management of knee osteoarthritis in Europe and internationally: a report from a task force of the European Society for Clinical and Economic Aspects of Osteoporosis and Osteoarthritis (ESCEO). *Semin Arthritis Rheum*. 2014;44(3):253–263.
5. Rillo O, Riera H, Acosta C, et al. PANLAR consensus recommendations for the management in osteoarthritis of hand, hip, and knee. *J Clin Rheumatol*. 2016;22(7):345–354.
6. McAlindon TE, Bannuru RR, Sullivan MC, et al. OARSI guidelines for the non-surgical management of knee osteoarthritis. *Osteoarthritis Cartilage*. 2014;22(3):363–388.
7. Zhang W, Nuki G, Moskowitz RW, et al. OARSI recommendations for the management of hip and knee osteoarthritis: part III: changes in evidence following systematic cumulative update of research published through January 2009. *Osteoarthritis Cartilage*. 2010;18(4):476–499.
8. Dai WL, Zhou AG, Zhang H, et al. Efficacy of platelet-rich plasma in the treatment of knee osteoarthritis: a meta-analysis of randomized controlled trials. *Arthroscopy*. 2017;33(3):659.e1–670.e1.
9. Pas HI, Winters M, Haisma HJ, et al. Stem cell injections in knee osteoarthritis: a systematic review of the literature. *Br J Sports Med*. 2017;51(15):1125–1133.
10. Chen B, Zhan H, Marszalek J, et al. Traditional Chinese medications for knee osteoarthritis pain: a meta-analysis of randomized controlled trials. *Am J Chin Med*. 2016;44(4):677–703.
11. Liu X, Machado GC, Eyles JP, et al. Dietary supplements for treating osteoarthritis: a systematic review and meta-analysis. *Br J Sports Med*. 2018;52(3):167–175.

CLINICAL PEARLS

- OA is a degenerative disorder of joints and is predominantly noninflammatory but can have inflammatory flares.
- Core treatments for all types include patient education on goals and self-management, multimodal exercise, and weight reduction for those overweight.
- Multidisciplinary treatment—providers, physical therapists, nutritionists, fitness trainers, nurse educators, complementary/alternative therapists—can optimize outcomes.
- Topical NSAIDs, exercise, and weight loss are first-line therapies.
- Opioids should be avoided.

OSTEOCHONDRITIS DISSECANS

Holly J. Benjamin, MD, FAAP, FACSM • Melissa Faubert, DO

BASICS

DESCRIPTION

- Osteochondritis dissecans (OCD) defined as a focal idiopathic alteration of subchondral bone with risk for instability and disruption of adjacent articular cartilage that may result in premature osteoarthritis
- It is classified into juvenile and adult forms, depending on the presence or absence of immature physes.
- Most commonly occurs at the posterolateral aspect of medial femoral condyle, talar dome, and humeral capitellum but can occur in all large joints

EPIDEMIOLOGY

- Incidence estimated to be 15 to 30/100,000 persons
- Predominantly males > female (4:1)
- Juvenile form most common
- Occurs typically in ages 12 to 19 yr but can occur at any age

ETIOLOGY AND PATHOPHYSIOLOGY

- Multiple hypotheses as to etiology—likely multifactorial and lacks consensus
- Most accepted hypothesis is repetitive microtrauma leads to microfractures, possibly resulting in focal ischemia and subsequent growth impairment:
  - This causes cartilage separation and fragmentation.
- Other hypotheses include single traumatic episode, genetic causes, inflammatory causes, and vascular abnormalities.

RISK FACTORS

ALERT

OCD in one joint is risk factor for contralateral involvement; 20–30% of patients with OCD of the knee have bilateral involvement.

- Sports involving jumping, pivoting, cutting movements
- Sports with repetitive loading of the elbows, such as baseball and gymnastics, are specific risk factors for OCD of the elbow.

GENERAL PREVENTION

- Using proper mechanics and avoiding overload especially with the elbow and capitellum in adolescent throwers
- Strength and joint stability training

DIAGNOSIS

HISTORY

- Insidious onset of symptoms
- Vague, poorly localized joint pain
- Varying levels of pain and stiffness
- May or may not report joint swelling
- May have sensation of locking or catching or giving way

PHYSICAL EXAM

- Effusion may be present.
- Decreased or painful range of motion (ROM)
- Poorly localized joint-line tenderness
- Mild antalgic gait in lower extremity OCDs
- Ipsilateral quad atrophy if symptoms in knee

DIFFERENTIAL DIAGNOSIS

- Fracture
- Ligamentous or cartilage injury
- Tendinosis
- Inflammatory arthropathy
- Mechanical issue (i.e., patellofemoral pain syndrome)
- Juvenile: apophyseal injury
- Adult: osteoarthritis

DIAGNOSTIC TESTS & INTERPRETATION

Initial Tests (lab, imaging)

- X-ray is first line for diagnosis due to radiographs being inexpensive and readily available (1)[B].
- Characteristic appearance on x-ray is a well-circumscribed lucent defect in subchondral bone that may or may not contain an internal bone density (2)[B]:
  - In children, these findings may reflect normal development of ossification centers (magnetic resonance imaging [MRI] can differentiate, whereas x-ray often cannot).
- MRI is preferred method for characterizing and staging OCD lesions.
- MRI staging classification (3)[A]:
  - Stage I: subchondral lesion of low signal intensity indicating subchondral compression fracture; stable
  - Stage II: hypointense rim on images indicating demarcation with or without partial separation of lesion; stable
  - Stage III: high signal intensity and underlying cystic changes indicative of instability with detached, nondisplaced fragment; unstable
  - Stage IV: complete dislocation of osteochondral fragment into the joint space; loose body may or may not be seen; unstable

Diagnostic Procedures/Other

- Arthroscopy is the gold standard for assessing OCD lesions (size, staging, stability, etc.) (4)[A]:
  - Grade I: stable lesions with continuous but softened area with intact cartilage
  - Grade II: lesions with partial discontinuity that are stable when probed
  - Grade III: lesions with complete discontinuity but not dislocated
  - Grade IV: empty defect or dislocated fragment
- However, arthroscopy is rarely performed as a diagnostic procedure but rather as a therapeutic procedure (see below).

TREATMENT

GENERAL MEASURES

- Early recognition of condition is important. If not treated, can lead to degenerative osteoarthritis.
- Juvenile (3,4)[A]:
  - When diagnosis is incidental, no specific treatment is needed, but patients should follow up until there is radiographic healing.
  - Most stable lesions can be treated conservatively with non–weight-bearing for 6 to 8 wk.
  - If repeat radiographs are stable and patient is pain free, they can bear weight as tolerated and start physical therapy with full return to activity at 3 to 4 mo.
  - Stable lesions that do not respond to conservative management after 6 mo usually proceed to surgical intervention.
  - Unstable lesions require surgical intervention.
- Adult (3,4)[A]:
  - Stage/grade I lesions are treated nonoperatively with activity modification.
  - Treatment of stage/grade II lesions is controversial; lower success rate with conservative treatment when symptomatic
  - Unstable lesions require surgical intervention.
  - Some OCDs are found in non–weight-bearing locations (e.g., posterior femoral condyle) and are asymptomatic; therefore, no surgical intervention is needed.

ISSUES FOR REFERRAL

Orthopedic referral is indicated for all patients with unstable OCD lesions, for adults with OCD, and for those juvenile or adult patients who fail conservative treatment.

ADDITIONAL THERAPIES

- Physical therapy may be initiated for conservatively managed patients. Stretching, ROM exercises, conditioning exercises, and strengthening are beneficial.
- Postoperative physical therapy can be tailored to the procedure.

SURGERY/OTHER PROCEDURES

- Patients with larger lesions, greater skeletal maturity, and high signal on MRI likely will do better with surgery.
- Arthroscopy has better outcomes than open procedures.
- Surgical options include (2)[B]:
  - Débridement, loose body removal, with or without marrow stimulation.
  - Fixation, with or without bone grafting.
  - Transarticular/retroarticular drilling.
  - Autologous chondrocyte implantation.
  - Osteochondral autograft/allograft transplantation.

ONGOING CARE

PROGNOSIS

- All patients with OCD lesions have increased risk for osteoarthritis, but risk decreases with proper healing.
- Groups who underwent fixation of OCD lesion had lower rates of osteoarthritis at 30 yr follow-up compared to drilling and allografts (3)[A].

REFERENCES

1. Zbojniewicz AM, Laor T. Imaging of osteochondritis dissecans. *Clin Sports Med*. 2014;33(2):221–250.
2. Bauer KL, Polousky JD. Management of osteochondritis dissecans lesions of the knee, elbow and ankle. *Clin Sports Med*. 2017;36(3):469–487.
3. Bruns J, Werner M, Habermann C. Osteochondritis dissecans: etiology, pathology, and imaging with a special focus on the knee joint. *Cartilage*. 2017;1947603517715736.
4. Accadbled F, Vial J, Sales de Gauzy J. Osteochondritis dissecans of the knee. *Orthop Traumatol Surg Res*. 2018;104(1S):S97–S105.

ADDITIONAL READING

Carey JL, Grimm NL. Treatment algorithm for osteochondritis dissecans of the knee. *Orthop Clin North Am*. 2015;46(1):141–146.

CLINICAL PEARLS

- Juvenile OCD patients with stable lesions require a period of non–weight-bearing and rest from activity for 3 to 4 mo.
- Patients should be pain free before return to sports.
- MRI is gold standard for staging and guides treatment plan.
- Unstable lesions or stable lesions that do not progress toward healing should be referred to orthopedic surgeon for arthroscopy.
- Juvenile OCD has a good potential for full recovery if treated appropriately but still may lead to early degenerative joint disease.
- Adult forms tend to be more complicated and often lead to early degenerative joint disease.

OSTEOMYELITIS

Dusty Marie Narducci, MD, Board Certified Family Medicine, CAQSM

BASICS

DESCRIPTION

- Broadly defined; recognizes the duration of the infection and whether suppuration or sclerosis of bone is present
- Progressive inflammatory destruction of bone with apposition of new bone usually secondary to infection
- Osteomyelitis occurs either as a result of contiguous spread of infection to bone, hematogenous dissemination, or direct inoculation of infection into the bone.
- Presently, there is no generally accepted, interdisciplinary classification of osteomyelitis.
- Acute osteomyelitis develops within 2 wk of disease onset:
  - Predominantly in children
  - Typically, the result of hematogenous dissemination
  - Metaphysis of long bones is the most commonly involved location.
- Subacute osteomyelitis presents within 1 to several months of disease onset:
  - Diagnosis difficult because characteristic signs and symptoms of acute form absent
  - Mimics other conditions (e.g., tumor either benign or malignant)
- Chronic osteomyelitis develops after a few months of disease onset:
  - May be recurrent or intermittent in presentation
  - Direct contamination frequent cause of chronic form (open fracture, penetrating wound, surgical manipulation)

EPIDEMIOLOGY

- Overall age and sex-adjusted annual incidence of osteomyelitis is ~22 cases per 100,000 person-years (1).
- Annual incidence higher for men than women and increased with age; no association with race
- Acute osteomyelitis occurs in ~8 of 100,000 children per year (1).
- Overall incidence higher in developing countries
- Contiguous spread of infection from decubitus ulcers and infected total joint arthroplasties more common in adults; trauma and related surgery in younger individuals
- Hematogenous dissemination more common in children (particularly age <5 yr)
- Special populations:
  - Annual incidence of osteomyelitis has increased due to high prevalence of diabetic patients.
  - Foot osteomyelitis among diabetic patients ~0.3% per year, lifetime risk of 4%
- Long-term recurrence rate of chronic osteomyelitis is 10–30%.
- In primary hip and knee replacements, early infections are expected in 0.5–2% of cases.
- Infectious complications occur in 5% of traumatic/orthopedic implants during the lifetime of the implant.
- Deep musculoskeletal infection incidence from open fracture is 25%.
- Vertebral osteomyelitis is rare occurring in 2–4% of cases; mortality is <5%.
- Morbidity significant:
  - Pain, disability, amputation, extension of infection, and sepsis
  - Residual neurologic deficits from vertebral osteomyelitis is <7%.
  - In long-standing infections, sinus tract formation may be associated with malignant transformation.
- Mortality low unless associated sepsis

ETIOLOGY AND PATHOPHYSIOLOGY

- Normal bone highly resistant to infection unless result of very large inocula, trauma, or presence of foreign bodies
- Categorized as acute, subacute, or chronic
- Biofilm formation: Microorganisms adhere to bone/devices, survive intracellularly in osteoblasts, express resistance to antimicrobial treatment, and form inflammatory markers (potent osteolytic factors) and phagocytes (generate toxic oxygen radicals and release enzymes that lyse surrounding tissues).
- Increased intramedullary pressure occurs in the bone marrow due to inflammatory exudate. Extension of exudate into the bone cortex can rupture the periosteum. Interruption of blood supply results in necrosis and subsequent new bone formation.
- Infectious agents include bacteria, mycobacteria, and fungi; may be monomicrobial or polymicrobial
- Routes of infection include hematogenous, contiguous focus, and direct inoculation.
- Primary hematogenous osteomyelitis occurs mainly in infants and children:
  - Sluggish circulation at highly vascular metaphyseal–physeal barrier predisposes vessels to thrombosis and bone to localized necrosis and bacterial seeding.
  - Metaphyseal arteries lack phagocytic lining cells, and sinusoidal veins (in growth plate) contain functionally inactive phagocytic cells.
  - Usually monomicrobial
- Simultaneous presence of microorganisms and necrotic bone (sequestra) is hallmark of chronic osteomyelitis.
- Bacterial osteomyelitis:
  - Age and inoculation method important factor in species prevalence
  - *Staphylococcus aureus* most common pathogen of acute and chronic hematogenous osteomyelitis in adults and children
  - In adults, *S. aureus* is the most common pathogen in bone and prosthetic joint infections.
  - Group A *Streptococcus*, *Streptococcus pneumoniae*, and *Kingella kingae* are the next most common pathogens in children.
  - Group B streptococcal infection occurs primarily in newborns.
  - Increasing methicillin-resistant *S. aureus* (MRSA)
  - Consider anaerobes if "fight bite" injury.
- Vertebral osteomyelitis:
  - Primarily in adults; rare
  - Involves two adjacent vertebrae and disk spaces between them
  - Focal neck or back pain, fever
- Fungal osteomyelitis:
  - Usually result of catheter-related complication, use of illicit drugs, or prolonged neutropenia
  - Common agents include coccidioidomycosis, blastomycosis, cryptococcosis, candidiasis, or sporotrichosis.
  - Most common presentation is a cold abscess overlying an osteolytic lesion.
- Tuberculosis osteomyelitis:
  - Any bone can be involved; usually occurs at a single site
  - Typically insidious onset, presenting as a "cold abscess" with swelling, erythema, pain, and little or no local warmth
- Fungal and mycobacterial infections rare and more common in immunosuppressed patients

- Subacute osteomyelitis:
  - Brodie abscess rare; 2% of all patients with osteomyelitis
  - Cavitary lesion in epiphysis or metaphysis characterized by small, localized lucency surrounded by reactive, dense-appearing bone
  - Usually of hematogenous origin but can occur in the setting of trauma; patients <25 yr of age
- Chronic osteomyelitis most likely *Staphylococcus epidermidis* or *S. aureus*, *Pseudomonas*, *Serratia*, *Escherichia coli*
- *Staphylococcus* and *Salmonella* predominate sickle cell disease.
- Osteomyelitis following trauma:
  - Develops as a result of open fractures or surgical treatment of closed fractures

RISK FACTORS

- Open or compound fracture
- Surgical manipulation (orthopedic, colorectal, genitourinary procedures)
- Intravenous (IV) drug abuse
- Immunosuppression (AIDS, chronic steroid use)
- Peripheral vascular disease/peripheral neuropathy (diabetes mellitus)
- Sickle cell disease
- Genitourinary or biliary tract infection
- Chronic joint disease
- Presence of prosthetic orthopedic device
- Low socioeconomic status
- Infancy
- Elderly
- Alcoholism
- History of tuberculosis (Pott disease)

GENERAL PREVENTION

- Timely diagnosis and treatment of primary infections to avoid seeding of bone
- Appropriate wound management
- Use of prophylactic antibiotics with injury or manipulative surgery; ideally within 6 hr (2)
- Tetanus immunization

DIAGNOSIS

HISTORY

- Children with acute hematogenous osteomyelitis may present with abrupt-onset high fever, chills, fatigue, irritability, lethargy, restricted motion and local pain, edema, erythema, and tenderness.
- In a young child, inability to get to seated position, limp, and refusal to walk may be observed if the spine, pelvis, or lower extremity is involved; pseudoparalysis if upper extremity
- Some children and most adults present with vague complaints, nonspecific pain of involved limb, and minimal if any temperature elevation or constitutional symptoms.
- Osteomyelitis due to contiguous focus often presents with painful or unstable joint and little or no fever.
- Subacute osteomyelitis presents with mild pain, minimal fever, and few constitutional symptoms.
- In chronic osteomyelitis, there is local bone loss, persistent drainage through fistulas or sinus tracts, nonhealing ulcers, recurrent pain, possibly low-grade fever, and mild systemic symptoms (i.e., chronic fatigue).
- Diabetic patients with a foot ulcer larger than 2 × 2 cm or if exposed bone is present, osteomyelitis is highly likely.
- Symptoms associated with vaso-occlusive crisis (VOC) and osteomyelitis are common in sickle cell patients.

PHYSICAL EXAM

- Fever (temperature >100.4°F) but not always present
- Tenderness to palpation, swelling, erythema, warmth over involved area
- Fluctuance
- Decreased use of extremity, refusal to bear weight
- Limited movement of adjacent joint
- Other possible foci of infection
- Sinus tract drainage
- Passive range of motion tolerated, unlike septic arthritis

DIFFERENTIAL DIAGNOSIS

- Acute leukemia
- Acute rheumatic fever
- Rheumatoid arthritis (adult or juvenile)
- Acute gout, pseudogout
- Cellulitis
- Malignant bone tumors (Ewing sarcoma, osteosarcoma)
- Septic arthritis
- Multiple myeloma (elderly)
- Sepsis
- Deep vein thrombosis, thrombophlebitis
- Intervertebral disk disorders
- Fracture
- Aseptic bone infarction
- Neuropathic joint disease (Charcot arthropathy)
- Transient synovitis
- Venous insufficiency

DIAGNOSTIC TESTS & INTERPRETATION

- Laboratory investigations can be helpful but generally lack specificity for osteomyelitis:
  - Complete blood count (CBC) may reveal elevated white blood cell (WBC) or left shift in acute osteomyelitis but frequently normal.
  - C-reactive protein (CRP) and erythrocyte sedimentation rate (ESR) almost always elevated but nonspecific tests
  - Changes in CRP detected sooner; CRP and procalcitonin (PCT) levels correlate with clinical response to therapy and may be used to monitor treatment; both return to near normal levels by day 7.
  - In chronic osteomyelitis, leukocytosis is uncommon; the ESR and/or CRP may be elevated or normal.
  - Persistent elevation of CRP and ESR "rules out" osteomyelitis.
  - Serum PCT levels may be useful to "rule-in" the diagnosis of osteomyelitis.
  - Decrease in ESR after treatment is a favorable prognostic indication; may remain elevated for up to 3 mo
- Superficial wound cultures do not contribute significantly to the diagnosis.
- Blood culture positive in 50% of cases:
  - May obviate the need for bone biopsy
  - More likely to be positive in vertebral disease and hematogenous spread involving the clavicle or pubis
- Bone biopsy can be achieved by percutaneous needle, radiographic-guided instruments, or open surgical procedure:
  - *Gold standard for guiding antibiotic therapy*; few studies have assessed treatment outcomes based primarily on bone biopsy results.
  - Send for Gram stain and culture (aerobic, anaerobic, mycobacterial, and fungal) and histopathology.
  - Open biopsy is preferred over needle biopsy.
  - Because the prevalence of diabetic foot osteomyelitis increases, the sensitivity of the test increases and the specificity of the test decreases.
- False-negative blood or biopsy cultures are common in patients on empiric antibiotic therapy; if possible, patients should discontinue antimicrobial therapy 2 wk before sample collection.
- If osteomyelitis is suspected in patients with at least 2 wk of symptoms, the initial imaging of choice is conventional radiographs.

- Radiographs:
  - Osseous changes usually appear 14 days after symptom onset when nearly 50% of the bone matrix is destroyed (3).
  - 80% of patient have normal radiographs in the first 2 wk of infection; bone marrow edema is the earliest pathologic finding and not visible on plain films.
  - Features include periosteal elevation and/or destruction of bone with radiolucency, fading cortical margins, and no surrounding reactive bone.
  - Chronic osteomyelitis demonstrates sequestrum (a focal sclerotic lesion with lucent rim).
- Magnetic resonance imaging (MRI):
  - MRI is the test of choice in patients with <2 wk of symptoms, normal radiographs, or suggestive radiographs without definitive features.
  - MRI effective in early detection (3 to 5 days of disease onset) and localization
  - Reported 90% sensitivity
  - MRI is superior to bone scintigraphy because it can also detect necrotic bone, sinus tracts, and abscesses.
- Computed tomography (CT):
  - If MRI is not available, CT is an appropriate alternative test.
  - Should be used only to determine the extent of osseous destruction (spinal vertebral lesions or other areas with complex anatomy, e.g., pelvis, sternum, calcaneus) in patients with contraindications to MRI or to guide biopsy
- Ultrasonography:
  - May show periosteal thickening and elevation, soft tissue abscess, or fluid collection. Provides direction for aspiration; may demonstrate changes earlier, but can't evaluate bone cortex
- Nuclear studies:
  - Radioisotope bone scan (triple phase with technetium-99m) sensitivity is comparable to MRI, but the specificity is poor; only to be used if metal hardware precludes MRI or CT
  - Positron emission tomography has the highest sensitivity and specificity (>90%) but is not widely available and expensive.

TREATMENT

- Consider issues related to débridement, antibiotic selection, and duration of therapy.
- Immobilization of the affected part, hydration, fever, and pain control
- Involvement of specialists (orthopedic surgeon, infectious disease specialist)
- Empiric treatment is guided by the age of the patient, severity of disease, and suspected organism(s):
  - If clinically possible, delaying antibiotics is recommended until microbial culture and sensitivity is available.
  - Empiric antibiotic regimens should cover MRSA: vancomycin or daptomycin or teicoplanin PLUS an agent with activity against gram-negative organisms (ciprofloxacin, ceftazidime, cefepime, levofloxacin); ceftaroline, telavancin, and linezolid are acceptable alternative agents.
  - Prescribe broad-spectrum antibiotics until lab results are known and then tailor to culture and sensitivities.
- Antibiotic selection:
  - In methicillin-susceptible *S. aureus* (MSSA), suspected first-line options include parenteral β-lactam antibiotics: (nafcillin, oxacillin) or cefazolin; alternatives ceftriaxone and vancomycin
  - Coagulase-negative staphylococci should be treated with vancomycin.
  - *S. aureus* with involvement of prosthetic material rifampin should be used as an adjunctive agent in combination with one or more anti-staphylococcal agents (rifampin should NOT be used as monotherapy, and the likelihood of toxicity and drug interactions should be considered) (2).
  - Gram-negative organisms, fluoroquinolones are the drug of choice; high bone penetration with oral form; alternative ceftazidime, cefepime
  - Diabetic foot infections or penicillin allergies, fluoroquinolones are an alternate option for staphylococcal infections
  - Sickle cell patients, use fluoroquinolones except in pediatric population. Alternative is 3rd-generation cephalosporin.
- Antibiotic duration in children (4):
  - Treatment of acute hematogenous osteomyelitis is typically much shorter than chronic osteomyelitis in adults.
  - Therapy with 4 days of parenteral antibiotics followed by oral antibiotics for a total of 4 wk seems to prevent recurrence in healthy children.
  - Immunocompromised children, the transition to oral antibiotics should be delayed, and treatment should continue for at least 6 wk based on clinical response
- Antibiotic duration in adults:
  - The optimal duration of therapy is not certain; total duration (IV and step-down to oral) is usually 6 wk.
  - Recommend treatment with IV antibiotics 6 wk from last débridement (2).
  - For chronic osteomyelitis, total treatment period of 4 to 8 wk, starting with IV antibiotics and transitioning to oral antibiotics in 2 to 6 wk
  - Long-term oral therapy (3 to 6 mo) may be warranted if orthopedic hardware is known or presumed to be infected.
  - If bone fully resected (amputation), antibiotic therapy can be discontinued when wounds heal without signs of infection.
- Surgery:
  - Indications for surgery include antibiotic failure, infected surgical hardware, and chronic osteomyelitis with necrotic bone and soft tissue; impending sinus formation, drainage into a synovial joint, and signs of subperiosteal pus or synovitis (indicating an acute component)
  - Surgical decompression may release intramedullary and subperiosteal pus.
- Hyperbaric oxygen (HBO) and negative pressure wound therapy (NPWT) may be a useful adjunctive therapy in patients with refractory osteomyelitis:
  - Theoretically, provides oxygen to promote collagen production, angiogenesis, synergistic antibiotic activity, and ultimately wound healing

- Osteomyelitis following trauma (5):
  - Initial management includes irrigation, débridement (routine cultures suggested only if subsequent débridement is performed, not needed in the setting of superficial débridement); administer antibiotics (ideally within 6 hr), tetanus immunization
  - Stabilization and union with internal or external fixation varies; once union is achieved, if clinically possible, hardware should be removed and additional débridement performed.
  - Duration of prophylactic antibiotics depends on classification of fracture; closed fractures require a single dose, whereas open fractures require antibiotics for 24 to 72 hr (prolonged prophylactic antibiotics do not reduce the risk of infection).
- Subacute osteomyelitis:
  - Brodie abscess respond well to surgical curettage of the abscess, cancellous bone grafting, and antibiotic therapy.
- Chronic osteomyelitis (6):
  - Remove infected prosthetic devices and hardware.
  - Treatment can be palliative or curative.
  - Curative: Débridement of all devitalized bone and soft tissue is essential for cure; amputation or reconstruction (prosthetic implant, arthrodesis, callus distraction, vascularized pedicle graft)
  - Palliative: débridement and drainage followed by antibiotic and analgesics
  - New treatment driven by genetic and molecular biology of the biofilm is promising.
- Fungal osteomyelitis: surgical débridement and antifungal chemotherapy
- Vertebral osteomyelitis:
  - If medical therapy fails, consider surgical intervention.
  - Percutaneous transpedicular débridement and discectomy by removing infected necrotic bone accelerates healing and prevents progression of bone destruction and deformity in the early stages.

ONGOING CARE

- Protection of the joint with traction or splinting and starting protected motion early is a consideration.
- Limitation of weight-bearing until x-ray evidence of defect's partial healing due to risk of collapse
- Closely monitor for signs of response to treatment (clinical and laboratory); consider serial weekly measurements of serum inflammatory markers (CRP, ESR); could be useful to determine need for extended antibiotic regimen
- Follow-up based on response to therapy and overall health of patient
- Radiologic healing is slower than clinical healing and usually occurs within 3 to 12 mo. Metaphyseal and epiphyseal cavities usually heal, leaving either a small area of sclerosis or a small, indistinct lucency in the cortex.
- The purpose of follow-up after a year is for assessment of bone growth and alignment; consider for at least 2 yr in subacute cases.

PROGNOSIS

Variable but markedly improved with timely diagnosis and aggressive treatment

COMPLICATIONS

- Include bone abscess, bacteremia, fracture, loosening of hardware, overlying cellulitis, and draining soft tissue tracts.
- Sinus tract formation may be associated with neoplasms, especially with long-standing infection:
  - Squamous cell carcinoma (Marjolin ulcer) most common tumor associated with chronic osteomyelitis; other tumors reported
  - Recalcitrant infection that does not respond should prompt biopsy evaluation for malignancy from multiple sites.
- Despite localized transgression of the epiphyseal plate by subacute osteomyelitis, growth disturbances are exceedingly rare.
- Most common complication is recurrence; despite débridement and antibiotics, recurrence rate of osteomyelitis in adults is ~30% at 12 mo; 50% when the infective organism is *Pseudomonas aeruginosa*
- Most recurrences occur within 6 mo, but recurrence after up to 18 mo has been reported.

REFERENCES

1. Kremers HM, Nwojo ME, Ransom JE, et al. Trends in the epidemiology of osteomyelitis: a population-based study, 1969 to 2009. *J Bone Joint Surg Am*. 2015;97(10):837–845.
2. Hatzenbuehler J, Pulling T. Diagnosis and management of osteomyelitis. *Am Fam Physician*. 2011;84(9):1027–1033.
3. Lee Y, Sadigh S, Mankad K, et al. The imaging of osteomyelitis. *Quant Imaging Med Surg*. 2016;6(2):184–198.
4. Peltola H, Pääkkönen M. Acute osteomyelitis in children. *N Engl J Med*. 2014;370(4):352–360.
5. Hoff WS, Bonadies JA, Cachecho R, et al. East Practice Management Guidelines Work Group: update to practice management guidelines for prophylactic antibiotic use in open fractures. *J Trauma*. 2011;70(3):751–754.
6. Walter G, Kemmerer M, Kappler C, et al. Treatment algorithms for chronic osteomyelitis. *Dtsch Arztebl Int*. 2012;109(14):257–264.

CLINICAL PEARLS

- The most common pathogen implicated in development of osteomyelitis in both children and adults is *S. aureus* (MRSA, MSSA).
- Often, abrupt high fever presents with acute hematogenous osteomyelitis. It is not uncommon to have no fever or a low-grade fever with the other forms of the disease.
- The preferred diagnostic criteria for osteomyelitis are a positive culture from bone biopsy and histopathology consistent with necrosis.
- Initial image of choice is plain radiographs; if <2 wk from the onset of symptoms, perform MRI (can detect osteomyelitic changes within 3 to 5 days and is superior to CT and bone scan).
- The development of malignancy should be considered in long-standing, recalcitrant infection that does not respond to treatment.

OSTEOPOROSIS

Julie M. Kerr, MD, CAQSM

BASICS

DESCRIPTION

- Systemic disorder characterized by decreased bone mass and microarchitectural deterioration of bone leading to bone fragility and increased susceptibility to fractures of the hip, spine, and wrist
- World Health Organization (WHO) definitions:
  - Osteopenia (low bone mass):
    - Bone mineral density (BMD) defined as T-score between −1.0 and −2.5 standard deviation (SD) below the mean of a young adult reference population on dual energy x-ray absorptiometry (DEXA) scan
  - Osteoporosis (decreased bone mass):
    - BMD T-score ≤2.5 SD below the mean of a young adult reference population
  - Severe osteoporosis: BMD T-score ≤2.5 SD below the mean of a young adult reference population with a history of fracture
  - In adolescents and young adults, definition is based on <2 SD below the mean Z-score based on age, *not* T-score.
- Classifications:
  - **Primary**: age-related (postmenopausal estrogen deficiency, age-related vitamin D deficiency)
  - **Secondary**: (drug or concurrent medical condition etiology)

EPIDEMIOLOGY

- Prevalence of osteoporosis will increase as the population ages.
- 9.9 million Americans have osteoporosis and 43.1 million have osteopenia. Lifetime risk of osteoporosis fracture is 1 of every 2 Caucasian women and 1 in 5 men; osteoporosis less frequent in African Americans, but those with osteoporosis have same elevated fracture risk as Caucasians

RISK FACTORS

- Female sex
- Race:
  - Non-Hispanic Caucasian race
  - Asian race
- Parental history of osteoporotic hip fracture
- Personal history of fracture
- Age 65 yr or older
- Low body weight (<58 kg [128 lb])
- Diet low in calcium; low in vitamins C, D, and K; and decreased copper, manganese, and zinc mineral content
- Estrogen deficiency: postmenopausal or premenopausal secondary to over exercising and/or eating disorder
- Sedentary lifestyle, lack of weight-bearing exercise
- History of falls
- Female athlete triad: low energy availability (EA) (with or without disordered eating), menstrual dysfunction, low BMD
- Medications: glucocorticoids, anticonvulsants, cancer chemo drugs, thyroid replacement drugs, proton pump inhibitors (PPIs)
- Excessive alcohol (>4 drinks per day; >2 drinks per day women) and active or passive tobacco use
- Other diseases: diabetes, hyperparathyroidism, hyperthyroidism, multiple myeloma, rheumatoid arthritis
- Impaired absorption of calcium, phosphate, and vitamin D from the gastrointestinal (GI) tract, as in inflammatory bowel disease, gastrectomy, celiac disease, jejunoileal bypass, or pancreatic insufficiency

GENERAL PREVENTION

- Identification and treatment of risk factors/secondary causes of osteoporosis (1)[A]
- Calcium and vitamin D supplementation recently controversial
- Correlation between calcium supplementation and cardiovascular (CV) risk but more research is needed
- Women's Health Initiative (WHI): no statistically significant effect on any CV outcome with combined 400 IU vitamin D and 1,000 mg calcium carbonate
- Current evidence supports the use of calcium plus vitamin D to reduce fracture risk in community-dwelling and institutionalized middle-aged to older adults (2)[A].
- Dietary intake of calcium not linked to CV risk (3)[A]
- Vitamin D deficiency associated with CV risk factors; supplementation associated with better survival (3)[C]

DIAGNOSIS

HISTORY

- General risk factor assessment
- Low trauma fracture at age 50 yr and above
- Historical height loss: peak height age 20—current height ≥4 cm
- Prospective height loss: previously documented height—present height ≥2 cm
- Evaluate Fracture Risk Assessment Tool (FRAX) 10-year fracture risk calculation for hip fracture and major osteoporotic fracture of spine, forearm, hip, and shoulder (http://www.NOF.org and http://www.shef.ac.uk/FRAX).

PHYSICAL EXAM

Silent disease, that is, not evident on exam unless advanced stage and subsequent fracture. Those with undiagnosed compression fractures may have tenderness to palpation in the midline of the spine.

DIAGNOSTIC TESTS & INTERPRETATION

- Assessment of biochemical markers of bone turnover: osteocalcin, total and bone-specific alkaline phosphatase useful in monitoring response to treatment
- Serum type I collagen propeptide, pyridinoline levels in blood and urine, and plasma tartrate-resistant acid phosphatase levels are markers used in research settings.
- DEXA measures bone mineral content of lumbar spine, femoral neck, and distal radius yielding BMD (g/cm^2) and is the basis of definition for osteoporosis according to WHO criteria.
- Vertebral fracture assessment (VFA) uses central DEXA of the thoracic and lumbar spine to assess for compression fractures; lower cost and radiation than plain radiographs of the spine
- Thoracic and lumbar spine films can be useful for identification of fracture and determination of significant arthritis that might falsely elevate T-score.

TREATMENT

Osteoporosis treatment reduces fracture risk and is recommended by the National Osteoporosis Foundation (NOF) for women and men with a personal history of a hip or vertebral fracture, a T-score ≤−2.5, or a combination of low bone mass (T-score −1 to −2.5) and a 10-yr probability of hip fracture of at least 3% or any major fracture of at least 20% as calculated by FRAX WHO Fracture Assessment Tool.

MEDICATION

First Line

- Bisphosphonates: most commonly prescribed therapy for the prevention and treatment of osteoporosis; inhibit both osteoblast and, to a greater extent, osteoclast activity, thus decreasing bone turnover and increasing BMD; decrease vertebral fracture 41–70%:
  - Adverse effects: GI: nausea, vomiting, abdominal pain, dyspepsia, esophagitis, reflux
  - Risk of osteonecrosis of jaw a rare complication:
    - Alendronate (Fosamax):
      - Decreases spine and hip fracture 50% over 3 yr

- Risedronate (Actonel):
  - Decreases nonvertebral fracture 36% over 3 yr
- Ibandronate (Boniva):
  - Has antifracture effectiveness in the spine only; intravenous (IV) 3 mg every 3 mo increases BMD or oral.
- Zoledronic acid (Reclast):
  - Decreased nonvertebral fracture 25% over 3 yr; IV 5 mg yearly
  - Cost for IV medications is high but may be indicated in high-risk women who cannot tolerate or are noncompliant with oral therapy due to pre- and postdose fasting and posture requirements.
- Selective estrogen receptor modulators: raloxifene (Evista):
  - Estrogen agonist activity in bone tissue and on lipids, with antagonist activity in breast and uterine tissue; especially useful in women at elevated risk for breast cancer
  - Decreases vertebral and nonvertebral fracture 30–50%
  - No hip fracture prevention
- Parathyroid hormone:
  - Teriparatide (Forteo):
    - Recombinant human parathyroid hormone with bone anabolic activity stimulating bone formation and inhibiting resorption
    - 20 μg subcutaneous (SC) daily for 2 yr
    - Indicated for postmenopausal women with severe bone loss, men with osteoporosis at elevated risk of fracture, and in persons not improved with bisphosphonate therapy
    - Decreases vertebral fracture 65–69%
    - Decreased nonvertebral fracture 35–40%
    - No hip fracture prevention (3)[A]

Second Line

- Calcitonin:
  - Antiresorptive treatment via osteoclast inhibition
  - Decreases occurrence of vertebral compression fractures by 30% but not nonvertebral or hip fractures
  - Women 5 yr postmenopausal if alternative treatments no suitable
  - 100 IU SC/intramuscular (IM) daily or every other day
  - 200 IU intranasal spray daily with 1,000 mg calcium and 400 IU vitamin D
  - Appears to reduce acute fracture pain
  - Possible association between malignancy and calcitonin-salmon use; reevaluate periodically (1,3)[A].
- Hormone therapy:
  - WHI: Estrogen, with or without progesterone, slightly reduces risk of hip and vertebral fractures, but benefit did not outweigh the increased risk of stroke, deep vein thrombosis (DVT), heart disease, and breast cancer even in women at elevated risk of fracture.

ALERT

U.S. Food and Drug Administration (FDA) recommends hormone replacement therapy for osteoporosis only in women with moderate or severe vasomotor symptoms using the lowest effective dose for the shortest time (1,3)[A].

- Denosumab:
  - Human monoclonal antibody inhibiting osteoclast bone resorption
  - Reduces risk of vertebral, nonvertebral, and hip fractures.
  - SC every 6 mo
  - High-risk women
  - Rebound increase in bone resorption and increase in vertebral fracture after treatment discontinued (4)[A]

ALERT

Exercise and balance therapy:

- Physical therapy and rehabilitation can reduce disability, improve strength, improve function of activities of daily living (ADLs), and decrease risk of falls.
- Weight-bearing exercise with additional resistance training can maintain bone mass and can help prevent falls when coupled with adequate dietary calcium and vitamin D intake.
- Fall prevention addressing vision deficits, balance and gait abnormalities, cognitive impairment, dizziness, and home safety assessment

ONGOING CARE

FOLLOW-UP RECOMMENDATIONS

Patient Monitoring

- Changes in BMD levels indicative of real biologic change can be measured after 1 yr of treatment with serial DEXA.
- Repeat BMD assessments every 2 yr per Medicare and NOF guidelines (1)[C].
- Changes in bone turnover marker levels in treated patients can be observed within 3 mo of treatment initiation. Suppression of bone turnover markers after 3 to 6 mo of treatment and increases after 1 to 3 mo of anabolic therapy have been predictive of BMD responses and fracture risk reduction (1)[A].
- T-score targets of >-2.5 reasonable in assessing efficacy of initial drug therapy or changing therapy but may not be applicable to all patients (5)[C]

REFERENCES

1. Cosman F, de Beur SJ, LeBoff MS, et al. Clinician's guide to prevention and treatment of osteoporosis. *Osteoporos Int*. 2014;25(10):2359–2381.
2. Duque G, Daly R, Sanders K, et al. Vitamin D, bones and muscle: myth versus reality. *Australas J Ageing*. 2017;36(Suppl 1):8–13.
3. Kling JM, Clarke BL, Sandhu NP. Osteoporosis prevention, screening, and treatment: a review. *J Womens Health (Larchmt)*. 2014;23(7):563–572.
4. Tsourdi E, Langdalh B, Cohen-Solal M, et al. Discontinuation of denosumab therapy for osteoporosis: a systematic review and position statement by ECTS. *Bone*. 2017;105:11–17.
5. Lewiecki EM. Osteoporosis: treat to target. *Curr Osteoporos Rep*. 2017;15(2):103–109.

ADDITIONAL READING

- Binkley N, Carter GD. Toward clarity in clinical vitamin D status assessment: 25(OH)D assay standardization. *Endocrinol Metab Clin North Am*. 2017;46(4):885–899.
- Harsløf T, Langdahl B. New horizons in osteoporosis therapies. *Curr Opin Pharmacol*. 2016;28:38–42.

CLINICAL PEARLS

- United States Preventive Services Task Force (USPSTF) recommends DEXA screening for women 65 yr and older.
- USPSTF recommends screening for postmenopausal women <65 yr at increased risk of osteoporosis, determined by clinical risk assessment tool.
- Insufficient evidence for screening in asymptomatic men
- All ethnic groups are at risk.
- Osteoporosis treatment reduces fracture risk and recommended for those with personal history of fracture and those at elevated risk as defined by the NOF.
- Optimal treatment duration unknown

OVERTRAINING SYNDROME

W. Scott Black, MD • Robert Hosey, MD, FACSM, CAQSM

BASICS

DESCRIPTION

- Overreaching:
  - The accumulation of training and/or nontraining stress, which results in a short-term decrease in performance capacity with or without related physiologic and psychological symptoms. Recovery of performance capacity and resolution of psychological symptoms can take several days to several weeks to occur (1,2). States of overreaching lie along a spectrum from functional (planned) overreaching in which the expected outcome is a positive adaptation or improvement in performance to nonfunctional overreaching (NFOR) in which the balance between training stress and recovery is disrupted, and a positive adaptation may not occur.
- Overtraining:
  - The accumulation of training and/or nontraining stress, which results in a long-term decrease in performance capacity with or without related physiologic and psychological symptoms. Recovery of performance capacity and resolution of psychological symptoms can take from several weeks to several months to occur. When being used to describe a clinical entity, this is often referred to as "overtraining syndrome" (OTS). Synonym(s) include "unexplained underperformance syndrome," "staleness," and "burnout" (1,2).

EPIDEMIOLOGY

- Functional overreaching is common and may be intentionally induced as part of a training regimen (1,2).
- The prevalence of NFOR and OTS is difficult to estimate given the somewhat vague nature of the symptoms and the lack of a widely accepted diagnostic test. Nevertheless, some studies have suggested a rate of NFOR/OTS of about 10% in athletes coming out of an intense training cycle (1). Other studies have noted a lifetime incidence of 30–60% in non-elite and elite endurance athletes, respectively (1).

ETIOLOGY AND PATHOPHYSIOLOGY

- Currently, there is no universally accepted hypothesis as to the cause of OTS.
- OTS likely represents the final common result of persistent, repetitive, or excessive activation of various allostatic mechanisms.
- Multiple pathophysiologic mechanisms have been proposed as causes for OTS: dysfunction of the autonomic nervous system (sympathetic or parasympathetic forms of OTS), hypothalamic dysfunction (hypothalamic–pituitary–adrenal axis and hypothalamic–pituitary–gonadal axis), muscle trauma with resulting cytokine-mediated systemic inflammation, reduced blood glutamine levels, decreased blood levels of branched-chain amino acids, and glycogen depletion (1,2,3).

RISK FACTORS

- Highly motivated athletes who respond to poor athletic performance by increasing training loads
- Athletes subjected to generic overload stimuli, without individualized training
- Additional "nonathletic" stressors (social, economic, scholastic, relationship, etc.)
- Nutritional deficiency/reduced energy availability

GENERAL PREVENTION

- Consensus at this time is that there is no effective treatment for OTS other than rest and recovery. Therefore, the emphasis should be on prevention (1,4).
- Daily training logs:
  - Helpful in determining the cumulative strain involved with training
  - To be useful in early detection of OTS, systematic documentation of subjective and objective factors must be completed at baseline (when the athlete has no signs or symptoms) and reevaluated regularly.
  - Although small daily variations occur in athletes, training logs can identify an individual athlete's abnormal response to training at an early stage.
  - Once identified, interventions can be made to prevent further deterioration of performance and normalization of subjective and objective criteria.
  - Training logs should include:
    - Daily workout schedule (including intensity, duration, and mode of training).
    - Rating of perceived exertion (RPE) for the *entire* training session on a specific day. This can be done using the modified (category ratio) Borg scale, which rates perceived effort from 0 (nothing at all) to 10 (almost maximal) (5).
    - The product of the session RPE and session duration can be recorded and represents an objective measurement of daily "training load" (5).
    - Some general description of sense of fatigue or overall state of well-being of the athlete.
- Proper coaching and training techniques:
  - Recognize overtraining early and intervene.
  - Avoid monotony in training.
  - Avoid punishing poor training performance with higher levels of training.
  - Training goals should be formulated on a week-to-week basis during times of increased training.
  - Training loads should display day-to-day variability.
  - Alternate hard day/easy day and include one rest day per week (hard day = RPE >5; easy day = RPE <5)
  - If athlete begins to show strain (performance decrements, increasing RPE at low-level training), reduce training to a lower level.
- Ensure adequate recovery:
  - Athletes should have no less than one passive rest day each week.
  - All athletes should be assessed for adequacy of sleep. Significant individual differences exist in the amount of sleep necessary for adequate recovery, so it is best to simply inquire if athletes feel well rested and energetic each day.
  - Screen for negative energy balance in athletes with signs/symptoms suggestive of NFOR/OTS.
  - Ensure adequate carbohydrate intake in line with current recommendations related to training volume and intensity.

DIAGNOSIS

- An algorithm to aid in the diagnosis of OTS in athletes has been proposed (1)[C].
- There is no single diagnostic test for OTS. Blood testing may be performed if clinically indicated to rule out organic disease/"other" causes of fatigue.
- Research generally supports the use of psychological testing in the evaluation of possible cases of OTS (1)[B].
- Profile of Mood States questionnaire may show an "inverse iceberg profile."
- Several sport-specific psychological evaluation tools are currently available: (i) Standardized Overtraining Questionnaire from the French Society for Sports Medicine, (ii) Recovery-Stress Questionnaire for Athletes (RESTQ-Sport), and (iii) Daily Analysis of Life Demands in Athletes (DALDA).

- Measurements of psychomotor speed (e.g., Stroop test) may show decrements from baseline early in NFOR (1)[B].
- A two-bout exercise test in which adrenocorticotropic hormone (ACTH) and prolactin are measured following two sequential maximum graded exercise tests separated by 4 hr has shown promise in being able to distinguish NFOR from OTS (6)[B].
- Reduced performance on speed-endurance or short, high-intensity exercise tests (decreased performance on time trials) is consistently found (1,2)[B].
- VO_2max may be reduced, but unchanged values are not unusual.
- Blood lactate at submaximal steady-state exercise and at maximal exercise may be reduced from baseline.
- Performance decrements may be seen when evaluating maximum sport-specific performance with increased perceived exertion at a given workload.
- Decreased coordination may be observed.

HISTORY

Consider:

- Current training load: intensity, frequency, duration, and/or mode of training
- Historical training load over past several months
- Any changes in "nonathletic" stressors (e.g., financial problems, family illness, relationship problems, scholastic concerns)
- Any changes in sleep pattern
- Recent exposure to infection
- Changes in menstruation
- Nutritional assessment

PHYSICAL EXAM

- Because OTS is a spectrum of diseases, the clinical presentation varies among individual athletes.
- Subjective complaints of fatigue or "heavy legs"
- Sleep disturbance
- Document temperature to rule out systemic infection.
- Evaluate resting heart rate and blood pressure (BP), including orthostatics.
- Head/eyes/ears/nose/throat exam to evaluate possible upper respiratory infection/infectious mononucleosis
- Neck exam for adenopathy or thyroid abnormalities
- Chest auscultation to evaluate for cardiopulmonary disease
- Abdominal examination to evaluate spleen and liver
- Neurologic examination to evaluate for neuromuscular disease

DIFFERENTIAL DIAGNOSIS

- Major depression or other psychological disorder
- Disordered eating pattern
- Organic disease (mononucleosis or other infections, hypothyroidism, anemia)
- Drug abuse
- Nutritional deficiencies
- Concussion

TREATMENT

- The primary treatment for OTS is relative or absolute rest, depending on the severity of overtraining (1)[C].
- During the rest period, the clinician should evaluate and manage any conditions that might be interfering with adequate recovery (sleep disturbance, nutritional deficiency, etc.).
- Mild cases may improve with a relative decrease in training load (frequency and/or intensity), an increase in rest between training sessions, and/or an increase in training variety (cross-training).
- More severe cases may need weeks to months of absolute rest. Occasionally, athletes never return to their previous level of function.
- It has been suggested that some of the newer antidepressant medications (selective serotonin reuptake inhibitors, noradrenaline reuptake inhibitors, combination serotonin and noradrenaline reuptake inhibitors) might offer a pharmacologic approach to the treatment of OTS (7). Although there may be a theoretical benefit if central nervous system (CNS) neurotransmitters are involved in the pathogenesis, there is no significant proven benefit for antidepressant medications for the management of OTS, and their use for this purpose would be strictly off-label. Antidepressant medications may cause problems with thermoregulation, so caution should be used when treating athletes who exercise in the heat (7).

REFERENCES

1. Meeusen R, Duclos M, Foster C, et al. Prevention, diagnosis, and treatment of the overtraining syndrome: joint consensus statement of the European College of Sport Science and the American College of Sports Medicine. *Med Sci Sports Exerc*. 2013;45(1):186–205.
2. Halson SL, Jeukendrup AE. Does overtraining exist? An analysis of overreaching and overtraining research. *Sports Med*. 2004;34(14):967–981.
3. Smith LL. Cytokine hypothesis of overtraining: a physiological adaptation to excessive stress? *Med Sci Sports Exerc*. 2000;32(2):317–331.
4. Lewis NA, Collins D, Pedlar CR, et al. Can clinicians and scientists explain and prevent unexplained underperformance syndrome in elite athletes: an interdisciplinary perspective and 2016 update. *BMJ Open Sport Exerc Med*. 2015;1(1):e000063.
5. Foster C. Monitoring training in athletes with reference to overtraining syndrome. *Med Sci Sports Exerc*. 1998;30(7):1164–1168.
6. Meeusen R, Nederhof E, Buyse L, et al. Diagnosing overtraining in athletes using the two-bout exercise protocol. *Br J Sports Med*. 2010;44(9):642–648.
7. Armstrong LE, VanHeest JL. The unknown mechanism of the overtraining syndrome: clues from depression and psychoneuroimmunology. *Sports Med*. 2002;32(3):185–209.

ADDITIONAL READING

- Cadegiani FA, Kater CE. Hormonal aspects of overtraining syndrome: a systematic review. *BMC Sports Sci Med Rehabil*. 2017;9:14.
- Kreher JB. Diagnosis and prevention of overtraining syndrome: an opinion on education strategies. *Open Access J Sports Med*. 2016;7:115–122.
- Meeusen R, Duclos M, Gleeson M, et al. Prevention, diagnosis and treatment of the overtraining syndrome. *Eur J Sport Sci*. 2006;6(1):1–14.

CLINICAL PEARLS

- Consensus at this time is that there is no effective treatment for OTS other than rest and recovery. Therefore, the emphasis should be on prevention.
- The primary treatment for OTS is relative or absolute rest, depending on the severity of overtraining.
- An algorithm to aid in the diagnosis of OTS in athletes has been proposed.
- There is no single diagnostic test for OTS.

PAGET-SCHROETTER SYNDROME

Misha Khalighi, MD • Chris Koutures, MD, FAAP

BASICS

DESCRIPTION

- Paget-Schroetter syndrome (PSS) is venous thrombosis resulting from chronic compression of the subclavian vein (1). Compression in an anatomically normal extremity occurs in extremes of shoulder abduction or external rotation (1).
- Thrombosis occurs within a triangular space bordered by the 1st rib, clavicle, and subclavius muscle/costoclavicular ligament (2).
- PSS is a subset of the venous thoracic outlet syndrome (VTOS) (1).
- Synonyms: effort thrombosis (1), primary VTOS (3).

EPIDEMIOLOGY

Incidence

- Rare syndrome that has been estimated to be about 1 to 2/100,000 people per year, which would translate to 3,000 to 6,000 incidences in the United States yearly (4).
- Mean age of presentation is early in the 3rd decade, and the male to female ratio is 2:1 (4).

ETIOLOGY AND PATHOPHYSIOLOGY

- PSS results from chronic or repeated compression of the subclavian vein within the thoracic outlet (2).
- Compression occurs inside of a triangular space (the venous thoracic outlet) formed by the 1st rib, clavicle, and the subclavius muscle or costoclavicular ligament (2).
- A narrow thoracic outlet for the subclavian vein increases the chances of compression of the vein, which can lead to stasis of venous blood flow as well as decreased mobility of the vein and subsequent increased susceptibility to trauma with arm use (5).
- A narrow venous thoracic outlet is further compressed when the arm is in abduction and/or external rotation (1).
- Repeated trauma to the vein leads to a cycle of endothelial injury causing intimal hyperplasia, inflammation, fibrosis, worsening stasis and compression of the vein (5), and increasing risk of thrombosis. Stretching of the vein as the arm moves can also cause small tears and further damage (3).

RISK FACTORS

- Anatomic variations of the size and position of the costoclavicular ligament or anterior scalene or subclavius muscle that cause a narrow outlet (2)
- Athletes who perform repeated overhead movement of the upper extremity such as throwing, swimming, and weight lifting (2)
- Occupations requiring repeated overhead movement (2)
- The role of thrombophilia is debated (2).

GENERAL PREVENTION

Early recognition of symptoms and detection of possible intermittent obstruction without thrombosis, which can increase risk of thrombus development (2)

COMMONLY ASSOCIATED CONDITIONS

43% of patients with VTOS had either occult 1st rib facture, irregular costochondral calcification, and/or osteophytic degeneration of the anterior portion of the 1st rib (6).

DIAGNOSIS

HISTORY

- Abrupt painful and swollen upper extremity with blue hue in a young athletic male (2)
- Symptoms typically occur within 24 hr of vigorous or heavy upper extremity activity (1).

PHYSICAL EXAM

- Visual inspection reveals asymmetric swelling and superficial venous engorgement of the upper arm (1,2).
- Axillary vein may be palpated has a hard, linear structure, which may represent extension of clotted vein (1).
- There are no specific physical exam tests to confirm diagnosis (1).

DIFFERENTIAL DIAGNOSIS

- Neurologic or arterial thoracic outlet syndrome
- Tumors of the head, neck, or arm, including Pancoast tumor
- Complex regional pain syndrome
- Lymphedema
- Secondary causes of thrombosis such as presence of central line, pacemaker lead, or thrombophilia

DIAGNOSTIC TESTS & INTERPRETATION

Initial Tests (lab, imaging)

- Urgent venous duplex ultrasound is recommended for initial diagnostic purposes because thrombolysis is optimal if performed within 2 wk (3)[B].
- If no thrombus is identified and concerned for intermittent occlusion, arm should be placed in abduction with assessment of flow through the subclavian and axillary veins (2)[C].

Follow-Up Tests & Special Considerations

Contrast venography is indicated for those with abnormal initial ultrasound and plans for endovascular intervention (2)[C].

TREATMENT

GENERAL MEASURES

- Anticoagulation, symptomatic treatment, and relief of extrinsic compression (2)
- Symptom relief requires pain control and compression (2).
- Catheter-directed thrombolysis provides short-term benefits (2).
- First rib resection and scalenectomy (FRRS) for complete decompression of the thoracic outlet (2)[C]

MEDICATION

Anticoagulation alone is not recommended due to a high rate of disability and recurrent thrombosis, and prolonged anticoagulation is lifestyle limiting (2)[B]. However, temporary anticoagulation will be necessary.

ISSUES FOR REFERRAL

Patients with suspected PSS should be referred immediately to a vascular specialist as rate of successful thrombolysis after 14 days or more of symptoms decreases significantly (2)[B].

SURGERY/OTHER PROCEDURES

- Currently, decompression of the thoracic outlet via 1st rib resection after thrombolysis or anticoagulation is generally considered the treatment of choice, however, some studies have disputed the need (4)[C].
- Multiple approaches to this have been developed (2).

COMPLEMENTARY & ALTERNATIVE MEDICINE

- Anticoagulation for 3 to 6 mo after thrombolysis and decompression is recommended, although some studies have advocated for limiting anticoagulation to 3 mo (4)[C].
- Passive range of motion should be initiated during anticoagulation to prevent stiffness (1).

ADMISSION, INPATIENT, AND NURSING CONSIDERATIONS

Inpatient management may be required for patients with severe symptoms, particularly if anticipating thrombolytic or surgical therapy.

ONGOING CARE

FOLLOW-UP RECOMMENDATIONS

- After surgical decompression, patients discharged on therapeutic anticoagulation, typically weight-based low-molecular-weight heparin (2).
- Follow-up venography should be performed 2 to 3 wk postoperatively (2)[C].
- Anticoagulation may be continued if vein has reoccluded or until patency achieved, up to 6 mo (2)[C].
- Angioplasty may be recommended for those with persistent intrinsic defects of the vein or those with chronic occlusion (2)[C].

Patient Monitoring

There is no standardized method of monitoring. Some monitor with ultrasound or venography postoperatively, with repeat ultrasound if there is any recurrence of symptoms (3,4)[C].

PATIENT EDUCATION

Recurrence is possible, some may argue, more commonly without decompressive surgery. Patients should be educated to return with any signs of recurrence.

PROGNOSIS

- The majority of literature regarding outcomes after treatment of PSS is based on uncontrolled, single-center series, making definitive data difficult to extrapolate (4).
- Prompt thrombolysis and 1st rib resection has been reported to lead to better outcomes (2)[C].
- For young athletes, return to play has been noted to be quicker with earlier intervention (1).

COMPLICATIONS

- Pulmonary embolism
- Postthrombotic syndrome
- Recurrent thrombosis (5)

REFERENCES

1. Mall NA, Van Thiel GS, Heard WM, et al. Paget-Schroetter syndrome: a review of effort thrombosis of the upper extremity from a sports medicine perspective. *Sports Health*. 2013;5(4):353–356.
2. Moore R, Lum YW. Venous thoracic outlet syndrome. *Vascular Medicine*. 2015;20(2):182–189.
3. Hangge P, Rotellini-Coltvet L, Deipolyi A, et al. Paget-Schroetter syndrome: treatment of venous thrombosis and outcomes. *Cardiovasc Diagn Ther*. 2017;7(Suppl 3):S285–S290.
4. Illig KA, Doyle AJ. A comprehensive review of Paget-Schroetter syndrome. *J Vasc Surg*. 2010;51(6):1538–1547.
5. Alla VM, Natarajan N, Kaushik M, et al. Paget-Schroetter syndrome: review of pathogenesis and treatment of effort thrombosis. *West J Emerg Med*. 2010;11(4):358–362.
6. Sheng G, Duwayri Y, Emery V, et al. Costochondral calcification, osteophytic degeneration, and occult first rib fractures in patients with venous thoracic outlet syndrome. *J Vasc Surg*. 2011;55(5):1363–1369.

CLINICAL PEARLS

- PSS is venous thrombosis of the subclavian/axillary vein caused by compression of the venous thoracic outlet in conjunction with chronic injury to the vein by repeated overhead arm activity.
- Definitive treatment of choice is still debated but currently consists of anticoagulation or thrombolysis, followed by decompressive surgery.
- Prognosis and treatment outcomes would best be assessed by prospective randomized trials which are lacking.

PANNER DISEASE AND OCD OF ELBOW CAPITELLUM

Holly J. Benjamin, MD, FAAP, FACSM

BASICS

Panner disease and osteochondritis dissecans (OCD), conditions of the pediatric elbow, are commonly the result of overuse, particularly in the young throwing athlete and gymnasts.

DESCRIPTION

Panner disease (osteochondrosis) and OCD of the capitellum are overuse injuries of the elbow found in children and adolescents (respectively) that involve disordered endochondral ossification of the humeral capitellum. They are generally considered different pathologic entities but may be a continuum of disordered endochondral ossification.

EPIDEMIOLOGY

- Occur most commonly in the dominant arm
- Boys affected more often than girls in both
- Panner disease occurs most commonly before the age of 10 yr.
- OCD of the capitellum mainly in adolescents:
  - Average patient age is between 12 and 17 yr.
- <5% are bilateral.
- OCD lesions of the capitellum are most common, but disorders of the radial head, trochlea, olecranon, and olecranon fossa are also described.

ETIOLOGY AND PATHOPHYSIOLOGY

- Panner disease:
  - Articular osteochondrosis
  - Articular chondrocyte viability may be compromised by repetitive compressive loading.
  - Ossific nucleus of capitellum has a tenuous blood supply, which may be vulnerable to stresses at the elbow.
- OCD of the elbow capitellum:
  - Disordered growth of articular cartilage and subchondral bone, resulting in spontaneous osteonecrosis and formation of osteochondral fragments
  - Histopathologic examination has failed to demonstrate inflammatory reaction.
  - Likely a result of repetitive compressive forces exerted across the radiocapitellar joint during a time of epiphyseal vulnerability

Genetics

A genetic predisposition has been hypothesized.

RISK FACTORS

- Precise etiology is not well established.
- Valgus stress results in lateral compression and shear forces applied to the radiocapitellar joint during the late cocking and early acceleration phases of throwing and racquet sports.
- Increased weight-bearing and axial impact loads across the upper extremity are seen in young gymnasts and weight lifters.
- Repetitive compressive forces may compromise vulnerable blood supply to capitellum and result in articular cartilage breakdown and fragmentation of subchondral bone.

GENERAL PREVENTION

- Proper throwing technique in overhead throwing athletes
- Adequate rest from activities that cause repetitive microtrauma to the lateral elbow
- Early evaluation of elbow pain in high-risk patients

DIAGNOSIS

HISTORY

- Often insidious onset of elbow pain with activity:
  - Acute, sudden onset is rare.
- Pain is relieved with rest.
- Pain is often lateral, but diffuse pain can occur.
- Restricted range of motion is common.
- Other symptoms: stiffness, swelling, clicking, catching, grinding, locking

PHYSICAL EXAM

- Tenderness over radiocapitellar joint
- Loss of extension; 15 to 30 degrees is common:
  - Loss of flexion less common
  - Pronation, supination usually unaffected
- Effusion may be present.
- Crepitus may be present with active or passive pronation and supination.
- Pain with radiocapitellar compression test:
  - Arm actively pronated and supinated with elbow fully extended

DIFFERENTIAL DIAGNOSIS

- Trochlear lesions (avascular necrosis, OCD of the elbow trochlea)
- Distal humerus fracture
- Posterolateral elbow impingement
- OCD of the radial head
- Angular deformity of the radial neck
- Ulnar collateral ligament (UCL) injury
- Tendinopathy

DIAGNOSTIC TESTS & INTERPRETATION

Initial Tests (lab, imaging)

- Labs not indicated unless other underlying etiology suspected (e.g., infectious, endocrine)
- Plain radiographs:
  - Obtain anteroposterior and lateral elbow radiographs:
    - May be compared to contralateral elbow to detect subtle changes of capitellum
    - Able to demonstrate interval healing
  - Panner disease: irregular epiphysis with fissuring, radiolucency, decreased size, flattened articular surface, sclerosis
  - OCD of capitellum:
    - Focal lucency in subchondral bone in anterolateral capitellum
    - Similar appearance to Panner disease; however; loose bodies and capitellar flattening more common in OCD
  - Low sensitivity to detect OCD and loose bodies; 66% and 57%, respectively
- Magnetic resonance imaging (MRI) (1):
  - Imaging modality of choice
  - Capable of detecting early lesions not visible on plain radiographs (bone edema)
  - Useful for lesion characterization of size and extent
  - Allows assessment of lesion stability and integrity of articular cartilage
  - Staging of osteochondral injury on MRI
  - Stage I: subchondral edema with articular cartilage injury only (x-rays often normal)
  - Stage II: cartilage injury with associated subchondral fracture and sclerosis without detachment (X-rays show sclerosis or various irregularities.)
  - Stage III: detached nondisplaced fragment with high signal around osteochondral fracture—nondisplaced (x-rays with lucency between OCD fragment and underlying bone)
  - Stage IV: displaced osteochondral fragment ± joint effusion with peripheral ring of fluid surrounding fragment and filling donor site (x-rays with lucency between OCD fragment and donor site)
  - Stage V: subchondral cyst formation with degenerative changes with unstable loose body (X-rays often show advanced degenerative changes.)
  - MRI also able to demonstrate interval healing and lesion resolution
- Computed tomography (CT) arthrography:
  - Useful for confirming presence of intra-articular loose bodies
  - Depicts cartilage integrity and fissuring
- Ultrasound (US):
  - Able to assess subchondral bone and overlying cartilage integrity
  - Can assess joint stability
  - Operator-dependent imaging modality
- Radionuclide bone scan:
  - Very sensitive but nonspecific for Panner disease and OCD of the capitellum
  - Limited usefulness in the diagnosis and staging of these conditions

Diagnostic Procedures/Other

Elbow arthroscopy allows direct visualization of the articular cartilage surface for staging:

- May fail to identify changes of the capitellum not evident at joint surface

TREATMENT

MEDICATION

Analgesics and nonsteroidal anti-inflammatory drugs (NSAIDs) may be used as necessary for pain relief.

ISSUES FOR REFERRAL

- Panner disease:
  - Persistent pain or symptoms despite appropriate conservative care
- OCD of the capitellum:
  - Persistent pain or symptoms despite appropriate conservative care
  - Symptomatic loose bodies
  - Articular cartilage fracture
  - Unstable, loose, or displaced osteochondral lesion

ADDITIONAL THERAPIES

Little evidence exists for duration of treatment, bracing, or physical therapy for these conditions:

- Panner disease:
  - Rest from offending activities and avoidance of radiocapitellar joint loading for 3 to 6 mo.
  - Nonoperative treatment provides excellent long-term prognosis.
  - Surgery rarely necessary
  - Similar natural history to Perthes disease in the hip
- OCD of the capitellum:
  - Rest from offending activities and avoidance of radiocapitellar joint loading for 3 to 6 mo:
    - Some advocate for hinged unloader elbow brace to avoid excessive valgus stress.
  - Nonoperative treatment for early, intact, and stable lesions in skeletally immature patients is recommended.
  - Conservative monitoring with serial radiographs is reasonable in skeletally immature patients, often with successful resolution of stable OCD lesions over a period of weeks to months.
  - Patients with stage III to IV lesions on MRI, particularly in the presence of a loose body, is an indication for early surgical referral.
  - In skeletally mature patients with symptomatic OCD, early referral for surgical consultation is preferred.

SURGERY/OTHER PROCEDURES

- Operative management is indicated for the following reasons (2)[C]:
  - Failure of appropriate conservative management
  - Mechanical symptoms
  - Intra-articular loose bodies
  - Unstable lesions
- Operative techniques vary, include the following:
  - Loose body or unstable fragment removal
  - In situ fixation of unstable osteochondral fragment
  - Chondroplasty
  - Autologous chondrocyte implantation
  - Osteochondral autograft transplantation system (OATS)
  - Subchondral drilling (microfracture)
  - Closing wedge osteotomy of the lateral epicondyle

ONGOING CARE

FOLLOW-UP RECOMMENDATIONS

Patient Monitoring

Return to activity:

- Gradual progressive return to activity and sports can begin after a period of rest when patient is asymptomatic.
- Physical therapy may begin when symptoms improve:
  - Range of motion, stretching, and gentle strengthening while avoiding radiocapitellar stress
- Evidence of healing should be seen on follow-up radiographs or MRI before return of elbow loading:
  - Serial radiographs performed at 6-wk intervals are useful to document healing or progression.
  - MRI follow-up 6 mo after initiation of conservative management to document lesion healing; consider imaging at 1 yr.
- Athlete should be monitored closely by health care team during return to sport:
  - Progress activity as tolerated, gradually increasing weight-bearing and load across lateral elbow.
  - Rest and resumption of activity avoidance if symptoms return
- For pitchers, recommend strict adherence to established pitch count recommendations.
- It is important to establish good core strength to improve sport mechanics and potentially decrease loading of the radiocapitellar joint.

PATIENT EDUCATION

- Instruct patients on importance of proper sport technique.
- Strict adherence to pitch counts upon return to pitching
- Reevaluation is necessary for return of elbow symptoms after return to sport.
- Consider activity modification to decrease elbow loading following recovery.

PROGNOSIS

- Favorable prognostic factors (3)[C]:
  - Open capitellar physis
  - Age <10 yr
  - Normal elbow range of motion
  - Absence of mechanical symptoms
  - Stable lesion with radiographic findings of subchondral lucency or flattening
- Poor prognostic factors:
  - Closed capitellar physis
  - Age >10 yr for Panner disease and skeletally mature elbow for OCD (stage I to III)
  - Loss of elbow extension
  - Mechanical symptoms
  - Unstable lesion or loose bodies (stage IV/V)
  - Large fragment involving >50% of capitellum

COMPLICATIONS

- Many patients will have persistent loss of extension despite good clinical outcome with return to sport.
- Early degenerative joint disease and continued symptoms of pain and stiffness are more likely in advanced cases.
- Some athletes have difficulty returning to high-risk weight-bearing or throwing sports.

REFERENCES

1. Kijowski R, De Smet AA. MRI findings of osteochondritis dissecans of the capitellum with surgical correlation. *AJR Am J Roentgenol*. 2005;185(6):1453–1459.
2. Baker CL III, Romeo AA, Baker CL Jr. Osteochondritis dissecans of the capitellum. *Am J Sports Med*. 2010;38(9):1917–1928.
3. Kobayashi K, Burton KJ, Rodner C, et al. Lateral compression injuries in the pediatric elbow: Panner's disease and osteochondritis dissecans of the capitellum. *J Am Acad Orthop Surg*. 2004;12(4):246–254.

ADDITIONAL READING

- Claessen FM, Louwerens JK, Doomberg JN, et al. Panner's disease: literature review and treatment recommendations. *J Child Orthop*. 2015;9(1):9–17.
- Churchill RW, Munoz J, Ahmad CS. Osteochondritis dissecans of the elbow. *Curr Rev Musculoskeletal Med*. 2016;9(2):232–239.
- Edmonds EW, Polousky J. A review of knowledge in osteochondritis dissecans: 123 years of minimal evolution from König to the ROCK study group. *Clin Orthop Relat Res*. 2013;471(4):1118–1126.
- Greiwe RM, Saifi C, Ahmad CS. Pediatric sports elbow injuries. *Clin Sports Med*. 2010;29(4):677–703.

CLINICAL PEARLS

- Panner disease and OCD of the elbow capitellum are common causes of elbow pain and disability in young adolescent athletes.
- Repetitive overuse of the elbow, such as in throwing sports, gymnastics, and weight lifting, are known risk factors.
- Clinical suspicion warrants evaluation with plain radiographs and MRI.
- Early, stable lesions that are treated with prompt rest and nonoperative treatment with favorable results and return to activity in skeletally immature patients
- Patients with advanced unstable lesions, loose bodies, mechanical symptoms, or failed conservative management are candidates for operative treatment as well as OCD patients who are skeletally mature.

PARONYCHIA

Holly J. Benjamin, MD, FAAP, FACSM • Yaqoob Syed, DO

BASICS

DESCRIPTION
- Inflammation of the folds of skin surrounding the fingernail or toenail
- May be acute (<6 wk) or chronic (>6 wk)
- Typically infectious but can be noninfectious
- System(s) affected: skin/exocrine
- Genetics: no known genetic pattern
- Synonym(s): eponychia; perionychia

EPIDEMIOLOGY
- Incidence/prevalence in United States: common
- Predominant age: all ages
- Predominant gender: female > male (3:1)

ETIOLOGY AND PATHOPHYSIOLOGY
- Acute: skin flora such as *Staphylococcus aureus*, *Streptococcus pyogenes*; oral flora such as *Eikenella corrodens*; anaerobic bacteria; viruses such as herpes simplex
- Acute flare on chronic: *Pseudomonas* spp.
- Chronic: irritants (chemicals) primary; *Candida albicans* secondary; less frequently, bacteria

RISK FACTORS
- Acute: trauma to skin surrounding nail, nail biting, finger sucking, manicures, retained foreign body, ingrown nails
- Chronic: frequent immersion of hands in water, diabetes mellitus, artificial nail placement
- Reported to be an adverse effect of certain drugs: antiretrovirals, systemic retinoids, epidermal growth factor receptor inhibitors, and cytotoxic chemo (1)
- May be considered work related in bartenders, waitresses, nurses, and others who often wet their hands

GENERAL PREVENTION
- Use moisturizing lotion after washing hands, avoid prolonged exposure to irritants, avoid nail trauma, keep nails short.
- Chronic: Avoid frequent wetting of hands. Wear rubber gloves with cloth liner, cut nails carefully.
- Good diabetic control

COMMONLY ASSOCIATED CONDITIONS
- Diabetes mellitus (1)
- May be associated with atopic dermatitis or psoriasis

DIAGNOSIS

- Special tests: digital pressure test to look for abscess
- Diagnostic procedures: can do ultrasound to look for abscess (2)[C], x-ray (XR) or magnetic resonance imaging (MRI) if atypical

PHYSICAL EXAM
- Separation of nail fold from nail plate
- Red, painful swelling of skin around nail plate
- Purulent and fluctuant
- Abscess may be present.
- Deformity of nail plate
- Green discoloration in nail (*Pseudomonas*) (2)

DIFFERENTIAL DIAGNOSIS
- Herpetic whitlow
- Felon
- Reiter disease
- Psoriasis
- Squamous cell carcinoma (chronic)

DIAGNOSTIC TESTS & INTERPRETATION
- Gram stain
- Culture and sensitivity
- Potassium hydroxide preparation plus fungal culture

TREATMENT

GENERAL MEASURES

- Depends on severity of inflammation and abscess formation
- Acute: warm compresses with warm water or antiseptic soaks and a topical antibiotic (triple antibiotic ointment)
- Chronic: avoid irritants, keep fingers dry (3).
- Base antibiotic treatment on local resistance patterns and culture, if applicable.

MEDICATION

First Line

- Acute (minimal inflammation and no abscess) (1):
  - Frequent soaks with warm water, aluminum acetate, vinegar, dilute povidone-iodine solution, or chlorhexidine
  - Topical antibiotics may be added (gentamicin, mupirocin, bacitracin).
- Acute (inflammation with abscess):
  - Amoxicillin-clavulanate 875/125 mg q12h
  - Clindamycin 300 to 450 mg q6h
  - Doxycycline 100 mg q12h
  - Trimethoprim-sulfamethoxazole 160 mg/800 mg q12h
  - Dicloxacillin 250 to 500 mg q6h
  - Cephalexin 500 mg q6–8h
  - Ciprofloxacin 500 to 750 mg q12h
- Chronic (4):
  - Topical corticosteroids q12–24h
  - Tacrolimus topical q12h
  - Fungus: topical imidazoles (clotrimazole, ciclopirox)
- Systemic (multiple fingers or toes):
  - Fluconazole (Diflucan) 200 mg/wk
  - Oral corticosteroids short course
- Viral: acyclovir 400 mg q8h
- Contraindications: allergy to medication

Second Line

Antipseudomonal drugs

SURGERY/OTHER PROCEDURES

- Incision and drainage (I&D) of abscess, if present
- Partial or complete nail removal if indicated

ONGOING CARE

FOLLOW-UP RECOMMENDATIONS

Full activity

Patient Monitoring

Routine follow-up until healed

DIET

- No special diet
- Zinc 20 mg daily supplementation may be helpful (2).

PATIENT EDUCATION

Chronic: Keep fingers dry.

PROGNOSIS

With adequate treatment and prevention, healing can be expected.

COMPLICATIONS

- Acute: subungual abscess
- Chronic: secondary ridging, thickening, and discoloration of nail, nail loss

REFERENCES

1. Shafritz AB, Coppage JM. Acute and chronic paronychia of the hand. *J Am Acad Orthop Surg*. 2014;22(3):165–174.
2. Leggit JC. Acute and chronic paronychia. *Am Fam Physician*. 2017;96(1):44–51.
3. Biesbroeck LK, Fleckman P. Nail disease for the primary care provider. *Med Clin North Am*. 2015;99(6):1213–1226.
4. Relhan V, Goel K, Bansal S, et al. Management of chronic paronychia. *Indian J Dermatol*. 2014;59(1): 15–20.

ADDITIONAL READING

Ritting AW, O'Malley MP, Rodner CM. Acute paronychia. *J Hand Surg Am*. 2012;37(5):1068–1070.

CLINICAL PEARLS

- Acute paronychia is usually bacterial and chronic paronychia is usually due to irritants.
- Diagnosis is based on history and physical.
- Treatment should start with warm compresses and I&D if an abscess is present.
- Antibiotics should cover methicillin-resistant *S. aureus* (MRSA) and be based on local resistance patterns.
- Topical corticosteroids or tacrolimus are first line for chronic paronychia.

PATELLAR DISLOCATION AND INSTABILITY

Aaron Gray, MD, CAQSM

BASICS

DESCRIPTION

- Patellar instability is defined as hypermobility of the patella in either the medial or lateral direction.
- Medial instability is extremely rare.
- Complete dislocation and subluxation represent variations in severity of instability.
- Acute dislocation typically occurs with a twisting injury and strong contraction of the quadriceps; rarely, it is due to direct trauma to the medial aspect of the patella.

EPIDEMIOLOGY

- Incidence of initial lateral patellar dislocation: 23.2 per 100,000 person-years
- Increased incidence in adolescents aged 14 to 18 yr of 147.7 per 100,000 person-years (1)

RISK FACTORS

- Prior history of subluxed or dislocated patella
- Recurrence rate 15–50% after initial dislocation
- Adolescent females
- Patella alta ("high-riding patella")
- Excessive genu valgum
- Weak vastus medialis
- Excessive tibial torsion
- Family history of patellar instability
- Trochlear dysplasia
- Lateralized tibial tuberosity
- Weak hip abductor and external rotator muscles
- Risk factors associated with developmental dysplasia (firstborn girl, high birth weight, deliver by cesarean section, breech delivery)

COMMONLY ASSOCIATED CONDITIONS

- Avulsion fracture of the superior medial pole of the patella
- Osteochondral fractures of the lateral femoral condyle or posterior patellar articular surface
- Tear of the medial patellofemoral ligament
- Concomitant major ligamentous or meniscal injury

DIAGNOSIS

Prehospital:

- Patient has severe pain and may have heard a pop at time of dislocation.
- Knee is usually held in 20 to 30 degrees of flexion, and patella is palpable laterally.
- Hemarthrosis causing an acutely swollen knee
- Tenderness to palpation over the medial edge of patella
- Tenderness just proximal to medial femoral epicondyle
- Consider subluxation if:
  - History is consistent of a dislocation, but pain and examination findings have resolved.
  - Look for patella alta (high-riding patella) or laterally displaced patella.

HISTORY

- Mechanism of injury?
- Initial or recurrent?
- History of previous knee injury or patellofemoral pain syndrome?
- Does your patella feel like it is slipping or moving laterally on certain movements?
- Do you have swelling?

PHYSICAL EXAM

- Immediately after dislocation, may show patella dislocated laterally and prominence medially due to uncovered medial femoral condyle
- Obvious effusion
- Tenderness most apparent over the medial edge of patella and lateral femoral condyle
- Limited range of motion with knee in extended position
- Fear of redislocation when knee is flexed
- Positive apprehension sign with movement of patella laterally
- Check anterior cruciate ligament (ACL) and meniscus, as up to 12% of patellar dislocations have associated major ligamentous or meniscal injury.
- "J" sign: Seated patient straightens the knee; the patella moves outward instead of straight upward.

DIFFERENTIAL DIAGNOSIS

- Subluxation versus dislocation
- Although history of patellar dislocation is fairly classic, consider other entities that cause early effusions or hemarthrosis (e.g., ACL tear, meniscal tear, and tibial plateau fractures).

DIAGNOSTIC TESTS & INTERPRETATION

- Standard anteroposterior, lateral, and "sunrise" views
- Sunrise view mandatory. Rule out presence of associated osteochondral fractures. Avulsion fracture or calcification along the medial edge of the patella is considered pathognomonic for patellar dislocation.
- Magnetic resonance imaging (MRI) is more informative than computed tomography (CT) for identifying patellar malalignment and can also evaluate articular cartilage.
- MRI finding of medial patellar facet contusion combined with lateral femoral condyle contusion is pathognomonic for patellar dislocation (2).

TREATMENT

GENERAL MEASURES

- If not reduced spontaneously, may require conscious sedation for pain control and muscle relaxation
- Alternatively, arthrocentesis performed with instillation of 10 to 15 mL of lidocaine and/or bupivacaine
- Extension of the leg with hip flexed (reduces tension of quadriceps tendon)
- Gentle pressure on patella directed lateral to medial
- Postreduction radiographs to confirm reduction and rule out fractures
- Examine anterior ACL and medial and lateral menisci to rule out accompanying tears.
- After reduction, rest, ice, focal compression, and elevation are indicated for the first 24 to 48 hr.
- Knee immobilization is maintained for ~2 to 3 wk, although early passive range of motion in terminal extension is allowed to minimize disuse atrophy.
- Hinged brace may be substituted for knee immobilizer as early as 1 wk and weight-bearing as tolerated.

MEDICATION

- Trial of nonsteroidal anti-inflammatory drugs (NSAIDs)
- Tylenol

ISSUES FOR REFERRAL

Orthopedic referral indicated if:

- Osteochondral fracture noted on either plain radiographs or MRI (2)
- Recurrent patellar dislocations despite adequate rehabilitation, especially in younger patients (<14 yr old), in whom recurrence rates can reach 60%
- Evidence of joint locking
- High-risk athlete participates in activities involving pivoting and is at increased risk of recurrent patellar dislocation.

ADDITIONAL THERAPIES

- A significant number of patients develop large hemarthrosis. Aspiration may be considered after 48 to 72 hr, both to relieve pain and to check for fat globules, which might help diagnose an occult osteochondral fracture.
- Isometric quadriceps exercises are begun as soon as possible, although it is often difficult and painful for the athlete to produce a contraction that involves the vastus medialis.
- Active range of motion exercises (closed chain) are started at 1 wk and physical therapy consultation given for quadriceps and lateral hip strengthening.
- Knee immobilizer or hinged brace is used for ambulation until 100 degrees of painless flexion is present, there is no effusion, and a normal heel-to-toe gait is possible.
- Immobilizer or hinged brace ultimately is replaced with a neoprene sleeve with a lateral buttress until normal, painless activities of daily living are possible.
- Rehabilitation alone appears to be effective as operative treatment that is followed by rehabilitation in children under 16 yr with patellofemoral instability (3)[A].

SURGERY/OTHER PROCEDURES

- Typically, patients who fail a conservative trial of ~6 mo become surgical candidates.
- Surgical management includes medial patellofemoral ligament reconstruction, proximal extensor mechanism realignment alone, or combined proximal and distal realignment.
- Isolated lateral retinacular release has no long-term benefit for patellar instability.
- Minimally invasive patellar realignment improves morbidity and recovery when compared with open realignments (4)[C].
- Operative treatment of acute patellar dislocations may have a lower rate of recurrent dislocation compared to nonoperative treatment but does not improve functional outcome scores (5)[A].

REFERENCES

1. Sanders TL, Pareek A, Hewett TE, et al. Incidence of first-time lateral patellar dislocation: a 21-year population-based study. *Sports Health*. 2018;10(2):146–151.
2. Jain N, Khan N, Fithian D. A treatment algorithm for primary patellar dislocations. *Sports Health*. 2011;3(2):170–174.
3. Palmu S, Kallio PE, Donell ST, et al. Acute patellar dislocation in children and adolescents: a randomized clinical trial. *J Bone Joint Surg Am*. 2008;90(3):463–470.
4. Andrish J. The management of recurrent patellar dislocation. *Orthop Clin North Am*. 2008;39(3):313–327.
5. Erickson BJ, Mascarenhas R, Sayegh ET, et al. Does operative treatment of first-time patellar dislocations lead to increased patellofemoral stability? A systematic review of overlapping meta-analyses. *Arthroscopy*. 2015;31(6):1207–1215.

ADDITIONAL READING

- Iobst CA, Stanitski CL. Acute knee injuries. *Clin Sports Med*. 2000;19(4):621–635.
- Roberts DM, Stallard TC. Emergency department evaluation and treatment of knee and leg injuries. *Emerg Med Clin North Am*. 2000;18(1):67–84.

CLINICAL PEARLS

- Patellar dislocation is a common diagnosis in an adolescent with knee effusion after twisting injury. Tenderness of the medial patella in this situation can suggest patella dislocation.
- Return to sports: There should be evidence of adequate healing (absence of sensations of instability, lack of effusion, and absence of pain on patellofemoral compression) and adequate function (able to perform rotational movements such as pivoting, cutting, and twisting without evidence of instability) for return to sports. Athlete may need McConnell taping or patellar stabilizing braces to accomplish this.

PATELLAR/QUADRICEPS TENDINOPATHY

Sean T. Bryan, MD, FAAFP, CAQSM • Isaac P. Syrop, MD

BASICS

DESCRIPTION

- Overuse syndrome of the patellar and/or quadriceps tendons/knee extensor mechanism complex
- Anterior knee pain worsened by activity such as jumping or running
- Also termed "jumper's knee"

EPIDEMIOLOGY

Prevalence

- Commonly seen in athletes who participate in sports with excessive jumping or running (volleyball, basketball, soccer, track and field)
- Prevalence is estimated to be 40–50% among high-level volleyball players and 35–40% among elite basketball players (1,2).
- Affects males and females equally

RISK FACTORS

- Participation in a sport with excessive "jumping" (volleyball, basketball)
- Risk increases with training volume and intensity (3).
- Poor flexibility of quadriceps and hamstrings
- Anatomic variants that can lead to abnormal repetitive biomechanical stresses such as patella alta, patella baja, or patellar malalignment/maltracking
- Use of a fluoroquinolone antibiotic within the past 90 days (4)
- Underlying connective tissue disease such as rheumatoid arthritis or ankylosing spondylitis (5)

ETIOLOGY AND PATHOPHYSIOLOGY

- Histopathology shows (6):
  - Collagen degeneration and disorganization/disruption of normal parallel arrangement of fibrils.
  - Microscopic to macroscopic intrasubstance tendon tears can occur.
  - Increase in mucoid ground substance.
  - Fibroblast proliferation.
  - Neovascularization.
  - Intratendinous calcifications with gritty toothpaste-like consistency can occur.
- More accurately termed tendinopathy which includes the full spectrum of disease from tendinitis (early stage lasting about 1 wk when inflammatory cells are present) to tendinosis (end stage after months to years when tendon is thickened and has central mucoid degeneration)

DIAGNOSIS

HISTORY

- Anterior knee pain exacerbated by activity or by prolonged knee flexion
- Participation in a sport with excessive jumping
- A progressive condition of anterior knee pain (Blazina classification) (7):
  - Phase 1: pain after activity
  - Phase 2: pain during and after activity not affecting performance
  - Phase 3: pain during and after activity impeding performance

PHYSICAL EXAM

- Patellar tendinitis: localized tenderness at the patellar tendon origin (inferior pole of the patella), patellar tendon midportion, and/or patellar tendon insertion (tibial tubercle)
- Quadriceps tendinitis: localized tenderness at the quadriceps tendon midportion and/or quadriceps tendon insertion (superior pole of the patella)
- Both: pain reproduced with extension of the knee versus resistance and/or with maximal stretching of the quadriceps
- Both: poor flexibility of the quadriceps and hamstrings

DIFFERENTIAL DIAGNOSIS

- Patellofemoral pain syndrome
- Hoffa disease (fat pad impingement)
- Osgood-Schlatter disease
- Sinding-Larsen-Johansson syndrome
- Chondromalacia patella/patellofemoral osteoarthritis
- Osteochondral lesions
- Patellar subluxation/dislocation
- Patellar stress fracture
- Patellar tendon rupture (partial or complete)
- Quadriceps tendon rupture (partial or complete)
- Lumbar radiculitis/radiculopathy involving the L3 and/or L4 nerve roots

DIAGNOSTIC TESTS & INTERPRETATION

- Patellar/quadriceps tendinitis remains a clinical diagnosis, and routine imaging is neither required nor recommended.
- Plain film radiographs may show occasional intratendinous calcification.
- Magnetic resonance imaging (MRI) may reveal increased signal within the patellar or quadriceps tendon and/or at the junction with the patella (6).
- Ultrasound (US) may reveal focal hypoechoic areas in the patellar or quadriceps tendon and/or neovascularization on color Doppler flow (6).
- The study of choice and relevance of abnormalities remain somewhat controversial.

TREATMENT

MEDICATION

- Conservative measures typically include relative rest (reduction in amount or intensity of training to achieve pain-free state), ice, acetaminophen, and/or nonsteroidal anti-inflammatory drugs (NSAIDs).
- NSAIDs are commonly used as analgesics and may be beneficial for acute symptoms; however, there is a lack of evidence showing benefits in chronic cases.
- Topical nitroglycerin (patches/ointments) have been shown to reduce pain during activities of daily living in the acute and chronic phases and may help enhance tendon forces in the chronic phase (8).

ADDITIONAL THERAPIES

- Mainstay treatment is stretching and strengthening exercises for the quadriceps to improve flexibility and stimulate tendon tissue repair via mechanotransduction (9).
- Eccentric strengthening exercises of the quadriceps, mainly single leg squats with a slow negative phase, have been shown to decrease pain and improve function in volleyball players after 3 mo and 12 mo, and doing these squats on a 25-degree decline board may provide additional clinical benefit at 12 mo in athletes participating with pain (10).
- Correction of biomechanical abnormalities (if possible) and/or training errors
- Wearing a patellar tendon strap has been shown to decrease localized tendon strain forces and may help reduce symptoms during sports participation (11).

SURGERY/OTHER PROCEDURES

- Iontophoresis/phonophoresis
- Percutaneous interventions for those who fail conservative therapy for >6 mo (under US guidance):
  - Needle tenotomy
  - Platelet-rich plasma (PRP)
  - Prolotherapy
  - Tendon scraping or hydrodissection, separating the peritenon/fat pad from the tendon, disrupting the neovessels and nerves
  - Ultrasonic tenotomy (Tenex procedure)
- Extracorporeal shock wave therapy (ECSWT) directed at areas of tendinopathy
- Open surgical tenotomy may be considered for patients who fail to respond to 6 mo of conservative measures and/or who fail to respond to the above-mentioned less invasive procedures.
- No randomized trials have been able to clearly demonstrate superior efficacy of one procedure or surgical technique over others.

ALERT
Steroid injections into a tendon should be avoided due to the risk of tendon rupture.

ONGOING CARE

Corticosteroid injections into the patellar tendon or quadriceps tendon should be avoided due to the theoretical increased risk of tendon rupture.

REFERENCES

1. Bahr R, Fossan B, Løken S, et al. Surgical treatment compared with eccentric training for patellar tendinopathy (jumper's knee). A randomized, controlled trial. *J Bone Joint Surg Am*. 2006;88(8):1689–1698.
2. Lian OB, Engebretsen L, Bahr R. Prevalence of jumper's knee among elite athletes from different sports: a cross-sectional study. *Am J Sports Med*. 2005;33(4):561–567.
3. Peers KH, Lysens RJ. Patellar tendinopathy in athletes: current diagnostic and therapeutic recommendations. *Sports Med*. 2005;35(1):71–87.
4. Hall MM, Finnoff JT, Smith J. Musculoskeletal complications of fluoroquinolones: guidelines and precautions for usage in the athletic population. *PM R*. 2011;3(2):132–142.
5. Matschke V, Jones JG, Lemmey AB, et al. Patellar tendon properties and lower limb function in rheumatoid arthritis and ankylosing spondylitis versus healthy controls: a cross-sectional study. *ScientificWorldJournal*. 2013;2013:514743.
6. Khan KM, Bonar F, Desmond PM, et al. Patellar tendinosis (jumper's knee): findings at histopathologic examination, US, and MR imaging. Victorian Institute of Sport Tendon Study Group. *Radiology*. 1996;200(3):821–827.
7. Blazina ME, Kerlan RK, Jobe FW, et al. Jumper's knee. *Orthop Clin North Am*. 1973;4(3):665–678.
8. Gambito ED, Gonzalez-Suarez CB, Oquiñena TI, et al. Evidence on the effectiveness of topical nitroglycerin in the treatment of tendinopathies: a systematic review and meta-analysis. *Arch Phys Med Rehabil*. 2010;91(8):1291–1305.
9. Khan KM, Scott A. Mechanotherapy: how physical therapists' prescription of exercise promotes tissue repair. *Br J Sports Med*. 2009;43(4):247–252.
10. Young MA, Cook JL, Purdam CR, et al. Eccentric decline squat protocol offers superior results at 12 months compared with traditional eccentric protocol for patellar tendinopathy in volleyball players. *Br J Sports Med*. 2005;39(2):102–105.
11. Lavagnino M, Arnoczky SP, Dodds J, et al. Infrapatellar straps decrease patellar tendon strain at the site of the jumper's knee lesion: a computational analysis based on radiographic measurements. *Sports Health*. 2011;3(3):296–302.

ADDITIONAL READING

- Everhart JS, Cole D, Sojka JH, et al. Treatment options for patellar tendinopathy: a systematic review. *Arthroscopy*. 2017;33(4):861–872.
- Schwartz A, Watson JN, Hutchinson MR. Patellar tendinopathy. *Sports Health*. 2015;7(5):415–420.

CLINICAL PEARLS

- Patellar/quadriceps tendinopathy remains a clinical diagnosis, and the mainstay of treatment is strengthening of the quadriceps muscles via one-legged squats emphasizing the eccentric (negative) phase for a prolonged period of time (6 mo to 1 yr) which promotes the slow and gradual process of microscopic tendon repair via mechanotransduction.
- Evidence suggests that topical nitroglycerin decreases pain in the acute and chronic phases of patellar tendinopathy and may help increase patellar tendon forces in the chronic phase.
- If the diagnosis is in question or if the patient is not responding to an appropriate course of conservative measures including eccentric quadriceps strengthening exercises, then patellar/quadriceps tendinopathy can be confirmed by either MRI or US.
- If the patient is not responding to an appropriate course of conservative measures after 6 mo and patellar/quadriceps tendinopathy is confirmed by either MRI or US, then ECSWT or minimally invasive US-guided procedures (percutaneous needle tenotomy [PNT], PRP, prolotherapy, or Tenex) or open surgical tenotomy can be considered.

PATELLAR/QUADRICEPS TENDON RUPTURE

Rathna R. Nuti, MD, CAQSM

BASICS

DESCRIPTION

- Partial or complete rupture of the patellar or quadriceps tendon
- Synonym(s): extensor mechanism disruption

EPIDEMIOLOGY

- In the general population, quadriceps tendon rupture is an uncommon injury (1).
- Quadriceps tendon ruptures tend to occur most commonly in the 6th and 7th decade with a male preponderance of 4 to 8:1 and ethnically with increased frequency in black Americans (2,3).
- Quadriceps tendon ruptures are twice as common in the nondominant limb, with bilateral ruptures reported at around 12% of all ruptures (3).
- Patellar tendon ruptures are infrequent events, usually seen in active under 40s male patients following direct or indirect trauma; often in the form of a sudden quadriceps contracture with the knee flexed at around 60 degrees (3)

ETIOLOGY AND PATHOPHYSIOLOGY

- Most commonly due to rapid, eccentric contraction of the myotendinous group with the knee in partial flexion and the foot planted (2)
- Patellar tendon ruptures usually are complete, occurring most commonly at the osseotendinous junction in athletic trauma versus midsubstance in those with systemic disease (3).
- Quadriceps tendon ruptures usually occur 1 to 2 cm from the superior patellar pole, with patients aged <40 yr having midsubstance tears and those >40 yr of age rupturing at the tendon-bone junction (3).
- Chronic tendinosis, corticosteroids, fluoroquinolones, and systemic disease change tendon structure, decreasing its failure point.

RISK FACTORS

- Trauma
- History of patellar/quadriceps tendinosis or patellar spurs
- High-power sports (e.g., high jump, basketball, weight lifting)
- Previous total-knee arthroplasty, anterior cruciate ligament (ACL) reconstruction using patellar autograft or excision of tendinosis
- Steroid injection in the patellar or quadriceps tendon
- Fluoroquinolone use in previous 6 mo
- Systemic lupus erythematosus
- Autoimmune inflammatory diseases
- Rheumatoid arthritis
- Diabetes mellitus
- Primary hyperparathyroidism
- Osteogenesis imperfecta
- Chronic kidney disease
- Uremia
- Obesity
- Tumors
- Gout

COMMONLY ASSOCIATED CONDITIONS

- Jumper knee/tendinopathy
- Patellar spurs
- Quadriceps injury

DIAGNOSIS

HISTORY

- Mechanism of injury: specifically jumping, stumbling, or slipping
- Hearing or feeling "pop" or tearing sensation
- Immediate, disabling pain
- Difficulty straightening or bearing weight on affected extremity
- Acute onset of swelling
- History of chronic patellar or quadriceps tendinosis
- History of steroid injection in tendon
- Recent fluoroquinolone use

PHYSICAL EXAM

- Acute knee pain
- Diffuse swelling or effusion
- Ecchymosis, possible hemarthrosis
- Audible sensation of crepitus
- Patella alta in complete patellar tendon rupture
- Patella baja in complete quadriceps tendon rupture
- Palpable defect (may be masked by swelling acutely or by scar tissue in delayed evaluation)
- Tenderness to palpation over patellar poles, retinaculum, or tibial tuberosity
- Inability to actively achieve full extension/having significant extension lag—may be able to mimic straight-leg raise by internal rotation of the hip due to contracting sartorius (1)
- Absence of/altered patellar tendon reflex
- Altered gait if able to bear weight
- Quadriceps atrophy (in chronic cases)

DIFFERENTIAL DIAGNOSIS

- Fracture
- Muscular strain (grade I or II)
- Patellar subluxation/dislocation
- Meniscal or ligamentous pathologies
- Osgood-Schlatter disease
- Sinding-Larsen-Johansson syndrome

DIAGNOSTIC TESTS & INTERPRETATION

- Laboratory studies are rarely indicated but, depending on history and physical exam, may be performed to evaluate for associated risk factors.
- Plain radiographs:
  - Diagnosis usually based solely on history, physical exam, and plain radiographs
  - Obtain anteroposterior, lateral, tunnel, and patellar (sunrise or merchant) views.
  - Contralateral films allow comparison of patellar height.
  - Superior or inferior patellar migration without fracture is conclusive for rupture; Insall-Salvati index <0.8 for patella baja (4)
  - Avulsion fractures may occur at the superior or inferior patellar poles or the tibial tuberosity.
  - Obliteration of the quadriceps shadow, suprapatellar soft tissue defect, or joint effusion (1)
  - Rule out tumor or fracture.
- Ultrasound (US):
  - High-resolution US shows hypoechogenicity in acute tears, tendon thickening, and heterogeneous echotexture in chronic tears (5).
  - Dynamic evaluation is more useful (6).
  - Inexpensive and high sensitivity

- Magnetic resonance imaging (MRI):
  - May be performed if diagnosis cannot be made by clinical and radiographic examination or clinically obtuse patient
  - Findings include tendon fiber disruption with associated edema or hemorrhage.
  - In-depth information regarding the extent of the rupture
  - Gold standard and high sensitivity
- Pathologic findings:
  - Pathologic changes usually are degenerative, including hypoxic degenerative tendinopathy, mucoid degeneration, tendolipomatosis, and calcifying tendinopathy.

TREATMENT

GENERAL MEASURES

- Immobilization of knee with straight-leg immobilizer, ice, elevation, and crutch-assisted ambulation in the immediate setting
- Immobilization and crutch use should be continued until evaluation and, if indicated, surgical intervention are completed.
- Incomplete tendon ruptures (3)[C]:
  - Most can be treated nonoperatively with immobilization and protected ambulation for 6 wk, followed by a hinged brace allowing active extension in situ until pain resolves (3).
  - Surgery is indicated for complete ruptures or for incomplete ruptures failing to respond to nonoperative treatment (3).

ISSUES FOR REFERRAL

Patients should be referred for orthopedic evaluation as soon as a patellar/quadriceps tendon rupture is suspected to decrease complications (3)[B].

SURGERY/OTHER PROCEDURES

- Surgery is necessary for all complete ruptures to restore the extensor mechanism of the knee; it is also indicated for partial ruptures failing nonoperative treatment (3).
- Repair should occur as soon as possible, preferably within 2 wk. Delays >6 wk complicate surgical intervention and lead to poorer outcomes (3)[B].
- The exact surgical intervention depends on which portion of the extensor mechanism was disrupted and the acuity of the injury.
- If ruptures are several months old, semitendinosus tendon or synthetic graft may be used in the repair.
- Postoperative rehabilitation (3,7)[C]:
  - Strict immobilization for 4 to 6 wk, followed by a further period of passive motion and eccentric exercises prior to allowing concentric exercises, aiming for full recovery by 4 to 6 mo (3,7)
  - Immediate start of isometric quadriceps exercises
  - Weeks 0 to 3: 0 to 45 degrees of active flexion and passive extension
  - Weeks 4 to 6: progression to 0 to 90 degrees of active flexion and passive extension
  - 6 wk onward: straight-leg raise exercises
  - 8 wk onward: stationary biking and water running
  - 3 mo onward: progressive quadriceps exercises
  - 4 mo onward: jogging
  - 9 mo onward: jumping and contact sports permitted
  - Comprehensive physical therapy program should be completed before return to athletics.

ONGOING CARE

PATIENT EDUCATION

- Reasonable function can be obtained in most individuals, especially in the acute tendon rupture that is repaired immediately.
- Most patients can return to their previous occupation but many have difficulty returning to their preinjury athletic level, particularly with quadriceps tendon ruptures.

PROGNOSIS

- Outcome after repair is closely related to the length of time between injury and repair, the quality of the preexisting tissues, and the tendon healing at the proper length and tension.
- If the tendon is repaired immediately, most patients experience nearly full return of knee motion.

COMPLICATIONS

- Loss of flexion is common after quadriceps tendon rupture.
- Extensor mechanism weakness
- Postoperative infection
- Degenerative change at the patellofemoral joint

REFERENCES

1. Gao X, Shao Z, Liu S, et al. A case report of spontaneous rupture of the quadriceps tendon. *Clin Case Rep*. 2017;5(9):1477–1481.
2. Perfitt JS, Petrie MJ, Blundell CM, et al. Acute quadriceps tendon rupture: a pragmatic approach to diagnostic imaging. *Eur J Orthop Surg Traumatol*. 2014;24(7):1237–1241.
3. Pengas IP, Assiotis A, Khan W, et al. Adult native knee extensor mechanism ruptures. *Injury*. 2016;47(10):2065–2070.
4. Ni Fhoghlu C, Ellanti P, Moriarity A, et al. MRI features of a quadriceps tendon rupture. *BMJ Case Rep*. 2015;2015:bcr2015209942.
5. Divani K, Subramanian P, Tsitskaris K, et al. Bilateral patellar tendon rupture. *JRSM Short Rep*. 2013;4(11):2042533313499557.
6. Phillips K, Costantino TG. Diagnosis of patellar tendon rupture by emergency ultrasound. *J Emerg Med*. 2014;47(2):204–206.
7. Ibounig T, Simons TA. Etiology, diagnosis and treatment of tendinous knee extensor mechanism injuries. *Scand J Surg*. 2016;105(2):67–72.

ADDITIONAL READING

- Greis PE, Holmstrom MC, Lahav A. Surgical treatment options for patella tendon rupture, part I: acute. *Orthopedics*. 2005;28(7):672–681.
- Ilan DI, Tejwani N, Keschner M, et al. Quadriceps tendon rupture. *J Am Acad Orthop Surg*. 2003;11(3):192–200.
- Kannus P, Józsa L. Histopathological changes preceding spontaneous rupture of a tendon. A controlled study of 891 patients. *J Bone Joint Surg Am*. 1991;73(10):1507–1525.
- White DW, Wenke JC, Mosely DS, et al. Incidence of major tendon ruptures and anterior cruciate ligament tears in US Army soldiers. *Am J Sports Med*. 2007;35(8):1308–1314.

CLINICAL PEARLS

- Rupture of the extensor mechanism is an uncommon yet disabling injury requiring prompt diagnosis and early surgical management.
- Suspect patellar or quadriceps tendon rupture in any patient with acute knee pain and inability to actively extend the knee.

PATELLOFEMORAL PAIN (PFP)

Kevin deWeber, MD, FAAFP, FACSM, RMSK • Vihangi Hindagolla, DO

BASICS

DESCRIPTION

- Overuse injury with pain located around or behind the patella
- Multifactorial in origin resulting in biomechanical changes in normal alignment of the patella
- Synonym(s):
  - Chondromalacia patella (term frequently used synonymously in older literature; a subset of anterior knee pain related to softening and damage to the articular cartilage)
  - Runner's knee
  - Patellar tracking dysfunction

EPIDEMIOLOGY

- Anterior knee pain represents 20–40% of all knee problems.
- Most common running injury presenting to a sports medicine clinic
- Incidence rate for amateur runners in general population is 1,080.5/1,000 person-years.
- Annual prevalence in general adult population is 22.7%; in adolescent population is 28.9%
- More common in females (2:1)

RISK FACTORS

- Recent increase or change in training/activity
- Increased joint overload with activities (i.e., running, squats, lunges)
- Deviations of normal rollover pattern of foot (i.e., excessive or insufficient pronation)
- Patellar hyper- or hypomobility
- Malalignment (i.e., increased femoral anteversion, inward-looking patella, external tibial torsion, pronated feet)
- Valgus/varus deformities of lower leg
- Strength imbalances in quads (i.e., vastus medialis oblique [VMO] deficit relative to vastus lateralis), hamstrings, and hip musculature
- Gluteus medius inhibition or dysfunction; leads to decreased hip control and greater femoral adduction and/or internal rotation
- Family history of patellofemoral or anterior knee pain
- Increased Q-angle formerly felt to be a significant risk factor, but multiple studies have not seen significant correlation when comparing symptomatic and asymptomatic individuals

COMMONLY ASSOCIATED CONDITIONS

- Chondral injury especially with history of blunt trauma
- Increased residual laxity or tearing of the medial patellar stabilizers with lateral dislocation of the patella
- Patellofemoral compartment osteoarthritis

DIAGNOSIS

HISTORY

- Recent changes in activity frequency, type, and intensity
- Increased duration of wear or changes to current exercise footwear
- Anterior knee pain after prolonged sitting ("theater sign"), squatting, running, climbing/descending stairs
- Insidious onset of anterior knee pain with activity
- In-line "giving way" of the knee secondary to pain and not due to ligamentous or tendinous deficiency
- Effusion is not a typical finding of patellofemoral pain (PFP). Its presence is likely, but not necessarily, related to other pathology.
- Any subluxation versus dislocation episodes and/or history of direct trauma
- Prior treatments, including nonsteroidal anti-inflammatory drugs (NSAIDs), taping, physical therapy, orthotics, injections, or surgery
- The presence of crepitus is not helpful to make a diagnosis because most healthy women and almost half of healthy men also have crepitus on exam.

PHYSICAL EXAM

- Physical examination tests have been reported to have sensitivities <50%, although specificity for some tests have ranged from 72% to 100% (1).
- Evaluate gait (Trendelenburg gait, quadriceps avoidance) and overall limb alignment (varus/valgus, leg length discrepancy), as mentioned in "Risk Factors."
- Dynamic testing with single and double leg squats to assess patellar motion
- Evaluate lumbar spine, core strength, and hips.
- Evaluate neurologic system.
- Note any atrophy of the lower extremity, especially VMO.
- Assess strength of gluteus medius using Trendelenburg test or side-lying hip abduction test.
- Examine flexibility of quadriceps (Thomas test), iliotibial band (Ober test), hamstring (popliteal angle test), hip (Thomas test), and gastrocsoleus (ankle range of motion).
- Assess for presence of crepitus or J-sign (abrupt lateral motion of patella with full extension) during active flexion and extension of the knee.
- Assess for patellar height: patella alta, patella baja, squinting patella, or grasshopper eyes (proximal and lateral patellar rotation).
- Rule out patellar and quadriceps tendinopathy, ligamentous instability, and meniscal pathology.
- Evaluate the prepatellar, infrapatellar, and pes anserine bursae and presence of joint effusion.
- Examine for patellar facet and retinaculi tenderness; tenderness over lateral retinaculum present in 90% of patients
- Evaluate patellar glide and apprehension:
  - Divide patella into four quadrants.
  - If unable to move >1 quadrant laterally or medially, this is suggestive of a tight medial or lateral retinaculum.
  - If able to translate >3 quadrants medially or laterally, suggestive of hypermobile patella; hypermobility usually seen with positive patellar apprehension as the patient senses impending patellar dislocation
- Perform patellar tilt test: With knee in full extension or 30 degrees of flexion, press posteriorly on medial aspect of patella. Lateral patella should translate anteriorly; if examiner cannot get the lateral border of patella to horizontal with posterior pressure on medial edge, suggestive of a tight lateral retinaculum

DIFFERENTIAL DIAGNOSIS

- Patellar or quadriceps tendinopathy
- Patellofemoral osteoarthritis
- Patellar instability with subluxation or dislocation
- Osteochondral defect of the trochlear or patellar surface
- Osteochondritis dissecans
- Iliotibial band syndrome
- Infrapatellar fat pad inflammation or impingement
- Synovial plica
- Retinacular strain
- Osgood-Schlatter apophysitis (proximal anterior tibia)
- Sinding-Larsen-Johansson apophysitis (inferior patellar pole)
- Referred pain from the hip, often affecting the anterior distal thigh and knee
- Multiple other sources of knee pain and arthritis (e.g., gout, infection, reflex sympathetic dystrophy, neuroma, or sickle cell disease)
- Pigmented villonodular synovitis

DIAGNOSTIC TESTS & INTERPRETATION

- Imaging studies are not required for an accurate diagnosis of PFP syndrome. Multiple studies have evaluated sulcus angle, patellar height (determined by Insall-Salvati index), patellar tilt (determined by Laurin angle), and patellar displacement (determined by Merchant angle) and have found no significant difference between symptomatic and asymptomatic patients (1)[A].
- Imaging studies are recommended if there is clinical suspicion of another diagnosis, or if a patient has failed initial conservative management. Most radiographs will appear normal. Any structural abnormalities may need to be addressed when determining the appropriate care plan for an individual patient.
- Computed tomography (CT), magnetic resonance imaging (MRI), or bone scintigraphy may be considered only in difficult cases to determine presence of additional pathology causing anterior knee pain or to assist with surgical options when conservative management has failed.

- Plain radiographs:
  - Anteroposterior bilateral standing: may show varus or valgus orientation of femur, knee, or tibia
  - Lateral view of affected knee: Evaluate for patellar height with Insall-Salvati ratio (patellar tendon length to patella length). Ratio <0.8 consistent with patella baja; ratio >1.2 consistent with patella alta
  - Merchant view of bilateral patellofemoral joints: will not distort trochlea/patella appearance. Evaluate for a shallow sulcus angle, subluxation degree, and femoral condyle appearance. Standing, loaded Merchant view is more accurate representation of joint kinematics.
  - Tunnel view if osteochondral deficit lesion suspected
- CT:
  - Useful to evaluate patellofemoral relationships (e.g., tilt and subluxation), especially in patients with suspected subluxation at <30 to 45 degrees of flexion that cannot be visualized well on plain film
  - Useful to evaluate intraosseous lesions and to plan selective surgical realignment procedures
- MRI:
  - Useful in evaluation of soft tissue, including patellofemoral cartilage, other articular cartilage, tendinopathy, and retinacula
  - Stages III and IV chondromalacia can be evaluated reliably with accuracy of 89%.

TREATMENT

GENERAL MEASURES

- There is no evidence that a single treatment modality works for all patients with patellofemoral syndrome. Limited evidence shows that some treatment modalities may work for some subgroups of patients with PFP (likely dependent on etiology) (2)[A].
- Because PFP is typically multifactorial in origin, adequate treatment should address multiple facets of care:
  - 80% of patients respond to conservative management.
  - Reduce activities that may have led to onset of symptoms, such as resistance training (lunges or full squats), increased mileage with running, or plyometric exercises.
  - Encourage relative rest using alternate exercises (i.e., pool running, bicycling, swimming, or using an elliptical trainer).
  - Evaluate footwear with focus on excessive deterioration, inadequate support, or excessive support.
  - Ice, compression, and elevation can help with acute pain control.
- Physical therapy is paramount, focusing on the physical findings or deficits seen for each individual patient (e.g., strength training for those with muscle weakness and flexibility training for those with decreased range of motion):
  - Strength training with focus on knee and hip exercises; especially knee extension, hip abduction, and external rotation
  - Flexibility training should address the hamstrings, quadriceps, hip flexors, iliotibial band, and gastrocsoleus.
  - Open versus closed kinetic chain training programs can lead to good functional outcomes.
  - Isokinetic exercise (variable resistance applied so movement remains at a constant speed) has positive effects on knee joint position sense, which in turn increases strength and work capacity.
- Physical therapy can reduce pain in short, medium and long terms, and improve function in medium and long terms (3)[A].
- Knee joint mobilization/manual therapy, when used as part of comprehensive approach, has shown to be effective compared to control group (4)[A].

MEDICATION

- Medication management should focus on pain control, not inflammation control.
- Acetaminophen or NSAIDs may be used initially to provide relief of pain symptoms during daily activities.
- Steroid injections are of limited value.
- Topical analgesics may be helpful for those with superficial hypersensitivity.

ADDITIONAL THERAPIES

- Orthotics: Off-the-shelf foot orthoses improve pain in the short term, but long-term benefits are uncertain (3,5)[A].
- Unproven and ineffective therapies:
  - Bracing/knee orthoses (e.g., dynamic brace, knee strap, knee sleeve): lack of evidence to support use (5)[A]
  - Electrophysical agents (e.g., ultrasound, phonophoresis, and laser therapy), while once widely used, are inappropriate and unproven (3)[A].
  - Patellar taping probably only has a placebo effect and, if used, should be combined with proven therapies as above (2,3,6)[A].
  - Acupuncture or dry needling to trigger points have uncertain effects (3)[A].

SURGERY/OTHER PROCEDURES

- Considered if identifiable lesion seen on imaging and if patient has not shown improvement after >6 mo of adequate conservative therapy
- Isolated lateral retinacular release of the patella has not been shown to provide long-term benefit for treatment of patellar instability but may be used along with proximal or distal realignment of the extensor mechanism.
- Patients with Q-angles >20 degrees plus abnormal congruence angles may undergo distal realignment procedures such as an anterior medial tibial tubercle transfer.
- Dislocators are operated on if symptoms of patellofemoral instability were present before their dislocation.
- Patellectomy and derotational osteotomies are last resorts.

REFERENCES

1. Haim A, Yaniv M, Dekel S, et al. Patellofemoral pain syndrome: validity of clinical and radiological features. *Clin Orthop Relat Res*. 2006;451:223–228.
2. Saltychev M, Dutton RA, Laimi K, et al. Effectiveness of conservative treatment for patellofemoral pain syndrome: a systematic review and meta-analysis. *J Rehabil Med*. 2018;50(5):393–401.
3. Collins NJ, Barton CJ, van Middelkoop M, et al. 2018 Consensus statement on exercise therapy and physical interventions (orthoses, taping and manual therapy) to treat patellofemoral pain: recommendations from the 5th International Patellofemoral Pain Research Retreat, Gold Coast, Australia, 2017. *Br J Sports Med*. 2018;52(18):1170–1178.
4. Jayaseelan DJ, Scalzitti DA, Palmer G, et al. The effects of joint mobilization on individuals with patellofemoral pain: a systematic review. *Clin Rehabil*. 2018;32(6):722–733.
5. Smith TO, Drew BT, Meek TH, et al. Knee orthoses for treating patellofemoral pain syndrome. *Cochrane Database Syst Rev*. 2015;(12):CD010513.
6. Logan CA, Bhashyam AR, Tisosky AJ, et al. Systematic review of the effect of taping techniques on patellofemoral pain syndrome. *Sports Health*. 2017;9(5):456–461.

ADDITIONAL READING

- Brushøj C, Hölmich P, Nielsen MB, et al. Acute patellofemoral pain: aggravating activities, clinical examination, MRI and ultrasound findings. *Br J Sports Med*. 2008;42(1):64–67.
- Gulati A, McElrath C, Wadhwa V, et al. Current clinical, radiological and treatment perspectives of patellofemoral pain syndrome. *Br J Radiol*. 2018;91(1086):20170456.
- Lattermann C, Toth J, Bach BR Jr. The role of lateral retinacular release in the treatment of patellar instability. *Sports Med Arthrosc Rev*. 2007;15(2):57–60.
- Lester JD, Watson JN, Hutchinson MR. Physical examination of the patellofemoral joint. *Clin Sports Med*. 2014;33(3):403–412.
- Smith BE, Selfe J, Thacker D, et al. Incidence and prevalence of patellofemoral pain: a systematic review and meta-analysis. *PLoS One*. 2018;13(1):e0190892.
- Thijs Y, Van Tiggelen D, Roosen P, et al. A prospective study on gait-related intrinsic risk factors for patellofemoral pain. *Clin J Sport Med*. 2007;17(6):437–445.

CLINICAL PEARLS

- Return to activity:
  - If patient has PFP during, immediately following, or the day after exercising:
    - Decrease activity. Avoid strength training exercises such as full squats and lunges.
    - Consider alternate activities, such as an elliptical trainer, bicycling, or swimming.
    - Runners who need to maintain running-specific conditioning, use a floatation belt for pool running.
- Physical therapy with a focus on knee and hip strength and lower extremity flexibility are proven effective and are mainstays of treatment.
- Foot orthoses can reduce short-term pain; patellar taping and knee bracing are unproven.
- 80% of patients respond to a nonoperative therapy, most within 4 wk; complete resolution of symptoms may take longer.

PECTORALIS MAJOR TENDON RUPTURE

Jeremy Schmitz, MD, ABFM • Kenneth P. Barnes, MD, MSc, CAQSM, FACSM

BASICS

DESCRIPTION

- Most commonly refers to complete avulsion of the pectoralis tendon at the humeral insertion (1)
- Ruptures at the myotendinous junction, muscle belly, or bony avulsion are possible but less likely (1).
- Associated with weight lifting (bench press) mostly but possible with falls as well as direct trauma to tendon (2)
- Pectoralis is a powerful adductor, internal rotator, and flexor of humerus.
- Main source of power to the torso during strenuous activity
- Two heads:
  - Superior/clavicular: originates at medial clavicle and upper sternum
  - Inferior/sternal: originates at distal sternum, external oblique fascia, costal cartilage of first 6 ribs
- Fibers converge, rotate 90 degrees, and insert lateral to bicipital groove on humerus.
- Inferior portion of the sternal head is most typically involved during an injury (1).
- Innervation: medial and lateral pectoral nerves
- Blood supply: pectoral branch of thoracoacromial artery

EPIDEMIOLOGY

- First reported in 1822 by P. Patissier
- Increasing incidence with increase in health and fitness activities

ETIOLOGY AND PATHOPHYSIOLOGY

- Stretching of the pectoralis major muscle during active eccentric contraction (1)
- Weight lifting (bench press specifically) is a common mechanism (1).
- Direct trauma to muscle in wrestling, rugby, and automotive accidents also reported (3)

RISK FACTORS

- Medications:
  - Steroid use: Studies have suggested that muscle strength increases disproportionately to tendon strength leaving it vulnerable to injury (4).
  - Corticosteroid injection: weakens tendon structure
- Systemic diseases: connective tissue disorders, collagen vascular disease, diabetes (5)
- Advanced age
- Disuse atrophy

DIAGNOSIS

HISTORY

- Men 20 to 40 yr of age (4)
- Usually report a pop or tearing in the shoulder (4)
- Complain of pain/weakness in chest or shoulder (3)

PHYSICAL EXAM

- Swelling and ecchymosis in anterior shoulder/chest most common (4)
- Loss of anterior axillary fold with an asymmetric muscle outline that is retracted medially is a useful diagnostic tool (4).
- Shoulder motion limited by pain
- Weakness in adduction and internal rotation

DIFFERENTIAL DIAGNOSIS

- Long head biceps subluxation
- Proximal humerus fracture
- Glenohumeral dislocation
- Rotator cuff tear

DIAGNOSTIC TESTS & INTERPRETATION

- Plain radiographs initially to rule out bony avulsions, fracture, or dislocations (4)[A]
- Characteristic finding on x-ray is soft tissue swelling and loss of pectoralis major shadow (4)[A].

- Ultrasound (US) can be useful adjunct to clinical exam when diagnosis is in doubt or an unacceptable delay to obtaining a magnetic resonance imaging (MRI) (4)[A].
- US findings will depend on location and time from injury, ranging from muscle fiber disruption that is hypoechoic with a mixed echogenic hematoma when acute to an anechoic fluid collection when chronic (1)[A].
- MRI is optimal. It assesses grade, muscle retraction, acuity, and presence of adhesions in chronic tears (4)[A].
- Standard MRI will not be sufficient. Dedicated sequence is required with axial slices extending superiorly from the quadrilateral space and inferiorly to the deltoid tuberosity with coronal oblique cuts (4)[A].

TREATMENT

- Acute treatment:
  - Analgesics
  - Ice
  - Sling immobilization
- Long-term care:
  - Tear type, patient age, activity level, and cosmetic desires determine care (4)[A].
  - Most partial tears, sternoclavicular tears, and muscle belly tears are treated nonsurgically (4)[A].
  - Complete sternal tears require surgical repair to restore function and strength (4)[A].
  - Nonsurgical treatment may be adequate in elderly/inactive population irrespective of type of tear (4)[A].

ONGOING CARE

- Nonsurgical treatment:
  - Begin shoulder mobilization and gentle stretching/strengthening when tolerated (4)[A].
  - Advance to resisted strengthening exercises at 6 to 8 wk postinjury (4)[A].
  - Unrestricted activity at 2 to 3 mo after injury (4)[A]
- Surgical management:
  - Provides best outcomes in terms of patient satisfaction, strength, cosmetic outcome, and return to sport (4)[A]
  - Acute repair within 3 wk is preferable (4)[A].
  - Delayed repairs do better than nonsurgical treatment (4)[A].

REFERENCES

1. Chiavaras MM, Jacobson JA, Smith J, et al. Pectoralis major tears: anatomy, classification, and diagnosis with ultrasound and MR imaging. *Skeletal Radiol*. 2015;44(2):157–164.
2. Hasegawa K, Schofer J. Rupture of the pectoralis major: a case report and review. *J Emerg Med*. 2010;38(2):196–200.
3. Dodds SD, Wolfe SW. Injuries to the pectoralis major. *Sports Med*. 2002;32(14):945–952.
4. Butt U, Mehta S, Funk L, et al. Pectoralis major ruptures: a review of current management. *J Shoulder Elbow Surg*. 2015;24(4):655–662.
5. Petilon J, Carr D, Sekiya J, et al. Pectoralis major muscle injuries: evaluation and management. *J Am Acad Orthop Surg*. 2005;13(1):59–68.

CLINICAL PEARLS

- Usually a complete avulsion of pectoralis major tendon at humerus
- Most commonly occurs during weight lifting; specifically bench press
- Patients may report a pop and present with swelling, ecchymosis, and palpable tendon deformity.
- MRI is gold standard for diagnosis.
- Type of tear, patient age, and activity level dictate treatment.
- Surgical repair provides best outcomes in terms of strength, return to play, and patient satisfaction.

PERIORBITAL AND ORBITAL CELLULITIS

Matthew Chung, DO • Mark D. Harris, MD, MPH, MBA, MDiv, FAAFP, CAQSM

BASICS

DESCRIPTION

- Periorbital (preseptal) cellulitis:
  - Infection or inflammatory process of the dermis anterior (superficial) to the orbital septum
  - Rarely progresses to orbital cellulitis (1)
- Orbital (postseptal) cellulitis:
  - Severe infection or inflammatory process of the fat and muscles posterior (deep) to the orbital septum
- Orbital septum (palpebral fascia):
  - Fascial extension down into the lower eyelid between the orbital rim periosteum and tarsal plate of the eyelid
  - Nearly impervious to the spread of infection into the orbit

EPIDEMIOLOGY

- More common in children than adults, based on retrospective cohort studies (2)
- Periorbital cellulitis:
  - Predominantly in children $<$5 yr
  - Incidence is roughly equal in males and females.
- Orbital cellulitis:
  - Mean age 7.5 yr in orbital cellulitis
  - Incidence is roughly 2:1 male to female ratio.

ETIOLOGY AND PATHOPHYSIOLOGY

- Prior to the introduction of *Haemophilus influenzae* type b (Hib) immunization, *H. influenzae* was the most common organism:
  - Migrant, not fully immunized or unvaccinated children are most at risk (3).
- Currently the most causative agents:
  - *Staphylococcus*:
    - Methicillin-sensitive *Staphylococcus aureus* (MSSA)
    - Methicillin-resistant *Staphylococcus aureus* (MRSA)
  - Streptococcal:
    - *Streptococcus pyogenes* (Group A)
    - *Streptococcus pneumoniae*
- Rare causes in case reports:
  - *Moraxella catarrhalis*
  - *Neisseria meningitidis*
  - *Mycobacterium marinum*
  - *Pseudomonas aeruginosa*
  - Chlamydia
- Periorbital cellulitis:
  - Progression of preexisting infections (4):
    - Conjunctivitis
    - Hordeolum (stye)
    - Dacryocystitis or dacryoadenitis (infection or inflammation of lacrimal duct or gland, respectively)
    - Upper respiratory infection
  - Superficial trauma:
    - Insect bite
    - Impetigo
    - Acne
    - Penetrating injury
  - Hematogenous dissemination (5):
    - Especially in children 3 to 36 mo due to pneumococcal bacteremia
- Orbital cellulitis:
  - Typically occurs by one of the following:
    - Spread of organisms from sinuses to orbital cavity (i.e., sinusitis); most common cause
    - Hematogenous dissemination
    - Direct/traumatic inoculation:
      - Surgical procedures
      - Orbital trauma
      - Dermoid cyst
      - Thyroid-associated ophthalmopathy
      - Herpes simplex
      - Chalazion

Genetics

No known genetic pattern

RISK FACTORS

Periorbital and orbital cellulitis precursors include:

- Upper respiratory tract infections:
  - Sinusitis or sinus disease (acute or chronic)
- Dental disease or surgery.
- Previous eye surgery.
- Trauma:
  - Scratches
  - Insect bites
- Compromised immunity.

GENERAL PREVENTION

- Avoiding periorbital skin trauma is important for prevention:
  - Protective goggles or other American National Standards Institute–approved eyewear may decrease risk.
- Vaccine coverage of common causative organisms:
  - Children who receive at least two Hib immunizations are unlikely to have Hib-related infection.
  - Pneumococcal conjugate vaccine

DIAGNOSIS

Clinical diagnosis is based on history, signs and symptoms, and neurologic exam. Early identification of orbital cellulitis is essential, as disease progression can lead to blindness, meningitis, or death.

HISTORY

- Periorbital cellulitis:
  - Pain
  - Conjunctivitis
  - Epiphora (excessive tearing)
  - Blurred vision
  - Fever
  - Recent or current upper respiratory infection
- Orbital cellulitis:
  - Above, plus:
    - Pain or decreased eye movement
    - Facial or dental surgery
    - Recent sinusitis
    - Other systemic infections

PHYSICAL EXAM

- Periorbital cellulitis:
  - Periorbital swelling, erythema, warmth, and tenderness
  - Normal vision
  - Full and painless extraocular muscle (EOM) range of motion
  - No proptosis
  - No afferent pupillary defect
- Orbital cellulitis:
  - Eyelid swelling (does not extend beyond orbital rim)
  - Proptosis (anterior bulging of eye from orbit)
  - Chemosis (swelling of conjunctiva)
  - Ophthalmoplegia (limited ocular motility)
  - Painful EOM
  - Decreased visual acuity

DIFFERENTIAL DIAGNOSIS

- Periorbital cellulitis:
  - Allergic reaction
  - Edema:
    - Hypoproteinemia or congestive heart failure
  - Orbital trauma
  - Dermoid cyst
  - Thyroid-associated ophthalmopathy
  - Herpes simplex
  - Chalazion
- Orbital cellulitis:
  - Cavernous sinus thrombosis
  - Orbital trauma
  - Thyroid-associated ophthalmopathy
  - Orbital myositis
  - Granulomatosis with polyangiitis
  - Idiopathic orbital inflammatory syndrome
  - Tumor:
    - Rhabdomyosarcoma, lymphoma, or leukemia

DIAGNOSTIC TESTS & INTERPRETATION

- Complete blood count (CBC):
  - Leukocytosis $>$15,000 can be associated with bacteremic periorbital cellulitis.
  - Left shift
- Blood culture if sepsis suspected
- Gram stain and culture of tissue aspirate or draining purulent material:
  - Surgical aspirates often have the best results.
- Lumbar puncture/cerebrospinal fluid evaluation if athlete appears markedly ill, has insufficient Hib immunization, or meningitis must be ruled out.
- Orbital, sinus, and facial computed tomography (CT) scan with contrast:
  - If clinical features cannot differentiate between periorbital and orbital cellulitis
  - If unable to perform complete physical exam secondary to patient discomfort
  - Clinical deterioration or failure to improve following 24 to 48 hr of parenteral antimicrobial therapy
- Magnetic resonance imaging (MRI):
  - May be needed to detect smaller abscesses
  - MR with venography or angiography to detect cavernous sinus thromboses

TREATMENT

Emergency department:

- Establish intravenous (IV) access, administer oxygen for serious complications, including sepsis, meningitis, and cavernous sinus thrombosis.
- Consider vancomycin in geographic areas with prevalent penicillin-resistant pneumococci or MRSA.
- Children with orbital cellulitis require:
  - Parenteral antibiotics.
  - CT scan.
  - Recommend Pediatric ophthalmologic and otolaryngology (ear, nose, and throat [ENT]) consultation (6).
  - Prompt surgery may be necessary.

MEDICATION

First Line

- Periorbital cellulitis:
  - There is no evidence that IV antibiotics are generally better than oral antibiotics (7).
  - Suspected MSSA or streptococcal spp (8):
    - Dicloxacillin:
      - Adults: 500 mg PO 4 times daily
      - Pediatrics: 25 to 50 mg/kg/day PO in 4 divided doses daily
    - Cephalexin:
      - Adults: 500 mg PO 4 times daily
      - Pediatrics: 25 to 50 mg/kg/day PO in divided doses daily

- Suspected MRSA:
  - Clindamycin:
    - Adults:
      - 600 mg IV q8h
      - 300 to 450 mg PO 4 times daily
    - Pediatrics:
      - 25 to 40 mg/kg/day IV in 3 divided doses
      - 30 to 40 mg/kg/day PO in 3 divided doses
  - Bactrim (trimethoprim and sulfamethoxazole):
    - 8 to 12 mg/kg/day (trimethoprim component) IV in 4 divided doses
    - 8 to 12 mg/kg/day (trimethoprim component) PO in in 2 divided doses

- Orbital cellulitis:
  - Hospitalize patients with suspected orbital cellulitis.
  - Empiric broad-spectrum antibiotic regimen that targets MRSA, streptococci, gram-negative organisms, and anaerobes
  - IV antibiotics:
    - Adults:
      - Vancomycin 15 to 20 mg/kg IV q8–12h, PLUS either:
        - Zosyn (piperacillin-tazobactam) 4.5 g IV q8h, OR
        - Ceftriaxone 2 g IV q24h AND metronidazole 1 g IV q12h
    - Pediatrics:
      - Vancomycin 15 mg/kg IV q8h, PLUS either:
        - Zosyn 300 mg (piperacillin component) IV in 3 divided doses daily, OR
        - Ceftriaxone 100 mg IV in 1 or 2 divided doses daily AND metronidazole 30 mg/kg IV in 4 divided doses daily
    - Penicillin allergy:
      - Adults:
        - Vancomycin (at above dose) PLUS
        - Ciprofloxacin 400 mg IV twice daily
        - Levofloxacin 500 to 750 mg IV once daily
      - Pediatrics:
        - Vancomycin (at above dose) PLUS
        - Ciprofloxacin 20 to 30 mg/kg IV in 2 divided doses daily (maximum of 1.5 g PO or 800 mg IV)
        - Levofloxacin 10 mg/kg every 12 hr (≥6 mo and <5 yr) or 10 mg/kg every 24 hr (≥5 yr)
        - NOTE: Fluoroquinolones have black box warning for tendinopathy/tendon rupture and are not considered first-line therapy in pediatrics due to potential for arthropathy. Consider infectious disease consultation before use in athletes or pediatric population.
  - Several studies have shown that oral and IV corticosteroids in conjunction with IV antibiotics have statistically significant earlier improvement in symptoms with shorter hospital stays (6,8).
- Penicillin allergy:
  - Type 1 anaphylaxis, urticarial or Stevens-Johnson syndrome (2):
    - Avoid all β-lactams.
  - Nonurticarial rash to penicillin:
    - Cephalosporin in controlled environment
- Optimal duration of therapy not determined (9):
  - One study revealed 14 (±3) days of IV antibiotics for periorbital cellulitis and 17 (±5) days for orbital cellulitis (10)
  - Typical course of 10 to 21 days, transition to oral therapy as symptoms resolve
- Complicated or no response to antibacterial regimen (11,12,13):
  - Prompt evaluation by ophthalmology or ENT for surgery
- Symptomatic treatments:
  - Sinus decongestion
  - Nasal sprays
  - Oral decongestants
  - Oral antihistamines

ISSUES FOR REFERRAL

Multidisciplinary management (2):

- Orbital cellulitis:
  - Adults: infectious disease, ENT, and ophthalmologist
  - Pediatrics: infectious disease, ENT, ophthalmologist, and pediatrician

SURGERY/OTHER PROCEDURES

Orbital cellulitis:

- Surgical intervention with the following (11):
  - Visual impairment
  - Progressive ophthalmoplegia
  - Larger abscess
  - Lack of clinical improvement following 24 hr of antibiotics

ADMISSION, INPATIENT, AND NURSING CONSIDERATIONS

- Most patients with orbital cellulitis should be admitted for IV antibiotics:
  - With significant clinical improvement, can transition to oral antibiotics
  - No improvement, repeat CT scan and surgical intervention
- Initial stabilization:
  - Adequate fluid resuscitation:
    - 500 cc or 20 cc/kg bolus for dehydration, sepsis, or hypotension
- Admission criteria:
  - Any signs of orbital cellulitis (4):
    - Outpatient treatment should only be attempted if the eye is at least 50% open and very close outpatient follow-up can be guaranteed (11).
  - Toxicity or systemic illness
  - Incomplete physical exam of eye
  - Clinical deterioration on oral antibiotics
  - Uncertainty that patient can get adequate care at home
- Discharge criteria:
  - No more than modest swelling, tolerating oral antibiotics well with progressive improvement, nontoxic appearance, and reliable caregivers
  - Monitor for progressive swelling, irritability, increased fever, or vision changes.

ONGOING CARE

FOLLOW-UP RECOMMENDATIONS

Return-to-play guidance:

- Athlete and medical personnel must be able to demonstrate the following:
  - Asymptomatic with normal physical exam
  - Must pass sport-specific functional assessment.
- Closely observe the athlete's performance in practice prior to clearing for competition.
- With any complications noted below, athlete should be cleared by appropriate specialist (14).

Patient Monitoring

Repeat imaging in patients with orbital cellulitis if there is any question about resolution following treatment.

COMPLICATIONS

- Blindness
- Cavernous sinus thrombosis
- Meningitis
- Subdural empyema
- Brain abscess

REFERENCES

1. Rashed F, Cannon A, Heaton PA, et al. Diagnosis, management and treatment of orbital and periorbital cellulitis in children. *Emerg Nurse*. 2016;24(1):30–35, quiz 37.
2. Atfeh MS, Khalil HS. Orbital infections: five-year case series, literature review and guideline development. *J Laryngol Otol*. 2015;129(7):670–676.
3. Amin N, Syed I, Osborne S. Assessment and management of orbital cellulitis. *Br J Hosp Med (Lond)*. 2016;77(4):216–220.
4. Howe L, Jones NS. Guidelines for the management of periorbital cellulitis/abscess. *Clin Otolaryngol Allied Sci*. 2004;29(6):725–728
5. Hauser A, Fogarasi S. Periorbital and orbital cellulitis. *Pediatr Rev*. 2010;31(6):242–249.
6. Pushker N, Tejwani LK, Bajaj MS, et al. Role of oral corticosteroids in orbital cellulitis. *Am J Ophthalmol*. 2013;156(1):178–183.e1.
7. Goldman RD, Dolansky G, Rogovik AL. Predictors for admission of children with periorbital cellulitis presenting to the pediatric emergency department. *Pediatr Emerg Care*. 2008;24(5):279–283.
8. Chen L, Silverman N, Wu A, et al. Intravenous steroids with antibiotics on admission for children with orbital cellulitis. *Ophthalmic Plast Reconstr Surg*. 2018;34(3):205–208.
9. Stevens DL, Bisno AL, Chambers HF, et al. Practice guidelines for the diagnosis and management of skin and soft tissue infections: 2014 update by the Infectious Diseases Society of America. *Clin Infect Dis*. 2014;59(2):e10–e52.
10. Gonçalves R, Menezes C, Machado R, et al. Periorbital cellulitis in children: analysis of outcome of intravenous antibiotic therapy. *Orbit*. 2016;35(4):175–180.
11. Nageswaran S, Woods CR, Benjamin DK Jr, et al. Orbital cellulitis in children. *Pediatr Infect Dis J*. 2006;25(8):695–699.
12. Botting AM, McIntosh D, Mahadevan M. Paediatric pre- and post-septal peri-orbital infections are different diseases: a retrospective review of 262 cases. *Int J Pediatr Otorhinolaryngol*. 2008;72(3):377–383.
13. Sciarretta V, Dematte M, Ferneti P, et al. Management of orbital cellulitis and subperiosteal orbital abscess in pediatric patients: a ten-year review. *Int J Pediatr Otorhinolaryngol*. 2017;96:72–76.
14. Cass S. Ocular injuries in sports. *Curr Sports Med Rep*. 2012;11(1):11–15.

CLINICAL PEARLS

- Orbital cellulitis is any infection/inflammatory process posterior to orbital septum and can be life-threatening, whereas periorbital cellulitis is anterior to orbital septum.
- Most common causative organisms currently are *Staphylococcus* and *Streptococcus* spp.
- If clinically unable to differentiate obtain orbital, sinus and facial CT with contrast or MRI
- Treatment of orbital cellulitis includes hospital admission and empiric IV antibiotics; optimal duration of therapy undetermined but should be driven clinically
- Close outpatient follow-up for orbital cellulitis with clearance by appropriate specialists prior to return to play

PERONEAL TENDON DISLOCATION/SUBLUXATION

Holly J. Benjamin, MD, FAAP, FACSM • Claire Gross, MD

BASICS

DESCRIPTION

- The lateral compartment of the ankle contains the peroneus longus (PL) and peroneus brevis (PB) tendons.
- The tendons lie posterior to the lateral malleolus in the retromalleolar groove within a single tendon sheath and are fixed in place by the superior peroneal retinaculum (SPR).
- The actions of PB and PL are ankle eversion and ankle plantarflexion and contribute to dynamic ankle stability.
- There are two categories of peroneal tendon subluxation/dislocation:
  - Anterior dislocation:
    - Disruption of the SPR allows the peroneal tendons to sublux or dislocate anteriorly.
    - Avulsion of the SPR from the lateral malleolus can occur during an acute, traumatic injury or from repetitive overuse.
  - Intrasheath subluxation:
    - The PB and PL tendons reverse positions within the common sheath, usually occurs with ankle circumduction, causing a snapping sensation.

EPIDEMIOLOGY

- Generally considered a rare injury in sports
- May be a missed injury in up to 40% of cases (1), can be misdiagnosed as a lateral ankle sprain
- Associated with calcaneal fractures (2)

ETIOLOGY AND PATHOPHYSIOLOGY

- Acute avulsion of the SPR is usually due to contraction during dorsiflexion of an everted foot or inversion of a dorsiflexed ankle.
- Chronic, atraumatic subluxation can also occur, related to anatomic variants and/or generalized ligamentous laxity.
- Originally described in ballet dancers
- Classically seen in sports such as skiing, football, ice skating, soccer, basketball rugby, and gymnastics

RISK FACTORS

- Anatomic variations may increase susceptibility:
  - A low-lying PB muscle belly intruding under the SPR
  - Presence of a peroneal quartus muscle, an accessory muscle, which, if present, lies within the retromalleolar groove with the peroneal tendons
  - Shallow, flat, or concave retromalleolar groove (up to 18% prevalence)
  - Excessive calcaneal varus
  - Pes cavus
  - Developmental absence of the SPR
- Generalized ligamentous laxity
- Contact sports
- Excessive push off and jump landing

COMMONLY ASSOCIATED CONDITIONS

- Conditions predisposing to hindfoot varus such as Charcot-Marie-Tooth
- Chronic ankle instability
- Calcaneal fractures (3–5% of calcaneal fractures) (2)

DIAGNOSIS

HISTORY

- Snapping or popping at time of injury over lateral ankle (1)
- High index of suspicion after trauma with lateral ankle pain
- Most common mechanism is contraction during dorsiflexion of an everted foot or inversion of a dorsiflexed ankle.
- History and initial physical exam may be indistinguishable from a lateral ankle sprain.
- Lateral ankle pain that localizes posterior or inferior to the lateral malleolus
- Lateral snapping or popping with walking or ankle circumduction, with or without history of ankle trauma
- May have previously treated for a lateral ankle sprain (3)[C]

PHYSICAL EXAM

- Acute injury may present with lateral ankle swelling and pain, resembling lateral ankle sprain or occurring in conjunction with an ankle sprain.
- Swelling and ecchymosis posterior to the lateral malleolus and may track along path of the tendons
- Tenderness to palpation over the tendons
- Resisted ankle dorsiflexion and eversion or ankle circumduction while compressing the tendons may reproduce subluxation or snap/click.
- Chronic ankle instability
- Excessive calcaneal varus in standing
- Generalized ligamentous laxity (1,3)[C]

DIFFERENTIAL DIAGNOSIS

- Peroneal strain, tendonitis, or tear
- Lateral ankle sprain
- Lateral ankle instability
- Ankle fracture
- Achilles tendinopathy
- Tarsal coalition
- Sinus tarsi syndrome
- Talar osteochondral lesion
- Sural neuritis

DIAGNOSTIC TESTS & INTERPRETATION

Initial Tests (lab, imaging)

- Radiographs:
  - Assess for associated fracture.
  - "Fleck sign" shows the avulsion of cortical bone from the lateral aspect of the lateral malleolus, indicative of SPR avulsion (1,3)[C].

- Computed tomography (CT):
  - May be obtained to evaluate the size and shape of the retromalleolar groove and for presurgical planning (1,3)[C]
- Ultrasound (US):
  - Dynamic real-time imaging can reveal the integrity of the SPR and can demonstrate subluxation out of the groove or intrasheath reversal of the peroneal tendons (positive predictive value [PPV] 100%).
  - Can see presence of the SPR if intact (4)[C]
- Magnetic resonance imaging (MRI):
  - Evaluates the integrity of the SPR
  - Elucidates the size and shape of the retromalleolar groove
  - Tendons will be out of place if frankly dislocated and not reduced but may appear to be in proper position if subluxation is not occurring at the time the image is obtained (1,3)[C].

Diagnostic Procedures/Other

- Tendoscopy of the peroneal tendons
- Performed for diagnostic and therapeutic purposes
- Findings at time of tendoscopy include:
  - SPR tear.
  - Low-lying PB muscle belly.
  - Peroneus quartus tendon.
  - Tendinosis.
  - Split tendon tears (5)[A].

TREATMENT

- Acute treatment:
  - Rest, ice, compression, and elevation (RICE)
  - Nonsteroidal anti-inflammatory drugs (NSAIDs)
  - Limit weight-bearing if painful; off-load as needed for pain-free ambulation.
  - Ankle bracing to limit the excursion of the foot and may decrease the episodes of painful subluxation
  - Activity modification to reduce the occurrence of subluxation in certain patients if the subluxation is activity specific
  - If symptoms are minimal, can try a J-shaped compression pad and lateral heel wedge
- Conservative treatment (1)[C]:
  - Immobilization 5 to 6 wk with below-knee casting or bracing with ankle in slight plantarflexion
  - Although this is the initial intervention, there is up to 50% failure of nonsurgical treatment with persistent pain, instability, and recurrent dislocation.
  - Physical therapy for biomechanical evaluation and ankle stabilization
  - Early referral for surgical evaluation is appropriate for athletes.
  - Recurring symptoms after a trial of conservative treatment are indications for surgical intervention.

SURGERY/OTHER PROCEDURES

- Surgical intervention is commonly required due to high incidence of recurrence with nonoperative treatment (1)[C].
- Many techniques exist; there are no studies comparing techniques (1,3)[C],(5)[A]:
  - Primary repair or reconstruction of the SPR
  - Deepening of the retromalleolar groove may be performed if required.
  - Resection of low-lying PB muscle belly or peroneus quartus (accessory muscle) may be performed if present.
  - Procedure may be open or tendoscopic.

ONGOING CARE

PROGNOSIS

- Recurrence rate 50–75% after conservative treatment (1)
- Recurrence rate 5–20% after surgical intervention (5)
- After surgery, resumption of daily activities after 3 to 4 mo, full athletic activity in 6 to 18 mo (3,5)

REFERENCES

1. Davda K, Malhotra K, O'Donnell P, et al. Peroneal tendon disorders. *EFORT Open Rev.* 2017;2(6):281–292.
2. Golshani A, Zhu L, Cai C, et al. Incidence and association of CT findings of ankle tendon injuries in patients presenting with ankle and hindfoot fractures. *AJR Am J Roentgenol.* 2017;208(2):373–379.
3. Saragas NP, Ferrao PN, Mayet Z, et al. Peroneal tendon dislocation/subluxation—case series and review of the literature. *Foot Ankle Surg.* 2016;22(2):125–130.
4. Pesquer L, Guillo S, Poussange N, et al. Dynamic ultrasound of peroneal tendon instability. *Br J Radiol.* 2016;89(1063):20150958.
5. Bernasconi A, Sadile F, Smeraglia F, et al. Tendoscopy of Achilles, peroneal and tibialis posterior tendons: an evidence-based update. *Foot Ankle Surg.* 2017:S1268-7731(17)30128-5. doi:10.1016/j.fas.2017.06.004.

CLINICAL PEARLS

- Peroneal subluxation can either be from SPR disruption leading to tendon dislocation over the lateral malleolus (anterior dislocation) or the two tendons subluxing over each other within the sheath (intrasheath dislocation).
- Lateral ankle pain due to acute peroneal dislocation is frequently misdiagnosed as a lateral ankle sprain.
- Conservative treatment is generally attempted initially, but recurrence rate is high, and surgical intervention is commonly required.

PES ANSERINE BURSITIS

Alecia Gende, DO • Britt Marcussen, MD, FAAFP, CAQSM

BASICS

DESCRIPTION

- Acute or chronic inflammatory condition that affects the medial aspect of the knee, specifically area of pes anserine bursa and pes anserine tendon
- The pes anserine bursa, located on anteromedial proximal tibia, buffers insertion of pes anserine tendon, a conjoining tendon of sartorius, gracilis, and semitendinosus muscles.
- Sartorius, gracilis, and semitendinosus are responsible for knee flexion and internal rotation of tibia and protect the knee against a valgus and rotary stress.
- Considered a bursitis but may be better understood as a tendinopathy because pes anserine tendon can be pain generator
- The pes anserine bursa, which is deep to the tendon, typically does not communicate with the knee joint.

EPIDEMIOLOGY

- Exact incidence and prevalence is unknown.
- Pes anserine bursitis has reported prevalence of 2.5% in patients with medial knee pain (1).
- In patients with knee pain or swelling and history of osteoarthritis (OA), the prevalence of pes anserine bursitis is increased (2).

ETIOLOGY AND PATHOPHYSIOLOGY

Exact etiology is unclear, but tendinopathy, friction on the bursa from repetitive stressors, valgus forces, or direct trauma to bursa maybe be causative.

RISK FACTORS

- Female
- Obesity
- OA of the knee
- Type 2 diabetes mellitus
- Long-distance runners

COMMONLY ASSOCIATED CONDITIONS

- Medial collateral ligament (MCL) pathology
- OA
- Obesity
- Pes planus
- Valgus knee deformity

DIAGNOSIS

HISTORY

- Gradual onset of symptoms
- Pain, tenderness, ± acute swelling within localized area of the tendon and bursa along the medial tibia
- Exacerbated by rising from a seated position and ascending or descending stairs
- May also present with vague medial knee pain

PHYSICAL EXAM

- Tenderness at the insertion of the pes anserine tendon at the proximal medial tibia, ~2 to 5 cm below the anteromedial joint line of the knee
- Rarely, crepitus of the bursa is palpated; more commonly the bursa is edematous.
- Pain occasionally is reproduced with resisted external rotation of the tibia and flexion of the knee or with McMurray test confusing picture of a meniscus pathology.
- Pain may also be reproduced when a valgus stress is applied. This may make it difficult to distinguish this problem from an MCL injury; however, MCL injuries are typically superior and posterior to this type of bursitis.
- Hamstring-popliteal angle can be measured to assess hamstring flexibility. Have the patient flex the hip to 90 degrees and then passively extend the leg. The angle is formed by a perpendicular line to the femoral shaft and the tibial shaft.
- Chronic cases are marked by local pain, swelling, and fullness at the site of the bursa.

DIFFERENTIAL DIAGNOSIS

- Stress fracture
- MCL injury
- OA
- Medial meniscus tear or cyst
- Tendinosis of sartorius, gracilis, or semitendinosus
- Medial plica and discoid medial meniscus
- Medial hamstring strain (semitendinosus)
- Patellofemoral pain syndrome
- Regional tumors, including villonodular synovitis, osteochondromatosis, and synovial sarcoma
- Prepatellar bursitis

DIAGNOSTIC TESTS & INTERPRETATION

Initial Tests (lab, imaging)

- Typically a clinical diagnosis; plain films are done to evaluate for bony pathology.
- Plain films may be normal or show signs of OA.
- Musculoskeletal (MSK) ultrasound (US) when skilled MSK ultrasonography available; demonstrates enlarged bursa and possible loculated fluid collection within bursa
- Magnetic resonance imaging (MRI) is performed to evaluate for other knee pathology (meniscus and MCL injuries) and may confirm diagnosis in refractory cases.

Diagnostic Procedures/Other

- Aspiration of the bursa is typically not required.
- In difficult cases, a local anesthetic block may be used to confirm the diagnosis. Relief of pain with the injection is diagnostic.

TREATMENT

The mainstay of treatment for patients with pes anserine bursitis is to reduce pain and inflammation through the following (3)[C]:

- Activity modification
- Hamstring stretching
- Closed kinetic chain quadriceps strengthening
- Anti-inflammatory medications
- Ice massage
- Use of a pillow between knees at night
- Address gait abnormalities.
- Older patients and those with chronic pain should be encouraged to maintain activity levels to prevent disuse atrophy.
- Weight loss

MEDICATION

First Line

Nonsteroidal anti-inflammatory drugs (NSAIDs) are recommended, including both nonselective NSAIDs as first line and the selective cyclooxygenase-2 (COX-2) inhibitors if there are tolerance issues (3)[C]. Topical NSAIDs should be tried before oral NSAIDs if possible.

Second Line

Corticosteroid injections are traditionally used as first- or second-line medications. Injection may be done by palpation or preferably US guided.

ALERT

Take caution to exclude medial tibial plateau stress fractures as etiology of pain prior to corticosteroid injections. Masking of stress fracture pain with injection may lead to adverse outcome.

ADDITIONAL THERAPIES

Modalities such as US, Kinesio Taping, and ice massage can be helpful in relieving pain in patients with pes anserine bursitis.

SURGERY/OTHER PROCEDURES

- Extracorporeal shock wave therapy is another alternative to injection.
- Surgery is a rare option in chronic cases and includes tendon débridement, bursectomy, and/or excision of bony exostoses.

ONGOING CARE

- In general, patients experience success with conservative treatments:
  - Hamstring strengthening
  - Quadriceps strengthening
  - Activity modification
  - Oral NSAIDs
  - Ice massage
- Most patients will experience alleviation of pain within 6 to 8 wk but may persist several months.

FOLLOW-UP RECOMMENDATIONS

Patients may return to their activities based on their level of pain and function.

PATIENT EDUCATION

- The following recommendations can be made to the patient:
  - Minimize the use of stairs and climbing.
  - Eliminate squatting.
  - Prevent direct pressure on the bursa by using a pillow between the legs at night.
  - Avoid crossing the legs.
- Patients and their coaches should be counseled on the gradual increase in activity based on symptoms.

PROGNOSIS

Pes anserine bursitis is usually a self-limiting condition, with few complications if the individual decides to participate through the pain. In general, pain resolves after 6 to 8 wk of conservative treatment (3)[C].

REFERENCES

1. Rennie WJ, Saifuddin A. Pes anserine bursitis: incidence in symptomatic knees and clinical presentation. *Skeletal Radiol*. 2005;34(7):395–398.
2. Uysal F, Akbal A, Gökmen F, et al. Prevalence of pes anserine bursitis in symptomatic osteoarthritis patients: an ultrasonographic prospective study. *Clin Rheumatol*. 2015;34(3):529–533.
3. Helfenstein M Jr, Kuromoto J. Anserine syndrome. *Rev Bras Reumatol*. 2010;50(3):313–327.

ADDITIONAL READING

- Khosrawi S, Taheri P, Ketabi M. Investigating the effect of extracorporeal shock wave therapy on reducing chronic pain in patients with pes anserine bursitis: a randomized, clinical-controlled trial. *Adv Biomed Res*. 2017;6:70.
- Saggini R, Di Stefano A, Dodaj I, et al. Pes anserine bursitis in symptomatic osteoarthritis patients: a mesotherapy treatment study. *J Altern Complement Med*. 2015;21(8):480–484.
- Sapp GH, Herman DC. Pay attention to the pes anserine in knee osteoarthritis. *Curr Sports Med Rep*. 2018;17(2):41.
- Sarifakioglu B, Afsar SI, Yalbuzdag SA, et al. Comparison of the efficacy of physical therapy and corticosteroid injection in the treatment of pes anserine tendino-bursitis. *J Phys Ther Sci*. 2016;28(7):1993–1997.

CLINICAL PEARLS

- Pes anserine bursitis and/or tendinopathy may be a cause of medial-sided knee pain.
- Diagnosis can be made with local tenderness over the bursa, located 2 to 5 cm distal to the joint line; a negative valgus stress test; and negative radiographs.
- Treat any underlying gait abnormalities; use activity modification, ice, NSAIDs, and possibly steroid injection to decrease pain and inflammation.

PHALANGEAL INJURIES

Jessalynn Adam, MD • Jeffrey C. Leggit, MD, CAQSM

BASICS

- Frequently dismissed as minor injuries and therefore may present as subacute or chronic injuries
- All finger phalangeal injuries require radiographic evaluation.
- Attempt to reduce dislocations immediately if neurovascular compromise is suspected.

DESCRIPTION

- Typically due to direct trauma (i.e., crushing injury to the distal phalanx with high likelihood of concomitant soft tissue injury such as nail bed trauma)
- Dislocations are inherently associated with ligament and tendon injuries.

EPIDEMIOLOGY

Prevalence

- Hand fractures represent 19–28% of all fractures.
- Account for 10–15% of all sports-related injuries
- Phalangeal fractures are the most common sports-related fractures in adolescents and adults.
- 50% of all hand fractures are distal phalanx fractures.
- The most frequent dislocation in the hand is a dorsal dislocation of the proximal interphalangeal (PIP) joint.

ETIOLOGY AND PATHOPHYSIOLOGY

Usually low-energy mechanism: fall, twisting or crush injury, or direct trauma

RISK FACTORS

Middle finger and thumb are the most commonly affected digits because they tend to be more exposed than the other digits.

COMMONLY ASSOCIATED CONDITIONS

- Soft tissue injury
- Nail bed trauma
- Tendon injuries:
  - Mallet finger, also known as "baseball finger": avulsion injury of the terminal portion of the common extensor tendon
  - Jersey finger: avulsion injury of the flexor digitorum profundus from the insertion on the distal phalanx. 75% of jersey finger injuries affect the ring finger.
- Central slip injuries
- Collateral ligament injuries
- Flexor pulley ruptures
- Dislocations—high risk for concomitant ligamentous injuries/disruptions

DIAGNOSIS

HISTORY

- Hand dominance
- Occupation and/or athletic position
- Environment surrounding injury (risk of infection)
- Mechanism of injury and hand position at time of injury:
  - Forceful passive flexion of distal phalanx suggests a mallet injury.
  - Forceful hyperextension of an actively flexed digit, such as while grabbing a player's jersey, suggests a jersey finger injury.
- Palpable or audible pop at the time of injury
- Associated symptoms of numbness or tingling suggest associated nerve injury.
- Swelling and ecchymosis suggest serious injury such as fracture, dislocation, or tendon rupture.

PHYSICAL EXAM

- Pain, swelling, focal tenderness, and ecchymosis are common findings.
- Subungual hematoma frequently encountered with distal phalanx fracture; presence of a subungual hematoma should prompt radiographic imaging.
- Gross deformity, such as a mallet deformity or evidence of open fracture
- Malrotation (flex distal interphalangeal (DIP) and PIP while keeping metacarpophalangeal (MCP) extended; all fingertips should point toward scaphoid tubercle; if they do not, malrotation is present)
- Scissoring (overlapping digits during midrange of active flexion/extension. Digits may realign in full flexion. Malformation is typically associated.)
- Interphalangeal joints allow flexion and extension with normal arc of motion from 0 to 120 degrees of extension. Thorough assessment of range of motion can help identify ruptured tendons.
- Volar plate provides block to hyperextension, and collateral ligaments provide lateral stability.
- Assess collateral ligament stability with stress testing in extension and 20 to 30 degrees of flexion:
  - Laxity >10 degrees in extension or >15 degrees in flexion is pathologic.
- Assess integrity of flexor and extensor tendons:
  - Inability to actively flex the distal phalanx at the DIP with the PIP joint in extension suggests a jersey finger injury.
  - Inability to actively extend the distal phalanx at the DIP, with passive extension at the DIP intact, suggests a mallet injury.
- Assess neurovascular status.

DIAGNOSTIC TESTS & INTERPRETATION

Initial Tests (lab, imaging)

- True posteroanterior (PA), lateral, and oblique radiographs before and after reduction
- Lateral radiographs are used to assess joint alignment. "Dorsal V sign" indicates subtle but significant subluxation of the joint (1).
- Oblique radiographs aid with diagnosis of phalangeal head fractures (2).
- Oblique or spiral fractures may be associated with shortening (3)[C].

Diagnostic Procedures/Other

Inspection of nail bed for suspected laceration or hematoma

TREATMENT

- Hand:
  - Nondisplaced extra-articular fractures:
    - Buddy tape nondisplaced fractures: Never leave 5th finger isolated and unprotected (remember to place absorptive padding between digits).
    - Drain subungual hematoma by trephination of the nail if >50% nail bed, and repair nail bed if lacerated.
    - Splint PIP joints in 45 to 60 degrees of flexion to avoid inadvertent trauma to fingers (2)[C].
    - Splint MCP joint in 70 to 90 degrees of flexion (2)[C].
    - Allow range of motion to prevent stiffness.
    - Oral analgesics
    - Pain decreases over 2 to 3 wk.

- Displaced intra-articular fractures of interphalangeal joint:
  - Closed reduction with longitudinal traction within 7 to 10 days following injury (4)[C]
  - Acceptable reduction is <2 mm of displacement or shortening, <15 degrees of angulation, and no rotational deformity (2)[C].
  - Refer to hand surgeon if >30% of volar intra-articular surface is involved (2)[C].
  - If unstable after closed reduction, then open reduction internal fixation is required (2)[C].
- Interphalangeal joint dislocations:
  - Digital or wing block anesthesia
  - Reduction of dorsal dislocations: longitudinal traction with gentle downward pressure on distal phalanx while stabilizing the proximal phalanx
  - Reduction of volar dislocations: longitudinal traction with gentle upward pressure on the distal phalanx while stabilizing the proximal phalanx
  - Volar and rotatory dislocations may not be reducible as the middle phalanx can "buttonhole" through the extensor mechanism (4).
  - Buddy tape to next digit for 3 to 4 wk (caution with 5th finger) (5)[C]
  - Immediate protected return to play is recommended for stable PIP joint dislocations.
  - Reduce and splint PIP fracture dislocation with dorsal subluxation in 30-degree flexion to block extension (6)[C].
  - Unstable reductions require surgical management.
- Extensor tendon injury: mallet finger:
  - Conservative management is preferred in almost all cases (7)[C].
  - Splint in the "intrinsic plus position" with the DIP joint in full extension for 6 to 8 wk at all times for both bony and soft tissue mallet injuries. Daily splint changes to assess skin integrity. DIP should not be allowed to flex at any time. Nighttime splinting and splinting during sports participation should continue for an additional 6 to 8 wk (7)[C].
  - Surgical management with reduction and fixation of the DIP is reserved for irreducible displaced injuries or injuries with significant joint incongruity, typically those involving >1/3 of the articular surface (2,7)[C].
- Flexor digitorum profundus injury: jersey finger:
  - Always require surgical repair
  - Urgency of repair depends on degree of tendon retraction. Type I injuries, in which the tendon retracts to the level of the distal palmar crease, should be surgically repaired within 1 wk. Tendon repair in type II or III injuries with lesser degree of tendon retraction can occur up to several weeks from the time of injury (7)[C].
  - Return to play typically between 2 and 3 months

- Foot:
  - Nondisplaced fracture:
    - Hard-sole shoe for toe fractures and weight-bearing as tolerated with crutches
  - Displaced fractures:
    - Short leg walking cast with toe platform

Pediatric Considerations

ALERT

Seymour fractures—distal phalanx fracture through the physis with concomitant nail bed trauma that occurs in the skeletally immature. It is an open fracture despite an often benign appearance. It is typically irreducible and requires open fracture reduction and nail bed repair. Skeletally immature athletes should not return to play until healing is certain due to risk to the growth plate.

SURGERY/OTHER PROCEDURES

- Unstable fractures
- Irreducible dislocations
- Condylar fractures of the proximal and middle phalanges
- Consider surgical referral for intra-articular fractures >30% surface area or fractures with >2-mm displacement.
- Flexor tendon injuries
- Open fractures other than nail bed or tufts

ONGOING CARE

- Buddy tape/splint simple fractures continuously for a minimum of 2 wk; protected return to play with splinting during sporting activities for another 4 wk
- For persistent mallet injuries with a deformity of >20 degrees, an additional 6 wk of splinting may be needed.
- Chronic mallet injuries can be successfully managed with up to 3 mo of splinting (7)[C].
- Soft shoe or splint for comfort

FOLLOW-UP RECOMMENDATIONS

Patient Monitoring

- Fractures that required reduction should be seen within 1 wk, and repeat radiographs should be obtained to check for fracture stability.
- Subungual hematoma: 24 hr

PROGNOSIS

Most heal well within 4 weeks but may develop stiffness.

COMPLICATIONS

- Chronic pain
- Chronic deformity: Even with ideal management of a mallet injury, a 5- to 10-degree extensor lag may persist. Untreated mallet injuries can lead to swan-neck deformity (7).
- Stiffness and loss of range of motion. The PIP joint is especially prone (4).

REFERENCES

1. Williams CS IV. Proximal interphalangeal joint fracture dislocations: stable and unstable. *Hand Clin*. 2012;28(3):409–416.
2. Hile D, Hile L. The emergent evaluation and treatment of hand injuries. *Emerg Med Clin North Am*. 2015;33(2):397–408.
3. Lee SG, Jupiter JB. Phalangeal and metacarpal fractures of the hand. *Hand Clin*. 2000;16(3):323–332.
4. Rosenbaum YA, Aman HM. Acute hand injuries in athletes. *Phys Sportsmed*. 2017;45(2):151–158.
5. Chen F, Kalainov DM. Phalanx fractures and dislocations in athletes. *Curr Rev Musculoskelet Med*. 2017;10(1):10–16.
6. Birman MV, Rosenwasser MP. Proximal interphalangeal joint fracture dislocations in professional baseball players. *Hand Clin*. 2012;28(3):417–420.
7. Yeh PC, Shin SS. Tendon ruptures: mallet, flexor digitorum profundus. *Hand Clin*. 2012;28(3):425–430.

ADDITIONAL READING

- Cheah AE, Yao J. Hand fractures: indications, the tried and true and new innovations. *J Hand Surg Am*. 2016;41(6):712–722.
- Rettig AC. Athletic injuries of the wrist and hand. Part I: traumatic injuries of the wrist. *Am J Sports Med*. 2003;31(6):1038–1048.
- Soubeyrand M, Biau D, Jomaah N, et al. Penetrating volar injuries of the hand: diagnostic accuracy of US in depicting soft-tissue lesions. *Radiology*. 2008;249(1):228–235.

CLINICAL PEARLS

- Obtain radiographs in all finger injuries before and after reduction.
- Mallet injuries are the most common closed tendon injury in the athlete, particularly baseball and softball athletes (7).
- Jersey finger injuries must be diagnosed early because all jersey finger injuries require surgical repair.
- Seymour fractures may appear benign but are open fractures and need to be recognized as such.
- Have a high suspicion for concomitant soft tissue injury; all dislocations have associated ligament and tendon injuries.
- Early mobilization is critical to reduce stiffness and loss or range of motion.

PHOTODERMATITIS

Jayson Loeffert, DO • Daniel Schlegel, MD, MHA • Matthew L. Silvis, MD

BASICS

- Photodermatitis is an abnormal skin reaction to light or ultraviolet (UV) rays.
- The reaction may be acute or chronic, allergy mediated, or irritative and often is associated with substances or conditions that create an increase in photosensitivity.

DESCRIPTION

- Light-induced eruptions seen in a pattern of photodistribution on the skin
- Exogenous:
  - Phototoxic reactions (nonallergic): result of acute toxic effect on skin by UV light alone (sunburn) or together with a photosensitizing substance; occurs in 100% of individuals if exposed to enough of the agent and light
  - Photoallergic eruptions (allergic, delayed hypersensitivity): a form of allergic dermatitis resulting from combined effects of a photosensitizing substance (drugs or chemical) plus UV light
- Endogenous:
  - Porphyria cutanea tarda: defect in uroporphyrinogen decarboxylase, inherited, and acquired types
  - Erythropoietic protoporphyria: autosomal dominant deficiency in ferrochelatase, diagnosed in childhood
- Idiopathic and immunologic:
  - Polymorphous light eruption: chronic, intermittent light-induced eruption with erythematous papules, urticaria, or vesicles owing to a certain threshold of UV light; presents in 20s and 30s; spring and summer most common
  - Chronic actinic dermatitis: lichenified papules or plaques on sun-exposed areas; pruritic; older adults
  - Solar urticaria: immunoglobulin E (IgE) formation with mast cell degranulation; urticaria minutes after sun exposure; disappears within hours
- Photoaggravated conditions:
  - Lupus erythematosus
  - Dermatomyositis
  - Atopic dermatitis
  - Seborrheic dermatitis
- UV radiation:
  - Both UVA and UVB are responsible for photodermatitis (light-induced eruptions); therefore, both UVA and UVB should be blocked during outdoor sport activities.
  - UVA range 320 to 400 nm: penetrates skin deepest; can penetrate window glass; 360-nm wavelength is peak for many photosensitizing drugs.
  - UVB range 290 to 320 nm: penetrates skin superficially; responsible for most acute skin erythema

EPIDEMIOLOGY

- Can affect patients from all backgrounds and races who are exposed to UV light
- Most frequently identified photoallergens by photopatch testing: medications, sunscreen agents, fragrances, and antiseptics

Incidence

Up to 29.7% of persons who use sensitizing agents will get a reaction.

Prevalence

Estimated 25% of Caucasians in the United States are Fitzpatrick skin type I or II and have an increased risk of sunburn with limited exposure.

ETIOLOGY AND PATHOPHYSIOLOGY

- Exogenous photosensitizers (over 300 drugs known):
  - Antiarrhythmics
  - Nonsteroidal anti-inflammatory drugs (NSAIDs)
  - Phenothiazines
  - Diuretics
  - Quinolones
  - Tetracyclines
  - Thiazides
  - Sulfonamides
  - Sulfonylureas
  - Oral contraceptives
  - Topicals: psoralens, coal tars, photoactive dyes (e.g., eosin, acridine orange)
- Phytophotosensitizing agents:
  - Citrus fruits (Rutaceae): lemon, lime, grapefruit; furocoumarins are more concentrated in the peel.
  - Fig (Moraceae)
  - Cayenne pepper, paprika, chili, tabasco (Solanaceae)
  - Nettle (Urticaceae)
- Photoallergens:
  - Antiseptics
  - Fragrances
  - Medications
  - Sunscreen filters

Genetics

- Skin types I and II will exceed sunburn threshold tolerance in 10 to 20 min of noontime summer sunlight.
- Other genetic conditions increase risk (e.g., xeroderma pigmentosa, porphyrias).

RISK FACTORS

Fitzpatrick skin types:

- Type I: never tan, always burn
- Type II: occasionally tan, usually burn
- Type III: usually tan, occasionally burn
- Type IV: easily tan, rarely burn
- Type V: brown skin
- Type VI: black skin

GENERAL PREVENTION

- Avoid sun from 10 AM to 2 PM when 2/3 of total daily UV radiation reaches the earth.
- Avoid being outdoors during high UV index days.
- Avoid indoor tanning beds.
- Use protective clothing: long sleeves, wide-brim hats, sunglasses. Consider UV protective clothing.
- Use tinted glass windows.
- Identify and avoid sun-sensitizing drugs and agents (see under "Etiology").
- Sunscreens:
  - No. 15 sun protection factor (SPF) or greater recommended
  - Apply 30 min before exposure and every 2 hr, especially after sweating and swimming.
  - 1 oz to cover whole body
  - Physical blocking agents: zinc oxide, titanium dioxide, iron oxide, kaolin
  - Sunscreen with ingredients that filter out both UVA and UVB rays recommended
- UVB filters:
  - Para-aminobenzoic acid (PABA) derivatives
  - Cinnamates
  - Salicylates
  - Octocrylene
- UVA filters:
  - Benzophenones
  - Avobenzone (Parsol 1789)
  - Anthranilates
- Physical blocking agents:
  - Iron oxide
  - Kaolin
  - Titanium dioxide
  - Zinc oxide
  - UV protective factor (UPF) clothing

DIAGNOSIS

HISTORY

- History of previous sun or UV light exposure
- Exposure to, or ingestion of, the many sun-sensitizing agents
- Family history of similar disorders
- Type of sunscreen and how the sunscreen has been used prior to reaction

PHYSICAL EXAM

- Phototoxic:
  - Erythema
  - With increasing severity: vesicles and bullae
  - Classic example: sunburn
  - Nails may exhibit onycholysis.
  - Chronic: epidermal thickening, elastosis, telangiectasia, and pigmentary changes
  - Sharp lines of demarcation between involved and uninvolved skin (sunlight exposure)
  - Phototoxic eruption owing to topicals: area of application
  - Usually develops minutes to hours after sun exposure
  - Hyperpigmentation may follow resolution.
  - Pain
- Photoallergic:
  - Papules with erythema and occasionally vesicles
  - Area exposed to light with less distinct borders
  - Usually delayed: 24 hr or more after exposure
  - May spread to unexposed areas
  - Pruritus
- Polymorphous light eruption:
  - Erythematous papules
  - Occasionally urticaria or vesicles
  - Scattered over sun-exposed areas with normal skin in between
  - Can spread to nonexposed areas
  - Often flares in spring or early summer
  - Desensitization affect (less over the course of the summer)
  - Burning or pruritus may precede lesions.

- Chronic actinic dermatitis:
  - Lichenified papules on sun-exposed areas in older person
  - Usually pruritic
  - Biopsy and phototesting confirm diagnosis.
- Solar urticaria:
  - Urticaria within minutes of UV exposure
  - Unidentified photosensitizing agent
  - Wheals itch and burn and disappear within hours
- Porphyria cutanea tarda:
  - Skin fragility
  - Blisters, crusts, milia
  - Mottled skin pigmentation
  - Hypertrichosis on periorbital area
- Erythropoietic protoporphyria:
  - Presents by age 2 yr
  - Child cries or screams in pain when exposed to sun.
  - Burning feeling, induration, and purpura
  - Waxy thickening of skin on knuckles

DIFFERENTIAL DIAGNOSIS

- Phototoxicity
- Photoallergic reaction
- Cellulitis
- Pityriasis rosea
- Viral exanthem
- Drug eruption
- Polymorphous light eruption
- Chronic actinic dermatitis
- Solar urticaria
- Porphyria
- Atopic dermatitis
- Seborrheic dermatitis
- Dermatomyositis
- Systemic lupus erythematosus
- Stevens-Johnson syndrome

DIAGNOSTIC TESTS & INTERPRETATION

Initial Tests (lab, imaging)

- Antinuclear antibody and other rheumatologic tests when systemic lupus erythematosus and dermatomyositis are suspected
- Check serum, urine, and stool porphyrin if porphyria is suspected.
- Drugs that may alter lab results: N/A
- Disorders that may alter lab results: N/A

Diagnostic Procedures/Other

- Photopatch test: Test a small patch of a potentially photosensitive substance on the skin to find out if this is the substance that caused the reaction. Examples of substances tested include medications, sunscreens or other lotions, fragrances, antiseptics, and plant products.
- Phototest: Test the skin for a photoreaction to UV light after normal diet and/or after ingestion of a possible photosensitizing agent such as an NSAID, a sulfa drug, a diuretic, or an oral contraceptive pill.
- Skin biopsy: used to determine the type of skin inflammation and the potential disease process or malignancy
- Pathologic findings:
  - Lymphohistiocytic dermal infiltrates and spongiosis seen in the more common condition of phototoxicity

TREATMENT

GENERAL MEASURES

- Avoid sunlight/limit exposure.
- Protective clothing/sunscreens
- Ice packs/cold water compresses

MEDICATION

- Drugs of choice for phototoxic and photoallergic reactions (1,2,3):
  - NSAIDs, topical or oral (e.g., diclofenac gel or oral 75 mg BID, ibuprofen, others)
  - Oral and topical corticosteroids have not been shown to be effective in mild or severe injury.
  - Antihistamines for pruritus (e.g., hydroxyzine 25 to 50 mg QID)
  - Sunscreens for prevention: Use broad-spectrum sunscreen to block both UVA and UVB.
- Treatment for polymorphous light eruption:
  - Desensitization with UVB or UVA (psoralen UVA [PUVA]) phototherapy for 15 min 2 to 3 times per week during the spring
  - Antimalarial drugs for protections during the spring and summer
  - Topical or oral steroids once the outbreak has occurred, continue 3 to 7 days
- Treatment for chronic actinic dermatitis:
  - Topical and oral corticosteroids
  - Topical tacrolimus
  - Low-dose PUVA
  - Mycophenolate mofetil
  - Cyclosporine
  - Azathioprine
- Treatment for solar urticaria:
  - Antihistamines
  - Low-dose PUVA
- Treatment for porphyria cutanea tarda:
  - Phlebotomy
  - Avoid hepatotoxins and iron.
  - Antimalarial drugs
- Treatment for erythropoietic protoporphyria:
  - β-Carotene
  - Narrowband UVB
  - PUVA
- Contraindications: Refer to manufacturer's profile for each drug.
- Precautions: PABA, benzophenones, and cinnamates may cause contact dermatitis. Also, if allergic to benzocaine, procaine, paraphenylenediamine, or sulfonamides, one may have allergy to PABA. Refer to manufacturer's profile for each drug.
- Significant possible interactions: Refer to manufacturer's profile for each drug.

ADDITIONAL THERAPIES

Long-term treatment:

- Sun and light radiation protection and avoidance
- Identification and avoidance of photo enhancing, sensitizing, and allergic substances

ONGOING CARE

FOLLOW-UP RECOMMENDATIONS

Avoid sunlight.

Patient Monitoring

Monitor as necessary for persistence or recurrence.

DIET

No special diet

PATIENT EDUCATION

- Avoidance of sunlight
- Avoidance of photosensitizing drugs
- Protective clothing, wide-brimmed hat
- Use sunglasses that wrap around and absorb UVA and UVB rays.
- Use lip balm sunscreens.
- Sunscreens:
  - SPF 15 to 30 with both UVA and UVB protection
  - Apply 15 to 30 min before exposure.
  - Reapply generously every 1 to 2 hr and especially after swimming or sweating.
  - Stress application to be sure to cover neck and ears (one study showed that 60% of people miss these areas).
  - Children:
    - Avoid midday sun.
    - For those <6 mo of age, use titanium dioxide, which is less likely to irritate the skin.
- Fingernail protection can prevent subungual damage.
- Photocontact allergy to sunscreen has been reported.

PROGNOSIS

Good with avoidance/protection measures

COMPLICATIONS

Geriatric Considerations

More likely to experience adverse reactions to causative drugs.

REFERENCES

1. Faurschou A, Wulf HC. Topical corticosteroids in the treatment of acute sunburn: a randomized, double-blind clinical trial. *Arch Dermatol*. 2008;144(5):620–624.
2. Martina E, Rosa L, Postacchini V, et al. Photoprotection and photodermatitis: a case. *Contact Dermatitis*. 2017;76(1):54–55.
3. Drucker A, Rosen C. Drug-induced photosensitivity: culprit drugs, management and prevention. *Drug Saf*. 2011;34(10):821–837.

ADDITIONAL READING

- Fitzpatrick TB, Johnson RA, Polano MK, et al. *Color Atlas and Synopsis of Clinical Dermatology: Common and Serious Diseases*. 2nd ed. New York, NY: McGraw-Hill; 1992:210–213.
- McKee PH, Calonje E, Granter SR. *Pathology of the Skin: With Clinical Correlations*. Vol 1. 3rd ed. New York, NY: Elsevier Mosby; 2005:630–633.
- Scalf LA, Davis MD, Rohlinger AL, et al. Photopatch testing of 182 patients: a 6-year experience at the Mayo Clinic. *Dermatitis*. 2009;20(1):44–52.
- Tyring SK, Lupi O, Hengge UR. *Tropical Dermatology*. New York, NY: Elsevier; 2006:441–443.

CLINICAL PEARLS

- Use sunscreens that block UVA and UVB rays.
- Consider phototoxic, photoallergic, or polymorphous light eruption as a diagnosis for any rash in sun-exposed areas.

PHYSEAL INJURIES IN CHILDREN: SALTER-HARRIS CLASSIFICATION

Rachel A. Coel, MD, PhD, FAAP, CAQSM

BASICS

DESCRIPTION

- In pediatric bone, the primary areas of growth include the physis and the epiphysis.
- Physeal injuries may occur in the skeletally immature population from acute trauma as well as from chronic overuse and repetitive loading, infections, or tumors.
- In 1963, Salter and Harris described a classification scheme for acute injuries to the physis (1)[C].
- Although most physeal fractures heal well, growth plate injuries can lead to complications including avascular necrosis, premature growth arrest, or angular deformities.

EPIDEMIOLOGY

- Occurs most commonly after 10 yr of age but can be seen in any skeletally immature patient
- Typical age range: 10 to 16 yr of age; median age: 13 yr (peak incidence: boys 14 yr, girls 11 yr)
- Predominant gender: boys > girls (~2:1)
- Most common time frame: spring through summer months (more outdoor playtime)
- Most common bone location: distal radial physis
- Most common reported type of physeal injury: Salter-Harris type II (75%) (Underdiagnosis of type I injuries is likely an explanation for preponderance of type II injuries.)

Prevalence

Current estimates suggest that from 15% to 30% of all pediatric fractures involve the physis.

ETIOLOGY AND PATHOPHYSIOLOGY

- There are two types of epiphyses: traction epiphyses (apophyses), where major tendons originate or insert into bone, and pressure epiphyses, at the ends of long bones.
- Traction epiphyses shape and strengthen bone but do not add longitudinal growth; hence, their injury typically does not cause longitudinal growth arrest.
- Pressure epiphyses add longitudinal growth to long bones.
- The physis, located between the epiphysis and the metaphysis of long bones, serves as the area of rapid longitudinal bone growth.
- Injury to the physis or pressure epiphyses may result in growth disturbance.
- The active physis consists of four zones of cells separated by cartilage matrix; the third zone (hypertrophic zone) is the area most susceptible to injury and cleavage.
- The epiphysis provides the nutrient blood supply to the physis; epiphyseal injury can cause disruption of normal growth and maturation owing to compromised vascular supply.
- The physis is surrounded peripherally by the groove of Ranvier and the ring of LaCroix, which add growth, strength, and stability to the growth plate (2)[C].

RISK FACTORS

- Skeletal immaturity
- Falls, especially while running or playing
- Competitive organized sports, especially contact sports
- Recreational sports, including skiing/snowboarding, skateboarding, and bicycling
- Overuse training activities that cause repetitive loading and stress, such as gymnastics, cheerleading, throwing, and running
- Invasive pathology, including osteomyelitis and tumors (3)[C]

GENERAL PREVENTION

- Monitor training demands, especially in young athletes during periods of heightened growth.
- Cross-training to avoid overuse and repetition
- Overtraining prevention: Alternate periods of heavy training with designated periods of rest.

DIAGNOSIS

Salter-Harris classification of epiphyseal plate injuries (1)[C]:

- Type I: injury including complete separation of epiphysis from metaphysis without bone fracture
- Type II: Separation occurs partially along physis and out through an associated metaphyseal bone fracture.
- Type III: intra-articular epiphyseal fracture extending out through partially separated physis
- Type IV: intra-articular epiphyseal fracture extending through the full thickness of physis and out through metaphyseal bone fracture
- Type V: severe crush injury at one area of physis
- Although cited less frequently, Peterson, Rang, and Ogden have subsequently proposed additional classifications of Salter-Harris fractures (2,4)[C].

HISTORY

- Fall onto an outstretched hand (FOOSH) is a common mechanism of distal radius growth plate injury (3,5)[C].
- Abduction, adduction, and twisting mechanisms are especially common in tibial physeal injuries and other lower extremity growth plate injuries (1,3,5)[C].
- Severe abduction or adduction mechanisms in the ankle or knee can cause type V crush injury to the physis (1,3,5)[C].
- Patient often reports "sprain" of a joint.
- Chronic stress injuries to the physis may present with a history of intense training with minimal rest or with overuse repetitive motion, such as baseball pitchers or gymnasts. Patients complain of focal pain at the area of the physis (5,6)[C].

PHYSICAL EXAM

- Swelling
- Angular or rotational deformity
- Ecchymosis
- Focal tenderness to palpation
- Limited range of motion due to pain or deformity
- Refusal to bear weight
- Salter-Harris type I injuries are often a clinical diagnosis owing to the radiolucent nature of physis on radiographs.

DIFFERENTIAL DIAGNOSIS

- Bone fractures
- Sprains: physeal injuries most commonly mistaken for sprains
- Ligamentous rupture
- Dislocation
- Infection (abscess, osteomyelitis)
- Tumor
- Renal failure
- Hypothyroidism
- Steroid treatment or chemotherapy
- Genetic disorder (achondroplasia)

DIAGNOSTIC TESTS & INTERPRETATION

- Initial approach:
  - Plain x-ray trauma series: typically three to four views of injured joint (anteroposterior [AP], lateral, and oblique) (6)[C]
  - Type I fractures and chronic stress injuries may appear as physeal widening, epiphyseal displacement, or irregularity and sclerosis at the metaphysis; however, no radiographic abnormality is common (3,4,6)[C].
  - Comparative plain films of the opposite side may be helpful (6)[C].
  - Stress radiography may worsen physeal injury and should be used with caution (5,6)[C].
  - Type II to IV fractures are usually evident on plain x-rays and demonstrate associated bone fracture lines or bone fragmentation (Thurstan Holland sign) (1,3,4)[C].
  - Evaluate fractures for angulation and displacement.
- Follow-up:
  - Growth recovery lines, or Harris lines, appear in the metaphysis on plain films typically 12 wk after trauma (6)[C].
  - If they are parallel to the epiphysis and extend entirely across the metaphysis, future growth disturbance is unlikely.
  - If they are angled, curved, or highly irregular, subsequent growth disturbance is more likely.
- Special considerations:
  - If growth plate injury is suspected but plain radiographs are negative, advanced diagnostic measures may be employed, such as computed tomography (CT) or magnetic resonance imaging (MRI). Other options include ultrasound (US) and bone scintigraphy (5,6)[C]. US can be helpful to identify Salter-Harris type I fracture because point of maximum tenderness can be determined using US location.
  - Further evaluation typically is advocated only if initial management of the injury will be altered by definitive radiographic diagnosis (5)[C].
  - MRI: preferred method; can identify intact versus separated growth plate, physeal bridging, growth arrest, and avascular necrosis as well as cartilage, ligamentous/tendinous, and soft tissue imaging (3,6)[C]
  - CT scan: useful in further defining known physeal injuries and aids in treatment planning, such as alignment and displacement of fractures at the articular surface, growth arrest, physeal bridging, and surgical planning (3,4,6)[C]
  - Lower extremity limb length discrepancy may be evaluated with CT scanogram or full-length hips-to-ankles standing AP x-ray (4)[C].

TREATMENT

Emergency department (ED) treatment:

- Nondisplaced or minimally displaced type I and II fractures: splint immobilization, ice, elevation, and sports medicine or pediatric orthopedics referral (5)[C]
- Type III and IV fractures: Obtain orthopedic consultation in ED owing to intra-articular fracture (5)[C].
- If diagnosed in ED, type V fractures require orthopedic consultation (5)[C].

MEDICATION

Pain management should be addressed (over-the-counter [OTC] versus prescription pain medications).

ADDITIONAL THERAPIES

- Diagnosed type I fractures: closed reduction and rigid immobilization (cast versus brace) for 3 to 4 wk
- Suspected type I fractures: immobilization for 1 to 2 wk, then reexamination and repeat radiographs for periosteal reaction. If healing reaction is evident, immobilize for 1 to 2 more wk. Alternatively, MRI, CT, or US imaging may be obtained to definitively identify physeal versus soft tissue injury (3,4)[C].
- Type II fractures: typically closed reduction and rigid immobilization with casting for 3 to 4 wk; if unstable, refer to orthopedic surgery (3,4)[C].
- Type III and IV fractures: Refer to orthopedic surgery; often require open reduction and internal fixation to ensure stability and joint surface congruity (1,3,4)[C]
- Diagnosed type V fractures: non–weight-bearing cast for 3 to 4 wk followed by another 2 to 3 wk of weight-bearing casting; refer to orthopedic surgery (1,3,4)[C].
- Late-diagnosis type V fractures: frequently a missed diagnosis acutely and diagnosed after growth disturbance has occurred; refer to orthopedic surgery (3,4)[C].
- Multiple attempts at reduction and reductions performed 7 days after the date of injury are not recommended owing to increased risk of physeal injury (1,3,4)[C].
- Consider bracing for sports activity for another 3 to 4 wk after initial rigid immobilization is complete and while the patient is in rehabilitation.
- Consider physical therapy prior to return to play for ankle and knee physeal injuries.

SURGERY/OTHER PROCEDURES

- May be required for significantly displaced or unstable type I or type II fractures or, more commonly, for intra-articular type III and IV fractures
- Operative techniques may be necessary to produce anatomical reduction and fixation of the fracture. Care is taken to minimize further trauma to the physis and surrounding blood supply (3)[C].
- Intra-articular fractures require anatomic alignment to maintain joint surface congruity. Surgical techniques should be considered if anatomic alignment cannot be obtained or maintained with conservative measures (3,4)[C].
- Surgery may also be indicated for growth complications after Salter-Harris fracture, including physeal bar or growth arrest leading to limb length discrepancy or angular deformity. CT scanning can be helpful for surgical planning. Effective surgical techniques may include epiphysiodesis (fusion of the growth plate), corrective osteotomy, physeal bone bar resection, lengthening, grafting, and use of spacers (3,4)[C].

ONGOING CARE

FOLLOW-UP RECOMMENDATIONS

Consider bracing for sports activity for another 3 to 4 wk after initial rigid immobilization is complete.

Patient Monitoring

ALERT

Patients, especially those with high-risk type II to V injuries, should be monitored for growth disturbance or deformity every 6 mo for the 1st yr after physeal injury.

Thereafter, patients should be reevaluated annually until skeletal maturity owing to risk of growth disturbance complications until adolescent growth spurt has been completed.

PATIENT EDUCATION

Patients and their parents should be informed of the risk of complications with growth plate injury, including late-onset avascular necrosis, growth arrest, or deformity.

PROGNOSIS

- Several studies suggest that Salter-Harris classification is not a reliable predictor of outcome (2)[C].
- Fracture displacement at time of injury, accuracy of reduction, specific physis of injury, and mechanism of injury may be the best predictors of physeal growth disturbance (2)[C].
- Estimates range from 30% to 75% of all physeal injuries lead to some type of growth disturbance or angular deformity (1,2,3,4,6)[C].
- However, current estimates predict only 1–10% of these patients demonstrate significant functional deficits requiring surgical intervention (2,6)[C].

ALERT

Typically, Salter-Harris type I and II fractures have a good to excellent prognosis. Types III and IV have a poorer prognosis, and type V injury invariably results in growth disturbance with the worst prognosis (1,3,5,6)[C].

- Younger children have a worse prognosis owing to longer duration of remaining growth that may be affected (1)[C].
- Decreased remodeling potential exists in older children nearing skeletal maturity (4)[C].
- Other indicators of poor prognosis include compromised epiphyseal blood supply, repeated or forceful manipulation of physis during reduction, and open physeal fracture (1,3,4)[C].

COMPLICATIONS

- Entrapment of periosteum within fracture site
- Partial or complete growth arrest/limb-length discrepancy
- Fibrous bone bar/physeal bridging
- Angular deformity
- Avascular necrosis
- Arthritis after intra-articular Salter-Harris III to IV fracture
- Regardless of age of onset of physeal injury, growth disturbances may not manifest until the adolescent growth spurt (5)[C].
- Risk of complications (3,4,5)[C]:
  - Greatest risk in early adolescence (pubescence) during periods of rapid growth
  - Increases with higher grade acute Salter-Harris injury (types III to V) (Type V has nearly 100% focal growth arrest rate.)
  - Increases with high-velocity, high-energy injury
  - Increases in lower extremity injury, especially distal femur (52% growth disturbance rate), proximal tibia, and distal tibia (43%) (3,4)[C]
  - Also may occur with chronic repetitive stress injury to physis

REFERENCES

1. Salter RB, Harris WR. Injuries involving the epiphyseal plate. *J Bone Joint Surg Am*. 1963;45:587–622.
2. Cepela DJ, Tartaglione JP, Dooley TP, et al. Classifications in brief: Salter-Harris classification of pediatric physeal fractures. *Clin Orthop Relat Res*. 2016;474(11):2531–2537.
3. Dover C, Kiely N. Growth plate injuries and management. *Orthopaedics and Trauma*. 2015;29(4):261–267.
4. Mallick A, Prem H. Physeal injuries in children. *Surgery*. 2016;35(1):10–17.
5. Perron AD, Miller MD, Brady WJ. Orthopedic pitfalls in the ED: pediatric growth plate injuries. *Am J Emerg Med*. 2002;20(1):50–54.
6. Nguyen JC, Markhardt BK, Merrow AC, et al. Imaging of pediatric growth plate disturbances. *Radiographics*. 2017;37(6):1791–1812.

SEE ALSO

Osgood-Schlatter Disease; Sever Disease/Calcaneal Apophysitis

CLINICAL PEARLS

- The Salter-Harris classification system of physeal injuries in children describes growth plate injuries by the level of involvement of the physis, the bone, and the joint.
- Growth plate injury can occur from both acute trauma and chronic stress as well as from infection or tumor.
- Although most physeal injuries have a favorable prognosis, up to 10% may result in significant growth arrest, angular deformity, or avascular necrosis.
- There are numerous prognostic indicators, such as age at onset of injury, location of injury, and severity of injury.
- Orthopedic surgery consultation is recommended for unstable, displaced, or angulated fractures and for growth complications.

PIGMENTED VILLONODULAR SYNOVITIS (PVNS)

Nancy White, MD • Fouad Sayde, MD, ABIM, FACP

BASICS

DESCRIPTION

- Pigmented villonodular synovitis (PVNS) is a proliferative disorder of the synovium.
- There are two forms described, localized and diffuse, which are likely both ends of a spectrum of the same disorder.
- The synovial lesions are composed of lipid-laden macrophages, giant cells, and hemosiderin.
- The knee is the most commonly involved joint.
- PVNS also can involve the hip, ankle, shoulder, and elbow.

EPIDEMIOLOGY

- Predominant age: most commonly seen in 3rd and 4th decades; can be seen in patients as young as 10 yr of age or as old as the 70 yr
- Incidence: 1.8/1 million (general population)
- Predominant gender: male = female

ETIOLOGY AND PATHOPHYSIOLOGY

- Etiology not fully understood; theories include the following:
  - Trauma and recurrent local hemorrhage to affected joint
  - Abnormal metabolic activity within the joint causing inflammatory response (macrophages, giant cells, hemosiderin)
  - Neoplastic process: Rare cases of malignant transformation have been reported.
- Synovial lesions contain lipid-laden macrophages, giant cells, hemosiderin, and stromal and fibroblast proliferation.
- There are two forms:
  - Localized PVNS:
    - Lesions are pedunculated/lobular and localized to one area of synovium.
    - Knee is the most common joint involved.
  - Diffuse PVNS:
    - Histology is similar to localized PVNS; however, involvement is noted throughout most or all of the involved joint, bursa, or affected tendon sheath.
    - Knee is the most commonly affected joint; however, can involve the hip, ankle, shoulder, and elbow.
    - More common than localized PVNS
    - Higher recurrence rate following treatment than local form
    - More destructive course and consequently leads to more end-stage joint disease than localized PVNS

Genetics

No genetic component

RISK FACTORS

Risk factors are unknown.

DIAGNOSIS

HISTORY

- Insidious onset
- History of associated trauma is unusual.
- Symptoms are often vague, may be intermittent, and are typically slowly progressive.
- Swelling and stiffness out of proportion to pain
- Monoarticular involvement is the norm, with the knee the most commonly involved joint.
- Localized PVNS symptoms most commonly involve locking/catching/instability; also can have pain/swelling
- Diffuse PVNS symptoms include insidious onset of pain, swelling, and stiffness (often mistaken for early arthritis, meniscal or ligamentous injuries).

PHYSICAL EXAM

- Localized PVNS:
  - Effusion
  - May have a palpable synovial mass:
    - Most common in anterior compartment of the knee (anterior horn of medial meniscus)
    - Infrapatellar fat pad, suprapatellar pouch, intercondylar notch, anterior horn of lateral meniscus also common
  - Tenderness to palpation
  - Loss of motion
- Diffuse PVNS:
  - Global effusion of joint
  - Decreased and often painful range of motion (ROM)
  - Tenderness to palpation

DIFFERENTIAL DIAGNOSIS

- Osteoarthritis: similar exam/radiographs, but PVNS does not have osteophytes
- Hemophilia: similar exam/radiographs but without history of hemophilia
- Synovial hemangioma: similar exam/radiograph but age of presentation different (PVNS 3rd to 4th decades, synovial hemangioma 1st to 3rd decades)
- Rheumatoid arthritis: similar exam/radiographs but PVNS monoarticular
- Tuberculous arthritis: similar exam but without periarticular osteoporosis/abscesses on radiographs/magnetic resonance imaging (MRI)
- Lipoma arborescens: similar exam and MRI findings, but lesions show low signal enhancement with contrast versus no enhancement

DIAGNOSTIC TESTS & INTERPRETATION

Initial Tests (lab, imaging)

- Plain radiographs:
  - Often are normal
  - May see periarticular erosions/subchondral cysts
  - Reciprocal erosions on opposite sides of the joint, with a preserved joint space, are highly suggestive of PVNS (1)[C].
- Computed tomography (CT) scan:
  - PVNS is a high-density soft tissue mass compared with skeletal muscle.
  - Bone erosion and cysts may be seen.
  - CT scan with contrast material displays the synovial changes.
- MRI:
  - Improved sensitivity/specificity for PVNS
  - Helps to determine extent of disease
  - Local PVNS: MRI reveals synovial nodular mass with bone erosion; T1/T2-weighted images show low signal owing to hemosiderin (1)[C].
  - Diffuse PVNS:
    - T1/T2-weighted images show diffuse mass/synovial thickening with periarticular "dark on dark" erosions.
    - Fat-suppressed images show high-signal synovial mass (hemosiderin deposits not seen).
    - Fast field echo shows hemosiderin deposits.
    - Thallium-201 uptake also useful

Diagnostic Procedures/Other

Aspiration/joint fluid evaluation:

- Blood-tinged aspirate is common, but aspirate may be clear.

ALERT
Blood-tinged aspirate without a history of trauma is highly suggestive of PVNS.

- Aspirate may show hemosiderin pigment and macrophages.

TREATMENT

- Surgery is treatment of choice.
- Localized PVNS: Arthroscopic partial synovectomy of lesion with margin of healthy synovium is recommended (2,3)[A]:
  - Lesions in anterior compartment allow for surgeon to use standard arthroscopy approach.
  - Lesions in posterior compartment require additional portals.
  - Recurrence rate is low.
- Diffuse PVNS: Arthroscopy is an option, but open arthrotomy is often selected:
  - Extent of disease, location of lesions, or surgeon's preference determine if arthroscopy or open arthrotomy is selected.
  - Open arthrotomy is recommended when lesion is posterior to posterior collateral ligament, extra-articular, or located within a cyst.
  - Complete synovectomy is treatment of choice.
- Radiation and immunotherapy may be combined with surgical techniques for extensive or recurrent disease (3)[A].
- Joint replacement also is considered for severe or recurrent disease where significant joint space narrowing is involved (1)[C].

ONGOING CARE

FOLLOW-UP RECOMMENDATIONS

Patient Monitoring

- No clear-cut guidelines
- Recurrence is common especially with diffuse PVNS.
- Consider monitoring with MRI.

COMPLICATIONS

- Recurrence
- Joint erosion
- End-stage joint disease as result of erosion

REFERENCES

1. Botez P, Sirbu PD, Grierosu C, et al. Adult multifocal pigmented villonodular synovitis—clinical review. *Int Orthop*. 2013;37(4):729–733.
2. Verspoor FG, Zee AA, Hannink G, et al. Long-term follow-up results of primary and recurrent pigmented villonodular synovitis. *Rheumatology (Oxford)*. 2014;53(11):2063–2070.
3. Mollon B, Lee A, Busse JW, et al. The effect of surgical synovectomy and radiotherapy on the rate of recurrence of pigmented villonodular synovitis of the knee: an individual patient meta-analysis. *Bone Joint J*. 2015;97-B(4):550–557.

ADDITIONAL READING

- Rodriguez-Merchan EC. Review article: open versus arthroscopic synovectomy for pigmented villonodular synovitis of the knee. *J Orthop Surg (Hong Kong)*. 2014;22(3):406–408.
- Tyler WK, Vidal AF, Williams RJ, et al. Pigmented villonodular synovitis. *J Am Acad Orthop Surg*. 2006;14(6):376–385.

CLINICAL PEARLS

- Insidious onset, not usually associated with trauma
- Symptoms can be vague with swelling and stiffness out of proportion to pain.
- Aspirate may be blood-tinged and show hemosiderin pigment and macrophages.
- MRI is most helpful; T1/T2-weighted images show diffuse mass/synovial thickening with periarticular "dark on dark" erosions with reciprocal erosions on opposite sides of the joint with preserved joint space.
- Synovectomy is treatment of choice.

PIP JOINT DISLOCATIONS

Jarrod Yamanaka, MD

BASICS

DESCRIPTION

- Dislocation of the proximal interphalangeal (PIP) joint
- Hinge joint allowing flexion and extension with little lateral movement because collateral ligaments are tight through entire range of motion (ROM) (1)
- Dislocations may be dorsal (most common), ventral, or rotary subluxation where the twisting injury to the finger causes buttonholing of the head of the proximal phalanx through a tear in the central slip and lateral band (2).
- Synonym(s): finger dislocation

EPIDEMIOLOGY

Most commonly injured joint in the hand (3)

RISK FACTORS

Playing sports, particularly contact and ball sports

GENERAL PREVENTION

Wear appropriate sport-specific padding and safety equipment when participating in sports or activities.

DIAGNOSIS

HISTORY

- Ascertain the direction of dislocation if already reduced.
- Determine mechanism: Dislocated finger may be due to forced hyperextension or hyperflexion of digit from traumatic athletic injury, entrapment of finger between objects, or a fall.

PHYSICAL EXAM

- Swelling and deformity if not already reduced by coach or friend
- Deformity will indicate direction of dislocation.
- Careful palpation about the joint to locate the most tender area can help to differentiate between injuries:
  - Volar tenderness: volar plate
  - Lateral joint line tenderness: collateral ligaments
  - Dorsal tenderness: central slip injury
- Neurologic examination before and after reduction: Check sensation in distal finger (radial and ulnar sides).
- Check extensor tendon function: Have patient actively extend PIP and distal interphalangeal (DIP) joints.
- If able to extend DIP but not PIP joint, consider central slip rupture, which may lead to a boutonnière deformity. Extended DIP and flexed PIP with late loss of DIP flexion is the most disabling problem.
- Check flexion:
  - Have patient actively flex PIP joint with other fingers held in extension.
  - Check DIP flexion with PIP held in extension.
  - If unable to flex DIP joint, consider flexor digitorum profundus rupture, which requires surgical consultation.
- Check collateral ligaments:
  - Apply radial and ulnar stress with PIP joint in full extension and 30 degrees of flexion.
  - Look for increased laxity, compare with other hand.
- Check volar plate:
  - Excessive hyperextension is consistent with volar plate injury.
  - If volar plate is unstable and not treated properly, it will lead to hyperextension of the PIP joint and flexion of DIP joint, a swan-neck deformity.

DIFFERENTIAL DIAGNOSIS

- Fracture-dislocation: Large dorsal fracture-dislocations can be missed, with the volar fracture involving >75% of joint surface with dorsal subluxation of the remaining portion of the middle phalanx (1)[C].
- Central extensor tendon rupture (boutonnière injury) of central slip allows lateral bands to slip below PIP joint and cause PIP flexion with DIP extension.

DIAGNOSTIC TESTS & INTERPRETATION

- X-rays: two views, including anteroposterior and lateral, before reduction if possible
- Oblique view if initial x-rays are negative but high suspicion of fracture
- Ensure joint congruity to rule out fracture-dislocation.
- May see small volar avulsion fracture
- With rotary subluxation, will see true lateral view of middle phalanx with oblique view of proximal phalanx, or vice versa

TREATMENT

- Determine stability: generally, fractures involving joint <30% stable, 30–50% borderline, >50% unstable.
- If stable, can proceed nonoperatively

- Dorsal dislocation: reduction:
  - If reduced before onset of swelling, reduction is easier.
  - Reduce with longitudinal traction and gentle pressure to the dorsal aspect of the midphalanx.
- Postreduction evaluation:
  - X-rays: two views if not already obtained
  - Rule out dorsal fracture-dislocation.
  - Check collateral ligament stability after reduction.
- Immobilization (2)[C]:
  - If dorsally dislocated and stable, simple, and reduced quickly, patient can continue sporting activity after "buddy taping" fingers if injury is to nondominant hand.
  - Stable: Splint for 1 to 2 wk in 15 to 20 degrees of flexion with a figure-of-eight (also may use extension block splint) until pain free. Often have volar plate injury; if so, consider splint in flexion for 4 to 5 wk.
  - Splint should include only PIP joint; may be dorsal or volar
  - "Buddy tape" for an additional 3 to 4 wk
  - Can treat with "buddy taping" alone for 3 to 6 wk if no volar plate injury
- Volar dislocation reduction (2)[C]:
  - Partial flexion, distal translation
  - Closed treatment if minimally displaced avulsion fracture
  - Avulsion fracture reduces with full extension.
- Postreduction evaluation (2)[C]:
  - X-rays: two views
  - Check collateral ligament stability after reduction.
- Immobilization (2)[C]:
  - Splint PIP joint in full extension for 6 wk (dorsal or volar splint) because central slip is often involved, DIP and metacarpophalangeal joints free.
  - Need to actively and passively flex DIP joint
  - Night splint for an additional 3 to 4 wk
  - Splint until full active extension of PIP joint and active flexion of DIP joint.
- Rotary subluxation: reduction:
  - Sometimes difficult to reduce closed
  - Closed reduction:
    - Digital block
    - Gentle traction with metacarpophalangeal and PIP joints at 90 degrees of flexion
    - Dorsiflex wrist (relaxes extensor mechanism)
    - Apply gentle rotatory and traction force.
- Postreduction evaluation:
  - X-rays: two views
  - Check collateral ligament stability after reduction.
- Immobilization: "buddy tape" after closed reduction

ADDITIONAL THERAPIES

Rehabilitation (2)[C]:

- Dorsal dislocation: Work on ROM when out of splint.
- Volar dislocation: Work on ROM of DIP and metacarpophalangeal joints while in splint.
- Rotary subluxation: Start active and passive ROM when out of splint; add resisted ROM when pain free, active and passive ROM.
- Refer to hand therapy if persistent stiffness.

SURGERY/OTHER PROCEDURES

- Unable to reduce closed
- Dorsal fracture-dislocation carries significant risk of long-term disability if treated improperly.
- Volar dislocation with significant avulsion fracture or fracture does not reduce with extension and carries high risk of disability if treated improperly (2)[C].

REFERENCES

1. Huq NS, Siddiqui F, Hossain S. Current concepts in treatment of fracture-dislocations of the proximal interphalangeal joint. *Plast Reconstr Surg*. 2015;136(6):851e–852e.
2. Saitta BH, Wolf JM. Treating proximal interphalangeal joint dislocations. *Hand Clin*. 2018;34(2):139–148.
3. Joyce KM, Joyce CW, Conroy F, et al. Proximal interphalangeal joint dislocations and treatment: an evolutionary process. *Arch Plast Surg*. 2014;41(4): 394–397.

ADDITIONAL READING

- Mangelson JJ, Stern P, Abzug JM, et al. Complications following dislocations of the proximal interphalangeal joint. *J Bone Surg Am*. 2013;95(14): 1326–1332.
- Pang EQ, Yao J. Anatomy and biomechanics of the finger proximal interphalangeal joint. *Hand Clin*. 2018;34(2):121–126.
- Skelley NW, McCormick JJ, Smith MV. In-game management of common joint dislocations. *Sports Health*. 2014;6(3):246–255.

CLINICAL PEARLS

- Return to play can be immediate with "buddy taping" or if able to play in splint.
- Volar lip fracture involves >20–70% of articular surface. Joint is unstable after reduction and requires referral.
- Recurrent dorsal dislocations occasionally can result in pseudo-boutonnière deformity. Treat with dynamic splinting.
- Early mobilization is key to preventing long-term stiffness.

PIRIFORMIS SYNDROME

Douglas Comeau, DO, CAQSM, FAAFP • Angelene M. Elliott, DO

BASICS

DESCRIPTION

- Sciatic nerve irritation as it courses underneath or through the piriformis muscle causing buttock pain with or without radiation into the leg
- The piriformis muscle acts as an external rotator in hip extension and an abductor in hip flexion.
- Piriformis muscle spasm or hypertrophy can occur in certain motions, such as running downhill or repetitive motions.
- Direct irritation of the sciatic nerve may be caused by inflammatory agents released from an injured piriformis muscle.
- Synonym(s): piriformis syndrome; sciatica; sciatic neuritis; "hip pocket neuropathy"; "wallet neuritis"; "pelvic outlet syndrome"; "deep gluteal syndrome"; "pseudosciatica"

EPIDEMIOLOGY

Incidence

- 6/100 cases of sciatica; 2.4 million cases per year (1)
- Mean age 38 yr old
- Predominant gender: female > male (6:1 in some trials)
- The incidence of piriformis syndrome is skewed secondary by the lack of evidence-based guidelines. The ratio is likely higher.

ETIOLOGY AND PATHOPHYSIOLOGY

- The piriformis muscle originates at the S2–S3 vertebrae, sacrotuberous ligament, and upper margin of the greater sciatic foramen.
- The piriformis muscle then passes through the greater sciatic notch, inserting on the greater trochanter.
- It is innervated by L5, S1, and S2.
- In hip extension, the piriformis serves as an external rotator.
- In hip flexion, it serves as a hip abductor.

RISK FACTORS

- In roughly 20% of the population, the sciatic nerve passes through the piriformis muscle, which may irritate the nerve and cause pain.
- Leg-length discrepancy may predispose a patient to development of symptoms.
- A Morton foot can predispose a patient from the change in ambulation.

GENERAL PREVENTION

- Maintaining an appropriate lumbar core stabilization can decrease the recurrence of symptoms.
- A core stabilization program includes the anterior pelvis, posterior back, and buttocks.

COMMONLY ASSOCIATED CONDITIONS

- Sciatica
- Gluteal strain

DIAGNOSIS

HISTORY

- Trauma to the gluteal region is seen in <50% of patients.
- Sitting on hard surfaces exacerbates pain.
- Location of referred pain; not likely piriformis syndrome if below the knee
- Complaint of pain with movements that cause external hip rotation
- Women may complain of dyspareunia.

PHYSICAL EXAM

- Cramping or aching pain in the buttock ± pain radiating into the hamstrings
- Sensation of "tight hamstrings"
- Point tenderness to deep palpation over any part of the piriformis muscle
- Pain increased with sitting
- Full range of motion and 5/5 strength in active and passive forward flexion and extension
- Negative stork test
- Negative straight-leg raise and negative flexion, abduction, and external rotation
- Buttock pain ± radiation to hamstrings produced by combination of hip flexion, adduction, and internal rotation; this maneuver stretches the piriformis muscle.
- Pace sign: weakness in resisted abduction and external rotation
- Tenderness to palpation over the piriformis muscle
- Sciatic notch tenderness
- Usually normal neurologic examination
- Pelvic and/or digital rectal examination elicits pain ipsilaterally proximal to the ischial tuberosity.
- A proposed clinical scoring system using history and exam may be helpful with sensitivity of 96.4% and specificity of 100% (2).

DIFFERENTIAL DIAGNOSIS

- Lumbar facet arthropathy
- Lumbar spondylolysis and spondylolisthesis
- Lumbosacral radiculopathy
- Myofascial pain
- Achilles tendinitis
- Cord tumor
- Spinal stenosis
- Aneurysm of the inferior or superior gluteal artery
- Fibrotic band around the sciatic nerve
- Hematoma
- Gluteal abscess
- Pelvic tumor
- Endometriosis and other pelvic diseases
- Bursitis: obturator internus, trochanteric or ischial

DIAGNOSTIC TESTS & INTERPRETATION

Initial Tests (lab, imaging)

- No laboratory tests are recommended in the workup.
- Diagnostic imaging is rarely helpful in confirming the diagnosis.
- Clinical history and physical examination are keys to diagnosing piriformis syndrome.
- Further diagnostic tests may be needed to rule out other potential diagnoses.
- Magnetic resonance imaging (MRI) and computed tomography (CT) scanning can be used if history and physical examination are not conclusive; two case reports supporting the use of magnetic resonance neurography to confirm diagnosis and verify effect of treatment (3)
- Atrophy or fibrous tissue replacement of the piriformis muscle on MRI or CT scan supports the diagnosis.
- Musculoskeletal ultrasound (US) demonstrating hypertrophy of the muscle is a newer radiologic technique that may be used in difficult cases.

Diagnostic Procedures/Other

Electromyography (EMG) findings of peronei and/or tibial H reflex prolongation in the adducted, internally rotated, flexed hip strongly anecdotally support the diagnosis in some studies; however, EMG is typically normal and not a recommended diagnostic tool.

TREATMENT

Emergency department (ED) treatment:

- Low back pain is one of the top 10 causes of acute emergency visits.
- Typically, a lumbar spine film will be taken and is negative.
- The patient should be treated with nonsteroidal anti-inflammatory drugs (NSAIDs) and muscle relaxants and sent for primary care and/or sports medicine follow-up.

MEDICATION

First Line

- NSAIDs for 10 to 4 days
- Short course of analgesics and/or muscle relaxants may be beneficial (4)[C].
- Ice
- Acetaminophen

ADDITIONAL THERAPIES

- Relative rest for a short period but should begin piriformis stretch and physical therapy as soon as possible
- Physical therapy incorporating stretching and strengthening of the piriformis muscle; also should incorporate correction of pelvic obliquities and leg-length discrepancies (4)[A]
- Deep muscle massage with US
- Long-term treatment:
  - Continued lumbar stabilization program
  - Continued piriformis stretching
- Injections:
  - With no improvement after conservative therapy, consider local injection of anesthetic (1–2% lidocaine hydrochloride ± bupivacaine 4 to 6 mL) with or without steroids (mixed evidence for use of steroids) under fluoroscopic or US guidance into the tender area within the piriformis muscle.
  - Botulinum toxin has shown benefit in randomized, double blind, controlled trials (5)[A] and nonrandomized, controlled trials (6)[C]. The mechanism of action would be decreasing the piriformis spasm by injecting botulinum.
- Surgery as indicated earlier for recalcitrant cases of piriformis syndrome

SURGERY/OTHER PROCEDURES

- If conservative treatment fails, surgical release of the piriformis muscle around the sciatic nerve should be used as a last resort. In these cases, surgery has a favorable outcome in the majority of cases (7).
- Patients with documented EMG nerve impairment have the best outcome after surgical release.

COMPLEMENTARY & ALTERNATIVE MEDICINE

- Osteopathic manipulative treatment (OMT) may be used in conjunction with physical therapy.
- Techniques include muscle energy technique and myofascial release to help with piriformis strengthening and stretching.

ADMISSION, INPATIENT, AND NURSING CONSIDERATIONS

A patient typically is admitted only if preoperative for surgical correction.

ONGOING CARE

FOLLOW-UP RECOMMENDATIONS

Patient Monitoring

- Initially, a patient should follow up with primary care or sports medicine 6 to 8 wk after starting physical therapy (8).
- On follow-up, close interaction should be maintained to ensure compliance with the home exercise program (lumbar stabilization).

PATIENT EDUCATION

- Patient education may include home exercise program handouts to ensure compliance.
- Showing the patient a diagram of the piriformis and its closeness to the sciatic nerve may help in patient recognition.

PROGNOSIS

- Prognosis is predicated on compliance with home exercise program and core stability.
- Although compliance with core stabilization cannot guarantee lifelong relief of symptoms, a stronger core can decrease the chance of recurrence.

COMPLICATIONS

- Complications typically occur without early diagnosis and treatment.
- Chronic low back pain may be debilitating and multifactorial.

REFERENCES

1. Siddiq MA, Hossain MS, Uddin MM, et al. Piriformis syndrome: a case series of 31 Bangladeshi people with literature review. *Eur J Orthop Surg Traumatol*. 2017;27(2):193–203.
2. Michel F, Decavel P, Toussirot E, et al. Piriformis muscle syndrome: diagnostic criteria and treatment of a monocentric series of 250 patients. *Ann Phys Rehabil Med*. 2013;56(5):371–383.
3. Yang HE, Park JH, Kim S. Usefulness of magnetic resonance neurography for diagnosis of piriformis muscle syndrome and verification of the effect after botulinum toxin type A injection: two cases. *Medicine (Baltimore)*. 2015;94(38):e1504.
4. Rouzier P. Piriformis syndrome. *The Sports Medicine Patient Advisor*. Amherst, MA: McKesson; 2004.
5. Fishman LM, Wilkins AN, Rosner B. Electrophysiologically identified piriformis syndrome is successfully treated with incobotulinum toxin A and physical therapy. *Muscle Nerve*. 2017;56(2):258–263.
6. Kirschner JS, Foye PM, Cole JL. Piriformis syndrome, diagnosis and treatment. *Muscle Nerve*. 2009;40(1):10–18.
7. Han SK, Kim YS, Kim TH, et al. Surgical treatment of piriformis syndrome. *Clin Orthop Surg*. 2017;9(2):136–144.
8. Jankovic D, Peng P, van Zundert A. Brief review: piriformis syndrome: etiology, diagnosis, and management. *Can J Anaesth*. 2013;60(10):1003–1012.

CLINICAL PEARLS

- Prevention: a strong core stabilization program to increase strength and range of motion
- Any activities that involve prolonged sitting (i.e., biking) should be avoided.
- Return to play: weight-bearing as tolerated 5 to 10 days after surgery with gradual return to full activity; avoidance of prolonged sitting for 4 to 6 wk after surgery is recommended.

PLANTAR FASCIITIS

Randall Burgett, DO • Douglas J. DiOrio, MD

BASICS

DESCRIPTION
- Degeneration and irritation of the plantar fascia origin at the medial calcaneal tuberosity on the anteromedial side of the heel and surrounding perifascial structures
- Synonym(s): enthesopathy of plantar fascia; plantar fasciosis

EPIDEMIOLOGY
- Plantar fasciitis accounts for 80% of patients with plantar heel pain.
- Occurs bilaterally in up to 33% of patients
- Estimated prevalence up to 10% of the general population
- Nearly 2 million patients receive treatment each year in the United States.
- In the running population, plantar fasciitis accounts for 10% of running injuries.
- Peak age of incidence is between 40 and 60 yr but can occur in adults of all ages.

ETIOLOGY AND PATHOPHYSIOLOGY
- Likely multifactorial
- ~50% of patients with plantar fasciitis will have heel spurs. Up to 19% of patients without plantar fasciitis will also have heel spurs. Heel spurs can occur with plantar fasciitis, but they are not the cause.
- Histologic findings include myxoid degeneration, microtears in the fascia, collagen necrosis, and angiofibroblastic hyperplasia.

RISK FACTORS
- Excessive torsion and hyperpronation with poor supporting footwear
- Poor shock dissipation with cavus foot
- Hindfoot valgus with pronation deformity
- Limited ankle dorsiflexion
- Varus knee alignment in runners
- Obesity and prolonged standing on hard surfaces
- Spiked athletic shoes

DIAGNOSIS

HISTORY
- Insidious and progressive pain in the inferior heel that can radiate across the medial side and less so to the lateral aspect
- Pain can involve both feet.
- Pain can be described as throbbing, searing, or piercing.
- Worst with first few steps out of bed in the morning
- Pain tends to lessen with gradually increased activity and worsens at the end of the day.
- Worsens after periods of prolonged standing or inactivity
- Pain exacerbated with walking barefoot, on toes, in dress shoes, on hard surfaces, or upstairs

PHYSICAL EXAM
- Tenderness localized to anteromedial aspect of the heel with palpation
- Tight Achilles heel cord
- Pes planus or pes cavus foot deformity
- Passive range of motion: hypermobility of subtalar joint, midtarsal joint, and first ray
- Pain with passive dorsiflexion of toes
- Gait evaluation: calcaneus everted at heel lift
- Palpable defect or loss of arch height may be seen if complete tear has occurred.

DIFFERENTIAL DIAGNOSIS
- Skeletal:
  - Calcaneal stress fracture
  - Bone contusion
  - Subtalar arthritis
  - Inflammatory arthropathies
  - Infections (osteomyelitis/subtalar pyarthrosis)
  - Neoplasm
- Soft tissue:
  - Intrinsic muscle strain (abductor hallucis, flexor digitorum brevis, quadratus plantae)
  - Plantar fibromatosis
  - Plantar fascia rupture
  - Achilles tendinitis
  - Posterior tibial tendinitis
  - Retrocalcaneal bursitis
  - Fat pad atrophy
- Neurologic:
  - Entrapment of branches of the posterior tibial nerve usually at or after passage through the posterior tarsal tunnel: medial plantar nerve, lateral plantar nerve, or medial calcaneal nerve
  - Radicular symptoms of L4–S1 (sciatic nerve)
  - Abductor digiti quinti nerve entrapment
  - Peripheral neuropathy

DIAGNOSTIC TESTS & INTERPRETATION
- Imaging plays a limited role in routine clinical evaluation and is rarely needed. Radiographic evaluation would be appropriate in patients who fail to improve with appropriate treatment in a reasonable amount of time or if patient presents with an atypical history or physical exam.
- X-rays may show calcifications in the soft tissues around the heel or osteophytes on the anterior calcaneus (i.e., heel spurs). Ultrasound (US) may show thicker heel aponeurosis.
- Triple-phase bone scan can differentiate between plantar fasciitis and a calcaneal stress fracture. A bone scan or magnetic resonance imaging (MRI) should be ordered when heel pain has not improved after 4 to 6 mo of nonsurgical treatment.

TREATMENT

- Initial treatment is conservative and consists of pain control, activity modifications, exercise therapy, shoe modifications, and weight loss.
- Avoidance of activities causing or exacerbating pain
- Avoid flat shoes and barefoot walking.
- Nonsteroidal anti-inflammatory drugs (NSAIDs) for analgesic effect
- Early morning stretching of heel cord as well as throughout the day
- High-load eccentric strength training has potential to improve symptoms faster than stretching (1)[B].
- Ice massage and deep friction massage of the arch and insertion
- Shoe inserts: prefabricated insoles (i.e., soft heel pads/Silastic), custom orthotics, or medial heel wedges
- Arch taping during athletic activities
- Motion-control shoes with rigid heel counters
- Posterior-tension night splints
- Supination strap
- Risk of fat pad atrophy must be noted. Benefits appear limited to the short term (4 to 12 wk) (2)[B].
- Autologous blood-derived products (platelet-rich plasma [PRP] regimen). Limited data comparing to placebo or conservative therapies. Meta-analysis suggested PRP was superior to corticosteroid injection and shock wave therapy at 3 and 6 mo follow-up (3)[A].
- Dexamethasone (Decadron) or acetic acid iontophoresis
- Physical therapy with plantar fascia: specific stretching and Achilles tendon stretching programs
- Extracorporeal shock wave therapy
- Walking cast
- Conservative therapy should be used for a minimum of 6 mo and, preferably, for 12 mo because >90% respond positively to nonsurgical management.

SURGERY/OTHER PROCEDURES

- Surgery can be considered after failure of extensive conservative therapy, even up to 2 yr: operative release of proximal fascia of deep abductor fascia
- Plantar fasciotomy can be either partial or complete and is a common surgical procedure for treating recalcitrant cases of plantar fasciitis.
- Postoperative therapy includes splint for 2 wk, mild stretching and ambulation with crutches and walking boot, pool running for 3 wk, and return to activity in 3 to 4 mo.

COMPLEMENTARY & ALTERNATIVE MEDICINE

- Acupuncture
- Direct myofascial release

REFERENCES

1. Rathleff MS, Mølgaard CM, Fredberg U, et al. High-load strength training improves outcome in patients with plantar fasciitis: a randomized controlled trial with 12-month follow-up. *Scand J Med Sci Sports*. 2015;25(3):e292–e300.
2. Schulhofer SD. Short-term benefits of ultrasound-guided corticosteroid injection in plantar fasciitis. *Clin J Sport Med*. 2013;23(1):83–84.
3. Hsiao MY, Hung CY, Chang KV, et al. Comparative effectiveness of autologous blood-derived products, shock-wave therapy and corticosteroids for treatment of plantar fasciitis: a network meta-analysis. *Rheumatology (Oxford)*. 2015;54(9):1735–1743.

ADDITIONAL READING

- Clanton TO, Porter DA. Primary care of foot and ankle injuries in the athlete. *Clin Sports Med*. 1997;16(3):453–466.
- Cole C, Seto C, Gazewood J. Plantar fasciitis: evidence-based review of diagnosis and therapy. *Am Fam Physician*. 2005;72(11):2237–2242.
- Lemont H, Ammirati KM, Usen N. Plantar fasciitis: a degenerative process (fasciosis) without inflammation. *J Am Podiatr Med Assoc*. 2003;93(3):234–237.
- McPoil TG, Martin RRL, Cornwall MW, et al. Heel pain—plantar fasciitis: clinical practice guidelines linked to the international classification of function, disability, and health from the orthopaedic section of the American Physical Therapy Association. *J Orthop Sports Phys Ther*. 2008;38(4):A1–A18.
- Neufeld SK, Cerrato R. Plantar fasciitis: evaluation and treatment. *J Am Acad Orthop Surg*. 2008;16(6):338–346.
- Williams SK, Brage M. Heel pain—plantar fasciitis and Achilles enthesopathy. *Clin Sports Med*. 2004;23(1):123–144.

CLINICAL PEARLS

- Initial treatment is conservative, focusing on high-load eccentric strength training.
- Surgery should only be considered after exhaustive conservative treatment of at least 6 mo to 1 yr has failed.
- A Cochrane review showed that corticosteroid injections improved plantar fasciitis at 1 mo but not at 6 mo when compared with control groups. In addition, the risk of fat pad atrophy (a devastating complication) likely outweighs the benefits of corticosteroid injection.

PNEUMOTHORAX AND HEMOTHORAX

Stephen Carek, MD • Daniel C. Herman, MD, PhD, FAAPMR, FACSM, CAQSM

BASICS

DESCRIPTION

- Air (pneumothorax), blood (hemothorax), or both (hemopneumothorax) in the pleural space between the lung and chest wall
- Tension pneumothorax: Progressive accumulation of air in the pleural space causing compression of mediastinal structures including heart and restricting venous return and the contralateral lung can lead to cardiac arrest.
- Pneumothorax can be categorized as:
  - Spontaneous: no obvious precipitating factor present; further divided into:
    - Primary: no apparent underlying pulmonary disease
    - Secondary: clinically apparent underlying disease (such as chronic obstructive pulmonary disease [COPD] or cystic fibrosis)
    - Catamenial: occurs in conjunction with menstruation
  - Nonspontaneous or traumatic: caused by trauma; can be further divided into:
    - Open: direct communication between the environment and pleural cavity through the chest wall, caused by sharp, penetrating trauma
    - Closed: Chest wall remains intact, caused by direct, blunt trauma.
  - Iatrogenic: secondary to a procedure such as transthoracic or transbronchial biopsy, subacromial injections, central line placement, pleural biopsy, or thoracentesis
- Synonym(s): collapsed lung

EPIDEMIOLOGY

- Rare, but potentially serious
- <4% of all sports injuries involve the chest or abdomen.

Incidence

- ~20,000 new cases of spontaneous pneumothorax are reported each year in the United States (1).
- Primary spontaneous pneumothorax affects ~9,000 persons in the United States each year.
- Exercise and sport accounts for <10% of reported cases of pneumothoraces (2).
- Predominant gender: male > female (6:1)

ETIOLOGY AND PATHOPHYSIOLOGY

- Spontaneous pneumothorax:
  - Theorized to be caused by the rupture of subpleural blebs
  - Rupture caused by increased intrathoracic pressure or shear force (coughing, straining, vomiting)
- Iatrogenic pneumothorax:
  - Caused by tear in visceral pleura resulting in air leak into the pleural space
- Hemothorax: caused by virtually any disruption of the tissues of the chest wall and pleura with subsequent bleeding
- Precipitating factors may include atmospheric pressure changes and exposure to loud music.

RISK FACTORS

- Tall, thin, young (20s to 40s), males
- Smoking
- Substance use such as heroin, ecstasy, marijuana, speed, and cocaine
- Congenital apical lung blebs
- Underlying lung disease (e.g., COPD, cystic fibrosis, tuberculosis [TB])
- Connective tissue disorder (Marfan)
- Homocystinuria
- Trauma, especially rib fractures (most commonly first 4 and last 2, multiple, or flail segments) or scapular fractures
- Preparticipation recommendations:
  - SCUBA contraindicated if history of spontaneous pneumothorax

GENERAL PREVENTION

- Avoid smoking and substance use.
- If history of pneumothorax, avoid SCUBA, contact sports, and trauma.

COMMONLY ASSOCIATED CONDITIONS

- COPD
- Cystic fibrosis
- Asthma
- Marfan syndrome

DIAGNOSIS

Prehospital:

- Initial evaluation should include vital sign assessment and auscultation in a quiet setting.

HISTORY

- Trauma to thoracic wall
- Persistent pain at injury site
- Shortness of breath
- Localized chest pain, especially on deep inspiration, frequently present: may radiate to neck, shoulder, back, or abdomen
- Dyspnea and/or tachypnea frequently present
- Up to 25% of patients may be asymptomatic.

PHYSICAL EXAM

- Decreased or absent breath sounds on affected side
- Decreased tactile fremitus on side of pneumothorax
- Unequal expansion of right and left sides of chest with inspiration
- Hyperresonance to percussion in the case of pneumothorax; dullness to percussion in the case of hemothorax
- In tension pneumothorax, tracheal deviation away from site of pneumothorax, neck vein distension, and laterally displaced cardiac impulse all may be present.
- Crepitation or subcutaneous (SC) emphysema may be present, especially in traumatic pneumothorax.
- Possible pallor or cyanosis (usually with tension pneumothorax)
- Tachycardia may be present.

DIFFERENTIAL DIAGNOSIS

- Chest wall/rib contusion
- Lung contusion
- Costochondral separation
- Muscle strain
- Fracture

DIAGNOSTIC TESTS & INTERPRETATION

Initial Tests (lab, imaging)

- Upright posteroanterior and lateral chest films:
  - Inspiratory and expiratory films have equal sensitivity in detecting pneumothoraces, so a standard inspiratory chest radiograph is sufficient in most cases (3).
  - Pneumothorax is demonstrated by a white visceral pleural line on the chest radiograph.
  - The visceral pleural line defines the interface of the lung and pleural air and is either straight or convex toward the chest wall with no pulmonary vessels usually visible beyond the visceral pleural edge.
- Rib x-rays on affected side
- CT scanning generally is not necessary unless abnormalities are noted on the plain chest radiograph that require further evaluation or poor chest tube placement is suspected (3).
- Ultrasound can be utilized to look for an absence of lung sliding and a loss of "comet-tail artifacts" (4).

Diagnostic Procedures/Other

- Electrocardiogram (ECG) often demonstrates right-axis deviation, decreased QRS amplitude, and precordial T-wave inversion.
- If hemodynamically unstable and findings are consistent with a pneumothorax (most likely tension pneumothorax), may consider emergency needle aspiration, which is both diagnostic and therapeutic
- Diagnosis is confirmed by rapid gush of air coming through the needle.

TREATMENT

GENERAL MEASURES

- Acute treatment:
  - Determine if patient is hemodynamically stable because primary job is to stabilize.
  - Airway, breathing, and circulation (ABCs) of basic life support, especially airway management
  - Determine diagnostic possibilities; transfer to hospital (x-ray) facility if suspicious for pneumothorax.
  - Semi-Fowler position
  - Supplemental oxygen
  - If unstable and/or findings consistent with a tension pneumothorax, emergency needle decompression (thoracostomy) should be performed.
  - Needle decompression is performed by inserting a large-caliber needle (usually 14 or 18 gauge), preferably with a catheter over needle, into the 2nd intercostal space at the midclavicular line just above the 3rd rib.
  - If catheter over needle, then remove needle and leave plastic sheath; may attach a syringe

- Flail chest may accompany rib fractures; if present, stabilize flail segment with manual pressure or a bulky dressing to the segment.
- Foreign body should not be removed until transferred to emergency room.
- If open pneumothorax, cover wound with three-sided occlusive dressing to create flap valve, prohibiting air entrance but allowing air to escape during exhalation.

- Emergency personnel:
  - Supplemental oxygen
  - Intravenous (IV) line placement
  - Transport to emergency facility
- Further treatment depends on patient characteristics and clinical circumstances:
  - When pneumothorax is small (<20%) tension-free pneumothorax (no mediastinal shift) and patient is hemodynamically stable, treat expectantly without chest tube and with supplemental oxygen and observation only (1)[C]:
    - Must be observed in the emergency department (ED) for at least 6 hr with follow-up films obtained before discharge showing no progression of pneumothorax and again in 12 to 48 hr (1)[C]
    - Exception is when associated with underlying lung disease: requires urgent and immediate treatment (1)[C]
  - When pneumothorax is large (>20%) and clinically stable, treat initially with pleural aspiration (1)[A]:
    - If aspiration fails, treat with closed thoracostomy chest tube insertion with Heimlich valve or, preferably underwater seal (1)[C].
  - In cases of recurrent primary spontaneous pneumothorax when patient is clinically stable, treat with video-assisted thoracoscopic surgery (VATS) after chest tube insertion.
  - If patient is clinically unstable, he or she should undergo chest tube insertion (1)[C]:
    - If the chest tube insertion is delayed, decompression can be performed as a bridge.
    - The chest tube can be connected to a water-seal device. Suction should be applied to the chest tube if the pneumothorax fails to resolve (1)[C].
- Chest tube size recommendations:
  - Patients who require mechanical ventilation or who may have a large air leak should be managed with a 24 to 32Fr chest tube.
  - All other patients who require chest tube insertion can be managed with a 16 to 22Fr chest tube or a ≤14Fr chest catheter.
- Hemothorax with even a small pneumothorax requires a chest tube to preclude development of "trapped lung," which eventually may require decortication.

MEDICATION

- Lidocaine (Xylocaine) 1% for chest tube insertion
- Oral or IV medication prior to chest tube insertion and after as needed for comfort
- May consider Tylenol #3 or other narcotic for oral use, especially around time of chest tube insertion

ISSUES FOR REFERRAL

Should refer to cardiothoracic surgeon in cases of persistent air leak or recurrent pneumothorax requiring further intervention

ADDITIONAL THERAPIES

Avoid chest binders, taping, and so forth, which tend to compromise deep inspiration and may contribute to the development of atelectasis.

SURGERY/OTHER PROCEDURES

- VATS:
  - Should consider, along with chest tube placement, if pleural aspiration alone is unsuccessful (1)[A]
  - Should perform in cases of recurrent primary spontaneous pneumothorax after chest tube insertion (1)[C]
  - Consider in patients being managed with a chest tube who have a persistent air leak (1)[C].
- Thoracotomy:
  - Alternative to VATS
  - Rarely necessary

ADMISSION, INPATIENT, AND NURSING CONSIDERATIONS

- Admission criteria:
  - Hemodynamically unstable
  - Tension pneumothorax and/or chest tube placement
  - Pneumothorax with >15–20% lung volume loss
  - All patients with secondary spontaneous pneumothorax
- Discharge criteria:
  - Resolution of pneumothorax with removal of chest tube
  - Chest tube can be removed when air leak has stopped and x-ray confirms lung expansion; usually within 24 to 72 hr
  - Repeat x-ray after removal of chest tube (prior to discharge) to check for recurrence

ONGOING CARE

FOLLOW-UP RECOMMENDATIONS

- Advise patient that pain likely will be present for at least 6 wk, especially if rib fracture produced the pneumothorax.
- May return to conditioning 3 to 4 wk after pneumothorax resolved, provided no evidence of pneumothorax on chest x-ray, with return to play soon after

Patient Monitoring

Recheck chest x-ray in 4 to 6 wk.

PATIENT EDUCATION

- Counsel on high risk of recurrence if spontaneous pneumothorax: For traumatic pneumothorax, there is no increased risk of recurrence compared with other types.
- Counsel against smoking.
- Air travel recommendations (5):
  - Commercial air travel is contraindicated in the presence of an acute, unresolved pneumothorax.
  - For commercial travelers, no travel for 2 to 3 wk after radiographic resolution of pneumothorax
  - May restrict air travel in persons with a history of pneumothorax with underlying lung disease
- SCUBA diving absolute contraindications:
  - A history of a spontaneous pneumothorax
  - Diving within 3 mo after any type of nonspontaneous pneumothorax
  - Expert divers with recurrent pneumothorax following a pleurectomy

PROGNOSIS

- Depends on type and extent: Small (<20%) usually resolves on own without treatment.
- When associated with underlying disease, even when small, is more serious and has a mortality rate of ~15%
- Recurrence rate is ~40% for both primary and secondary pneumothoraces (2).
- Most recurrences occur within 1.5 to 2 yr; recurrence is at its highest likelihood in the first few months after the initial pneumothorax (6).
- For traumatic pneumothorax, there are no data to suggest that there is an increased risk of recurrence with or without return to play (6).
- Recurrence rate increases with each recurrence.
- Most recurrences are seen on the same side but not always.

COMPLICATIONS

Recurrence: If it occurs, consider VATS pleurodesis or thoracotomy.

REFERENCES

1. Baumann MH, Strange C, Heffner JE, et al. Management of spontaneous pneumothorax: an American College of Chest Physicians Delphi consensus statement. *Chest*. 2001;119(2):590–602.
2. Tschopp JM, Bintcliffe O, Astoul P, et al. ERS task force statement: diagnosis and treatment of primary spontaneous pneumothorax. *Eur Respir J*. 2015;46(2):321–335.
3. Choi W. Pneumothorax. *Tuberc Respir Dis (Seoul)*. 2014;76(3):99–104.
4. Husain LF, Hagopian L, Wayman D, et al. Sonographic diagnosis of pneumothorax. *J Emerg Trauma Shock*. 2012;5(1):76–81.
5. Hu X, Cowl CT, Baqir M, et al. Air travel and pneumothorax. *Chest*. 2014;145(4):688–694.
6. Putukian M. Pneumothorax and pneumomediastinum. *Clin Sports Med*. 2004;23(3):443–454.

ADDITIONAL READING

- Bintcliffe O, Maskell N. Spontaneous pneumothorax. *BMJ*. 2014;348:g2928.
- Soundappan S, Holland A, Browne G. Sports-related pneumothorax in children. *Pediatr Emerg Care*. 2005;21(4):259–260.

CLINICAL PEARLS

Return to activity:

- Return to play: 3 to 6 wk
- Air travel: contraindicated until 2 to 3 wk after chest tube removal (only if repeat x-ray shows resolution of pneumothorax)
- SCUBA diving: contraindicated if history of spontaneous pneumothorax

POPLITEAL (BAKER) CYST

Samuel J. Galloway, MD • David E.J. Bazzo, MD, FAAFP, CAQSM

BASICS

DESCRIPTION

- Cystic enlargement of the gastrocnemius-semimembranosus bursa, located on the medial side of the popliteal fossa between the medial head of the gastrocnemius and the semimembranosus tendon:
  - Primary cysts arise with no communication into the joint (more common in children).
  - Secondary cysts are associated with communication between the bursa and joint capsule (more common in the adult population).
- Originally reported by Robert Adams in 1840, described in detail and named by William Baker in his article published in 1877

EPIDEMIOLOGY

Prevalence

- Most prevalent cyst/soft tissue mass in the posterior knee
- In adults, prevalence has been reported with ranges from 4% to 40%, although most studies report prevalence closer to 5% (1):
  - Varies depending on type of imaging used and population sampled
  - Peak age in adults is 35 to 70 yr, whereas in pediatrics is 4 to 7 yr (2).
- No consistent significant gender difference

ETIOLOGY AND PATHOPHYSIOLOGY

- Association of popliteal cysts with intra-articular knee pathology originally described by Baker in 1877
- Result from communication between the gastrocnemius-semimembranosus bursa and joint capsule (in secondary cysts)
- A valve-like structure between the joint space and bursa results in one-way flow of synovial fluid into the bursa, leading to cyst formation:
  - Valve is open when the knee is in flexion and closed when the knee is in extension due to tension from semimembranosus and gastrocnemius.
- Intra-articular knee pressure is negative during partial flexion (minus 6 mm Hg) and positive during extension (16 mm Hg) (2).
- Intra-articular knee pathology results in increased production of synovial fluid, which accumulates in the bursa leading to popliteal cyst.
- Intra-articular bodies may make their way into the cyst.

Genetics

No known genetic factors; consider underlying causes (e.g., rheumatoid arthritis).

RISK FACTORS

- Intra-articular knee pathology
- History of trauma

GENERAL PREVENTION

Avoid knee trauma.

COMMONLY ASSOCIATED CONDITIONS

- In adults, most commonly associated with intra-articular pathology of the knee, resulting from increased production of synovial fluid:
  - Meniscal pathology (most commonly tears of the posterior horn of medial meniscus)
  - Osteoarthritis/rheumatoid arthritis
  - Anterior cruciate ligament tear
  - Other joint disease: infectious arthritis, pigmented villonodular synovitis
- In pediatrics, cysts are most commonly a primary process and do not communicate with the joint space and are not associated with intra-articular pathology.

DIAGNOSIS

HISTORY

- Most are small, asymptomatic, and discovered incidentally on imaging.
- Symptoms, if present, include posterior knee pain, swelling, palpable mass, or knee stiffness.
- Patients may only present with symptoms of associated intra-articular knee pathology.
- Patients may present with leg swelling, calf pain, and positive Homans sign due to compression of adjacent structures or cyst rupture.

PHYSICAL EXAM

- May or may not have palpable medial popliteal mass depending on size
- Knee should be examined from full extension to at least 90 degrees of flexion.
- Tense cyst with knee in extension softens or decreases in size with knee flexion (Foucher sign):
  - Change in findings related to knee position helps to differentiate popliteal cyst from solid masses.
- May have physical findings of cyst compression on surrounding structures (see "Complications")

DIFFERENTIAL DIAGNOSIS

- Deep vein thrombosis (DVT)
- Popliteal artery aneurysm
- Solid tumors (lipoma, sarcoma, etc.)
- Other cystic structures (ganglion cyst, meniscal cyst, myxoid tumors)

DIAGNOSTIC TESTS & INTERPRETATION

Initial Tests (lab, imaging)

- Ultrasonography is the initial imaging modality of choice (3)[C]:
  - 100% ability to diagnose but lacks specificity to differentiate from other conditions
  - Inexpensive, noninvasive, no radiation exposure, and can be performed in the office
  - Can reliably detect cysts >1 to 2 cm in size
  - Can differentiate cyst from solid mass
  - Doppler can help to differentiate from popliteal artery aneurysm.
  - Allows for good visualization of cyst in relation to surrounding structures
- Plain radiographs are often helpful to evaluate for other associated joint pathology:
  - May be able to see loose bodies in cyst if present
- Magnetic resonance imaging (MRI) is the gold standard for diagnosis and can better delineate the cyst as well as evaluate internal derangement of the knee that is not able to be visualized with ultrasound (3)[C].

Diagnostic Procedures/Other

Arthrography with contrast or contrast + air can be useful for diagnosis; however, less common now with availability of MRI (4):

- Can be helpful for visualizing ruptured cyst with tracking of leaked contrast
- May result in false-positive due to distension of the joint capsule or enlargement of a normal bursa due to injection of fluid volume (2)

Test Interpretation

Fluid aspirate can be sent for cellular studies to rule out infectious, inflammatory, or gouty causes.

TREATMENT

GENERAL MEASURES

- Management of underlying joint pathology, if present, is necessary; otherwise, there is a very high rate of cyst recurrence.
- Asymptomatic cysts that were an incidental finding on evaluation of the knee for other reasons do not require any treatment (2)[C].
- When symptomatic and without vascular or neural compression, initial treatment should be nonoperative for >6 wk; rehab directed toward maintaining knee flexibility (3)
- Intra-articular corticosteroid injections have been shown to decrease the size and symptoms associated with cysts.
- Direct cyst aspiration and corticosteroid injection were found to be superior to intra-articular approach, but both can be beneficial (5)[B].
- If the cyst does not communicate directly with the joint space, direct aspiration and injection of corticosteroid is necessary.

ISSUES FOR REFERRAL

Symptomatic cysts not improved with conservative measures should be referred for surgical management.

SURGERY/OTHER PROCEDURES

- Surgical excision should be reserved for cases resistant to initial therapy that continue to be symptomatic or limit mobility:
  - Also should be considered initially for cysts compressing surrounding structures (3)[C]
- Intra-articular knee pathology should be addressed during surgical management of cyst; if this is not corrected, recurrence rates have been reported at 63% (6)[A].
- Several different surgical approaches have been described, with success rates of 85–98% (6)[A]:
  - Most common approaches are direct posterior and posteromedial.
  - Cyst either fully excised or communication with knee joint surgically closed

ONGOING CARE

FOLLOW-UP RECOMMENDATIONS

Monitor for symptom improvement after treatment initiated; follow up as needed if cyst recurs.

PATIENT EDUCATION

Discuss pathophysiology of cyst formation and options for management, including both conservative and surgical.

PROGNOSIS

- Many cysts are asymptomatic, discovered incidentally, and do not require any intervention.
- Most cysts in pediatrics do not require intervention and resolve spontaneously.
- Most will improve with treatment of underlying joint pathology.
- Cysts have been shown to decrease in size and symptoms with corticosteroid injection.
- Cysts often recur in patients with underlying joint pathology that is not adequately treated.
- Surgery is very effective, but not definitive, and cysts may recur despite full excision.

COMPLICATIONS

- Cyst rupture or dissection
- Enlarged cyst may compress adjacent vein, resulting in pseudothrombophlebitis or thrombophlebitis with symptoms of leg swelling and erythema.
- Compression of tibial nerve may result in neuropathy, plantar foot numbness, or gastrocnemius atrophy.
- Compression of popliteal artery may lead to limb claudication or ischemia.
- Compartment syndrome may result from cyst rupture, which requires emergent management.

REFERENCES

1. Sanchez JE, Conkling N, Labropoulos N. Compression syndromes of the popliteal neurovascular bundle due to Baker cyst. *J Vasc Surg*. 2011;54(6):1821–1829.
2. Handy JR. Popliteal cysts in adults: a review. *Semin Arthritis Rheum*. 2001;31(2):108–118.
3. Frush TJ, Noyes FR. Baker's cyst: diagnostic and surgical considerations. *Sports Health*. 2015;7(4):359–365.
4. Fritschy D, Fasel J, Imbert JC, et al. The popliteal cyst. *Knee Surg Sports Traumatol Arthrosc*. 2006;14(7):623–628.
5. Bandinelli F, Fedi R, Generini S, et al. Longitudinal ultrasound and clinical follow-up of Baker's cysts injection with steroids in knee osteoarthritis. *Clin Rheumatol*. 2012;31(4):727–731.
6. Zhou X, Li B, Wang J, et al. Surgical treatment of popliteal cyst: a systematic review and meta-analysis. *J Orthop Surg Res*. 2016;11:22.

ADDITIONAL READING

- Acebes JC, Sánchez-Pernaute O, Díaz-Oca A, et al. Ultrasonographic assessment of baker's cysts after intra-articular corticosteroid injection in knee osteoarthritis. *J Clin Ultrasound*. 2006;34(3):113–117.
- Angoules AG. Baker's cyst rupture may mimics deep vein thrombosis. *Emerg Med (Los Angel)*. 2012;2:e108.
- Hayashi D, Roemer FW, Dhina Z, et al. Longitudinal assessment of cyst-like lesions of the knee and their relation to radiographic osteoarthritis and MRI-detected effusion and synovitis in patients with knee pain. *Arthritis Res Ther*. 2010;12(5):R172.

CLINICAL PEARLS

- Many cysts are asymptomatic and discovered incidentally on imaging. These can be managed expectantly.
- In adults, most popliteal cysts are associated with intra-articular joint pathology. In pediatrics, most cysts are primary and not related to any underlying pathology.
- Ultrasound is the initial imaging modality of choice; MRI is the gold standard for diagnosis.
- Initial treatment for symptomatic popliteal cysts should be conservative treatment options or cyst and/or knee arthrocentesis with corticosteroid injection.
- Cysts that do not respond to conservative measures should be referred for surgical management.

POPLITEAL ARTERY ENTRAPMENT SYNDROME

Bittu Kuruvilla, MD, FAAPMR, CAQSM • Timothy Tiu, MD, FAAPMR, CAQSM

BASICS

DESCRIPTION

- Anatomic abnormality in popliteal artery entrapment syndrome (PAES) was first described in 1879 by Anderson Stuart, a 64-yr-old medical student, during anatomy dissections (1).
- Arterial insufficiency from external compression of the popliteal artery by surrounding musculotendinous structures (2):
  - Can have concurrent compression of popliteal vein and/or tibial nerve (2)

EPIDEMIOLOGY

- True incidence unknown (3)
- Prevalence ranges from 3.5% in cadaver studies to 0.6% (3,4).
- May be the underlying cause of claudication symptoms in young athletes in up to 60% of cases (3)
- Most frequently occurs in young men with well-developed muscles (athletes, military) (1).
- Occurs bilaterally in 29–67% cases (1)
- Average age: 32 yr (2)
- Male: female ratio ranges from 2:1 to 15:1 (1,3).

ETIOLOGY AND PATHOPHYSIOLOGY

- Two types:
  - Anatomic variations:
    - Congenital deviation of popliteal artery
    - Embryologic anomaly of musculotendinous structures surrounding popliteal artery (1)
  - Functional entrapment:
    - Popliteal artery compression demonstrated with stress maneuvers in symptomatic individuals but without any apparent anatomic abnormalities (1,3).
    - Associated with hypertrophy of the medial gastrocnemius, plantaris, and soleus (5)
- Progressive neovascularization, inflammatory cell infiltration, and vessel wall disruption leads to arterial wall fibrosis and replacement with collagen scar tissue (3):
  - Begins in adventitia (stage 1), then the media (stage 2), and finally the intima (stage 3) (3)
  - Progressive fibrosis of arterial wall leads to intraluminal stenosis, poststenotic dilation, and true aneurysm formation (3,4).
  - Intimal fibrosis results in thrombogenic flow surface, causing formation of mural thrombus (3).
  - Development of arterial occlusion in the diseased vessels occurs in a slow and chronic nature, allowing for the creation of collateral vessels (4).

RISK FACTORS

- Active individuals, without any atherosclerotic risk factors, who participate in activities involving excessive ankle dorsiflexion and plantar flexion (football, basketball, soccer, running on inclines, marching up/down hills) (6)
- Functional entrapment typically affects young, athletic women (average age 26 yr) (5,7).
- Anatomic entrapment typically affects middle-aged men (average age 46 yr) (5,7).

DIAGNOSIS

HISTORY

- Leg (calf or anterolateral compartment) and foot pain/claudication (deep ache or cramping) (5,6):
  - Symptoms are related to the degree of popliteal artery compression (6).
- Pain typically occurs suddenly after intense exercises involving the lower limbs and resolves quickly once activity ceases (3,6,7).
- Claudication may occur paradoxically with walking, rather than running, due to prolonged gastrocnemius contraction with walking (6).
- Paresthesia of foot occurs sometimes (3):
  - Repeated injury of tibial nerve during ankle dorsiflexion can cause paresthesia (4).
  - Paresthesia more common in PAES than chronic exertional compartment syndrome (5).
- Other symptoms: coldness, blanching and numbness of the calf/foot (3)
- Must ascertain details of training regimen, surface conditions, and shoe wear to rule out other common causes of leg/foot pain (6).

PHYSICAL EXAM

- If patent popliteal artery, generally will have normal physical exam at rest (6)
- Exam components:
  - Palpation of bones and soft tissues of the leg/foot for tenderness:
    - May elicit tenderness in calf only after exercise (6)
  - Evaluation for localized or diffuse edema
  - Palpation of bilateral dorsalis pedis and posterior tibial artery pulses for reduction in pulse volume between limbs (6):
    - Must be performed in neutral position and with stress maneuvers (6)
    - Stress maneuvers:
      - Passive ankle dorsiflexion with knee extended
      - Active plantar flexion with knee extended
      - Causes tension on gastrocnemius and induces external compression
- Stress ankle brachial index (ABI):
  - May be normal at rest (2)
  - Decrease in ABI during plantar flexion or post-exercise is indicative of vascular pathology (2).

DIFFERENTIAL DIAGNOSIS

- Chronic exertional compartment syndrome
- Muscle strains (gastrocnemius, soleus, plantaris)
- Tendinopathy
- Medial tibial stress syndrome
- Stress fracture
- Nerve entrapment (common peroneal nerve, superficial peroneal nerve, saphenous nerve)
- Arteritis (Buerger disease)
- Neurogenic claudication

DIAGNOSTIC TESTS & INTERPRETATION

Initial Tests (lab, imaging)

- Duplex ultrasound (DUS): commonly used for initial investigation (2):
  - Allows for anatomic evaluation with B-mode images as well as provides analysis of arterial flow during dynamic/stress maneuvers (4)
  - Initial imaging of artery done with leg in neutral position to evaluate for intimal changes, stenosis, or aneurysm, and evaluate velocity/waveform of arterial flow (8)
  - Repeat evaluation to be done after stress maneuvers with ankle plantarflexed against resistance (8):
    - Repeated plantar flexion until patient symptomatic may be needed (8)
    - All portions of popliteal artery must be assessed (above knee joint to below knee joint) (8).
  - Diagnostic sonographic finding: complete obstruction of flow within the popliteal artery (2)
  - Concurrent popliteal vein entrapment can be evaluated by squeezing calf to evaluate for normal venous flow (2).
  - Drawbacks: can overdiagnose occlusion
- Magnetic resonance imaging (MRI) and magnetic resonance angiogram (MRA):
  - Combination of stress positional T2-weighted MRI and MRA useful for visualization of anatomy in popliteal fossa and providing accurate arterial imaging (7)
  - Dynamic MRI/MRA imaging has been attempted but may result in motion artifact (7):
    - Patient asked to dorsiflex and plantarflex ankle with maximal exertion while T2-weighted 2D steady state axial images across popliteal region is obtained (8)
    - Patient to dorsiflex and plantarflex until pain is reproduced and then asked to maximally plantarflex while contrast MRA performed (8).
  - Drawbacks:
    - False-negative results can occur with <50% stenosis due to decreased spatial resolution of MRA (7).
    - Expensive (8)
    - Dynamic MRI/MRA imaging may result in motion artifact due to difficulty in maintaining muscle contraction during imaging (7).
- Computed tomography angiography (CTA):
  - Alternative diagnostic modality to MRA (2):
    - Less costly than MRI/MRA
  - Drawback: exposure to ionizing radiation
- Arteriography:
  - Gold standard test for PAES (6,7)
  - Can confirm diagnosis if PAES suspected on MRI/MRA (6)
  - Should be performed bilaterally after exercise or with provocative maneuvers (may be normal when ankle in neutral position) (6)
  - Drawbacks:
    - Invasive: involves placement of catheter and injection of radio-opaque contrast into artery of interest (6).
    - Exposure to ionizing radiation (6)
- Bone scans and radiography can be used to rule out stress fractures.

Follow-Up Tests & Special Considerations

- Median of three diagnostic evaluations needed before diagnosis (2)
- 1/3 to 1/2 of asymptomatic individuals can demonstrate popliteal artery narrowing or occlusion with resisted ankle dorsiflexion or plantar flexion (3).

Test Interpretation

PAES classification (2,3):

- Type 1: Popliteal artery passes medially and deep to normal medial head of gastrocnemius.
- Type II: Medial head of gastrocnemius inserts more laterally than usual resulting in the normally oriented popliteal artery to pass medial to the muscle.
- Type III: Medial head has accessory slip arising laterally, which compresses the popliteal artery.
- Type IV: Popliteal artery is compressed by running deep to popliteus muscle or by anomalous fibrous band.
- Type V: entrapment of popliteal vein
- Type IV: functional entrapment without any anatomic abnormality

TREATMENT

SURGERY/OTHER PROCEDURES

- Surgery advised in all cases for which PAES is confirmed to prevent long-term arterial damage (3,6)
- Entrapment types I to V:
  - If undamaged popliteal artery and stage 1 (early) disease:
    - Surgical exploration with division and resection of entrapment mechanism (medial head of gastrocnemius, abnormal muscle slips or tendinous bands) to restore normal arterial flow provides excellent outcomes (3,6).
    - For intermittent occlusion, timely musculotendinous release of popliteal artery has superior outcomes (2).
  - If any occlusion, stenosis or aneurysm: Placement of saphenous vein graft with division of any entrapment mechanism is recommended (3,6).
- Functional entrapment (type VI):
  - If no alternative explanations present for cause of symptoms, surgical treatment with division of origin medial head of gastrocnemius and resection of 1 cm of proximal muscle (3)
  - Resection of soleus fascia band distally, rather than myectomy of medial head of gastrocnemius, may provide adequate relief without muscle compromise in higher level athletes (7).
  - Botulinum toxin injections to area of hypertrophied muscle may provide same benefit as myotomy (7).
  - If evidence of arterial degeneration, vascular reconstruction is needed.

ONGOING CARE

PROGNOSIS

- PAES is generally considered progressive if left untreated (3):
  - Can result in eventual complete obstruction of popliteal artery causing risk of severe leg ischemia, disability, or limb loss (1)
  - Distal embolization of mural thrombus to peripheral vessels can occur, causing acute ischemia (4).
- Rate of arterial wall degeneration may depend on degree of compression and magnitude of compression rather than duration of compression (3).
- Poor medium-term patency if popliteal occlusion is treated with thrombolysis, angioplasty, or thrombectomy with patching (3)
- With acute occlusion, thrombolysis, and angioplasty alone have high risk of reocclusion and will not be effective without addressing underlying cause of entrapment:
  - Once thrombosis or aneurysm has occurred, arterial degeneration is severe and artery not salvageable (3).
- Excellent 10-yr patency with aneurysm repair or treatment of occlusion with saphenous vein bypass graft (3)
- Excellent results with myotomy for type VI entrapment (3)

REFERENCES

1. Tsilogianni Z, Grapatsas K, Papanikolaou Z, et al. Popliteal artery entrapment syndrome: a common cause of a rare clinical entity—critical leg ischemia in the young. *Mil Med*. 2014;179(1):e124–e126.
2. Hameed M, Coupland A, Davies AH. Popliteal artery entrapment syndrome: an approach to diagnosis and management. *Br J Sports Med*. 2018;52(16):1073–1074.
3. Levien L. Popliteal artery entrapment syndrome. *Semin Vasc Surg*. 2003;16(3):223–231.
4. Baltopoulos P, Filippou DK, Sigala F. Popliteal artery entrapment syndrome: anatomic or functional syndrome? *Clin J Sport Med*. 2004;14(1):8–12.
5. Turnipseed W. Functional popliteal artery entrapment syndrome: a poorly understood and often missed diagnosis that is frequently mistreated. *J Vasc Surg*. 2009;49(5):1189–1195.
6. Edwards PH Jr, Wright ML, Hartman JF. A practical approach for the differential diagnosis of chronic leg pain in the athlete. *Am J Sports Med*. 2005;33(8):1241–1249.
7. Joy S, Raudales R. Popliteal artery entrapment syndrome. *Curr Sports Med Rep*. 2015;14(5):364–367.
8. Williams C, Kennedy D, Bastian-Jordan M, et al. A new diagnostic approach to popliteal artery entrapment syndrome. *J Med Radiat Sci*. 2015;62(3):226–229.

ADDITIONAL READING

- Clemens M, Scott D, Watson J, et al. A diagnostic evolution: surgical experience with popliteal artery entrapment syndrome at a military tertiary referral center. *Ann Vasc Surg*. 2015;29(6):1078–1083.
- Hislop M, Brideaux A, Dhupelia S. Functional popliteal artery entrapment syndrome: use of ultrasound guided Botox injection as a non-surgical treatment option. *Skeletal Radiol*. 2017;46(9):1241–1248.
- Isner-Horobeti M, Muff G, Masat J, et al. Botulinum toxin as a treatment for functional popliteal artery entrapment syndrome. *Med Sci Sports Exerc*. 2015;47(6):1124–1127.
- Kwon Y, Kwon T, Gwon J, et al. Anatomical popliteal artery entrapment syndrome. *Ann Surg Treat Res*. 2018;94(5):262–269.
- Lejay A, Delay C, Georg Y. Five year outcomes of surgical treatment for popliteal artery entrapment syndrome. *Eur J Vasc Endovasc Surg*. 2016;51(4):557–564.
- Skeik N, Thomas TM, Engstrom BI, et al. Case report and literature review of popliteal artery entrapment syndrome. *Int J Gen Med*. 2015;8:221–225.

CLINICAL PEARLS

- Sudden onset of claudication symptoms in young adult with no atherosclerotic risk factors is highly suggestive of PAES (3).
- Isolated popliteal artery aneurysm or occlusion in young and physically active individuals should be considered due to PAES or cystic adventitial disease unless otherwise proven (3).
- If diagnosed early, PAES is the most common surgically correctable cause of leg claudication in young adults.
- No current evidence to suggest that surgical intervention is needed for asymptomatic patients with "functional entrapment" noted only on imaging studies without any anatomic abnormalities, given this likely represents a physiologic rather than pathologic finding (5)

POPLITEAL TENDONITIS

Laura Lintner, DO, CAQSM • Joshua Dilley, MD

BASICS

DESCRIPTION

- The popliteus muscle originates at the lateral condyle and travels underneath the biceps femoris tendon and lateral collateral ligament (LCL). It inserts on the posteromedial surface of the tibia and forms the floor of the popliteus fossa (1).
- Often, a popliteofibular ligament is also present. This anchors the early popliteus tendon to the proximal aspect of the fibula (2).
- The femoral origin of the popliteus is consistently anterior and distal to the femoral attachment of the LCL.
- The primary function of the popliteus muscle is internal rotation and stabilization of the tibia on the femur while walking (3).
- May help prevent forward translation of the femoral condyle relative to the lateral tibial plateau during downhill running
- Popliteal tendonitis is a cause of posterolateral knee pain due to inflammation of the popliteus tendon that connects the lateral femoral condyle to the proximal tibia.

EPIDEMIOLOGY

Rare, uncommon

ETIOLOGY AND PATHOPHYSIOLOGY

- May occur as overuse injury or acutely in case of trauma
- Popliteus tendonitis occurs due to repetitive stress on the popliteal tendon from training on inclined surfaces. Downhill running places stress on the popliteal tendon as it attempts to prevent forward displacement of the femoral condyle relative to the lateral tibial plateau.
- Mechanism of injury can be due to direct stretch or when overused to maintain posterolateral stability (3).
- There have been rare cases reported of acute calcific tendinopathy of the popliteus tendon.
- Case report of a cyamella (sesamoid bone) within the popliteus muscle causing popliteal tendonitis (4)

RISK FACTORS

- May be associated with pes planus due to increased external rotation of the tibia
- Long distance runners, especially those training on inclined surfaces
- Quadriceps weakness

GENERAL PREVENTION

- Appropriate warm-up before sports participation
- Avoid overtraining and running on incline or uneven surfaces.
- Consider foot orthoses for pes planus.
- Maintain good quadriceps strength.

COMMONLY ASSOCIATED CONDITIONS

True rupture of the popliteus tendon commonly occurs in combination with other posterior lateral corner injuries (3).

DIAGNOSIS

HISTORY

- Commonly presents with lateral knee pain when the knee is partially flexed 15 to 30 degrees while weight-bearing or when sitting cross legged
- Severe lateral knee pain accompanied by swelling (2)
- Pain during the initial swing phase of the gait (3)
- History of running, walking, or backpacking downhill (5)
- May describe trauma to the knee (hyperextension or direct force to anteromedial knee)

PHYSICAL EXAM

- Tenderness to palpation of posterolateral knee
- Gait analysis with posterior knee pain reported in initial swing phase
- Stable ligamentous exam with hemarthrosis could indicate rupture of the popliteus tendon (3).
- Posterolateral knee pain with resisted internal and external rotation of the tibia
- Figure-4 position: Have the patient flex, abduct, and externally rotate their hip so the ankle on the side of their affected knee rests on the contralateral knee (cross-legged position). Tenderness elicited particularly around the tendon insertion on the lateral femoral condyle may suggest popliteal tendonitis.
- Test the strength of the popliteal muscle by having the patient resist internal rotation of the tibia with their knee flexed at 90 degrees (Garrick test). Pain elicited with this maneuver suggests popliteal pathology.

DIFFERENTIAL DIAGNOSIS

- Posterior cruciate ligament injury
- Posterolateral corner injury
- Popliteal (Baker) cyst
- Hamstring strain
- Semimembranosus tendinopathy

DIAGNOSTIC TESTS & INTERPRETATION

- Can be a clinical diagnosis or diagnosis of exclusion
- X-rays are usually normal but may demonstrate calcifications on the lateral aspect of the knee (in the case of acute calcific popliteal tendinopathy).
- Ultrasound may demonstrate tendon hypoechogenicity, swelling, and increased Doppler signal.
- Magnetic resonance imaging (MRI) may demonstrate inflammation and edema surrounding the popliteus muscle.
- Arthroscopy alone may be inadequate for diagnosis due to poor visualization of the musculotendinous junction and femoral insertion (3); however, this can be valid diagnostic option in recalcitrant cases.

TREATMENT

GENERAL MEASURES

- Treatment plan for isolated popliteal tendon rupture has not been formalized (3)[C].
- Usually conservative with ice, rest, and nonsteroidal anti-inflammatory drugs (NSAIDs) for pain
- Avoid activity that aggravates pain (walking/running downhill) for at least 6 wk.
- Gradual return to activity
- Due to the rarity of an isolated popliteal tendon avulsion, consensus is not clear on conservative versus surgical management, as both have demonstrated success.

ISSUES FOR REFERRAL

- Ruptured tendon or calcific tendonitis
- Failed conservative treatment

MEDICATION

- Encourage patient to purchase shoes with good support.
- Orthotics may provide benefit to those with hyperpronation.

ADDITIONAL THERAPIES

- Physical therapy, including shock wave therapy, ultrasonography, dry needling, and massage are additional treatment options.
- Physical therapy may provide benefit through hamstring stretching and eccentric quadriceps strengthening (6)[C].

SURGERY/OTHER PROCEDURES

- Corticosteroid injections have shown benefit to those who do not respond to conservative therapy.
- Surgery may be performed for an avulsed tendon or if with failure to respond to conservative therapy for >6 mo.

Geriatric consideration

In elderly patients, surgery is indicated only when the knee is locked; potentially, this could be accomplished with simple resection (3).

ONGOING CARE

FOLLOW-UP RECOMMENDATIONS

- Treatment plan has not been formalized for isolated popliteal tendonitis (3).
- Consider follow-up after initial 6-wk conservative management for overuse popliteal tendonitis.
- Consider more immediate follow-up and management for acute popliteal pathology.

PATIENT EDUCATION

- Counsel on need for rest and compliance with physical therapy treatment.
- If recalcitrant, may require more invasive treatment options

PROGNOSIS

With proper treatment, activity adjustments, and biomechanical adjustments, the prognosis of popliteal tendonitis should follow a general pattern of healing for inflammatory tendon injury.

COMPLICATIONS

- Acute calcific tendonitis
- Tendon rupture

REFERENCES

1. Jadhav SP, More SR, Riascos RF, et al. Comprehensive review of the anatomy, function, and imaging of the popliteus and associated pathologic conditions. *Radiographics*. 2014;34(2):496–513.
2. Doucet C, Gotra A, Reddy SMV, et al. Acute calcific tendinopathy of the popliteus tendon: a rare case diagnosed using a multimodality imaging approach and treated conservatively. *Skeletal Radiol*. 2017;46(7):1003–1006.
3. English S, Perret D. Posterior knee pain. *Curr Rev Musculoskelet Med*. 2010;3(1–4):3–10.
4. Rehmatullah N, McNair R, Sanchez-Ballester J. A cyamella causing popliteal tendonitis. *Ann R Coll Surg Engl*. 2014;96(1):91E–93E.
5. Mayfield GW. Popliteus tendon tenosynovitis. *Am J Sports Med*. 1977;5(1):31–36.
6. Nyland J, Lachman N, Kocabey Y, et al. Anatomy, function, and rehabilitation of the popliteus musculotendinous complex. *J Orthop Sports Phys Ther*. 2005;35(3):165–179.

ADDITIONAL READING

- Petsche TS, Selesnick FH. Popliteus tendinitis: tips for diagnosis and management. *Phys Sportsmed*. 2002;30(8):27–31.
- Tennent TD, Goradia VK. Arthroscopic management of calcific tendinitis of the popliteus tendon. *Arthroscopy*. 2003;19(4):E35.

CLINICAL PEARLS

- Popliteal tendonitis is a rare cause of posterolateral knee pain most likely to occur in long distance runners or hikers (especially after significant downhill activity).
- In the case of acute pain over the posterolateral knee, acute calcific popliteal tendonitis or popliteal tendon rupture should be considered.
- The general treatment for popliteal tendonitis is rest, ice, anti-inflammatory medication, and avoidance of painful activity. Physical therapy for proper knee function, and lower extremity flexibility and strengthening, can assist in improvement.
- Gradual return to activity
- Recalcitrant cases could benefit from advanced imaging and possible cortisone injection or arthroscopic evaluation.

POSTERIOR CRUCIATE LIGAMENT (PCL) TEAR

Priscilla Tu, DO, FAAFP, FAOASM, DABMA • Briana Beach, DO

BASICS

DESCRIPTION

Rupture of any or all parts of the posterior cruciate ligament (PCL) of the knee (anterolateral portion and posteromedial portion)

EPIDEMIOLOGY

Incidence

- All knee injuries in general population 3% (1)
- Knee injuries in trauma patients 37% (1)
- Knee injuries in athletes <2%, although may be underreported and/or underdiagnosed (1)
- Of all PCL injuries, 45% are vehicular trauma and 40% from sport (2).
- 48% of patients will have combined ligament injuries (2).

RISK FACTORS

- Contact sports, especially American football
- Other sports, specifically soccer, skiing, and wrestling

COMMONLY ASSOCIATED CONDITIONS

- Anterior cruciate ligament (ACL) tear
- Lateral or medial collateral ligament tears
- Meniscal derangement
- Posterolateral corner injury
- Tibial plateau fractures
- Bony avulsions at the insertions of the cruciate ligament
- Avulsion fracture at the tibial tubercle
- Fibular head fracture
- Chondral injury
- Posterior knee subluxation or dislocation caused by hamstring force in the PCL-deficient knee

DIAGNOSIS

HISTORY

- "Dashboard injury": traumatic injury often seen in motor vehicle accidents, with posteriorly directed force to the anterior proximal tibia in a flexed knee (1)
- Similar mechanism to preceding in sports, particularly in American football and wrestling, resulting from an opponent's hit to lower leg driving tibia backward and rupturing PCL (2)
- Often in sports, fall onto flexed knee, particularly with foot plantarflexed
- Less commonly, cutting, twisting, and hyperextension injury in sports; often accompanied by other ligament injuries
- Unlike ACL injuries, often do not report hearing or feeling a "pop" or "tear" (3)
- Acute injuries:
  - Pain in the posterior knee
  - Pain with kneeling
  - Feeling of instability
- Chronic injuries:
  - Vague anterior knee pain
  - Pain with or inability to descend inclines/stairs, deceleration, or running at full stride

PHYSICAL EXAM

- Rapid onset (within few hours) of swelling and tenderness in knee
- May have difficulty walking or walk with slight limp
- Anterior patellar contusions may be seen.
- Posterior knee or popliteal ecchymosis may be found.
- Neurovascular examination:
  - Perform neurovascular examination before other provocative tests.
  - Important to determine and document associated nerve damage or vascular injury (particularly popliteal artery injury)

ALERT
If combined with an ACL injury, assume vascular injury, perform ankle-brachial index, and, if low stat, referral to vascular surgeon.

- Comprehensive knee examination:
  - Rule out dislocation.
  - Rule out other ligament or meniscus injuries.
- Posterior drawer test:
  - 90% sensitive and 99% specific for diagnosing PCL tears (4)
  - Perform with the patient supine and knee flexed at 90 degrees and hip flexed at 45 degrees.
  - Examiner stabilizes foot.
  - A posteriorly directed force is applied to the proximal tibia to elicit abnormal posterior tibial translation.
  - Posterior translation of 0 to 5 mm (grade 1), 5 to 10 mm (grade 2), and >10 mm (grade 3)
  - A secondary grading scale of the amount of posterior translation of the tibial plateau in relation to femoral condyles can also be used:
    - Grade A: plateau anterior to condyle
    - Grade B: plateau flush to condyle
    - Grade C: plateau posterior to condyle (5)
- Posterior sag test:
  - Perform with the patient supine and knee flexed at 90 degrees and hip flexed at 45 degrees.
  - Examiner stabilizes both heels.
  - Observe the knee from lateral perspective.
  - Normally, the tibial plateau sits ~1 cm anterior to the femoral condyles.
  - An abnormal contour, or sag, of the tibial plateau in relation to the femoral condyles is consistent with PCL deficiency.
- Quadriceps active test:
  - Perform with the patient supine and knee flexed at 90 degrees and hip flexed at 45 degrees.
  - Examiner stabilizes the foot, and the patient attempts to extend the knee while the examiner applies a counter force against the ankle.
  - Patient also may be asked to activate quadriceps by sliding foot down the table.
  - In a PCL-deficient knee, the posteriorly subluxed tibia will translate anteriorly with quadriceps activated.
- Dynamic posterior shift test:
  - Patient is supine with knee and hip flexed at 90 degrees.
  - Examiner slowly extends knee.
  - With a PCL tear, there will be "clunk" near full extension when the posteriorly subluxed tibia is reduced.

DIFFERENTIAL DIAGNOSIS

- ACL tear
- Tibial or fibular fracture
- Medial or lateral collateral ligament tear
- Meniscal derangement
- Posterolateral corner injury
- Knee and/or patella dislocation

DIAGNOSTIC TESTS & INTERPRETATION

- Radiographic evaluation with anteroposterior (AP), lateral, sunrise, and tunnel views to rule out bony avulsions, other fractures, or patellar subluxations
- Oblique views are sometimes helpful to rule out tibial plateau fractures.
- Flexion weight-bearing posteroanterior and patellar radiographs can help to distinguish early degenerative changes from chronic PCL deficiencies.
- Stress radiographs: 8 mm or more posterior tibial translation is indicative of complete PCL tear.
- Magnetic resonance imaging (MRI):
  - Reported to be up to 100% sensitive and specific in evaluating an acute complete PCL rupture
  - The healing process in chronic PCL injuries may mask the degree of tear on MRI.
  - No specific bone bruising pattern with PCL tears on MRI, but medial compartment bruising is associated with PCL–posterolateral corner injuries (3).
  - Also can evaluate other soft tissue pathology of the affected knee.

TREATMENT

GENERAL MEASURES

- Acute treatment:
  - Ice
  - Compression
  - Elevation
- Immobilization:
  - Partial weight-bearing
  - Possible immobilization in full extension for grade 3 lesions

ISSUES FOR REFERRAL

- Early orthopedic referral except in uncomplicated, isolated grade 1 and 2 lesions
- Early physical therapy referral may be beneficial because loss of proprioception and sprint speed are major problems with return to play.

ADDITIONAL THERAPIES

- Physical therapy
- No one protocol has been proven to have better outcomes than another (6).
- General concepts of nonoperative rehab programs:
  - Multiphase with time-specific and objective finding–related phases
  - Progressive weight-bearing
  - Quadriceps strengthening
  - Immobilization initially, with progressive addition of flexion until full range of motion (ROM) achieved
  - Functional PCL brace may be useful but not proven effective (6).

SURGERY/OTHER PROCEDURES

Indications include (6):

- Associated bony avulsion fractures.
- Multiple ligament injuries.
- Persistent pain in grade 3 lesions.
- Chronic symptomatic instability with activities of daily living or with sports.
- Acute grade 3 injury in young, active patient.

ONGOING CARE

COMPLICATIONS

- Nonoperative:
  - Chronic PCL laxity
  - Progressive medial compartment and patellofemoral degenerative changes
  - Increased risk of meniscal tears, articular cartilage injury with chronic PCL insufficiency
- Operative:
  - Most common: residual laxity
  - Iatrogenic neurovascular injury (especially of the popliteal artery)
  - Loss of motion
  - Infection
  - Medial femoral condyle osteonecrosis
  - Anterior knee pain
  - Painful hardware

REFERENCES

1. Wind WM Jr, Bergfeld JA, Parker RD. Evaluation and treatment of posterior cruciate ligament injuries: revisited. *Am J Sports Med*. 2004;32(7):1765–1775.
2. McAllister DR, Petrigliano FA. Diagnosis and treatment of posterior cruciate ligament injuries. *Curr Sports Med Rep*. 2007;6(5):293–299.
3. LaPrade CM, Civitarese DM, Rasmussen MT, et al. Emerging updates on the posterior cruciate ligament: a review of the current literature. *Am J Sports Med*. 2015;43(12):3077–3092.
4. Montgomery SR, Johnson JS, McAllister DR, et al. Surgical management of PCL injuries: indications, techniques, and outcomes. *Curr Rev Musculoskelet Med*. 2013;6(2):115–123.
5. Voos JE, Mauro CS, Wente T, et al. Posterior cruciate ligament: anatomy, biomechanics, and outcomes. *Am J Sports Med*. 2012;40(1):222–231.
6. Pierce CM, O'Brien L, Griffin LW, et al. Posterior cruciate ligament tears: functional and postoperative rehabilitation. *Knee Surg Sports Traumatol Arthrosc*. 2013;21(5):1071–1084.

ADDITIONAL READING

- Ahn JH, Lee SH, Choi SH, et al. Evaluation of clinical and magnetic resonance imaging results after treatment with casting and bracing for the acutely injured posterior cruciate ligament. *Arthroscopy*. 2011;27(12):1679–1687.
- Petrigliano FA, McAllister DR. Isolated posterior cruciate ligament injuries of the knee. *Sports Med Arthrosc Rev*. 2006;14(4):206–212.

CLINICAL PEARLS

- Posterior drawer is the most sensitive and specific test for PCL. If it shows >10 mm of posterior translation, have a high suspicion for posterolateral corner injury (4).
- In isolated grade 1 and 2 PCL tears, uncomplicated patients may be able to return to play with knee brace within 2 to 4 wk depending on the sport.
- In grade 3 injuries, uncomplicated patients may take up to 3 mo of rehabilitation before return to play.
- MRI is the imaging of choice for acute injuries, but stress radiographs may be more beneficial for chronic injuries.

POSTERIOR INTEROSSEOUS NERVE SYNDROME

Bjorn Allan Jacobson, MD • Richard Okragly, MD

BASICS

DESCRIPTION

- A peripheral nerve syndrome occurring in the extensor compartment of the forearm secondary to extrinsic compressive or intrinsic inflammatory processes
- Presenting as a painful spontaneous weakness of the extensor muscles supplied by the posterior interosseous nerve (PIN) without sensory deficits

EPIDEMIOLOGY

- Incidence reported as 3 per 100,000 people annually, although likely underestimated owing to underreporting and misdiagnosis
- Dominant arm is involved twice as much as the nondominant arm.
- More common in manual laborers, body builders, racquet sports
- Male > female (2:1)

RISK FACTORS

- Microtrauma from overuse/repetitive pronation and supination (usually strenuous activity)
- Trauma (Monteggia or radial head fractures)
- Autoimmune inflammatory disease (rheumatoid synovitis, Parsonage-Turner syndrome)
- Space-occupying lesions (lipoma, neuroma, ganglion, fibroma)
- Iatrogenic (elbow/forearm surgery)

ALERT

Extracorporeal compression (tight arm bands, e.g., holding a rifle sling wrapped around the forearm for prolonged periods, as seen in military recruits)

GENERAL PREVENTION

Avoidance of preventable risk factors

ETIOLOGY AND PATHOPHYSIOLOGY

- The PIN is a deep motor branch off of the radial nerve originating just proximal to the lateral epicondyle, coursing along the dorsal surface of the radius/interosseous membrane under the arcade of Frohse entering the forearm between the two heads of supinator and eventually dividing into medial and lateral branches innervating extensor carpi ulnaris, extensor digitorum communis, extensor digitorum minimi and abductor pollicus longus, extensor pollicus longus, extensor pollicis brevis, and extensor indicis proprius, respectively (1).
- Potential sites of extrinsic mechanical compression include the extensor carpi radialis brevis (ECRB), arcade of Frohse (fibrous arch formed by the superficial proximal supinator 3 to 5 cm distal to the lateral epicondyle), leash of Henry (recurrent radial vessels fanning out across the PIN at the level of the radial neck), and proximal > distal edge of the supinator (1).
- Net effect is a magnitude- and duration-dependent nerve ischemia reducing the capacity of the axons to transmit action potentials (1).

DIAGNOSIS

HISTORY

- Identifiable risk factor related to overuse usually present
- Progressive weakness of thumb, fingers, and wrist extension
- Pain in the forearm/wrist dependent on site of PIN pathology
- No sensory deficits

PHYSICAL EXAM

- In severe/chronic cases, forearm atrophy may be present.
- Sensation intact
- Weakness/inability to extend wrist in neutral or ulnar deviation, however able to extend wrist in radial deviation owing to preservation of ECRB/extensor carpi radialis longus (ECRL)
- Weakness/inability to extend fingers/thumb at the metacarpophalangeal joint
- Tenderness on deep palpation along proximal radius
- Resisted wrist supination or middle finger extension can provoke pain.

DIFFERENTIAL DIAGNOSIS

- Other radial nerve pathology:
  - Radial nerve palsy
  - Radial tunnel syndrome (lateral forearm pain only without neurologic deficits)
  - Wartenberg syndrome (sensory only, no motor)
- Cervical (C7) radiculopathy
- Lateral epicondylitis (tennis elbow)
- Forearm extensor tendon rupture

DIAGNOSTIC TESTS & INTERPRETATION

Initial Tests (lab, imaging)

- Plain radiographs: obtained to exclude osseous pathology
- Ultrasound (US; preferred imaging modality): can identify structural changes to the PIN including pathologic enlargement, site of entrapment with dynamic testing, and potentially secondary changes to distal structures; also can identify space-occupying lesions (2)[C]
- Magnetic resonance imaging (MRI): not always indicated but can demonstrate PIN neuritis, muscular denervation, and other pathology helpful in the event surgical intervention needed

Diagnostic Procedures/Other

Electromyography (EMG)/nerve conduction velocity studies (NCVS): used to identify anatomical location of nerve injury and exclude cervical radiculopathy, brachial plexopathy, or other polyneuropathy; findings:

- Normal sensory nerve action potentials (SNAPs)
- Slowed conduction velocity, prolonged distal latency, reduced amplitude compared to unaffected side
- Needle examination reveals membrane instability/abnormal spontaneous activity with positive sharp waves and fibrillations.
- Triceps, brachioradialis, and ECRB/ECRL are spared.
- Serial exams can document recovery (every 3 to 6 mo) (3)[C].

TREATMENT

- Guided by etiology
- Conservative management almost always first line:
  - Rest/activity modification/physical therapy
  - Anti-inflammatory medication
  - Immobilization
- Emergency department (ED) treatment:
  - Immobilize with a cock-up wrist splint.

MEDICATION

First Line

Nonsteroidal anti-inflammatory drugs (NSAIDs) (4)[C]:

- Use PRN as initial treatment in conjunction with activity modification.

Second Line

Corticosteroid injection (4)[C]:

- Placement dependent on location of pathology, usually 3 to 4 cm distal to lateral epicondyle
- Doses and types of corticosteroids vary but can include 1 cc of local anesthetic with 1 cc of corticosteroid.

ISSUES FOR REFERRAL

- Refractory cases (3 mo without improvement)
- Progressive symptoms despite conservative treatment

ADDITIONAL THERAPIES

Physical therapy that includes:

- Range of motion exercises that increase strength, endurance, and postural awareness
- Progressive strengthening and modified work-simulated tasks
- Application of heat and/or US
- Massage
- Duration of therapy varies from 1 to 6 mo.
- If severe, a dynamic splint is needed to hold the fingers in extension.
- Occupational therapy

SURGERY/OTHER PROCEDURES

Surgical decompression may be necessary in refractory cases or if an identifiable compressive lesion is present to avoid irreversible nerve/muscle damage.

ONGOING CARE

FOLLOW-UP RECOMMENDATIONS

Follow-up and physical therapy postoperatively to prevent contractures and stiffness

PROGNOSIS

Prognosis for full recovery is generally good with mean duration of symptoms around 3 to 4 mo.

REFERENCES

1. Sigamoney KV, Rashid A, Ng CY, et al. Management of atraumatic posterior interosseous nerve palsy. *J Hand Surg Am*. 2017;42(10):826–830.
2. Kim Y, Ha DH, Lee SM. Ultrasonographic findings of posterior interosseous nerve syndrome. *Ultrasonography*. 2017;36(4):363–369.
3. Bevelaqua AC, Hayter CL, Feinberg JH, et al. Posterior interosseous neuropathy: electrodiagnostic evaluation. *HSS J*. 2012;8(2):184–189.
4. Moradi A, Ebrahimzadeh MH, Jupiter JB. Radial tunnel syndrome, diagnostic and treatment dilemma. *Arch Bone Jt Surg*. 2015;3(3):156–162.

ADDITIONAL READING

Wheeless CR III. Posterior interosseous nerve compression syndrome. Wheeless' Textbook of Orthopaedics. www.wheelessonline.com. Updated January 21, 2013. Accessed September 24, 2018.

CLINICAL PEARLS

- History of repetitive forearm pronation/supination with key exam findings of forearm pain, extensor weakness, and normal sensation
- Good prognosis with activity modification and conservative management; surgery rarely needed

POSTEROLATERAL CAPSULAR TEAR

James M. Daniels, MD, MPH, RMSK, FAAFP, FACOEM, FACPM • Cesar Arguelles, MD, CAQSM • Johnny Tenegra, MD, MS

BASICS

DESCRIPTION

- The posterolateral corner (PLC) was once referred to as "the dark side of the knee" due to the limited understanding of the structures and how to treat them (1).
- An isolated injury of PLC is rare (2).
- Clinically important because it can complicate the treatment of other ligament injuries—anterior cruciate ligament (ACL) and posterior cruciate ligament (PCL).
- PLC laxity is more common than initially believed as it is associated with cruciate ligament injuries (missed diagnosis is common cause of ACL reconstruction failure).
- There are 10 main anatomic structures that make up the PLC of the knee:
  - Static structures:
    - Lateral cruciate ligament (LCL)
    - Popliteus tendon (PT)
    - Popliteus ligament
    - Lateral capsule
    - Arcuate ligament (variable)
    - Fabellofibular ligament and fibula (variable)
  - Dynamic structures:
    - Biceps femoris
    - Popliteus muscle
    - Iliotibial (IT) tract
    - Lateral head of gastrocnemius
- Recent studies noted three primary stabilizers of the lateral knee in the PLC:
  - Fibular collateral ligament (FCL): originates femoral lateral condyle and inserts (after combining with the biceps femoris to form the conjoint tendon) onto the anterior aspect of the fibula. It serves as the primary varus stabilizer of the knee in late knee flexion.
  - PT: Its femoral attachment is the most anterior aspect of the PLC. Before this, it courses through a sulcus which includes a small tunnel through the lateral meniscus. It becomes the popliteus muscle which inserts into the posterior aspect of the tibia. This structure resists external rotation of the knee.
  - Popliteofibular ligament (PFL). This ligament acts like a sling to hold the popliteus muscle/tendon complex down against the posterior lateral portion of the tibia. It is a varus stabilizer of the knee in extension. It has two divisions: the anterior and the more robust posterior. They wrap around the musculotendinous junction of the popliteus muscle/tendon and then inserts onto the fibular styloid process.
- Grading of PLC injuries is done in full knee extension and then with 30 degrees of knee flexion; this can be affected by presence of effusion or pain.
- Place a varus stress with knee in extension; if opens up over 4 mm compared to opposite side, impacts the PCL tear
- Then test at 30 degrees and compare to other side. If point of care ultrasound (POCUS) is available, it adds accuracy to exam.

EPIDEMIOLOGY

- Most PLC injuries are associated with ACL or PCL injuries. Only 28% of PLC occur in isolation. An isolated injury is one of the least common traumatic problems of the knee (<2% of all ligament injuries to the knee).
- The main reason this injury has to be considered is that failure to diagnose a PLC injury in patients with ACL or PCL injuries can lead to graft failure and/or premature arthritis of the knee.

ETIOLOGY AND PATHOPHYSIOLOGY

- Associated with an acute episode of injury. If this is not part of the history, doubt the diagnosis of PLC injury.
- High-velocity injury:
  - Falls, land on fully extended lower extremity
  - Knee then "fails" in varus, hyperextended position then buckles
- Any knee hyperextension injury (contact and noncontact)
- Knee dislocation
- High-velocity varus blow to anteromedial aspect of knee
- Varus blow to flexed knee
- All these patients *must* have a neuro (fibular nerve) exam, specifically "toe raise."
- All these patients *must* have a vascular exam; "two-second" capillary refill and palpitation of posterior tibialis, dorsalis pedis pulse

RISK FACTORS

- Female gender
- Sports competition (vs. practice)
- Contact sports
- American football
- Prior knee or ankle injury

COMMONLY ASSOCIATED CONDITIONS

- ACL tears
- PCL tears
- Knee dislocation
- Lateral meniscus tear
- Fibular nerve injury
- Vascular injury to popliteal artery
- Bone contusion

Geriatric Considerations

PLC injuries can be associated with tibial plateau fractures in osteopenic elderly patients. They may be weight-bearing despite of severe injury and knee effusion. In this group of patients with these clinical findings, the clinician should have an increased index of suspicion. Even if x-ray is negative, a computed tomography (CT) will often show the fracture.

Pediatric Considerations

Salter-Harris (SH) fracture of tibia can occur. The definition of type I SH fracture is tenderness over physis and "negative" original radiograph. PLC injuries are more posterior and proximal than joint line on palpation.

DIAGNOSIS

HISTORY

- Not as common in pediatric or geriatric population
- Any injury that may hyperextend, externally rotate, or force the tibia into varus angle can injure the PLC (1)[A].
- A posterolateral blow to the anteromedial portion of the tibia (1)[A]
- Contact and noncontact; low or high velocity (1)[A]
- Important to obtain the mechanism of injury to a hyperextended knee or knee dislocation (1)[A]
- Difficult to make diagnosis without some type of history of trauma (1)[A]
- Chronic injury may present with gait issues or difficulty using stairs (1)[A].
- Often have instability symptoms with full knee extension (1)[A]
- Often associated with other injuries; most common is with ACL and then PCL; may also injure common fibular nerve or blood supply from geniculate artery

PHYSICAL EXAM

- Primary trauma evaluation: airway, breathing, circulation
- Neuro: especially fibular nerve great toe extension, ankle dorsiflexion
- Vascular: dorsalis pedis, posterior tibialis
- Effusion/pain has a big effect on musculoskeletal (MSK) exam.
- Ottawa Rules for radiographic evaluations are very helpful; if the patient flunks Ottawa Rules, very low chance of acute PLC injury:
  - Ottawa Knee Rules: Obtain radiographs if:
    - 55 yr of age or older.
    - Isolated tenderness over patella.
    - Tenderness over head of fibula.
    - Inability to flex knee to 90 degrees.
    - Inability to bear weight four steps.
- Because PLC injuries rarely occur in isolation, other injuries should be evaluated. If no end point on any ligament test or if more than one ligament is lax, assume knee dislocation and treat as such:
  - *ACL*—Lachman, pivot shift
  - *PCL*—prominent tibial plateau, posterior sag test, quad active flexion test
  - *LCL*—varus force to knee in full extension. If opens up >10 degrees difference from other knee, suspect both PCL and LCL injury would be at very high risk for PLC injury. If opens up 30 degrees, suspect LCL only.
- Use of POCUS allows more precise measurement (2)[C].
- Tests more specific for PLC:
  - These maneuvers are not well studied, but when used in an additive fashion (all negative or positive), they are useful in ruling out/in PLC injury (2)[C].
  - *External rotation recurvatum test*: Some literature state that this test is inconsistent, but with an added modification, it is useful, and when present, also should make one suspicious for an ACL tear. Patient is in supine position; the examiner stabilizes the femur by pushing downward in the quadriceps area just proximal to the patella. With the other hand, the examiner grasps the patient's great toe and lifts. A measurement is taken from the heel of the raised leg and the table. The opposite leg is also tested, and any difference over a centimeter indicates a positive test (2)[B]. A recent study discovered that only 10% of PLC injuries had a positive test, but a positive test had a good predictive value for patients with both PLC and ALC tears (1)[B].

- *Dial test*: Patient is in prone position. The examiner grabs the patient's forefoot while allowing their heels to touch. The knees are flexed 30 degrees, then externally rotated by the examiner. The knees are then flexed 90 degrees, and the same test is done. If there is >10 degrees difference with the other knee at either position, result is a positive test. If the difference is at 30 degrees of flexion, it implicates the PLC. If the difference is 90 degrees of flexion, it implicates both the PLC and the PCL (1,3)[B]. Recently, this test's ability to diagnose minor injuries has been called into question (1)[B].
- *Reverse pivot shift test*: essential component of the PLC evaluation, positive predictive value 68%, and negative predictive value 89%. Patient should be in supine position with knee flexed 90 degrees. The lateral joint line is palpated, and the knee is slowly extended while the examiner places a valgus force and external rotation on the tibia. As approximately 30 to 40 degrees of flexion if the knee subluxes, it indicates a positive test (1)[B].
- *Posterolateral drawer test*: a difficult test to learn. Only positive with high-grade PLC injury. Patient supine with knee flexed 90 degrees, foot flat on table. Examiner places a posterior, external rotation force on the proximal tibia. If the tibial tuberosity rotates in reference to the femur, it is a positive test (1)[B].

DIFFERENTIAL DIAGNOSIS

- ACL tear
- PCL tear
- Knee dislocation
- Tibial plateau fracture
- Growth plate injury
- Bone contusion
- Lateral meniscus tear
- IT band subluxation at knee
- Fibular nerve injury
- Vascular injury to geniculate artery system (2,3)[B]

DIAGNOSTIC TESTS & INTERPRETATION

- Ottawa or Pittsburgh Knee Rules
- Anteroposterior (AP), lateral, sunrise views
- Varus stress views, if injury is chronic:
  - This is to evaluate if there is enough deformity to justify wedge osteotomy. 4-mm difference from opposite side indicates severe PLC tear and possible PCL injury.
- POCUS; some authors routinely scan all of their ACL injuries to rule out injury to popliteus and LCL. The PFL is more difficult to scan.
- Magnetic resonance imaging (MRI) is the gold standard for diagnosis of PLC injury because it also evaluates cruciate ligament injuries.

ALERT

On radiographs, look for arcuate sign, an avulsion fracture for the fibular head associated with PLC injury and ACL injury, and the Segond fracture, avulsion fracture from lateral tibial plateau associated with ACL injury.

TREATMENT

- Because an isolated injury of the PLC is extremely rare and most PLC injuries are associated with multiple ligament injuries to the knee, some authors, including our faculty, promote treating all of these injuries as grade III, with immobilization, non–weight-bearing, and close (within 48 hr) follow-up with an orthopedic surgeon (1,2)[C].
- Table 1 describes the grades of injury and their specific treatments.

Grade	Definition	Amount of Ligament Pathology	Treatment
Grade I	0–5 mm of lateral opening	Minimal ligament disruption	Hinge brace Crutches Allow knee flexion Exercise, weight-bearing 4–5 wk
Grade II	5–10 mm of lateral opening	Moderate ligament disruption	Crutches Knee immobilizer Non–weight-bearing × 3 wk Then treat like grade I
Grade III	>10 mm of lateral opening	Severe ligament disruption (no end point)	Immobilizer Non–weight-bearing Crutches Orthopedic referral

ALERT

Grading can be difficult without experience and POCUS, and a good working relationship (or phone consult) with an experienced orthopedic surgeon is very helpful. It is perfectly fine to treat all of these injuries as a grade III, especially if other injuries, (i.e., ACL, PCL, meniscus) are suspected.

ADDITIONAL THERAPIES

- In addition to repairing other ligaments (ACL, PCL, etc.), the PLC can be repaired with graft augmentation and fibular head stabilization suing suture anchors and screws if the patient is seen within 2 wk of the injury; otherwise, PLC reconstruction is needed.
- PLC reconstruction is used for most grade III injuries and even for lower grade injuries because there is evidence that reconstruction has better outcomes than repair (1,2)[B].

ONGOING CARE

COMPLICATIONS

- Fibular nerve injury
- Vascular injury
- Physical injury
- Multiple ligament injury
- If ACL or PCL is repaired and PLC injury is missed, early arthritis and graft failure occur.
- Arthrofibrosis (1,2,3)[B]

REFERENCES

1. Chahla J, Moatshe G, Dean CS, et al. Posterolateral corner of the knee: current concepts. *Arch Bone Jt Surg*. 2016;4(2):97–103.
2. Pacheco RJ, Ayre CA, Bollen Sr. Posterolateral corner injuries of the knee: a serious injury commonly missed. *J Bone Joint Surg Br*. 2011;93(2):194–197.
3. Schweller EW, Ward PJ. Posterolateral corner knee injuries: review of anatomy and clinical evaluation. *J Am Osteopath Assoc*. 2015;115(12):725–731.

ADDITIONAL READING

- Geiger D, Chang E, Pathria M, et al. Posterolateral and posteromedial corner injuries of the knee. *Radiol Clin North Am*. 2013;51(3):413–432.
- Sekiya JK, Swaringen JC, Wojtys EM, et al. Diagnostic ultrasound evaluation of posterolateral corner knee injuries. *Arthroscopy*. 2010;26(4):494–499.
- Stiell IG, Greenberg GH, Wells GA, et al. Prospective validation of a decision rule for the use of radiography in acute knee injuries. *JAMA*. 1996;275(8):611–615.
- Stoller DW. The Knee. In: *Stoller's Atlas of Orthopaedics and Sports Medicine*. Philadelphia, PA: Wolters Kluwer/Lippincott Williams & Wilkins; 2008:261–424.
- Vinson EN, Major NM, Helms CA. The posterolateral corner of the knee. *AJR Am J Roentgenol*. 2008;190(2):449–458.

CLINICAL PEARLS

- PLC injuries are often associated with other ligament injuries.
- Always perform a neurovascular check:
  - Foot dorsiflexion
  - Palpate dorsalis pedis pulse.
  - Posterior tibial pulse
- Look for Segond and arcuate fractures.
- Evaluate whole knee (i.e., Ottawa Rules good start looking for other pathology).
- Because this injury is often associated with multiligament pathology, some clinicians consult orthopedic surgery on every suspected case.

PREGNANCY IN SPORTS

David E. Olson, MD, CAQSM, FACSM • Priya Nagarajan, DO • Mark L. Nelson, MD

BASICS

American College of Obstetricians and Gynecologists (ACOG) 2002 recommendations for exercise in pregnancy:

- Women without contraindications should and can safely participate in aerobic and strength exercise when pregnant.
- In the absence of either medical or obstetrical complications, pregnant women should participate in 30 min or more of moderate intensity exercise on most, if not all, days of the week. There is no evidence that this is detrimental to the woman or fetus if the pregnancy is uncomplicated.
- A thorough clinical evaluation should be performed prior to the initiation of any exercise program. In the absence of contraindications, regular and moderate intensity exercise is advised. Women should be counseled on warning signs of when to stop exercise.
- Avoid activities with a high risk of falling or trauma such as hockey, soccer, basketball, gymnastics, horseback riding, downhill skiing, racquet sports, and scuba diving. Women should avoid exercises where they will be in the supine position or exposed to prolonged motionless standing.
- Women who plan to exercise at altitudes of >6,000 feet should be made aware of signs of altitude sickness.
- Recommended exercises include walking, hiking, jogging/running, aerobic dance, swimming, cycling, rowing, cross-country skiing, and dancing.
- Athletes participating in National Collegiate Athletic Association (NCAA) or professional sports may continue to participate in sports during the early phases of pregnancy. However, they should be made aware of the risks and benefits of continued participation in high-level sports and they should be monitored more closely.
- As pregnancy progresses, athletic performance tends to decline. The physical demands of high-intensity training should be balanced with close monitoring of body temperature, hydration status, and weight. Patients engaged in high-intensity training should be seen more frequently than their routine prenatal visits.
- Gradual resumption of exercise in the postpartum period is advised.
- Return to physical activity after pregnancy has been associated with decreased incidence of postpartum depression if the exercise is felt to be stress relieving (1,2,3).

ETIOLOGY AND PATHOPHYSIOLOGY

- Thermoregulation:
  - In active nonpregnant women, exercise can elevate body temperature >103°F (39.2°C). Current recommendations are that core body temperature should not rise >1.5°C above resting temperature or >38.9°C during exercise in pregnancy (4,5).
  - Studies show that women appear well protected against hyperthermia even during prolonged exercise when the intensity is low. However, nearly all previous studies have been performed in women who trained prior to the study, and no prospective trials exist that focus primarily on the risk of elevated temperatures. Also, no human study has elicited an increase of >1.1°C in maternal core temperature during pregnancy in response to exercise (4,6,7,8).
- Metabolic changes:
  - Utilization of glucose is of potential concern for the fetus. However, no studies have shown an actual decrease in fetal growth during exercise because there is likely increased glucose delivery after exercise, and women who exercise may have an increased placental size. Regular aerobic exercise has been shown to lower fasting and postprandial glucose concentrations in several small studies of previously sedentary individuals with gestational diabetes mellitus (GDM) (2,7,9,10).
- Lower back and pelvic pain:
  - These symptoms are commonly associated with hormonal change. The increased levels of estrogen and relaxin in pregnancy lead to increased ligamentous laxity associated with back and pelvic pain.
  - Symptoms may be exacerbated with weight-bearing and activity.
  - Sitting, rest, and recumbency often ameliorate symptoms, and good results have been seen following acupuncture and use of a pelvic binder.
  - Hyperlordosis of pregnancy is associated with ligamentous laxity.
  - Pubic symphysis pain is caused by widening of the pubic symphysis due in part to the effects of relaxin:
    - Rupture of the pubic symphysis is a rare complication.
    - Treatment of this is generally conservative.
    - Consideration of operative intervention is needed if diastasis is >4 cm.
- Careful monitoring of women who become pregnant within a few months of anterior cruciate ligament (ACL) reconstruction is recommended (11).
- Cardiopulmonary changes:
  - Cardiac output may increase up to 40% by as early as 24 weeks' gestation.
  - After 30 weeks' gestation, cardiac output is greatly influenced by body position. Specifically, a recumbent position may decrease cardiac output.
  - Decreased splanchnic blood flow may result from the effects of exercise potentially compromising uterine or umbilical artery blood flow:
    - Doppler ultrasound (US) has shown no change in perfusion to either artery.
    - An increase in fetal heart rate (FHR) may occur during maternal exercise.
    - A small percentage of fetuses have developed bradycardia or decelerations in response to maternal exercise. Episodes of bradycardia resolved within 2 min and were not thought to be substantial enough to result in fetal hypoxia. Additionally, there were no identifiable adverse birth outcomes (12).
    - Iron supplementation is advised. It is not uncommon for a pregnant female to have a hemoglobin of 12.5 m/dL or less (2,7).

GENERAL PREVENTION

- Warning signs to terminate exercise while pregnant (1,3,4):
  - Vaginal bleeding
  - Dyspnea prior to exertion
  - Dizziness
  - Headache
  - Chest pain
  - Muscle weakness
  - Calf pain or swelling
  - Preterm labor
  - Decreased fetal movements
  - Amniotic fluid leakage
- Absolute contraindications to exercise in pregnancy (1,3,4):
  - Incompetent cervix
  - Intrauterine growth restriction (IUGR)
  - Multiple gestations (more than triplets)
  - Persistent 2nd- or 3rd-trimester bleeding
  - Placenta previa after 25 to 28 wk of gestation
  - Preeclampsia
  - Pregnancy-induced hypertension (HTN)
  - Premature labor during current or prior pregnancy
  - Premature rupture of membranes
  - Risk of premature labor

COMMONLY ASSOCIATED CONDITIONS

- Orthopedic considerations during pregnancy include:
  - Soft tissue swelling in the 2nd and 3rd trimesters; this may manifest as carpal tunnel syndrome (CTS):
    - Elevated prolactin, fluid retention, and hand positioning during nursing may worsen symptoms.
  - de Quervain tenosynovitis and meralgia paresthetica, neuropathy of the lateral femoral cutaneous nerve, are often seen.
  - Symptoms from nerve compression syndromes typically resolve after pregnancy and should be treated conservatively.
  - Night splints can relieve CTS, and steroid injections are useful in patients with recalcitrant symptoms. Similar treatments are recommended for de Quervain patients. For patients with meralgia paresthetica, loose-fitting clothes, positional changes, and activity modification often relieve symptoms.
- In late pregnancy and after delivery, transient changes in cortisol and clotting factors can lead to femoral head osteonecrosis:
  - Symptoms can include antalgic gait, pain at rest, and painful range of motion.
  - Treatment consists of restricted weight-bearing; avoid surgery until after delivery.

- Transient osteoporosis of pregnancy should be suspected in any patient with an antalgic gait and complaints of pain with activity, with minimal pain at rest (5,6,9):
  - Usually presents in the 3rd trimester and plain anteroposterior (AP) radiographs with appropriate shielding often show diffuse osteopenia of the pelvis:
    - Magnetic resonance imaging (MRI) may show high-intensity signal in the bone marrow on T2 images.
  - Treatment consists of protected weight-bearing. Use of calcitonin is controversial but may shorten the duration of symptoms; bisphosphonate exposure during gestation may lead to decreased fetal bone growth.
  - Transient osteoporosis of pregnancy usually results in a self-limited course with no long-term sequelae; however, failure to properly diagnose could lead to fracture.
  - Serial exams are important to distinguish between these conditions. The clinician should try to avoid unnecessary radiographs because hip pain is common in pregnancy.

ONGOING CARE

Specific sport recommendations include (12):

- Stationary upright cycling is recommended by the Society of Obstetricians and Gynecologists of Canada (SOGC) and American College of Sports Medicine (ACSM):
  - FHR and maternal temperature are not negatively affected. However, there may be more variability of FHR and maternal temperature with higher intensity and longer duration exercise.
  - No negative fetal outcomes have been reported.
  - Cycling for 30 min at a maternal heart rate around 140 beats per min (bpm) or exercising for 15 min at a rate of 155 bpm is recommended.
- Swimming is an optimal exercise during pregnancy due to buoyant effects and the thermally conductive properties of water. It is recommended by ACOG, SOGC, and ACSM:
  - Baseline FHR may be less affected by swimming than cycling (1,3,10).
- Many women use walking as a primary means of exercise throughout pregnancy:
  - Walking is recommended by ACOG, SOGC, and ACSM. It increases maternal sense of well-being and decreases physical complaints.
  - It has not been shown to have a negative effect on maternal weight gain or on labor outcomes (12).
- Weight-training exercises and physical therapy have been recommended by ACOG to help maintain posture and prevent low back pain:
  - No incidents of adverse effects have been reported with light to moderate weight training with free weights or weight machines.
  - Moderate strength conditioning has been shown to be safe in a healthy pregnancy with no obvious positive or negative effects; minimal FHR changes from baseline and fetal wakefulness is increased.
  - Avoid weight training in the supine position late in gestation (10,12).
- SCUBA diving is not endorsed by the ACOG:
  - Those who dive frequently and professionally are at 3 to 6 times greater risk for spontaneous abortion, IUGR, and fetal malformation (1,12).
- High-altitude exercise: Few cases of injury have been reported with exercises such as skiing, hiking, mountain biking, and running:
  - Pregnancy complications such as low birth weight occur at a higher rate at altitudes >10,000 feet. SOGC has suggested women to modify or avoid mountain climbing all together. Cycling with short bursts of moderate to high intensity at altitude levels of 6,000 and 7,300 feet have been reported without injury to mother or fetus (10,12).
  - Sports with abdominal trauma risk from contact or falling such as downhill skiing, water skiing, horseback riding, road cycling, surfing, basketball, racquet sports, ice hockey, soccer, and gymnastics are discouraged (3,12).
- Running can become uncomfortable later in gestation:
  - Jogging is supported by ACOG. It may enhance placental growth, indicating a healthy pregnancy outcome (11).
- Women who continue to exercise throughout pregnancy generally maintain their training regimens and level of fitness. Among these women, cardiovascular risk level generally continues well below levels among the general populace and women who temporarily stopped exercise during pregnancy (10,11).

REFERENCES

1. Committee on Obstetric Practice. ACOG committee opinion. Exercise during pregnancy and the postpartum period. Number 267, January 2002. American College of Obstetricians and Gynecologists. *Int J Gynaecol Obstet*. 2002;77(1):79–81.
2. Artal R, O'Toole M. Guidelines of the American College of Obstetricians and Gynecologists for exercise during pregnancy and the postpartum period. *Br J Sports Med*. 2003;37(1):6–12.
3. Kramer MS, McDonald SW. Aerobic exercise for women during pregnancy. *Cochrane Database Syst Rev*. 2006;(3):CD000180.
4. Olson DA, Sikka RS, Hayman J, et al. Exercise in pregnancy. *Curr Sports Med Rep*. 2009;8(3):147–153.
5. Ritchie JR. Orthopedic considerations during pregnancy. *Clin Obstet Gynecol*. 2003;46(2):456–466.
6. Artal R, Fortunato V, Welton A, et al. A comparison of cardiopulmonary adaptations to exercise in pregnancy at sea level and altitude. *Am J Obstet Gynecol*. 1995;172(4, Pt 1):1170–1178.
7. Clapp JF III. Exercise during pregnancy. A clinical update. *Clin Sports Med*. 2000;19(2):273–286.
8. Soultanakis-Aligianni HN. Thermoregulation during exercise in pregnancy. *Clin Obstet Gynecol*. 2003;46(2):442–455.
9. Borg-Stein J, Dugan SA, Gruber J. Musculoskeletal aspects of pregnancy. *Am J Phys Med Rehabil*. 2005;84(3):180–192.
10. Clapp JF III. Long-term outcome after exercising throughout pregnancy: fitness and cardiovascular risk. *Am J Obstet Gynecol*. 2008;199(5):489.e1–489.e6.
11. Guerra JJ, Steinberg ME. Distinguishing transient osteoporosis from avascular necrosis of the hip. *J Bone Joint Surg Am*. 1995;77(4):616–624.
12. Blecher AM, Richmond JC. Transient laxity of an anterior cruciate ligament-reconstructed knee related to pregnancy. *Arthroscopy*. 1998;14(1):77–79.

ADDITIONAL READING

- Cunningham FG, Gant NF, Leveno KJ, eds., et al. *Williams Obstetrics*. 21st ed. New York, NY: McGraw-Hill; 2001:109–195.
- Drinkwater B, Artal R. Heat stress and pregnancy. In: Mittlemark R, Drinkwater B, eds. *Exercise in Pregnancy*. Baltimore, MD: Williams and Wilkins; 1991.

CLINICAL PEARLS

- Positive effects of exercise during pregnancy include potential risk reduction for development of GDM, pregnancy-induced HTN, and preeclampsia; also, a decrease in postpartum depression symptoms and decreased incidence of urinary incontinence
- Exercise during pregnancy does not increase the risk for preterm birth.
- The cardiovascular benefits of exercise are the same for pregnant women as they are for nonpregnant women.
- Exercise in morbidly obese women may have a preventative effect on the development of GDM.
- All pregnant women should be evaluated for medical and/or obstetrical contraindications prior to beginning an exercise regimen (1,3,4).
- Recreational and competitive athletes with uncomplicated pregnancies should remain active. They should be monitored by regular prenatal visits unless participating in high-intensity exercise.
- Sedentary individuals without contraindications should be encouraged to begin exercising for the health benefits.
- Women with an increased risk for preterm labor or fetal growth restriction should be advised to reduce their activity in the 2nd and 3rd trimesters.
- Women participating in higher intensity sports should be monitored closely throughout their pregnancy.

PRONATOR SYNDROME

Kevin E. Burroughs, MD, CAQSM

BASICS

Seyffarth first described compression of the median nerve as it passes through the pronator teres just distal to the elbow in 1951 (1,2).

DESCRIPTION

- Classically, entrapment of the median nerve occurring between the humeral and ulnar heads of the pronator teres muscle, or at a tight fibrous arch proximally between the heads of the flexor digitorum superficialis, the sublimis arch
- However, can also occur at the ligament of Struthers, the lacertus fibrosus, or due to an accessory head of the flexor pollicis longus
- Compression between the heads of the pronator teres muscle is the most common etiology, with the sublimis arch the second most common.
- Synonym(s): lacertus fibrosus syndrome; pronator teres syndrome; sublimis bridge syndrome

EPIDEMIOLOGY

- Relatively uncommon but should be considered in any patient with carpal tunnel symptoms or volar hand numbness
- Carpal tunnel syndrome (CTS) is responsible for >90% of cases of median nerve entrapment neuropathies.

Prevalence

- Usually presents in the 5th decade and 4 times more common in women
- Delay in diagnosis ranging from 9 mo to 2 yr

ETIOLOGY AND PATHOPHYSIOLOGY

- In >80% of individuals, the pronator teres arises from two heads, superficial (humeral) and deep (ulnar), and the median nerve travels between as it enters the antecubital area.
- Variants have been demonstrated where the nerve travels posterior to both heads, under a single head, or pierces the superficial head.
- Compression can occur proximally in individuals with a supracondyloid process. This is an anomalous bone spur on the anteromedial distal 1/3 of the humerus and occurs in 1% of people of European ancestry.

RISK FACTORS

- Repetitive occupational pronation/supination
- Acute forceful pronation or wrist flexion
- Weight lifters with hypertrophied pronator-flexor mass

DIAGNOSIS

HISTORY

- Typically, patients complain of an aching or fatigue-like pain in proximal forearm. Other symptoms may include occasional hand pain, dysesthesias of the radial 3 1/2 digits, and cramping in the hand (writer's cramp).
- Many report an increase in pain with exercise or an increase in activity.
- Frank hand weakness occurs only in long-standing or severe cases.
- Motor and sensory symptoms can be poorly defined.
- Onset typically is insidious, but a specific event may cause a sudden increase in pain.
- Typically, pain does not occur at night, as it would with CTS.

PHYSICAL EXAM

- Thickened or hypertrophied pronator muscle mass
- Tenderness or positive Tinel sign proximal and lateral to the proximal edge of the pronator muscle typical. Compression at this site causes pain or paresthesias radiating to the palm and/or radial 3 1/2 digits within 30 sec of compression.
- May have weakness or atrophy of the hand intrinsics innervated by the median nerve (LOAF muscles): lumbricals (first two on radial side of hand), opponens pollicis, abductor pollicis brevis, and flexor pollicis brevis
- May have weakness of the extrinsic finger flexors, wrist flexors, and pronator quadratus

ALERT

Pronator syndrome should not have a Tinel sign at the wrist nor reproduction of symptoms with nerve compression testing at the wrist.

- Tests of Spinner can determine location of median nerve entrapment:
  - Pain or paresthesia reproduced with resisted flexion of the forearm in a position of >120 degrees of elbow extension, maximal supination: lacertus entrapment of median nerve
  - Reproduction of pain or paresthesia with resisted pronation (forearm in neutral) as the elbow is extended: pronator entrapment of median nerve
  - Reproduction of symptoms with resisted proximal interphalangeal (PIP) joint flexion of the middle finger with forearm fully supinated and elbow extended: flexor digitorum superficialis entrapment of median nerve (caution, can be present with CTS as well)

DIFFERENTIAL DIAGNOSIS

- CTS (common): Double crush phenomena can occur where both CTS and pronator syndrome appear in same arm up to 6%. Consider possibility particularly in those with failed CTS surgery (3).
- C6 or C7 radiculopathy (common)
- Anterior interosseous syndrome (Kiloh-Nevin syndrome) (uncommon, motor function affected, *not sensory symptoms*)
- Thoracic outlet syndrome (rare)
- Neuralgic amyotrophy (brachial neuritis, Parsonage-Turner syndrome) (rare)

DIAGNOSTIC TESTS & INTERPRETATION

Initial Tests (lab, imaging)

- Plain radiographs of the elbow rule out bone involvement such as a supracondyloid process (exostosis that attaches to ligament of Struthers).
- Magnetic resonance imaging (MRI):

P

ALERT
The median nerve often is poorly depicted at the elbow due to the minimal amount of perifascial fat in this region; MRI is not indicated for the diagnosis of pronator syndrome but may be used for excluding other etiologies. The nerve can look normal at the site of entrapment.

- The pronator teres and other muscles innervated by the median nerve distal to the site of the lesion may show abnormally high signal intensity on T2-weighted fat-suppressed, STIR (short TI inversion recovery), or T1-weighted images, or atrophy in more advanced cases (4)[C].

Diagnostic Procedures/Other

Electrodiagnostic testing:

- Needle electromyography (EMG) is the most helpful to identify evidence of denervation, but findings may not be present prior to 4 to 6 wk after symptoms begin.
- Nerve conduction may be normal despite compressive pathology because only 7–31% of patients show abnormal nerve conduction velocity (NCV) findings that support the clinical diagnosis (2).

ALERT
In the electrodiagnostic evaluation of CTS, EMG of muscles innervated by the median nerve proximal to the wrist should be performed to decrease unnecessary carpal tunnel surgeries.

TREATMENT

GENERAL MEASURES

- Small studies show a wide range of improvement in nonsurgical interventions, but no randomized trials have been performed; up to 3 to 6 mo of conservative treatment recommended (2)[C]
- Rehabilitation is the initial treatment and can be summarized using the acronym APORIM:
  - *A*ctivity modification: avoidance of provocative activities
  - *P*rotection from external compression
  - *O*rthoses: Night splints to prevent excessive elbow flexion can be considered.
  - *R*ehabilitation: Assess proximal and distal kinetic chain (shoulder girdle and wrist) for strength, flexibility, and movement; forearm flexor muscle stretching, nerve-gliding exercises
  - *I*njections can be considered at point of compression, but exercise caution to avoid direct injection into nerve bundle.
  - *M*edication: nonsteroidal or steroid anti-inflammatory medications

SURGERY/OTHER PROCEDURES

- Surgical management is controversial unless there is a clear compressive area discovered.
- If conservative measures fail, or if muscle atrophy or denervation occurs, one should consider exploration and release of all potential sites of entrapment.
- For a proven supracondyloid process, excision of the bone prominence and release of the ligament of Struthers should provide resolution.
- Surgical approaches vary, but most recommend complete decompression of the median nerve in the upper forearm:
  - In retrospective studies, approximately 80% of patients, there was complete or partial resolution of symptoms with open surgical decompression (1)[B].
  - A small study of 13 patients showed all patients with improvement in subjective symptoms following endoscopic release (5)[C].

ONGOING CARE

Postsurgical intervention, active range of motion as early as postoperative day 2, with full return to activity by 6 to 8 wk (1)[C]

REFERENCES

1. Rodner CM, Tinsley BA, O'Malley MP. Pronator syndrome and anterior interosseous nerve syndrome. *J Am Acad Orthop Surg*. 2013;21(5):268–275.
2. Strohl AB, Zelouf DS. Ulnar tunnel syndrome, radial tunnel syndrome, anterior interosseous nerve syndrome, and pronator syndrome. *J Am Acad Orthop Surg*. 2017;25(1):e1–e10.
3. Hsiao CW, Shih JT, Hung ST. Concurrent carpal tunnel syndrome and pronator syndrome: a retrospective study of 21 cases. *Orthop Traumatol Surg Res*. 2017;103(1):101–103.
4. Carpenter EL, Bencardino JT. Focus on advanced magnetic resonance techniques in clinical practice: magnetic resonance neurography. *Radiol Clin North Am*. 2015;53(3):513–529.
5. Lee AK, Khorsandi M, Nurbhai N, et al. Endoscopically assisted decompression for pronator syndrome. *J Hand Surg Am*. 2012;37(6):1173–1179.

ADDITIONAL READING

- Bencardino JT, Rosenberg ZS. Entrapment neuropathies of the shoulder and elbow in the athlete. *Clin Sports Med*. 2006;25(3):465–487, vi–vii.
- Tetro AM, Pichora DR. High median nerve entrapments. An obscure cause of upper-extremity pain. *Hand Clin*. 1996;12(4):691–703.
- Werner CO, Rosén I, Thorngren KG. Clinical and neurophysiologic characteristics of the pronator syndrome. *Clin Orthop Relat Res*. 1985;(197):231–236.

CLINICAL PEARLS

- Tinel test and other compression tests of the median nerve at the wrist level should be absent.
- Symptoms of pronator syndrome typically do not occur at night. Also, wrist splints typically do not improve symptoms.
- Prognosis usually depends on the severity of median neuropathy. Worse prognosis with extensive axon loss and atrophy. Expect some reinnervation of distal musculature once the median nerve is free from compromising structures.

PROTEINURIA IN SPORTS

Mario Gutierrez, MD • Gerardo Vazquez, MD, CAQSM • Justin M. Wright, MD, CAQSM

BASICS

DESCRIPTION

- Proteinuria is defined as the excretion of >150 mg/day of urinary protein (1).
- Macroalbuminuria implies a loss of >300 mg/day, microalbuminuria a loss of 30 to 300 mg/day (2).
- Present in 17% of asymptomatic individuals (1)
- Exercise-induced proteinuria (3):
  - Transient increase in urine protein following exercise; resolves over 24 to 48 hr
  - Relatively common, benign finding
  - Proteinuria related more to exercise intensity than duration
  - Due to increased glomerular permeability and decreased tubular resorption of protein as a result of reversible physiologic change in the kidney
  - May also be due to a decrease in the intravascular volume from acute dehydration in athletes partaking in severe or extreme exercise
  - No known long-term sequelae

EPIDEMIOLOGY

- Proteinuria seen in up to 17% of asymptomatic individuals in general population (1)
- In the athletic population, prevalence between 18% and 100%, depending on type of activity and intensity (3)
- Seen in activities with higher exercise intensity, such as boxing, wrestling, gymnastics, football, and rowing
- Also seen in long-distance running, swimming, and track

ETIOLOGY AND PATHOPHYSIOLOGY

- Factors underlying exercise-induced proteinuria include local vascular changes, local hypoxia, lactate accumulation, oxidant stress, hormonal changes, and a general septic reaction (2,4).
- Proteins seen in the urine include:
  - Plasma proteins such as albumin, transferrin, kappa, and lambda chains.
  - Tubular proteins such as secretory immunoglobulin A (IgA), Tamm-Horsfall protein.
- Three categories of proteinuria (3):
  - Glomerular:
    - Increased filtration of macromolecules across the glomerular capillary wall
    - Permeability affected by increased organic acid production, renin-angiotensin system, prostaglandins, and catecholamine activation
    - Urine protein components similar to plasma proteins
    - Seen with mild-to-moderate exercise
  - Tubular:
    - Decreased resorption of filtered proteins
    - Presence of low-molecular-weight proteins
    - Due to saturation of reabsorbing mechanisms caused by a higher quantity of proteins filtered at the glomerular level
    - Seen in strenuous exercise in combination with glomerular proteinuria
  - Overflow:
    - Increased production of low-molecular-weight proteins (e.g., multiple myeloma)
    - Unless preexisting condition is present, not seen in exercise-induced proteinuria

DIAGNOSIS

The history and physical are important to differentiate benign and transient exercise-induced proteinuria from pathologic causes of proteinuria.

HISTORY

- Exercise type, intensity, and duration
- Prior history of renal disease
- Underlying conditions that may cause proteinuria
- History of recent illness
- Family history of renal disease

PHYSICAL EXAM

Identifying signs of underlying renal disease or process, including (5)[C]:

- Elevated blood pressure (BP)
- Peripheral edema
- Flank pain
- Abdominal bruits

DIFFERENTIAL DIAGNOSIS

- Transient proteinuria:
  - Orthostatic proteinuria:
    - Elevated protein excretion in upright position, with normal excretion in recumbent position
    - Most common cause of proteinuria in children (6)
    - Diagnosis made by collecting urine throughout the day and then again in the morning after recumbent all night. If orthostatic proteinuria is present, protein level in overnight sample will be within normal limits. Elevated protein in overnight sample should prompt workup for persistent proteinuria (1,5)[C].
  - Fever
  - Stress
  - Pregnancy
  - Seizures
- Glomerular causes (e.g., minimal change disease, membranous glomerulonephritis)
- Tubular causes (e.g., hypertensive nephrosclerosis)
- Overflow (e.g., multiple myeloma, hemoglobinuria)
- Postrenal causes in patients with inflammation of the urinary tract (e.g., urinary tract infection (UTI), nephrolithiasis, tumors)

DIAGNOSTIC TESTS & INTERPRETATION

- Urinalysis/dipstick:
  - Inexpensive, quick screening test for proteinuria
  - Standard dipstick test measures albumin concentration via a colorimetric reaction.
  - False-positive results seen with alkaline urine; highly concentrated urine; gross hematuria; presence of certain medications (penicillin, sulfonamides, tolbutamide); and the presence of pus, semen, or vaginal secretions
  - False-negative results seen with dilute urine or when urine proteins are nonalbumin or low-molecular-weight
  - In exercise-induced proteinuria, dipstick may become positive within 30 min of onset of exercise and is positive for 24 to 48 hr.
  - Usually no >2+ on dipstick
  - For dipstick-positive proteinuria lasting >48 hr after a period of rest, further workup is required (3,5)[C].
- Further workup (3,5)[C]:
  - Blood urea nitrogen and creatinine
  - Complete blood count (CBC)
  - 24-hr urine collection for creatinine and total protein or spot protein-to-creatinine ratio
- Imaging not routinely used in exercise-induced proteinuria
- For persistent proteinuria or suspicion of renal parenchymal disease, a renal ultrasound (US) should be performed (5)[C].
- Dimercaptosuccinic acid (DMSA) scan is the preferred study to detect renal scarring (6)[C].

TREATMENT

GENERAL MEASURES

- Exercise-induced proteinuria is transient and self-limited; no specific therapy indicated
- For underlying renal disease, treatment aimed at specific cause
- Screening for proteinuria during sports preparticipation physical examination (PPE) is not recommended.

ISSUES FOR REFERRAL

Evaluation by nephrologist should be considered for:

- Persistent proteinuria, especially in patients >30 yr.
- Elevated serum creatinine.
- Evidence of underlying medical disease or glomerular process.

ONGOING CARE

PROGNOSIS

There is no evidence that suggests these athletes are at increased risk for chronic renal disease or have any reason to limit their physical activity.

REFERENCES

1. Carroll MF, Temte JL. Proteinuria in adults: a diagnostic approach. *Am Fam Physician*. 2000;62(6):1333–1340.
2. Shephard RJ. Exercise proteinuria and hematuria: current knowledge and future directions. *J Sports Med Phys Fitness*. 2016;56(9):1060–1076.
3. Bellinghieri G, Savica V, Santoro D. Renal alterations during exercise. *J Ren Nutr*. 2008;18(1):158–164.
4. Saeed F, Naga Pavan Kumar Devaki P, Mahendrakar L, et al. Exercise-induced proteinuria? *J Fam Pract*. 2012;61(1):23–26.
5. Kane SF, Cohen MI. Evaluation of the asymptomatic athlete with hepatic and urinalysis abnormalities. *Curr Sports Med Rep*. 2009;8(2):77–84.
6. Leung AKC, Wong AH, Barg SS. Proteinuria in children: evaluation and differential diagnosis. *Am Fam Physician*. 2017;95(4):248–254.

CLINICAL PEARLS

- Exercise-induced proteinuria is transient, lasting 24 to 48 hr.
- Repeat testing in 48 hr after a period of rest to ensure clearance of protein.
- Persistent proteinuria requires workup for underlying renal disease.

PSEUDOANEMIA

Amity Tung, MD

BASICS

DESCRIPTION

- Dilutional phenomenon in endurance athletes leading to hemoglobin and hematocrit values that are lower than normal limits
- Technically, not a true "anemia" because athletes tend to have increased total mass of red blood cells in circulation, compared to sedentary individuals (1)
- Caused by plasma volume expansion by 10–20% with little change in red cell numbers (i.e., oxygen-carrying capacity) (2)
- Contributing factors include:
  - Exercise-induced release of aldosterone, renin, and vasopressin.
  - Increased size of vascular bed owing to muscle hypertrophy.
  - Retention of crystalloids and colloids governed by hormones.
  - Oxidative stress and release of chemical factors that alter red blood cell structure and function (3).
- Theoretically, this increased blood volume decreases viscosity, thereby maximizing stroke volume, cardiac output, and subsequent oxygen delivery (4).
- Hemodilution occurs over the 48 hr after every episode of endurance exercise and may persist for as long as 1 wk after discontinuing training (2).
- If training continues, red cell mass will catch up with plasma volume expansion over the span of few weeks, causing hemoglobin and hematocrit values to normalize.
- Synonym(s): sports anemia; athletes' pseudoanemia; dilutional pseudoanemia

EPIDEMIOLOGY

Incidence

- Elite athletes involved in endurance training
- Previously sedentary individuals starting an exercise program
- Athletes increasing intensity of training

DIAGNOSIS

HISTORY

Check exercise schedule, type of training activity, and occurrence of any symptoms.

PHYSICAL EXAM

- Hemoglobin levels 13 to 14 g/100 mL in men and 11 to 12 g/100 mL in women; dose-response relationship between amount/intensity of exercise and hemoglobin drop (5)
- Elite endurance athletes have a greater degree of dilutional pseudoanemia than moderate-endurance athletes.
- Females are more likely than males to have iron deficiency anemia with sports ± presence of pseudoanemia.
- No particular symptoms or physical findings
- Laboratory studies are performed if etiology is unclear or symptoms are present.
- Normal mean corpuscular volume

- No hematuria or hemoglobinuria on urinalysis
- Normal bilirubin and haptoglobin
- Ferritin may be lower in endurance athletes, owing to the same relative dilutional effect; values often <60 μg/L, occasionally <30, but <15 = iron deficiency (6)

DIFFERENTIAL DIAGNOSIS

- Iron deficiency anemia
- Gastrointestinal (GI) bleeding
- Hematuria
- Foot-strike hemolysis
- Hemolysis due to muscle contraction compressing capillaries (7)

TREATMENT

- Rule out iron deficiency anemia.
- Self-limited condition; indices return to pretraining levels after training is discontinued.
- Normal physiologic response; no treatment required

REFERENCES

1. Mairbäurl H. Red blood cells in sports: effects of exercise and training on oxygen supply by red blood cells. *Front Physiol*. 2013;4:332.
2. Eichner ER. Sports medicine pearls and pitfalls: nature's anticoagulant. *Curr Sports Med Rep*. 2009;8(1):2–3.
3. Liu CH, Tseng YF, Lai JI, et al. The changes of red blood cell viscoelasticity and sports anemia in male 24-hr ultra-marathoners. *J Chin Med Assoc*. 2018;81(5):475–481.
4. El-Sayed MS, Ali N, El-Sayed Ali Z. Haemorheology in exercise and training. *Sports Med*. 2005;35(8): 649–670.
5. Chatard JC, Mujika I, Guy C, et al. Anaemia and iron deficiency in athletes. Practical recommendations for treatment. *Sports Med*. 1999;27(4):229–240.
6. Bärtsch P, Mairbäurl H, Friedmann B. Pseudo-anemia caused by sports. *Ther Umsch*. 1998;55(4):251–255.
7. Chiu YH, Lai JI, Wang SH, et al. Early changes of the anemia phenomenon in male 100-km ultramarathoners. *J Chin Med Assoc*. 2015;78(2):108–113.

ADDITIONAL READING

- Balaban EP. Sports anemia. *Clin Sports Med*. 1992;11(2):313–325.
- Raunikar RA, Sabio H. Anemia in the adolescent athlete. *Am J Dis Child*. 1992;146(10):1201–1205.
- Watts E. Athletes' anaemia. A review of possible causes and guidelines on investigation. *Br J Sports Med*. 1989;23(2):81–83.
- Weight LM, Darge BL, Jacobs P. Athletes' pseudoanemia. *Eur J Appl Physiol Occup Physiol*. 1991;62(5):358–362.

CLINICAL PEARLS

With pseudoanemia, iron supplementation does not affect occurrence or improve lab values, nor is it necessary unless there is a coexisting iron deficiency anemia.

PULMONARY CONTUSION

Douglas Comeau, DO, CAQSM, FAAFP • Angelene M. Elliott, DO

BASICS

- The clinical syndrome, following blunt chest trauma of chest pain and respiratory difficulty, with or without hemoptysis, confirmed by findings on chest radiographs (CXRs) or other imaging:
  - Specific symptoms may include persistent and progressive shortness of breath, tachypnea, or decreasing pulse oximetry.
  - CXR or computed tomography (CT) demonstrates focal or diffuse infiltrates that *do not conform* to pulmonary lobes or segments.
  - Typically, manifests within hours of injury, peak at 72 hr and resolves within 7 days (1)
- Although rarely reported in sports, the true incidence is not well-known:
  - Seven case studies since 1997 (2,3,4,5,6)
  - Most of the literature reviews severe trauma and injury, such as motor vehicle accidents, that generally require more intervention than those reported in sports.
- Although pulmonary contusion is dramatic in presentation, athletes appear to recover and return to play within 1 wk limited primarily by chest wall pain rather than respiratory status.

DESCRIPTION

- Blunt trauma to the chest causing disruption of alveolar capillary interface, resulting in collection of blood, edema, and protein in the interstitium and alveoli
- Clinical diagnosis is suggested by hemoptysis or progressive respiratory distress and confirmed by imaging.
- Synonym(s): bruised lung

EPIDEMIOLOGY

- In contact sports, chest wall contusions occur frequently and are managed by athletic trainers without being reported.
- There are only seven sport-reported cases of pulmonary contusion in the literature since 1997 (2,3,4,5,6).
- In all comers to an emergency department (ED) during the 1990s (7):
  - 26% of rib fractures are associated with pulmonary contusion.
  - 32% are associated with hemothorax/pneumothorax.

ETIOLOGY AND PATHOPHYSIOLOGY

Blunt trauma to the chest causing disruption of alveolar capillary interface, resulting in collection of blood, edema, and protein in the interstitium and alveoli which can lead to bronchospasm, increase in production and decrease of clearance of mucus, and decrease in production of surfactant, resulting in possible pulmonary dysfunction like ventilation/perfusion mismatch, increase in intrapulmonary shunt, increase in lung fluid, and loss of lung compliance. This results in damaged lung that is unable to exchange gas effectively in respiration.

RISK FACTORS

- Collision/contact sports
- Sports with high speeds or where the athlete is airborne:
  - Cycling, equestrian, winter sports, auto and motorcycle racing, extreme sports, and so forth

GENERAL PREVENTION

Use protective equipment and padding appropriate for the activity, such as seat restraints in motor sports to prevent ejection:

- Padding may diffuse force on impact.
- Padding after the injury can decrease pain of subsequent impacts.

COMMONLY ASSOCIATED CONDITIONS

- Chest wall contusion
- Rib fracture
- If high-velocity trauma, intra-abdominal organ injury may occur.

DIAGNOSIS

Diagnosis is suspected when an athlete sustains a blunt trauma to the chest and has respiratory difficulty:

- Hemoptysis after an injury is highly suggestive of a pulmonary contusion.

HISTORY

- Blunt nonpenetrating trauma
- Chest wall contusion is often the initial diagnosis.
- Hemoptysis may be present, but its absence does not rule out a contusion.
- Pain in the shoulder or scapular angle suggests abdominal or diaphragmatic injury.
- If fever is present, consider infectious differential.
- Consider pulmonary parenchymal contusion when dyspnea is progressive over hours or days or if hemoptysis occurs.
- Nasal or facial trauma supports consideration of epistaxis as the etiology of bleeding possibly instead of pulmonary injury in the absence of obvious chest trauma.
- High-energy/velocity injuries should increase suspicion for associated injuries.

PHYSICAL EXAM

- High-velocity/energy injuries should prompt full trauma evaluation:
  - Both primary and secondary surveys should be performed in these cases.
- Dyspnea or tachypnea must be present for diagnosis, unless hemoptysis occurs.
- Palpable and pleuritic chest wall pain are present due to the impact force required to produce a pulmonary contusion.
- Arm or trunk movement may worsen chest pain.
- Dyspnea may persist after rest.
- Chest wall region is tender.
- Ecchymosis usually will not be present initially, but crepitus or more severe point tenderness often is present when ribs are fractured.
- Auscultation is generally normal:
  - Consider hemopneumothorax if abnormal lung sounds are present.
- Inspect and record naso-oropharyngeal findings, as hemoptysis may be reported later:
  - Note any evidence of bleeding in the nose or mouth.
  - Evaluate nose and posterior pharynx for sites of bleeding, as nasal trauma or bites of cheeks or tongue are more common than pulmonary contusion as the source of blood in suspected hemoptysis.
- Clear cervical (C)-spine and other abdominal injuries in the presence of significant blunt trauma to the chest.
- Record serial vital signs/exams if athlete is unable to return to play to observe for deterioration:
  - Pulse oximetry <91% suggests contusion with arteriovenous (AV) shunting.
- Abdominal examination for tenderness or guarding is critical:
  - Penetrating injury occurring anteriorly at rib interspace 5 or below may penetrate the abdomen.
- Observe the chest closely for paradoxical movement of a segment of ribs indicative of flail chest.

DIFFERENTIAL DIAGNOSIS

- Pulmonary emboli
- Traumatic pneumothorax or hemothorax
- Diaphragmatic, splenic, or hepatic injury
- Pulmonary laceration or hematoma
- Spontaneous pneumothorax
- Rib fracture or contusion
- Naso-oropharyngeal trauma
- Tracheobronchial mucosal avulsion
- Epistaxis

DIAGNOSTIC TESTS & INTERPRETATION

Initial Tests (lab, imaging)

- Decreasing pulse oximetry (<91%) suggests pulmonary contusion with AV shunting:
  - Consider pneumothorax with low pulse oximetry as well.
- Posterior, anterior, and lateral CXR:
  - May not be required for chest pain in absence of dyspnea or hemoptysis.
  - Rib films do not contribute to management in absence of pulmonary symptoms or clinical flail fracture.
  - Clinically significant hemopneumothorax and pneumothorax can generally be ruled out with negative radiographs; however, additional imaging should be considered based on the mechanism of injury and clinical findings, as normal radiographs do not definitively exclude underlying lung injury.
- Posterior, anterior, and lateral CXR reveals peripheral infiltrate in area of trauma when significant contusion occurs:
  - Generally seen within 6 hr but may take up to 48 hr for radiographic changes
  - The infiltrate may not correlate to lobular architecture.
  - Enlargement in x-ray in first 24 hr is generally a poor prognostic finding.
- CT and other imaging will be guided by the clinical picture:
  - CT might be useful to determine the need for mechanical ventilation and likelihood of pneumonia or acute respiratory distress syndrome (ARDS).
  - Ventilation/perfusion scan may show matched ventilation/perfusion defect, unlike pulmonary embolus, which shows ventilation/perfusion mismatch.
- Chest ultrasound (US) may be comparable to CT for pulmonary contusion.
- Follow-up imaging guided by clinical symptoms and severity of injury:
  - Isolated contusion in the athlete generally does not require repeat radiographs.
  - Consider if symptoms are not resolving over 5 to 7 days or worsen.

Diagnostic Procedures/Other

If hemoptysis is recurrent over >48 hr, bronchoscopy may be considered, depending on clinical status (8):

- Hemoptysis should generally clear within 1 wk.

TREATMENT

- Prehospital:
  - Primary on-field concerns:
    - Multiple cites of trauma in motor sports or high-velocity sports (downhill skiing) should be stabilized and transported immediately by emergency services to a designated trauma center:
      - Primary concerns with severe trauma are airway, breathing, and circulation.

- Evaluate for C-spine injury; immobilize as indicated.
- Expose by removing equipment as needed.
- Report any increase in dyspnea; may need support, oxygen, and ventilation
– Mild to moderate injuries may be observed on site and reevaluated frequently for signs of decompensation.
– Transport for worsening symptoms:
  - Dyspnea and tachypnea are the most important signs of deterioration.
- ED treatment:
  – In cases of multiple trauma due to motor vehicle accident or high-velocity impact, general trauma protocols should be followed.
  – In contact sports, trauma with isolated pulmonary contusion may be treated with observation and minimal support as needed:
    - Pain medication
    - Oxygen
  – Penetrating injuries and flail chest are associated with a much higher risk of complications, including the need for mechanical support.

MEDICATION

- Acetaminophen and nonsteroidal anti-inflammatory drugs (NSAIDs) can be used as first line for mild to moderate pain:
  – Consider avoiding NSAIDs in patients with hemoptysis.
- Narcotic pain medications may be needed in more severe cases:
  – Monitor use closely, as these may cause respiratory depression.

ADDITIONAL THERAPIES

- Isolated pulmonary contusion in stable patients does not require additional treatment:
  – Rest from strenuous exercise as needed to allow pulmonary healing
- Additional supportive and treatment measures will be dictated by the severity of injuries:
  – Pulmonary toilet
  – Chest tube may be required emergently if hemopneumothorax is present.
- Light exercise or walking promotes deep breathing and retards atelectasis.
- When asymptomatic, begin stepwise return to play as tolerated by symptoms.
- Rib taping and other attempts at immobilization are generally not effective and should be used with caution, as they could possibly increase the risk of atelectasis and pneumonia.

ADMISSION, INPATIENT, AND NURSING CONSIDERATIONS

- Admission criteria:
  – Traumatic injuries requiring stabilization and support
  – Patient with respiratory difficulty and oxygen saturations <90%
  – Patients with uncontrolled pain
- Special considerations:
  – Rib fractures can be associated with severe blunt trauma, but these cases generally involve high-energy mechanism.
  – Flail chest is a rare but serious complication requiring hospitalization to observe for pulmonary deterioration and need for intubation with respiratory support.
  – Pulmonary laceration:
    - Transfer of energy from the chest wall; shear forces often are generated that can tear the lung.
    - Most lacerations heal without complications, but elastic recoil of the lung may extend the laceration to form a pulmonary pseudocyst, which may result in infection, abscess, hemoptysis, air leak, adult respiratory distress syndrome, and death.
    - One case report in soccer player
  – Airway avulsion or rupture:
    - Most common site is within 2.5 cm of the carina between tracheal rings.
    - Findings include subcutaneous (SC) emphysema and hemoptysis.
  – Isolated pneumothorax is uncommon with blunt trauma due to dense fibroconnective tissue surrounding carina and mainstem bronchi.
- Discharge criteria:
  – Stable patients can be discharged home with observation and instructions to return for worsening symptoms:
    - Pain controlled
    - No significant dyspnea
    - Stable oxygen saturation on room air:
      - No consensus but generally >90% for an otherwise healthy individual

ONGOING CARE

Return to play (2,3)[C]:

- Simple chest wall contusions:
  – Same day
  – Athlete must be nondyspneic, able to perform usual movements as required for the sport, and able to tolerate pain without narcotics or local anesthetic.
  – On return to play, rib pads, flak jacket, or equestrian chest protector may decrease discomfort and reinjury during contact.
  – Remove from activity for recurrent dyspnea; consider CXR.
- Pulmonary contusions:
  – Field-side diagnosis with hemoptysis or persistent pain precludes return to that contest.
  – Athlete may return to full activity at 1 wk if they tolerate progressive training without dyspnea, hemoptysis, or limited performance after the last episode.
  – After strenuous exercise is tolerated for 48 hr and athlete is able to perform at a level appropriate for contact sports, return to play in contact sports may be allowed.

FOLLOW-UP RECOMMENDATIONS

- Report any deterioration in performance or dyspnea.
- Pulmonary consultation for bronchoscopy if hemoptysis persists

PROGNOSIS

- Most isolated pulmonary contusions will resolve without complication.
- Chest wall pain usually persists for 6 wk but generally will not interfere with function.
- Isolated pulmonary contusion in young, healthy patients is not associated with mortality.

COMPLICATIONS

- Posttraumatic empyema
- ARDS (strong association if Thoracic Trauma Severity score at admission >13) (9)[C]
- Pneumonia
- Factors associated with a poor outcome in severe pulmonary contusion (multiple traumas/motor vehicle accident):
  – Poor outcome = death, prolonged hospitalization >7 days, severe complications (pneumonia, empyema, atelectasis requiring bronchoscopy or bronchopleural fistula):
    - Pulmonary contusion on admission CXR
    - Three or more rib fractures
    - Chest tube insertion
    - Hypoxia on admission (PO_2 <70 torr)

REFERENCES

1. Cohn SM, Dubose JJ. Pulmonary contusion: an update on recent advances in clinical management. *World J Surg*. 2010;34(8):1959–1970.
2. Lively MW, Stone D. Pulmonary contusion in football players. *Clin J Sport Med*. 2006;16(2):177–178.
3. Meese MA, Sebastianelli WJ. Pulmonary contusion secondary to blunt trauma in a collegiate football player. *Clin J Sport Med*. 1997;7(4):309–310.
4. Gillespie H, Sisson R, DiFiori JP. Pulmonary contusion in a football player. *Curr Sports Med Rep*. 2013;12(2):57–58.
5. Milne LW. Thoracic trauma in polo: two cases and a review of the literature. *J Emerg Med*. 2011;40(4):410–414.
6. Lively M. Pulmonary contusion in a collegiate diver: a case report. *J Med Case Rep*. 2011;5:362.
7. Ziegler DW, Agarwal NN. The morbidity and mortality of rib fractures. *J Trauma*. 1994;37(6):975–979.
8. Bidwell JL, Pachner RW. Hemoptysis: diagnosis and management. *Am Fam Physician*. 2005;72(7):1253–1260.
9. Daurat A, Millet I, Roustan J, et al. Thoracic trauma severity score on admission allows to determine the risk of delayed ARDS in trauma patients with pulmonary contusion. *Injury*. 2016;47(1):47–153.

ADDITIONAL READING

Dubinsky I, Low A. Non-life-threatening blunt chest trauma: appropriate investigation and treatment. *Am J Emerg Med*. 1997;15(3):240–243.

CLINICAL PEARLS

- Blunt thoracic trauma with high-energy mechanism should always prompt a thorough evaluation, as pulmonary contusions and rib fractures are commonly associated with significant internal injuries:
  – This is in contrast to most sports-related injuries, which are usually lower energy and are generally associated with good outcomes.
- Significant morbidity in clinically stable patients has not been reported. One episode of hemoptysis in an asymptomatic athlete will likely not recur and imaging is not required. Pulmonary dysfunction associated with a contusion may take 24 to 48 hr to develop as fluid accumulates in the air spaces. Serial reevaluations daily may be needed to detect worsening tachypnea and tachycardia. Get emergency follow-up evaluation if delayed deterioration occurs rapidly.
- Future ability to play is only as limited by chest wall pain. Return to peak conditioning depends on ability to reach maximum exertion effort. Involuntary guarding of pleuritic pain during healing may delay recovery to peak form for up to 6 wk.

QUADRICEPS CONTUSION

Sarah Merrill, MD, CAQSM • Kinshasa Morton, MD, CAQSM • Jason P. Womack, MD

BASICS

DESCRIPTION

- The quadriceps extends the knee and stabilize the pelvis and patella during the gait cycle. The muscles also work with the hamstrings to coordinate the movements of kicking, jumping, and running (1,2).
- Quadriceps contusions occur when traumatic thigh injury causes muscle fiber damage and capillary rupture, leading to subsequent bleeding into the quadriceps muscle tissue (1). These are common sports-related injuries, seen most frequently in high-impact sports, such as rugby, soccer, or football (3,4).
- Recurrent quadriceps contusions predispose to more severe injury and development of complications (2,4).
- Delay in onset of therapy leads to a higher percentage of complications and delay in recovery (1,2).
- Synonym(s): Charley horse; thigh bruise; dead leg; quadriceps hematoma

EPIDEMIOLOGY

- Thigh injuries account for 14% of all lower extremity sports-related injuries in high school sports (3,5).
- Muscle contusion injuries are second only to strain injuries as a major cause of morbidity in the modern athlete (1,2).
- Incidence varies by sport, with contact sports having higher incidence of these injuries (3).
- Quadriceps strains and contusions account for approximately 40% of all injuries in high-level soccer players (3).

RISK FACTORS

- Direct trauma to the middle portion of the quadriceps muscle belly, given the increased vascularity at that point (1,5)
- Inappropriately sized, thinly cushioned, or nonuse of thigh pads (1)
- Associated medical problems that increase the risk of bleeding (such as liver disease, coagulopathies, etc.) increase the risk of quadriceps contusion (3,5).

COMMONLY ASSOCIATED CONDITIONS

- Quadriceps strain
- Femur or patellar fracture
- Myositis ossificans traumatica (MOT)
- Acute compartment syndrome (ACS) of anterior thigh

DIAGNOSIS

HISTORY

- Patient or athlete will often describe a distinct injury or trauma to the thigh occurring during a high-impact collision with opponent or sports equipment (1).
- Pain is typically immediate and significant, and visible swelling may be quickly apparent (1).

PHYSICAL EXAM

- Inspection:
  - May ambulate with antalgic gait or has reluctance to bear weight (1,5)
  - May have area of ecchymosis at trauma site (1,5)
  - Swelling in the anterior thigh, which may extend to proximal knee (5):
    - Patients with severe quadriceps contusions may get knee effusion without intra-articular pathology.
- Palpation:
  - Tense and tender to palpation over area of direct injury; most commonly anterior lateral thigh (1,5)
- Range of motion (ROM):
  - Reduced ability to actively flex the knee (1,5)
- Strength:
  - Reduced ability to perform straight leg raise (1,5)
  - Reduced ability to perform knee extension against resistance (1,5)
- Sensation:
  - Sensation deficits along anterolateral thigh (1,5)
- Grading of contusions:
  - Mild: normal gait, localized tenderness, active ROM (AROM) knee flexion >90 degrees (1)
  - Moderate: antalgic gait, swollen and tender mass in quadriceps, AROM knee flexion 45 to 90 degrees (1)
  - Severe: severely antalgic gait, visibly swollen and tender mass, AROM knee flexion >45 degrees (1)

ALERT

- ACS: Elevated pressure within the anterior thigh compartment due to bleeding causes impaired blood flow to tissues and eventually ischemia (6):
  - Can occur from similar mechanisms to quadriceps contusion (6)
  - Surgical emergency and must be quickly identified by rapid swelling, pain out of proportion to exam, decreased sensation and pulses (6)
  - If there is concern, athlete needs to be evaluated in emergency department (ED) with compartment testing (6).

DIFFERENTIAL DIAGNOSIS

- Femur fracture or contusion
- Quadriceps tendon rupture
- Quadriceps strain or muscle tear
- Patellar fracture
- Referred lumbosacral radiculopathy
- Bony or soft tissue tumor
- Meralgia paresthetica
- Morel-Lavallée lesion

DIAGNOSTIC TESTS & INTERPRETATION

- Diagnosis can typically be made clinically with a thorough history and physical exam (1,2,4).
- Radiographs:
  - Usually normal but helpful in identifying for fractures (1,2)
- Musculoskeletal (MSK) ultrasound:
  - Can be used to diagnose hematomas and rule out associated muscle tears or tendon ruptures (2,4,6)
  - Contusions appear as a focal loss of muscle fibrillary architecture with a heterogenous region of increased echogenicity, which may cross fascial boundaries (2,4,6).
  - Serial ultrasounds can assess size of resolving contusion at future visits (2,6).
- Magnetic resonance imaging (MRI):
  - Not necessary but can be used if ultrasound is not available or inconclusive (2,4,5)
  - Can reliably detect and grade quadriceps contusions (2,4,5)

TREATMENT

GENERAL MEASURES

- RICE therapy—rest, ice, compression, and elevation to limit the severity of contusion (1,4,5):
  - Rest reduces retraction of ruptured myofibrils, preventing large gaps in the muscle (4).
  - Icing associated with smaller hematoma formation, less inflammation, and early muscle regeneration (4)
  - Compression reduces intramuscular bleeding (4).
  - Elevation reduces interstitial fluid accumulation (swelling) (4).
- Initially, the knee should be immobilized in an elastic wrap or hinged knee brace at 120 degrees of flexion for 24 hr to limit hematoma formation (1,4).

- Subacute treatment (after first 24 hr):
  - Discontinue immobilization and begin stretching (1):
    - Passive flexion with goal of 120 degrees of pain-free flexion (1,5)
    - Begin active quadriceps stretching and strengthening exercises once pain decreases and motion improves (1).
  - Strengthening should progress from isometric to isotonic to isokinetic training (4).
- Long-term treatment/rehabilitation:
  - May return to sports-specific training when:
    - ROM on injured quadriceps side and uninjured side are equal (1,4).
    - Use of injured quadriceps is pain free with basic movement (1,4).
  - Prior to return to sport, player should be fitted for oversized quadriceps pad (1):
    - Helps to protect from recurrent injury, which could lead to MOT
    - Wear for 3 to 6 mo or until end of season.

MEDICATION

- Nonsteroidal anti-inflammatory drugs (NSAIDs) can be used for the first 1 to 7 days, depending on the severity of the injury (1,4).
- For severe injuries, NSAIDs may prevent development of MOT, although further studies need to be done to determine the most appropriate dose and choice of NSAID (1).

ISSUES FOR REFERRAL

Isolated quadriceps contusions rarely require referral. Indications for referral include complications such as myositis ossificans, tendon rupture, fracture, or compartment syndrome (1,4,5).

SURGERY/OTHER PROCEDURES

- Aspiration should be reserved for large hematomas or those that clearly restrict motion. If indicated, aspiration should be performed within the 1st wk of injury (2,4,6).
- Steroid injections are not recommended for treatment of these injuries (1,4).
- Surgery is rarely, if ever, indicated (1,4).

COMPLEMENTARY & ALTERNATIVE MEDICINE

- Massage and muscle manipulation should be avoided in the acute phase because these can worsen underlying injury (4,5).
- It is unclear whether protective equipment can reduce the incidence of this type of injury (1).

ONGOING CARE

FOLLOW-UP RECOMMENDATIONS

- Athletes should follow up approximately every 2 wk to assess ongoing ROM and strengthening (2).
- Serial ultrasounds can also be performed at these visits to document resolution of hematoma and early signs of MOT (2).

PROGNOSIS

- Quadriceps contusions typically resolve over the course of 3 to 10 wk, depending on severity (1). With appropriate rehabilitation, patients and athletes can expect to regain full strength and ROM (1).
- Athletes should adhere to a functional progression of sport-specific activities as part of their rehabilitation. They should have symmetric, pain-free ROM and at least 85% strength recovery prior to return to sport (1).

COMPLICATIONS

MOT: benign heterotopic calcification of the traumatic hematoma (4):

- Suspect MOT when lesions persist longer than 2 wk or get worse over time (1,4).
- Early signs of myositis ossificans may be identifiable on MSK ultrasound (1). At later stages, it can be seen on radiographs and MRI3.
- Risk increases with larger contusions (1).
- Athletes with MOT who have persistent pain and limited motion may have the heterotopic bone removed when it has matured, at least 12 mo after the initial injury (1,4).

REFERENCES

1. Kary J. Diagnosis and management of quadriceps strains and contusions. *Curr Rev Musculoskelet Med*. 2010;3(1–4):26–31.
2. Pasta G, Nanni G, Molini L, et al. Sonography of the quadriceps muscle: examination technique, normal anatomy, and traumatic lesions. *J Ultrasound*. 2010;13(2):76–84.
3. Fernandez WG, Yard EE, Comstock RD. Epidemiology of lower extremity injuries among U.S. high school athletes. *Acad Emerg Med*. 2007;14(7):641–645.
4. Järvinen TA, Järvinen TL, Kääriäinen M, et al. Muscle injuries: optimising recovery. *Best Pract Res Clin Rheumatol*. 2007;21(2):317–331.
5. Trojian TH. Muscle contusion (thigh). *Clin Sports Med*. 2013;32(2):317–324.
6. Purohit NB, King LJ. Ultrasound of lower limb sports injuries. *Ultrasound*. 2015;23(3):149–157.

ADDITIONAL READING

- Aronen JG, Garrick JG, Chronister RD, et al. Quadriceps contusions: clinical results of immediate immobilization in 120 degrees of knee flexion. *Clin J Sport Med*. 2006;16(5):383–387.
- Diaz JA, Fischer DA, Rettig AC, et al. Severe quadriceps muscle contusions in athletes. A report of three cases. *Am J Sports Med*. 2003;31(2):289–293.
- Hayashi D, Hamilton B, Guermazi A, et al. Traumatic injuries of thigh and calf muscles in athletes: role and clinical relevance of MR imaging and ultrasound. *Insights Imaging*. 2012;3(6):591–601.
- How MI, Lee PK, Wei TS, et al. Delayed presentation of compartment syndrome of the thigh secondary to quadriceps trauma and vascular injury in a soccer athlete. *Int J Surg Case Rep*. 2015;11:56–58.
- Weiss NA, Johnson J, Anderson S. Morel-Lavallee lesion initially diagnosed as quadriceps contusion: ultrasound, MRI, and importance of early intervention. *West J Emerg Med*. 2015;16(3):438–441.

CLINICAL PEARLS

- Quadriceps contusions are caused by blunt trauma to the quadriceps muscle belly and area graded according to size and loss of function.
- Ultrasound is the imaging modality of choice for diagnosis as well as ongoing assessment.
- Initially, the knee should be immobilized with an elastic wrap or hinged knee brace in 120 degrees of flexion for 24 hr. After that, athlete can proceed with graduated flexibility and strengthening protocol.
- Think MOT when a quadriceps contusion is not improving as expected over 2 to 3 wk.

QUADRICEPS TEAR

Jason P. Womack, MD • Kinshasa Morton, MD, CAQSM

BASICS

Quadriceps strains are graded based on the degree of injury:

- Grade I: stretch injury of muscle fibers
- Grade II: partial tearing of muscle fibers
- Grade III: complete tear of muscle fibers:
  - Grade III tears most commonly involve the distal rectus femoris muscle.
  - Grade III tears may involve complete rupture of the extensor mechanism if the distal quadriceps tendon is involved (1).
  - Proximal ruptures may involve avulsion of anterior inferior iliac spine (AIIS).

EPIDEMIOLOGY

- Rectus femoris is the most common location of clinically significant quadriceps strains (2):
  - Majority of injuries around the muscle body along the central tendon, with distal and proximal injuries being rare (3)
- Represents 10% of injuries to soccer players (4)
- Proximal rupture/avulsion is rare:
  - More commonly seen in adolescent, kicking athletes
- Distal quadriceps rupture is a rare event:
  - 88% of ruptures occur in those >40 yr of age.

ETIOLOGY AND PATHOPHYSIOLOGY

- Commonly affects athletes with repetitive functional overloading of the extensor mechanism in an eccentric fashion:
  - The dominant kicking leg is at risk for quadriceps strain (4).
- National Collegiate Athletic Association (NCAA) injury surveillance saw highest rates in men's and women's soccer from 2009 to 2015 (6).

RISK FACTORS

Distal tendon rupture (5):

- Age >40 yr
- Hemodialysis patients
- Anabolic steroid use
- Diabetes
- Gout
- Hyperparathyroidism
- Hypocalcemia

DIAGNOSIS

HISTORY

- Strain to quadriceps muscle is most commonly associated with kicking, jumping, sprinting, or change in direction.
- Pain is often immediate.
- May lead to local pain and swelling
- Strains are a noncontact injury. History of contact leads to diagnosis of quadriceps contusion.

PHYSICAL EXAM

- Appearance:
  - There may be swelling and possibly ecchymosis around the area of injury.
- Palpation:
  - Tenderness, spasm, or both at the area of muscle injury
  - A defect in the muscle tissue may be felt in grade III strains.
  - In distal quadriceps ruptures, the intercondylar notch may be palpated because the quadriceps tendon is not present.
- Range of motion:
  - The extensor mechanism must be evaluated in all knee and quadriceps injuries.
  - Inability of any active extension of the knee is concerning for quadriceps rupture.
  - Strains show pain with active extension and passive knee flexion.

ALERT

Lack of active extension of the knee should raise concern of complete tendon rupture that requires prompt diagnosis and surgical consultation.

- Strength exam:
  - Weakness and/or painful knee extension secondary to the injured muscle tissue is common.
- Neurologic exam:
  - Sensation and reflexes are intact:
    - No reflex will be present in complete rupture.

DIFFERENTIAL DIAGNOSIS

- Quadriceps tendonitis
- Quadriceps contusion
- Patellar tendinitis
- Patellofemoral pain syndrome
- Patellar dislocation/subluxation
- Sinding-Larsen-Johansson disease
- Myositis ossificans

DIAGNOSTIC TESTS & INTERPRETATION

- Plain radiographs:
  - Not helpful in the diagnosis of acute quadriceps strain
  - A history of an old quadriceps strain with reaggravation may suggest myositis ossificans that would be visualized on plain radiographs.
  - Radiographs should be obtained in the skeletally immature with proximal pain to rule out avulsion fracture.
  - Complete ruptures may show patella baja on lateral views.
- Magnetic resonance imaging (MRI):
  - Not necessary in quadriceps strain, but will show edema and possible defects in the musculature (3)
  - Proximal ruptures may show avulsion of the AIIS and degree of retraction from the pelvis.
- Ultrasound (US):
  - Partial tearing:
    - Hypoechoic cleft seen in the muscle belly adjacent to the central tendon
    - Scanning in the long and short axis helps to determine the extent of the strain.
  - Complete rupture:
    - Complete discontinuity noted on scanning in the long axis

TREATMENT

GENERAL MEASURES

- Grade I and II injuries are treated in a similar fashion with rest, ice, compression, and pain control.
- Gentle stretching as permitted to maintain range of motion
- Early surgery is indicated for complete distal rupture:
  - Proximal rupture/avulsion may be treated nonoperatively.
  - Recovery of range of motion with stretching
  - Exercise to regain strength of the quadriceps and hamstring tendons.
  - Padding could be worn to protect the injured portion of the quadriceps musculature.

MEDICATION

- Nonsteroidal anti-inflammatory drugs (NSAIDs).
  - NSAIDs may be used acutely to help with pain.
- Controversy exists as to whether NSAIDs delay healing and collagen formation.

ALERT

Be careful if there is a suspected quadriceps contusion because NSAID use could theoretically increase bleeding. Conversely, early use of indomethacin in high-risk quadriceps contusions may reduce the risk of heterotopic bone formation.

ADDITIONAL THERAPIES

- If hematoma is discovered, aspiration can be considered.
- Platelet-rich plasma injections are often considered for faster resolution of muscle injuries, but evidence to support its use is lacking.

ISSUES FOR REFERRAL

Prompt surgical referral and surgery is indicated for quadriceps rupture at the patellar insertion.

SURGERY/OTHER PROCEDURES

- Acute rupture of the distal quadriceps tendon:
  - Requires prompt surgical repair
  - Time from injury to repair is the greatest determinant of outcome in athletes with quadriceps tendon ruptures. Repair within 2 to 3 wk yields significantly better outcomes (1)[C].
  - End-to-end repairs and tendon-to-bone repairs are used, depending on the level of the rupture.
- Proximal avulsion of the AIIS:
  - Vast majority are successfully treated nonoperatively.
  - Surgery to reattach the avulsed AIIS may be successful treatment if there is continued pain, disability, or both after conservative measures have failed.
- Intrasubstance rectus femoris grade III strains:
  - Removal of the tear may benefit those who continue to have pain or dysfunction after physical therapy.

ONGOING CARE

Return to play:

- When quadriceps has 120 degrees of flexion
- No signs of quadriceps weakness
- May take days to months based on the degree of injury

COMPLICATIONS

- Myositis ossificans—rare after noncontact injury but has been reported and can lead to prolonged pain or dysfunction
- Missed distal ruptures can lead to complicated surgical procedure and complicated postsurgical courses.

REFERENCES

1. Ibounig T, Simons TA. Etiology, diagnosis and treatment of tendinous knee extensor mechanism injuries. *Scand J Surg*. 2016;105(2):67–72.
2. Mendiguchia J, Alentorn-Geli E, Idoate F, et al. Rectus femoris muscle injuries in football: a clinically relevant review of mechanisms of injury, risk factors and preventive strategies. *Br J Sports Med*. 2013;47(6):359–366.
3. Brukner P, Connell D. "Serious thigh muscle strains": beware the intramuscular tendon which plays an important role in difficult hamstring and quadriceps muscle strains. *Br J Sports Med*. 2016;50(4):205–208.
4. Ekstrand J, Hägglund M, Waldén M. Epidemiology of muscle injuries in professional football (soccer). *Am J Sports Med*. 2011;39(6):1226–1232.
5. Gao X, Shao Z, Liu S, et al. A case report of spontaneous rupture of the quadriceps tendon. *Clin Case Rep*. 2017;5(9):1477–1481.
6. Eckard TG, Kerr ZY, Padua DA, et al. Epidemiology of quadriceps strains in National Collegiate Athletic Association Athletes, 2009–2010 through 2014–2015. *J Athl Train*. 2017;52(5):474–481.

ADDITIONAL READING

Kary JM. Diagnosis and management of quadriceps strains and contusions. *Curr Rev Musculoskelet Med*. 2010;3(1–4):26–31.

CLINICAL PEARLS

- Quadriceps strains are common in sports with kicking and other eccentric quadriceps loads.
- Be sure to rule out quadriceps tendon rupture by examining an intact extensor mechanism.

RADIAL TUNNEL SYNDROME

Katherine M. Pohlgeers, MD, MS, CAQSM

BASICS

DESCRIPTION

- Intermittent compression of the radial nerve through the radial tunnel is thought to be the pathologic basis for radial tunnel syndrome (RTS).
- The condition is not associated with extensor muscle weakness, and due to the fact that the diagnosis is clinical, the existence of RTS remains controversial (1).
- There is some discussion about whether RTS and posterior interosseous nerve (PIN) syndrome are two separate entities or a continuum of the same condition:
  - The presence of weakness is common with PIN.
  - In contrast, RTS typically presents as a pure pain syndrome without any objective clinical muscular weakness (2).
- RTS was first discovered when physicians were unable to relieve discomfort in patients with lateral epicondylitis. These two syndromes may also exist concurrently, in which case they are often confused and misdiagnosed, with patients presenting with epicondylitis that can exacerbate symptoms of RTS (3).

EPIDEMIOLOGY

Incidence

The disease is more prevalent in women ages 30 to 50 yr (1) and accounts for an estimated 2.97 per 100,000 cases of radial neuropathy in men and 1.42 per 100,000 of new cases in women (3).

ETIOLOGY AND PATHOPHYSIOLOGY

Anatomically, the radial tunnel is approximately 5 cm long and begins as the radial nerve courses past the radiocapitellar joint. Compression can occur at the following sites (4):

- Lateral elbow joint in radial head (osteoarthritis of fibrous bands anterior to the radiocapitellar joint or synovitis of the radiocapitellar joint)
- Leash of Henry (an arcade of anastomosing branches of the recurrent radial artery)
- Fibrous edge of the extensor carpi radialis brevis (ECRB)
- The arcade of Frohse (most common area of compression)
- Distal edge of radial tunnel (1)

RISK FACTORS

- History of a previous surgical intervention in ipsilateral upper extremity is a common finding in RTS (1).
- Trauma and heavy manual labor, especially in patients that perform effort-intensive forearm extensions in pronation or supination (1) as well as repetitive use of the index and middle fingers during activities such as computer mouse use(3)
- Other causes include idiopathic entrapment, lipomas, cysts, or rheumatoid synovitis (3).

DIAGNOSIS

HISTORY

- Lateral elbow pain and forearm pain that may radiate distally to the wrist and dorsum of the fingers
- Aggravated pain at night that may interfere with sleeping (1)
- Typically, do not have paresthesias, but instead, characteristic pain at the area of entrapment
- Pain often worsens with rotational movements of the forearm (4).

PHYSICAL EXAM

- Often, provocative maneuvers that can be used to aid in the diagnosis of RTS are also positive in patients with lateral epicondylosis, which is a closely associated differential diagnosis.
- Pressure that is applied over a patient's lateral forearm approximately 3 to 5 cm distal to the elbow (over the supinator muscle) with the wrist in full supination should reproduce pain (pronation during this maneuver should relieve the pain) (4).
- Positive Tinel sign at the radial tunnel (2)
- Symptoms are exacerbated with resisted supination, resisted extension of the wrist, and resisted middle finger extension (middle finger test) (1).

DIFFERENTIAL DIAGNOSIS

- Lateral epicondylitis
- PIN syndrome
- Osteoarthritis of the radiocapitellar joint
- Impingement of the articular branch of the radial nerve
- Synovitis of the radiocapitellar joint
- A muscle tear of the ECRB
- Posterior plica impingement
- Brachial plexus injury
- Biceps tendon pathology (1)

DIAGNOSTIC TESTS & INTERPRETATION

Initial Tests (lab, imaging)

- Shoulder and cervical radiographs can be helpful to exclude other pathologies.
- The validity of magnetic resonance imaging (MRI) studies is controversial, but in some cases, they may show muscle edema or atrophy along the distribution of the radial and PINs (1)[C].

Diagnostic Procedures/Other

- Electromyography and nerve conduction velocity results are typically normal and generally not useful (1)[C].
- Local anesthetic injection into the radial tunnel can be used to differentiate RTS from epicondylitis (3)[C].

TREATMENT

- Nonoperative approaches are considered first-line treatment (1,4)[C]:
  - Immobilization of the wrist with splinting or casting
  - Anti-inflammatory medication
  - Ultrasound massage
  - Radial nerve block (1)
  - Steroid injections
  - Physical therapy which may include nerve-gliding exercises, ultrasonographic therapy, heat/cold modalities (4)
- Operative treatment should be considered in patients that have failed conservative treatments for at least 3 mo (3)[C]:
  - The decompression is performed for the radial nerve and both of its branches: the PIN and superficial branch of the radial nerve (SBRN).
  - Surgery has been found to diminish pain and symptoms completely in 67–93% of patients (1).
  - Regardless of the surgical approaches, release of the nerve from the arcade of Frohse and ligating the radial recurrent blood vessels are essential.
  - The transbrachioradialis and anterior approaches are the most commonly used approaches today (1).
  - Patients with isolated RTS and no concurrent compressive neuropathy or tendinopathy have more favorable outcomes compared with patients with associated conditions (4).

ONGOING CARE

- Return to activity should be undertaken slowly as symptoms improve.
- Rehabilitation program should be continued for both nonoperative and postoperative patients.

REFERENCES

1. Moradi A, Ebrahimzadeh MH, Jupiter JB. Radial tunnel syndrome, diagnostic and treatment dilemma. *Arch Bone Jt Surg*. 2015;3(3):156–162.
2. Kane SF, Lynch JH, Taylor JC. Evaluation of elbow pain in adults. *Am Fam Physician*. 2014;89(8):649–657.
3. Kaswan S, Deigni O, Tadisina KK, et al. Radial tunnel syndrome complicated by lateral epicondylitis in a middle-aged female. *Eplasty*. 2014;14:ic44.
4. Strohl AB, Zelouf DS. Ulnar tunnel syndrome, radial tunnel syndrome, anterior interosseous nerve syndrome, and pronator syndrome. *J Am Acad Orthop Surg*. 2017;25(1):e1–e10.

CLINICAL PEARLS

- Entrapment of the deep branch of the radial nerve within the radial tunnel
- Diagnosis is based completely on clinical examination, leading to some skepticism of the actual prevalence.
- No motor deficits
- Often misdiagnosed as lateral epicondylitis
- Nonoperative treatment is preferred (nonsteroidal anti-inflammatory drugs [NSAIDs], physical therapy, injections); however, surgery is a viable option for those who are refractory to conservative measures.

RENAL TRAUMA

Angelina R. Edwards, MD • David S. Edwards, MD, CAQSM

BASICS

Genitourinary (GU) trauma comprises approximately 10% of all trauma but is relatively infrequent in sport-related injury. The most commonly injured organ is the kidney (1,2).

EPIDEMIOLOGY

- Renal trauma occurs in 5% of all trauma cases and in 8–10% of patients with abdominal trauma (3).
- Over the last two decades, incidence is rising due to motor vehicle collisions (MVC), particularly in young men (mean age 30.8 yr) (2).
- Pediatric consideration: Trauma registry data indicate that 80–90% of renal injuries occur in children with 6.6% of cases secondary to sport (62% of these occur in football), 51% of cases due to bicycling or falls, and 6% of cases due to other team sports:
  - Approximately 10% of blunt trauma in children includes renal involvement (2).
- Renal injuries are divided into renal laceration, renal contusion, and renal vascular injury (4,5).

ETIOLOGY AND PATHOPHYSIOLOGY

- The major mechanisms that generate renal injury are blunt, iatrogenic during an interventional procedure, or intraoperative (4).
- The most common causes of renal injury are blunt trauma to the abdomen or back/flanks, especially with rapid deceleration as occurs in MVC, contact/collision sports, or fall from a height.
- Penetrating injuries can cause up to 20% of renal injuries in urban areas (1).

RISK FACTORS

- Pediatric consideration: Children and adolescents are at increased risk due to greater kidney size relative to body size, less protection from ribs and perinephric fat, and weaker abdominal muscles (2,6).
- Risk factors are heavily dependent on patient population and location and are seen in a variety of sports from equestrian events to snow sports or use of all-terrain vehicles (2,6).

COMMONLY ASSOCIATED CONDITIONS

- Lower rib fractures
- Thoracolumbar vertebral fractures
- Intra-abdominal visceral injury

DIAGNOSIS

HISTORY

- Typical mechanisms include direct impact to the abdomen or flank, blow to the back, fall from a height, and rapid deceleration (1).
- Often, there is history of gross hematuria, which may be related to exercise in the absence of an obvious traumatic event (6).
- In cases of penetrating trauma, the type or caliber of weapon or blade size can be helpful.
- A history of underlying renal abnormality can increase the risk of injury (5).
- In the absence of trauma: Hematuria suggests nephrolithiasis or infection, whereas painless hematuria in an adult could indicate bladder cancer (5).

PHYSICAL EXAM

- Determine the stability of the patient with attention to primary survey, secondary survey, and vital signs, particularly blood pressure (BP):
  - Pediatric consideration: Hypotension may not correlate with degree of hypovolemia in children, so serial physical exams, BP measurements, and labs are essential (2,6).
- Inspect for ecchymosis or hematoma to the abdomen and/or flanks.
- Inspect for penetrating injury to the abdomen, flanks, or lower chest.
- Palpate ribs and thoracolumbar spine for tenderness, crepitance, or step-offs.
- Auscultate then palpate the abdomen for signs of visceral injury or peritonitis.

DIFFERENTIAL DIAGNOSIS

Hematuria: renal contusion; renal infarction; renal laceration; nephrolithiasis; exercise-induced trauma to the bladder, urethra, or prostate; urinary tract infection; malignancy

DIAGNOSTIC TESTS & INTERPRETATION

- Obtain basic labs with emphasis on hematocrit, creatinine, and urinalysis with microscopy.
- Increased creatinine suggests baseline renal impairment.
- Gross hematuria is present in 95% of renal trauma.
- Microscopic hematuria:
  - Three or more red blood cells (RBCs) per high-power field (HPF) in adults
  - Five or more RBCs per HPF in children (>50 RBCs per HPF in children per some sources)
- Neither degree nor absence of hematuria predicts severity of injury.
- The preferred imaging modality is computed tomography (CT) of abdomen and pelvis with intravenous (IV) contrast and with immediate and delayed images (5)[C]:
  - Renal imaging during the focused assessment with sonography in trauma is limited by inability to detect depth of laceration and inability to differentiate extravasated blood from urinoma.
- Indications for CT abdomen and pelvis with IV contrast include:
  - Gross/microscopic hematuria (may be absent in 25–50% of ureteropelvic junction injuries) (5)[B].
  - Hypotension (systolic BP <90 mm Hg) (5)[B].
  - History or physical exam consistent with renal injury (even in the absence of hematuria) (5)[C].
  - Suspicion of renal injury or multiorgan trauma.
- Indications for delayed contrast-enhanced CT (excretory phase imaging 5 to 10 min after contrast):
  - Evaluate the collecting system:
    - Parenchymal laceration (superficial <1 cm vs. deep >1 cm, can be poorly enhancing due to clotted blood and may mask a urine leak)
    - Perirenal hematoma (crescentic if small, lens-shaped/biconvex if large, enters perinephric space if capsule is lacerated) versus urinoma
- If too unstable for CT, consider intraoperative "single shot" IV pyelogram (5)[C]:
  - Identifies a functional contralateral kidney
  - Provides staging information on the renal pelvis and ureter
- The American Association for the Surgery of Trauma (AAST) grading system correlates well with CT findings and need for surgery and should be used to grade severity. Grade 2 or higher is considered a "major" injury (3):
  - Grade 1: contusion or subscapular hematoma (75–85% of renal trauma) (3)
  - Grade 2: cortical renal laceration <1 cm and lack of urinary extravasation on excretory phase CT imaging or perirenal hematoma that is nonexpanding
  - Grade 3: deep renal laceration extending to the medulla, without urinary extravasation
  - Grade 4: laceration extending through the collecting system with extravasation, vascular injury or segmental infarction, hilum preserved, contained hematoma
  - Grade 5: shattered or fractured kidney or hilar avulsion and devascularization

TREATMENT

- The approach to renal injuries has changed over time, from aggressive surgical interventions to more conservative, nonoperative observational or endovascular management (1).
- Typically conservative in 95% of cases:
  - Prehospital/sidelines evaluation: primary survey, secondary survey if feasible, urgent transport via ambulance
  - Emergency department: primary and secondary survey if not already done, close hemodynamic monitoring, labs, imaging, IV resuscitation, and consultation with trauma and/or urology colleagues
  - Inpatient ward versus intensive care unit: depending on clinical status:
    - Noninvasive if hemodynamically stable (5)[B]
    - Hemodynamic monitoring
    - Bed rest until macroscopic hematuria clears
    - Serial examination and hemoglobin/hematocrit measurement
    - Broad spectrum IV antibiotics can be used if there is damage to the collecting system/urine leak, perinephric abscess, and/or concern for infected retroperitoneal hematoma in the setting of devitalized tissue, bowel or pancreatic injury, comorbidities, or immunosuppression (3).
  - Conservative care for:
    - Grades 1 to 2: differentiate contusion from segmental infarction on CT (5)[B]
    - Grade 3: if hemodynamically stable (5)[B]

SURGERY/OTHER PROCEDURES

- There is a 64% rate of nephrectomy when renal injuries are explored surgically, regardless of the indication for exploration (3):
  - Goal of surgery is to control hemorrhage and salvage kidney function.
  - Indications for surgery:
    - Hemodynamic instability (5)[B]
    - Renal pedicle avulsion
    - Expanding, noncontained retroperitoneal hematoma
    - Persistent urinary leak
    - Worsening abdominal exam in children
- Endovascular management (4):
  - Transcatheter arterial angioembolization (TAE), with or without placement of stents/grafts, is becoming the preferred management of traumatic arterial injuries in those who are hemodynamically stable, without other indication for exploratory laparotomy.
  - Indication for endovascular management:
    - Diagnostic angiography and selective embolization of parenchymal injuries
    - Stenting of renal arterial thrombosis
    - Segmental arterial injuries
  - May prevent nephrectomy in 78% of grade 4 and 83% of grade 5 renal injuries (4)
  - Grades 4 and 5 lesions may require a second endovascular intervention to treat recurrent bleeding.
  - Postembolization syndrome:
    - Common side effect following TAE
    - Constellation of fever, abdominal pain, paralytic ileus with nausea and vomiting, leukocytosis
    - Severity of symptoms is dependent on the volume of infarcted tissue.
    - Moderate hematuria can occur depending on degree of infarction.
    - Treatment is supportive, and duration is self-limited, resolving in a few days.
- Urinary drainage performed only in the presence of complications such as fever, increased pain, ileus, fistula, or infection (5)[C]

ONGOING CARE

FOLLOW-UP RECOMMENDATIONS

- Follow-up CT scan if any clinical signs of complications (5)[C]
- Follow-up CT scan after 48 hr indicated if deep injury or grades 4 to 5 injury (5)[C]
- Complications occur in 3–33% of renal trauma, especially with higher grade injuries, and include:
  - The leading complication is extravasation of urine and infection of this urinoma:
    - Small urinomas often reabsorb spontaneously.
    - Perinephric abscess is best treated by percutaneous drainage.
  - Early (acute, $<$1 mo): worsening flank pain, uncontrolled bleeding, abdominal distention
  - Late:
    - Page kidney phenomenon/arterial hypertension (up to 40% of cases): extrinsic compression of renal parenchyma leading to intrarenal ischemia and activation of the renin-angiotensin system
    - Hypertension and renal impairment develop and can occur in native kidneys and renal allografts.
    - Hydronephrosis, stones, chronic pyelonephritis
- Outpatient follow-up: low-grade injury typically in 3 mo for physical exam, urinalysis, measurement of electrolytes and creatinine, serial BP (5)[C]
- Considerations in renal transplant patients:
  - Kidney transplant remains an ideal treatment for end-stage renal disease, and although transplant patients make up a small percentage of trauma patients, large outcome data is lacking.
  - Retrospective reviews have challenged the common presumption among physicians that trauma patients with organ transplants do worse than nontransplanted patients.
  - Trauma registries show rare direct renal allograft injuries, few acute kidney injury events, and no greater infection risk from traumatic injury.
  - An increased risk of posttrauma rejection was observed, perhaps due to trauma-related activation of the immune system, triggering a proinflammatory state.
  - Transplant trauma patients should be assessed by a transplant surgeon as soon as possible, and graft function should be closely followed, with input by the transplant nephrologist, during the hospitalization and after discharge.

REFERENCES

1. Anselmo da Costa I, Amend B, Stenzl A, et al. Contemporary management of acute kidney trauma. *J Acute Dis*. 2016;5:29–36.
2. Bernard J. Renal trauma: evaluation, management, and return to play. *Curr Sports Med Rep*. 2009;8(2):98–103.
3. Cimbanassi S, Chiara O, Leppaniemi A, et al. Nonoperative management of abdominal solid-organ injuries following blunt trauma in adults: results from an international consensus conference. *J Trauma Acute Care Surg*. 2018;84(3):517–531.
4. Loffroy R, Chevallier O, Gehin S, et al. Endovascular management of arterial injuries after blunt or iatrogenic renal trauma. *Quant Imaging Med Surg*. 2017;7(4):434–442.
5. Morey A, Brandes S, Dugi D III, et al. Urotrauma: AUA guideline. *J Urol*. 2014;192(2):327–335.
6. Nicola R, Menias C, Mellnick V, et al. Sports-related genitourinary trauma in the male athlete. *Emerg Radiol*. 2015;22(2):157–168.

ADDITIONAL READING

Medical conditions affecting sports participation. American Academy of Pediatrics Committee on Sports Medicine and Fitness. *Pediatrics*. 1994;94(5):757–760.

CLINICAL PEARLS

- AAST grades 1 to 3 injuries have a low risk of complications with no need for follow-up CT scan in the setting of ongoing clinical improvement.
- The leading vascular injury due to blunt trauma is renal artery occlusion, manifesting as a well-defined segmental or global absence of parenchymal enhancement on CT scan. Collateral perfusion can create the "cortical rim sign" within 8 hr of trauma.
- Regardless of the grade of injury, nonoperative management, including observation, supportive therapy, and endovascular interventions, in hemodynamically stable patients, is favored over surgical intervention.
- Participation in contact or collision sport in the athlete with a single kidney is controversial. Please see the "Additional Reading" section for details.
- Although no consensus statement exists for return to play, athletes should not return to play until hematuria has resolved. For those in contact sports with grades 1 to 3 injuries, 2- to 6-wk recovery time is reasonable. For those with more extensive injuries, more prolonged recovery on the order of 6 to 12 mo may be required before returning to contact sports.

RETINAL DETACHMENTS AND TEARS

Giselle Aerni, MD • Robert L. Howard, MA, ATC

BASICS

DESCRIPTION

- Retinal detachment occurs when the neurosensory layer of the retina separates from the underlying retinal pigment epithelium.
- Three distinct classifications of retinal detachments:
  - Rhegmatogenous retinal detachment (RRD)
  - Tractional retinal detachment (TRD)
  - Exudative retinal detachment (ERD)
- RRD:
  - Occurs when a break in the sensory retina allows fluid from the vitreous to enter the subretinal space
- TRD:
  - Occurs because of contraction of fibrovascular or fibrotic tissue pulling the sensory retina off of the pigment epithelium
- ERD:
  - Abnormal collections of fluid are produced below the retina, separating the layer of the retina.

EPIDEMIOLOGY

- RRD is the most common type.
- Incidence increases with age.
- Male greater than female
- Occurs in 5–25% of patients with Marfan syndrome

ETIOLOGY AND PATHOPHYSIOLOGY

- RRD occurs as a result of either structural or developmental abnormalities of the eye or trauma:
  - High myopia
  - Lattice degeneration
  - Posterior vitreous detachment (PVD)
  - Trauma is less common etiology, however, produces more retinal dialysis and giant tears.
- TRD:
  - Diabetic retinopathy
  - Proliferative vitreoretinopathy
  - Retinopathy of prematurity
  - Sickle cell retinopathy
  - Toxocariasis
- ERD arises from transudative fluid:
  - Tumors of the choroid or retina
  - Inflammatory disorders such as Coats or Harada disease
  - Central serous retinopathy
  - Hypertensive retinopathy
  - Toxemia of pregnancy

RISK FACTORS

- Myopia
- Cataract surgery
- Aphakia
- Trauma
- Retinal detachment in fellow eye
- Glaucoma
- Vitreoretinal tufts: caused by focal areas of vitreous traction
- Meridional folds: redundant retina
- Family history of retinal detachment

GENERAL PREVENTION

- Early identification of retinal tears and treatment may prevent progression to retinal detachment and significant vision loss.
- Protective eyewear may prevent traumatic RRD.

DIAGNOSIS

HISTORY

- Floaters
- Flashes of light
- Sudden loss of vision
- Expanding shadow
- Progressive peripheral visual field defect
- May be asymptomatic

PHYSICAL EXAM

- Visual acuity and visual field testing:
  - May be decreased depending on location of tear/detachment
- Pupil exam:
  - May have relative afferent pupillary defect
- Dilated funduscopic exam:
  - RRD:
    - Mobile, convex retina
    - Retinal tears
    - Subretinal fluid does not shift with changes in head position.
    - Pigmented cells within the vitreous ("tobacco dust")
    - Vitreous hemorrhage
    - Chronic RRD: pigmented demarcation lines, intraretinal cysts, static retinal folds
  - TRD:
    - Smooth elevated retina
    - Fibrovascular proliferation
  - ERD:
    - Smooth elevated retina
    - Subretinal fluid shifts with changes in head position.
- Depressed peripheral retinal exam:
  - Indirect ophthalmoscopy using pressure to depress sclera in order to examine the peripheral retina for tears

DIFFERENTIAL DIAGNOSIS

- Senile retinoschisis
- Juvenile retinoschisis
- Choroidal detachment
- Vitreous hemorrhage
- Vitreous inflammation (e.g., *Toxoplasma* chorioretinitis)
- Ocular lymphoma
- Intraocular foreign body

DIAGNOSTIC TESTS & INTERPRETATION

B-scan ultrasound:

- Smooth, convex, mobile retina visualized as hyperechoic lesion in vitreous cavity
- In ERD, hyperechoic areas will shift with head movement.
- In TRD, will have tented appearance with vitreous adhesions

TREATMENT

ISSUES FOR REFERRAL

- Urgent ophthalmologic consultation
- A retina specialist ultimately will need to care for the patient if retinal detachment is present.

SURGERY/OTHER PROCEDURES

- PVD management:
  - Most patients who present with PVD and do not have any retinal breaks or tears require only reassurance and education.
  - Full dilated exam with indirect ophthalmoscopy at least twice during the 6 wk following onset of symptoms
- Retinal detachment repair is trending toward less invasive techniques with greater preference for vitrectomy over scleral buckling or pneumatic retinopexy (1)[C].
- RRD:
  - Vitrectomy and scleral buckling have similar outcomes (2,3,4)[B],(5)[A].
  - Pneumatic retinopexy is a simple and cost-effective treatment for uncomplicated RRD (6)[B].
  - RRDs that do not yet involve the macula ("macula on") require repair within 24 to 48 hr.
  - RRDs involving the macula ("macula off") may be repaired within 2 to 4 days because there is no evidence that urgent repair affects the outcome (7)[C].
- TRD:
  - Vitreoretinal surgery to release traction if necessary
  - Observation unless macula is threatened or combined traction-rhegmatogenous detachment develops
- ERD:
  - Identify and treat etiology; surgical repair is not recommended in most cases.

ADMISSION, INPATIENT, AND NURSING CONSIDERATIONS

- Bed rest prior to surgery
- Postoperatively, if intraocular gas has been used, the patient may need specific head positioning and may need to avoid all air travel or high altitudes.

ONGOING CARE

PROGNOSIS

RRD:

- Pneumatic retinopexy leads to successful retinal attachment 70–80% of the time after one procedure (8)[A]:
  - In cases of failure, treat with scleral buckle placement and/or vitrectomy.
- Scleral buckle placement is successful 80–90% of the time after one procedure (8)[A]:
  - Failed cases usually are treated with vitrectomy.
- Vitrectomy has an 80–90% success rate after one surgery (8)[A]:
  - In failed cases, more extensive vitreoretinal procedures are required.
- Virtually, all patients age >50 yr will develop progressive cataract following vitrectomy.

REFERENCES

1. Williams PD, Hariprasad SM. Evolving trends in primary retinal detachment repair: microincisional vitrectomy and the role of OCT. *Ophthalmic Surg Lasers Imaging Retina*. 2014;45(4):268–272.
2. Chang JS, Marra K, Flynn HW Jr, et al. Scleral buckling in the treatment of retinal detachment due to retinal dialysis. *Ophthalmic Surg Lasers Imaging Retina*. 2016;47(4):336–340.
3. Cankurtaran V, Citirik M, Simsek M, et al. Anatomical and functional outcomes of scleral buckling versus primary vitrectomy in pseudophakic retinal detachment. *Bosn J Basic Med Sci*. 2017;17(1):74–80.
4. Lindsell LB, Sisk RA, Miller DM, et al. Comparison of outcomes: scleral buckling and pars plana vitrectomy versus vitrectomy alone for primary repair of rhegmatogenous retinal detachment. *Clin Ophthalmol*. 2016;11:47–54.
5. Sun Q, Sun T, Xu Y, et al. Primary vitrectomy versus scleral buckling for the treatment of rhegmatogenous retinal detachment: a meta-analysis of randomized controlled clinical trials. *Curr Eye Res*. 2012;37(6):492–499.
6. Dhami A, Shah KK, Ratra D. Pneumatic retinopexy outcomes as primary or secondary surgical option for treating rhegmatogenous retinal detachment. *Indian J Ophthalmol*. 2018;66(3):420–425.
7. Wykoff CC, Flynn HW Jr, Scott IU. What is the optimal timing for rhegmatogenous retinal detachment repair? *JAMA Ophthalmol*. 2013;131(11):1399–1400.
8. Hatef E, Sena DF, Fallano KA, et al. Pneumatic retinopexy versus scleral buckle for repairing simple rhegmatogenous retinal detachments. *Cochrane Database Syst Rev*. 2015;(5):CD008350.

ADDITIONAL READING

- Lee T, Chen Y, Kuo H, et al. Retinal detachment associated with basketball-related eye trauma. *Am J Ophthalmol*. 2017;180:97–101.
- Read SP, Young RC, Flynn HW Jr. Outcomes in bullous retinal detachment. *Am J Ophthalmol Case Rep*. 2016;6:18–20.
- Yokoyama S, Kojima T, Mori T, et al. Clinical outcomes of endoscope-assisted vitrectomy for treatment of rhegmatogenous retinal detachment. *Clin Ophthalmol*. 2017;11:2003–2010.

CLINICAL PEARLS

- Concern for retinal tear or detachment should prompt urgent ophthalmology consultation.
- Although trauma is an uncommon etiology, protective eyewear may help to prevent traumatic causes of retinal detachment.
- Return to play:
  - The injured eye should feel comfortable and have adequate return of vision.
  - Eye protectors must be worn.

RHABDOMYOLYSIS

Vijay Jotwani, MD

BASICS

DESCRIPTION

- The breakdown and necrosis of skeletal muscle with subsequent release of intracellular contents, such as myoglobin and creatine phosphokinase (CK)
- A combination of myoglobinuria, hypovolemia, and aciduria may lead to acute renal disease.
- Can be result of trauma/crush injury or as a result of training error where exertion persists beyond the point of fatigue (exertional rhabdomyolysis [ER]), often due to novel activity

EPIDEMIOLOGY

- Occurs in up to 85% of trauma patients
- 10–50% of patients with rhabdomyolysis will develop acute renal failure (ARF).
- ~26,000 people are affected in the United States each year (1).
- Exact incidence of ER is unknown but is likely comparable to military reports of 0.3–3%.

ETIOLOGY AND PATHOPHYSIOLOGY

- Muscle damage and/or necrosis that results in elevation in CK levels, electrolyte disturbances, and renal compromise as a result of:
  - Trauma/crush injuries (motor vehicle accidents, fall from seizure or stroke, struggle against restraints, abuse, prolonged tourniquet)
  - ER occurs due to exercise past the point of fatigue.
- Skeletal muscle necrosis occurs due to an increase in intracellular calcium resulting in rupture of the cellular membrane.
- Cell damage results in the release of intracellular contents including myoglobin, which is nephrotoxic. Myoglobin can be detected in the urine and causes darkening of urine color.
- Skeletal muscle damage also results in release of potassium, which can trigger arrhythmia and sudden death.

Genetics

Metabolic myopathies:

- Considered in recurrent cases or persistent CK elevation or kidney injury >2 wk (1)
- Inherited disorders:
  - McArdle disease
  - Carnitine palmitoyltransferase deficiency
  - Fatty acid oxidation deficiency
  - Aconitase deficiency
  - Myoadenylate dehydrogenase deficiency
  - Mitochondrial myopathies
  - Muscular dystrophy

RISK FACTORS

- Sudden increase in exercise intensity and repetitive muscular loading
- Inadequate conditioning
- Poor hydration
- Exercise in high heat or humidity
- Stimulant and supplement use (phentermine, creatine)
- High body mass
- High-risk medication or drug use (cocaine, amphetamines, alcohol, nonsteroidal anti-inflammatory drugs [NSAIDs], antihistamines, statins, etc.)
- Ongoing infection/exercise while febrile
- Sickle cell trait
- Heritable muscle enzyme deficiencies
- The majority of U.S. military cases occurred between June and August in black, non-Hispanic males <20 yr of age (2).

DIAGNOSIS

- Symptoms of muscle injury along with an increase in CK levels used to make the diagnosis. Typical threshold is a CK level 5 to 10 times the upper limit of normal (~1,000 IU/L) (1)[C].
- Symptoms include muscle pain, swelling, and weakness. Other general symptoms may include malaise, fever, tachycardia, nausea.
- History and physical are insensitive in making the diagnosis and a high level of suspicion is needed for athletes with risk factors above.
- *Serum CK level must be checked if any clinical suspicion exists* (2)[C].
- Serum electrolytes, BUN, creatinine, calcium, and liver enzyme levels should be obtained:
  - Urine dipstick that is positive for heme but absent for RBCs suggests rhabdomyolysis (myoglobinuria):
    - Because of rapid urinary excretion of myoglobin, up to 26% of patients with rhabdomyolysis have negative urine dipstick.

HISTORY

- Wide range of severity of symptoms
- Classic triad of symptoms: muscle pain, weakness, and dark urine (seen in <10% of patients)
- General symptoms may include malaise, fever, tachycardia, nausea/emesis.
- ER typically due to error in training and will occur soon after exertion of increased intensity (i.e., early season training sessions/"two a days," new, intense, and group-based exercise programs, punishment-based workouts).

PHYSICAL EXAM

- Muscle tenderness, swelling, or weakness (proximal upper and lower extremities, calves, and lower back are most commonly involved)
- Change in urine color; orange to cola-colored to black (not a reliable finding occurring in as few as 25% of cases)
- Visible crush injury in traumatic rhabdomyolysis
- Patient may be either alert or obtunded.
- Hypovolemic state, dry mucous membrane, poor skin turgor, tachycardia, hypotension
- Hypothermia/hyperthermia
- Decreased urine output

DIFFERENTIAL DIAGNOSIS

The following conditions can also cause muscle pain or swelling:

- Muscle strain
- Delayed onset muscle soreness
- Muscle infection
- Sickle cell crisis
- Nontraumatic myopathies
- Hypercalcemia/hyperparathyroidism
- Hypo/hyperthyroidism
- Renal failure
- Tumor

DIAGNOSTIC TESTS & INTERPRETATION

Initial Tests (lab, imaging)

- CK levels are the most sensitive; CK-MM isoenzyme is most elevated.
- CK rise of 5 to 10 times normal upper limit (~1,000 IU/L) concerning for rhabdomyolysis
- CK levels rise within 12 hr, typically peak in 1 to 4 days, and gradually return to normal over days to weeks.

ALERT

CK levels can rise well above levels of 100,000 IU/L, but severity of CK rise does not necessarily correlate to presence of myoglobinuria or severity of renal failure.

- Physical exertion can increase CK levels without rhabdomyolysis as well:
  - Black military recruits had a mean rise in CK to 1,226 IU/L at day 7 of basic training (but range as high as 35,000) without rhabdomyolysis (2).
  - Study of ultra-marathoners found a mean CK increase to 2,400 IU/L also without symptoms of rhabdomyolysis.
- Urine dipstick will show blood but no RBCs due to myoglobinuria.
- Serum and urine myoglobin levels useful in acute phase but have short half-life and may return to normal within 6 to 8 hr
- Metabolic profile to check for hyperkalemia, hypocalcemia, hyperphosphatemia, hyperuricemia
- Toxicology screen in absence of physical injury
- Prothrombin time/partial thromboplastin time, platelet count, fibrinogen, fibrin-split products if disseminated intravascular coagulopathy is suspected
- Magnetic resonance imaging (MRI) is sensitive in visualizing muscle injury but is not typically obtained because it does not affect treatment.

Diagnostic Procedures/Other

Forearm ischemic test:

- To differentiate genetic causes of rhabdomyolysis
- Performed after rhabdomyolysis is resolved
- Obtain baseline ammonia and lactic acid levels.
- Inflate sphygmomanometer to >200 mm Hg.
- Patient performs hand-grip exercises to fatigue.
- Cuff is removed and serial blood tests are drawn.
- Minimal or no rise in lactic acid suggests carbohydrate metabolism disorder or McArdle disease.
- Delayed rise or no rise in the ammonia level suggests myoadenylate deaminase deficiency.
- Normal rise in ammonia and lactic acid levels suggests the presence of a disorder of lipid metabolism.

TREATMENT

- Aggressive fluid resuscitation is paramount to limiting renal compromise.
- Prehospital:
  - Need for rapid extrication in case of crush injury
  - Early intravenous (IV) fluids to prevent complications (hypovolemia, ARF, hyperkalemia, etc.)
- Emergency department (ED) treatment:
  - Directed toward treating or reversing the underlying cause of rhabdomyolysis
  - Prevent ARF:
    - Immediate IV isotonic saline
    - Bicarbonate administration can be considered for alkalization of urine to decrease myoglobin toxicity to renal tubules (3)[C].
    - Mannitol following IV saline promotes diuresis, acts as renal vasodilator, and may act as free-radical scavenger, but clinical effects are unproven.
    - Furosemide administration is controversial.
  - Hyperkalemia: IV fluid, sodium bicarbonate, dextrose, insulin, telemetry monitor/electrocardiogram
  - Drug overdose: activated charcoal, lavage, antidote
  - Infection: broad-spectrum antibiotics
  - Compartment syndrome: fasciotomy (compartment pressure >35 mm Hg)
  - Neuroleptic malignant syndrome: dantrolene, bromocriptine
  - Need for hemodialysis: refractory to treatment, hyperkalemia, hyperphosphatemia, hyperuricemia, volume overload, overdose

MEDICATION

Medication guidelines (1,3):

- Administer IV isotonic saline at 400 to 2,000 mL/hr initially followed by maintenance at 120 to 400 mL/hr (3).
- Goal: to achieve urine output of 200 to 300 mL/hr until myoglobinuria resolves

First Line

IV fluids: isotonic saline

Second Line

- Addition of potassium chloride, bicarbonate, and mannitol has been recommended but has unproven benefit.
- Furosemide administration is controversial.

ADMISSION, INPATIENT, AND NURSING CONSIDERATIONS

- Initial stabilization:
  - Airway, breathing, and circulation (ABCs)
  - Immobilization of trauma/crush injuries
  - IV fluids for hypotension and hypovolemia
- Admission criteria:
  - Because it is impossible to predict which patients will develop complications, all patients with significant elevated CK or suspicion for rhabdomyolysis should be admitted.
  - Admit to telemetry-monitored bed for patients with electrolyte abnormalities.
  - Admit to intensive care unit bed for patients who might require hemodialysis or closer fluid and electrolyte monitoring.
  - Consider nephrology consultation if significant or persisting renal injury is noted.
  - CK levels should be reevaluated at least once daily (2)[C].
- IV fluids:
  - Plasma volume resuscitation with isotonic saline is first-line treatment.
- Nursing:
  - Monitor input/output closely with attention to urinary output.
- Discharge criteria:
  - No specific CK level is necessary for discharge, but level should be decreasing before considering discharge (3).
  - Myoglobinuria, when present, should be resolved.
  - Stable electrolytes and adequate renal function required before discharge from hospital
  - Patient should demonstrate tolerance for PO hydration. Patient should follow-up within 1 wk after discharge.

ONGOING CARE

- Underlying cause of rhabdomyolysis should be determined if etiology was not discovered during hospital stay.
- Genetic testing and muscle biopsy should be considered when suspicion for underlying genetic conditions.
- Medications, if implicated, should be stopped.
- Metabolic-modifying supplements and enhancing agents should be stopped.
- Activity modification if exercise induced

FOLLOW-UP RECOMMENDATIONS

- No evidence-based guidelines exist for return to exercise after ER (2).
- Return-to-play considerations:
  - Symptoms should be completely resolved.
  - Blood work should be trending toward normal limits.
  - Myoglobinuria should be resolved.
  - Infection and fever should be resolved.
  - Examination should demonstrate normal muscle strength and resolution of muscle pain.
  - Gradual return to exercise should first begin in cool, controlled environments to allow acclimatization before moving outdoors (4).
  - Return to exercise should begin with low-impact aerobic activities involving concentric muscle contractions and gradually advance toward higher impact resistance and eccentric exercise (4).

Patient Monitoring

Initially, patient should be monitored clinically at regular short intervals with close physician follow-up.

DIET

- Education should be provided about hydration.
- Specific diet recommendations may be considered for specific myopathies.

PATIENT EDUCATION

Prevention strategies for return to sports after rhabdomyolysis:

- Appropriate hydration counseling should be provided.
- Gradual return to exercise may include acclimatization.
- Return to exercise should begin with mild to moderate intensity.
- Athlete should be advised to stop activity if he or she experiences similar symptoms and physician should be contacted immediately.

COMPLICATIONS

- Early complications:
  - Hyperkalemia
  - Hypocalcemia
  - Cardiac arrhythmia
  - Cardiac arrest
  - Compartment syndrome
- Late complications (past 12 hr):
  - ARF with oliguria
  - Hypercalcemia
  - Disseminated intravascular coagulation
  - Compartment syndrome

REFERENCES

1. Hummel K, Gregory A, Desai N, et al. Rhabdomyolysis in adolescent athletes: review of cases. *Phys Sportsmed*. 2016;44(2):195–199.
2. Tietze D, Borchers J. Exertional rhabdomyolysis in the athlete: a clinical review. *Sports Health*. 2014;6(4):336–339.
3. Manspeaker S, Henderson K, Riddle D. Treatment of exertional rhabdomyolysis in athletes: a systematic review. *JBI Database System Rev Implement Rep*. 2016;14(6):117–147.
4. Schleich K, Slayman T, West D, et al. Return to play after exertional rhabdomyolysis. *J Athl Train*. 2016;51(5):406–409.

CLINICAL PEARLS

- Consider rhabdomyolysis in any athlete with muscle pain, swelling, or weakness or following significant trauma.
- ER is a preventable condition that occurs secondary to training error when exertion persists beyond fatigue.
- CK elevation >5 times the upper limit and symptoms of muscle injury are required for diagnosis, but CK levels can vary significantly amongst cases and can also be elevated in cases of asymptomatic physical exertion.
- Inpatient monitoring of kidney function and IV fluid administration is required for treatment.
- Discharge from hospital can be made when CK and creatinine values are trending toward normal, and return to sport must be gradual and individualized.

RHEUMATOID ARTHRITIS IN SPORTS

Kenneth P. Barnes, MD, MSc, CAQSM, FACSM • Shane Hudnall, MD, CAQSM

BASICS

Chronic systemic inflammatory autoimmune disorder that primarily affects the small joints of the body causing a symmetric polyarthritis

DESCRIPTION

- Polyarthritis most commonly affecting the joints of the wrist, the proximal interphalangeal (PIP) and metacarpophalangeal (MCP) joints of the hands, and the metatarsophalangeal (MTP) joints of the feet
- Less commonly affects cervical spine (although higher risk of atlantoaxial instability than general population), ankles, knees, hips, elbows, and shoulders
- Extra-articular manifestations: anemia, rheumatoid nodules (20–30%), pleuritis, pericarditis, entrapment neuropathies (carpal tunnel syndrome), episcleritis and scleritis (<1%), splenomegaly, renal disease, interstitial lung fibrosis, pericarditis, interstitial lung disease, vasculitis, Sjögren syndrome, Felty syndrome (rheumatoid arthritis [RA], splenomegaly, neutropenia)

EPIDEMIOLOGY

Incidence

- Annual incidence roughly 3/10,000
- Prevalence overall 1%; varies from 0.1% to 5% based on ethnic background
- Predominant gender: female > male (2 to 5:1; increases in patients >60 yr)
- Mean age of onset is 52 yr.
- Peak age of onset is between 35 and 70 yr, although possible in all ages.

ETIOLOGY AND PATHOPHYSIOLOGY

- Characterized by the presence of pannus (a proliferative mass of inflammatory vascularized tissue that may erode bone or cartilage)
- Macrophages produce cytokines (e.g., tissue necrosis factor α [TNF-α]), which produce many of the systemic features (e.g., fatigue, weight loss, elevated C-reactive protein [CRP] and erythrocyte sedimentation rate [ESR], and joint damage).

RISK FACTORS

- Female gender (Pregnancy and oral contraceptive use may be protective.)
- Nulliparity
- Family history (identical twins 3 to 4 times more likely to share disease than fraternal twins)
- Human leukocyte antigen (HLA)-DR4 (also tend to have more severe disease)
- Cigarette smoking
- Silica or asbestos exposure
- Electrical workers
- Wood workers

DIAGNOSIS

HISTORY

- Clinical diagnosis: usually symmetric synovitis (warmth, swelling, tenderness) of small joints (MCPs, PIPs, MTPs, wrists) with morning stiffness >1 hr that improves with activity
- Progression to joint destruction and deformities (ulnar deviation at MCPs, volar subluxation at MCPs and wrists, swan-neck, and/or boutonnière deformities of fingers)
- Constitutional symptoms are very common (e.g., low-grade fever, fatigue, myalgia, weight loss).
- American Rheumatism Association (ARA) criteria (4 or more for >6 wk):
  - Morning stiffness
  - Symmetric arthritis
  - Arthritis in 3+ joints
  - Involvement of hand joints
  - Rheumatoid nodules
  - Serum rheumatoid factor positive
  - Radiographic changes
- Note that ~25% of patients have monoarticular involvement at initial presentation.
- Extra-articular manifestations (e.g., chest pain, shortness of breath, skin changes, nodules, dry eyes or mouth)

PHYSICAL EXAM

- Examine joints thoroughly for synovitis (warmth, swelling, tenderness, erythema).
- Look for deformities (swan-neck, boutonnières, ulnar deviation of digits/wrists, volar subluxation at MCP or wrist)
- Nail fold infarcts
- Splinter hemorrhages
- Rheumatoid nodules
- Splenomegaly
- Pericardial rub
- Pleural effusions

DIFFERENTIAL DIAGNOSIS

- Systemic lupus erythematosus (SLE)
- Osteoarthritis (typically involves distal interphalangeals, knees, hips)
- Reactive arthritis
- Lyme disease
- Gout
- Pseudogout
- Polymyalgia rheumatica
- Hypothyroidism
- Hypertrophic osteoarthropathy
- Colitis
- Ankylosing spondylitis

DIAGNOSTIC TESTS & INTERPRETATION

- Joint fluid exam most helpful: >10,000 white blood cells (WBCs) with neutrophilic predominance characteristic but nondiagnostic
- Rheumatoid factor positive >80% of the time but is not sufficient for diagnosis or to rule out diagnosis; if positive, more likely to have severe disease and extra-articular involvement than if was negative
- Antinuclear antibodies (ANAs) also not diagnostic
- ESR and CRP not specific but may be elevated
- Complete blood count (CBC): anemia: hemoglobin generally >9; level correlates with disease severity, leukocytosis, thrombocytosis.
- Abnormal liver function tests: low albumin: directly linked to disease severity; elevated alkaline phosphatase
- Anticyclic citrullinated peptide (anti-CCP) antibodies: sensitivity of 67%, specificity of 95% for diagnosis of RA
- X-rays: erosions or bony decalcification in wrist or posteroanterior hand radiographs
- Early: Obtain posteroanterior view of hands and wrists, anteroposterior view of both feet for future comparison of bony destruction.
- Computed tomography (CT) scan, magnetic resonance imaging (MRI), and ultrasound (US) much more sensitive for detecting early signs of damage and revealing erosions or edematous bony lesions (that were not seen on plain radiography)

TREATMENT

- Nonpharmacologic treatment:
  - Patient education, relative rest, routine exercise, physical and occupational therapy, cognitive-behavioral therapy, dietary therapy
  - Cognitive-behavioral therapy and self-management educational interventions have been shown to reduce pain and disability.
  - Strength training has been shown to improve strength and function in early RA without adversely affecting disease activity.
  - Aerobic exercise improves pain scores and quality of life at least in the short term (1)[A].
  - Occupational therapy hand exercise programs in RA improved hand function out to 12 mo (2)[A].
  - Fish oil at 5.5 g daily added to methotrexate + sulfasalazine + hydroxychloroquine resulted in quicker remission or low disease activity (3)[A].
  - Limit and treat cardiovascular risk factors (smoking, hyperlipidemia, hypertension, diabetes) given RA increases risk of atherosclerotic disease.
- Pharmacologic treatment:
  - Disease-modifying antirheumatic drugs (DMARDs) monotherapy preferred in patients who have never taken one before regardless of disease activity
  - Review specific side-effect profiles and monitoring parameters for medications.

MEDICATION

- Analgesia: nonsteroidal anti-inflammatory drugs (NSAIDs) helpful in controlling pain and inflammation, improving daily function, but they do not alter natural course of disease:
  - High-dose aspirin (12 to 16 tabs/day) or ibuprofen (2,400 mg/day)
- DMARDs: Many of these agents inhibit progression of erosive disease; offer to all patients as early as possible in disease course; divided into nonbiologic and biologic agents
- Nonbiologic agents:
  - Methotrexate most commonly used nonbiologic agent and is generally preferred; takes effect as early as 4 wk; not to take in pregnancy; monitor for hematologic, hepatic, or pulmonary side effects (use folic acid supplementation 1 mg daily with methotrexate):
    - If fails, combine therapy with other DMARDs (methotrexate + sulfasalazine + hydroxychloroquine) or a biologic agent with or without methotrexate (4)

- Sulfasalazine
- Hydroxychloroquine
- Minocycline
- Azathioprine
- Gold
- Biologic agents:
  - Effective at modifying disease and preventing erosions but increased risk of infection
  - Tuberculosis skin test prior to initiation because it can reactivate mycobacterial infections
  - As general rule, do not combine biologic agents with one another.
  - Etanercept: inhibits action of TNF-α; subcutaneous (SC) injection 50 mg every week or 25 mg twice weekly
  - Infliximab: antibody to TNF-α; periodic intravenous (IV) infusion
  - Other biologic agents include adalimumab, rituximab, anakinra, abatacept, certolizumab pegol, and golimumab.
- Corticosteroids:
  - Oral, IV, and intra-articular forms
  - Prednisolone <7.5 mg/day is relatively safe; greater doses should be used only for short periods of time.

ADDITIONAL THERAPIES

Consider total joint replacement for severe disability or pain that is unresponsive to medical therapy.

ONGOING CARE

PATIENT EDUCATION

- Exercise and increase in activity are associated with decreased level of pain, increased function, and better outcomes in patients with RA (best data shown for whole-body low-intensity group and individual exercise).
- Athletes with a history of cervical spine involvement need flexion/extension radiographs of C1 and C2 to assess risk of motion (atlantoaxial instability) and subsequent spinal cord injury.
- Generally can play most sports, although contact sports and sports with a trampoline confer much greater risk and may be discouraged
- Athletes with ocular involvement should be screened by ophthalmologist before being allowed to play; may need eye protection
- If have systemic idiopathic (juvenile) RA or HLA-B27–associated RA, must have cardiovascular assessment

PROGNOSIS

- Clinical course and severity highly variable, ranging from insidious onset, slowly progressive disease with little destruction of joint spaces and few deformities (majority of cases), to a rapidly progressive disease leading to severe bony destruction and deformities (roughly 10–15%)
- Poor prognostic factors:
  - Functional limitation
  - Extra-articular disease
  - Rheumatoid factor positivity or anti-CCP antibody positive
  - Bony erosions by x-ray
  - Cigarette smoking

COMPLICATIONS

- 50% increased risk of cardiovascular disease death in those with RA
- Increased risk of stroke (especially ischemic) with RA
- 70% higher risk for developing infection (most likely related to immune dysfunction)
- Increased likelihood to develop lymphoma; correlates directly with RA disease severity

REFERENCES

1. Baillet A, Zeboulon N, Gossec L, et al. Efficacy of cardiorespiratory aerobic exercise in rheumatoid arthritis: meta-analysis of randomized controlled trials. *Arthritis Care Res (Hoboken)*. 2010;62(7):984–992.
2. Lamb SE, Williamson EM, Heine PJ, et al. Exercises to improve function of the rheumatoid hand (SARAH): a randomized controlled trial. *Lancet*. 2015;385(9966):421–429.
3. Proudman SM, James MJ, Spargo LD, et al. Fish oil in recent onset rheumatoid arthritis: a randomized, double-blind controlled trial within algorithm-based drug use. *Ann Rheum Dis*. 2015;74(1):89–95.
4. Singh JA, Saag KG, Bridges SL Jr, et al. 2015 American College of Rheumatology guideline for the treatment of rheumatoid arthritis. *Arthritis Rheumatol*. 2016;68(1):1–25.

ADDITIONAL READING

- Aviña-Zubieta JA, Choi HK, Sadatsafavi M, et al. Risk of cardiovascular mortality in patients with rheumatoid arthritis: a meta-analysis of observational studies. *Arthritis Rheum*. 2008;59(12):1690–1697.
- Baecklund E, Iliadou A, Askling J, et al. Association of chronic inflammation, not its treatment, with increased lymphoma risk in rheumatoid arthritis. *Arthritis Rheum*. 2006;54(3):692–701.
- Bradley LA, Young LD, Anderson KO, et al. Effects of psychological therapy on pain behavior of rheumatoid arthritis patients. Treatment outcome and six-month followup. *Arthritis Rheum*. 1987;30(10):1105–1114.
- Doran MF, Crowson CS, Pond GR, et al. Frequency of infection in patients with rheumatoid arthritis compared with controls: a population-based study. *Arthritis Rheum*. 2002;46(9):2287–2293.
- Goekoop-Ruiterman YP, de Vries-Bouwstra JK, Allaart CF, et al. Clinical and radiographic outcomes for four different treatment strategies in patients with early rheumatoid arthritis (the BeSt study): a randomized, controlled trial. *Arthritis Rheum*. 2005;52(11):3381–3390.
- Häkkinen A, Sokka T, Kotaniemi A, et al. A randomized two-year study of the effects of dynamic strength training on muscle strength, disease activity, functional capacity, and bone mineral density in early rheumatoid arthritis. *Arthritis Rheum*. 2001;44(3):515–522.
- Nadareishvili Z, Michaud K, Hallenbeck JM, et al. Cardiovascular, rheumatologic, and pharmacologic predictors of stroke in patients with rheumatoid arthritis: a nested, case-control study. *Arthritis Rheum*. 2008;59(8):1090–1096.
- Nishimura K, Sugiyama D, Kogata Y, et al. Meta-analysis: diagnostic accuracy of anti-cyclic citrullinated peptide antibody and rheumatoid factor for rheumatoid arthritis. *Ann Intern Med*. 2007;146(11):797–808.
- Østergaard M, Hansen M, Stoltenberg M, et al. New radiographic bone erosions in the wrists of patients with rheumatoid arthritis are detectable with magnetic resonance imaging a median of two years earlier. *Arthritis Rheum*. 2003;48(8):2128–2131.
- Ottawa Panel. Ottawa Panel evidence-based clinical practice guidelines for therapeutic exercises in the management of rheumatoid arthritis in adults. *Phys Ther*. 2004;84(10):934–972.
- Rantalaiho V, Korpela M, Hannonen P, et al. The good initial response to therapy with a combination of traditional disease-modifying antirheumatic drugs is sustained over time: the eleven-year results of the Finnish rheumatoid arthritis combination therapy trial. *Arthritis Rheum*. 2009;60(5):1222–1231.
- Saag KG, Teng GG, Patkar NM, et al. American College of Rheumatology 2008 recommendations for the use of nonbiologic and biologic disease-modifying antirheumatic drugs in rheumatoid arthritis. *Arthritis Rheum*. 2008;59(6):762–784.
- Smolen JS, Landewé R, Bijlsma J, et al. EULAR recommendations for the management of rheumatoid arthritis with synthetic and biological disease-modifying antirheumatic drugs: 2016 update. *Ann Rheum Dis*. 2017;76(6):960–977. doi:10.1136/annrheumdis-2016-210715.
- Solomon DH, Goodson NJ, Katz JN, et al. Patterns of cardiovascular risk in rheumatoid arthritis. *Ann Rheum Dis*. 2006;65(12):1608–1612.
- Terslev L, Torp-Pedersen S, Savnik A, et al. Doppler ultrasound and magnetic resonance imaging of synovial inflammation of the hand in rheumatoid arthritis: a comparative study. *Arthritis Rheum*. 2003;48(9):2434–2441.
- van der Heijde DM. Overview of radiologic efficacy of new treatments. *Rheum Dis Clin North Am*. 2004;30(2):285–293.
- Warsi A, LaValley MP, Wang PS, et al. Arthritis self-management education programs: a meta-analysis of the effect on pain and disability. *Arthritis Rheum*. 2003;48(8):2207–2213.
- Wasserman AM. Diagnosis and management of rheumatoid arthritis. *Am Fam Physician*. 2011;84(11):1245–1252.
- Zintzaras E, Voulgarelis M, Moutsopoulos HM. The risk of lymphoma development in autoimmune diseases: a meta-analysis. *Arch Intern Med*. 2005;165(20):2337–2344.

CLINICAL PEARLS

RA can go into remission; must have 5+ to qualify for >2 mo: <15 min morning stiffness, no fatigue, no joint pain, no joint tenderness or pain with activity, no soft tissue swelling, ESR <30 in women or <20 in men

ROTATOR CUFF TEARS

Kenneth Bielak, MD, FACSM, FAAFP, CAQSM

BASICS

DESCRIPTION

- Partial or complete tears or disruption of any one or combination of the four rotator cuff muscles of the glenohumeral joint
- Supraspinatus and infraspinatus muscle-tendon complexes are the most common tears.
- Rotator cuff muscles are the supraspinatus, infraspinatus, teres minor, and subscapularis muscles.

EPIDEMIOLOGY

- Rare in young athletes
- More common in athletes >40 yr of age, especially those with a history of many years of repetitive overhead sports
- More common than osteoarthritis (Shoulder is the only joint where soft tissue often wears out before joint.)

RISK FACTORS

- Older-than-40-yr "weekend warrior" with years of repetitive overhead use (e.g., swimming, tennis, volleyball, gymnastics, weight lifting, and throwing sports)
- Previous trauma
- Sports with potential fall risk, such as equestrian, skiing, and body surfing

ETIOLOGY AND PATHOPHYSIOLOGY

- Can present following specific trauma (acute traumatic tear)
- Usually degenerative (chronic impingement syndrome), especially in older athlete with overarm sports
- Asymptomatic tears are more prevalent with age >40 yr.

DIAGNOSIS

HISTORY

- Mechanism of injury:
  - Acute traumatic events such as a fall, direct blow, or forceful boxing punch
  - Traumatic hyperextension of abducted arm
  - Traumatic external or internal rotation of abducted arm
  - Anterior dislocation

ALERT
Chronic overhead arm use may develop insidiously.

ALERT
Nocturnal pain and pain on sleeping on the affected side are common.

- Pain location can be variable (anterior, lateral, or posterior shoulder).
- Pain may radiate to elbow.
- Pain typically is aggravated with reaching motions: laterally (abduction), toward the back (internal rotation) and/or overhead.

PHYSICAL EXAM

- Diminished range of motion (ROM)
- Pain with arm abduction, especially at 80 to 120 degrees of arc (1)[B]
- Atrophy of cuff muscles, especially if chronic
- Crepitus of supraspinatus muscle during abduction
- Rotator cuff muscle weakness
- Drop-arm test is positive for partial-thickness tear (14.3% sensitive, 88.4% specific) and full-thickness tear (34.9% sensitive, 87.5% specific) (1)[B]:
  - Arm is passively abducted to 90 degrees.
  - Patient is instructed to slowly return the arm to the side.
  - Severe pain or inability to do so is positive test for a torn rotator cuff complex.
- Empty can test is positive for large or full-thickness tears of supraspinatus (88% sensitive, 70% specific) (2)[B]:
  - Resistance applied to arm abducted 90 degrees, angled 30 degrees anteriorly with a medially rotated forearm (thumbs down, "empty can")
  - Test is positive for inability to do so or severe pain.
- Test external rotation (infraspinatus/teres minor) strength (partial tear, 19.4% sensitive, 68.9% specific; full tear 50.5% sensitive, 84% specific) (1)[B]:
  - Perform test with elbow flexed 90 degrees at the side.
- Lift-off lag test (subscapularis): inability to lift the dorsum of the hand off the back hip
- Internal rotation lag test (modified lift-off test): Inability to maintain lift-off position and springs back (toward the back) is more accurate (3)[B], with 97% sensitivity and 83% specificity (4)[A].
- External rotation lag test (inability to maintain position of full external rotation) has sensitivity of 47% and specificity of 94% (4)[A].
- Significant pain with internal rotation can preclude an accurate test.
- Poor scapular stability is often present.
- Anterior glenoid-humeral laxity may be noted.
- Comprehensive testing of active and passive ROM, strength testing, and adequate neurovascular testing are recommended.

ALERT
In a multicenter review, the authors found that anatomic features defining the severity of atraumatic rotator cuff tears are not associated with the pain level. Factors associated with pain are comorbidities, lower education level, and race (4)[C].

DIFFERENTIAL DIAGNOSIS

- Rotator cuff strains
- Glenoid labrum tear
- Subluxation or unstable shoulder
- Subacromial impingement
- Isolated bicipital tendinitis
- Acromioclavicular joint disorders
- Glenohumeral arthritis
- Rare subacromial abscess or tumors
- Adhesive capsulitis
- Cervical radiculopathy can radiate to the shoulder.

DIAGNOSTIC TESTS & INTERPRETATION

Initial Tests (lab, imaging)

- Plain radiographs, although not specific for rotator cuff tears, may show some findings that are suggestive:
  - Calcifications along the tendons of the rotator cuff muscle (repetitive/chronic injury)
  - Subacromial osteophytes (may predispose to tears)
  - Superior or anterior migration of the humeral head (indicates full-thickness tear) (5)[B]
- Magnetic resonance imaging (MRI) demonstrates an 80–97% sensitivity in detecting full-thickness rotator cuff tears. Partial tears are more difficult to detect, with a sensitivity of 67–89%. This improves if fat suppression is used (6)[B].
- One caution is the use of MRI evaluation in patients with severe osteoarthritis of the glenohumeral joint as one study suggests that although MRI is highly sensitive, it has a low positive predictive value and moderately low specificity and accuracy in detecting full-thickness rotator cuff tears in patients with severe glenohumeral osteoarthritis (7)[C].
- 40% asymptomatic >50 yr old have full rotator cuff tear (8,9)[B].
- 60% asymptomatic >60 yr old have partial or full rotator cuff tear (8)[B].
- One other study differs slightly on asymptomatic tears: 26–56% asymptomatic tears age: 63.1 ± 9 yr
- Double-contrast arthrotomography (DCAT) is 100% sensitive and 94% specific in diagnosing complete rotator cuff tears but is much less sensitive for partial tears; probably more appropriate when concern for instability rather than pain alone

- Ultrasound (US) advantages are inexpensive and can localize areas of tenderness and dysfunction with patient present and in dynamic examination (technician dependent) (10)[B]. One study found no statistically significant difference between US and MRI in detection of rotator cuff tears of any type (11)[C].

ALERT

Diagnostic accuracy of shoulder US when evaluating rotator cuff tears can reach 91–100% for partial- and full-thickness tears detection, respectively, having been reported to be as accurate as MRI in experienced hands (12)[C].

Diagnostic Procedures/Other

Diagnostic injection: Subacromial bursa injection (10 mL of 1% lidocaine) may distinguish minor impingement and tendinosis from distinct tears of the rotator cuff (no pain relief or strength improvement from the injection).

TREATMENT

GENERAL MEASURES

- Acute treatment
- Analgesia:
  - Nonsteroidal anti-inflammatory drugs (NSAIDs) are the drugs of choice initially, but long-term use prior to operative repair can result in inferior long-term outcomes (13)[C].
  - More potent analgesics should rarely be necessary temporarily to relieve nocturnal symptoms.
- Immobilization: Sling may provide some relief for the acutely injured shoulder, but limit to initial 2 to 3 wk as needed.
- Subacromial corticosteroid injection may provide short term (<8 wk) limited pain benefit (14)[C].

ADDITIONAL THERAPIES

- Prolonged rehabilitation emphasizing increased ROM and strengthening is indicated for a partial tear.
- Normalizing scapulothoracic stabilization and posterior capsular flexibility with a 1:1 strength ratio for rotator cuff to anterior/middle cuff deltoid muscle
- *Future considerations as more research is published*:
  - A small study found that prolotherapy using dextrose solution reported excellent or good outcomes in 53 patients (92.9%) compared to 56.8% in the control group of 25 patients with partial tears (15)[C].
  - One author's review suggests of the myriad options being currently trialed that the platelet-rich plasma (PRP) fibrin matrix version holds the greatest promise for improving clinical success after rotator cuff tendon repair (16)[C].
  - Steroid injections are indicated for bursitis and/or tendinitis to reduce inflammation and have been used successfully and without compromise to tendon repairs 6 wk out from repair (17)[C].

SURGERY/OTHER PROCEDURES

- For complete tears, surgery may be warranted in the young patient or active athlete.
- Early operative repair provides the best chance for functional recovery. Severely retracted tendons/muscles create additional challenges to the surgeon for optimal recovery (18)[C].

ONGOING CARE

FOLLOW-UP RECOMMENDATIONS

Orthopedic surgeon referral encouraged for acute full-thickness tears early and partial tears after failed conservative therapy

PATIENT EDUCATION

Overhead athletes undergoing surgical repair may require 6 mo or longer before being able to return to full active sports participation.

REFERENCES

1. Park HB, Yokota A, Gill HS, et al. Diagnostic accuracy of clinical tests for the different degrees of subacromial impingement syndrome. *J Bone Joint Surg Am*. 2005;87(7):1446–1455.
2. Holtby R, Razmjou H. Validity of the supraspinatus test as a single clinical test in diagnosing patients with rotator cuff pathology. *J Orthop Sports Phys Ther*. 2004;34(4):194–200.
3. Hertel R, Ballmer FT, Lombert SM, et al. Lag signs in the diagnosis of rotator cuff rupture. *J Shoulder Elbow Surg*. 1996;5(4):307–313.
4. Hermans J, Luime JJ, Meuffels DE, et al. Does this patient with shoulder pain have rotator cuff disease?: the rational clinical examination systematic review. *JAMA*. 2013;310(8):837–847.
5. Dunn WR, Kuhn JE, Sanders R, et al. Symptoms of pain do not correlate with rotator cuff tear severity: a cross-sectional study of 393 patients with a symptomatic atraumatic full-thickness rotator cuff tear. *J Bone Joint Surg Am*. 2014;96(10):793–800.
6. Weiner DS, Macnab I. Superior migration of the humeral head. A radiological aid in the diagnosis of tears of the rotator cuff. *J Bone Joint Surg Br*. 1970;52(3):524–527.
7. Burks RT, Crim J, Brown N, et al. A prospective randomized clinical trial comparing arthroscopic single- and double-row rotator cuff repair: magnetic resonance imaging and early clinical evaluation. *Am J Sports Med*. 2009;37(4):674–682.
8. Sershon RA, Mather RC, Sherman SL, et al. Low accuracy of interpretation of rotator cuff MRI in patients with osteoarthritis. *Acta Orthop*. 2013;84(5): 479–482.
9. Moosikasuwan J, Miller T, Burke B. Rotator cuff tears: clinical, radiographic, and US findings. *Radiographics*. 2005;25(6):1591–1607.
10. Mall NA, Kim HM, Keener JD, et al. Symptomatic progression of asymptomatic rotator cuff tears: a prospective study of clinical and sonographic variables. *J Bone Joint Surg Am*. 2010;92(16): 2623–2633.
11. Teefey SA, Middleton WD, Yamaguchi K. Shoulder sonography. State of the art. *Radiol Clin North Am*. 1999;37(4):767–785.
12. Elmorsy A, Keightley A, Flannery M. Accuracy of ultrasonography (US) and magnetic resonance imaging (MRI) in detection of rotator cuff tears in district general hospital. *Pol J Radiol*. 2017;82:634–637.
13. Corazza A, Orlandi D, Fabbro E. Dynamic high-resolution ultrasound of the shoulder: how we do it. *Eur J Radiol*. 2015;84(2):266–277.
14. Inderhaug E, Kollevold KH, Kalsvik M, et al. Preoperative NSAIDS, non-acute onset and long-standing symptoms predict inferior outcome at long-term follow-up after rotator cuff repair. *Knee Surg Sports Traumatol Arthrosc*. 2017;25(7):2067–2072.
15. Cook T, Minns Lowe C, Maybury M, et al. Are corticosteroid injections more beneficial than anaesthetic injections alone in the management of rotator cuff-related shoulder pain? A systematic review. *Br J Sports Med*. 2018;52(8):497–504.
16. Seven MM, Ersen O, Akpancar S, et al. Effectiveness of prolotherapy in the treatment of chronic rotator cuff lesions. *Orthop Traumatol Surg Res*. 2017;103(3):427–433.
17. Barber FA. Platelet-rich plasma for rotator cuff repair. *Sports Med Arthrosc Rev*. 2013;21(4): 199–205.
18. Kim IB, Jung DW. An intra-articular steroid injection at 6 weeks postoperatively for shoulder stiffness after arthroscopic rotator cuff repair does not affect repair integrity. *Am J Sports Med*. 2018;46(9):2192–2202.

ADDITIONAL READING

Rashid M, Cooper C, Cook J, et al. Increasing age and tear size reduce rotator cuff repair healing rate at 1 year. *Acta Orthop*. 2017;88(6):606–611.

CLINICAL PEARLS

- Diagnostic accuracy of shoulder US when evaluating rotator cuff tears can reach 91–100% for partial- and full-thickness tears detection, respectively, having been reported to be as accurate as MRI in experienced hands.
- Surgery is an option, especially for the young and/or active athlete, and should be considered early on for diagnosis of complete tears of the rotator cuff.
- Rehabilitation of a partial tear of the rotator cuff is a prolonged process that may take months to return to preinjury status.

SCAPHOLUNATE DISSOCIATION

Benjamin D. Brusch, MD • Robert L. Jones, MD, CAQSM

BASICS

DESCRIPTION

Scapholunate (SL) dissociation may be more accurately characterized as a spectrum of SL instability resulting from a tear of the SL interosseous ligament (SLIL). Concomitant or subsequent injury to secondary ligamentous restraints alter the biomechanics of the wrist, resulting in progressive carpal instability and leading to a predictable pattern of debilitating, degenerative changes of the wrist (1,2).

EPIDEMIOLOGY

- Most common ligamentous instability of the wrist (2)
- Frequently associated with a distal radius fracture
- Precise epidemiologic data is lacking.

ETIOLOGY AND PATHOPHYSIOLOGY

- Often a fall on an outstretched hand with hyperextension, ulnar deviation, and supination (1,2)
- Axial compression can drive the capitate between the scaphoid and lunate (1).
- Repetitive motion after an isolated SLIL injury may produce attritional changes in the secondary stabilizers leading to their eventual failure, thus completing the SL dissociation (1,2).
- May also result from repetitive minor trauma

RISK FACTORS

Active individuals who have ulnar-negative variance; shorter distal ulna compared with the radius on a neutral anteroposterior (AP) radiograph of the wrist (measured from the articular surface of the ulna to the lunate fossa of the radius)

DIAGNOSIS

- Early diagnosis and surgery offers the best chance for successful outcome (1,3).
- There are different levels of injury, which can be classified by increasing severity of wrist instability (1,2,3,4):
  - Occult instability: isolated tear or attenuation of a portion of the SLIL. There is no radiologic evidence of SL widening, and wrist pain is usually only with mechanical loading.
  - Dynamic instability: subtotal or complete tear of the SLIL, including the dorsal portion, with a partial secondary ligament injury; may have normal static radiographs, but instability will be apparent on stress radiographs
  - SL dissociation: involves a complete tear of the SLIL with additional tear of one or more secondary ligaments. SL widening is apparent on static radiographs (>3 mm).
  - Dorsal intercalated segment instability (DISI): term used to describe the shifted positions of the bones of the carpus, as viewed on lateral radiograph, due to lack of association between the lunate and scaphoid (1). Abnormalities include flexion of the scaphoid, extension of the lunate and triquetrum, and dorsal and proximal translation of the distal carpal row.
  - SL advanced collapse (SLAC): end stage of the spectrum of instability (1). There is predictable and progressive degeneration and arthritis of the carpus due to the irreversible postural changes of the scaphoid, capitate, and lunate.

HISTORY

- Patient may report a fall or sudden load applied to the wrist but may not recall any specific fall or injury.
- Pain or swelling in the dorsal wrist (1,2)
- Pain or weakness with hyperextension and loading of the wrist

ALERT

May not seek immediate care because initial injury seems too trivial

- Subacutely, there may be symptoms of painful popping or clicking with activities, or decreased grip strength (1).
- Later on, limited motion may be a complaint (4).

PHYSICAL EXAM

- In the acute setting, pain may be poorly localized about the periscaphoid area. Swelling may be diffuse or localized to the SL region (2).
- In the subacute setting, there is usually well-localized tenderness about the scaphoid and dorsal SL interval (distal to Lister tubercle).
- The patient may have weakness of grip and pinch strength (2).
- Watson scaphoid shift test should be performed:

ALERT

Patient places wrist in ulnar deviation, and the physician puts dorsal pressure on the palmar scaphoid tubercle with the thumb. The physician then radially deviates the patient's wrist. Relief of thumb pressure will allow the scaphoid to reduce, often with an audible or palpable clunk. Pain with a clunk may represent SL instability.

- Compare to the contralateral side as false positives occur frequently (1).
- The shift test may become negative in chronic cases as arthritis stabilizes the scaphoid.

DIFFERENTIAL DIAGNOSIS

- Scaphoid or other carpal fracture
- Lunotriquetral instability
- Radial styloid or distal radius fracture
- Synovitis
- Radioscaphoid impingement
- Occult ganglion cyst
- Triangular fibrocartilage complex tear
- Osteoarthritis or rheumatoid arthritis
- Kienböck disease

DIAGNOSTIC TESTS & INTERPRETATION

Initial Tests (lab, imaging)

- Imaging should be obtained in individuals with appropriate history and positive scaphoid shift test.
- Initial plain films should include AP, lateral, and stress views.
- Radiographs of the opposite wrist should always be obtained for comparison (2)[C].
- Normal static and stress films in the acute setting do not always rule out serious injury because it may take time for instability to develop (4)[C].
- By the time frank dissociation is present on static films, significant damage is already present (1).
- Key findings on the lateral film (wrist in neutral):
  - SL angle >70 degrees is considered highly suggestive of diagnosis (normal 30 to 60 degrees) (1,2,3,5).
  - Radiolunate angle exceeding 15 degrees indicates DISI (1,2).
- Key findings on the AP film:
  - Scaphoid ring sign: Distal scaphoid tubercle is superimposed on the scaphoid waist when scaphoid is flexed >70 degrees (1).

ALERT
Gap >3 mm (2,3,4) between scaphoid and lunate on AP is indicative of SL dissociation with 97% specificity (4).

ALERT
"Pencil grip posteroanterior (PA)" is the most useful stress view (2,3)[C]. It profiles the SL joint and demonstrates pathologic SL widening (>3 mm) under axial loaded conditions (2)[C]. Additional stress view could include AP in ulnar deviation (3).

- Radiography has a sensitivity of 57–81% and specificity of 73–98% (4).
- Cineradiography (functional fluoroscopy) has a sensitivity of 86–96% and specificity of 80–97% (4).
- CT arthrography has been reported as having a sensitivity of 80–100%, whereas magnetic resonance (MR) arthrography has a sensitivity of 85–100%; both have a specificity of 80–100% (4). Traction MR arthrography has been proposed to have greater sensitivity and specificity (3).
- Traditional arthrography is limited by its static nature and the high prevalence of degenerative tears, which are often asymptomatic and bilateral (1,2).
- Static imaging modalities are felt to often miss early cases of instability when intervention may be most effective.
- The dorsal SL ligament can be assessed with ultrasound.
- Wrist arthroscopy remains the gold standard for diagnosis (1,3,4,5).

Diagnostic Procedures/Other

Arthroscentesis indicating hemarthrosis may be helpful in the acute setting when initial imaging is negative, but clinical suspicion remains high (2)[C].

TREATMENT

- Treatment must be predicated by the patient's symptoms and clinical exam, not imaging.
- Management of injuries may depend on age, sport, position, level of competition, and schedule (3)[C].

ALERT
The treatment is most often surgical, so do not delay referral.

- The goal of surgery is to restore carpal kinematics to arrest the degenerative process (3).
- Emergency department (ED) treatment:
  - Stabilize with a thumb spica splint.
  - Refer for appropriate follow-up.

MEDICATION

Nonsteroidal anti-inflammatory drugs (NSAIDs) or acetaminophen for pain

ADDITIONAL THERAPIES

- Occult instability may be successfully treated with immobilization for 4 to 6 wk followed by therapy (3)[C].
- There has been some success with casting, splinting, NSAIDs, and therapy without surgical intervention for dynamic instability (2)[C]. This would include a short arm cast for 4 to 6 wk, followed by removable splint for active range of motion (ROM) exercises and gentle strengthening across the wrist.
- All treatment courses should be followed by rehabilitation consisting of strengthening and proprioceptive training (3)[C].

SURGERY/OTHER PROCEDURES

- In general, unstable wrists should undergo surgical repair as soon as possible if the athlete desires to return to play. The procedures performed are dictated based on the timing and severity of the wrist instability.
- Occult instability:
  - There has been some success with arthroscopic débridement with or without pinning, but usually this is treated with conservative measures (3)[C]. There is also some evidence for K-wire fixation and/or electrocautery for electrothermal collagen shrinkage following arthroscopic débridement (1,3)[C]. However, the mechanism for pain reduction is felt to be a result of denervation rather than mechanical stabilization.
- Acute, dynamic instability:
  - Usually require early surgical intervention
  - Some will use closed reduction and K-wire fixation, attempting to allow the torn ligaments to heal (1,5)[C]. Otherwise, attempt is made to repair the damaged ligaments before they degenerate (3,5)[C].
- Subacute or chronic injuries:
  - Typically require ligament reconstruction (3)[C]
- Chronically injured wrists with fixed deformity such as DISI or SLAC:
  - Salvage procedures are sometimes needed to alleviate pain (1)[C].
- A salvage procedure is performed to restore alignment, improve load distribution, and attempt to slow degenerative changes. Unfortunately, salvage procedures are likely to indicate the end of an athletic career (3)[C].
- Salvage procedures may include scaphoid excision, carpal fusion, or proximal row carpectomy (1)[C].

ONGOING CARE

FOLLOW-UP RECOMMENDATIONS

- Following repair, immobilize the wrist for 8 wk and then slowly rehab.
- Decisions about return to play must be individualized based on sport-specific demands and competition level.
- In general, an athlete may return after demonstrating progression in strength and ROM in a supervised rehabilitation program.
- Physical therapy should be performed within pain tolerance.
- Avoid power gripping and weight-bearing exercises of the upper extremity.
- Gentle putty or sponge gripping can help improve grasp strength.

COMPLICATIONS

- Injury has the potential to be career ending (3).
- Arthritis of the wrist, which can be severe and debilitating

REFERENCES

1. Manuel J, Moran SL. The diagnosis and treatment of scapholunate instability. *Orthop Clin North Am*. 2007;38(2):261–277.
2. Kitay A, Wolfe SW. Scapholunate instability: current concepts in diagnosis and management. *J Hand Surg Am*. 2012;37(10):2175–2196.
3. Morrell NT, Moyer A, Quinlan N, et al. Scapholunate and perilunate injuries in the athlete. *Curr Rev Musculoskelet Med*. 2017;10(1):45–52.
4. Cheriex KCAL, Sulkers GSI, Terra MP, et al. Scapholunate dissociation; diagnostics made easy. *Eur J Radiol*. 2017;92:45–50.
5. Geissler WB, Burkett JL. Ligamentous sports injuries of the hand and wrist. *Sports Med Arthrosc Rev*. 2014;22(1):39–44.

CLINICAL PEARLS

- Most common ligamentous injury of the wrist
- Normal static and stress films in the acute setting do not always rule out serious injury.
- Radiographs of the contralateral side should always be obtained.
- Early diagnosis and treatment can avoid potentially career-ending, lifelong morbidity.

SCHEUERMANN'S KYPHOSIS

David McClaskey, MD, ATC

BASICS

DESCRIPTION
- Juvenile osteochondrosis of the spine
- Scheuermann kyphosis is rigid and most commonly affects the thoracic spine.
- Vertebrae grow unevenly with regard to the sagittal plane (posterior angle is greater than the anterior), resulting in the signature "wedging" shape of the vertebrae, causing kyphosis.
- Defined by anterior wedging ≥5 degrees in three or more adjacent vertebral bodies
- Type I—thoracic spine only, apex of curve T7–T9
- Type II—lower thoracic and lumbar spine involvement

EPIDEMIOLOGY
Prevalence
- 1–8% in the United States (1)
- Most common age of diagnosis is 12 to 17 yr; male to female ratio is at least 2:1.

ETIOLOGY AND PATHOPHYSIOLOGY
- Results from mechanical stress on a weakened vertebral endplate
- The vertebral endplate is weakened due to defective growth, likely from predisposing genetic defects. Hormonal abnormalities are postulated to contribute as well.
- Defective endplate may also affect the health of the adjacent intervertebral disc, resulting in early disc disease.

Genetics
- Suspected autosomal dominant inheritance
- Seen more commonly in monozygotic twins
- Heritability (percentage of all cases that can be attributed to genetics) is 74% (2,3).

RISK FACTORS
- Repetitive strain (particularly with flexion/extension) from strenuous sports or manual labor may increase or accelerate the severity of the kyphosis.
- Contribution of elevated body mass index (BMI) to this condition is not well defined.

COMMONLY ASSOCIATED CONDITIONS
- Scoliosis
- Cervical or lumbar hyperlordosis (compensatory curvature due to the thoracic kyphosis)
- Spondylolysis
- The above conditions occur in up to 1/3 of patients with Scheuermann kyphosis.

DIAGNOSIS

HISTORY
- Affected patient will present with cosmetic deformity, back pain, and hamstring tightness.
- Thoracic kyphosis may produce pain at the thoracic spine and/or result in strain on the cervical or lumbar spine.
- Pain is typically insidious with no traumatic event.
- The pain worsens with activity and improves with rest.
- Cosmetic deformity may be noticed by parents or during school-based screenings, preparticipation examinations, or routine wellness exams.
- A family history of Scheuermann kyphosis may be present in most cases.

PHYSICAL EXAM
- Spinal range of motion should be carefully evaluated and documented in all planes of motion.
- Physical exam shows a rigid, hyperkyphotic curve that is accentuated with forward bending (roundback).
- The kyphosis does not resolve with postural maneuvers (extension, lying supine, prone, etc.). The kyphosis cannot be consciously corrected.
- Loss of vertebral height, thus appearing shorter
- May result in kyphoscoliosis, scoliosis, or cervical/lumbar hyperlordosis
- Patients typically have tight hamstrings to compensate for excessive lumbar curvature.
- Excessive curvature (>100 degrees) may cause restrictive lung disease, which can be confirmed with pulmonary function tests.
- Rarely, may cause neurologic deficits, therefore, a complete neurologic exam is warranted
- Look for findings that may suggest other causes of kyphosis, such as marfanoid body habitus, hypermobile joints (Marfan or Ehlers-Danlos syndrome), cafe-au-lait spots (neurofibromatosis), etc.

DIFFERENTIAL DIAGNOSIS
- Postural kyphosis (improves with postural maneuvers)
- Ankylosing spondylitis
- Scoliosis
- Neuromuscular disorders
- Ehlers-Danlos syndrome
- Marfan syndrome
- Rickets
- Congenital kyphosis (Klippel-Feil syndrome, vertebral anomalies (V), anal atresia (A), cardiac malformations (C), tracheo-oesophageal fistula (TE), renal dysplasia (R) and limb abnormalities (L) syndrome)

DIAGNOSTIC TESTS & INTERPRETATION
Initial Tests (lab, imaging)
- X-rays:
  - Anteroposterior (AP)/lateral radiographs confirm the diagnosis, demonstrating kyphosis >40 degrees, or anterior wedging ≥5 degrees in three or more adjacent vertebral bodies (3)[B].
  - Cobb angle is used to measure angle of kyphotic deformity; this angle is the intersection of the lines drawn from the endplates of the terminal vertebrae, which are most tilted toward each other.
  - Sagittal balance can also quantify spinal deformity by measuring the horizontal distance between the center of C7 and the superior endplate of S1 on a lateral radiograph. An abnormal balance (plumb line passing more than 2 cm in front of, or behind, the posterosuperior S1 body) is predictive of dysfunction.
  - May show signs of an irregular vertebral endplate, including Schmorl nodes, loss of disc space height, spondylolysis, or spondylolisthesis (3)[B]
  - Schmorl nodes are the herniation of the nucleus pulposus through the vertebral end plate into the body of the adjacent vertebra.
- Magnetic resonance imaging (MRI):
  - Useful for evaluating disc and spinal cord abnormalities in the presence of neurologic deficits
  - Can be used for preoperative planning

TREATMENT

GENERAL MEASURES
- Majority of cases treated with nonoperative management
- Physical therapy:
  - Focuses on stretching and strengthening of the paraspinal and hamstring musculature as well as postural control
  - Manual medicine may have a role in treatment among providers who are familiar with treating this condition.

- Lifestyle modification:
  - Avoidance of sports or exercises that places excessive pressure on the spine, such as weight lifting or rugby
  - OK to participate in athletics if kyphosis is nonpainful and being treated nonoperatively
- Bracing:
  - Painful, mild to moderate kyphosis can be treated with bracing for 12 to 24 mo.
  - Most effective in the skeletally immature patient
  - Bracing may effectively slow progression but may not resolve the kyphosis (1)[B].
  - Types of braces: Milwaukee brace, kyphologic brace, thoracolumbosacral orthosis-style Boston brace
  - Efficacy of braces is limited by compliance; requires the patient to wear up to 18 to 20 hr/day
- Emotional support:
  - Spinal deformity may negatively impact self-esteem and body image, particularly because this condition occurs during adolescence.
  - Treatment is time-consuming and may significantly impact daily activities.
  - Options for support groups and therapy should be explored and offered.

MEDICATION

First Line

Nonsteroidal anti-inflammatory drugs (NSAIDs) or acetaminophen is typically used for pain control.

ISSUES FOR REFERRAL

Referral for surgical correction should be considered for the following cases (4)[B]:

- Persistent or worsening symptoms despite conservative management
- Progressive kyphosis >70 degrees despite conservative management
- Unacceptable cosmetic deformity
- Pulmonary compromise (restrictive lung defect) secondary to kyphosis
- Patient/parent preference

SURGERY/OTHER PROCEDURES

- Significant variability among threshold to treat surgically
- Curve magnitude typically exceeds 70 to 80 degrees among surgical candidates, but decision to operate is individualized and influenced by maturity, level of pain, response to conservative measures, and patient/parent preference (5)[B].
- Surgery involves release of spine structures, correction of the kyphosis, and arthrodesis.
- Arthrodesis may occur through combined anterior-posterior or posterior-only approach.
- Even with surgery, the kyphosis may progress over time, both in the fusion as well as at the levels above or below the fusion (junctional kyphosis) (6)[B].
- Risks of surgery include postoperative infection, neurologic injury, and reoperation. Risks are increased when more levels are fused.

ONGOING CARE

FOLLOW-UP RECOMMENDATIONS

- A sports medicine or spine specialist should follow patients every 4 to 6 mo to monitor progression, particularly during skeletal maturation.
- Serial imaging should be performed at 6 to 12 mo intervals until skeletally mature; can perform in shorter intervals if the kyphosis is progressive and the patient is skeletally immature

PATIENT EDUCATION

- Kyphosis <60 degrees generally has few long-term complications.
- Athletic activity is allowed for patients with nonpainful kyphosis in nonoperative treatment. Given the potential for progression, high-impact or sports that strain the spine should be avoided.

PROGNOSIS

- The majority of patients maintain high functional scores with conservative treatments.
- A high incidence of back pain is reported among patients long term with both conservative and surgical treatments (6).
- Kyphosis <60 degrees generally has few long-term complications.

COMPLICATIONS

- Untreated Scheuermann kyphosis may result in a higher risk of back pain and lower quality of life in the later adult years.
- Restrictive lung disease may occur with severe kyphosis (>100 degrees).
- Surgical complications include junctional kyphosis, neurologic complications, hardware failure, infection, and lung or kidney injury (4).

REFERENCES

1. Etemadifar MR, Jamalaldini MH, Layeghi R. Successful brace treatment of Scheuermann's kyphosis with different angles. *J Craniovertebr Junction Spine*. 2017;8(2):136–143.
2. Damborg F, Engell V, Nielsen J, et al. Genetic epidemiology of Scheuermann's disease. *Acta Orthop*. 2011;82(5):602–605.
3. Gokce E, Beyhan M. Radiological imaging findings of Scheuermann disease. *World J Radiol*. 2016;8(11):895–901.
4. Lonner BS, Newton P, Betz R, et al. Operative management of Scheuermann's kyphosis in 78 patients: radiographic outcomes, complications, and technique. *Spine (Phila Pa 1976)*. 2007;32(24):2644–2652.
5. Polly DW Jr, Ledonio CG, Diamond B, et al. What are the indications for spinal fusion surgery in Scheuermann kyphosis? [published online ahead of print January 30, 2017]. *J Pediatr Orthop*. doi:10.1097/BPO.0000000000000931.
6. Graat H, Schimmel J, Hoogendoorn R, et al. Poor radiological and good functional long-term outcome of surgically treated Scheuermann patients. *Spine (Phila Pa 1976)*. 2016;41(14): E869–E878.

ADDITIONAL READING

- Palazzo C, Sailhan F, Revel M. Scheuermann's disease: an update. *Joint Bone Spine*. 2014;81(3):209–214.
- Ristolainen L, Kettunen JA, Heliövaara M, et al. Untreated Scheuermann's disease: a 37-year follow-up study. *Eur Spine J*. 2012;21(5):819–824.

CLINICAL PEARLS

- Scheuermann kyphosis is distinguished as a rigid kyphosis that does not resolve with postural maneuvers and most commonly affects the thoracic spine.
- The majority of cases are treated successfully with conservative management. Surgical considerations are influenced not only by the degree of kyphosis (typically >70 degrees) but also by individual patient considerations, including maturity, pain, response to conservative measures, and patient or parent preference.
- The kyphosis may progress despite bracing and surgical management.
- Mild-moderate kyphosis <60 degrees has fewer long-term complications than more severe kyphosis.

S

SCIATICA

Dhiren J. Naidu, MD, FRCPC, Dip. Sport Med.

BASICS

- Sciatica is referred to in the medical literature as lumbosacral radicular syndrome, radiculopathy, or nerve root pain.
- The classic description of sciatica or radiculopathy is compromise of a spinal nerve with resultant pain, weakness, and/or sensory impairment in the distribution of the affected nerve root (1).
- Sciatica pain radiates from the lower back into the leg. It usually radiates below the knee into the foot.
- Sciatica should not be confused with mechanical lower back pain because pain is typically worse in the leg than the back.

DESCRIPTION

- Radicular pain in the distribution of a lumbosacral nerve root (L4, L5, S1, S2, or S3), usually producing symptoms along the posterior or lateral aspect of the lower extremity and extending to the ankle or foot (1)
- It is typically described as a burning-type pain with numbness and tingling being common.
- Weakness can occur in the myotomal distribution depending on severity of nerve root compression (1).

EPIDEMIOLOGY

- Lower back pain is extremely common in the general population and the athletic population (e.g., football, gymnastics, tennis).
- General population: 5% annual occurrence; 60–90% lifetime incidence (2):
  - Men and women equally affected
  - Common reason to visit primary care physician
  - Leading cause of job-related disability in the United States
- Sciatica:
  - Sciatica is a common cause of pain and disability but less common than lower back pain.
  - Occurs in approximately 5% of the population (2)
  - 10–25% of people have >6 wk of symptoms.
  - In males, typically occurs in their 40s
  - In females, typically occurs in their 50s to 60s
  - L5 and S1 are the most common nerve roots involved (90%).

ETIOLOGY AND PATHOPHYSIOLOGY

The usual etiology of sciatic or radicular pain is the result of direct mechanical compression to the affected nerve root by a disk herniation and/or from chemical irritation of the nerve root by chemical substances, commonly referred to as radiculitis (1).

RISK FACTORS

Occupations or activities that require repetitive lifting, flexion, or rotation movements. These may occur in laborers or dancers and golfers.

COMMONLY ASSOCIATED CONDITIONS

- Cauda equina syndrome
- Urinary retention
- Motor loss
- Intractable pain

DIAGNOSIS

HISTORY

- Determine mechanism of injury.
- Onset of pain can be variable from immediate (acute) or over days (subacute).
- Pain is described as sharp, "electrical," burning, or as a numbness or tingling.
- Pain is located in the leg more than the lower back.
- Usually, unilateral pain
- Pain is worse in the morning.
- Pain is aggravated by flexion-based activities, rotation, prolonged sitting, Valsalva maneuvers (coughing, sneezing, straining with bowel movement), and occasionally with prolonged standing.
- Alleviating factors include extension-based postures, lying in prone position,
- Radiation of pain is into the buttock and leg in a posterolateral distribution to the foot.
- Rule out any red flags, which, if positive, warrant further investigations.
- The red flags for lower back pain include:
  - Age <20 yr or >50 yr.
  - Pain persists >6 wk.
  - History or signs and symptoms of infection.
  - History of cancer or immunosuppression.
  - Unexplained weight loss.
  - Severe worsening or atypical pain.
  - Significant trauma.
  - Intravenous (IV) drug use.
  - Abdominal pain.
  - Significant neurologic deficit.
  - Neurologic bowel/bladder dysfunction.
  - Saddle anesthesia.
- Evaluate and manage any positive red flags.
- Determine if any constitutional symptoms are present.
- Psychosocial issues that may add to symptoms and prolong pain

PHYSICAL EXAM

- Inspection may reveal fasciculations if there is motor weakness or muscle atrophy in long standing conditions.
- Range of motion is restricted into flexion and rotation; usually, extension is comfortable and may relieve pain.
- Sensation is decreased or lost in a dermatomal pattern:
  - Sensory loss:
    - L4: anteromedial leg, medial malleolus
    - L5: lateral lower leg, web space on dorsum of foot between the great and 2nd toes
    - S1: back of lower leg, lateral aspect of heel
- Strength is decreased in a myotomal pattern:
  - Motor weakness:
    - L4: ankle dorsiflexion
    - L5: big toe extension
    - S1: ankle plantar flexion
- Reflexes are absent or decreased:
  - Reflexes:
    - L4: patellar tendon (knee jerk)
    - L5: none
    - S1: Achilles tendon (ankle jerk)
- Straight-leg raise (SLR): Patient is in supine position, and the examiner passively raises fully extended leg. A positive test is reproduction of leg pain at approximately 30 degrees of flexion.
- Crossed SLR: Raising the contralateral leg results in reproduction of leg pain on the affected (opposite) side.
- Seated SLR: performed while patient is sitting with knees flexed to 90 degrees; passive extension of the knee reproduces radicular leg pain (modification of SLR).
- Slump test: performed with patient sitting with hands behind back, then patient flexes spine (slumps), followed by neck flexion. The examiner places hand on top of head, and patient extends knee. A positive test is if radicular leg pain occurs in the slumped position and decreases when patient moves out of neck flexion. This test has limited sensitivity and specificity in patients with a disc herniation.
- Examination to include rectal tone and anal sensation in setting of suspected cauda equina syndrome or spinal cord injury
- Vascular examination to include peripheral pulses

DIFFERENTIAL DIAGNOSIS

- Ankylosing spondylitis
- Cauda equina syndrome
- Extrinsic nerve compression, for example, from wallet or prolonged cycling
- Facet arthropathy
- Pathologic, traumatic, or osteoporotic compression fracture
- Herniation of the nucleus pulposus
- Infection, for example, osteomyelitis, epidural abscess
- Neoplasm, primary or metastatic

- Osteoarthritis of hip or spine
- Trochanteric bursitis
- Tarsal tunnel syndrome
- Paget disease
- Piriformis syndrome
- Sacroiliitis
- Spinal stenosis
- Spondylolisthesis
- Synovial cyst
- Trauma, for example, hematoma, musculoligamentous strain, fracture
- Nonspinal causes, for example, abdominal aortic aneurysm, herpes zoster, hip arthritis or bursitis, iliotibial band syndrome, psychogenic, vascular claudication

DIAGNOSTIC TESTS & INTERPRETATION

- X-rays: Anteroposterior and lateral radiographs of lumbar sacral spine usually are not indicated unless red flags are present (see "History").
- Magnetic resonance imaging (MRI): imaging of choice with excellent sensitivity. Consider ordering if red flags are present, especially in the setting of:
  - Suspected cauda equina syndrome.
  - Neurologic deficits.
  - Suspected malignancy or history of malignancy.
  - Suspected infection or abscess.
  - 6 wk of failed conservative therapy for sciatica.
- Computed tomography (CT) scan is the study of choice for identifying bony vertebral injuries. It should also be used if an MRI is contraindicated (i.e., if hardware, pacemaker present).
- Ultrasound or a CT scan of the abdomen: to evaluate for abdominal pathologies, such as an abdominal aortic aneurysm
- Electrodiagnostic studies: Nerve conduction studies and electromyography (EMG) can localize a specific level of injury. It is helpful to differentiate between a peripheral nerve and nerve root injury. It can also differentiate between acute or chronic injury (denervation vs. reinnervation).

TREATMENT

GENERAL MEASURES

- 6 wk of conservative management should be tried before obtaining imaging or invasive procedures, unless red flags are present or develop (3).
- Acute low back pain: Avoid inactivity; sciatica: activity level not found to make a difference (4)
- Nonsteroidal anti-inflammatory drugs (NSAIDs): show global improvement compared to placebo, however, has increased side effects (5)
- Oral steroids: A short 5-day course seems to improve function but not pain (6).
- Physical therapy to teach core stability. Core stability is adversely affected in patients with lumbosacral radiculopathy (7).
- Physical therapy directed toward restoring motor or strength deficits (7)
- For the best physical therapy outcomes, both aerobic conditioning and core strengthening are essential.
- Epidural steroid injections provide short-term improvement in pain but do not affect long-term outcomes. They may also serve as a preoperative assessment tool (8).
- Surgery should be considered for people failing to respond to conservative management for 6 wk. Surgery more reliably alleviates leg pain than back pain (3).
- Patients with lumbar disk herniations that are not responding to conservative management should be considered for lumbar decompression and discectomy (3).
- In the absence of severe intractable pain, neurologic deficits, and/or severe disease, surgery should be avoided.

COMPLEMENTARY & ALTERNATIVE MEDICINE

- Education and exercises and yoga are beneficial for patients with lower back pain (7).
- Manual spine treatment is helpful in acute, nonradicular lower back pain (7).
- Acupuncture is supported as an adjuvant treatment in the management of lower back pain (7).

ONGOING CARE

PATIENT EDUCATION

- Weight loss is beneficial.
- Aerobic exercise and core stability are the mainstays of an exercise-based treatment approach.
- Stay active (4).
- Avoid long-term pain medication.
- Stop smoking.

PROGNOSIS

- Acute pain is almost always self-limited.
- Estimated recovery time: 75–90% by 6 wk (2)

REFERENCES

1. Kennedy D, Noh M. The role of core stabilization in lumbosacral radiculopathy. *Phys Med Rehabil Clin N Am*. 2011;22(1):91–103.
2. Konstantinou K, Dunn KM. Sciatica: review of epidemiological studies and prevalence estimates. *Spine (Phila Pa 1976)*. 2008;33(22):2464–2472.
3. Bruggeman AJ, Decker RC. Surgical treatment and outcomes of lumbar radiculopathy. *Phys Med Rehabil Clin N Am*. 2011;22(1):161–177.
4. Dahm KT, Brurberg KG, Jamtvedt G, et al. Advice to rest in bed versus to advice to stay active for acute low-back pain and sciatica. *Cochrane Database Syst Rev*. 2010;(6):CD007612.
5. Rasmussen-Barr E, Held U, Grooten W, et al. Nonsteroidal anti-inflammatory drugs for low back pain with sciatica. *Cochrane Database Syst Rev*. 2016;(10):CD012382.
6. Goldberg H, Firtch W, Tyburski M, et al. Oral steroids for acute radiculopathy due to a herniated lumbar disk: a randomized clinical trial. *JAMA*. 2015;313(19):1915–1923.
7. Carneiro KA, Rittenberg JD. The role of exercise and alternative treatments for low back pain. *Phys Med Rehabil Clin N Am*. 2010;21(4):777–792.
8. Leung SM, Chau WW, Law SW, et al. Clinical value of transforaminal epidural steroid injection in lumbar radiculopathy. *Hong Kong Med J*. 2015;21(5):394–400.

ADDITIONAL READING

Kreiner DS, Hwang SW, Easa JE, et al. An evidence-based clinical guideline for the diagnosis and treatment of lumbar disc herniation with radiculopathy. *Spine J*. 2014;14(1):180–191.

CLINICAL PEARLS

- Sciatica is referred to as a lumbar radiculopathy and occurs from impingement on a nerve root, usually from a disc herniation.
- Obtaining a history focusing on the red flags is of prime importance to rule out more emergent conditions that require urgent imaging and medical attention.
- Conservative management is the mainstay of early treatment.
- Surgical referral is warranted if symptoms persist for >6 wk despite conservative management.
- Most radiculopathies improve by 6 wk.

SCOLIOSIS

Erin S. Barnes, MD • Mark E. Lavallee, MD, CSCS, FACSM

BASICS

Not a diagnosis but a description of a structural change in anatomy

DESCRIPTION

- Three dimensional deformity of the spine, characterized by lateral curvature of the spine measuring >10 degrees of curvature by Cobb angle, accompanied by rotation
- Three categories:
  - *Neuromuscular scoliosis* develops in patients with neurologic or musculoskeletal abnormalities and may be structural or nonstructural.
  - *Congenital scoliosis* is usually evident before adolescence and is a result of congenital asymmetry in the vertebrae.
  - *Idiopathic scoliosis* is a diagnosis of exclusion; infantile (0 to 3 yr) and juvenile (4 to 9 yr) are considered early onset, and children 10 yr and older are considered to have adolescent idiopathic scoliosis (AIS).
- AIS is the most common type of idiopathic scoliosis (80–85%).

EPIDEMIOLOGY

- Worldwide prevalence of AIS with curvature exceeding 10 degrees estimated between 2% and 4%
- Female to male ratio ranges from 1.5:1 to 3.0:1 and increases with age.
- Girls are at greater risk of curve progression and have a higher prevalence of curves with greater Cobb angles than boys.
- Only 10% of adolescents with AIS require treatment: 0.3% of the population.

Prevalence

- Cobb angle 10 to 19 degrees: 2–3%
- Cobb angle 20 to 29 degrees: 0.3–0.5%
- Cobb angle >40 degrees: ≤0.1%

ETIOLOGY AND PATHOPHYSIOLOGY

- By definition, AIS causes are unknown.
- *Genetic*: positive familial history for scoliosis in 30% (not predictive for severity)
- *Connective tissue disorder*: Platelet calmodulin levels may be predictive of curve progression.
- *Neurologic*: most widely supported theory, with abnormalities noted in vestibular, ocular, proprioceptive, and vibratory functions
- *Hormonal*: lower levels of melatonin secreted from pineal body in those with AIS:
  - Growth-stimulating hormone is more of an influential factor than etiologic factor studies.

Genetics

- Greater concordance rate in the incidence of scoliosis in monozygotic twins versus dizygotic twins
- Chromosomes 8, 9, 17, and 19 have been identified as having genetic loci for AIS.
- Inheritance pattern is not known.
- Expression of familial AIS may be linked to the X chromosome, with a dominant inheritance pattern.

RISK FACTORS

- Etiology of AIS is unclear at this time.
- Believed to be multifactorial
- Genetic contribution supported by twin and family history studies
- Other proposed factors: growth hormone secretion, connective tissue structure, paraspinal musculature, vestibular function, melatonin secretion, platelet microstructure

GENERAL PREVENTION

- None
- Benefit of preclinical detection not proven at this time
- U.S. Preventive Services Task Force recommends against the routine screening of asymptomatic adolescents for idiopathic scoliosis.

DIAGNOSIS

- *Neuromuscular scoliosis*: occurs in patients with neurologic or musculoskeletal conditions; may be seen with cerebral palsy, myelomeningocele, muscular dystrophy, or leg length discrepancy
- *Congenital scoliosis*: occurs from vertebral asymmetry secondary to congenital abnormalities, such as hemivertebrae, wedge vertebrae, failure of segmentation. This usually manifests before adolescence.
- *Idiopathic scoliosis*: no definite etiology:
  - Age 0 to 3 yr: infantile
  - Age 4 to 9 yr: juvenile
  - Age ≥10 yr: adolescent
- Criteria for AIS:
  - Age ≥10 yr
  - Curvature of spine in coronal plane that has a Cobb angle of ≥10 degrees
  - Exclusion of neuromuscular and congenital causes
  - Exclusion of leg length discrepancy (>8 mm)
- Prehospital:
  - Identify underlying etiologies.
  - Assessment of the curve clinically
  - Determine need for radiographs.
  - Determine risk of progression.

HISTORY

Consider:

- Onset: Consider when first noted, by whom, rate of worsening, previous treatment, associated signs or symptoms, familial history, and so forth.
- Rate of progression: Rapid progression is suggestive of a nonidiopathic cause.
- Pain: Patients with idiopathic scoliosis should not have pain, unless curve is >40.
- Night pain: If pain, consider tumor.
- Neuromuscular etiology? Bowel or bladder problems? Muscle weakness? Headache? Neck pain?
- Neurologic symptoms increase likelihood of nonidiopathic causes.
- Does the patient have difficulty breathing? Severe thoracic scoliosis may affect respiratory function.
- Has the pubertal growth spurt started? Important for determining remaining linear growth and need for intervention.
- Has menarche occurred? Pubertal growth spurt occurs just before menarche.
- Is there a history of lower limb fracture, joint infection, or arthritis? This may result in a leg length discrepancy.
- Is there a family history of scoliosis? A family history may suggest AIS.
- Other signs or symptoms?
- Review of systems (especially neurologic)

PHYSICAL EXAM

- Plot height and weight on growth curve.
- Spine inspection: Head should be balanced in line over the center of the sacrum.
- Assess Tanner stage (risk for progression is greatest during the pubertal spurt).
- Tanner grade 2 precedes the onset of pubertal growth spurt in boys. Tanner 2 follows the onset of pubertal growth spurt in girls.
- General inspection to look for skin changes, such as café au lait spots, pigmentation, or other signs of neurofibromatosis, for example, dysraphic signs (hairy patches, etc.)
- Assess for maturity, hyperelasticity, contracture, and congenital anomalies.
- Assess for deformity, symmetry of spine, symmetry of iliac crests, shoulders and trunk, including decompensation, abnormalities of thoracic kyphosis, or cervical or lumbar lordosis.
- The Adam forward bending test is used to look for rib or paraspinous elevations; demonstrates rotational component
- Assess for leg length discrepancy, congenital anomalies, and neurologic abnormalities (including abdominal reflex).
- *Findings:*
  - Crankshaft phenomenon: progressive deformity resulting from continued growth of the anterior aspect of the spine after posterior arthrodesis
  - Patient with open triradiate cartilage, younger age, and Risser 0 at the time of posterior fusion are at greater risk for developing crankshaft phenomenon.
  - If seen, may need to consider anterior fusion in addition to revision of the posterior fusion
- *Physical examination tools:*
  - Scoliometer: To measure trunk rotation, an angle of 7 degrees generally corresponds to Cobb angle of 20 degrees.
  - Important note: Not all patients with radiographic scoliosis have trunk rotation.
- Plumb line testing: Drop a line from C7 to demonstrate pelvic deviation.
- Abnormal abdominal reflex: may suggest intraspinal pathology, including syrinx

DIFFERENTIAL DIAGNOSIS

- Scoliosis: neuromuscular, congenital, idiopathic
- Postural abnormalities
- Leg length discrepancy

DIAGNOSTIC TESTS & INTERPRETATION

- Usually not helpful unless used to rule out associated metabolic conditions
- Pulmonary function testing is useful preoperatively.
- Plain standing full-length posteroanterior (PA) and lateral scoliosis films on a long 3-foot x-ray cassette
- Direction of curve labeled by convexity (left thoracic curves have been associated with nonidiopathic causes)
- Location is identified by vertebra that is most deviated and rotated from midline.
- Cobb angle: formed by the intersection of a line parallel to the superior end plate of the most cephalad vertebra that has the greatest tilt with the line parallel to the inferior end plate of the most caudal vertebra of the curve
- Skeletal maturity assessment using x-rays aids in determining time of treatment.
- Curve patterns are classified according to the Risser and Sanders classification systems.
- *Risser staging*: visual grading of the degree of ossification and fusion of the iliac apophysis (lower Risser grade indicates more growth remaining); simple with validated reliability, but multiple limitations have been identified

- Sanders Skeletal Maturity Staging System: a more reliable measure using hand and wrist PA radiograph to classify skeletal maturity in eight stages (1)[A]
- Magnetic resonance imaging (MRI) is not routinely necessary but indicated in patients with neurologic symptoms, early age of onset with rapid progression, and for abnormalities found on plain radiographs.

TREATMENT

Concepts for treatment are based on the severity of the deformity present and on the likelihood of progression:

- *Risk for progression:*
  - Skeletal maturity and curve magnitude are the two strongest predictors of curve progression in AIS.
  - Curve magnitude: Initial Cobb angles of 20 to 29 degrees are more likely to increase by at least 5 degrees.
  - Skeletal maturity (remaining growth potential): for example, the lower the Risser sign, the greater the risk for progression
  - Gender: Females have a 3- to 10-fold increased risk for progression.
  - Curve pattern: Double and thoracic curves have a 3-fold increased risk of progression.
- *Guidelines for management*:
  - Options for treatment include observation, bracing, and surgery.
  - Patients with trunk rotation <7 degrees are followed every 6 mo, and standing full-length PA views are repeated if trunk rotation increases.
  - Cobb angles <20 degrees may be observed every 6 to 8 mo; younger children and patients with curves closer to 20 degrees should be followed more frequently.
  - Scoliosis-specific exercises indicated if Cobb 15 to 20 degrees
  - Risser sign 0 to 2 with Cobb 20 to 29 degrees should be followed closely and braced if angle increases by 5 degrees or more over 3 to 6 mo.
  - Risser sign 0 to 2 with Cobb angles of 30 to 40 degrees should be braced.
  - Risser sign 0 to 2 with Cobb angles between 40 degrees and 50 degrees may be braced or considered for surgery.
  - Risser sign 0 to 2 with Cobb angle >50 degrees at time of diagnosis typically require surgical evaluation and intervention.
  - Risser sign ≥3 should be followed for at least 1 yr past skeletal maturity with radiographs every 6 to 9 mo.
  - Skeletally mature with Cobb angles <40 degrees can be reassured and discharged.
  - Skeletally mature with Cobb angles between 40 and 50 degrees are managed on an individual basis.

GENERAL MEASURES

- Therapy recommendation:
  - Physiotherapeutic scoliosis-specific exercises (PSSE) 2 to 7 times weekly in skeletally immature patients with Cobb angle >15 degrees. PSSE can be used in conjunction with corrective bracing in progressive curves (2)[A].
- Bracing recommendation:
  - Only indicated for skeletally immature
  - Brace criteria are currently based on low sensitivity Risser classifications.
  - Sanders Maturity Scale correlates with rapid growth phase and curve progression and has greater reliability, but no treatment criteria have been defined (3)[B].
  - Indicated if patient has a Risser sign of 0 to 3 and a Cobb angle of 30 to 60 degrees at time of diagnosis
  - Indicated if patient has Risser sign of 0 to 2 and has progression of 5 degrees or more over 6- to 8-mo period of observation; no need for bracing if skeletally mature
  - Rigo Cheneau de-rotational type braces provide corrective forces in multiple planes, addressing both Cobb angle and spinal rotation. These braces are useful to treat many curves (4)[B].
  - Rigo Cheneau type thoracic lumbar sacral orthosis (TLSO) and the cervico-thoraco-lumbar-sacral orthosis (Milwaukee brace) are both indicated for curves with apex above T8 and double thoracic curves.
  - Braces should be worn for 23 hr/day until the end of growth. Effectiveness of bracing diminishes if worn <18 hr daily.
  - After discontinuation of brace, monitor patient every 6 to 8 mo. Patients may benefit from continued Schroth-style physical therapy.

ISSUES FOR REFERRAL

- Trunk rotation angle >7 degrees and inability to assess Cobb angle
- Cobb angle between 20 degrees and 29 degrees in premenarchal girls and boys 12 to 14 yr of age
- Cobb angle >30 degrees in any patient
- Progression of Cobb angle of ≥5 degrees in any patient
- Surgical referral for skeletally immature patients with curves ≥50 degrees

SURGERY/OTHER PROCEDURES

- Posterior spinal fusion (PSF) with instrumentation using segmental rods and bone grafting
- Anterior spinal fusion and PSF needed at times to prevent the anterior spine from continuing to grow after the PSF (crankshaft phenomenon)
- Bony fusion is paramount; pseudoarthrosis or failure to fuse is a complication of surgery.
- Sports restriction for 9 to 12 mo following surgery and the surgeon must clear for contact sports

ONGOING CARE

FOLLOW-UP RECOMMENDATIONS

- Follow up 2 yr after onset of skeletal maturity.
- Skeletally mature patients do not need routine follow-up if Cobb angle <40 degrees; beyond 40 degrees should be individualized.
- Back pain associated with idiopathic scoliosis:
  - Pain in 23% of patients at time of initial evaluation (additional 9% during follow-up)
  - Of those with back pain, only 9% found to have identifiable cause, such as spondylolysis, Scheuermann, syrinx, disk herniation, tumor, and tether cord.
- Increased suicidal thoughts and self-image concerns among patients; address on individual basis.
- Pregnancy does not impact curve progression, nor does curve progression affect pregnancy outcome.

PROGNOSIS

- Risk of curve progression is related to patient's maturity (Risser sign, menarcheal status) and to the size of the curve.
- Curves I <20 to 25 degrees have a low risk of progression, even if patient is Risser 0 or Risser I.
- Curves 25 to 45 degrees have higher risk of progression, particularly in the immature.
- Curves >45 to 50 degrees have much higher risk of progression, regardless of maturity.
- Overall, good prognosis for the majority of patients

COMPLICATIONS

- Reduced pulmonary function for patients with thoracic curves >60 degrees
- Progression of lumbar curves >50 degrees in adult life with degenerative disk disease and pain
- Psychosocial factors
- No increased mortality rates compared with general population

REFERENCES

1. Sitoula P, Verma K, Holmes L Jr, et al. Prediction of curve progression in idiopathic scoliosis: validation of the Sanders Skeletal Maturity Staging System. *Spine (Phila Pa 1976)*. 2015;40(13):1006–1013.
2. Schreiber S, Parent EC, Khodayari Moez E, et al. Schroth physiotherapeutic scoliosis-specific exercises added to the standard of care lead to better Cobb angle outcomes in adolescents with idiopathic scoliosis—an assessor and statistician blinded randomized controlled trial. *PLoS One*. 2016;11(12):e0168746.
3. Vira S, Husain Q, Jalai C, et al. The interobserver and intraobserver reliability of the Sanders classification versus the Risser stage. *J Pediatr Orthop*. 2017;37(4):e246–e249.
4. Minsk MK, Venuti KD, Daumit GL, et al. Effectiveness of the Rigo Chêneau versus Boston-style orthoses for adolescent idiopathic scoliosis: a retrospective study. *Scoliosis Spinal Disord*. 2017;12:7.

ADDITIONAL READING

- Bettany-Saltikov J, Turnbull D, Ng SY, et al. Management of spinal deformities and evidence of treatment effectiveness. *Open Orthop J*. 2017;11:1521–1547.
- Horne JP, Flannery R, Usman S. Adolescent idiopathic scoliosis: diagnosis and management. *Am Fam Physician*. 2014;89(3):193–198.
- Negrini S, Donzelli S, Aulisa AG, et al. 2016 SOSORT guidelines: orthopaedic and rehabilitation treatment of idiopathic scoliosis during growth. *Scoliosis Spinal Disord*. 2018;13:3.

CLINICAL PEARLS

- If any of the signs mentioned are seen in conjunction with significant back pain, an x-ray or referral is indicated. The scoliometer is also a useful tool in screening patients.
- Scoliosis associated with osteoid osteoma is the suggested diagnosis for children who present with scoliosis and back pain that occurs especially at night and is relieved with aspirin.
- Scoliosis is not preventable. Wearing heavy backpacks, calcium deficiency, or poor posture is not related to deformity development.

SCUBA DIVING INJURIES: DECOMPRESSION SICKNESS AND ARTERIAL GAS EMBOLISM

Joseph E. Allen, MD, MS, FAAFP, CAQSM

BASICS

DESCRIPTION

- Decompression sickness and arterial gas embolism are adverse medical conditions, which may manifest in the self-contained underwater breathing apparatus environment, due to sudden changes in ambient pressure.
- DCS and AGE have collectively been described as forms of dysbarism, or decompression illness (DCI).
- Ambient gases (mainly nitrogen) present in the atmosphere are diffused throughout the human body and distributed via the circulatory system into tissues and organs.
- In the SCUBA diver, ambient pressure increases with increasing underwater depth, compressing gases, and further diffusing them into solution and bodily tissues.
- As a diver ascends from depth, the reverse process occurs, and nitrogen gas reexpands, diffusing back into tissues via circulation, and eventually decompresses through the lungs.
- Rapid ascent or decompression can result in trapping/coalition/expansion of nitrogen bubbles in the tissues, joints, and vasculature causing pathologic illness (DCS).
- In severe cases (AGE), nitrogenous bubble formation can obstruct circulatory flow causing cerebral, spinal cord, or cardiac ischemia with associated inflammatory vascular response, rupture of pulmonary alveoli or pulmonary embolism, and other associated pathologic end organ damage.
- DCS may be subdivided into two categories:
  - *Type I* DCS: manifest by milder symptoms of musculoskeletal pain, dermatologic rash, and vague constitutional symptoms. Extreme fatigue may be a prelude to a more severe DCI.
  - *Type II* DCS: characterized by moderate to severe neurologic impairment, cardiorespiratory dysfunction, and vestibular symptoms (1)
- AGE: a central nervous system (CNS) or cardiac injury as a consequence of pulmonary barotrauma, whereby air released from over-pressurized alveoli enters the pleural space (pneumothorax), mediastinum (pneumomediastinum), interstitium, and pulmonary capillary circulation, with subsequent access to systemic circulation
- Nitrogen gas bubbles returning to the heart may also reach the arterial circulation paradoxically via patent foramen ovale (PFO) or a right-to-left shunt, which can then embolize and obstruct cardiac or cerebral circulation (1).
- Type II DCS and AGE present similar symptoms and are best differentiated by time of onset.
- AGE symptoms from lung overexpansion typically present *immediately* or within minutes after resurfacing, whereas DCS symptoms usually develop *hours to days* after diving.
- Synonym(s): the bends; air embolism; caisson disease; decompression illness

EPIDEMIOLOGY

- The incidence rate of DCI is estimated between 0.02% and 0.03% per dive (2). Divers Alert Network (DAN) estimates 2.0 to 4.0 per 10,000 person-dives in the recreational community (1). Based on international dive surveys, minor incidents occur at a rate of 1.3% of all dives (3).
- Predominant age is young adulthood 20 to 29 yr, and predominant sex is male.

RISK FACTORS

- Inexperience
- Fatigue
- Hypovolemia/dehydration
- Poor physical conditioning
- Obesity
- Acute illnesses (ear, nose, and throat [ENT]; pulmonary; or gastrointestinal [GI])
- Chronic obstructive pulmonary disease (COPD) or poorly controlled asthma (increases risk for pulmonary barotrauma) (2,4)
- Previous history of cerebral, spinal, inner ear, or cutaneous DCI
- Migraine with aura (MWA)
- PFO
- Atrial septal defect (ASD)
- Panic or anxiety while diving
- Rapid ascent from depth
- Holding breath during ascent
- Omitted decompression stops
- Prolonged dive at depth of >33 feet sea water (>10 m sea water or 2 ATA)
- Multiple/repetitive dives
- Cold water, rough sea, or strong current dives
- Free diving (breath-hold diving)
- Inadequate rest/recovery between dives
- Strenuous physical activity while diving (commercial diving), tunnel, bridge, or oil platform work (caisson disease)
- Elevated body temperature
- Strenuous exertion after diving
- Flying <24 hr after SCUBA diving
- Inadequate aircraft cabin pressurization when flying

GENERAL PREVENTION

- Maintain adequate hydration.
- Do not dive under the influence of alcohol, drugs, or sedative medication.
- Ensure dive equipment is in good condition and proper working order.
- Ensure adequate wet suit protection for projected water immersion temperatures.
- Always dive with a partner (dive buddy).
- Do not dive with sinus or ear infection, eustachian tube dysfunction, or inability to effectively perform Valsalva maneuver.
- Do not dive with poorly controlled asthma or other upper respiratory illness.
- Do not dive with any ongoing or active GI disturbance.
- Use a dive computer to control exposure and ensure performance of adequate safety stops.
- Avoid holding breath during ascent.
- High-oxygen/low-nitrogen dive breathing gas mixture, or nitrox, may decrease tissue uptake of nitrogen but may also increase potential for oxygen toxicity at shallower depth.
- Use of closed-circuit oxygen rebreather (O2-CCR) apparatus (5)
- Wait 24 hr after diving before flying or traveling to higher altitudes.

DIAGNOSIS

HISTORY

- Determine time of onset of symptoms and any change in type or severity of symptoms.
- Obtain an independent account from a dive buddy or dive instructor, particularly if altered consciousness or mental status was impaired.
- Information from a dive computer (if the patient was equipped with one) may help to determine recent dive history, dive profile, and rate of ascent.
- Determine history of diving followed by exposure to altitude or past history of DCI.
- Note any significant past medical history of asthma, COPD, seizures, cardiac abnormality, prescription medications, recreational drug, or alcohol use.

PHYSICAL EXAM

- General manifestations of gas deposition in the CNS may mimic a transient ischemic attack (TIA), cerebrovascular accident (CVA), or seizure (epilepsy): manifest by confusion, personality changes, altered level of consciousness, delirium, numbness, weakness, aphasia, paresthesias, rapidly ascending paraplegia, or paralysis.
- Bubble formation in the inner ear can cause tinnitus (ringing sensation), sensorineural hearing loss, and dysequilibrium, with associated nausea, vomiting, ataxia and nystagmus (the staggers).
- Cardiac findings include tachy- or bradyarrhythmia, signs of myocardial infarction, or congestive heart failure.
- Pulmonary examination may detect decreased breath sounds or deviated trachea (pneumothorax), tachypnea, cough, wheeze, rales (the chokes), and decreased oxygen saturation with pulse oximetry.
- Joints may exhibit erythema and edema of periarticular surfaces, vague soreness, muscle weakness or fatigue, and pain with movement.
- Gas deposition in soft tissues may manifest as urticaria, mottled skin rash (cutis marmorata), or subcutaneous emphysema.

DIFFERENTIAL DIAGNOSIS

- Near drowning and hypoxic brain injury
- CVA
- Migraine
- Middle ear or sinus barotrauma with cranial nerve compression

- Inner ear barotrauma
- Seizure (hypoglycemia, epilepsy) and postictal state
- Spinal cord compression (disc herniation, hematoma, or tumor)
- Guillain-Barré syndrome
- Multiple sclerosis
- Transverse myelitis
- Acute myocardial infarction
- Cold water immersion pulmonary edema
- Contaminated breathing gas (carbon monoxide)
- Urticaria/anaphylaxis
- Seafood toxin poisoning (ciguatera, puffer fish, paralytic shellfish, sea snake envenomation)
- Malingering

DIAGNOSTIC TESTS & INTERPRETATION

- Chest radiography to assess for pneumothorax, mediastinal emphysema, and heart enlargement
- Chest computed tomography (CT) to screen pulmonary emboli (PE)
- CT scan or magnetic resonance imaging (MRI) to diagnose cerebral or spinal cord abnormalities
- Transesophageal bubble contrast echocardiogram to detect PFO
- Nonacute plain radiography, scintigraphy, MRI, and ultrasound of long bones and joints if dysbaric osteonecrosis is suspected

TREATMENT

- To locate the nearest hyperbaric oxygen therapy (HBOT) resources, access the DAN emergency hotline (+1-919-684-9111).
- DCS type I: Mild cases of DCS type I may be treated by breathing 100% oxygen via a nonrebreather mask. Consider HBOT if conservative measures fail to alleviate symptoms (1)[C].
- DCS type II: recompression therapy in a hyperbaric oxygen chamber. HBOT involves compression of nitrogen gas bubbles underlying the symptoms of DCS, whereas oxygen administered replaces nitrogen in the circulatory system. Nitrogen gas diffuses out of affected tissues over time, alleviating the symptoms of DCS.
- Treatment is typically administered based on the U.S. Navy Treatment Table 6 (TT6), which lasts approximately 4.5 hr.
- Significant improvement of symptoms soon after arrival to a depth of 60 feet (2.8 ATA) supports the diagnosis of DCS.
- Treatment tables may be modified to extend protocol or repeated until symptoms completely resolve.
- AGE: Check for spontaneous breathing and circulation. If necessary, call 911 and initiate cardiopulmonary resuscitation (CPR) per American Heart Association CPR protocol. Administer 100% oxygen via a nonrebreather mask if available. Access the nearest emergency room facility via emergency medical services (EMS).
- Once stabilized, assess for hypoglycemia, CVA, spinal cord trauma, and PE/pneumothorax. Initiate correction of any volume deficit with isotonic intravenous (IV) fluid resuscitation. Prepare for transfer to a hyperbaric oxygen chamber facility.
- Initiate HBOT using U.S. Navy TT6 protocol (100% oxygen at 2.8 ATA).
- If symptoms do not improve significantly at the standard 2.8 ATA, TT6 may be modified by an extended initial 30-min period of 50% oxygen at 6 ATA. Treatment is continued until symptoms resolve or plateau (6)[C].

ADDITIONAL THERAPIES

- Diazepam 5 to 15 mg IV may be considered for inner ear bends to alleviate symptoms of nausea and vomiting associated with severe vertigo.
- Deep venous thrombosis (DVT) prophylaxis may be indicated for patients immobilized by severe CNS bends.
- Avoid nonsteroidal anti-inflammatory drugs (NSAIDs) administration to patients with pain symptoms of DCS until hyperbaric treatment has been initiated.
- Fever in a patient with DCS should be worked up to rule out source of infection because hyperthermia may adversely affect prognosis.
- Additional resources:
  – International DAN (iDAN +1-919-684-9111)

ONGOING CARE

FOLLOW-UP RECOMMENDATIONS

- Patients may be discharged home if minor cutaneous symptoms are present and the patient responded to conservative therapy administered in the emergency department.
- Follow-up should be made with a physician knowledgeable in dive medicine.
- Wait 24 hr before flying after SCUBA diving.
- Exposure to altitude can precipitate relapse of DCS symptoms post-HBOT. If possible, postpone travel for 3 days at sea level after reaching a clinical plateau.
- In-flight oxygen supplementation may prevent DCS relapse.
- Type I DCS: 2 wk is recommended before returning to diving.
- Type II DCS with minor neurologic symptoms: 6 wk is recommended before return to diving.
- Type II DCS with severe neurologic symptoms: Diving is no longer recommended (1,6)[C].

PROGNOSIS

- The prognosis is excellent for early symptomatic recognition and timely treatment.
- Delay in treatment of severe symptoms negatively affects outcome.
- Rehabilitation of the injured diver may continue to improve residual sequelae by continuing hyperbaric treatment for up to 2 yr.

COMPLICATIONS

- Oxygen toxicity
- Transient myopia due to ocular lens oxygen toxicity (older patients), which may resolve in 4 to 6 wk
- Sensorineural hearing loss
- Dysbaric osteonecrosis
- Residual neurologic deficits in CNS bend (46–75%), despite comprehensive treatment.
- Permanent paralysis may occur if recompression is not initiated promptly.
- Residual paralysis may occur even in adequately treated patients if initial presentation is severe.

REFERENCES

1. Pollock NW, Buteau D. Updates in decompression illness. *Emerg Med Clin North Am*. 2017;35(2):301–319.
2. Klapa S, Meyne J, Kähler W, et al. Decompression illness with hypovolemic shock and neurological failure symptoms after two risky dives: a case report. *Physiol Rep*. 2017;5(6):e13094.
3. Eichhorn L, Leyk D. Diving medicine in clinical practice. *Dtsch Arztebl Int*. 2015;112(9):147–158.
4. Lawrence CH, Chen IY. The effect of scuba diving on airflow obstruction in divers with asthma. *Diving Hyperb Med*. 2016;46(1):11–14.
5. Wingelaar TT, van Ooij PAM, van Hulst RA, et al. Oxygen toxicity and special operations forces diving: hidden and dangerous. *Front Psychol*. 2017;8:1263.
6. U.S. Navy. *U.S. Navy Diving Manual, Volume 1: Diving Principles and Policies, Revision 7*. Washington, DC: Naval Sea Systems Command; 2016.

ADDITIONAL READING

Divernet: http://www.divernet.com/medical-health/

CLINICAL PEARLS

- DCS and AGE occur when compressed dissolved nitrogen gas reexpands into tissues and circulation as a result of rapid ascent from underwater depth.
- DCS should lead the differential diagnosis in any individual with recent history (hours to days) of SCUBA diving who presents with associated clinical symptomatology.
- AGE should be suspected in divers who surface with immediate signs of severe neurologic or cardiopulmonary pathology.
- AGE is associated with PFO and/or persistent cardiac septal defects.
- HBOT is the definitive treatment for DCS and AGE.
- HBOT is contraindicated with an unresolved pneumothorax.
- Proper diagnosis of DCS is supported if the patient's symptoms improve within a relatively short period of time after recompression.
- U.S. Navy TT6 is the preferred protocol for HBOT treatment.

SEIZURES AND EPILEPSY IN SPORTS

Nilesh Shah, MD, FAAFP, CAQSM • Chad J. Giles, DO

BASICS

DESCRIPTION

- A seizure is an abnormal paroxysmal electrical discharge in the brain, usually with mental status changes.
- Individuals who have two unprovoked seizures that occur >24 hr apart are deemed to have epilepsy.
- Status epilepticus: one continuous seizure lasting >5 min or two or more seizures between which there is no full return of consciousness
- Seizure types:
  - Generalized: sudden onset involving an altered level of consciousness, usually bilateral and symmetrical
  - Partial: either simple (no alteration of consciousness) or complex (alteration/loss of consciousness often with semipurposeful inappropriate movements)
- Synonym(s): convulsions, fits, attacks, spells

EPIDEMIOLOGY

- Incidence of seizure disorders in developed countries is approximately 50 per 100,000 persons per year (1).
- Prevalence of active epilepsy is 5 to 10 per 1,000 persons in most areas (1).
- >10% of the population will have at least one seizure during their lifetime.
- ~3% will have epilepsy by age 70 yr.
- 100,000 new cases of epilepsy per year in the United States, many in pediatric patients (2)
- 70–80% of patients with epilepsy will go into remission (2).

RISK FACTORS

- Family history
- Cerebrovascular disease
- Brain tumors
- Alcohol or drug abuse
- Previous head injury
- Malformations of cortical development
- Infections
- Abnormal early neurologic development

GENERAL PREVENTION

- Exercise may decrease seizure frequency.
- Sufficient and regular sleep (3)
- Limiting alcohol intake (3)
- Adhering to antiepileptic drug (AED) therapy (3)

COMMONLY ASSOCIATED CONDITIONS

- Behavioral problems (personality disorders)
- Hematologic disorders (sickle cell disease, porphyria, and antiphospholipid syndrome)
- Learning disabilities
- Migraine headaches
- Mood disorders (anxiety/depression)
- Psychiatric conditions
- Systemic autoimmune conditions (systemic lupus erythematosus [SLE])

DIAGNOSIS

HISTORY

- Convulsions (focal or generalized)
- Change in muscle tone
- Decreased level of consciousness
- Staring spells
- Loss of control of bowel or bladder
- Postictal confusion
- Postictal psychosis
- Todd paralysis
- Actual account by first-hand observer is extremely helpful or smartphone video.
- Previous history of seizure
- Previous history of head trauma
- Medications
- Social/family history

PHYSICAL EXAM

- Fever: suggests infectious etiology
- Focal neurologic deficit: possible localized trauma or tumor
- Meningismus: may be present in meningitis
- Papilledema: secondary to increased intracranial pressure
- Tongue biting (low sensitivity, high specificity)
- Look for injuries that may have occurred during the seizure.
- Look for evidence of acutely increased intracranial pressure, such as pupillary dilatation or posturing, indicating an emergency.
- Expect postictal confusion that gradually clears after a seizure.

DIFFERENTIAL DIAGNOSIS

- Alcohol withdrawal
- Arteriovenous malformation
- Electrolyte abnormalities (hypoglycemia, hyponatremia)
- Fever
- Hepatic failure
- Illicit drug use/abuse/withdrawal
- Infection
- Intracranial swelling/second-impact syndrome
- Primary/secondary brain tumor
- Posttraumatic (impact) seizure
- Stroke
- Syncope
- Uremia
- Vascular disease

DIAGNOSTIC TESTS & INTERPRETATION

Initial Tests (lab, imaging)

- Electrolytes, including glucose, calcium, magnesium, and phosphorus
- Renal/liver function tests, including ammonia level
- Complete blood count (CBC), urinalysis
- Blood/urine toxicology
- Anticonvulsant level(s): Inadequate levels are a significant cause of recurrent seizures.
- Computed tomography (CT) or magnetic resonance imaging (MRI) indicated for individuals with first-time seizure to evaluate for structural brain abnormality
- CT scan: rules out acute bleeding or intracranial masses
- MRI: may better define posterior fossa tumors, vascular abnormalities, and temporal lobes
- Electroencephalography (EEG): may define true seizure activity and focus, although a negative EEG result does not rule out seizure disorder. Sometimes, a sleep-deprived EEG may be required.

Diagnostic Procedures/Other

- Electrocardiogram (ECG): evaluates for cardiogenic causes of hypoxia-related seizure
- Spinal tap to rule out infectious etiology, elevated intracranial pressure, some congenital etiologies

TREATMENT

GENERAL MEASURES

- Supportive: airway, breathing, and circulation (ABCs)
- Roll patients with active tonic-clonic seizures on their side in the "recovery position."
- Do *not* use bite block or tongue depressor.
- Keep area clear: Ensure that the patient does not injure self or others.
- If in the setting of trauma, stabilize C-spine.
- Transfer to emergency department (ED) if the patient has no known seizure disorder:
  - ED treatment:
    - Immediate ED treatment includes benzodiazepines or other AEDs if patient is in status epilepticus.
    - Workup as above for etiology
    - Consider neurology consultation.

MEDICATION

- If no reversible cause is found, place patient on AEDs.
- A number of drugs are available.
- Use depends on etiology of seizures.
- Most AEDs are approved by the National Collegiate Athletic Association (NCAA) and International Olympic Committee (IOC).

First Line

- Benzodiazepines for status epilepticus
- Common AEDs: levetiracetam, fosphenytoin/phenytoin, and valproic acid

Second Line

Depends on etiology of seizure

ISSUES FOR REFERRAL

Neurology:

- First-time unprovoked seizure
- Initiation of AEDs
- Outpatient EEG

ADMISSION, INPATIENT, AND NURSING CONSIDERATIONS

- Hospitalization recommended for immediate care of uncontrolled seizures
- Abnormal mental status associated with seizures
- Ongoing studies (i.e., sleep study or 24-hr EEG monitoring)

- Need for intravenous (IV) access:
  - Ongoing IV drug administration
  - Correction of electrolyte abnormalities
  - Correction of dehydration

ONGOING CARE

FOLLOW-UP RECOMMENDATIONS

Patient Monitoring

Monitor levels of AEDs, especially in first couple months of training.

PATIENT EDUCATION

- People with chronic diseases, including epilepsy, should be encouraged to exercise, as should the general population. The mental and physical advantages of regular exercise are regarded as highly beneficial to a group that is normally sedentary, overweight, and with higher rates of depression (4)[C].
- Recommendations with respect to fitness to participate in a specific sport should consider the probability of a seizure occurring, the seizure type, the usual timing of seizure occurrence, and other factors (5)[C].
- International League Against Epilepsy (ILAE) proposed sports be classified into three categories based on potential risk of injury/death should a seizure occur (5)[C]:
  - Group 1 sports (no significant additional risk to person with epilepsy or bystanders):
    - Athletics
    - Bowling
    - Most collective contact sports (judo, wrestling, etc.)
    - Collective sports on the ground (baseball, basketball, cricket, field hockey, football, soccer, rugby, volleyball, etc.)
    - Cross-country skiing
    - Curling
    - Dancing
    - Golf
    - Racquet sports (squash, table tennis, tennis, etc.)
  - Group 2 sports (moderate risk to persons with epilepsy but no risk for bystanders):
    - Alpine skiing
    - Archery
    - Athletics (pole vault)
    - Biathlon, triathlon, modern pentathlon
    - Canoeing
    - Collective contact sports involving potentially serious injury (e.g., boxing, karate, etc.)
    - Cycling
    - Fencing
    - Gymnastics
    - Horse riding (e.g., olympic equestrian events—dressage, eventing, show jumping, etc.)
    - Ice hockey
    - Shooting
    - Skateboarding
    - Skating
    - Snowboarding
    - Swimming
    - Water skiing
    - Weight lifting
  - Group 3 sports (high risk to persons with epilepsy and, for some sports, also risks for bystanders):
    - Aviation
    - Climbing
    - Diving (platform, springboard)
    - Horse racing (competitive)
    - Motor sports
    - Parachuting (and similar sports)
    - Rodeo
    - Scuba diving
    - Ski jumping
    - Solitary sailing
    - Surfing, windsurfing
- One or more acute symptomatic seizures:
  - Group 1 sports permitted
  - Group 2 and 3 sports at neurologist discretion
- Single unprovoked seizure:
  - Group 1 sports permitted after medical/neurologic assessment
  - Group 2 and 3 sports after seizure free for 12 mo
- Sleep-related seizures only:
  - Group 1 sports permitted
  - Group 2 sports at neurologist discretion or after 12 mo follow-up if seizures confirmed to be exclusively associated with sleep and sports does not involve alterations in the sleep-wake cycle
  - Group 3 sports generally barred
- Seizures without impaired awareness:
  - Group 1 sports permitted
  - Group 2 sports at neurologist discretion or after 12 mo follow-up if seizure occurs exclusively without impairment of awareness
  - Group 3 sports generally barred
- Seizures with impaired awareness:
  - Group 1 sports permitted
  - Group 2 sports at neurologist discretion
  - Group 3 sports generally barred
- Resolved epilepsy (age-dependent epilepsy syndrome past applicable age, seizure free for 10 yr, and off antiseizure medications for at least 5 yr):
  - Group 1, 2, and 3 sports permitted
- Medication withdrawal:
  - Group 2 or 3 sports are not permitted for 6 mo.
  - If seizure reoccurs, group 2 and 3 sports are not permitted for a period of 3 mo after previously effective treatment is reinstated and no further seizures.

PROGNOSIS

Prognosis is generally excellent with well-controlled seizures.

COMPLICATIONS

- Exercise at high altitudes (>2,000 m) can predispose to hypoxia and induce seizures.
- Hyperhydration (consumption that outpaces demand) in combination with sodium loss can result in hyponatremic seizures.
- AED side effects may include impaired concentration or coordination.
- Certain AEDs can predispose athletes to heat-related illness and hyperthermia which is a known seizure trigger.

REFERENCES

1. Sander JW. The epidemiology of epilepsy revisited. *Curr Opin Neurol*. 2003;16(2):165–170.
2. Arida RM, Cavalheiro EA, da Silva AC, et al. Physical activity and epilepsy: proven and predicted benefits. *Sports Med*. 2008;38(7):607–615.
3. Nashef L, Capovilla G, Camfield C, et al. Transition: driving and exercise. *Epilepsia*. 2014;55(Suppl 3): 41–45.
4. Pimentel J, Tojal R, Morgado J. Epilepsy and physical exercise. *Seizure*. 2015;25:87–94.
5. Capovilla G, Kaufman KR, Perucca E, et al. Epilepsy, seizures, physical exercise, and sports: a report from the ILAE Task Force on Sports and Epilepsy. *Epilepsia*. 2016;57(1):6–12.
6. Dimberg EL, Burns TM. Management of common neurologic conditions in sports. *Clin Sports Med*. 2005;24(3):637–662.

ADDITIONAL READING

- Cantu RV. Epilepsy and athletics. *Clin Sports Med*. 1998;17(1):61–69.
- Fountain NB, May AC. Epilepsy and athletics. *Clin Sports Med*. 2003;22(3):605–616.
- Howard GM, Radloff M, Sevier TL. Epilepsy and sports participation. *Curr Sports Med Rep*. 2004;3(1):15–19.
- Knowles BD, Pleacher MD. Athletes with seizure disorders. *Curr Sports Med Rep*. 2012;11(1):16–20.
- Miele VJ, Bailes JE, Martin NA. Participation in contact or collision sports in athletes with epilepsy, genetic risk factors, structural brain lesions, or history of craniotomy. *Neurosurg Focus*. 2006;21(4):E9
- Sirven JI, Varrato J. Physical activity and epilepsy: what are the rules? *Phys Sports Med*. 1999;27(3):63–70.

CLINICAL PEARLS

- In general, individuals with epilepsy or new onset seizure disorder should avoid high-risk activities such as scuba diving, skydiving, and group 3 sports.
- There is no definitive evidence of any relationship between repetitive minor head injury and deterioration of the epileptic patient; therefore, most collision/contact sports are acceptable (but no boxing). Swimming is acceptable with a certified lifeguard who should be made aware of the situation. Motor sports should be undertaken only by individuals with well-controlled seizures. Sports in which falling is a potential (e.g., gymnastics, rock climbing, hang gliding) should be judged on an individual basis based on the type and frequency of seizure.
- Sports need not be avoided for children who experience seizures. Improving overall health may reduce the number of seizures experienced by a child. He or she also may benefit from the increased self-esteem and social integration available with participation in sports. Children will obtain all the physiologic benefits of exercise, including increased cardiovascular fitness, increase muscle strength, and weight control.
- The following questions need to be asked when deciding if participation in sports is OK (6)[C]:
  - Are there any other impairments that modify the athlete's participation (i.e., ventricular shunts or vascular malformations)? What type of seizures occur? How often do seizures occur?
  - Do AEDs significantly impair the athlete's perception and alertness?
  - Overall, the decision is individualized, but the physiologic and psychological benefits of sport and exercise usually far outweigh the risk to athletes or their competitors.

SEPTIC ARTHRITIS AND BURSITIS

Kevin B. Gebke, MD • Matthew Rachwalski, DO

BASICS

DESCRIPTION

- Infection of articular joint(s) or bursae with a bacterial, mycobacterial, spirochetal, fungal, or viral source
- Usually acute, but bursitis can be chronic
- May be an indication of systemic infection
- Synonym(s): infectious arthritis; purulent synovitis; infectious bursitis

EPIDEMIOLOGY

- Incidence 2 to 6 cases per 100,000 person/year
- Monoarticular or oligoarticular pattern for acute bacterial infection, chronic mycobacterial infection, or fungal infection
- Acute polyarticular involvement usually signifies disseminated neisserial infection or acute hepatitis B.
- Septic arthritis from gonorrhea now very rare
- Olecranon and prepatellar bursae most common

RISK FACTORS

- Soft tissue/joint penetration or recent surgery
- Trauma, including repetitive microtrauma (bursitis)
- Abnormal joint architecture (rheumatoid arthritis [RA], osteoarthritis [OA], joint replacement)
- Intravenous (IV) drug abuse, alcoholism
- Intravascular devices, urinary catheters
- Sexually active person at risk for sexually transmitted infections (STIs) (rare etiology)
- Significant comorbid diseases (diabetes, malignancy, hepatic failure, sickle cell disease, immunocompromised states)
- Young age, elderly

DIAGNOSIS

HISTORY

- Rapid onset (1 to 2 wk) in septic arthritis; may have rapid or insidious onset with septic bursitis
- Single joint involvement in >85% of patients
- Most commonly involves knee (50%) > hip > shoulder, ankle, wrist, or elbow joints
- Hematologic spread: presence of infection leading to bacterial seeding of joint (Skin infection, pneumonia, pyelonephritis are commonly the source.)

PHYSICAL EXAM

- Various degrees of pain in region of joint or bursa
- Swelling (bursitis) or joint effusion (arthritis)
- Decreased range of joint motion (especially with septic arthritis may not have with bursitis)
- Localized or systemic fever
- Concomitant urethral discharge
- Erythema and tenderness to palpation of affected joint or bursa
- Intravenous drug abuse often develop bacterial arthritis in axial joints, such as the sternoclavicular and sternomanubrial joint and may develop bacterial arthritis as a consequence of infective endocarditis.
- Rare cutaneous lesions (infective endocarditis, Lyme disease, meningococcal infection, gonorrhea)

DIFFERENTIAL DIAGNOSIS

- Cellulitis
- Osteomyelitis
- Gout
- Pseudogout (calcium pyrophosphate deposition disease)
- RA
- Juvenile RA
- Rheumatic fever
- Lyme disease
- Spondyloarthropathy (Reiter syndrome, psoriatic arthritis, ankylosing spondylitis, irritable bowel disease)
- Sarcoidosis, amyloidosis
- Synovitis
- Synovial papilloma
- AIDS

DIAGNOSTIC TESTS & INTERPRETATION

- Laboratory evaluation of joint or bursal aspirate is gold standard for diagnosis. Collect prior to starting antibiotics (1,2)[C],(3)[A].
- Complete blood count (CBC), blood cultures, erythrocyte sedimentation rate, C-reactive protein, blood cultures × 2 (2)[C]
- Contaminated overlying tissue (i.e., cellulitis) should be avoided during arthrocentesis or bursal aspiration.
- Synovial or bursal fluid aspirate should be sent for white blood cell (WBC) count and differential, Gram stain and examination for crystals, and culture (aerobic/anaerobic bacteria, mycobacteria and fungi). Order polymerase chain reaction (PCR) testing for Lyme disease if high suspicion (2)[C].
- In acute septic arthritis, synovial WBC counts typically average 50,000 WBC/mL with >90% neutrophils (2)[C],(4)[B],(5)[A]
- In prosthetic joint infections, synovial WBC counts may be as low as 1,100 WBC/mL with >64% neutrophils.

- Plain radiographs initially may be normal, osteopenia first radiologic sign, and then diffuse joint space narrowing.
- Ultrasound (US) is useful for identifying hip effusions.
- Computed tomography (CT) visualizes bone edema, bone erosions, and sclerosis.
- Magnetic resonance imaging (MRI) better for detection joint effusion and differentiate between bone and soft tissue infections
- Bone scan is indicated for identification of region affected by inflammatory process.

TREATMENT

- Septic bursitis:
  - Most common organisms include *Staphylococcus aureus* (80%), β-hemolytic *Streptococcus*, and *Staphylococcus epidermidis* (3,6)[B].
  - With repetitive microtrauma and hematogenous seeding may broaden coverage.
  - Primary therapy includes penicillinase-resistant penicillins (nafcillin or dicloxacillin). If allergic, then use Bactrim or clindamycin (1)[A].
  - No consensus on duration but generally 10 to 14 days
  - Hospitalization for parenteral therapy is required when signs of systemic or bony extension of infection are observed.
  - Surgical intervention includes endoscopic versus open bursectomy; reserved for persistent infection despite antibiotic treatment, presence of foreign body, or underlying osteomyelitis (6)[B]
- Septic arthritis:
  - Empiric IV broad-spectrum antibiotic should be initiated based on Gram stain result (5)[B].
  - If Gram stain shows gram-positive cocci, treat with vancomycin (2)[C].
  - If Gram stain shows gram-negative cocci or bacilli, treat with a 3rd-generation cephalosporin such as ceftriaxone. If *Pseudomonas* is suspected, then start 4th-generation cephalosporin such as cefepime. If β-lactam allergy, then use aztreonam or ciprofloxacin (2)[C].
  - If Gram stain negative, start vancomycin in immunocompetent and add 3rd-generation cephalosporin in immunocompromised and at risk for STIs (2)[C].
  - Infection eradication is complicated by the presence of joint prostheses, and removal of the prosthesis may be necessary (5)[B].
  - No indication for intra-articular antibiotics (4)[C]
  - No consensus on duration of antibiotic therapy, Infectious Diseases Society of America (IDSA) recommends 4-wk course of parenteral therapy in *S. aureus* and gram-negative bacilli infections (5)[C].
  - Patients treated for gonorrhea also should receive doxycycline 100 mg PO BID × 7 days to cover possible concurrent *Chlamydia* infection.
  - Longer treatment is required for joints affected by arthritis.
  - Surgical intervention via arthroscopic lavage or arthrotomy is indicated only if needle drainage is ineffective (fluid loculation or inaccessible joint).
  - After initial joint drainage, therapeutic response monitored with serial synovial fluid analysis

ONGOING CARE

- Complete resolution and restoration of joint function is the goal.
- Possible adverse outcomes include death, impaired joint function (e.g., decreased motion, fusion, dislocation), septic necrosis, sinus formation, ankylosis, osteomyelitis, synovitis, and limb length changes.

FOLLOW-UP RECOMMENDATIONS

- Recurrent arthrocentesis is recommended as joint fluid reaccumulates to rule out persistent/recurrent infection.
- Regular office visits are recommended after hospital discharge for reevaluation and early recognition of persistent or new problems.
- Prosthesis replacement is possible in the future after clearance of infection.

REFERENCES

1. Khodaee M. Common superficial bursitis. *Am Fam Physician*. 2017;95(4):224–231.
2. Horowitz DL, Katzap E, Horowitz S, et al. Approach to septic arthritis. *Am Fam Physician*. 2011;84(6):653–660.
3. Lieber SB, Fowler ML, Zhu C, et al. Clinical characteristics and outcomes of septic bursitis. *Infection*. 2017;45(6).781–786.
4. Hyung CJ, Burke LA, Lee M. Septic arthritis. *Hosp Med Clin*. 2014;3(4):494–503.
5. García-Arias M, Balsa A, Mola EM. Septic arthritis. *Best Pract Res Clin Rheumatol*. 2011;25(3):407–421.
6. Hanrahan JA. Recent developments in septic bursitis. *Curr Infect Dis Rep*. 2013;15(5):421–425.

CLINICAL PEARLS

- Septic arthritis is considered an emergency, and prompt drainage and administration of IV antibiotics can prevent joint damage.
- Knee joint is most common, although axial joints more common in IVDA.
- Complete restoration of joint function is expected if early diagnosis and treatment occur before articular damage is seen.
- Sign of hip infection, more common in children, is hip held in flexed and externally rotated position.

SESAMOID DYSFUNCTION AND FRACTURE

Laura M. Distel, MD, CAQSM • James R. Borchers, MD, MPH

BASICS

- Anatomy:
  - Two sesamoid bones: the larger tibial (medial) sesamoid and fibular (lateral) sesamoid
  - Located on the plantar side of the 1st metatarsophalangeal (MTP) joint, just proximal to the metatarsal head, embedded within the flexor hallucis brevis tendon and connected by the intersesamoid ligament
  - The sesamoids' articular surfaces are located dorsally and articulate with the plantar facets on the 1st metatarsal head.
  - Blood supply is usually from a single artery, with a lack of significant secondary blood supply (which increases risk for nonunion of fractures) (1).
  - Can have multiple ossification centers that may lead to a bipartite sesamoid, which can be difficult to distinguish from an acute fracture (1)
  - Vitally important in the biomechanics of the foot
  - When the 1st MTP joint dorsiflexes, the sesamoids are pulled distally, covering and protecting the plantar surface of the 1st metatarsal head and absorbing the weight-bearing forces on the medial aspect of the forefoot.
  - Flexor hallucis brevis provides the active plantarflexion force at the 1st MTP joint, but the sesamoid complex provides an increased mechanical advantage in plantarflexion.
- Sesamoid function:
  - Protects the tendon of the flexor hallucis longus
  - Absorbs a majority of the weight on the medial aspect of the forefoot:
    - Sesamoid bones bear up to 3 times body weight during normal gait.
    - Medial (or tibial) sesamoid bears the majority of this weight and thus is at higher risk for injury.
  - Dissipates the forces on the metatarsal head
  - Increases the power of the flexor hallucis brevis and thus plantarflexion (1)

DESCRIPTION

- Stress fractures:
  - Most common sesamoid pathology (1)
  - More common in athletes than in general population (2)
- Sesamoiditis:
  - General term that encompasses multiple conditions including osteonecrosis, chondromalacia, or inflammatory changes (1)
  - Usually involves the medial (tibial) sesamoid (1)
- Acute fracture:
  - Typically caused by forced dorsiflexion (1)
  - Often, a transverse fracture line is seen on imaging with sharp edges (3).

EPIDEMIOLOGY

- Sesamoiditis is seen more commonly in young, active adults.
- Stress fractures are more common in athletes.

RISK FACTORS

- Repetitive, forceful dorsiflexion, or loading (pushing off) of the MTP joint
- At-risk sports include dancing (especially ballet), running, gymnastics, volleyball, basketball, high-impact aerobics, and soccer (1).
- Asymmetrical sesamoids
- Overpronation (3)
- Playing on artificial turf (1)
- Wearing shoes without adequate forefoot support (i.e., high heels)

GENERAL PREVENTION

- Wearing shoes with adequate forefoot support
- Use of orthotics to offload the 1st MTP joint

DIAGNOSIS

HISTORY

- Gradual onset of pain on the plantar surface of the 1st hallux
- Pain with dorsiflexion or weight-bearing (1)
- Unilateral symptoms are typical.
- Pain typically is located at the medial sesamoid.
- Acute fracture usually occurs with a history of hyperextension injury of the big toe (1).

PHYSICAL EXAM

- Tenderness with direct palpation of the sesamoids ± swelling or ecchymosis
- Pain with resisted plantarflexion of the 1st hallux
- Pain with passive dorsiflexion of the 1st MTP
- Pain with "pushing off" while walking or running
- Decreased range of motion and/or strength of the 1st MTP
- Occasional erythema or swelling of the sesamoids
- An enlarged bursa on the plantar surface may be present.
- Presence of significant pes cavus, pes planus, or cock-up deformity of the hallux

DIFFERENTIAL DIAGNOSIS

- Turf toe
- Flexor hallucis longus tendonitis
- Hallux rigidus
- Hallux valgus
- Neuroma
- Metatarsalgia
- Osteochondritis (more common in young women)
- Osteoarthritis or inflammatory arthritis
- Osteonecrosis
- Avascular necrosis of the sesamoids
- Neoplasm
- Nerve impingement (less common)
- Nonunion of a sesamoid fracture

DIAGNOSTIC TESTS & INTERPRETATION

- X-ray examination of the foot should include weight-bearing anteroposterior, lateral, medial, and lateral oblique views. Comparison views of the contralateral foot may be helpful (2)[A].
- If possible, an axial view of the 1st MTP joint in dorsiflexion, known as the "sesamoid view" (2)[A]:
  - Presence of a bilateral bipartite sesamoid is more likely a normal variant rather than an acute fracture; acute fractures are almost always unilateral.
  - A partitioned sesamoid may be seen in ~11% of the population (4).
  - 85% of bipartite sesamoids are bilateral (1).
  - An acutely fractured sesamoid is characterized by sharp, irregular edges, comminution, or widely spaced fragments in contrast to the sclerotic edges of a nonunion or the smooth edges of a bipartite sesamoid (1,3).
  - Magnetic resonance imaging (MRI) or bone scan are helpful in differentiating sesamoid injuries from normal bipartite variant because they can detect soft tissue or bony edema before radiographically evident (1,5).
- Computed tomography (CT) or single-photon emission computed tomography (SPECT) are more specific for sesamoid fractures (3,5)[C].

TREATMENT

- Sesamoiditis or stress fracture/nonunion:
  - Initially, conservative therapy is recommended for at least 4 to 6 wk (1,5,6)[A]:
    - Relative rest with immobilization by offloading the 1st MTP complex with orthotics or rocker sole shoes (forefoot unloader shoe), a dancer's pad, or metatarsal bar; taping the great toe in plantarflexion may be considered for severe symptoms (5,6)[A].
    - Ice
    - Pain control (oral nonsteroidal anti-inflammatory drugs [NSAIDs] or other analgesics) (5)[C]
    - Rarely, injections with corticosteroids can be considered (6).
    - Avoid wearing high-heeled shoes (5).
  - Long-term treatment includes:
    - Correction of any mechanical abnormalities with the use of taping, orthotics, or a stiff-soled shoe to limit dorsiflexion of the 1st MTP joint.
    - Eliminating or minimizing the stressing activity (1)[C].
    - Surgery, usually to excise the sesamoid, to treat prolonged symptoms despite several months of conservative management (see below).
- Acute fractures:
  - Non–weight-bearing immobilization with a short leg cast/ankle foot orthosis (AFO) for 6 to 8 wk, followed by protected weight-bearing in cast/AFO for 4 to 6 additional weeks (2)[A]
  - Open reduction and internal fixation or percutaneous fixation are surgical options (2,3,5)[A].

SURGERY/OTHER PROCEDURES

Surgical options are available for prolonged symptoms if nonoperative treatment fails, but mechanical defects can lead to long-term problems:

- Sesamoidectomy (surgical excision) (1)[A]:
  - Most common procedure for sesamoid pathology
  - Can be partial or complete
  - Can result in overload of the metatarsal head or flexor hallucis longus tendon
  - Excision of both sesamoids generally is not recommended owing to development of cock-up deformity and biomechanical morbidity (1).
  - Promising data for high rate of return to play to previous level of athletic activity (3,5)[C]
- Curettage and bone grafting (1)
- Shaving of the sesamoid (1)

ONGOING CARE

- Custom orthotics ± cutouts for the sesamoid bones (3)
- Short-leg walking cast can be considered for recalcitrant cases (1).
- Corticosteroid injection into the sesamoid area can be considered with caution.

FOLLOW-UP RECOMMENDATIONS

- Periodic follow-up every 4 to 8 wk until the patient is asymptomatic
- Continued modification of activities and use of orthotics
- Referral to orthopedic surgeon or podiatrist if symptoms persist >6 mo

PROGNOSIS

- Conservative management generally is successful in treating most sesamoid pathology.
- More severe cases that require surgical intervention are at risk for iatrogenic complications.

COMPLICATIONS

- Nonunion of fractures
- Development of stress fractures or avascular necrosis in untreated sesamoiditis

REFERENCES

1. Dedmond BT, Cory JW, McBryde A Jr. The hallucal sesamoid complex. *J Am Acad Orthop Surg*. 2006;14(13):745–753.
2. Mittlmeier T, Haar P. Sesamoid and toe fractures. *Injury*. 2004;35(Suppl 2):SB87–SB97.
3. Ribbans WJ, Hintermann B. Hallucal sesamoid fractures in athletes: diagnosis and treatment. *Sports Orthop Traumatol*. 2016;32(3):295–303.
4. Yammine K. The sesamoids of the feet in humans: a systematic review and meta-analysis. *Anat Sci Int*. 2015;90(3):144–160.
5. York PJ, Wydra FB, Hunt KJ. Injuries to the great toe. *Curr Rev Musculoskeletal Med*. 2017;10(1):104–112.
6. Mayer SW, Joyner PW, Almekinders LC, et al. Stress fractures of the foot and ankle in athletes. *Sports Health*. 2014;6(6):481–491.

CLINICAL PEARLS

- Medial sesamoid is injured most commonly.
- Acute fractures are almost exclusively unilateral.
- Bilateral bipartite sesamoids are usually benign.
- Tenderness over the sesamoids or pain with dorsiflexion that improves with non–weight-bearing should arise suspicion for sesamoid pathology.
- Nonoperative treatment, especially immobilization, is the mainstay of therapy.
- Sesamoidectomy is the most common surgical procedure to treat chronic symptoms.

SEVER DISEASE/CALCANEAL APOPHYSITIS

Stephen M. Simons, MD, FACSM • Ryan Sorell, MD

BASICS

DESCRIPTION

- Sever disease, also known as *calcaneal apophysitis*, is an overuse syndrome and one of the most common causes of late childhood and adolescent heel pain.
- This traction apophysitis is the foot equivalent to Osgood-Schlatter disease.
- Synonym(s): calcaneal apophysitis

EPIDEMIOLOGY

Incidence

- Typically occurs during an adolescent growth spurt
- Most common activities are ones requiring repetitive running or jumping (track, basketball, soccer, gymnastics).
- Occurrence in general population: 3.7/1,000 individuals age 6 to 17 yr old
- Predominant age: described most often between the ages of 9 and 12 yr; most frequent at age 11 yr in girls and at age 12 yr in boys
- Predominant gender: male > female
- Occurs bilaterally in just over 60% of cases

ETIOLOGY AND PATHOPHYSIOLOGY

- The posterior calcaneus develops as a secondary ossification center.
- This secondary ossification center provides attachment for the achilles tendon.
- During a growth spurt, bone growth greater than the ability of the muscle-tendon unit to sufficiently stretch creating increased tension
- The apophysitis is the weakest point of the chain.
- Repetitive stress results in microtrauma and chronic irritation leading to thickening and pain.
- Ongoing stress may lead to stress fracture of the body of the calcaneus.
- The calcaneal physis typically closes between the ages of 12 and 15 yr.

RISK FACTORS

- Adolescent growth spurt
- Increased or excessive sport and play activity without period of rest
- Tight gastrocsoleus complex
- Weak ankle dorsiflexors
- Biomechanical factors such as genu varum and forefoot varus
- Poor-quality or worn-out athletic shoes
- Poorly cushioned or low-heeled shoes such as soccer, baseball, track, or cycling cleats
- Running on hard surfaces
- High-impact sports

DIAGNOSIS

HISTORY

- An 8- to 13-yr-old child presents with heel pain worsened with increased activity (1)[C].
- Recent growth spurt coincides with vigorous sport or play activities (1)[C].
- Sports requiring a lot of running and jumping activities are particularly prone to cause this overuse syndrome (2)[C].
- Pain is typically unilateral but may be bilateral and is often relieved with rest (2)[C].
- The pain may become severe enough to stop sport activity and even require crutch walking (2)[C].

PHYSICAL EXAM

- Signs and symptoms include:
  - Intermittent or continuous posterior heel pain (1)[C].
  - No swelling.
  - No ecchymoses or skin changes.
- Physical examination includes the following:
  - Pain with single-heel rise test (Sever sign) (3)[C]
  - Tenderness with medial and lateral compression of the calcaneus (heel squeeze test) (2,3)[C]
  - Tenderness at Achilles insertion on heel (2,3)[C]
  - Heel cord inflexibility with sometimes <10 degrees of dorsiflexion
  - Biomechanical contributors such as forefoot varus, hallux valgus, pes cavus, and pes planus (1)[C]

DIFFERENTIAL DIAGNOSIS

- Nerve entrapment (plantar)
- Neuroma (plantar)
- Plantar fasciitis (plantar)
- Heel pad syndrome (plantar)
- Calcaneal stress fracture (plantar)
- Peroneal tendinopathy (midfoot/lateral)
- Sinus tarsi syndrome (midfoot/lateral)
- Tarsal tunnel syndrome (midfoot/medial)
- Achilles tendinopathy (posterior)
- Haglund deformity (posterior)

DIAGNOSTIC TESTS & INTERPRETATION

- Radiographs may show fragmentation, sclerosis, and increased density of the apophysis, but these radiographic changes can be normal (2,4)[C].
- Imaging is not necessary to make this clinical diagnosis but may be helpful to rule out other causes of heel pain (2,4)[C].

TREATMENT

- Rest or reduce activity to a pain tolerance level (2,5)[C].
- Ice (2)[C]
- Nonsteroidal anti-inflammatory drugs (NSAIDs) for pain control (2)[C]
- Heel lifts (2,5)[C]
- Shock-absorbing heel inserts (2,5)[C]
- Gastrocsoleus stretching exercises: knee straight and knee flexed stretch with the heel maintained on the floor or ground (2,5)[C]
- Eccentric calf strengthening exercises (2,5)[C]
- If not responsive to conservative treatment, a short leg cast or boot walker or even immobilization may be necessary (2)[C].

ADDITIONAL THERAPIES

- Strengthening of the quadriceps and gastrocsoleus to better equip these muscle groups to act as shock absorbers (2,5)[C]
- Strengthening of the foot dorsiflexors
- Good-quality shoe with adequate shock absorption and firm heel counter (2,5)[C]
- The use of heel raises over prefabricated orthoses may have a relative advantage in the first 2 mo of treatment, but there is no difference in pain or impact at 12 mo (5)[C].
- Off-the-shelf orthoses are much more cost-effective and can be tried first before custom orthoses are considered. Time to symptom resolution varies, but symptoms abate totally with skeletal maturity (2)[C].
- No reports of long-term sequelae from Sever disease (2)[C]

SURGERY/OTHER PROCEDURES

Not indicated

ONGOING CARE

FOLLOW-UP RECOMMENDATIONS

Referral/disposition necessary only when clinician is uncertain of diagnosis

COMPLICATIONS

Persistent pain that does not respond to conservative measures may indicate there is a calcaneal stress fracture and may require a 3- to 4-wk period of immobilization (4)[C].

REFERENCES

1. Micheli LJ, Ireland ML. Prevention and management of calcaneal apophysitis in children: an overuse syndrome. *J Pediatr Orthop*. 1987;7(1):34–38.
2. Hendrix CL. Calcaneal apophysitis (Sever disease). *Clin Podiatr Med Surg*. 2005;22(1):55–62.
3. Perhamre S, Lazowska D, Papageorgiou S, et al. Sever's injury: a clinical diagnosis. *J Am Podiatr Med Assoc*. 2013;103(5):361–368.
4. Rachel JN, Williams JB, Sawyer JR, et al. Is radiographic evaluation necessary in children with a clinical diagnosis of calcaneal apophysitis (Sever disease)? *J Pediatr Orthop*. 2011;31(5):548–550.
5. Uvelli K, Neher JO, Safranek S. Treatment for calcaneal apophysitis. *Am Fam Physician*. 2017;96(2):126–127.

ADDITIONAL READING

Tu P. Heel pain: diagnosis and management. *Am Fam Physician*. 2018;97(2):86–93.

S

CLINICAL PEARLS

- Conservative therapy remains the mainstay of treatment.
- Diagnosis should be made clinically without radiography unless signs and symptoms are atypical.
- Total rest may hasten the recovery from this heel pain but may not be necessary.
- Reducing the amount of activity may allow sports participation without worsening the heel pain and increase patient buy-in.
- Current evidence does not suggest any long-term sequelae.

SHOULDER INSTABILITY, ANTERIOR

Michael Seth Smith, MD, CAQSM, PharmD • Kristy Smith, MD

BASICS

DESCRIPTION

- A symptomatic anteroinferior subluxation or dislocation of the glenohumeral (GH) joint
- Synonym(s): GH dislocation; GH subluxation; dead-arm syndrome

EPIDEMIOLOGY

- One of the most commonly dislocated joints in the body due to its significant mobility. In a study of 8,056 dislocations, 45% involved the GH joint.
- Anterior traumatic dislocation accounts for 96% of all GH dislocations.

ALERT

Recurrence rate for athletes age <25 yr is >85% in those who have suffered an initial traumatic event.

RISK FACTORS

- History of previous dislocation
- Younger patients
- Athletes participating in repetitive overhead sports (i.e., throwing/volleyball) or contact sports (i.e., football, wrestling, ice hockey)

DIAGNOSIS

HISTORY

- Patients usually give a history of prior dislocation/subluxation event. The symptoms will be reported to occur when the arm is placed in the provocative position of abduction and external rotation.
- Patients also may complain of a "dead arm," which typically occurs with subluxation.

PHYSICAL EXAM

- Patients note the feeling of impending dislocation with the arm in a provocative position. Pain itself is generally not a sign of pure instability.
- A thorough exam of the cervical spine, proximal humerus, and scapula should be performed when evaluating anyone with shoulder pain. If multidirectional instability is suspected, an assessment of ligamentous laxity should be addressed. A complete neurologic exam should be performed to identify any central or peripheral neuropathy.
- Apprehension test: Arm is placed at 90 degrees of abduction and gently externally rotated. A sense of "impending" dislocation is regarded as a positive test.
- Relocation test: During the apprehension test, a posteriorly directed force is applied to the proximal humerus with the scapula stabilized by the examiner's opposite hand. If symptoms abate, the test result is positive.
- Load and shift test: The patient is seated while the examiner stabilizes the scapula with one hand and with the thumb and forefinger of the free hand on the proximal humerus attempts to sublux the head anteriorly and posteriorly. In general, this test works better with thinner patients and requires a fair amount of patient relaxation.

DIFFERENTIAL DIAGNOSIS

- Diagnoses that can mimic anterior instability include multidirectional instability, acromioclavicular instability, superior labrum anterior and posterior (SLAP) lesions, biceps tendon subluxation, and subscapularis tear.
- One should always rule out referred pain from the cervical spine.

DIAGNOSTIC TESTS & INTERPRETATION

- Imaging studies should include orthogonal views to rule out associated bony injuries and to ensure that the humeral head is located within glenoid.
- Radiography: The initial series includes an anteroposterior (AP), true shoulder AP, axillary lateral, and scapular Y. Additional views, if necessary, may include the West Point view (good for identifying a bony Bankart/anteroinferior glenoid rim fracture) and Stryker notch view (good for identifying a Hill-Sachs lesion/posterolateral humeral head compression fracture).
- Velpeau view (if required to stay in sling) if initial radiographs are inconclusive or patient is unable to be appropriately positioned for axillary radiograph
- Postreduction views are necessary for the acute treatment of a shoulder dislocation to ensure relocation and assess for possibility of a fracture.
- Magnetic resonance imaging (MRI) can identify rotator cuff tears, biceps abnormalities, and occasionally lesions associated with humeral avulsion of the GH ligament. Because of the normal variation of the labrum and GH ligaments, most studies overestimate the frequency of labral tears. Use of arthrogram with MRI increases sensitivity and specificity in evaluation of labral tears.

TREATMENT

GENERAL MEASURES

- Nonoperative management in young, active patients is associated with a high incidence of recurrent instability but can be considered in older/low-demand patients or in-season athletes waiting for surgical evaluation after completion of their season. Motion control braces can limit abduction and external rotation and decrease the position of vulnerability for instability events (1,2,3)[C].
- Early treatment consists of brief immobilization, followed by early protected range of motion (ROM) and strengthening. The anterior capsular structures must be protected throughout rehabilitation, and therefore, all stressors to the anterior structures should be limited.
- Rotator cuff strengthening: Initial strengthening should begin in the plane of the scapula. Internal and limited-range external rotation exercises can start with light free weights or TheraBand.
- Scapular stabilization: Exercises include rowing, modified push-ups with maximal protraction, scaption (elevation of the humerus in external rotation in the scapular plane), modified flies, and press-ups (later stage).

SURGERY/OTHER PROCEDURES

- Indications for surgery: rotator cuff tear >50%, Hill-Sachs lesion >25%, glenoid defect >20%, failure to return to activities after nonoperative therapy (2,3)[C]
- Relative indications for surgery: first-time dislocations in young (<30 yr) athletes or laborers, >2 dislocations in one season, participation in overhead or contact sports, bony Bankart lesion, significant glenoid bone loss (2,3)[C]
- Surgical techniques for the management of anterior shoulder instability are evolving. Both soft tissue (arthroscopic or open Bankart repair) and bone augmentation (Latarjet) procedures exist. Multiple factors will be considered when deciding on which surgical procedure to perform: possible pathology of labrum or rotator cuff, extent of bony Bankart of the glenoid or Hill-Sachs injury of the humeral head, and desired postsurgical activities (1,2,3)[C].
- Decreasing risk of recurrent instability while maximizing ROM is the ultimate goal of surgical stabilization (1,2,3)[C].

ONGOING CARE

FOLLOW-UP RECOMMENDATIONS

- Any patient with recurrent anterior dislocations or a young, athletic, first-time dislocator should discuss surgical options with a qualified sports medicine physician.
- Any patient failing nonoperative modalities also should be referred for surgical evaluation.

REFERENCES

1. Carpinteiro EP, Barros AA. Natural history of anterior shoulder instability. *Open Orthop J*. 2017;11:909–918.
2. Elsenbeck MJ, Dickens JF. Return to sports after shoulder stabilization surgery for anterior shoulder instability. *Curr Rev Musculoskelet Med*. 2017;10(4):491–498.
3. Pickett A, Svoboda S. Anterior glenohumeral instability. *Sports Med Arthrosc Rev*. 2017;25(3):156–162.

ADDITIONAL READING

- Bankart AS. Recurrent or habitual dislocation of the shoulder-joint. *Br Med J*. 1923;2(3285):1132–1133.
- Bedi A, Ryu RK. The treatment of primary anterior shoulder dislocations. *Instr Course Lect*. 2009;58:293–304.
- Cave EF, Burke JF, Boyd RJ. *Trauma Management*. Chicago, IL: Year Book Medical; 1974.
- Iannotti JP, Williams GR. *Disorders of the Shoulder: Diagnosis and Management*. Philadelphia, PA: Lippincott Williams & Wilkins; 1999.
- Jobe FW, Pink MM. *Operative Techniques in Upper Extremity Sports Injury*. St. Louis, MO: Mosby; 1996.
- Kazár B, Relovszky E. Prognosis of primary dislocation of the shoulder. *Acta Orthop Scand*. 1969;40(2):216–224.
- Ludewig PM, Reynolds JF. The association of scapular kinematics and glenohumeral joint pathologies. *J Orthop Sports Phys Ther*. 2009;39(2):90–104.
- Neviaser RJ, Neviaser TJ, Neviaser JS. Anterior dislocation of the shoulder and rotator cuff rupture. *Clin Orthop Relat Res*. 1993;(291):103–106.
- Ochoa E Jr, Burkhart SS. Glenohumeral bone defects in the treatment of anterior shoulder instability. *Instr Course Lect*. 2009;58:323–336.
- Rowe CR, Patel D, Southmayd WW. The Bankart procedure: a long-term end-result study. *J Bone Joint Surg Am*. 1978;60(1):1–16.

CLINICAL PEARLS

- Young athletes, particularly those participating in overhead or contact sports, continue to be at increased risk of anterior shoulder instability.
- Recurrent instability is common after the initial episode.
- Primary surgical stabilization should be considered after the first dislocation in the young athlete in a high-risk activity/sport.

S

SHOULDER INSTABILITY, MULTIDIRECTIONAL

David E.J. Bazzo, MD, FAAFP, CAQSM • Tara Robbins, MD

BASICS

DESCRIPTION

- Multidirectional instability (MDI) is an increase in glenohumeral translation in more than one direction causing either subluxation (any partial loss of normal articulation) or dislocation (a complete loss of glenohumeral articulation) in more than one direction, such as anterior, inferior, and posterior but rarely superior.
- The extent of laxity can be described objectively by the measured amount in millimeters of which the humeral head can be translated on the glenoid. Some individuals may be symptomatic with minimal millimeters of laxity, whereas others may have minimal symptoms with significant (3+) laxity.
- Hallmark pathology of MDI is a large, patulous inferior capsule, although this is not always the case.

EPIDEMIOLOGY

- MDI is much more common than previously realized but still represents <5% of all shoulder instability.
- Most patients are in their 3rd decade of life but range in age from teenagers to middle age.

ETIOLOGY AND PATHOPHYSIOLOGY

Etiology is thought to be multifactorial, with current theories focusing on anatomic, biochemical, and neuromuscular abnormalities:

- Anatomic:
  - Patients with MDI have been shown to have a large, patulous inferior pouch and wide rotator interval that are both common manifestations of inferior instability.
  - Pathologic changes in labral height and Bankart lesions also are observed in patients with MDI (1).
- Biochemical:
  - Patients with MDI have been shown to have alterations in the type and quantity of collagen, specifically types III and IV collagen, as seen in Ehlers-Danlos syndrome (1).
- Neuromuscular:
  - Loss of strength or neuromotor coordination of rotator cuff and scapular stabilizing muscles also contributes to MDI.
  - Recent studies have shown that when compared with controls, patients with MDI have altered functioning of the musculature of the shoulder girdle and the dynamic stabilizers of the glenohumeral joint during movement.
  - Loss of proprioception also can contribute to MDI because proprioceptive feedback is important in maintaining stability.
  - It still needs to be elucidated whether the proprioceptive defect is a cause or effect of the instability (1).

RISK FACTORS

- Repetitive microtrauma (especially overhead motion): butterfly and backstroke swimmers, gymnasts, baseball pitchers, weight lifters, and racquet sports
- Generalized ligamentous hyperlaxity

DIAGNOSIS

HISTORY

- MDI is associated with recurrent or "low-energy" trauma.
- Unilateral versus bilateral shoulder problems: 30–70% of patients with MDI have symptoms in the opposite shoulder as well.
- MDI of the humeral head reduces spontaneously or is self-reduced.
- Previously unsuccessful shoulder reconstruction for presumed unidirectional instability may indicate MDI.
- Most common complaint is vague pain radiating to the deltoid insertion, initially occurring after activity and progressing to pain at rest, and in late stages, patients may develop night pain.
- Transient neurologic symptoms, such as numbness ("dead arm") or tingling owing to transient subluxation, usually affecting ulnar > median nerve distribution
- Inferior instability: pain, numbness, tingling while carrying a briefcase or heavy suitcase; this is caused by traction on the brachial plexus.
- Posterior instability: pain while arm in forward-flexed, internally rotated position (e.g., pushing open a heavy door, performing push-ups or bench press, blocking in football, or during pull-through phase of rowing stroke)
- Anterior instability: pain with arm in overhead, abducted, externally rotated position (e.g., during windup or early acceleration of a throw)

PHYSICAL EXAM

- Often, general ligamentous laxity is present (e.g., thumb to forearm); elbow hyperextension, metacarpophalangeal joint hyperextension, genu recurvatum, patellofemoral subluxation (40–75%)
- Sulcus test involves inferior traction on the arm while at the side. Inferior translation of at least 1 to 2 cm causing concavity of skin inferior to acromion (positive sulcus sign) indicates inferior instability.
- Anterior and posterior load and shift test and/or drawer test usually result in anterior and posterior displacement (graded trace to III). Always remember to stabilize the scapula with one hand while the patient remains in either a seated or supine position.
- Apprehension test involves placing the shoulder in the position of instability (throwing position: abduction and external rotation for anterior instability; adduction, flexion, and internal rotation for posterior instability). A positive test is seen when the patient senses pending subluxation or has involuntary guarding. It is apprehension, not pain, which is most reliable in confirming shoulder instability.
- Relocation test involves relief of apprehension and symptoms when applying a stabilizing counterforce (posterior force on humeral head for anterior instability; anterior force on humeral head for posterior instability) to the arm in the provocative position with the scapula stabilized.
- Cervical range of motion, upper extremity strength, sensory function (including axillary nerve), and reflexes also should be evaluated.
- Muscle guarding may make the examination difficult, and repeat exams may be necessary for confirmation of diagnosis.

DIFFERENTIAL DIAGNOSIS

- Unilateral instability (anterior, posterior, inferior)
- Acute dislocation or subluxation
- Voluntary dislocator
- Primary impingement
- Thoracic outlet syndrome
- Cervical disc disease
- Brachial plexitis
- Connective tissue disorder (i.e., Ehlers-Danlos syndrome)

DIAGNOSTIC TESTS & INTERPRETATION

- MDI is a clinical diagnosis based on the history and physical exam; orthogonal plain radiographs should be obtained to evaluate for bony defects such as Bankart and Hill-Sachs lesions as well as glenoid dysplasia.
- Stryker notch: patient supine, cassette under shoulder, arm flexed, palm to head, elbow pointing straight upward, beam 10 degrees cranially centered over coracoid; reported to show defect in 90% of 20 patients studied
- Axillary view: clear delineation of glenoid-humerus relationship; evaluation of anteroposterior displacement of humeral head on glenoid and Hill-Sachs lesions as well as larger glenoid rim and humeral head compression fractures
- West Point view (reverse axillary lateral): patient placed prone on table, involved shoulder placed on raised (8 cm) pad, head and neck rotated away, cassette against superior aspect of shoulder, beam centered at axilla with 25 degrees down/25 degrees medial angulation; allows view of anteroinferior glenoid rim; this view is usually used for traumatic anterior dislocations.
- More sophisticated imagery is now accepted as routine preoperatively or for persistent symptoms. Most shoulder surgeons prefer a magnetic resonance imaging (MRI) arthrogram to help detect capsular redundancy, but MRI remains more useful in ruling out other pathology.

TREATMENT

GENERAL MEASURES

- Analgesia: Nonsteroidal anti-inflammatory drugs (NSAIDs) can decrease pain acutely, but long-term analgesic usage typically is not necessary.
- Reduction: typically, reduce spontaneously or self-reduce
- Immobilization:
  - May consider short-term immobilizing with a sling for up to 3 wk in younger patients (<30 yr of age) with an acute, initial dislocation. There has not been a well-demonstrated association between length of immobilization and recurrence.
  - Immobilization for recurrent dislocators is of less value.
  - Use caution in immobilizing older patients who are more likely to develop adhesive capsulitis.

ADDITIONAL THERAPIES

- First-line treatment is prolonged course of physical therapy/independent exercise program with emphasis on strengthening anterior deltoid and rotator cuff muscles for at least 6 mo and probably up to 1 yr. Symptomatic relief is gradual:
  - Traditionally two phases have been suggested: Phase I focuses on strengthening the anterior deltoid and rotator cuff muscles and usually lasts 6 to 12 wk. Phase II focuses on continuing to strengthen deltoid and rotator cuff muscles with the addition of strengthening scapular stabilizers and improving proprioception (1)[B].
  - Proprioceptive and plyometric training aimed at rehabilitating the sensorimotor system in recurrent instability has been reported more recently (2)[B].
  - Watson program is a six-stage program lasting 3 to 6 mo. It focuses on developing scapula and humeral head control prior to progression of exercises into increasing range of motion (arc of motion from 0 to 40 degrees abduction initially with progression to 90 degrees abduction) and is completed with functional and sports-specific exercises (3,4)[B].
  - Most patients will begin to improve within 3 mo of physical therapy (5)[B].
- It is important to continue a maintenance exercise program indefinitely.
- If patient is pain free with normal strength after 6 mo, prior activity may be resumed.
- May need to change prior activity (i.e., a butterfly stroke swimmer may need to choose a different stroke, or a pitcher may need to change his or her delivery or position)

SURGERY/OTHER PROCEDURES

- Surgery is indicated only for symptomatic, painful shoulders after the patient fails aggressive, prolonged physical therapy (usually minimum 6 mo) (1)[C].
- MDI is managed differently than management after unilateral anterior shoulder dislocation because the etiology may be related to a connective tissue disorder more often than injury.
- ~10–13% of patients require bilateral surgical repair.
- Laxity alone is not a typical indication for surgery.
- Some authorities advocate earlier surgery if there is a documented glenohumeral ligament avulsion on MRI arthrogram.
- Neer et al. described the open inferior capsular shift repair technique with good success in 1974, and it continues to be a reasonable choice of surgical interventions for MDI.
- Several arthroscopic approaches have been described, including transglenoid capsular shift and capsular plication with bone anchors and adjunctive thermal capsulorrhaphy and/or rotator interval closure. The arthroscopic techniques produce clinical results equivalent or superior to open techniques. Arthroscopic treatment results in less surgical time and presumed less morbidity (1)[B].
- Arthroscopic pancapsular capsulorrhaphy (APC) with suture anchors has been shown to result in improved function, low complication, and low revision rates (6)[B].
- Thermal capsulorrhaphy (capsular shrinkage through laser or radiofrequency energy) has been used to treat shoulder instability for centuries; however, clinical studies have not shown favorable results. In isolated thermal capsulorrhaphy, a high failure rate and complications of glenohumeral chondrolysis and axillary nerve injuries have been reported. However, thermal capsulorrhaphy may be useful as adjunctive therapy (5)[B].
- Note: Probably the earliest "sports surgery" was thermal capsulorrhaphy for anterior instability in ancient Egypt, where warriors with instability were treated with a hot poker to thermally shrink anterior structures to try to allow them to throw a spear.

ONGOING CARE

FOLLOW-UP RECOMMENDATIONS

- Most patients with MDI should be referred for physical therapy. Patients who fail physical therapy can be referred to an orthopedist for consideration of surgical treatment.
- Resumption of full sports generally is 6 mo. If surgery is required, then postoperative immobilization with a sling is typically for 3 to 6 wk, with early supervised range of motion exercises. Light sports and throwing can start at ~4 mo postoperatively if strength is at least 90% and full range of motion is achieved.

REFERENCES

1. Bahu MJ, Trentacosta N, Vorys GC, et al. Multidirectional instability: evaluation and treatment options. *Clin Sports Med*. 2008;27(4):671–689.
2. Bateman M, Smith BE, Osborne SE, et al. Physiotherapy treatment for atraumatic recurrent shoulder instability: early results of a specific exercise protocol using pathology-specific outcome measures. *Shoulder Elbow*. 2015;7(4):282–288.
3. Watson L, Warby S, Balster S, et al. The treatment of multidirectional instability of the shoulder with a rehabilitation program: part 1. *Shoulder Elbow*. 2016;8(4):271–278.
4. Watson L, Warby S, Balster S, et al. The treatment of multidirectional instability of the shoulder with a rehabilitation programme: part 2. *Shoulder Elbow*. 2017;9(1):46–53.
5. Miniaci A, Codsi MJ. Thermal capsulorrhaphy for the treatment of shoulder instability. *Am J Sports Med*. 2006;34(8):1356–1363.
6. Raynor MB, Horan MP, Greenspoon JA, et al. Outcomes after arthroscopic pancapsular capsulorrhaphy with suture anchors for the treatment of multidirectional glenohumeral instability in athletes. *Am J Sports Med*. 2016;44(12):3188–3197.

ADDITIONAL READING

- Caprise PA Jr, Sekiya JK. Open and arthroscopic treatment of multidirectional instability of the shoulder. *Arthroscopy*. 2006;22(10):1126–1131.
- Foster CR. Multidirectional instability of the shoulder in the athlete. *Clin Sports Med*. 1983;2(2):355–368.
- Mahaffey BL, Smith PA. Shoulder instability in young athletes. *Am Fam Physician*. 1999;59(10):2773–2782.
- Misamore GW, Sallay PI, Didelot W. A longitudinal study of patients with multidirectional instability of the shoulder with seven- to ten-year follow-up. *J Shoulder Elbow Surg*. 2005;14(5):466–470.
- Schenk TJ, Brems JJ. Multidirectional instability of the shoulder: pathophysiology, diagnosis, and management. *J Am Acad Orthop Surg*. 1998;6(1):65–72.
- Yamaguchi K, Flatow EL. Management of multidirectional instability. *Clin Sports Med*. 1995;14(4):885–902.

CLINICAL PEARLS

- First-line treatment is prolonged course of physical therapy/independent exercise program with emphasis on strengthening anterior deltoid and rotator cuff muscles for at least 6 mo and probably up to 1 yr. Symptomatic relief is gradual.
- Surgery is indicated only for symptomatic, painful shoulders after the patient fails aggressive, prolonged physical therapy (usually minimum 6 mo).

SINDING-LARSEN-JOHANSSON SYNDROME

Ian D. McKeag, MD, MS • Christopher P. Lake, MD • Timothy Ryan Draper, DO, ABFM, CAQSM

BASICS

DESCRIPTION

- Sinding-Larsen-Johansson Syndrome (SLJ) is a condition considered to be a chronic overuse injury caused by excessive and repetitive traction applied to the patella by the patellar tendon (i.e., jumping). Forces exerted gradually avulse the inferior pole of the patella at the apophysis:
  - Pain and swelling at the lower pole of the patella
  - Ossicle formation or fragmentation of inferior patellar pole on radiographs
- System: musculoskeletal
- Synonym: patellar apophysitis

EPIDEMIOLOGY

Incidence

Child and adolescent boys and girls with increased rate with those participating in organized sports

Prevalence

- A relatively common cause of anterior knee pain in adolescents (1)[B]
- Cause of nearly 10% of all anterior knee pain in high school–aged females; only 3% in middle school (2)[B]

ETIOLOGY AND PATHOPHYSIOLOGY

- Traction apophysitis with reactive calcification of the partially avulsed proximal patellar tendon
- Etiology unknown. Most common understanding of inciting factor is repetitive microtrauma.
- 4-fold increased risk in athletes with early sports specialization (1)[B]

Genetics

None

RISK FACTORS

- Early sports specialization (1)[B]
- Participation in jumping and kneeling sports (volleyball, basketball) (2)[B]
- Shortened/tight hamstring tendons; increased posterior tibial slope (3)[C]

GENERAL PREVENTION

- Avoid sports specialization (1)[B].
- Avoid high intensity and repetitive quadriceps loading.
- Preseason muscular and flexibility training to help avoid sudden increases in training load

COMMONLY ASSOCIATED CONDITIONS

- Osgood-Schlatter disease
- Spastic lower extremities (cerebral palsy)

DIAGNOSIS

HISTORY

- Gradual and progressive pain at the inferior pole of the patella
- Pain exacerbated with kneeling and exercise, especially with jumping activities

PHYSICAL EXAM

- Tenderness to palpation at the inferior pole of the patella
- Swelling at inferior patellar pole and the absence of a knee effusion
- Worsening pain with knee loading and/or prolonged knee flexion of the effected knee
- Erythema may be present at inferior patellar pole.
- Functional testing: Single-leg squat and knee extension against resistance may reproduce pain.

DIFFERENTIAL DIAGNOSIS

- Patellofemoral pain syndrome
- Patellar tendinitis
- Chondromalacia patellae
- Patellar sleeve fracture
- Osgood-Schlatter disease
- Infrapatellar bursitis
- Superficial patellar bursitis
- Osteochondroma
- Tibial fracture
- Patellar tendon lipoma

DIAGNOSTIC TESTS & INTERPRETATION

Initial Tests (lab, imaging)

- Diagnosis can be made clinically and imaging is not always necessary.
- Plain radiographs: fragmentation and/or irregular calcification of the ossification centers and calcification of the inferior pole of the patella
- Ultrasound: fragmentation of the inferior patellar pole, insertional patellar tendon thickening, and infrapatellar bursitis

Follow-Up Tests & Special Considerations

- Ultrasound can be considered for monitoring.
- Follow-up x-rays are typically unnecessary.

TREATMENT

GENERAL MEASURES

- Nearly all cases can be treated nonoperatively with conservative management and rest.
- Avoidance of aggravating activities, such as running, kneeling, squatting, jumping, and stair climbing

MEDICATION

First Line

- Relative rest and activity modification, typically for 2 to 3 days
- Compressive knee sleeve or tension band
- Stretches
- Ice
- Nonsteroidal anti-inflammatory drugs (NSAIDs)

ISSUES FOR REFERRAL

- Chronic pain
- Acute muscle weakness or atrophy
- Acute knee pain with inability to extend knee

ADDITIONAL THERAPIES

- Physical therapy for core strengthening, specifically with the quadriceps and hip flexors
- Stretching exercises, with ideal focus on the hamstrings (3)[C]

SURGERY/OTHER PROCEDURES

- For chronic pain and recurrence despite conservative measures, surgical intervention can be considered (4)[C].
- Necrotic area may be present in portion of patellar tendon, in which excision has been reported to be clinically successful in treatment (4)[C].

COMPLEMENTARY & ALTERNATIVE MEDICINE

- Very brief knee immobilization for the most severe cases (rare)
- Patellar banding with activity

ADMISSION, INPATIENT, AND NURSING CONSIDERATIONS

No urgent admission and inpatient treatment is needed for this condition.

ONGOING CARE

FOLLOW-UP RECOMMENDATIONS

- Continue with core strengthening exercises.
- Proper quadriceps and hamstring stretching and warm up prior to activity or competition

Patient Monitoring

Monitor for any recurrent signs of anterior knee pain after resuming activity.

PATIENT EDUCATION

Sports specialization in one sport has been found to be associated with increased risk of developing this condition, especially in adolescent females, compared to multisport athletes.

PROGNOSIS

- Spontaneous resolution typically occurs within 12 to 18 mo (5)[C].
- Complete resolution closely associated with skeletal maturity, patellar ossification, and apophyseal closure (5)[C]

COMPLICATIONS

In some instances, surgery is required if the skeletally mature ossicles become painful.

REFERENCES

1. Hall R, Barber Foss K, Hewett TE, et al. Sports specialization's association with an increased risk of developing anterior knee pain in adolescent female athletes. *J Sport Rehabil*. 2015;24(1):31–35.
2. Barber Foss KD, Myer GD, Hewett TE. Epidemiology of basketball, soccer, and volleyball injuries in middle-school female athletes. *Phys Sportsmed*. 2014;42(2):146–153.
3. Patel DR, Villalobos A. Evaluation and management of knee pain in young athletes: overuse injuries of the knee. *Transl Pediatr*. 2017;6(3):190–198.
4. Kajetanek C, Thaunat T, Guimaraes T, et al. Arthroscopic treatment of painful Sinding-Larsen-Johansson syndrome in a professional handball player. *Orthop Traumatol Surg Res*. 2016;102(5):677–680.
5. Valentino M, Quiligotti C, Ruggirello M. Sinding-Larsen-Johansson syndrome: a case report. *J Ultrasound*. 2012;15(2):127–129.

ADDITIONAL READING

- Draghi F, Danesino GM, Coscia D, et al. Overload syndromes of the knee in adolescents: sonographic findings. *J Ultrasound*. 2008;11(4):151–157.
- Duri ZA, Patel DV, Aichroth PM. The immature athlete. *Clin Sports Med*. 2002;21(3):461–482.

CLINICAL PEARLS

- Common cause of anterior knee pain without effusion in children/adolescents
- Diagnosis is typically made clinically, and imaging is not always necessary.
- Conservative measures, including relative rest, NSAIDs, physical therapy, and stretching, tend to resolve most cases of this condition.

SINUS TARSI SYNDROME

Timothy Dekker, MD • Krishna Israni, MD, MS, BS • George G.A. Pujalte, MD, FACSM

BASICS

Sinus tarsi syndrome is persistent, anterolateral ankle pain, often associated with previous ankle injury (1).

DESCRIPTION

- Sinus tarsi is the lateral extension of the tarsal canal formed by the sulcus of the talus and calcaneus (2).
- Within the sinus tarsi are the talocalcaneal interosseous ligament; cervical ligament; the subtalar joint capsule; synovium; and the medial, intermediate, and lateral roots of the inferior extensor retinaculum (2):
  - Talocalcaneal interosseous ligament is involved in movements of the subtalar joint (2). It functions to maintain apposition of the talus and calcaneus in all positions (2). Its rich innervation suggests that the sinus tarsi may be susceptible to neurogenic inflammation and may be a center of articular nociception (2).

EPIDEMIOLOGY

- Patients with sinus tarsi syndrome are usually between their 3rd and 4th decades of life (3).
- Often associated with dancers, volleyball players, basketball players, overweight individuals, and patients with foot deformities, usually flexible flat feet (4)

ETIOLOGY AND PATHOPHYSIOLOGY

- Soft tissue inversion injuries of the ankle most commonly involve the ligamentous structures of the lateral aspect of the ankle and sinus tarsi (5).
- Posttraumatic fibrotic changes in the wall and surrounding tissue of veins, causing disturbance of venous outflow and increased intrasinusal pressure, may be a factor in the pathogenesis of sinus tarsi syndrome (6).
- Sinus tarsi is not only a talocalcaneal joint space with interosseous ligaments but also a source of nociceptive and proprioceptive information on the movements of the foot and ankle (2).
- Sinus tarsi syndrome may result from disorders of nociception and proprioception of the foot (2).

RISK FACTORS

Forefoot and calcaneal valgus, mechanical factors predisposing to supination ankle injuries, may lead to sinus tarsi syndrome after such injuries (7). In the majority of cases, the lateral ankle pain follows a history of an inversion ankle sprain (6).

COMMONLY ASSOCIATED CONDITIONS

- 70% of cases are posttraumatic.
- 30% can be attributed to causes including systemic disease, structural abnormalities, and soft tissue masses, such as ganglions (8).

DIAGNOSIS

Four clinical characteristics have been used to describe and diagnose the syndrome (3)[A]:

- Pain at the lateral opening of the sinus tarsi, increasing with pressure, usually ceasing at rest
- Perception of instability of the rear foot on uneven ground
- Marked reduction of pain and discomfort following an injection of local anesthetic into the sinus tarsi
- Clinical and stress radiographic examination showing no or minimal instability

HISTORY

- Deep aching, throbbing, or sharp pain within the sinus tarsi may be associated with a sense of rear foot instability. Pain over the lateral part of the ankle and hindfoot, over the sinus tarsi, is often the primary complaint, but because the synovitis and the associated fibrotic tissues take time to develop, athletes with injuries to the subtalar joint may not initially have symptoms that are localized to the sinus tarsi (1). A previous sprain or other injury is often the inciting event:
  - Initial injury may have responded to conservative therapies, but recurrent pain or pain settling into the sinus tarsi may be experienced with activities of daily living.
- Can result in severe pain and instability of the ankle and the subtalar joints, particularly in athletes (5)
- Pain and paresthesia may also be felt over the dorsolateral aspect of the foot (9). Intermittent pain often radiates into the leg, with resulting paresthesia over the distal aspect of the foot (9). Swelling may and may not be present.
- Patients most often complain of "ankle" pain, when in reality, the pain is emanating from the subtalar area. When asked to identify the site of maximal tenderness, patients often point directly to the sinus tarsi region.
- Pain may involve the anterior and lateral ankle, although this pain is less intense.
- The perception of ankle symptoms may be secondary to previous trauma, referred pain, or an altered gait in an attempt to reduce pain.

PHYSICAL EXAM

- Diagnosis is often clinical; tenderness over the sinus tarsi often leads to the diagnosis of sinus tarsi syndrome.
- Pain over the sinus tarsi at the end range of ankle plantar flexion with foot supination is typical (1).
- Discomfort usually worsens with pressure over the lateral opening of the sinus tarsi, becoming more severe with the foot in varus position (6).
- Symptoms are usually alleviated when the foot is immobilized in a valgus position (6).
- Injury to the ligaments may result in laxity of the joints of the ankle complex; neuromuscular deficits are also likely to occur due to the injury to the nervous and musculotendinous tissue (10).
- Neuromuscular deficits may be manifested as impaired balance, reduced joint position sense, slower firing of the peroneal muscles on inversion, slowed nerve conduction velocity, impaired cutaneous sensation, strength deficits, and decreased dorsiflexion range of motion (10).
- Assessment of patients with lateral ankle sprain must address not only joint laxity and swelling but also should include examination for neuromuscular deficits (2).

DIFFERENTIAL DIAGNOSIS

- Peripheral mononeuropathies
- Radiculopathy
- Lateral ankle sprain
- Anterolateral soft tissue impingement
- Bifurcate ligament injury
- Stress fractures of the cuboid, talus, or calcaneus (11)

DIAGNOSTIC TESTS & INTERPRETATION

Initial Tests (lab, imaging)

- Radiologic examination usually will not reveal a bone lesion or any insufficiency of the ankle ligaments, and dynamically, there is usually no restriction of talocalcaneonavicular joint range of motion (6).
- Magnetic resonance imaging (MRI), with or without arthrography, can lead to better definition of abnormalities in the sinus tarsi and tarsal canal (8).
- Single photon emission computed tomography/computed tomography (SPECT/CT) can be used in those with contraindication to MRI. It is found to have sensitivity and specificity of 95% and 83%, respectively (12).

Diagnostic Procedures/Other

- Pain and functional instability in the region have been found to be reduced for a few hours after the injection of a local anesthetic into the opening of the sinus tarsi (7).
- A reduction in electrical activity or complete electrical silence of both the peroneus brevis and longus muscles have been noted on electromyographic studies (2).

TREATMENT

- Relative rest, avoidance of aggravating activities, and use of nonsteroidal anti-inflammatory drugs (NSAIDs) as needed for pain may give temporary relief.
- Orthotics may be used to address forefoot valgus and calcaneal valgus, mechanical factors predisposing to supination ankle sprains (7)[B].
- Conservative treatment includes corticosteroid injections, immobilization in a cast, application of local anti-inflammatory gels or local irritants such as capsaicin, and systemic drugs aimed at reducing neuralgic pain.
- When there is ankle instability or feeling of giving way, physical therapy should be tried first. Physical therapy should include balance and proprioceptive (13)[B].
- Other methods such as mobilization, friction massage and deep massage using ultrasound, soft laser, transcutaneous electrical stimulation, or any other method of deep massage
- Athletic training footwear is also a consideration, and recommendation includes those with a straight last, a firm heel counter, and rigid material through the midsole (13)[B].
- Corticosteroid injections mixed with local anesthetics have been shown to be effective (12)[A].
- Conservative treatment has been shown to be effective in up to 2/3 of patients (3)[A]. There seem to be no clear studies that delineate the length of time conservative measures should be tried, and the determination appears to be on a case-to-case basis for the most part, although, in our practice, a time frame of 4 to 6 wk is the most commonly used length of time for any conservative treatment chosen and applied to sinus tarsi syndrome.

MEDICATION

- A local anesthetic injection may be given as initial treatment for the pain of sinus tarsi syndrome; may also be diagnostic (5)[B]
- A mixed local anesthetic and corticosteroid injection may also be given as treatment for the pain of sinus tarsi syndrome, with 5 to 6 injections at weekly intervals usually sufficient (3,5)[B].

ISSUES FOR REFERRAL

Referral to orthopedic surgery may be appropriate after failure of conservative measures (5)[B].

SURGERY/OTHER PROCEDURES

Surgical treatment of sinus tarsi syndrome may involve excision of the lateral half of the sinus tarsi contents, followed by below-knee casting for 3 wk and physical therapy (5)[B].

ONGOING CARE

FOLLOW-UP RECOMMENDATIONS

Postoperatively, patients may be immobilized with a walking caliper for around 4 wk, then made to undergo physical therapy, usually for another 4 to 6 wk (3)[A].

PROGNOSIS

- 2/3 of sinus tarsi syndrome cases respond to conservative treatment.
- In the remaining 1/3 of cases, surgical intervention has been shown to cure or improve 90% of patients (3).
- A 15-yr retrospective study on conservative treatment of sinus tarsi syndrome showed that most of these patients eventually required surgical intervention after nonoperative treatment failed to alleviate their symptoms, whereupon long-term follow-up revealed relief from pain after surgery (14).

COMPLICATIONS

- Sinus tarsi syndrome responds well to therapeutic interventions, often mixed local anesthetic and corticosteroid injections (12).
- Should surgery be required, there are usually few postoperative complications (1,15).
- The most common reported complication from surgical intervention is a transient neurapraxia involving branches of the superficial peroneal nerve (16).

REFERENCES

1. Helgeson K. Examination and intervention for sinus tarsi syndrome. *N Am J Sports Phys Ther*. 2009;4(1):29–37.
2. Akiyama K, Takakura Y, Tomita Y, et al. Neurohistology of the sinus tarsi and sinus tarsi syndrome. *J Orthop Sci*. 1999;4(4):299–303.
3. Taillard W, Meyer JM, Garcia J, et al. The sinus tarsi syndrome. *Int Orthop*. 1981;5(2):117–130.
4. Herrmann M, Pieper KS. Sinus tarsi syndrome: what hurts? [in German]. *Unfallchirurg*. 2008; 111(2):132–136.
5. Mabit C, Boncoeur-Martel MP, Chaudruc JM, et al. Anatomic and MRI study of the subtalar ligamentous support. *Surg Radiol Anat*. 1997;19(2):111–117.
6. Schwarzenbach B, Dora C, Lang A, et al. Blood vessels of the sinus tarsi and the sinus tarsi syndrome. *Clin Anat*. 1997;10(3):173–182.
7. Duddy RK, Duggan RJ, Visser HJ, et al. Diagnosis, treatment, and rehabilitation of injuries to the lower leg and foot. *Clin Sports Med*. 1989;8(4):861–876.
8. Dozier TJ, Figueroa RT, Kalmar J. Sinus tarsi syndrome. *J La State Med Soc*. 2001;153(9):458–461.
9. Giorgini RJ, Bernard RL. Sinus tarsi syndrome in a patient with talipes equinovarus. *J Am Podiatr Med Assoc*. 1990;80(4):218–222.
10. Rab M, Ebmer J, Dellon AL. Innervation of the sinus tarsi and implications for treating anterolateral ankle pain. *Ann Plast Surg*. 2001;47(5):500–504.
11. Shear MS, Baitch SP, Shear DB. Sinus tarsi syndrome: the importance of biomechanically-based evaluation and treatment. *Arch Phys Med Rehabil*. 1993;74(7):777–781.
12. Zwipp H, Swoboda B, Holch M, et al. Sinus tarsi and canalis tarsi syndromes. A post-traumatic entity [in German]. *Unfallchirurg*. 1991;94(12): 608–613.
13. Yamashita MH. Evaluation and selection of shoe wear and orthoses for the runner. *Phys Med Rehabil Clin N Am*. 2005;16(3):801–829.
14. Kuwada GT. Long-term retrospective analysis of the treatment of sinus tarsi syndrome. *J Foot Ankle Surg*. 1994;33(1):28–29.
15. Oloff LM, Schulhofer SD, Bocko AP. Subtalar joint arthroscopy for sinus tarsi syndrome: a review of 29 cases. *J Foot Ankle Surg*. 2001;40(3):152–157.
16. Frey C, Feder KS, DiGiovanni C. Arthroscopic evaluation of the subtalar joint: does sinus tarsi syndrome exist? *Foot Ankle Int*. 1999;20(3):185–191.

S

ADDITIONAL READING

- Mann R, Coughlin MJ. Athletic injuries to the soft tissues of the foot and ankle. In: Mann RA, ed. *Surgery of the Foot and Ankle*. 6th ed. St. Louis, MO: Mosby; 1993:1165–1166.
- Schnirring-Judge M, Perlman M. Chronic ankle conditions. In: Banks AS, Downey MS, Martin DE, et al, eds. *McGlamry's Comprehensive Textbook of Foot and Ankle Surgery*. Vol 1. 3rd ed. Philadelphia, PA: Lippincott Williams & Wilkins; 2001:1091–1092.

CLINICAL PEARLS

- Sinus tarsi syndrome is persistent, anterolateral ankle pain, often associated with previous ankle injury, most common in individuals aged 20 to 40 yr; previous ankle inversion injury; and forefoot deformities making them more prone to pronation.
- Diagnostic requirements include pain at the lateral opening of the sinus tarsi, perception of instability, relief following an injection of local anesthetic into the sinus tarsi, and clinical and stress radiographic examination showing no or minimal instability.
- Imaging does not usually reveal an injury to the bone or soft tissue of the sinus tarsi but may help show abnormalities in the anatomy of the sinus tarsi leading them to have sinus tarsi syndrome.
- Conservative therapy is first-line treatment and includes relative rest, orthotics, NSAIDs, and corticosteroid injections, followed by physical therapy to improve instability.
- Referral to an orthopedic surgeon is reasonable if conservative therapy fails, occurs in up to 1/3 of patients.

SLAP TEARS

Marjorie Delo, MD, CAQSM, RMSK

BASICS

DESCRIPTION

- Superior labrum anterior-to-posterior (SLAP) tears are a type of tear of the fibrocartilaginous glenoid labrum.
- The glenoid labrum deepens the bony socket providing stability to the glenohumeral joint as well as serving as an attachment site for glenohumeral ligaments and the long head of the biceps tendon (LHBT).
- The LHBT attaches to the superior aspect of the labrum and the supraglenoid tubercle.
- SLAP tears involve the superior labrum biceps tendon complex.
- The most common cause of SLAP tears is sports injury.

ETIOLOGY AND PATHOPHYSIOLOGY

The majority of SLAP tears are likely multifactorial. Etiologies include:

- Traction during the deceleration phase of throwing.
- Posteroinferior capsular contractures increasing shear forces on the LHBT.
- Torsional forces through the "peel-back" mechanism of the biceps insertion on the superior labrum during the cocking phase.
- Labral degeneration from compressive grinding forces due to altered shoulder mechanics.
- Acute traumatic events such as direct blows or forceful traction.

RISK FACTORS

- Athletes engaging in repetitive throwing or overhead sports
- Acute injury such as a fall on an outstretched hand (FOOSH) or traction injury to the arm
- Degenerative tearing or fraying from general aging >40 yr

GENERAL PREVENTION

Some experts feel that posterior capsular stretching may decrease the incidence of SLAP tears (1)[C].

COMMONLY ASSOCIATED CONDITIONS

- Rotator cuff pathology
- Glenohumeral instability

DIAGNOSIS

HISTORY

- Typical complaint is deep shoulder pain with a decrease in sports performance.
- Symptoms intensify with lifting overhead or in the cocking position.
- Mechanical symptoms may be present like locking, popping, or grinding.
- A sense of instability may be present.
- Symptoms can be similar to those with other shoulder pathology; it is important to maintain a degree of suspicion for labral injury.

PHYSICAL EXAM

- Comprehensive evaluation of glenohumeral and scapulothoracic range of motion (ROM)
- Glenohumeral joint stability evaluation
- The literature has found exam tests for SLAP tears have poor diagnostic accuracy. A combination of tests increases sensitivity and specificity.
- The following tests were found to have the highest pooled diagnostic odds ratio in a recent large meta-analysis (2)[A].
- Compression rotation test: With the patient supine, the shoulder is abducted to 90 degrees and compression is applied to the joint. The test is positive if there is pain, clicking, or catching.
- Yergason test: The patient is seated with the elbow in flexion and the forearm neutral. Active elbow flexion and forearm supination is resisted by the examiner. The test is positive if it reproduces pain along the proximal biceps.
- Anterior apprehension: With the patient supine, the elbow is flexed to 90 degrees, and the shoulder abducted to 90 degrees. The examiner then externally rotates the shoulder. The test is positive if the patient has apprehension or pain.
- Crank test: With the patient seated, the shoulder is elevated to 160 degrees in the scapular plane and compression is applied to the joint. The test is positive if there is pain, clicking, or catching.

DIFFERENTIAL DIAGNOSIS

- Rotator cuff tear
- Rotator cuff impingement syndrome
- Chronic acromioclavicular joint pain
- Refractory bicipital tendonosis
- Symptomatic glenohumeral instability

DIAGNOSTIC TESTS & INTERPRETATION

Initial Tests (lab, imaging)

- Plain radiographs are usually normal.
- Nonenhanced magnetic resonance imaging (MRI) can show the anatomy of the labral biceps complex but is not as sensitive for superior labral detachments.
- Gadolinium-enhanced MRI increases the accuracy of identifying superior labral pathology (3)[A].
- 3T magnets are superior in the diagnosis of superior labral tears.
- Arthroscopy is the gold standard for diagnosis.

Test Interpretation

The majority of SLAP tears can be classified by the original Snyder classification:

- Type I: fraying of the superior labrum but no detachment of the biceps insertion
- Type II: detachment of the biceps tendon from the supraglenoid tubercle
- Type III: bucket handle tear of a meniscoid-type superior labrum
- Type IV: superior labral detachment that extends into the substance of the biceps tendon
- There are several variations that could be subcategorized within these types.

TREATMENT

GENERAL MEASURES

- Stable labral tears without mechanical symptoms may be successfully treated nonoperatively with nonsteroidal anti-inflammatory drugs (NSAIDs) and physical therapy.
- Therapy should include posterior capsular stretches, rotator cuff and scapular stabilization, and ROM exercises.
- Shoulder exercises should be supplemented with core and lower extremity strengthening in the throwing or overhead athlete (1)[B].
- Return to play can be graduated as tolerated.

ISSUES FOR REFERRAL

If an athlete or patient cannot progress after 3 to 6 mo, operative intervention should be considered.

SURGERY/OTHER PROCEDURES

- Unstable SLAP tears require arthroscopic surgery.
- Young (age is surgeon dependent) active patients often undergo primary SLAP repair.
- Older patients with chronic symptoms or degenerative labral tissue may undergo débridement or biceps tenodesis (4)[C].

ONGOING CARE

FOLLOW-UP RECOMMENDATIONS

- After surgical repair, time is needed for healing and recovery prior to the reinitiation of physical therapy.
- A throwing program can usually start within 3 to 4 mo of surgery.
- Return to full throwing may take 9 to 12 mo.

PROGNOSIS

- Nonsurgical treatment is normally recommended first; however, opinions vary on the success of this regimen.
- Studies demonstrate difficulty achieving a high return to play rate in elite athletes even after surgical repair (5)[B].
- Return-to-play rates are affected by concomitant rotator cuff pathology.
- Biceps tenodesis has demonstrated positive results in the general population.

COMPLICATIONS

- Breakage or dislodgement of nonabsorbable anchors
- Foreign body reaction to surgical anchors

REFERENCES

1. Fedoriw WW, Ramkumar P, McCulloch PC, et al. Return to play after treatment of superior labral tears in professional baseball players. *Am J Sports Med*. 2014;42(5):1155–1160.
2. Gismervik SØ, Drogset JO, Granviken F, et al. Physical examination tests of the shoulder: a systematic review and meta-analysis of diagnostic test performance. *BMC Musculoskelet Disord*. 2017;18(1):41.
3. Symanski JS, Subhas N, Babb J, et al. Diagnosis of superior labrum anterior-to-posterior tears by using MR imaging and MR arthrography: a systematic review and meta-analysis. *Radiology*. 2017;285(1):101–113.
4. Calcei JG, Boddapati V, Altchek DW, et al. Diagnosis and treatment of injuries to the biceps and superior labral complex in overhead athletes. *Curr Rev Musculoskelet Med*. 2018;11(1):63–71.
5. Smith R, Lombardo DJ, Petersen-Fitts GR, et al. Return to play and prior performance in Major League Baseball pitchers after repair of superior labral anterior-posterior tears. *Orthop J Sports Med*. 2016;4(12):2325967116675822.

ADDITIONAL READING

Somerville LE, Willits K, Johnson AM, et al. Clinical assessment of physical examination maneuvers for superior labral anterior to posterior lesions. *Surg J (N Y)*. 2017;3(4):e154–e162.

CLINICAL PEARLS

- SLAP tears are injuries to the superior labrum biceps tendon complex.
- Type II tears are the most common and are seen in overhead or throwing athletes.
- MR arthrogram is the diagnostic study of choice to evaluate for a SLAP lesion.
- Some athletes may do well with conservative rehabilitation; however, if symptoms persist after 3 to 6 mo, surgical consultation should be obtained.

SLIPPED CAPITAL FEMORAL EPIPHYSIS

Vicki R. Nelson, MD, PhD • W. Franklin Sease Jr., MD, FAAFP, FACSM

BASICS

DESCRIPTION

- A disorder of unknown cause in which the proximal femoral epiphysis (head of the femur) begins to "fall off or slip off" the femoral neck
- The slippage occurs at the epiphyseal plate, which begins to weaken as it matures.
- There are four presentation patterns for slipped capital femoral epiphysis (SCFE):
  - Preslip
  - Acute
  - Acute on chronic
  - Chronic
- SCFEs are classified based on the intensity and duration of symptoms present as well as the radiographic findings.

EPIDEMIOLOGY

- The disorder affects 0.2 to 10/100,000 children (1).
- Predominant age: The mean age at which it occurs is 12 yr in girls and 13.5 yr in boys. Age decreases with increasing obesity.
- The disorder is bilateral in 18–63% of affected children.
- The disorder frequently occurs in two distinct body types: (i) slender, tall, rapidly growing boys and (ii) large, obese boys ± undeveloped sexual characteristics. The second body type is more prevalent than the first.
- Pacific Islanders have the highest incidence, followed by African Americans, Hispanics, Native Americans, Americans, and children of Indonesian/Malay descent.

ETIOLOGY AND PATHOPHYSIOLOGY

- Biomechanical and biochemical factors play a role in SCFE.
- Biomechanical factors include obesity, femoral retroversion, and increased physeal obliquity.
- Biochemical factors include increased growth hormone during puberty, which increases the height of the zone of hypertrophy, and increased testosterone, which decreases physeal strength.

RISK FACTORS

- Rapid growth spurt
- Obesity
- Endocrine disorders that weaken the physis, particularly in preadolescent children
- Radiation therapy and renal failure
- Obesity

COMMONLY ASSOCIATED CONDITIONS

- Obesity
- Hypothyroidism
- Multiple endocrine neoplasia syndrome, type 2
- Panhypopituitarism
- Renal failure
- Radiation therapy

DIAGNOSIS

- Determined by history, physical examination, and pelvis anteroposterior (AP) and frog-leg lateral view radiographs.
- It is important to always examine both sides owing to possibility of bilateral disease (1).
- Acute SCFE: sudden onset severe pain usually of <3 wk duration that prevents weight-bearing. Usually associated with trauma. Joint effusion and no metaphyseal remodeling. Examination reveals external rotational deformity, shortening of the affected limb, decreased range of motion at the hip, and severe pain with attempted manipulation.
- Acute on chronic SCFE: history of at least 3 wk of hip pain and/or limp with a sudden increase in pain and inability to bear full weight. Patients usually have a joint effusion and metaphyseal widening.
- Chronic SCFE: Vague intermittent symptoms of hip, thigh, or knee pain, worsened by activity and relieved by rest. Exam reveals antalgic gait and even a Trendelenburg or waddling depending on whether unilateral or bilateral. Often the affected foot is turned outward. Often pain with internal rotation, abduction, and flexion of the hip with reduced movement in these planes. Metaphyseal modeling is present but no effusion.

PHYSICAL EXAM

- A common presenting complaint is hip pain and a limp (antalgic gait). Trendelenburg test is positive when the patient stands on the affected leg and a downward pelvic tilt occurs due to hip weakness on the affected side (2). Pain is typically located in the groin area and commonly presents as referred medial knee pain ± thigh pain.
- Pain can be gradual in onset, and symptoms occur even when minimal displacement is present or can be acute and dramatic with sudden severe hip or knee pain and inability to bear weight.
- The physical exam reveals tenderness over the hip joint capsule, and an external rotation deformity of the lower extremity may be present.
- There is restricted hip motion, especially internal rotation, abduction, and forward flexion.
- The hip tends to rotate externally and abduct as it is flexed (Whitman sign).
- In chronic late presenting cases, the affected leg may be 1 to 3 cm shorter than the normal leg, and the thigh muscles may be atrophied.

DIFFERENTIAL DIAGNOSIS

- Avascular necrosis/Legg-Calvé-Perthes disease (in younger age range)
- Septic arthritis
- Transient synovitis
- Iliac apophysitis or apophyseal avulsion fracture at avulsion anterior inferior iliac spine (AIIS) and avulsion anterior superior iliac spine (ASIS)
- Femoral cutaneous nerve entrapment (more common in muscular girls)
- Proximal femur fracture
- Avascular necrosis
- Juvenile rheumatoid arthritis
- Legg-Calvé-Perthes disease (in younger age range)

DIAGNOSTIC TESTS & INTERPRETATION

- AP pelvis and frog-leg lateral radiograph views confirm the diagnosis. The affected side always should be compared with the unaffected leg. Up to 10% of SCFE patients have normal radiographs initially:
  - AP pelvis can be useful to measure "Klein" line which is a line parallel to superior femoral neck and should interest with ~1/3 of the epiphysis.
  - The sensitivity and reliability is improved by measuring the epiphyseal width lateral to Klein line, which if differing by 2 mm (0.079 inch) or more between hips suggests the diagnosis of SCFE.
- Magnetic resonance imaging (MRI) is useful for detecting preslips that may be symptomatic but have normal radiographs.
- Computed tomography (CT) is occasionally useful for grading chronic slips.
- The capital epiphysis is seen to displace posteriorly and downward, whereas the femoral neck displaces upward and anteriorly. In some patients, displacement is not obvious, but the physeal plate is widened (preslipping stage).
- Classification is based on the severity of the slip. Type 1 slips involve <33% of the width of the femoral epiphysis. Type 2 involves a 33–50% slip, and a type 3 involves >50% of the width of the femoral epiphysis.

TREATMENT

GENERAL MEASURES

- Orthopedic referral should be made immediately upon diagnosis (3).
- Patients should be made non–weight-bearing.

SURGERY/OTHER PROCEDURES

- Surgical stabilization is the mainstay of treatment for all types of slippages (1).
- Current controversy exists surrounding the need for prophylactic surgical stabilization of the unaffected contralateral side. This is due to the prevalence of bilateral SCFE and inability to predict who will develop bilateral disease (3).

ADMISSION, INPATIENT, AND NURSING CONSIDERATIONS

- Acute treatment involves cessation of weight bearing and surgical stabilization.
- A displaced epiphysis may require reduction before fixation.
- In the preslip phase, with widening of the physeal plate evident on radiographs, in situ operative fixation is recommended.
- Weight-bearing begun at 6 wk postoperatively.

ONGOING CARE

FOLLOW-UP RECOMMENDATIONS

- Orthopedic referral should be made immediately on diagnosis.
- Patients should be made non–weight-bearing if the diagnosis is suspected.

PROGNOSIS

- Prognosis is usually good, except in patients with acute traumatic separation.
- Slight shortening of the leg of <1.25 cm may result, along with a mild external rotation deformity.
- The internal fixation devices are removed after the physeal plate closes in 1 to 2 yr.
- In acute traumatic separations, avascular necrosis of the femoral head is a common complication, and this usually results in severe arthritis of the hip.
- Another complication is acute cartilage necrosis or lysis of the articular cartilage of the hip joint. A painful fibrous ankylosis of the hip joint is frequently the end result.

REFERENCES

1. Peck DM, Voss LM, Voss TT. Slipped capital femoral epiphysis: diagnosis and management. *Am Fam Physician*. 2017;95(12):779–784.
2. Frank JS, Gambacorta PL, Eisner EA. Hip pathology in the adolescent athlete. *J Am Acad Orthop Surg*. 2013;21(11):665–674.
3. Peck K, Herrera-Soto J. Slipped capital femoral epiphysis: what's new? *Orthop Clin North Am*. 2014;45(1):77–86.

ADDITIONAL READING

Armstrong AD, Hubbard MC. *Essentials of Musculoskeletal Care*. 5th ed. Rosemont, IL: American Academy of Orthopedic Surgeons; 2016.

S

CLINICAL PEARLS

- SCFE can present unilaterally or bilaterally with only knee or thigh pain; not all cases have hip pain.
- All adolescent patients with thigh or hip pain should get x-rays. The recommended radiographs are AP and frog-leg lateral pelvis views, not individual hip radiographs.
- Treatment includes non–weight-bearing status and immediate referral for surgical stabilization.

SNAPPING SCAPULA AND WINGING OF THE SCAPULA

Joseph Chorley, MD, FAAP, FACSM, CAQSM

BASICS

DESCRIPTION

Snapping scapula syndrome (SSS) is a disorder of the scapulothoracic articulation resulting in crepitation that may or may not be painful. It can be the result of anatomic impediment to normal scapular motion from weakness, inflexibility, or inadequate proprioception of 1 or more of the 17 muscles that insert on the scapula. Winging scapula (WS) results from a nerve injury, usually of the long thoracic nerves (LTN) or spinal accessory nerves (SAN). This results in profound weakness of the serratus anterior or trapezius muscles, respectively, producing functional shoulder pain and dysfunction.

EPIDEMIOLOGY

Incidence

- SSS is relatively common.
- Altered scapular position and motion has been reported in 68–100% of patients with shoulder injuries.

Prevalence

- SSS:
  - Relatively common
  - Altered scapular position and motion has been reported in 31% of asymptomatic individuals.
- WS:
  - Rare
  - LTN palsy has been reported 15/7,000 electromyography (EMG) patients, 1/38,500 orthopedic patients, 3/12,000 neurologic evaluations.
  - SAN palsy prevalence is difficult to assess.

ETIOLOGY AND PATHOPHYSIOLOGY

- SSS:
  - Anatomic (1):
    - Thoracic rib disorders (fracture with prominent callus or displacement)
    - Thoracic spine disorder (costovertebral dysfunction, scoliosis, Scheuermann kyphosis)
    - Scapular disorders (fracture with prominent callus or displacement, hooked superior medial edge [Luschka tubercle], osteochondroma)
    - Soft tissue tumor (elastofibroma)
  - Inadequate strength, flexibility, and proprioception:
    - Weakness (mostly in serratus anterior, middle and lower trapezius)
    - Inflexibility (mostly in pectoralis minor, levator scapulae, and upper trapezius)
    - Abnormal firing patterns associated with repetitive motion (asymmetric strength training, throwing mechanics, swimming technique, etc.) may lead to bursitis in 1 of the 6 bursae.
- WS:
  - Blunt trauma:
    - LTN: sudden depression of the shoulder
    - SAN: blow over the posterior cervical triangle
  - Sports related: archery, ballet, baseball, basketball, bowling, football, golf, gymnastics, hockey, soccer, tennis, weight lifting, wrestling
  - Iatrogenic:
    - LTN: chiropractic manipulation, crutches, surgery
    - SAN: surgery to the neck area
  - Other: postviral, exposure to toxin or drugs, muscular dystrophy

DIAGNOSIS

HISTORY

- SSS:
  - Mechanical sensation, with or without pain, usually along the medial scapular border (superior > inferior > middle)
  - Classic anterior impingement complaints (pain with overhead activities)
  - Involved in higher incident sports (baseball, swimming, tennis)
- WS:
  - LTN: shoulder pain that usually is more toward the upper medial scapula. It may occur a few weeks after onset of palsy when the trapezius starts to stretch from the unopposing serratus anterior. Severe pain may occur with postviral neuritis. Burning neuralgic pain at the inferior scapular pole may occur with acute trauma.
  - SAN: stiffness, heaviness, pain, and weakness, especially with overhead activities or prolonged exertion

PHYSICAL EXAM

- Cervical spine evaluation, including range of motion of the cervical spine, strength, sensation, deep tendon reflexes in the upper extremity, Spurling maneuver
- Spine and shoulder inspection: standing and forward flexed, analyzing for asymmetry and posture
- Scapular position:
  - SSS (may be normal scapular position with classic "teenager posture" with rounded shoulders, dynamic thoracic kyphosis, forward flexed head, and suboccipital extension)
  - LTN (scapula is superior and adducted medially)
  - SAN (drooping shoulder with scapula abducted laterally)
- Scapular winging tests:
  - LTN (entire medial scapula will protrude with shoulder forward flexion [FF] or wall push-up)
  - SAN (superior medial scapula will laterally displace causing downward rotation with shoulder abduction or resisted external rotation; no winging with shoulder FF)
- Range of motion deficit:
  - LTN (<120 degrees of FF and 110 degrees of abduction)
  - SAN (normal FF and <90 degrees of abduction)
- Scapular motion with shoulder movement (2,3):
  - Lateral scapular slide test: Patient will place the (i) arms in the resting position, (ii) hands on iliac crest, (iii) and shoulders at 90 degrees abduction in the scapular plane. Distance from the inferior scapular pole to a fixed point on the midline thoracic spine (usually spinous process of T9) is measured in each position. Scapular dyskinesis is diagnosed when there is 1.5 cm difference from the opposite side.
  - Scapular assistance tests: Perform the classic Neer impingement test, which is painful.
  - Repeat the test with the examiner holding the superior medial scapula down (assisting serratus anterior) and gliding the inferior scapular pole medially (assisting the lower trapezius), and the pain will not be provoked.
  - Repeat the test with the examiner holding the medial scapula retracted, and the pain will not be provoked.
  - Scapular dyskinesis classification (SSS) based on scapular prominence at rest and with lateral scapular slide test:
    - Inferior medial
    - Entire medial
    - Superior medial and superior translation
    - Slightly lower (normal in the dominant arm)

DIFFERENTIAL DIAGNOSIS

- Cervical discogenic neuropathy
- Thoracic outlet syndrome
- Rotator cuff tear
- Glenohumeral instability
- Suprascapular nerve entrapment
- Primary neuromuscular disease
- Neurofibromatosis
- Primary pulmonary pathology

DIAGNOSTIC TESTS & INTERPRETATION

Initial Tests (lab, imaging)

- Radiographs of the cervical spine, shoulder, chest, and ribs will usually be normal.
- Computed tomography (CT) scans and magnetic resonance imaging (MRI) are rarely necessary unless concern about bone or soft tissue masses. Isolated left thoracic scoliosis should be evaluated with cervical spine MRI secondary to its association with congenital anomalies (syringomyelia, Arnold-Chiari malformations).

Diagnostic Procedures/Other

EMG is the only definitive diagnostic test for nerve dysfunction and muscle paralysis associated with WS. Abnormalities, such as resting denervation potentials, decreased motor unit recruitment, and polyphasic motor unit potential with volitional activities. EMG does not correlate with clinical improvement and cannot be used to predict extent of recovery (4)[C].

TREATMENT

GENERAL MEASURES

Emergency department (ED) treatment (5)[C]:

- Acute injury may result in WS, but the symptoms of pain and nerve dysfunction may not present for a few weeks.
- Avoiding painful activities, especially overhead activities, is important.
- Brief sling immobilization may be necessary for pain control.

MEDICATION

- Analgesic medications may be necessary for acute injuries and severe pain, like with postviral neuritis.
- Subacromial bursa steroid injection and oral anti-inflammatories may be used with SSS in order to decrease pain while physical therapy is retraining normal muscle firing patterns.

ADDITIONAL THERAPIES

- SSS (treat the etiology) (1)[C]:
  - Anatomic lesions (fracture callus, fracture displacement, mass lesion): assessment for surgical consultation, depending on their contribution to the pain and dysfunction
  - Thoracic dysfunction: Thoracic scoliosis and Scheuermann kyphosis may require bracing and surgery. Segmental thoracic dysfunction (resulting in malalignment) may benefit from manual manipulation followed by stabilization rehabilitation.
  - Scapular dyskinesis: requires an astute clinician to direct the subtle relationships that need to be restored (6). Outlined below are the most common components of most scapular dyskinesis:
    - Release the muscular and capsular restrictions:
      - Glenohumeral posterior capsule tightness with decrease internal rotation can be improved using the side lying "sleeper stretch."
      - Pectoralis minor muscular shortening can be improved with the patient supine with a towel roll under thoracic spine and a steady posteriorly directed force on the anterior shoulder. This can also be accomplished by soft tissue mobilization by physical therapy or lying prone on a lacrosse ball located at the pectoralis minor.
      - Scapular restrictions can be improved with manual mobilization techniques to improve scapular upward rotation and retraction/protraction.
    - Improve muscular strength and scapular force couples:
      - Early rehabilitation will include closed chain exercises like low, middle, and high rows, and advancing to "scapular clocks," "wall washes," and "punches."
      - When a stable scapular base is achieved, open chained exercises can be incorporated (classic rotator cuff with increasing abduction, scapular four directions against manual resistance).
      - "Push-ups with a plus" are effective in strengthening serratus anterior and plyometrics, and proprioceptive neuromuscular facilitation will complete most of this phase of rehab.
      - Return to activity: Correcting technique, overload, and other problems in the kinetic chain are important as return to activity is considered. Incorporating the new biomechanics into often-entrenched biomechanics takes time and an astute team, including the coach, patient, therapist, and clinician.
- WS (5)[C]:
  - LTN: 75% will respond to conservative management but will take anywhere from 6 to 24 mo. There are some that do not improve serratus anterior firing but improve their function by muscular compensation with other scapulothoracic stabilizers (usually trapezius):
    - In the early phase of rehabilitation, avoid further injury by limiting any overhead or painful activities.
    - As pain decreases, progress to gentle range of motion of the shoulder and scapula to avoid adhesive capsulitis. Avoid stretching the serratus anterior muscle by limiting passive scapular retraction.
    - As the serratus strength improves, shoulder girdle strengthening exercises can be started. Reducing the amount of winging during rehab and everyday activities is important during conservative treatment.
    - Scapular bracing may help but is often restrictive and has poor compliance. Doing rehab while lying supine will stabilize the winged scapula.
  - SAN: Conservative management is not as effective. A trial of protection, bracing, and progression as above is advised for 6 to 12 mo.

SURGERY/OTHER PROCEDURES

- WS: If symptoms continue despite compliant conservative management for 12 (SAN) to 24 mo (LTN), surgical intervention must be considered. Dynamic muscle transfer procedures show improved function, fewer symptoms of pain and winging, and are replacing many of the older procedures (5)[C].
- SSS: Surgical management is reserved for patients with impinging anatomic structures and recalcitrant bursitis that are not responding to conservative management (7).

REFERENCES

1. Martin RM, Fish DE. Scapular winging: anatomical review, diagnosis, and treatments. *Curr Rev Musculoskelet Med*. 2008;1(1):1–11.
2. Forthomme B, Crielaard JM, Croisier JL. Scapular positioning in athlete's shoulder: particularities, clinical measurements and implications. *Sports Med*. 2008;38(5):369–386.
3. Kibler WB, McMullen J. Scapular dyskinesis and its relation to shoulder pain. *J Am Acad Orthop Surg*. 2003;11(2):142–151.
4. Seror P, Lenglet T, Nguyen C, et al. Unilateral winged scapula: clinical and electrodiagnostic experience with 128 cases, with special attention to long thoracic nerve palsy. *Muscle Nerve*. 2018;57(6):913–920.
5. Didesch JT, Tang P. Anatomy, etiology, and management of scapular winging [published online ahead of print October 3, 2018]. *J Hand Surg Am*. 2018. doi:10.1016/j.jhsa.2018.08.008.
6. Osias W, Matcuk GR Jr, Skalski MR, et al. Scapulothoracic pathology: review of anatomy, pathophysiology, imaging findings, and an approach to management. *Skeletal Radiol*. 2018;47(2):161–171.
7. Menge TJ, Horan MP, Tahal DS, et al. Arthroscopic treatment of snapping scapula syndrome: outcomes at minimum of 2 years. *Arthroscopy*. 2017;33(4):726–732.

CLINICAL PEARLS

- Scapular dyskinesis should be considered in patients with shoulder pain. Whether it is a primary cause or a secondary problem, it is an important component of restoring shoulder function.
- LTN: 75% will respond to conservative management but will take anywhere from 6 to 24 mo. There are some that do not improve serratus anterior firing but improve their function by muscular compensation with other scapulothoracic stabilizers (usually trapezius).
- CT scans and MRI are rarely necessary unless concern about bone or soft tissue masses. Only definitive test is EMG.

SPINAL STENOSIS

Stephen Rohrer, DO, FAOASM

BASICS

DESCRIPTION

- Stenosis of the spinal canal is defined as narrowing of the available space within the spinal canal causing impingement on the neural and/or vascular elements of the spine.
- A general consensus defines cervical spinal stenosis as an anteroposterior diameter of <13 mm from C3–C7.
- Spinal stenosis is also divided into congenital and acquired forms.
- It appears to affect men more than women (1).

EPIDEMIOLOGY

- Most often occurs in the lumbar spine but can occur in the cervical (C)-spine
- Rarely occurs in the thoracic spine

Incidence

The absolute incidence of spinal stenosis is unknown, but lumbar spinal stenosis is an increasing cause of disability in older patients.

ETIOLOGY AND PATHOPHYSIOLOGY

Spondylosis, or degenerative arthritis affecting the spine, is the most common cause of lumbar spinal stenosis and typically affects individuals age >60 yr.

Genetics

Genetics play a role in some cases of spinal stenosis in conditions such as spondyloarthropathies, dwarfism, and spina bifida.

RISK FACTORS

- Degenerative changes in the intervertebral disks, ligaments, and facet joints as well as osteophyte formation surrounding the canal
- Older age
- Spondylitic disease of the spine may contribute to stenosis.

GENERAL PREVENTION

- Degenerative changes may not be able to be prevented, but symptom severity may be limited by maintaining a healthy back.
- Core strengthening, appropriate flexibility and posture, and maintaining a healthy body weight may slow the progression of symptoms.

COMMONLY ASSOCIATED CONDITIONS

- Degenerative arthritis
- Disk bulging
- Facet osteophytes
- Ligamentum flavum hypertrophy
- Spondylolisthesis

DIAGNOSIS

HISTORY

- Typically, the earliest complaint is back pain.
- Bilateral leg pain often involving the buttocks and thighs and spreading toward the feet
- The pain may be described as burning, cramping, or dull fatigue.
- Classically, the symptoms of lumbar canal stenosis worsen with ambulation or standing and are relieved by sitting and forward bending.
- In severe late-stage cases where the sacral roots are impinged, visceral disturbance may manifest with urinary incontinence.
- The history for cervical spinal stenosis may include transient quadriplegia after a tackle or just bilateral "stingers" (numbness and pain down both arms).

PHYSICAL EXAM

- A broad-based gait is often present.
- Abnormal Romberg test
- The spine must be examined for abnormal curvature or limitation in range of motion (ROM).
- Commonly, flexion relieves symptoms, and extension is painful.
- The back should be examined for tenderness, which may suggest a fracture, neoplasm, or infection.
- The straight-leg test should be done to rule out disk herniation. Generally, patients with lumbar spinal stenosis do not have a positive straight-leg test.
- A femoral stretch test, where the knee is flexed in a prone position, may elicit pain in patients with spinal stenosis at L3–L4.
- The physical examination also should include an examination of the skin, nails, and distal pulses of the feet to evaluate for possible vascular claudication. Patients with vascular claudication often will have pallor, nail dystrophy, absence of hair, and distal pulses in their feet. Popliteal and femoral pulses need to be examined.
- Cervical spinal stenosis requires a careful active ROM exam of the neck and an upper extremity neurologic exam.

DIFFERENTIAL DIAGNOSIS

- Vascular claudication
- Space-occupying lesion such as a neoplasm
- Herniated disk
- Trauma, for example, compression fracture
- Degenerative subluxation of the vertebrae (spondylolisthesis)
- Infectious process, for example, discitis or epidural abscess
- Spear tackler's spine:
  - Developmental narrowing of the cervical spinal canal
  - Straightening or reversal of the normal cervical lordotic curve
  - Preexisting minor posttraumatic x-ray evidence of bony or ligamentous injury
  - Documentation of using spear-tackling techniques

DIAGNOSTIC TESTS & INTERPRETATION

- Plain films are not diagnostic but may demonstrate degenerative spine disease or spondylosis.
- In the C-spine, a vertebral canal–vertebral body ratio under 0.8 was defined by Torg as spinal stenosis. The Torg ratio, however, is not used exclusively to evaluate cervical spinal stenosis. Even though it carries about a 93% sensitivity, it leads to many false-positive results and has a poor positive predictive value for predicting cervical cord neurapraxia (2)[C].

- Computed tomography (CT) scans ± intrathecal contrast material injection (CT myelogram) may demonstrate encroachment of the canal by osteophytes, hypertrophied lamina, or other degenerative changes.
- Magnetic resonance imaging (MRI) is currently the preferred method to establish a diagnosis and exclude other conditions. MRI is both noninvasive and visualizes the soft tissue structures that may be obstructing the canal (3)[B].

TREATMENT

GENERAL MEASURES

- Nonsurgical management of lumbar stenosis may be attempted initially in patients who do not have severe pain or significant weakness. Patients on warfarin, sodium, chronic anticoagulants, or those who have severe risks for complications with decompressive surgery may not be candidates for invasive procedures.
- Nonsteroidal anti-inflammatory drugs (NSAIDs) and exercises may provide some relief for patients with lumbar spinal stenosis. Flexion exercises that reduce lumbar lordosis are especially useful.
- Morbidly obese patients should be encouraged to lose weight.
- Research is limited to suggest support for or against specific nonsurgical approaches, but studies are currently ongoing.
- Prehospital:
  - Management of acute symptomatic cervical spinal stenosis after trauma includes stabilization of the spine with a cervical collar and transport to an emergency setting.

MEDICATION

There is little evidence that pharmacologic therapy provides long-term relief in spinal stenosis (3)[B].

ADDITIONAL THERAPIES

- Epidural steroid injections may provide short-term relief (2 to 3 wk), but long-term efficacy results are conflicting (3)[B].
- 6 wk of physical therapy is as effective as initially undergoing decompression surgery (4).

SURGERY/OTHER PROCEDURES

- Typically, multilevel decompressive laminectomies are needed because the canal stenosis often occurs at multiple levels.
- Multilevel laminotomies, foraminotomies, and even decompression of the lateral recesses may be alternative methods of treatment.
- Most patients with radiographic and clinical evidence of spinal stenosis get significant long-term relief from decompressive surgery.
- *Acupuncture may provide pain relief, but further research is needed to validate the efficacy.*

COMPLEMENTARY & ALTERNATIVE MEDICINE

- In a Cochrane review, spinal manipulation appears to be as effective as other common therapies for chronic low back pain, such as exercise, standard medical care, or physical therapy (5)[B].
- Lumbosacral corset bracing may provide symptomatic relief *without the complications of surgery* (4).

ONGOING CARE

PROGNOSIS

- According to the North American Spine Society, patients followed for 2 to 10 yr with mild to moderate stenosis have a 20–40% chance of requiring surgical intervention.
- Of those who do not have surgery, 50–70% will have improvement in their pain (3)[C].

REFERENCES

1. Gross AR, Hoving JL, Haines TA, et al. A Cochrane review of manipulation and mobilization for mechanical neck disorders. *Spine (Phila Pa 1976)*. 2004;29(14):1541–1548.
2. Torg JS, Guille JT, Jaffe S. Injuries to the cervical spine in American football players. *J Bone Joint Surg Am*. 2002;84-A(1):112–122.
3. Snyder DL, Doggett D, Turkelson C. Treatment of degenerative lumbar spinal stenosis. *Am Fam Physician*. 2004;70(3):517–520.
4. Zania F, Tomkins-Lane C, Carragee E, et al. Surgical versus nonsurgical treatment for lumbar spinal stenosis. *Spine (Phila Pa 1976)*. 2016;41(14):E857–E868.
5. Rubinstein SM, van Middelkoop M, Assendelft WJ, et al. Spinal manipulative therapy for chronic low-back pain. *Cochrane Database Syst Rev*. 2011;(2):CD008112.

ADDITIONAL READING

- Alvarez JA, Hardy RH Jr. Lumbar spine stenosis: a common cause of back and leg pain. *Am Fam Physician*. 1998;57(8):1825–1834, 1839–1840.
- Atlas SJ, Delitto A. Spinal stenosis: surgical versus nonsurgical treatment. *Clin Orthop Relat Res*. 2006;443:198–207.
- Bronfort G, Nilsson N, Haas M, et al. Non-invasive physical treatments for chronic/recurrent headache. *Cochrane Database Syst Rev*. 2004;(3):CD001878.
- Cantu RC. The cervical spinal stenosis controversy. *Clin Sports Med*. 1998;17(1):121–126.
- Garfin SR, Herkowitz HN, Mirkovic S. Spinal stenosis. *J Bone Joint Surg Am*. 1999;81(4):572–586.
- Lurie J, Tomkins-Lane C. Management of lumbar spinal stenosis. *BMJ*. 2016;352:h6234.
- Martinelli TA, Wiesel SW. Epidemiology of spinal stenosis. *Instr Course Lect*. 1992;41:179–181.
- Matz P, Meagher R, Lamer T, et al. *Clinical Guidelines for Multidisciplinary Spine Care: Diagnosis and Treatment of Degenerative Lumbar Spondylolisthesis*. 2nd ed. Burr Ridge, IL: North American Spine Society; 2014.

CLINICAL PEARLS

- Experience with the National Center for Catastrophic Sports Injury Research suggests that athletes with significant cervical spinal stenosis are at increased risk of quadriplegia and should not participate in contact or collision sports. Referral to a spine specialist is indicated for competitive athletes wishing to return to play.
- To evaluate a patient with surgical hardware for spinal stenosis, CT myelogram is the preferred imaging modality.

SPLENIC CONTUSION AND RUPTURE

Fernando Enrique Hernandez, MD • David S. Edwards, MD, CAQSM

BASICS

DESCRIPTION

- The spectrum of splenic trauma consists of contusion, hematoma, laceration, and rupture.
- Most commonly associated with blunt abdominal trauma in contact or collision sports
- Also noted with falls during rigorous activity or less commonly penetrating abdominal injuries

EPIDEMIOLOGY

- Sequela from splenic injury is the leading cause of preventable mortality in sports-related abdominal blunt force trauma (1).
- Blunt trauma requiring emergency laparotomy varies from 6.9% to 66.7% among trauma centers (2).

ETIOLOGY AND PATHOPHYSIOLOGY

Mechanism may be obvious from high-speed trauma or varied to include seemingly innocuous events in case reports such as impact from a surfboard, falling onto a football, or being hit by a lacrosse ball (3).

RISK FACTORS

The pediatric patient is more susceptible due to less protection offered by a smaller rib cage relative to the size of the organ and a more compliant rib cage that transmits energy from trauma to underlying viscera (3).

COMMONLY ASSOCIATED CONDITIONS

- Rib fractures
- Thoracolumbar vertebral fractures
- Other intra-abdominal visceral injury

DIAGNOSIS

HISTORY

- Blunt, splenic injury can occur through a variety of mechanisms.
- An underlying inflamed spleen can manifest with history of antecedent upper respiratory tract infection, fevers, or easy bruising/bleeding in the days prior to injury (3).
- Left upper quadrant pain is often accompanied by referred left shoulder pain (Kehr sign) because intra-abdominal bleeding causes irritation of the diaphragm.

PHYSICAL EXAM

- Determine the stability of the patient with attention to primary survey, secondary survey, and vital signs, particularly hypotension (systolic <90 mm Hg), orthostatic hypotension, tachycardia, and tachypnea:
  - Pediatric considerations: Hypotension may not correlate with degree of hypovolemia in children, so serial physical exams, blood pressure (BP) measurements, and labs are essential.
  - Neurologic status, beware altered mentation
  - Beware signs of poor perfusion to extremities
- Inspect for ecchymoses or hematoma of the abdomen with close attention to discoloration of the periumbilical area (Cullen sign) or flank (Turner sign) that are consistent with intra-abdominal bleeding; may take up to 24 hr to develop
- Inspect for penetrating injury to the abdomen, flanks, or lower chest.
- Palpate ribs and thoracolumbar spine for tenderness, crepitus, or step-offs.
- Auscultate and then palpate the abdomen for signs of visceral injury or peritonitis.
- Spleen exam in the stable, cooperative patient with no neck or spine injury:
  - Place the patient in the right lateral decubitus position, permitting gravity to anteriorly displace the spleen.
  - Ensure that the patient's hips and knees are flexed to relax the abdominal muscles.
  - Proceed with gentle palpation during deep inspiration.
- Palpation of the spleen over 2 cm below the left costal margin is an abnormal finding in adults.

DIFFERENTIAL DIAGNOSIS

- Rib fracture
- Diaphragmatic injury
- Thoracic aorta rupture
- Peritonitis due to liver injury or ruptured hollow viscus
- Rectus sheath hematoma (3)
- Spontaneous splenic rupture secondary to splenomegaly associated with infectious mononucleosis
- Splenomegaly with rupture secondary to:
  - Congestion: liver disease
  - Infiltration: amyloidosis; hematologic malignancies such as leukemia, lymphoma, myeloproliferative disorder
  - Inflammation: acute or chronic such as HIV, tuberculosis, parasitic diseases
  - Extramedullary hematopoiesis

DIAGNOSTIC TESTS & INTERPRETATION

- Complete blood count (CBC)
- Serum electrolytes
- Type and screen or type and crossmatch (hemodynamically unstable patient in preparation for transfusion).
- Serial hemoglobin and hematocrit (suspected evolving bleed; 48 to 72 hr postinsult)
- Diagnostic peritoneal lavage (DPL) may reveal hemoperitoneum (but not the source) and is not advised in the stable patient (3).
- Thoracic and pelvic x-ray upon initiation of secondary survey during emergent care (3)
- For the hemodynamically stable patient with blunt splenic injury and no peritonitis, the preferred imaging modality is computed tomography (CT) of abdomen and pelvis with intravenous (IV) contrast (1)[B]:
  - Contrast extravasation ("blush") alone is not an absolute indication for surgery or angiography (1)[C].
  - Focal accumulation of contrast in the parenchyma suggests a contained vascular injury.
- For the hypotensive patient (systolic BP <90 mm Hg), splenic imaging during the focused assessment with sonography in trauma (FAST) is warranted:
  - Higher false-negative rate in children (4)
- The American Association for the Surgery of Trauma (AAST) Spleen Injury Scale:
  - 1994: widely used to grade severity
    - Location of hematoma or laceration
    - Percent of spleen damaged
    - Involvement of hilar vessels
  - Advance grade I for multiple injuries up to grade III
  - Some patients will require emergent surgery without preoperative grading.
  - Grade I:
    - Hematoma–subcapsular, <10% surface area (SA)
    - Laceration–capsular tear, extension into parenchyma <1 cm
  - Grade II:
    - Hematoma–subcapsular (10–50% SA) and/or intraparenchymal, <5 cm diameter
    - Laceration–capsular tear, extension into parenchyma 1 to 3 cm, spares trabecular vessels
  - Grade III:
    - Hematoma–subcapsular (>50% SA or expanding), ruptured hematoma in subcapsular or intraparenchymal location, intraparenchymal hematoma ≥5 cm or expanding
    - Laceration–extension into parenchyma >3 cm or involving trabecular vessels
  - Grade IV:
    - Laceration–extension into segmental or hilar vessels, major devascularization >25% of spleen
  - Grade V:
    - Laceration–shattered spleen
    - Vascular–extension into hilar vessels, devascularized spleen

- The World Society of Emergency Surgery (WSES) classification system:
  - Defines spleen injuries associated with blunt or penetrating trauma as minor, moderate, or severe
  - Advantages:
    - Incorporates the AAST grading system
    - Accounts for hemodynamic status
    - Applicable to pediatric and adult populations
  - Minor spleen injury: WSES class I:
    - Correlates with AAST I and II in a hemodynamically stable patient
    - CT scan advised
  - Moderate spleen injury: WSES II:
    - Correlates with AAST III in a hemodynamically stable patient
    - CT scan advised
  - Moderate spleen injury: WSES III:
    - Correlates with AAST IV and V in hemodynamically stable patient
    - CT scan advised
  - Severe spleen injury: WSES IV:
    - Correlates with AAST I to V in any hemodynamically unstable patient
    - CT scan is not recommended.

TREATMENT

- The approach to blunt splenic injuries has changed over time from aggressive surgical interventions to more conservative, nonoperative management (NOM) or endovascular management.
- Regarding age stratification for current treatment guidelines, pediatric patients are identified as <15 yr of age and adults >15 yr of age (3).
- Typically conservative in 75–93% of children and 35–65% of adults (2):
  - Prehospital/sidelines evaluation: primary survey, secondary survey if feasible, urgent transport via ambulance
  - Emergency department: primary and secondary survey if not already done, close hemodynamic monitoring, labs, imaging, IV resuscitation, consultation with trauma surgery, and perhaps interventional radiology colleagues
  - Arrange for urgent transport to a higher level of care if unable to provide close monitoring, serial assessment, and an operative room in the event of laparotomy (2)[B].
  - Inpatient ward versus intensive care unit (ICU): depending on clinical status:
    - Hemodynamic monitoring
    - Serial physical examination and hemoglobin measurement
    - No guidelines at this time regarding optimal timing for deep venous thrombosis (DVT) prophylaxis
    - Consider ICU admission and critical care consultation for:
      - Transfusion requirement.
      - "Blush" on CT, grade IV and V injuries.
  - Exam significant for hemodynamic instability or diffuse peritonitis warrants urgent laparotomy (2)[A].
  - Conservative care for:
    - Hemodynamically stable patient without peritonitis, isolated splenic injury (2)[B]
- Angiography/angioembolization:
  - Indications:
    - Consider for all blunt or penetrating spleen injury in the hemodynamically stable patient without peritonitis (4).
    - AAST ≥3, "blush," moderate hemoperitoneum, clinical evidence of ongoing bleeding (3)
  - Complications: 20% of patients (2):
    - Failure to control bleed
    - Missed injuries
    - Splenic abscess
    - Postembolization syndrome (PES) presenting in 90% of pediatric cases. Symptoms consist of abdominal pain, nausea, ileus, and fever; self-limited with spontaneous resolution in 6 to 9 days (3)

ONGOING CARE

FOLLOW-UP RECOMMENDATIONS

- Reimaging need/frequency determined by response to resuscitation, persistent abdominal pain, persistent evidence of systemic inflammatory response syndrome (SIRS), drop in hemoglobin (3)[C]
- Complications:
  - Delayed rupture (within 4 to 8 days) in 1–8% of adults and 0.5–7.5% of children (4)
  - Splenic pseudocyst
  - Overwhelming postsplenectomy infection (OPSI)—50% mortality:
    - Encapsulated organisms: *Streptococcus pneumoniae*, *Neisseria meningitidis*, *Haemophilus influenzae* type B (Hib)
    - Parasites: malaria, *Babesia*
    - Others: *Capnocytophaga canimorsus* from dog/human bites
- Outpatient follow-up: Immunizations are administered at 14 days postsurgery but should be given prior to hospital discharge if follow-up reliability is questioned.
- Immunizations to consider in asplenic patients as per Centers for Disease Control (CDC) guidelines are:
  - Seasonal influenza vaccine yearly.
  - Tdap vaccine.
  - Hib vaccine.
  - Pneumococcal vaccines (PCV13 and PPSV23).
  - Meningococcal vaccines against all three serogroups (B, C, and Y).
  - Zoster vaccine in adults >60 yr of age.
  - Human papillomavirus (HPV) vaccine series in men until 21 yr of age and women until 26 yr of age.
  - Measles, mumps, rubella (MMR) vaccine.
  - Varicella vaccine.
- Consider tailored antibiotic prophylaxis regimens in high-risk asplenic patients (3):
  - <6 yr of age
  - >50 yr of age
  - Inadequate response to pneumococcal vaccine
  - History of previous invasive pneumococcal disease
  - Malignancy or ongoing immunosuppression
- There are no evidence-based guidelines for return to sport. Follow-up imaging in the stable, recovering athlete is not routinely performed due to radiation risk and because clinical healing precedes radiographic healing. Some elite athletes with splenectomy have returned to full sport in as little as 3 wk. Light activity can begin at 2 wk with full activity in 6 wk in AAST grade I and II injuries receiving NOM. Most injuries take 2 to 2.5 mo to heal (3).

REFERENCES

1. Juyia R, Kerr H. Return to play after liver and spleen trauma. *Sports Health*. 2014;6(3):239–245.
2. Stassen NA, Buhllar I, Cheng JD, et al. Selective nonoperative management of blunt splenic injury: an Eastern Association for the Surgery of Trauma practice management guideline. *J Trauma Acute Care Surg*. 2012;73(5 Suppl 4):S294–S300.
3. Coccolini F, Montori G, Catena F, et al. Splenic trauma: WSES classification and guidelines for adult and pediatric patients. *World J Emerg Surg*. 2017;12:40.
4. Gannon EH, Howard T. Splenic injuries in athletes: a review. *Curr Sports Med Rep*. 2010;9(2):111–114.

ADDITIONAL READING

- Crichton J, Naidoo K, Yet B, et al. The role of splenic angioembolization as an adjunct to nonoperative management of blunt splenic injuries: a systematic review and meta-analysis. *J Trauma Acute Care Surg*. 2017;83(5):934–943.
- El-Matbouly M, Jabbour G, El-Menyar A, et al. Blunt splenic trauma: assessment, management and outcomes. *Surgeon*. 2016;14(1):52–58.

CLINICAL PEARLS

- Splenic contusion and rupture occur in a variety of sports and can be subtle initially. Consider spleen injury in the differential of patients with abdominal pain.
- "Delayed rupture" of the spleen can occur several days after initial injury. A high index of suspicion is essential.
- Evidence-based guidelines regarding return to play are lacking; however, most patients require 8 to 10 wk for full recovery. Return to play is ultimately determined by managing physician.

SPONDYLOARTHROPATHIES (SERONEGATIVE RA)

Brent H. Messick, MD, MS, FAAFP, CAQSM • Kevin E. Burroughs, MD, CAQSM

BASICS

DESCRIPTION

- Spondyloarthropathy (SpA) is a term applied to the clinical, radiologic, and immunogenetic features shared by a group of diseases that include:
  - Ankylosing spondylitis (AS).
  - Reactive arthritis (ReA).
  - Psoriatic arthritis (PsA).
  - Arthritis associated with inflammatory bowel disease (IBD).
  - Juvenile onset spondyloarthritis.
  - Undifferentiated spondyloarthropathy (USpA):
    - These conditions are variably associated with the human leukocyte antigen B27 (HLA-B27). Individuals with these conditions frequently exhibit overlapping clinical and radiologic features.
- Synonym(s): seronegative spondyloarthropathies; HLA-B27–related SpA

EPIDEMIOLOGY

- AS and USpA are the most common types of SpA.
- AS and ReA are more common in males.
- SpA is seen in all age groups, but most cases present at 20 to 50 yr of age.

Incidence

ReA incidence: 3–8% (1)

Prevalence

- SpA: 0.5–2% of the Caucasian population
- AS: 1 to 2/1,000
- ReA: 1/1,000
- PsA develops in 5% of patients with psoriasis.

ETIOLOGY AND PATHOPHYSIOLOGY

- Most cases of SpA are associated with HLA-B27.
- ReA is triggered by an infectious agent (*Yersinia*, *Escherichia Coli*, *Shigella*, *Salmonella*, *Campylobacter*, *Chlamydia*, and others) (1,2).

RISK FACTORS

- Male
- Caucasian
- Unprotected sex
- Positive family history
- ReA is significantly increased in persons with HIV.
- More common in patients who were not breast fed

Genetics

- HLA-B27 positivity:
  - AS 90–95%
  - ReA 80%
  - USpA 70%, PsA 40%
  - IBD associated 30%
- 8% of Caucasians and 4% of African Americans are HLA-B27 positive.
- <20% of HLA-B27–positive individuals will develop SpA.

DIAGNOSIS

- There are several criteria for research purposes, including European Spondyloarthropathy Study Group (ESSG) and Amor. Recently, the Assessment of Spondyloarthritis International Society (ASAS) criteria was shown the be the most specific (3).
- ASAS criteria:
  - Sacroiliitis on imaging plus one of the following or HLA-B27 and two of the following:
    - Sausage digit
    - Psoriasis—family history of SpA
    - Inflammatory back pain
    - Nonsteroidal anti-inflammatory drugs (NSAIDs) good response
    - Enthesitis
    - Arthritis
    - Crohn/colitis—elevated C-reactive protein (CRP)
    - HLA-B27
    - Uveitis

HISTORY

- Inflammatory back pain:
  - Insidious onset of low back pain before the age of 40 yr
  - Morning stiffness (>30 min)
  - Often associated with night pain
  - Persists for >3 mo
  - Improved with exercise and NSAIDs (inflammatory vs. mechanical back pain)
- Other joint or enthesis involvement; eye, bowel, skin, mucous membrane, gut, genitourinary symptoms

PHYSICAL EXAM

- Low back pain at night with prominent early morning stiffness (sacroiliitis, spondylitis)
- Peripheral joint pain and swelling (often lower limb and asymmetric)
- Pain and inflammation at the insertion of tendons or ligaments (enthesitis), sausage digits (dactylitis)
- Ocular: conjunctivitis, iritis
- Gastrointestinal (GI): oral ulcerations, gut inflammation
- Skin and nails: psoriasis, keratoderma blennorrhagica, psoriatic nail dystrophy
- Genitourinary: urethritis, cervicitis, circinate balanitis
- Constitutional: fever and weight loss (ReA)
- Lumbar spine: restricted range of motion:
  - Schober test: Mark the spinous process of L5 and make a mark 10 cm above that point. Ask the patient to bend forward. The distance between the two points should increase by >5 cm in a normal subject.
- Peripheral joints: tender and/or warm
- Enthesitis: tenderness around the heel (Achilles or plantar fascia)
- Skin and nails: psoriatic nail changes and plaques (scalp, extensor surface of knees)

DIFFERENTIAL DIAGNOSIS

- Rheumatoid arthritis
- Osteoarthritis
- PsA
- Seronegative arthritis
- Gout
- Septic (gonococcal) arthritis
- Sarcoidosis

DIAGNOSTIC TESTS & INTERPRETATION

- Elevated erythrocyte sedimentation rate (ESR) or CRP
- Elevated white blood cells (WBCs) in peripheral and synovial fluid:
  - Note: These studies have poor sensitivity and specificity.
- Joint space narrowing, signs of inflammation, multiple joint involvement, and distal involvement in the hands and feet with added features of bone proliferation suggest seronegative SpA:
  - Differentiation of these relies on the distribution of radiographic abnormalities and clinical information.
- Peripheral arthritis with soft tissue swelling, juxtaarticular osteopenia, joint space narrowing, and erosions
- Areas of periostitis or osteitis are not uncommon (PsA, ReA).
- PsA:
  - Typically involves the hands, wrists, and feet; bilateral or unilateral, symmetric or asymmetric
  - Involvement of several joints in a single digit produces the classic "sausage digit."

- – Irregular and indistinct appearance of marginal bone about the joint, characterized as "fuzzy" or "whiskering"; may also see one side of joint thinned, the other broad ("pencil in cup")
  - – In foot sclerosis, enthesitis, periostitis, and soft tissue swelling can give an "ivory phalanx" appearance.
  - – At the sacroiliac (SI) joint, advanced changes are usually bilateral and show bone erosions and narrowing to the point of fusion.
- ReA:
  - – Similar features to PsA
  - – Lower extremity involvement more common than upper. Sausage digit and pencil-in-cup deformities can also occur.
  - – In the spine, large, comma-shaped, paravertebral ossification may also be seen.
- AS:
  - – More commonly involves the axial skeleton, although peripheral joints can be affected
  - – The spine findings are characterized by osteitis, syndesmophyte formation, facet inflammation, and eventual facet joint and vertebral body fusion (bamboo spine of AS).
  - – SI joint disease is bilateral and symmetric and typically precedes spine involvement.
  - – Magnetic resonance imaging (MRI) may detect up to 75% of early sacroiliitis not seen on plain radiography.
  - – Spine involvement is centered at the thoracolumbar or lumbosacral junction. Focal areas of osteitis become sclerotic and are termed *the shiny corner sign*.
  - – Ultrasound may show areas of abnormal vascularization of the entheses.

TREATMENT

- The goal of treatment is to reduce pain and stiffness and maintain posture and function.
- Eye, skin, genitourinary, and bowel involvement should be treated accordingly.
- Patients with spondylitis should engage in a lifelong program of exercise to preserve posture and mobility.
- Antibiotic therapy is indicated for proven acute bacterial infections but does not reduce arthritis.

MEDICATION

First Line

NSAIDs and topical/intra-articular steroids for acute pain

Second Line

- Sulfasalazine for patients that do not respond to NSAIDs (4)[A]
- Disease-modifying antirheumatic drugs: Adalimumab, certolizumab, etanercept, golimumab or infliximab, and methotrexate are used for chronic pain and inflammation (4).
- Pamidronate for refractory cases (4)[C]

ISSUES FOR REFERRAL

Referral to an ophthalmologist for ocular symptoms because these may require additional treatments

ADDITIONAL THERAPIES

- Joint splinting and rest may be indicated for acute flares.
- Physical therapy and home exercise plans

SURGERY/OTHER PROCEDURES

Joint arthroplasty may be required for those with severe peripheral joint disease.

REFERENCES

1. Denison HJ, Curtis EM, Clynes MA, et al. The incidence of sexually acquired reactive arthritis: a systematic literature review. *Clin Rheumatol*. 2016;35(11):2639–2648.
2. Townes JM, Deodhar AA, Laine ES, et al. Reactive arthritis following culture-confirmed infections with bacterial enteric pathogens in Minnesota and Oregon: a population-based study. *Ann Rheum Dis*. 2008;67(12):1689–1696.
3. Chung HY, Lau CS, Wu KP, et al. Comparison of performance of the Assessment of SpondyloArthritis International Society, the European Spondyloarthropathy Study Group and the modified New York criteria in a cohort of Chinese patients with spondyloarthritis. *Clin Rheumatol*. 2011;30(7):947–953.
4. Zochling J, van der Heijde D, Burgos-Vargas R, et al. ASAS/EULAR recommendations for the management of ankylosing spondylitis. *Ann Rheum Dis*. 2006;65(4):442–452.

ADDITIONAL READING

- Akgul O, Ozgocmen S. Classification criteria for spondyloarthropathies. *World J Orthop*. 2018;2(12): 107–115.
- Buckton KE, Jacobs PA, Court Brown WM, et al. A study of the chromosome damage persisting after x-ray therapy for ankylosing spondylitis. *Lancet*. 1962;2(7258):676–682.
- Callhoff J, Sieper J, Weiß A, et al. Efficacy of TNFα blockers in patients with ankylosing spondylitis and non-radiographic axial spondyloarthritis: a meta-analysis. *Ann Rheum Dis*. 2015;74(6):1241–1248.
- Kataria RK, Brent LH. Spondyloarthropathies. *Am Fam Physician*. 2004;69(12):2853–2860.
- Mandl P, Navarro-Compán V, Terslev L, et al. EULAR recommendations for the use of imaging in the diagnosis and management of spondyloarthritis in clinical practice. *Ann Rheum Dis*. 2015;74(7): 1327–1339.
- Montoya J, Matta NB, Suchon P, et al. Patients with ankylosing spondylitis have been breast fed less often than healthy controls: a case-control retrospective study. *Ann Rheum Dis*. 2016;75(5): 879–882.
- Olivieri I, Salvarani C, Cantini F, et al. Ankylosing spondylitis and undifferentiated spondyloarthropathies: a clinical review and description of a disease subset with older age at onset. *Curr Opin Rheumatol*. 2001; 13(4):280–284.
- Oostveen J, Prevo R, den Boer J, et al. Early detection of sacroiliitis on magnetic resonance imaging and subsequent development of sacroiliitis on plain radiography. A prospective, longitudinal study. *J Rheumatol*. 1999;26(9):1953–1958.
- Ramiro S, Stolwijk C, van Tubergen A, et al. Evolution of radiographic damage in ankylosing spondylitis: a 12 year prospective follow-up of the OASIS study. *Ann Rheum Dis*. 2015;74(1):52–59.

CLINICAL PEARLS

- In most patients, the initial episode of ReA is short-lived and settles within weeks to months.
- Some may go on to experience recurrent attacks, and these occur more frequently in HLA-B27–positive individuals.
- >30%, however, develop a chronic arthritis.

SPONDYLOLYSIS AND SPONDYLOLISTHESIS

Bittu Kuruvilla, MD, FAAPMR, CAQSM • Timothy Tiu, MD, FAAPMR, CAQSM

BASICS

DESCRIPTION

- From Greek, spondylo (vertebra) + lysis (loosening), or listhesis (slippage)
- Spondylolysis:
  - Involves a defect in the pars interarticularis of the vertebral complex
  - Usually an acquired stress fracture or stress reaction of the lower lumbar spine (L-spine)
- Can be unilateral or bilateral (1). Spondylolisthesis:
  - Results from displacement of a vertebral body on the subjacent vertebra. Defect may be secondary to fracture, arthrosis, or systemic disease.
  - Vertebral translation can be a source of pain, radiculopathy (spinal nerve injury), or spinal cord injury.

EPIDEMIOLOGY

- Spondylolysis and spondylolisthesis are the most common causes of back pain in children and adolescents >10 yr old (2).
- Spondylolysis:
  - Most common cause of significant back pain in athletes
  - Most commonly involves L5 (85–95% of cases) and L4 (5–15% of cases) (1)
  - Prevalence: 6–8% in general population and up to 63% in certain sports involving repetitive flexion, extension, and rotation (2,3,4)
  - Highest incidence in sports emphasizing extension activities
  - Rare in children <5 yr old and usually does not develop after age 20 yr (2)
  - Seen most commonly in adolescent male athletes
  - Male:female ratio is 2:1 (1).
- Spondylolisthesis:
  - Most common segment involved is the L5–S1 level, followed by L4–L5.
  - Prevalence: up to 25% in Eskimo (Inuits) population, 6% in Caucasians, and 2–3% in African Americans (4)
  - Incidence of isthmic spondylolisthesis: 4.4% at age 6 yr and 6% at age 14 yr (5)

ETIOLOGY AND PATHOPHYSIOLOGY

- Spondylolysis:
  - May be either an overuse injury (continued microtrauma to pars interarticularis from repetitive spinal flexion, extension and rotation, and shear forces to the L-spine) or a traumatic fracture
  - Shear forces on the normal lumbar lordosis are increased in extension and accentuated by combined extension and lateral side bending.
- Spondylolisthesis:
  - Isthmic (spondylolytic) spondylolisthesis:
    - Listhesis caused by breakdown/fracture of bilateral pars interarticularis
    - Most common cause of listhesis in patients <50 yr old, representing up to 50% in some series
    - Most common cause of listhesis in athletes
    - Has the lowest rate of progression (1)
    - Usually occurs at L5–S1
  - Dysplastic (congenital) spondylolisthesis:
    - Caused by failure of development of the superior facets
    - Represents 20% of all cases of listhesis
    - Major slippage can occur.
    - Has the highest rate of progression (1)
    - Usually occurs at L5–S1
  - Degenerative spondylolisthesis:
    - Caused by facet joint osteoarthritis, degenerative disk disease, and ligamentum flavum hypertrophy
    - Most common cause of listhesis in patients >50 yr old
    - Typically occurs at L4–L5
    - Major cause of spinal stenosis
    - Has higher incidence of cauda equina or nerve root compression
  - Traumatic spondylolisthesis:
    - Disruption of the posterior elements of the neural arch other than pars (pedicles or lamina)
    - Requires large force (also likely to have other fractures)
  - Pathologic spondylolisthesis:
    - Due to osteoporosis, rheumatoid arthritis, tumor, or infection

RISK FACTORS

- Genetics:
  - 14–70% of patients with isthmic spondylolisthesis reported to have first-degree relatives with spondylolisthesis (4). Spondylolysis is reported in up to 69% of family members of patients with spondylolysis (2).
- Sports involving extreme spinal motion, especially repetitive hyperextension and rotational movements (e.g., football linemen, diving, Olympic weight lifting, wrestling, rowing, gymnastics, throwing sports, and high jump in track and field)
- Adolescent growth spurts (fatigue fractures)
- Anatomic variations: spina bifida occulta, transitional vertebrae, elongated pars interarticularis, scoliosis
- Biomechanics: increased lumbar lordosis and/or increased pelvic inclination (contributed to by tight hip flexors and weak abdominal muscles), increased hamstring tightness

DIAGNOSIS

- Classification of spondylolisthesis by direction:
  - Anterolisthesis (most common): forward slippage of superior vertebra over inferior vertebra
  - Retrolisthesis: backward slippage of superior vertebra over inferior vertebra
- Grading of spondylolisthesis (Meyerding classification) (1):
  - Displacement of cranial vertebral body relative to caudal as visualized on lateral x-ray:
    - Grade I: <25%
    - Grade II: 25–50%
    - Grade III: 50–75%
    - Grade IV: 75–100%
    - Grade V: >100%; also termed spondyloptosis

HISTORY

- Spondylolysis:
  - Usually asymptomatic and may be found incidentally on radiographic examination
  - If symptomatic, most commonly complain of insidious onset of low back pain (3)
  - Pain is usually worse with activity, especially spine flexion and extension/lateral side bending.
  - Pain may radiate into the buttocks or posterior thigh (3), but patients rarely experience radicular signs or symptoms.
  - May note increase in symptoms with an increase in intensity or volume of training. Should not usually report numbness, paresthesias, weakness, bowel or bladder changes, gait disturbance, or constitutional symptoms (fever, weight loss, night pain, or rashes).
- Spondylolisthesis:
  - Low back pain is most common symptom (may be intermittent). If symptomatic, pain typically chronic and mild; pain more commonly acute with traumatic
  - Over half of symptomatic individuals report sciatica or radicular symptoms (usually after longstanding back pain).
  - May have cauda equina or claudication symptoms

PHYSICAL EXAM

- Symptomatic patient may be tender to palpation of the paraspinal musculature or affected spinal level.
- Can exhibit hamstring tightness (crouch gait) and hyperlordosis
- May exhibit limited range of motion and pain with extension
- Some suggest performing the "stork" test or single leg lumbar hyperextension test:
  - Ipsilateral back pain when a patient stands on one leg and hyperextends the back may indicate active spondylolysis (not sensitive or specific for spondylolysis).
- If significant listhesis is present (≥ grade III), may appreciate a step-off when palpating the spinous processes
- Gait abnormality
- Neurologic findings are rare.

DIFFERENTIAL DIAGNOSIS

- Infection
- Tumor
- Herniated nucleus pulposus
- Mechanical low back pain
- Spinal stenosis

DIAGNOSTIC TESTS & INTERPRETATION

- Plain films:
  - Anteroposterior (AP) and lateral views (for spondylolisthesis) and oblique views (for spondylolysis)
  - Addition of oblique views for spondylolysis may not improve diagnostic detection of spondylolysis in adolescents (3).
  - May be normal in the acute or subacute stage
  - Standing lateral x-ray can help with grading of listhesis.
  - Flexion/extension views (standing or recumbent) are used to assess for stability (3):
    - Not typically obtained in the adolescent athlete
  - Weight-bearing x-rays may worsen the apparent slip by up to 25%.
  - Oblique films may allow visualization of the "Scotty dog"; a radiolucent line through the "dog's neck" may represent a defect through the pars interarticularis (2).
  - Indirect sign of spondylolysis on AP view include lateral deviation of the spinous process and sclerosis of the contralateral pedicle (2).
- On standing AP view, an "inverted Napoleon hat sign" can be seen with large (grade IV/V) slips, representing the radiographic appearance of spondyloptosis. This increases risk of cauda equina syndrome. Triple-phase bone scan:
  - Used to evaluate the acuity of the injury
  - Can demonstrate defects unseen on plain x-ray
  - Can be positive as soon as 48 to 72 hr after injury
  - High false-positive rate in older patients, especially those with significant osteoarthritis of the L-spine
  - Not recommended in asymptomatic patients or in patients with symptoms >1 yr

- Single photon emission computed tomography (SPECT) scan:
  - Improves resolution of planar bone scans (allows for precise localization)
  - Most sensitive tool in diagnosing spondylolysis (3)
  - May be more helpful in demonstrating stress reactions at the pars
  - Advantage: may help delineate the acute "hot" lesion with potential to heal versus more chronic "cold" lesion that may not heal or progress to a fibrous union:
    - Pars defect on imaging with normal SPECT scan indicates inactive healed lesion or nonunion (3).
  - Disadvantage: may not be widely available, much greater radiation exposure than computed tomography (CT) scans (3), and cannot distinguish spondylolysis from facet spondylosis, infection, or osteoid osteoma
- CT scan:
  - Best to visualize spondylolysis with pars fracture
  - Can delineate neural compression
  - Useful after SPECT to help stage and determine treatment stratification
  - Reverse gantry thin-cut CT used at the level seen on SPECT scan to define morphology of defect
  - Advantage: visualization of bony anatomy, assessment of healing at later interval (6 mo)
  - Disadvantage: radiation exposure (50 times plain films), not reliable to distinguish between active and inactive lesions
- Magnetic resonance imaging (MRI):
  - Sagittal T1-weighted images are best for seeing pars defects (2). Fluid-sensitive sequences (short tau inversion recovery [STIR] or fat-saturated T2 weighted) may reveal early stress reaction or pars defect (2).
  - May help detect early pars stress fractures missed on plain x-ray (5).
  - Advantages: lack of radiation, ability to detect other pathology (discitis, disk pathology, tumor), good to evaluate nerve root compression (2), able to detect early pars stress reactions that cannot be seen on x-ray or CT
  - Needed if cauda equina symptoms present
  - Disadvantages: unable to determine if lesion is improving or worsening (2), can miss detecting spondylolysis (3), and may see false positives in younger patients secondary to normal bone marrow edema
  - If negative results when MRI used as initial diagnostic test, further radiographic follow-up should be performed (3).

TREATMENT

GENERAL MEASURES

- Goal is to return the athlete to pain-free participation in sports along with the prevention of further slippage and spondylolisthesis.
- Spondylolysis:
  - Cessation of sports for 3 mo is effective nonoperative treatment for symptomatic spondylolysis in young athletes (compliance is important) (6)[C].
  - Nonoperative treatment of activity restriction and bracing for up to 6 mo for acute spondylolysis results in successful pain relief in >80% of athletes (7).
  - Bracing:
    - Controversial
    - Can reduce gross body motion but is ineffective in controlling the lower lumbar intervertebral segments (most common location of spondylolysis) (6)
    - Satisfactory outcomes can be achieved with or without bracing (6).
    - Most suggest using the brace if initial conservative management fails.
    - Reported duration is variable (6 wk to 6 mo).
    - If used, should continue until patient is asymptomatic with all activities
    - Positive x-ray and negative bone scan demonstrates a chronic injury that usually does not need bracing.
  - For lesions with chronic features on CT, healing is unlikely; however, rest should continue until full resolution of symptoms (8).
  - Surgical intervention is indicated only for individuals who have failed >6 mo conservative management (9) or for advanced cases causing neural compromise.
  - Surgical intervention can include direct repair of the pars interarticularis (Buck screw, Scott wiring technique, and Morscher hook screw) or posterolateral fusion (4).
  - Direct pars repair may facilitate higher return to play (RTP) rates because it preserves spinal motion (7).
- Spondylolisthesis:
  - Low-grade slips (grades I and II) can often be treated conservatively (1).
  - For slips higher or equal to grade III, decision to treat surgically is controversial (1).
  - Higher grade listhesis (>50%), high slip angle (>55 degrees), slip progression, or any neurologic findings should be evaluated by a surgeon.
  - For cases of higher grade listhesis with canal stenosis, surgical intervention has been shown to provide longer lasting relief (10).
  - Standard surgical intervention for canal compromise is decompressive laminectomy with fusion (10).
  - Postoperative casting/bracing is not generally indicated.
  - Return to noncontact sports permissible

ADDITIONAL THERAPIES

Physical therapy:

- Initial treatment will include modalities followed by strengthening activity.
- Typical rehabilitation includes hamstring/hip stretching and core strengthening (low back, hip, and abdominal musculature) (3).
- Water therapy, including water running, is very helpful when available.
- Aerobic conditioning with progression to sport-specific drills

ONGOING CARE

FOLLOW-UP RECOMMENDATIONS

- Monitor symptoms, gait abnormalities, and radiographic progression of spondylolisthesis.
- In the skeletally immature, monitoring is more important because changes are common during growth (8).
- X-rays: data on the timing and frequency of follow-up x-rays are not clear. Some recommend plain x-ray every 6 to 12 mo in skeletally immature (8).
- Risk factors to consider when assessing for slip progression of listhesis:
  - Clinical factors: age (10 to 15 yr), gender (female), recurrent symptoms, and postural deformity (gait disturbances)
  - Radiographic factors: type of slip (dysplastic spondylolisthesis), high-grade slip (grade III/IV) that show progression, and high slip angle (5)

PROGNOSIS

- Most young athletes with symptomatic spondylolysis are successfully managed nonoperatively (3).
- Most patients with acute spondylolysis eventually will have mild to no symptoms with conservative treatment.
- Nonsurgical and surgical treatments of young athletes with symptomatic spondylolysis have shown high levels of RTP at 92.2% and 90.3%, respectively; however, surgery has associated risks (9).
- Progression of listhesis uncommon after age 20 yr, after ossification of growth plate (1)
- Progression of spondylolysis most likely in adolescents <16 yr old (2)
- Following fusion for spondylolysis/spondylolisthesis, return to noncontact sport permissible; however, there are varying opinions among surgeons regarding returning to contact sports (4)

REFERENCES

1. Gagnet P, Kern K, Andrews K, et al. Spondylolysis and spondylolisthesis: a review of the literature. *J Orthop*. 2018;15(2):404–407.
2. Leone A, Cianfoni A, Cerase A, et al. Lumbar spondylolysis: a review. *Skeletal Radiol*. 2011;40(6):683–700.
3. Koerner J, Radcliff K. Spondylolysis in the athlete. *Oper Tech Sports Med*. 2013;21(3):177–184.
4. Alfieri A, Gazzeri R, Prell J, et al. The current management of lumbar spondylolisthesis. *J Neurosurg Sci*. 2013;57(2):103–113.
5. Tallarico RA, Madom IA, Palumbo MA. Spondylolysis and spondylolisthesis in the athlete. *Sports Med Arthrosc Rev*. 2008;16(1):32–38.
6. El Rassi G, Takemitsu M, Glutting J, et al. Effect of sports modification on clinical outcome in children and adolescent athletes with symptomatic lumbar spondylolysis. *Am J Phys Med Rehabil*. 2013;92(12):1070–1074.
7. Cook R, Hsu W. Return to play after lumbar spine surgery. *Clin Sports Med*. 2016;35(4):609–619.
8. Standaert CJ, Herring SA. Expert opinion and controversies in sports and musculoskeletal medicine: the diagnosis and treatment of spondylolysis in adolescent athletes. *Arch Phys Med Rehabil*. 2007;88(4):537–540.
9. Overley SC, McAnany SJ, Andelman S, et al. Return to play in adolescent athletes with symptomatic spondylolysis without listhesis: a meta-analysis. *Global Spine J*. 2018;8(2):190–197.
10. Weinstein JN, Lurie JD, Tosteson TD, et al. Surgical compared with nonoperative treatment for lumbar degenerative spondylolisthesis. Four-year results in the Spine Patient Outcomes Research Trial (SPORT) randomized and observational cohorts. *J Bone Joint Surg Am*. 2009;91(6):1295–1304.

CLINICAL PEARLS

- Initial imaging for suspected spondylolysis or spondylolisthesis, in the absence of neurologic abnormalities, should be x-ray with AP and lateral views.
- SPECT scan is the most sensitive imaging modality in diagnosing spondylolysis; however, radiation exposure from SPECT surpasses that of CT (3).
- Bilateral spondylolysis can potentially progress to isthmic spondylolisthesis.
- Pars defect on x-ray with normal SPECT scan indicates inactive healed lesion or nonunion (3).
- Use of bracing for conservative management of spondylolysis is controversial. Most recommend using brace if initial conservative management fails.
- Important to assess for neurologic deficits in athletes with spondylolysis and spondylolisthesis

SPORTS HERNIAS

Warren Young, MD, FAAP • William W. Briner Jr., MD, FACSM, FAAFP, CAQSM

BASICS

DESCRIPTION

- The sports hernia is a syndrome of chronic pain owing to weakness or injury to the posterior inguinal canal, conjoined tendon, common adductor origin, external oblique aponeurosis, and/or rectus abdominis (1)[C].
- Typically described as an activity-related pain of either insidious or acute onset, predominantly in the lower abdominal or groin area with no other obvious pathology, such as a hernia, to explain the symptoms (2)[C]
- Historically considered to be an early direct inguinal hernia, but recent evidence shows that no true hernia exists. Therefore, the term *sports hernia* may in fact be considered a misnomer.
- Synonym(s): athletic pubalgia; sportsman's hernia; Gilmore groin; inguinal disruption; inguinal-related groin pain; footballer's groin; hockey groin syndrome

EPIDEMIOLOGY

Incidence

- Unknown
- Male predominance: accounts for >90% of cases
- Most common in soccer players but also described in football, hockey, baseball, and rugby players
- Mostly diagnosed in professional or high-level school athletes but increasingly also in recreational athletes

ETIOLOGY AND PATHOPHYSIOLOGY

Pathogenesis is unclear but:

- May be related to overuse with underlying muscle strength, balance, stability, or endurance inequality between a weaker abdominal musculature and a stronger hip adductor muscle group, leading to increased stress to inguinal wall structures.
- Posterior inguinal canal weakness seen in 85% of surgical cases.
- Multiple injured structures are often seen operatively, including:
  - Distal rectus abdominis.
  - Conjoint tendon.
  - External oblique aponeurosis.
  - Inguinal ligament.
  - Adductor longus muscle/tendon.

RISK FACTORS

Activities with sudden acceleration and deceleration, kicking, cutting, twisting, and turning

GENERAL PREVENTION

- Strength and conditioning programs that stress flexibility, core strength, and sport-specific movements have been suggested.
- There may be a strength imbalance of musculature below the pubic symphysis over muscles above, so abdominal oblique and rectus strengthening may be beneficial; however, research is currently lacking (1)[C].

COMMONLY ASSOCIATED CONDITIONS

- Groin pain is often multifactorial.
- High rate of coexisting adductor longus tendinosis and femoro-acetabular impingement (FAI)

DIAGNOSIS

HISTORY

- Activity-related lower abdominal and proximal adductor-related pain with quick acceleration, deceleration, kicking, twisting, or lateral movement
- Often occurs in soccer players from hard or long kicks
- Relieved with rest but returns with resumption of sports
- Often gradual in onset but may occur after sudden tearing sensation
- Early in course, pain is felt after activity or toward the end of activity.
- As condition progresses, pain is more severe and occurs earlier in activity. Decreased ability to twist, turn, or stride out is observed.
- Later in course, pain occurs with running and may progress to affect daily activities.
- Usually unilateral but may radiate to uninvolved side or scrotum.
- Exacerbated by sudden movements, sit-ups, coughing/sneezing, Valsalva maneuver
- Ask about hip joint–related mechanical symptoms including catching, locking, and giving way.

PHYSICAL EXAM

- Inversion of scrotal skin and palpation along inguinal canal is the essential physical exam technique.
- Diagnosis of sports hernia may be made if at least three of the following five signs exist (2)[C]:
  - Pinpoint tenderness to the pubic tubercle at conjoint tendon insertion
  - Tenderness over deep inguinal ring
  - Pain and/or dilation of the external ring with no palpable hernia
  - Pain at origin of adductor longus tendon
  - Dull diffuse groin pain often radiating to perineum and inner thigh or across the midline
- Complete exam for other causes of groin pain should be performed (3)[C]:
  - Hip adductor origin tenderness AND pain with resisted adduction suggest adductor-related groin pain.
  - Tenderness at pubic symphysis suggests pubic-related groin pain.
  - Pain with resisted hip flexion AND/OR stretching of hip flexors suggests iliopsoas-related groin pain.
  - Hip joint–related groin pain may elicit pain with passive range of motion (ROM); flexion, adduction, and internal rotation (FADIR); and flexion, abduction, external rotation (FABER) tests.
- Careful hip/genitourinary exam should be performed.

DIFFERENTIAL DIAGNOSIS

- Inguinal or femoral hernia
- Hip adductor strain
- Rectus abdominis strain
- FAI
- Osteitis pubis
- Bursitis
- Snapping hip syndrome
- Femoral neck stress fracture
- Pubic ramus fracture
- Hip apophysitis or avulsion fracture
- Nerve entrapment:
  - Obturator
  - Ilioinguinal
  - Genitofemoral
  - Iliohypogastric
- Referred pain from lumbar spine or sacroiliac joint
- Intra-articular hip pathology
- Testicular/ovarian pathology
- Spondyloarthropathy
- Lymphadenopathy

DIAGNOSTIC TESTS & INTERPRETATION

- Diagnostic imaging tests are not specific for sports hernia. Most will have no pathologic findings.
- Magnetic resonance imaging (MRI) is the advanced imaging modality most commonly performed.
- MRI may identify injury to structures associated with sports hernia and is also helpful to identify associated muscle, tendon, intra-articular pathology, or occult stress fracture.
- Plain radiographs can evaluate for fractures, degenerative disease, FAI, dysplasia, pubic symphysis asymmetry.
- Bone scan/computed tomography (CT) scan may identify stress fractures, osteitis pubis.
- Dynamic ultrasound may visualize posterior inguinal wall insufficiency, but it is highly operator dependent.
- Herniography is not recommended due to invasive nature and complication risk.

TREATMENT

GENERAL MEASURES

- Nonoperative treatment should be attempted prior to surgical consideration.
- Nonsurgical rehabilitation treatment:
  - Initial 6- to 8-wk period of rest with supportive care (nonsteroidal anti-inflammatory drugs [NSAIDs], ice, heat) followed by a 6-wk rehabilitation program with gradual return to sports activity
  - Initial focus on hip adductor stretching, then advancing to eccentric strengthening of abdominal oblique, rectus abdominis, and adductors, and then progressing to sports-specific functional exercise
  - Entire process may take as long as 2 to 3 mo.
- Ultrasound-guided injection to rectus abdominis insertion, conjoint tendon, or adductor tendon may be considered, but there is limited evidence for its efficacy.

SURGERY/OTHER PROCEDURES

- Surgery should be considered if nonoperative treatment fails after 3 or more months.
- Herniorrhaphy is the definitive treatment.
- Surgical techniques vary, but general principles are the repair of injured structures and decreasing tension.
- Open or laparoscopic surgical techniques have both been reported to be effective at similar rates.
- Laparoscopic technique theoretically allows for quicker recovery.
- Time to full return to sports ranges from 4 to 12 wk depending on type of surgery.
- Postsurgery: 80–95% rate of return to prior level of activity

REFERENCES

1. Elattar O, Choi H, Dills VD, et al. Groin injuries (athletic pubalgia) and return to play. *Sports Health*. 2016;8(4):313–323.
2. Sheen AJ, Stephenson BM, Lloyd DM, et al. "Treatment of the sportsman's groin": British Hernia Society's 2014 position statement based on the Manchester Consensus Conference. *Br J Sports Med*. 2014;48(14):1079–1087.
3. Weir A, Brukner P, Delahunt E, et al. Doha agreement meeting on terminology and definitions in groin pain in athletes. *Br J Sports Med*. 2015;49(12):768–774.

ADDITIONAL READING

- Khan W, Zoga A, Meyers WC. Magnetic resonance imaging of athletic pubalgia and the sports hernia: current understanding and practice. *Mag Reson Imaging Clin N Am*. 2013;21(1):97–110.
- Meyers WC, McKechnie A, Philippon MJ, et al. Experience with "sports hernia" spanning two decades. *Ann Surg*. 2008;248(4):656–665.

CLINICAL PEARLS

- A sports hernia is a weakness or injury of the posterior inguinal canal with no protrusion of bowel into the canal.
- There is no palpable hernia on exam.
- Symptoms are likely to resolve with prolonged rest. However, symptoms often recur with resumption of activity.
- Imaging for sports hernia is nonspecific and is primarily to rule out other causes of chronic groin pain.
- Surgery is indicated for failed nonoperative treatment.
- Groin pain is often multifactorial. Coexisting causes of groin pain such as FAI and adductor longus tendinosis should be concurrently addressed for best outcomes.

STERNOCLAVICULAR JOINT INJURY

Douglas Comeau, DO, CAQSM, FAAFP • Angelene M. Elliott, DO

BASICS

- The sternoclavicular joint (SCJ) is a saddle-type joint that participates in all movements of the upper extremity.
- The SCJ provides free movement of the clavicle in nearly all planes.
- The joint is weakest inferiorly and reinforced superiorly, anteriorly, and posteriorly by the interclavicular, anterior, and posterior sternoclavicular and costoclavicular ligaments.

DESCRIPTION

- SCJ injuries are graded into three types:
  - Grade I: incomplete tear or stretching of the sternoclavicular and costoclavicular ligaments; joint stability and minimal pain
  - Grade II: complete tear of the sternoclavicular ligament and a partial tear of the costoclavicular ligament secondary to an anterior or posterior subluxation of the clavicle from the manubrium; pain and swelling of joint with mild deformity
  - Grade III: complete rupture of the sternoclavicular and costoclavicular ligaments; massive pain, swelling, and deformity
- The ligaments and capsule of the SCJ contribute to its stability, making it one of the least dislocated joints in the body.
- Dislocations are primarily due to trauma from vehicular or athletic injuries (>80%); congenital dislocations are extremely rare.

EPIDEMIOLOGY

Incidence

- 1% of all dislocations; 3% of shoulder-girdle lesions (1)
- Overall incidence is higher in males than in females.
- Incidence is increased in young adult males.

ETIOLOGY AND PATHOPHYSIOLOGY

- *Anterior dislocation* is much more common than posterior dislocation (9:1 ratio):
  - Caused by an anterolateral force compressing the shoulder that rotates the shoulder backward and transmits stress to the joint
- *Posterior dislocation* is caused either from a direct anterior-to-posterior blow to the medial clavicle or from a posterolateral force compressing the shoulder followed by forward rolling.
- *Posterior dislocation is a surgical emergency and has an estimated 25% complication rate*:
  - Compression of trachea, esophagus, and great vessels in the mediastinum demand immediate reduction.

DIAGNOSIS

- Elicit mechanism of injury, time from injury, and initial symptoms.
- Respiratory, neurologic, and vascular assessments mandatory
- Appropriate analgesia for patient comfort

HISTORY

- Mechanism of injury: Direct trauma (motor vehicle accident, athletic injury), falls, and dislocations can also be secondary to congenital, degenerative, and inflammatory processes.
- Symptoms: chest and/or shoulder pain exacerbated by arm movement or by lying down, dyspnea, dysphagia, or paresthesias

PHYSICAL EXAM

- Patient presents with the affected arm foreshortened and supported across the chest by opposite hand.
- Inability to abduct or externally rotate the affected arm because of severe pain over sternoclavicular junction
- In *anterior dislocation*, medial end of the clavicle is visibly prominent, palpable, and may be fixed or mobile.
- In *posterior dislocation*, loss of normal inner prominence of the clavicular head may be masked by significant local swelling:
  - Head tilted toward injured side because of spasm of the sternocleidomastoid muscle
  - Venous congestion in the neck or upper extremities, diminished pulses on affected extremity, shortness of breath, hoarseness, dysphagia, or signs of shock may suggest life-threatening impingement of the posteriorly displaced clavicle on vascular structures in the mediastinum.
- Check vital signs and perform a complete neurovascular examination of the affected extremity.

Pediatric Considerations

- True dislocations of the SCJ are extremely rare in children because of the strong ligamentous attachments about the medial physis.
- The medial physeal growth plates of the clavicles may not be radiographically apparent until age 18 yr and generally fuse between ages 22 and 25 yr. It is the last physis to close.
- Presumed SCJ dislocations are often actually fractures through the medial physis.
- In patients <25 yr of age, SCJ dislocations are classified as Salter-Harris type I or type II fractures.

DIFFERENTIAL DIAGNOSIS

- Sternoclavicular sprain/subluxation
- Medial clavicle fracture
- Rib fracture
- Septic joint
- Osteoarthritis

DIAGNOSTIC TESTS & INTERPRETATION

- Routine radiographs can be difficult to interpret and may appear normal.
- In patients with posterior dislocations, a plain chest radiograph is needed to rule out possible pneumothorax.
- Rockwood view (serendipity view): a specialized view that allows for better visualization of the position of the medial clavicle:
  - X-ray beam aimed at manubrium in a 40 degrees caudal tilt
- Point of care ultrasound can be useful, especially for prompt diagnosis in posterior dislocations (2).
- Magnetic resonance imaging (MRI) can be used to distinguish a dislocation from a physeal injury in children and young adults.
- Computed tomography (CT) scan is the best study to evaluate the SCJ:
  - Useful in the emergency department (ED) when plain films are inconclusive
  - Accurately differentiates fractures from dislocations
  - Demonstrates the position of the medial end of the clavicle in relation to the structures in the mediastinum
  - Shows detailed anatomy of the structures of the thoracic outlet and mediastinum

TREATMENT

Pediatric Considerations

- During childhood, the medial physeal growth plate of the clavicle provides 80% of longitudinal bone growth.
- Fractures in the medial clavicle have tremendous capability for healing and remodeling.
- Nonunion and significant malunion rarely occur.
- Anteriorly displaced fractures of the medial clavicle that mimic SCJ dislocation can be placed in a figure-8 splint without reduction.
- Posteriorly displaced fractures uniformly require reduction and should be considered a surgical and orthopedic emergency.

- Prehospital:
  - The close proximity of the sternum and clavicle to vital structures of the neck and chest predispose patients with SCJ injuries to additional severe and life-threatening injuries.
  - Airway, breathing, and circulation (ABCs) must first be addressed in these patients.
  - Vital signs and an initial neurovascular examination should be completed.
  - For patients with isolated SCJ injuries, the affected extremity should be splinted and immobilized to stabilize the joint and minimize pain prior to transport to the hospital.
- ED treatment:
  - Grade I and II usually with conservative treatment (immobilization or early functional therapy) (3)
  - Grade III usually closed reduction and immobilization versus open reduction and internal fixation (3)
  - *Anterior dislocations* may be reduced in the ED (4)[A].
  - Conscious sedation is necessary for pain control and muscle relaxation.
  - A rolled towel is placed between the shoulder blades in the supine position:
    - Longitudinal traction is applied to the ipsilateral arm in the extended position with the shoulder abducted at 90 degrees.
    - An assistant can maintain gentle inward pressure over the displaced medial end of the clavicle.
    - After reduction, immobilization is achieved using a well-padded figure-8 dressing.
    - Many anterior dislocations remain unstable after reduction; however, open reduction and internal fixation is rarely indicated, as the deformity is mainly cosmetic without functional loss.
  - *Posterior dislocations* require prompt reduction, best achieved in the operating room (OR) under general anesthesia (4)[A]:
    - If an appropriate surgeon is not immediately available to reduce a posterior dislocation in the OR, reduction may be attempted in the ED to relieve serious airway, neurologic, or vascular compromise.
    - After adequate sedation, a small incision is made directly over the medial head of the clavicle.
    - A sterile towel clamp can carefully be used to encircle the medial clavicular head and gentle anterior traction applied to reduce the dislocation.
    - A surgical consultant should subsequently evaluate the patient.

MEDICATION

Anti-inflammatory agents and analgesics are the drugs of choice to decrease inflammation and reduce pain:

- Acetaminophen: 500 to 1,000 mg q6–8h PRN
- Ibuprofen: 400 to 800 mg q4–8h PRN with meals
- Acetaminophen 300 mg with codeine: 30 mg q6h PRN
- Propoxyphene and acetaminophen: 1 to 2 tablets q4h PRN
- Hydrocodone and acetaminophen: 1 to 2 tablets q4–6h PRN

ADMISSION, INPATIENT, AND NURSING CONSIDERATIONS

- Initial stabilization:
  - Patients in respiratory distress require endotracheal intubation and immediate reduction.
  - Emergent reduction is also needed in patients with hoarseness, dysphagia, or neurovascular compromise (upper extremity weakness, paresthesia, diminished pulses, signs of shock).
  - *Patients with posterior dislocations represent true orthopedic and surgical emergencies*, and appropriate consults should be obtained promptly.
  - Appropriate analgesia (e.g., narcotics or nonsteroidal anti-inflammatory drugs [NSAIDs]) necessary for pain control
- Admission criteria:
  - All posterior dislocations of the SCJ require admission for prompt reduction in the OR and evaluation for potential intrathoracic complications.
- Discharge criteria:
  - Anterior dislocations of the SCJ that can be reduced and splinted, in the absence of neurovascular compromise, may be discharged with appropriate orthopedic follow-up.

ONGOING CARE

FOLLOW-UP RECOMMENDATIONS

Patient Monitoring

- Patients with sprains should initially restrict activity, and depending on the amount of pain or discomfort, a sling can be used for immobilization.
- Reductions performed in the ED require stabilization of the affected shoulder with a soft figure 8 or sling; immobilization for 4 wk.
- Anterior dislocations should restrict activity and follow up with their physician as directed.
- Patients with posterior dislocations who are discharged home should return for medical care if they exhibit symptoms of mediastinal injury.

PROGNOSIS

Prognosis depends on extent and type of joint damage, but most patients have adequate upper extremity function following SCJ injuries.

COMPLICATIONS

- Tracheal rupture
- Pneumothorax
- Laceration of superior vena cava
- Occlusion of the subclavian artery
- Recurrent dislocation
- Deformity

REFERENCES

1. Boesmueller S, Wech M, Tiefenboeck TM, et al. Incidence, characteristics, and long-term follow-up of sternoclavicular injuries: an epidemiologic analysis of 92 cases. *J Trauma Acute Care Surg*. 2016;80(2):289–295.
2. Bengtzen RR, Petering RC. Point-of-care ultrasound diagnosis of posterior sternoclavicular joint dislocation. *J Emerg Med*. 2017;52(4):513–515.
3. Groh GI, Wirth MA. Management of traumatic sternoclavicular joint injuries. *J Am Acad Orthop Surg*. 2011;19(1):1–7.
4. Cope R, Riddervold HO, Shore JL, et al. Dislocations of the sternoclavicular joint: anatomic basis, etiologies, and radiologic diagnosis. *J Orthop Trauma*. 1991;5(3):379–384.

ADDITIONAL READING

- Bicos J, Nicholson GP. Treatment and results of sternoclavicular joint injuries. *Clin Sports Med*. 2003;22(2):359–370.
- Cope R. Dislocations of the sternoclavicular joint. *Skeletal Radiol*. 1993;22(4):233–238.
- Gardner MA, Bidstrup BP. Intrathoracic great vessel injury resulting from blunt chest trauma associated with posterior dislocation of the sternoclavicular joint. *Aust N Z J Surg*. 1983;53(5):427–430.
- Gobet R, Meuli M, Altermatt S, et al. Medial clavicular epiphysiolysis in children: the so-called sterno-clavicular dislocation. *Emerg Radiol*. 2004;10(5):252–255.
- Lewonowski K, Bassett GS. Complete posterior sternoclavicular epiphyseal separation. A case report and review of the literature. *Clin Orthop Relat Res*. 1992;(281):84–88.
- Winter J, Sterner S, Maurer D, et al. Retrosternal epiphyseal disruption of medial clavicle: case and review in children. *J Emerg Med*. 1989;7(1):9–13.

CLINICAL PEARLS

- SCJ injuries are graded (I, II, III) based on severity of tearing of associated ligaments.
- Dislocations are usually from trauma (direct blows/falls). Anterior dislocation is most common. Posterior dislocations are less common but require prompt reduction and is a surgical emergency.
- Physical exam may show swelling and deformity of SCJ, and athlete may have restricted shoulder motion in abduction and external rotation.
- Treatment for grade I and II is usually conservative. Grade III injuries may require surgery.

STRESS FRACTURES

Nicholas M. Cardinale, MD

BASICS

A stress fracture (SF) is damage to bone caused by repetitive loading that exceeds healing capacity. SF injury can range from a mild periosteal reaction to a displaced fracture. SFs are grouped as low or high risk. Low-risk stress fractures (LRSFs) occur in the pelvis, femoral shaft (FSSF), posteromedial tibia, fibula, metatarsal shafts, cuboid, calcaneus, and cuneiform. These can be treated nonoperatively. High-risk stress fractures (HRSFs) involve the femoral neck (FNSF), anterior tibial shaft (ATSF), patella, medial malleolus, 2nd metatarsal base, proximal 5th metatarsal, sesamoids, tarsal navicular, and talus. HRSFs have a greater risk of complications. Early advanced imaging and specialty referral is recommended; operative treatment is indicated in some cases. SFs occur in the pelvis and lower extremities in military recruits, endurance athletes, dancers, soccer, and basketball players. SFs may also occur in the spine and upper extremities in certain sports (e.g., football, gymnastics).

EPIDEMIOLOGY

Incidence

- Highest in female military recruits 21% (1)
- Incidence varies with activity/sport.

Prevalence

- >10% of all sports injuries (1,2)
- 90% involve the lower extremity (3).
- Tibia, tarsals, and metatarsals are the most common sites (4).

ETIOLOGY AND PATHOPHYSIOLOGY

- Repetitive load plus inadequate rest
- Bone resorption is faster than bone formation.
- Microfractures lead to cortical break.
- Anatomical sites of HRSFs have reduced vascularity and bear high tensile load.

Genetics

Genes that regulate bone remodeling have shown an association with SFs in recent studies. More research is needed to establish a clear genetic link.

RISK FACTORS

- Female gender
- Female body mass index (BMI) <19
- Late menarche ≥15 yr
- Prior SF
- Extreme pes cavus or planus
- >5 degrees knee valgus/external rotation (ER)
- Inadequate caloric intake
- Excessive caffeine, alcohol, or tobacco use
- Amenorrhea/oligomenorrhea
- Osteopenia
- Chronic corticosteroid use
- Rapid increase in training volume
- Recreational runners >25 miles per week
- Poor footwear
- Running on hard surfaces
- Low 25-hydroxyvitamin D
- Low testosterone (males)

GENERAL PREVENTION

- Adequate calories and nutrition
- 1,500 to 2,000 mg calcium and 800 IU vitamin D per day
- Screen for female athlete triad.
- Padded insoles and orthotics (military recruits)
- Replace footwear after 6 mo or 300 miles.
- Limit training increase to 10% per week (intensity, duration, frequency).

COMMONLY ASSOCIATED CONDITIONS

- Female athlete triad
- Chronic corticosteroid use
- Osteopenia/osteoporosis
- Amenorrhea/oligomenorrhea

DIAGNOSIS

HISTORY

- Insidious local pain from repetitive activity
- Worse with continued activity
- Pain at rest (e.g., night pain)
- Assess risk factors and training history (miles per week, intensity, frequency).
- Assess for prior history of SF.
- Nutrition history (dairy intolerance), reduced calorie intake, weight loss
- Menstrual irregularity or amenorrhea
- Corticosteroid use
- Osteopenia/osteoporosis

PHYSICAL EXAM

- Direct bony tenderness ± edema
- Palpate for callus or bony step off.
- Limp/pain on weight-bearing
- Pain with axial compression
- Tender "N" spot (dorsal central third of the navicular bone between the anterior tibial and hallucis longus tendons) suggestive of SF
- Calcaneal squeeze test: simultaneous pressure on the medial and lateral aspects of calcaneus, pain suggestive of SF
- Fulcrum test: pain at the site with bending the long bone over a table edge or examiner's leg or forearm; useful for tibial and FSSF
- Log roll test: Passive internal rotation (IR)/ER of the thigh elicits groin pain in an FNSF.
- Patellar-pubic percussion test: Place stethoscope on the ipsilateral pubic tubercle and percuss the ipsilateral patella or use a tuning fork; the sound is reduced on the side in which an FNSF is present.
- Flamingo test: Patient stands on the affected side. A positive test is indicated by pain in the location of the SF; useful for FNSF, FSSF, lower leg, and sacral SF
- Tuning fork test: pain when applying a 128-Hz tuning fork over the site of suspected SF; useful for tibia and fibula SFs
- Assess lower extremity alignment and foot type that would predispose to SF.

DIFFERENTIAL DIAGNOSIS

- Muscle strain/tendinopathy
- Fasciitis/periostitis
- Exertional compartment syndrome
- Nerve/artery entrapment
- Bone tumor
- FNSF may mimic adductor or hip flexor strain.
- ATSF can be confused with shin splints.
- Medial tibial SF can mimic anserine bursitis.

DIAGNOSTIC TESTS & INTERPRETATION

Initial Tests (lab, imaging)

- X-rays:
  - Initial test, low cost and available. Sensitivity is only 10–56% (4,5).
  - Repeat x-ray (2 to 3 wk) is 30–70% sensitive; lucency or callus formation visible
- Bone scan:
  - 74–100% sensitive but less specific and can be falsely positive with infection or tumor (4)
  - Time-consuming (3 to 4 hr) and radiation exposure (5)
- Computed tomography (CT) scan:
  - Less sensitive than bone scan or magnetic resonance imaging (MRI) and involves significant radiation
  - Bone scan combined with single photon emission CT may be more accurate than MRI for pars interarticularis SF (4).
- Diagnostic ultrasound:
  - May be useful for superficial structures like metatarsals with a sensitivity of 83% and specificity of 75% in small studies (4)
- MRI:
  - The gold standard with a sensitivity of 86–100% and specificity of 100% (1). Is preferred over bone scan (4,5). T1 images show a fracture line; T2 and Short tau inversion recovery images show marrow edema.
  - Excludes other diagnoses and can grade severity which can aid in prognosis (3)

- Obtain labs based on clinical suspicion of nutritional, endocrine, and metabolic factors.
- 25-OH vitamin D3, complete blood count (CBC), chem 7, calcium, thyroid-stimulating hormone (TSH), albumin, prealbumin, phosphate, and parathyroid hormone
- Females with menstrual dysfunction: follicle-stimulating hormone (FSH), luteinizing hormone (LH), estradiol, testosterone, human chorionic gonadotropin (HCG)
- Dexamethasone suppression test if excess cortisol suspected

Follow-Up Tests & Special Considerations

- X-rays are useful in follow-up to demonstrate callus formation and union.
- CT provides greater detail to assess healing.
- Bone scan remains positive for over a year and is not useful for follow-up.
- MRI may show positive findings after the patient is asymptomatic.

Diagnostic Procedures/Other

A bone biopsy may sometimes be obtained to differentiate tumor from SF.

TREATMENT

GENERAL MEASURES

- Stop the offending activity.
- Use a cast, pneumatic boot, rigid sole shoe, or crutches to ensure pain-free relative rest.
- A compression boot for tibial SFs leads to earlier return to play (4)[A].
- Allow progressive weight-bearing based on symptomatic improvement.

MEDICATION

- Acetaminophen and nonsteroidal anti-inflammatory drugs (NSAIDs) for pain
- Use NSAIDs cautiously due to potential inhibition of bone healing.
- Bisphosphonates are controversial for treatment and not recommended for prevention (1,4)[B].

ISSUES FOR REFERRAL

- Urgent orthopedic/sports medicine consultation for HRSFs
- Early advanced imaging of HRSFs is needed to avoid complications and provide timely surgery if needed.

ADDITIONAL THERAPIES

- Electromagnetic or ultrasonic bone stimulation may be considered for recalcitrant cases, but evidence is lacking for efficacy (4)[B].
- Extracorporeal shock wave therapy (ESWT) has shown benefit in small studies (randomized controlled trial [RCT] and case series) (6)[B].
- Gait training may help runners reduce impact which may help prevent SFs.

SURGERY/OTHER PROCEDURES

- FNSF tension side (superolateral femoral neck) requires emergent surgical fixation.
- Compression side involving <50% of the width of the inferomedial neck can be treated with prolonged weight-bearing rest (average of 12 wk to return to sport) (1,2,3).
- ATSF has a high rate of nonunion, and surgery is recommended if 3 to 6 mo of conservative treatment has failed.
- Navicular SFs are often treated surgically in elite athletes, but outcomes are comparable with nonoperative treatment (2)[B].
- Proximal 5th metatarsal SFs involving zones 2 or 3 (distal to the tuberosity) benefit from surgical fixation with reduced complications and earlier return to sport (2)[A].

ONGOING CARE

FOLLOW-UP RECOMMENDATIONS

- Athletes are typically followed every 2 to 4 wk to assess for symptomatic improvement and allow a gradual increase in weight-bearing. A progressive jogging protocol can be used for return to sport.
- Follow-up imaging is used in HRSFs and complicated cases. Athletes with LRSFs may be followed on the basis of clinical signs and symptoms without repeat imaging.

DIET

- Adequate calories, protein, and carbohydrates for age; body type and sport
- Daily calcium 2,000 mg and vitamin D 800 IU
- 50,000 IU vitamin D weekly ×12 if deficient

PATIENT EDUCATION

- Athletes should understand their individual intrinsic and extrinsic risk factors and modify when possible. Individualize training to reduce injury and optimize performance.
- Do not ignore pain symptoms and resist overtraining.

PROGNOSIS

- Excellent for most if treated early with adequate weight-bearing rest
- Poor for ATSF with evidence of cortical disruption (dreaded black line)
- Completed FNSF can be associated with long-term morbidity and disability.

COMPLICATIONS

Complete fracture, delayed union, nonunion, avascular necrosis

REFERENCES

1. DeFroda SF, Cameron KL, Posner M, et al. Bone stress injuries in the military: diagnosis, management, and prevention. *Am J Orthop (Belle Mead NJ)*. 2017;46(4):176–183.
2. McInnis KC, Ramey LN. High-risk stress fractures: diagnosis and management. *PM R*. 2016;8 (Suppl 3):S113–S124.
3. Robertson GA, Wood AM. Lower limb stress fractures in sport: optimising their management and outcome. *World J Orthop*. 2017;8(3):242–255.
4. Patel DS, Roth M, Kapil N. Stress fractures: diagnosis, treatment, and prevention. *Am Fam Physician*. 2011;83(1):39–46.
5. Nye NS, Covey CJ, Sheldon L, et al. Improving diagnostic accuracy and efficiency of suspected bone stress injuries. *Sports Health*. 2016;8(3): 278–283.
6. Leal C, D'Agostino C, Gomez Garcia S, et al. Current concepts of shockwave therapy in stress fractures. *Int J Surg*. 2015;24(Pt B):195–200.

ADDITIONAL READING

- Reiman MP, Mather RC III, Cook CE. Physical examination tests for hip dysfunction and injury. *Br J Sports Med*. 2015;49(6):357–361.
- Varley I, Greeves JP. Functional polymorphisms in the P2X7 receptor gene are associated with stress fracture injury. *Purinergic Signal*. 2016;12(1): 103–113.
- Zhao L, Chang Q, Huang T, et al. Prospective cohort study of the risk factors for stress fractures in Chinese male infantry recruits. *J Int Med Res*. 2016;44(4):787–795.

CLINICAL PEARLS

- Diagnosis is based on high index of suspicion, risk factors, and clinical findings. Negative x-rays do not exclude SFs.
- Obtain urgent advanced imaging in patients with antalgic gait and clinical findings consistent with a HRSF. Use of an algorithm may aid the diagnostic approach.
- MRI is the advanced imaging study of choice.
- HRSFs warrant orthopedic or sports medicine specialty evaluation.
- High-demand athletes may benefit from early surgery to ensure a more rapid return to play.

SUBCONJUNCTIVAL HEMORRHAGE

Holly Beach, MD, CAQSM

BASICS

DESCRIPTION

- Rupture of small vessels leading to an accumulation of blood in the subconjunctiva, the potential space between the conjunctiva and the sclera
- Synonym(s): conjunctival hemorrhage

EPIDEMIOLOGY

One of the most frequently encountered eye problems in primary care offices; accounted for 2.9% of visits to outpatient eye clinics in one study

RISK FACTORS

- Sudden increase in ocular pressure, which may result from coughing, sneezing, vomiting, or straining
- Uncontrolled hypertension (HTN)
- Acute conjunctivitis
- Vigorous eye rubbing
- Aspirin or other anticoagulant use
- Underlying hematologic or systemic disease

DIAGNOSIS

HISTORY

- No visual changes
- Eye trauma, including rubbing
- Use of aspirin or other anticoagulant
- Medical conditions leading to increased intraocular pressure or straining, including uncontrolled HTN, constipation, prostatic hypertrophy, cough, sneezing, and vomiting (1)[C]
- Exercise or activities involving exertional straining (i.e., weight lifting)
- Diagnosis of or symptoms suggestive of bleeding disorders, such as easy bruising, menorrhagia, and so forth

PHYSICAL EXAM

- Asymptomatic
- Extreme redness of eye without change in vision
- Extensive subconjunctival hemorrhage may cause a protruding sac of blood, possibly beyond the lid margin.
- Bright red area of blood, either focally or diffusely in potential space under conjunctiva
- Blood pressure (BP) measurement to evaluate for uncontrolled HTN
- Stigmata of bleeding or other hematologic disorders (petechiae, bruising, etc.)
- Associated signs suggestive of acute hemorrhagic conjunctivitis

DIFFERENTIAL DIAGNOSIS

- Acute hemorrhagic conjunctivitis: a highly contagious disease caused by enterovirus 70 and coxsackievirus A24. Pain, photophobia, blurred vision, and epiphora develop acutely, with 80% developing bilateral disease within 24 hr (2). Ocular signs may include subconjunctival hemorrhage as well as discharge, punctate corneal epithelial keratitis, and lid edema. Patients also may complain of fever, headache, upper respiratory infection symptoms, myalgia, and may have tender preauricular lymphadenopathy. Symptoms usually resolve without treatment over 5 to 7 days, with persistent subconjunctival hemorrhages resolving over an additional few weeks (3).
- Scleral rupture should be suspected in a post-traumatic patient with a bullous subconjunctival hemorrhage, especially in the presence of blood in the vitreous, decreased intraocular pressure, or a shallow anterior chamber.
- Orbital hemorrhage may present with massive subconjunctival hemorrhage as well as proptosis and limitation of extraocular movements, usually after trauma.
- Infrequently, adenoviral conjunctivitis, bacterial conjunctivitis, and even allergic conjunctivitis may present with an associated subconjunctival hemorrhage.

TREATMENT

GENERAL MEASURES

- Reassurance. No analgesia; condition is self-limited.
- Condition is nonpainful; the presence of pain should alert examiner to a more serious condition (4)[C].
- Topical steroids are contraindicated, especially with suspicion of acute hemorrhagic conjunctivitis, due to risk of clinical deterioration and permanent side effects.

ADDITIONAL THERAPIES

- Again, reassurance: Hemorrhages usually resolve spontaneously in 1 to 3 wk.
- Further treatment should be directed at reduction of risk factors and treatment of any identified underlying etiology (bleeding problems, HTN).
- Treat secondary bacterial conjunctivitis and allergic conjunctivitis, as indicated.

ONGOING CARE

FOLLOW-UP RECOMMENDATIONS

- Consider ophthalmology consultation if history of ocular trauma is present or in the presence of associated ocular injury (5)[C].
- Consider hematology consultation if hemorrhages are idiopathic and recurrent.

REFERENCES

1. Sahinoglu-Keskek N, Cevher S, Ergin A. Analysis of subconjunctival hemorrhage. *Pak J Med Sci*. 2013;29(1):132–134.
2. Wright PW, Strauss GH, Langford MP. Acute hemorrhagic conjunctivitis. *Am Fam Physician*. 1992;45(1):173–178.
3. Cronau H, Kankanala RR, Mauger T. Diagnosis and management of red eye in primary care. *Am Fam Physician*. 2010;81(2):137–144.
4. Micieli J, Easterbrook M. Eye and orbital injuries in sports. *Clin Sports Med*. 2017;36(2):299–314.
5. Tarlan B, Kiratli H. Subconjunctival hemorrhage: risk factors and potential indicators. *Clin Ophthalmol*. 2013;7:1163–1170.

ADDITIONAL READING

- Fukuyama J, Hayasaka S, Yamada K, et al. Causes of subconjunctival hemorrhage. *Ophthalmologica*. 1990;200(2):63–67.
- Goroll AH, May LA, Mulley AG, eds. *Primary Care Medicine: Office Evaluation and Management of the Adult Patient*. Philadelphia, PA: Lippincott; 1995.
- Kaimbo Wa Kaimbo D. Epidemiology of traumatic and spontaneous subconjunctival haemorrhages in Congo. *Bull Soc Belge Ophthalmol*. 2009;(311):31–36.
- Mimura T, Usui T, Yamagami S, et al. Subconjunctival hemorrhage and conjunctivochalasis. *Ophthalmology*. 2009;116(10):1880–1886.
- Pavan-Langston D, ed. *Manual of Ocular Diagnosis and Therapy*. 4th ed. Boston, MA: Little, Brown; 1996.

CLINICAL PEARLS

- Most cases resolve completely over the course of 1 to 3 wk (3).
- Only recurrent or persistent cases require evaluation by an ophthalmologist (1).

SUBUNGUAL EXOSTOSIS AND HEMATOMA

Daniel C. Herman, MD, PhD, FAAPMR, FACSM, CAQSM • Glenn H. Sapp II, MD

BASICS

DESCRIPTION

- Subungual exostosis: a chronic, benign, and osteocartilaginous growth from the distal phalanx's terminal tuft that commonly causes pain and/or deformity of the nail
- Subungual hematoma: an acute, traumatic subungual collection of blood appearing as a red, blue, or black discoloration, usually caused by a direct, blunt impact or chronic, repetitive stresses to the distal phalanx
- Synonym(s) for subungual hematoma: tennis toe; jogger's toe; sportsman's toe

EPIDEMIOLOGY

Subungual exostosis:

- Relatively uncommon (1)
- Typically, present during the 2nd and 3rd decades of life (1)
- No gender preference (1)
- Most commonly affects the great toe but may also occur at the lesser toes or fingers (1)

ETIOLOGY AND PATHOPHYSIOLOGY

- Subungual hematomas are seen more commonly in sports that require frequent pivoting, abrupt stops, or repetitive kicking (e.g., basketball, handball, racquet sports, soccer, football, running).
- Repeated contact of the toes with the front of the shoebox causes toenail dyshesion and subsequent hemorrhage (2).
- If the activity continues, it may lead to chronic nail dystrophy, nail loss, and callus formation of the tip of the toe (2).
- Trauma (e.g., fingertip slammed in a car door, hammer blow, or blunt trauma)

RISK FACTORS

The cause of subungual exostosis is currently unknown. The suggested causal factors include local trauma, irritation, chronic infection, or hereditary abnormality (1).

GENERAL PREVENTION

Subungual hematoma:

- Wearing well-fitted, task-appropriate footwear with a snug midfoot and a wide toe box (e.g., steel-toed shoes for construction workers)
- Using orthotic devices to prevent foot sliding
- Maintaining toenails trimmed straight across without curved edges

DIAGNOSIS

HISTORY

- Subungual exostosis: typically weeks to months history of toenail pain, a localized mass or swelling in the toenail, or shoe wear discomfort. Previous history may include trauma or infection (1,3).
- Subungual hematoma: an acute history of digital trauma with resultant nail discoloration and pain. Inquiry into participation in athletic activities and physical exertion may help ascertain inciting event (4).
- Other pertinent history includes whether the discoloration was present at birth or acquired.
- A medication history to identify drugs that may contribute to abnormal nail pigmentation or increased the risk of bleeding (4)

PHYSICAL EXAM

- Subungual exostosis:
  - Presence of a firm mass noted at the distal portion of the terminal phalanx
  - Pain is typically elicited on direct palpation.
  - Exostosis may protrude superiorly causing an onycholysis (elevated nail plate) or onychodystrophy (deformity or discoloration of the nail) (1).
  - Gait may be affected secondary to pain and swelling related to the exostosis.
- Subungual hematoma:
  - Collection of blood that appears as a reddish to blackish pigmentation, under the nail with or without edema/erythema
  - The pigment in a subungual hematoma is homogenous in distribution, whereas melanocytic lesions have cellular inclusions (4).
  - Observe for any extension of discoloration from under the nail plate into the proximal nail fold and nail matrix (Hutchinson melanotic whitlow sign); suspect subungual melanoma.
  - Variable pain presentation that can range from painless to extreme throbbing
  - Examine all 20 nail units, periungual skin, and oral mucosa for additional lesions (for signs of Peutz-Jeghers syndrome or Laugier-Hunziker syndrome) (4)[C].
  - May note a callus on the skin distal to the affected nail
  - Toes most likely affected in a sport-specific pattern are:
    - "Tennis toe": more commonly lateral nail of the hallux or 2nd toe, depending on which is longer.
    - "Jogger's toe": 2nd through 5th toes.
    - Kicking sports: 2nd or 3rd toe.

DIFFERENTIAL DIAGNOSIS

- Subungual exostosis (1):
  - Subungual osteochondroma: Histologically, exostosis has a fibrocartilage cap, and the osteochondroma has hyaline cartilage that is confluent with the underlying trabecular and cortical bone (1).
  - Fibroma
  - Subungual verruca vulgaris
  - Subungual squamous cell carcinoma
  - Glomus tumor
  - Enchondroma protuberans
  - Multiple exostosis: Consider an autosomal-dominant multiple exostosis syndrome.
- Subungual hematoma (4):
  - Subungual benign and malignant tumors (e.g., melanoma)
  - Onychomycosis
  - Glomus tumor
  - Subungual exostosis

DIAGNOSTIC TESTS & INTERPRETATION

Initial Tests (lab, imaging)

- Subungual exostosis:
  - Radiographs are the main diagnostic tool if a hard subungual mass is noted on examination.
  - Imaging will differentiate subungual exostosis, osteochondroma, and enchondroma (which can rarely affect the distal phalanx).
  - Radiographically, an exostosis appears as a pedunculated radiopaque mass on the dorsomedial surface of the distal phalanx. An exostosis also lacks clear contiguity of the medullary cavity and cortex, unlike an osteochondroma (5).
- Subungual hematoma:
  - Anteroposterior, lateral, and oblique radiographs should be obtained when a hematoma involves ≥50% of the visible nail to assess for fracture (6)[C].

Diagnostic Procedures/Other

A chronic nontraumatic lesion or a patient with a history of melanoma each may require a biopsy of the underlying nail matrix and/or nail bed to rule out a pigmented lesion (4)[C].

TREATMENT

- Subungual exostosis:
  - Excision of the tumor
- Subungual hematoma:
  - Immediate elevation and application of ice or immersion in ice water may reduce pain and bleeding.
  - An acute subungual hematoma can be evacuated by puncturing the nail plate overlying the hematoma using thermal cautery, laser, or a drill (i.e., 18-gauge needle, scalpel blade, dental bur) (6)[C].
  - Evacuation is performed by directing the preferred heated trephine perpendicular to the nail plate overlying the hematoma; slow and gentle pressure is applied until blood is expressed from the nail plate.
  - Nail removal if the normal architecture of the nail plate or its surrounding structures has been damaged (6)[C]
  - Wound and laceration repair if needed. Prophylactic antibiotics are not recommended (6)[C].

ISSUES FOR REFERRAL

Chronic nail lesions, patients with history of melanoma, and pigmented lesions involving the periungual should be referred for evaluation for the possibility of a subungual melanoma.

ONGOING CARE

FOLLOW-UP RECOMMENDATIONS

Further evaluation with radiographs (exclude exostosis) and possibly a biopsy are required when a suspected subungual hematoma does not grow out distally as the nail plate grows or if there is a recurrence of the hematoma (4).

PATIENT EDUCATION

Subungual hematoma:

- To prevent infection following a trephination of the hematoma, instruct the patient on proper wound care, including:
  - Observing and reporting any signs of infection.
  - Keeping the area clean and dry.
  - Avoidance of swimming, hot tub, and whirlpool use.
- Inform the patient that they may eventually lose the affected nail and a new nail will grow out, typically within 2 to 6 mo.
- Wear well-fitted footwear with a snug midfoot and a wide toe box.
- Keep nails trimmed.
- Orthotic devices if appropriate

PROGNOSIS

Prognosis for both a subungual exostosis and a hematoma is excellent.

COMPLICATIONS

- A recurrence of the exostosis secondary to an incomplete excision
- Onychodystrophy, the discoloration or malformation of a nail, may result from disruption of nail bed and matrix (1).
- Infection following excision of a subungual exostosis or an evacuation of a subungual hematoma
- Recurring subungual hematomas of the same nail bed secondary to repetitive trauma may predispose the nail bed to onychomycosis.

REFERENCES

1. DaCambra MP, Gupta SK, Ferri-de-Barros F. Subungual exostosis of the toes: a systematic review. *Clin Orthop Relat Res*. 2014;472(4):1251–1259.
2. Cordoro KM, Ganz JE. Training room management of medical conditions: sports dermatology. *Clin Sports Med*. 2005;24(3):565–598.
3. Başar H, Inanmaz ME, Başar B, et al. Protruded and nonprotruded subungual exostosis: differences in surgical approach. *Indian J Orthop*. 2014;48(1):49–52.
4. Braun RP, Baran R, Le Gal FA, et al. Diagnosis and management of nail pigmentations. *J Am Acad Dermatol*. 2007;56(5):835–847.
5. Murphey MD, Choi JJ, Kransdorf MJ, et al. Imaging of osteochondroma: variants and complications with radiologic-pathologic correlation. *Radiographics*. 2000;20(5):1407–1434.
6. Patel L. Management of simple nail bed lacerations and subungual hematomas in the emergency department. *Pediatr Emerg Care*. 2014;30(10):742–748.

CLINICAL PEARLS

- Remember that not all dark patches under the nail are subungual hematomas. Consider the diagnosis of melanoma and other tumors when the history of trauma and the physical examination are not consistent with a simple subungual hematoma.
- Chronic subungual hematomas can be a manifestation of child abuse. If history and exam are suspicious, please notify a member of social services if warranted.

SUDDEN CARDIAC ARREST: COMMOTIO CORDIS

Elizabeth A. Williams, DO

BASICS

ALERT

Early resuscitation with automated external defibrillator (AED)/defibrillation improves survival.

DESCRIPTION

Commotio cordis (CC), Latin for "disturbance of the heart," is blunt, nonpenetrating trauma to the precordium, which results in an irregular heart rhythm such as ventricular tachycardia or ventricular fibrillation (VF). This is a rare event but must be considered secondary to its lethal nature.

EPIDEMIOLOGY

- This condition occurs primarily in young males, with the highest incidence in sports such as baseball and hockey, although it has been reported in nearly all sports. It may occur in any sport when the sports person (male/female) is struck in the precordial region with a firm object such as a ball, puck, other player, and so on.
- CC was first described in 1763.
- More than half of reported cases occurred during competitive sporting events.
- The mean age is 15 ± 9 yr.
- 95% of cases were male (1).
- Youth baseball accounts for most of the cases.

Incidence

- 60–75% of reported CC events involve sports.
- Occurs mostly in competitive sports, with highest incidence in youth baseball
- Highest incidence of CC is seen in youth baseball with pitches of standard baseballs thrown at speeds between 30 and 50 mph.
- Velocities above and below this range did not seem to carry the same risk; faster speeds incurred risk of contusio cordis.

Prevalence

- There has been an increase in reported cases. The CC registry has >200 cases, and only 5 cases were reported prior to 1983 (1).
- Historically low prevalence (prior to 1983) possibly due to lack of recognition/underreporting
- 53% of cases occur during organized competitive sports, with total of 77% occurring with all sports participation.
- Estimated 10 to 20 per year

ETIOLOGY AND PATHOPHYSIOLOGY

- Several variables must combine for an impact to result in CC: type (size and hardness) of projectile, force of projectile, location of impact, and timing of impact in the cardiac cycle.
- Impact to the precordium during the vulnerable period of the repolarization upslope of the T wave (10 to 30 ms before the T-wave peak) may lead to VF. VF is the most common initial rhythm in CC (2).
- Low-energy impact directly over the heart, specifically over the center of the left ventricle (LV), carries the highest risk. Blows at noncardiac sites does not carry the same risk.
- Causative theories on predisposition to VF/CC include rapid rises in LV pressures to forces between 250 and 450 mm Hg that may potentiate the associated arrhythmia. Stretch channels may be activated due to associated myocardial stretch with impact, and potassium adenosine triphosphate channel activation has been implicated (2).
- Sympathetic activation occurring during sports participation may increase the likelihood of CC, but this has not been substantiated in research studies.

Genetics

- No specific genes or genetic conditions have been attributed to the condition.
- It is unclear why there is a male predilection for this condition. One possibility is increased male relative to female participation in competitive youth baseball.

RISK FACTORS

- Participation in competitive sports
- Maron et al. found a significantly increased risk of death when CC occurred during recreational activities or normal daily activities as compared to occurrence in organized competitive sports (1).
- Harder projectiles used in certain sports
- Smaller round objects (size of a golf ball) had greater risk of inducing VF than a larger object (size of a baseball), and the flat objects of equal weight did not induce VF (3).
- Younger age: postulated that younger people are at greater risk due to the increased compliance of their chest wall
- Prolonged corrected Q-T interval (QTc) may increase susceptibility.
- African Americans are 8 times less likely to survive when compared to white counterparts (1).

GENERAL PREVENTION

- The U.S. Consumer Product Safety Commission recommends use of softer "safety baseballs" to reduce the risk of soft tissue trauma. These "safety baseballs" reduced the risk of onset of VF after precordial impact in a swine model study, and there is a linear correlation between CC events and the relative hardness of a baseball (4)[B]. Safety balls may decrease the risk but do not eliminate it.
- Kumar et al. demonstrated that more effective chest protectors could be developed. In a swine model, they demonstrated reduced incidence of VF from 54% to 5% for certain chest protectors. The advancement of materials is believed to contribute to improved performance (5). The performance of the newer materials will need further evaluation once used in sport. Previously available barriers were shown to have little protective benefit.
- National Operating Committee on Standards for Athletic Equipment (NOCSAE) updated its criteria for testing chest guards in February of 2018 in attempts to produce more effective chest protectors.
- Changes in coaching techniques to eliminate chest blocking are theorized to potentially reduce CC events.
- Public health measures, such as youth, parents, and coaches learning cardiopulmonary resuscitation (CPR), and the increased availability and use of AED may provide the biggest impact on improving CC outcomes, recognizing this does not prevent CC.

COMMONLY ASSOCIATED CONDITIONS

- Contusio cordis (myocardial contusion with tissue damage)
- Rule out other causes of sudden cardiac death (SCD) causing arrhythmia such as hypertrophic cardiomyopathy (HCM).

DIAGNOSIS

HISTORY

Witnessed trauma to the precordium followed by collapse should elicit suspicion of CC:

- There may be a delay from impact to collapse.

PHYSICAL EXAM

- In the setting of collapse, any physical exam should be focused on brief assessment of pulse and, if absent, initiating CPR with use of AED as soon as possible. CC is a diagnosis made based on witnessed precordial blow and confirmed by AED recognition of subsequent arrhythmia.

- There are no specific labs/imaging tests to aid in diagnosis.
- Note: There may be a brief period of consciousness after impact and before collapse; must maintain a high level of suspicion
- Pathologic findings:
  - Autopsy is notable for absence of any significant cardiac or thoracic injury.

DIFFERENTIAL DIAGNOSIS

- HCM
- Anomalous coronary artery
- Long QT syndrome
- Wolff-Parkinson-White syndrome
- Arrhythmogenic right ventricle dysplasia
- Brugada syndrome
- Dilated cardiomyopathy
- Ruptured/dissected aorta
- Severe aortic valve stenosis
- Mitral valve prolapse
- Coronary artery disease
- Asthma
- Heat stroke
- Drug abuse

TREATMENT

Treatment consists of immediate institution of basic life support (BLS)/advanced cardiac life support (ACLS) protocols, including implementation of an AED. Early defibrillation is critical to survival with CC. Increased survival if defibrillated within 3 min of collapse. Survival has been reported up to 58% most likely due to increased availability of AEDs (1)[C].

ADDITIONAL THERAPIES

All CC survivors should be referred to a cardiologist for a complete cardiac evaluation to investigate for structural heart disease (i.e., electrocardiogram [ECG], echocardiogram, cardiac magnetic resonance imaging [MRI], ambulatory ECG monitoring, stress testing). Additional testing to investigate for Brugada and long QT syndromes with pharmacologic testing is case dependent (6)[C].

ONGOING CARE

FOLLOW-UP RECOMMENDATIONS

Patient Monitoring

- All patients should be admitted to the hospital for observation and monitoring after the event.
- Patients should be followed after discharge to assess for potential cardiac or neurologic deficit.

PATIENT EDUCATION

- An individual athlete's susceptibility to CC should be considered in any return to play decisions regarding contact sports.
- Decisions are made on a case-by-case basis, with consideration given to residual cardiac deficit, neurologic deficit, or other morbidity. Cardiology consultation should be involved in these decisions (6)[C].
- Maron et al. demonstrated that 71% of CC survivors achieved complete physical recovery.

PROGNOSIS

- CC is a condition that carries a grave prognosis. Despite use of BLS/ACLS protocols, the condition is often lethal.
- Use of an AED has been found to be an independent predictor of survival (1).
- Sustaining blunt cardiac trauma while participating during organized competitive sporting activity was found to be an independent predictor of survival (1).

COMPLICATIONS

- Neurologic impairment may occur secondary to cerebral hypoperfusion.
- Cardiac sequela resulting in decreased left ventricular ejection fraction

REFERENCES

1. Maron BJ, Haas TS, Ahluwalia A, et al. Increasing survival rate from commotio cordis. *Heart Rhythm*. 2013;10(2):219–223.
2. Krexi L, Sheppard MN. Blow/trauma to the chest and sudden cardiac death: commotio cordis and contusio cordis are leading causes [published online ahead of print January 1, 2018]. *Med Sci Law*. doi:10.1177/0025802418754961.
3. Kalin J, Madias C, Alsheikh-Ali AA, et al. Reduced diameter spheres increases the risk of chest blow-induced ventricular fibrillation (commotio cordis). *Heart Rhythm*. 2011;8(10):1578–1581.
4. Doerer JJ, Haas TS, Estes NA III, et al. Evaluation of chest barriers for protection against sudden death due to commotio cordis. *Am J Cardiol*. 2007; 99(6):857–859.
5. Kumar K, Mandleywala S, Gannon M, et al. Development of a chest wall protector effective in preventing sudden cardiac death by chest wall impact (commotio cordis). *Clin J Sport Med*. 2017;27(1):26–30.
6. Link MS, Estes NA III, Maron BJ, et al. Eligibility and disqualification recommendations for competitive athletes with cardiovascular abnormalities: Task Force 13: commotio cordis: a scientific statement from the American Heart Association and American College of Cardiology. *Circulation*. 2015;132(22):e339–e342.

ADDITIONAL READING

- Alsheikh-Ali AA, Madias C, Supran S, et al. Marked variability in susceptibility to ventricular fibrillation in an experimental commotio cordis model. *Circulation*. 2010;122(24):2499–2504.
- Huis In 't Veld MA, Craft CA, Hood RE. Blunt cardiac trauma review. *Cardiol Clin*. 2018;36(1):183–191.
- Link MS. Commotio cordis: ventricular fibrillation triggered by chest impact-induced abnormalities in repolarization. *Circ Arrhythm Electrophysiol*. 2012; 5(2):425–432.
- Link MS, Maron BJ, Wang PJ, et al. Upper and lower limits of vulnerability to sudden arrhythmic death with chest-wall impact (commotio cordis). *J Am Coll Cardiol*. 2003;41(1):99–104.
- Maron BJ, Doerer JJ, Haas TS, et al. Sudden deaths in young competitive athletes: analysis of 1866 deaths in the United States, 1980–2006. *Circulation*. 2009; 119(8):1085–1092.
- Palacio LE, Link MS. Commotio cordis. *Sports Health*. 2009;1(2):174–179.
- Sharma N, Andrews S. Commotio cordis. *Br J Hosp Med (Lond)*. 2009;70(1):48–49.
- The National Registry of Sudden Death in Young Athletes: www.suddendeathathletes.org

S

CLINICAL PEARLS

- Witnessed precordial impact to a young athlete with resultant distress/collapse should elicit consideration of CC. Immediate institution of BLS/ACLS protocols with use of AED provides the best chance of survival.
- Use of age-appropriate safety baseballs has been shown to reduce CC events.
- Chest wall protective devices should be used in high-risk positions (catchers/goalies) but have not been proven to prevent CC. Newer materials show promise of being more effective in prevention of CC based on animal models.
- Thorough evaluation of all CC survivors should be undertaken, with return to play considerations made on a case-by-case basis.
- Awareness and availability of AED has increased survival rate; nevertheless, there is still a high mortality rate.

SUPERFICIAL RADIAL NERVE (WARTENBERG DISEASE)

Timothy Ryan Draper, DO, ABFM, CAQSM • Karl B. Fields, MD, CAQ

BASICS

DESCRIPTION

- Compression mononeuropathy of the superficial branch of radial nerve in the distal forearm
- Radial nerve, arises from C5–C8, provides motor function to the extensors of the forearm, wrist, and fingers and motor function for supinators of forearm. Superficial radial nerve (SRN) provides sensory function to posterior forearm via posterior cutaneous nerve and the web of skin between the thumb and index finger.
- SRN becomes susceptible to injury as it passes beneath the tendon of the Brachioradialis, and, pierces the deep fascia.
- Synonym(s): Wartenberg syndrome entrapment; cheiralgia paresthetica; prisoner's palsy; handcuff disease; radial sensory nerve entrapment

EPIDEMIOLOGY

- The incidence is not known.
- It is rare, although often is not recognized.
- More common in women

RISK FACTORS

- Wrist compression (i.e., tight bands, tape, watches, archery guards, gloves, or straps of a racquetball racquet, cast, soft tissue mass)
- Direct trauma in contact sports
- Laceration and postsurgical injury
- Sports involving repetitive pronation and supination at the wrist (e.g., batting, throwing, and rowing)

COMMONLY ASSOCIATED CONDITIONS

de Quervain syndrome

DIAGNOSIS

HISTORY

- Determine whether pain or sensory deficit is the primary symptom. If pain is the main complaint, then de Quervain syndrome seems a more likely diagnosis (1)[C].
- Duration of symptoms
- Location of symptoms
- Characteristics of symptoms to suggest sensory involvement

PHYSICAL EXAM

- Symptoms primarily limited to the dorsoradial aspect of the distal forearm and hand (wrist, hand, dorsal thumb, and index finger)
- Paresthesias (numbness and tingling)
- Hyperesthesia
- Less commonly, pain or burning
- Positive Tinel sign along the radial aspect of the midforearm
- Wrist flexion, ulnar deviation, and pronation place traction on the nerve and increase symptoms.
- Sensation deficit on the dorsoradial aspect of the forearm and/or hand
- Finkelstein test typically negative, as opposed to de Quervain syndrome, which usually has positive Finkelstein test
- With SRN injury, pain can be present with thumb abduction and adduction, differentiating this from de Quervain syndrome in which extension and flexion create more symptoms.
- Diagnostic nerve block to the cutaneous nerve in the proximal forearm just distal to the cubital crease and adjacent to the cephalic vein may help define its contribution to any pathology.
- Lidocaine test: This test is effective because the terminal branch of the lateral antebrachial cutaneous nerve (LACBN) often shares distribution with the SRN, its compression can mimic that involving the SRN.
- Nerve conduction study (NCS) may be useful for diagnosis (2)[C].
- The most common technique records the sensory nerve action potentials from the web space between the thumb and index finger with stimulation originating in the distal forearm.
- Ideally, it is preferable to perform NCS on both the SRN and the LACBN (3)[C].
- Sensory action potential, conduction velocity, and amplitude are decreased.
- Motor testing of radial nerve is normal.

DIFFERENTIAL DIAGNOSIS

- de Quervain syndrome
- Intersection syndrome
- Lateral antebrachial cutaneous neuropathy
- Thumb carpometacarpal arthritis
- C6 radiculopathy

TREATMENT

GENERAL MEASURES

- Almost all patients do well with conservative treatment.
- Remove constricting bands/devices.
- Avoid repetitive trauma to the area. Consider padding the area if unable to avoid trauma during the athletic season.
- Avoid repetitive pronation, wrist flexion, and ulnar deviation.
- Thumb spica splint for brief period of immobilization may be needed.
- Nonsteroidal anti-inflammatory drugs (NSAIDs)
- Steroid injection and anesthetic in the area of maximum pain can be helpful.
- Desensitization
- No information exists about neuropathic pain agents, and use of vitamin B_6 is anecdotal.

COMPLEMENTARY & ALTERNATIVE MEDICINE

No studies of acupuncture or other alternative products reported

SURGERY/OTHER PROCEDURES

If conservative treatment fails, then surgical decompression should be considered (4)[C].

REFERENCES

1. Dang AC, Rodner CM. Unusual compression neuropathies of the forearm, part I: radial nerve. *J Hand Surg*. 2009;34(10):1906–1914.
2. Cho NS, Kim KH, Park BK, et al. Superficial radial sensory neuropathy: medial and lateral branch injury. *Muscle Nerve*. 2016;53(5):690–693.
3. Kon T, Suzuki C, Hotta R, et al. Utility of nerve conduction studies for diagnosis of injury to the medial branch of the superficial radial nerve. *eNeurologicalSci*. 2017;8:38–39.
4. Spies CK, Unglaub F, Müller LP, et al. Endoscopically assisted release of the superficial radial nerve. *Arch Orthop Trauma Surg*. 2015;135(5):737–741.

ADDITIONAL READING

- Anto C, Aradhya P. Clinical diagnosis of peripheral nerve compression in the upper extremity. *Orthop Clin North Am*. 1996;27(2):227–236.
- Nuber GW, Assenmacher J, Bowen MK. Neurovascular problems in the forearm, wrist, and hand. *Clin Sports Med*. 1998;17(3):585–610.
- Plancher KD, Peterson RK, Steichen JB. Compressive neuropathies and tendinopathies in the athletic elbow and wrist. *Clin Sports Med*. 1996;15(2):331–371.
- Terrono AL, Millender LH. Management of work-related upper-extremity nerve entrapments. *Orthop Clin North Am*. 1996;27(4):783–793.

CLINICAL PEARLS

- If the symptoms are present >3 days, the neurapraxic injury may require up to 3 mo to reach maximum improvement.
- The splint usually needs to be worn 2 to 4 wk or until symptoms resolve.
- The protective padding needs to be worn until symptoms resolve or if engaging in sports with repetitive forearm trauma.

SUPRASCAPULAR NERVE PALSY

Philip H. Cohen, MD, CSQSM • James C. Puffer, MD

BASICS

EPIDEMIOLOGY

- Relatively uncommon; true incidence unknown
- May occur in up to 45% of international-level volleyball players (1)
- Ganglion cyst found at spinoglenoid notch in 1% of cadavers in one study
- Spinoglenoid ligament present in 50–60% of shoulders
- Suprascapular neuropathy in 7% of athletes with peripheral nerve injuries (1,2)

RISK FACTORS

- More common in volleyball players and overhead throwing athletes, possibly owing to traction injury or scar formation from overuse
- May be particularly associated with "floating serve" in volleyball, which requires intense eccentric contraction of infraspinatus to decelerate the arm and stabilize the shoulder; this can stretch the suprascapular nerve across the lateral edges of the scapular spine.
- Sudden downward depression of shoulder (traction injury to nerve near plexus origin)
- Compression by ganglion cyst, tumor, posttraumatic calcification, vascular malformation, or ligament at scapular or spinoglenoid notch
- Direct trauma (e.g., scapular fracture)
- Iatrogenic injury (e.g., during repair of massive rotator cuff tear, superior labrum anterior and posterior [SLAP] tear, distal clavicle excision, or reverse total shoulder arthroplasty)
- Possible traction injury caused by retraction of massive rotator cuff tear (1,2,3)

ETIOLOGY AND PATHOPHYSIOLOGY

- Suprascapular nerve arises from the upper trunk of the brachial plexus at Erb point, carrying fibers from the C5 and C6 nerve roots with variable contributions from C4.
- It crosses the posterior triangle of the neck, runs deep to the trapezius, and passes under the transverse scapular ligament via the scapular notch.
- Crossing the supraspinatus fossa, it sends two branches to the supraspinatus and sensory branches to the acromioclavicular and glenohumeral joints.
- The nerve makes a sharp turn around the spinoglenoid notch and passes into the infraspinatus fossa, where its branches terminate.
- Three main sites of injury:
  - Scapular notch
  - Spinoglenoid notch
  - Near the origin from the upper trunk of brachial plexus (1,2,3)

DIAGNOSIS

HISTORY

- Traumatic versus atraumatic? May yield clues to mechanism of injury; traction injury caused by blunt trauma has a good prognosis.
- Painful versus painless? Painless weakness suggests distal lesion.
- Overhead-throwing athlete? If yes, this may increase risk of suprascapular nerve lesion.

PHYSICAL EXAM

- Signs and symptoms depend on level of injury.
- If proximal, may have posterior/lateral shoulder pain along with weakness and atrophy of supraspinatus and infraspinatus
- If lesion is distal to sensory branches at spinoglenoid notch, painless, isolated infraspinatus atrophy and weakness of external rotation may be seen.
- Inspection is key. Look for supraspinatus and/or (especially) infraspinatus atrophy.
- Rule out cervical radiculopathy and other cervical (C)-spine pathology (complete neck exam, including the Spurling maneuver).
- External rotation testing against resistance to evaluate infraspinatus strength
- Jobe test to evaluate supraspinatus strength
- Complete neurologic examination to determine type, origin, and extent of injury; note that deep tendon reflexes should not be affected in isolated suprascapular neuropathy.
- Thorough shoulder examination to evaluate for associated injury
- Tenderness to palpation at scapular notch present in up to 77% of patients
- Cross-body adduction test (forward flexed arm externally rotated and adducted across body) puts tension on suprascapular nerve at spinoglenoid notch; may help to differentiate from rotator cuff lesion
- Injection into scapular notch may help to determine source of pain but is rarely necessary.

DIFFERENTIAL DIAGNOSIS

- Cervical radiculopathy
- Brachial plexopathy/"stinger"
- Rotator cuff tendonitis/tear
- Labral pathology
- Parsonage-Turner syndrome/neuritis

DIAGNOSTIC TESTS & INTERPRETATION

Initial Tests (lab, imaging)

- Plain films of the neck and shoulder evaluate for bony abnormalities.
- 30-degree cephalic tilt view helps to visualize the scapular notch; obtain especially if scapular fracture (1,3,4).
- 3.0 T magnetic resonance neurography (MRN) may now be noninvasive gold standard because it can image the nerve directly as well as compressive lesions (tumors, cysts) and mimics (C-spine disease causing radiculopathy, brachial neuritis/plexopathy, rotator cuff tear with fibrofatty replacement, etc.) (4).
- Ultrasound (US) can be useful in detecting compressive lesions affecting the suprascapular nerve; it also can be quickly used to evaluate the rest of the shoulder girdle during the same exam. However, it is extremely operator dependent (1).

Diagnostic Procedures/Other

- Electromyography of entire shoulder girdle
- Nerve conduction velocity studies from Erb point to the supraspinatus, with comparison to unaffected side (1,3)
- Wait minimum 3 to 4 wk after onset of complaint before neurodiagnostics because false-negative results may occur if done earlier.

TREATMENT

Unless there is a well-defined lesion causing suprascapular nerve compression, nonoperative therapy is recommended (1,3),(5,6)[B]. This includes:

- Rest from overhead movements/throwing/exacerbating activities.
- Physical therapy to strengthen external rotation and stabilize scapula.
- Nonsteroidal anti-inflammatory drugs (NSAIDs) or analgesics if warranted.

SURGERY/OTHER PROCEDURES

- If labral tear with associated ganglion cyst causes symptoms, repair/débridement of labral tear may allow cyst to resolve, thereby relieving pressure on the suprascapular nerve (1,3),(5,6)[B].
- US- or computed tomography (CT)-guided cyst aspiration has been reported.
- Repair of massive rotator cuff tear may relieve traction on suprascapular nerve (3).

ONGOING CARE

COMPLICATIONS

- Ganglion cysts at the spinoglenoid notch may be secondary to labral injuries, especially SLAP lesions.
- Secondary impingement may develop owing to loss of supraspinatus/infraspinatus function.

REFERENCES

1. Safran MR. Nerve injury about the shoulder in athletes, part 1: suprascapular nerve and axillary nerve. *Am J Sports Med*. 2004;32(3):803–819.
2. Toth C. Peripheral nerve injuries attributable to sport and recreation. *Neurol Clin*. 2008;26(1):89–113.
3. Kostretzis L, Theodoroudis I, Boutsiadis A, et al. Suprascapular nerve pathology: a review of the literature. *Open Orthop J*. 2017;11:140–153.
4. Ahlawat S, Wadhwa V, Belzberg AJ, et al. Spectrum of suprascapular nerve lesions: normal and abnormal neuromuscular imaging appearances on 3-T MR neurography. *AJR Am J Roentgenol*. 2015;204(3):589–601.
5. Memon M, Kay J, Ginsberg L, et al. Arthroscopic management of suprascapular neuropathy of the shoulder improves pain and functional outcomes with minimal complication rates. *Knee Surg Sports Traumatol Arthrosc*. 2018;26(1):240–266.
6. Momaya AM, Kwapisz A, Choate WS, et al. Clinical outcomes of suprascapular nerve decompression: a systematic review. *J Shoulder Elbow Surg*. 2018;27(1):172–180.

CLINICAL PEARLS

- Return to play depends on severity and cause of the neuropathy. As strength increases and atrophy and symptoms resolve, a gradual return to play may be initiated.
- Return of muscle strength usually occurs over time once the cause of the injury has been treated. However, especially with long-standing, severe lesions, muscle atrophy may not fully resolve.

SURFER'S EAR

Matthew J. Jepson, MD, MS • Tenley Murphy, MD, FAAFP, CAQSM • Jason J. Stacy, MD

BASICS

- Surfer's ear, or external auditory exostosis, is a benign overgrowth of the temporal bone in the external auditory meatus that occurs after prolonged exposure to cold water.
- Patients are usually asymptomatic but may present with recurrent ear infections, conductive hearing loss, and/or pain.

DESCRIPTION

- Benign overgrowth of temporal bone into external auditory meatus
- Usually bilateral
- May have multiple exostoses in a canal
- Occurs after prolonged exposure to cold water

EPIDEMIOLOGY

Rates are highly correlated with time spent in the associated activities. Typically, condition becomes symptomatic after 5 to 7 yr of surfing or other cold-water activities with development of exostoses in 90% of cold-water surfers at 10 yr (1,2).

Prevalence

Prevalence increases with time spent in the associated activities. Surfers have higher rates of exostoses with increasing years of surfing experience (3).

ETIOLOGY AND PATHOPHYSIOLOGY

Regular irritation of the auditory meatus by exposure to cold water was implicated in the causation of exostoses. Increasing size of exostoses can lead to recurrent infections, conductive hearing loss, and/or pain.

RISK FACTORS

- Occurs after prolonged and/or repetitive exposure to cold water (1,3)
- Most common in surfing; also seen in kayaking, white water rafting, diving (breath holding and scuba), and so on (4)

GENERAL PREVENTION

- Best method of prevention is molded earplugs worn during activity.
- Special headbands that cover ears are also preventive.
- Earplugs and headbands may be used in combination.

COMMONLY ASSOCIATED CONDITIONS

- Otitis externa
- Furunculosis
- Acute cellulitis
- Rare: perichondritis, chondritis, bullous myringitis

DIAGNOSIS

- Visual diagnosis during otoscopic exam
- Weber and Rinne test to evaluate for conductive hearing loss

HISTORY

Key points:

- Amount of cold-water exposure
- Use of preventive aids
- Previous surgeries
- Presence of recurrent infections or progressive hearing loss

DIFFERENTIAL DIAGNOSIS

- Fibrous dysplasia
- Otitis externa
- Acute otitis media
- Cholesteatoma
- Osteoma
- Mastoiditis
- Referred pain
- Temporomandibular joint syndrome

TREATMENT

MEDICATION

Medications typically are not needed, unless to treat related bacterial infection or cerumen impaction.

ISSUES FOR REFERRAL

- Referral to audiology to establish degree of hearing loss
- Referral to ear, nose, and throat (ENT) specialist indicated for recurrent infections, pain, or hearing loss (5)[B]

SURGERY/OTHER PROCEDURES

- Surgery is definitive care for exostoses.
- Reserved for severe, symptomatic cases; presence of exostoses without symptoms would not necessitate surgical intervention.
- Several approaches are used; postauricular is the most common and seems to minimize complications (5)[B].
- Transcanal approaches are being revisited because the use of an endoscope allows for this lower morbidity approach while lowering risk of damage to the tympanic membrane or facial nerve (6)[C].
- If hearing loss is present, generally, there is a good response to surgery with restored hearing.
- Some patients require repeated surgeries if cold-water exposure continues (usually after ≥5 yr of additional exposure).

ONGOING CARE

PROGNOSIS

Correctable with surgery but may recur with continued exposure

REFERENCES

1. Alexander V, Lau A, Beaumont E, et al. The effects of surfing behaviour on the development of external auditory canal exostosis. *Eur Arch Otorhinolaryngol*. 2015;272(7):1643–1649.
2. Chaplin JM, Stewart IA. The prevalence of exostoses in the external auditory meatus of surfers. *Clin Otolaryngol Allied Sci*. 1998;23(4):326–330.
3. Lennon P, Murphy C, Fennessy B, et al. Auditory canal exostoses in Irish surfers. *Ir J Med Sci*. 2016;185(1):183–187.
4. Sheard PW, Doherty M. Prevalence and severity of external auditory exostoses in breath-hold divers. *J Laryngol Otol*. 2008;122(11):1162–1167.
5. House JW, Wilkinson EP. External auditory exostoses: evaluation and treatment. *Otolaryngol Head Neck Surg*. 2008;138(5):672–678.
6. Kozin ED, Remenschneider AK, Shah PV, et al. Endoscopic transcanal removal of symptomatic external auditory canal exostoses. *Am J Otolaryngol*. 2015;36(2):283–286.

ADDITIONAL READING

Cooper A, Tong R, Neil R, et al. External auditory canal exostoses in white water kayakers. *Br J Sports Med*. 2010;44(2):144–147.

CLINICAL PEARLS

- Benign bony overgrowth of the temporal bone into the external auditory meatus
- Causes repeated ear infections, hearing loss, or pain in surfers (or other cold-water athletes)
- Preventable with earplugs and/or headbands
- Surgery is definitive treatment when hearing loss is present.

S

SWIMMING-INDUCED PULMONARY EDEMA (SIPE)

James Suchy, MD • Caitlyn C. Mooney, MD, FAAP, CAQSM

BASICS

DESCRIPTION

- Acute onset of respiratory symptoms, such as dyspnea, cough, chest pain/tightness, hemoptysis with potential for respiratory failure due to the leakage of fluid from the pulmonary capillaries into the alveoli, during physical activity in water
- SIPE can range in severity from mild symptoms that quickly self-resolve to potentially life-threatening respiratory failure.
- Synonym: immersion pulmonary edema (IPE)

EPIDEMIOLOGY

Incidence

- First described in healthy scuba divers in the 1980s
- Hundreds of cases involving triathletes, swimmers, snorkelers, free divers, and scuba divers have been reported in the scientific literature.
- A rise in case reports occurred in conjunction with the recent surge in popularity of triathlon and open water swimming events.
- Estimates of SIPE incidence vary considerably.
- Some consider SIPE to be the most common cause of death during diving and triathlons.
- Precise incidence and mortality rate unknown because SIPE episodes are misattributed to near and fatal drowning (with similar post mortem findings)
- Possible underreporting of mild cases (symptoms mistaken for overexertion)
- 1.1% of scuba divers have history consistent with SIPE.
- 1.4% of triathletes have reported symptoms highly suggestive of SIPE (1).
- 72.4% of triathlon-associated deaths from 2008 to 2015 occurred during the swimming component (2).
- SIPE may be a significant cause of these deaths because a greater than expected proportion of these triathletes had left ventricular hypertrophy (LVH), a marker of SIPE susceptibility (2).

ETIOLOGY AND PATHOPHYSIOLOGY

- Pathophysiology of disease poorly understood with need for ongoing research
- SIPE appears to be caused by a diverse set of factors, and there is great variability in circumstances in those who experience SIPE.
- There is some thought that a combination of factors are typically required, which overcome the body's ability to compensate and thus results in the development of pulmonary edema.
- SIPE is multifactorial with environmental and anatomic factors collectively causing overwhelming leakage of fluid from the pulmonary capillaries into the alveoli.
- Pulmonary edema occurs when fluid accumulates in the lung interstitium and alveoli secondary to extravasation from pulmonary vasculature.
- Pulmonary edema occurs due to an imbalance in (Starling) forces across the alveolar membrane resulting in a net influx of fluid into the alveoli, thus capillary hydrostatic pressure overcomes the plasma oncotic pressure.
- Factors that increase the hydrostatic pressure include increased external pressures, increased central blood volume, changes in pulmonary resistance, and increased cardiac output.
- Factors increasing central blood volume:
  - Water immersion at depth increases hydrostatic pressure on the extremities.
  - Cold water causing peripheral vasoconstriction to maintain core body temperature
  - Tight wet suits compressing the extremities
  - Excessive prehydration, increasing overall blood volume (particularly in triathletes concerned about dehydration during competition and scuba divers believing it will protect them from decompression illness)
- Factors increasing pulmonary resistance:
  - Cold water causing peripheral vasoconstriction and thus increased afterload on the ventricle
  - Reduced diastolic relaxation (often from long-standing hypertension) causing increased pulmonary resistance in the lungs
  - Exercise causing increased cardiac-filling pressures
  - Breathing against a negative pressure relative to the pressure at the lung centroid (snorkels and scuba diving breathing equipment)
- Additionally, damage to the capillary membrane may also create a leaky membrane that may also contribute.
- Together, these factors, which increase central blood volume and pulmonary resistance, result in increased hydrostatic pressure and subsequent alveolar edema.

RISK FACTORS

- Hypertension
- Preexisting cardiopulmonary disease
- Pulmonary hypertension
- LVH
- Cold water
- Exercise/exertion
- Age
- Female sex
- Depth of immersion
- Elevated negative inspiratory pressure
- Emotional stress
- Overhydration
- Tight-fitting wet suit
- *Note*: SIPE occurs even among otherwise healthy and well-conditioned athletes (3,4).

GENERAL PREVENTION

- Diving instructors, swimming event organizers, and medical staff, along with participants, should be aware of the signs of SIPE and risk in even otherwise healthy, experienced athletes.
- Medical risk factors for SIPE, including hypertension and cardiovascular disease, thus optimization of these conditions is recommended.
- Athletes can focus on reduction of modifiable risk factors:
  - Avoid overhydration prior to immersion.
  - Wear a properly fitted wet suit.
  - Minimize race anxiety and overexertion.
  - Warm-up swim prior to any event to acclimate to water temperature and exercise
- Sildenafil and nifedipine have shown benefit for prevention of SIPE recurrence in investigational studies potentially by reducing pulmonary artery pressures; off-label use (5)

DIAGNOSIS

The diagnostic hallmark of SIPE is complete resolution of symptoms within 24 to 48 hr (6).

HISTORY

- Acute onset of symptoms either during or immediately following exertion in water activities, swimming, or diving
- Symptoms may include dyspnea, cough, chest pain/tightness, and hemoptysis.

- No history of water aspiration (Near-drowning presents with similar symptoms, signs, and radiographic findings.)
- Returned to surface at a safe rate (divers)
- Swimmers and triathletes may report dyspnea above normal exertion levels.
- Divers may report malfunctioning breathing equipment, when it's in fact perfectly fine.
- Other early indicators in divers are using their own or a companion's secondary air supply or flushing a closed-circuit system.

PHYSICAL EXAM
- Hypoxemia
- Abnormal airway sounds to auscultation, such as crackles, rales, wheezing

DIFFERENTIAL DIAGNOSIS
- Near/fatal drowning
- Pulmonary decompression sickness
- Pulmonary overinflation syndrome
- Respiratory tract infection
- Exercise-induced bronchospasm or asthma exacerbation
- Exercise-induced pulmonary edema
- Congestive heart failure
- Noncardiogenic pulmonary edema
- Cardiopulmonary arrest

DIAGNOSTIC TESTS & INTERPRETATION
- Radiographic findings consistent with pulmonary edema or pleural effusions (bilateral or unilateral)
- Chest x-ray is usually sufficient for diagnosis.
- Ultrasound and chest computed tomography (CT) scan can be useful for detecting small accumulations of pleural fluid.
- Rule out other acute cardiopulmonary disease with chest x-ray, electrocardiogram (ECG), cardiac enzymes, and echocardiogram.

TREATMENT

GENERAL MEASURES
- Normalize the environment by stopping activity, removing the patient from the water, placing them in a warm environment, and sitting them upright if conscious (all of which reverse the common physiologic causes of SIPE).
- Provide supplemental oxygen, if needed.
- Don't provide fluids.
- Should be monitored by medical staff until complete resolution of symptoms

MEDICATION
First Line
- Diuretics (i.e., Lasix [Furosemide]):
  - Usually not required because pulmonary fluid will leave through natural diuresis in healthy individuals
- Vasodilators

ADMISSION, INPATIENT, AND NURSING CONSIDERATIONS
- Patients experiencing SIPE should be evaluated in the emergency department to rule out other possible causes of respiratory symptoms.
- Acute respiratory failure requiring supplemental oxygen necessitates hospital admission.
- Rare cases of SIPE with severe pulmonary edema and respiratory failure may require intensive care unit (ICU) admission for continuous positive airway pressure (CPAP) or mechanical ventilation to treat pulmonary edema.

ONGOING CARE

FOLLOW-UP RECOMMENDATIONS
- Recurrent episodes of SIPE are known to occur.
- Approximately a 17% recurrence rate (likely underestimated given fear of swimming again)
- Following resolution of symptoms, patients should undergo evaluation for predisposing risk factors, particularly underlying cardiopulmonary disease. (This workup may include ECG, echocardiogram, and cardiac stress testing.)
- Correction of a reversible cardiopulmonary disease may reduce risk of recurrence.

PATIENT EDUCATION
- Counsel patients on the potential for recurrence of SIPE.
- Discussion of return to play is dependent on patient's overall health, results of cardiopulmonary workup, severity of the SIPE episode, and planned future activities:
  - For example, an otherwise healthy, young warm-water diver with a mild case of SIPE would be less concerning than an older cold-water diver with heart failure who required hospitalization.
- Some patients choose to return to swimming or diving despite high risk.
- Patients resuming activity should be counseled preventively on warning signs and instructed to cease activity and exit the water if even mild symptoms, such as uncharacteristic shortness of breath or persistent cough, occur.

PROGNOSIS
- Most events are self-limited with complete resolution of presenting signs and symptoms within 24 to 48 hr following normalization of physiologic environment.
- However, SIPE can be life-threatening either directly due to pulmonary edema causing acute respiratory failure or resultant drowning while in respiratory distress.

REFERENCES

1. Miller CC III, Calder-Becker K, Modave F. Swimming-induced pulmonary edema in triathletes. *Am J Emerg Med*. 2010;28(8):941–946.
2. Moon RE, Martina SD, Peacher DF, et al. Deaths in triathletes: immersion pulmonary oedema as a possible cause. *BMJ Open Sport Exerc Med*. 2016;2(1):e000146.
3. Gempp E, Demaistre S, Louge P. Hypertension is predictive of recurrent immersion pulmonary edema in scuba divers. *Int J Cardiol*. 2014;172(2):528–529.
4. Peacher DF, Martina SD, Otteni CE, et al. Immersion pulmonary edema and comorbidities: case series and updated review. *Med Sci Sports Exerc*. 2015;47(6):1128–1134.
5. Moon RE, Martina SD, Peacher DF, et al. Swimming-induced pulmonary edema: pathophysiology and risk reduction with sildenafil. *Circulation*. 2016;133(10):988–996.
6. Grünig H, Nikolaidis PT, Moon RE, et al. Diagnosis of swimming induced pulmonary edema—a review. *Front Physiol*. 2017;8:652.

CLINICAL PEARLS

- Recent increases in the popularity of water immersion events have increased our awareness of SIPE as a potential cause of morbidity and mortality in water athletes.
- There are steps that can be taken to decrease severity if condition is identified.
- SIPE is likely due to multiple factors but may occur in completely healthy individuals during exertional activities in water.
- SIPE is initially treated by stopping activity, removing the patient from the water, and placing them upright in a warm environment.
- Assess for underlying cardiopulmonary disease in those with a history of SIPE.
- There is a risk of SIPE recurrence and death due to respiratory failure.

SYNCOPE IN SPORTS

Elizabeth A. Williams, DO

BASICS

ALERT
Need to differentiate cardiac syncope (CS) from noncardiac syncope (NCS) due to increased risk of sudden cardiac death with CS

DESCRIPTION

- Syncope: sudden loss of postural tone with loss of consciousness (LOC) due to global cerebral hypoperfusion and spontaneous recovery
- Exercise-related syncope (ERS): syncope occurring during exertion

EPIDEMIOLOGY

- Syncope is a common occurrence, especially in young females and is usually due to a benign etiology.
- Important to differentiate between syncope occurring *during* exertion, postexertional syncope (immediately after exertion), and nonexertional syncope as their underlying etiology and risk to the individual are drastically different.

ALERT
One study showed that 50% of syncope that occurred during exertion was due to underlying cardiac pathology, therefore with increased risk of sudden cardiac death (1).

Incidence

- Most syncopal events are not related to exertion:
  - Colivicchi et al. showed of ~7,500 athletes (mean age 16 yr old), 6.2% self-reported syncope within the past 5 yr. Of those with syncope, 87% were unrelated to exercise, 12% were postexertional, and ~1% occurred while exercising (2).
- Postexertional collapse: most common reason medical attention is sought after marathon/ultramarathon; 59–85% of all visits to medical tent after those races (3)

Prevalence

To date, there is no major epidemiologic study investigating syncope in athletes.

ETIOLOGY AND PATHOPHYSIOLOGY

- Syncope is due to decreased cerebral perfusion (specifically to the reticular activating system in the brainstem).
- Causes of syncope vary with general categories, including cardiac, neurogenic, metabolic, psychogenic, and unknown etiology (1).
- NCS pathophysiology is incompletely understood (4).
- Postexertional collapse: collapse and occasionally syncope after a period of exercise, usually after endurance activities (3):
  - Collapse/syncope due to transient postural hypotension due to venous pooling of blood from loss of muscle pump in legs after the athlete stops moving in conjunction with altered cardiac baroreflex and decreased peripheral resistance (3,4)
- Hyperthermic collapse: collapse with or without complete LOC due to prolonged exertion and decreased cardiac output due to dehydration (body temp >104°F), part of the heat illness spectrum
- Orthostatic hypotension: decrease of systolic blood pressure (SBP) >20 mm Hg or diastolic blood pressure (DBP) >10 mm Hg within 3 min of position change:
  - Increased susceptibility in middle-aged and older athletes possibly due to volume depletion and decreased vasomotor tone (1)

Genetics

Depends upon the etiology for syncope, for example:

- Hypertrophic cardiomyopathy (HCM): autosomal dominant inheritance
- Long QT syndrome (LQTS): three main types (LQTS1, LQTS2, and LQTS3); predominantly inherited autosomal dominant, rarely autosomal recessive
- Clinical suggestion of inheritable susceptibility to vasovagal syncope, although a specific gene has not yet been identified

RISK FACTORS

- CS: underlying condition that increases risk
- NCS: dehydration, strong emotional response, inadequate fueling, environmental conditions
- Medications such as macrolide antibiotics, antihistamines/decongestants, recent illness (5)

GENERAL PREVENTION

- NCS:
  - Hydration
  - Proper fueling
  - Continued movement immediately after an endurance event and proper cool down
  - Dressing appropriately for climate and ideally time for climate acclimation
- CS:
  - Identifying those at risk and implementing treatment strategy

DIAGNOSIS

HISTORY

Detailed history is critical to determining etiology:

- Obtain details from witness if available about events surrounding the syncopal episode such as muscle activity, tongue biting, loss of bladder control, time duration of LOC (usually brief, a few seconds):
  - Myoclonus can occur independently of seizure.
- Determine if prodromal symptoms were present such as lightheadedness, dizziness, tunnel vision, nausea, and so forth:
  - Syncope with prodrome more likely to be NCS as an individual senses the episode coming and is able to protect themselves (i.e., arms out or slumping to ground)
  - Syncope without prodromal state is more concerning for CS. Lack of prodrome increases risk of injury as individual is unable to place themselves into a more protective position.
- Determine circumstances surrounding syncope:
  - Was the athlete still exercising (suggestive of CS) or was it after exercise (suggestive of NCS)?
  - Was syncope triggered by loud noise or cold water (suggestive of CS, specifically LQTS)?
- Evaluate mentation status after regaining consciousness (i.e., groggy vs. mentally sharp):
  - NCS: tend to be very fatigued/groggy after event
  - CS: can be alert immediately following event
- Obtain details of family history (5)[B].

PHYSICAL EXAM

- Sideline/in the field assessment:
  - Rapidly assess for consciousness and pulse. If no pulse, start cardiopulmonary resuscitation (CPR) and rapid use of automated external defibrillator (AED).
  - If remains unconscious/unstable, rapid transfer to emergency room.
  - Assess for trauma.
  - If regains consciousness:
    - Check blood pressure on both arms.
    - Assess patient while he/she is supine with legs elevated (3).
    - Consider rectal temperature (if concern for hyperthermia, must have rectal temperature; oral/temporal temperature is not adequate).
    - Full neurologic evaluation
- In-office evaluation postsyncope:
  - Vital signs, including orthostatic vital signs
  - Cardiac auscultation:
    - Standing, supine, and supine with Valsalva
    - Murmurs
    - Irregular pulse
  - Neurologic evaluation
  - Evaluate for Marfan stigmata.

DIFFERENTIAL DIAGNOSIS

- CS (usually occurs during exertion):
  - Anomalous coronary artery
  - Arrythmogenic right ventricular cardiomyopathy (ARVC)
  - Brugada syndrome
  - Catecholaminergic polymorphic ventricular tachycardia (CPVT)
  - Coronary artery disease
  - HCM
  - LQTS
  - Myocarditis
  - Right ventricular outflow tract ventricular tachycardia
  - Severe aortic valve stenosis
- NCS (usually occurs after exertion or unrelated to exertion):
  - Drug abuse
  - Heat stroke
  - Hypoglycemia
  - Hyponatremia
  - Orthostatic hypotension
  - Seizure
  - Vasovagal syncope

DIAGNOSTIC TESTS & INTERPRETATION

Initial Tests (lab, imaging)

- Electrocardiogram (ECG) (5)[B]
- Lab work: comprehensive metabolic panel (CMP), complete blood count (CBC), thyroid-stimulating hormone (TSH), finger glucose test:
  - Additional labs based on differential (i.e., troponin if concerned for cardiac ischemia)
- Orthostatic vital signs

Follow-Up Tests & Special Considerations

- CS:
  - Echocardiogram
  - Holter monitor/event recorder
  - Consider the following after consultation with sport cardiologist:
    - Cardiac magnetic resonance imaging (MRI) with gadolinium
    - Exercise treadmill testing
    - Electrophysiology (EP) testing
    - Genetic testing (LQTS, Brugada syndrome, HCM)
- NCS:
  - If history is consistent with noncardiac etiology, usually no additional testing required, although may obtain addition testing if portions of history are concerning (4)

TREATMENT

GENERAL MEASURES

- For safety, all athletes with syncope or near syncope should be restricted from sports until further evaluation is completed (6)[B].
- If immediate reversible etiologies are identified, proceed with treating identified condition (i.e., hypoglycemia, hyponatremia, heat stroke).
- Treatment of CS depends on etiology.
- All syncope occurring during exertion should be restricted from sports until evaluation is completed (6)[B]:
  - CS: Restriction from sport is dictated base on underlying condition (6)[C].
  - NCS: Athlete is able to return to sports after "measures are demonstrated to prevent recurrent syncope" (6)[C].
  - Syncope of unknown etiology: advised to refrain from sporting events that may place themselves and others at risk should they syncopize. Water-based sports could be an example (6)[C].

MEDICATIONS

- Dictated by underlying etiology for cause of syncope
- Refractory cases of vasovagal syncope could consider midodrine or fludrocortisone (5)[B].

ISSUES FOR REFERRAL

- All syncopal events occurring during exercise should be evaluated by a sports medicine team.
- If doubt about etiology, consider referral for further evaluation by sports cardiologist and or an electrophysiologist.
- Recurrent postexertional collapse and concern for nutritional status and then consider referral to dietitian to work with athlete about proper fueling and hydration

ONGOING CARE

DIET

- Encourage proper fueling prior to exertion to ensure adequate fuel for activity. Nutrition plans will vary with the athlete but allow for adequate time for athlete to adjust to the fueling plan.
- Encourage proper hydration techniques will vary depending on event, environmental climate, and athlete.

PATIENT EDUCATION

- Discuss with athlete importance of continued movement after races and cool down, proper fueling leading up to event, hydration.
- Hydration strategies especially for endurance events
- Proper clothing for the climate— especially important for endurance athletes
- Education about syncopal warning signs and how to protect themselves if they develop:
  - Counter maneuvers in patients with prodrome can be helpful in preventing syncope (5)[B].
- AED operation and locations of AEDs
- Awareness of emergency action plans (EAP) and practice of EAPs

PROGNOSIS

- Postexertional collapse usually has excellent prognosis with implementation of activity modification (i.e., proper cool down and continued movement immediately after event).
- CS return to play is debated; decisions regarding return to play need to be based on joint decision-making by all stakeholders involved.
- CS: Access to AED is imperative if returning to sport.

COMPLICATIONS

- Potential for trauma from syncope
- Neurologic impairment may occur secondary to cerebral hypoperfusion if prolonged decreased blood flow due to nonperfusing cardiac rhythm.
- Possible cardiac sequela depending on underling etiology

REFERENCES

1. Vettor G, Zorzi A, Basso C, et al. Syncope as a warning symptom of sudden cardiac death in athletes. *Cardiol Clin*. 2015;33(3):423–432.
2. Colivicchi F, Ammirati F, Santini M. Epidemiology and prognostic implications of syncope in young competing athletes. *Eur Heart J*. 2004;25(19):1749–1753.
3. Asplund CA, O'Connor FG, Noakes TD. Exercise-associated collapse: an evidence-based review and primer for clinicians. *Br J Sports Med*. 2011;45(14):1157–1162.
4. Bader YH, Link MS. Syncope in the athlete. *Cardiac Electrophysiol Clin*. 2013;5(1):85–96.
5. Shen W, Sheldon R, Benditt D, et al. 2017 ACC/AHA/HRS guideline for the evaluation and management of patients with syncope: a report of the American College of Cardiology/American Heart Association Task Force On Clinical Practice Guidelines and the Heart Rhythm Society. *Circulation*. 2017;136(5):e60–e122.
6. Zipes DP, Link MS, Ackerman MJ, et al. Eligibility and disqualification recommendations for competitive athletes with cardiovascular abnormalities: Task Force 9: arrhythmias and conduction defects: a scientific statement from the American Heart Association and American College of Cardiology. *J Am Coll Cardiol*. 2015;66(21):2412–2423.

ADDITIONAL READING

- Ackerman MJ, Zipes DP, Kovacs RJ, et al. Eligibility and disqualification recommendations for competitive athletes with cardiovascular abnormalities: Task Force 10: The cardiac channelopathies: a scientific statement from the American Heart Association and American College of Cardiology. *J Am Coll Cardiol*. 2015;66(21):2424–2428.
- American College of Cardiology. 36th Bethesda Conference eligibility recommendations for competitive athletes with cardiovascular abnormalities. *J Am Coll Cardiol*. 2005;45(8):1312–1375.
- Maron B, Levine B, Washington R, et al. Eligibility and disqualification recommendations for competitive athletes with cardiovascular abnormalities: Task Force 2: preparticipation screening for cardiovascular disease in competitive athletes: a scientific statement from the American Heart Association and American College of Cardiology. *Circulation*. 2015;132(22):e267–e272.
- Maron B, Udelson J, Bonow R, et al. Eligibility and disqualification recommendations for competitive athletes with cardiovascular abnormalities: Task Force 3: hypertrophic cardiomyopathy, arrhythmogenic right ventricular cardiomyopathy and other cardiomyopathies, and myocarditis: a scientific statement from the American Heart Association and American College of Cardiology. *Circulation*. 2015;132(22):e273–e280.

CLINICAL PEARLS

- Differentiating CS from NCS is key in determining next steps in evaluation and return-to-play decision making.
- If concern for CS, consult with sports cardiology if available.
- Return-to-play decisions after a syncopal episode should be made using the joint decision model.
- Have EAP documented and practiced regularly with all responsible parties involved.

TARSAL TUNNEL SYNDROME/POSTERIOR TIBIAL NERVE ENTRAPMENT

Stephen M. Simons, MD, FACSM • Jordan F. Geroski, DO

BASICS

DESCRIPTION

- A compression neuropathy which causes pain and/or paresthesia along the medial ankle and plantar foot secondary to entrapment of the posterior tibial nerve or one of its branches as it passes through the tarsal tunnel on the medial side of the ankle
- Synonym(s): posterior tibial nerve entrapment

EPIDEMIOLOGY

- Unknown
- Likely underdiagnosed or misdiagnosed due to low clinician suspicion
- Women > men
- More common in athletes and individuals with prolonged weight-bearing

ETIOLOGY AND PATHOPHYSIOLOGY

- Tarsal tunnel is formed by the distal tibia anteriorly, talus and calcaneus laterally, and the flexor retinaculum (laciniate ligament) medially. The flexor retinaculum forms the roof of the tunnel. Contents of the tunnel include the posterior tibial nerve, tibial artery and vein, the flexor hallucis longus (FHL), flexor digitorum longus (FDL), and posterior tibial tendons (PTTs).
- The tibial nerve branches within the tarsal tunnel into medial and lateral plantar nerves and the medial calcaneal nerve.
- The medial plantar nerve provides sensation to the plantar medial foot and the medial 3.5 toes.
- The lateral plantar nerve provides sensation to the lateral plantar foot and the lateral 1.5 toes.
- The medial calcaneal nerve provides sensation to the posterior and medial aspects of the heel.
- Tarsal tunnel entrapment can be differentiated into distal and proximal syndromes based on whether the tibial nerve itself is compressed (proximal) or a terminal branch is compressed (distal).

RISK FACTORS

- Decreased volume or increased pressure within the tarsal tunnel
- Hypertrophy of or within the tarsal tunnel (e.g., flexor retinaculum, abductor hallucis muscle)
- Space-occupying lesions (e.g., ganglion or lipoma, bone spurs, osteophytes)
- Tenosynovitis
- Local trauma
- Prior surgery in the area
- Scar tissue formation
- Abnormal foot/ankle mechanics (e.g., pes planus)
- Hindfoot deformities (e.g., heel valgus or varus)
- Repetitive activity
- Weight gain
- Lower extremity edema
- Accessory muscles (e.g., accessory soleus)
- Systemic diseases (e.g., diabetes)

DIAGNOSIS

HISTORY

- Tarsal tunnel syndrome (TTS) presents with a nonspecific, highly variable clinical picture.
- History of trauma or repetitive activity (e.g., running)
- Numbness, tingling, and burning to the medial aspect and plantar surface of the foot; can include calf symptoms and radiation to the toes
- Foot cramping in the medial longitudinal arch
- Typically unilateral
- Symptoms typically worsen throughout the day.
- Prolonged standing or walking often exacerbates the symptoms.
- Rest may alleviate the symptoms.
- Habit of removing shoes to obtain relief
- Patients lack morning pain and often lack heel pain.
- Nocturnal pain may awaken the patient, especially after excessive activity.

PHYSICAL EXAM

- Numbness/tingling that progresses to a burning sensation at the plantar aspect of the foot; intermittent initially; can become constant
- Plantar foot pain accentuated by walking and foot dorsiflexion
- Nocturnal pain often relieved with walking
- Pain worse at the end of the day
- Occasional fusiform swelling over the nerve course
- Motor weakness or loss as late finding: poor prognostic indicator
- Muscle fasciculations
- Pain radiation proximally into the midcalf during percussion over the tunnel (Valleix phenomenon)
- Inspect for biomechanical abnormalities such as excessive heel varus or valgus positioning.
- Observe for swelling.
- Observe for toe contractures, which can occur late.
- Palpate for soft tissue thickening or lesions; light touch–induced paresthesias
- Diminished pinprick sensation to plantar foot
- Intrinsic muscle weakness, although possibly present, is difficult to assess.
- Atrophy of abductor hallucis or abductor digiti minimi as a late finding
- Tinel sign: paresthesia during percussion over the tunnel
- Cuff sign: pain with pneumatic pressure device around leg
- Dorsiflexion-eversion test: pain elicited when placing the foot in maximum dorsiflexion and eversion and then maximally dorsiflexing the metatarsophalangeal joints and holding this position for 5 to 10 sec
- Trepman test: maximal plantar flexion and inversion
- Triple compression stress test: combination of Tinel test and Trepman test for 30 sec

DIFFERENTIAL DIAGNOSIS

- Plantar fasciitis
- Calcaneal bursitis or spurs
- Tendinitis/tenosynovitis (FHL, PTT, FDL)
- Nerve root avulsions
- Osteomyelitis
- Morton metatarsalgia
- Heel pad atrophy
- Nerve entrapment at more proximal locations (e.g., beneath the piriformis muscle, posterior knee or fibula)
- Peripheral vascular disease, including popliteal artery entrapment
- Peripheral neuropathy
- Systemic disease (e.g., diabetes, vitamin B_{12} deficiency, Reiter disease, rheumatoid arthritis, gout)
- Bony abnormalities (e.g., degenerative changes, previous fractures, calcaneal stress fracture)
- L3–S1 radiculopathies

DIAGNOSTIC TESTS & INTERPRETATION

- Plain x-ray and computed tomography (CT) scan to rule out morphologic or structural abnormalities (1)[C]
- Magnetic resonance imaging (MRI) is gold standard for evaluating compression of the tunnel due to soft tissue structures such as anomalous or hypertrophied muscles, ganglion cysts, and/or tumors (1)[C].
- Electrodiagnostic studies to rule out proximal nerve pathology causing a double crush syndrome (2)[C]
- Electromyography (EMG) to evaluate for motor latencies; has a high false-positive rate when evaluating intrinsic foot muscles (2)[C]
- Nerve conduction studies (NCSs) evaluating for sensory action potentials may increase sensitivity but are best for adjunctive assessment for confirmation of diagnosis as often yield false-negative results (1)[C].
- Ultrasound (US) to evaluate enlarged tibial nerve cross-sectional area (CSA). Imaging was positive for TTS in patients whose within tunnel CSA was 19 mm^2 (61% sensitivity, 88% specificity) and/or within-tunnel-to-proximal tunnel CSA ratio >1 (74% sensitivity, 100% specificity) (3)[B].

TREATMENT

GENERAL MEASURES

Conservative treatments are recommended prior to NCSs or surgical interventions (1)[C]:

- Acute treatment:
  - Custom orthotics with arch support
  - Immobilizing braces
  - Muscular stretching and strengthening of the lower leg and foot musculature
  - Acupuncture
  - Transcutaneous electrical nerve stimulation (TENS)
  - Corticosteroid injections
- Long-term treatment:
  - Activity modification
  - Weight loss for obese patients
  - Optimize proper gait biomechanics.
  - Surgery

MEDICATION

- Nonsteroidal anti-inflammatory drugs (NSAIDs)
- Corticosteroid injection
- Tricyclic antidepressants (4)[C]
- Vitamin B complex supplementation

ISSUES FOR REFERRAL

- Indicated for acute cases with space-occupying lesions, patients who present with obvious muscle atrophy, and cases which do not respond to conservative management
- Best surgical results in patients with tumor or coalition
- Surgical referral should be considered for patients recalcitrant to a high-quality nonoperative treatment program.

ADDITIONAL THERAPIES

- Ice
- Relative rest
- Discontinued use of any external compression (e.g., shoes, clothing)
- Rehabilitation:
  - Aimed at controlling pain, edema, and inflammation (1)[C]
  - Optimize proper biomechanics.
  - Strengthen foot intrinsic and extrinsic muscles.

SURGERY/OTHER PROCEDURES

- Endoscopic tarsal tunnel decompression allows for earlier mobilization and may cause less soft tissue trauma and scarring (5)[A].
- Flexor retinaculum release
- Surgical decompression of the tibial nerves and its branches
- Fascial release of the abductor hallucis muscle
- Cryosurgery can be performed; however, further research is needed (1)[C].
- Postoperative physical therapy is aimed at controlling pain, edema, and inflammation.

ONGOING CARE

FOLLOW-UP RECOMMENDATIONS

Patient Monitoring

Higher cutaneous pressure thresholds. Periodically repeating basic sensory testing throughout the treatment course allows for monitoring of the patient's condition (1)[C].

COMPLICATIONS

- Poor nerve recovery outcomes are more likely when surgical intervention is delayed for >10 mo (1).
- Untreated patients risk permanent nerve damage resulting in persistent pain, motor deficits, and potentially plantar ulcerations and complex regional pain syndrome.
- Recurrence of symptoms following surgical release is likely secondary to inadequate initial decompression (5)[A].

REFERENCES

1. McSweeney SC, Cichero M. Tarsal tunnel syndrome—a narrative literature review. *Foot (Edinb)*. 2015;25(4):244–250.
2. Pomeroy G, Wilton J, Anthony S. Entrapment neuropathy about the foot and ankle: an update. *J Am Acad Orthop Surg*. 2015;23(1):58–66.
3. Tawfik EA, El Zohiery AK, Abouelela AA. Proposed sonographic criteria for the diagnosis of idiopathic tarsal tunnel syndrome. *Arch Phys Med Rehabil*. 2016;97(7):1093–1099.
4. Gulur P, Soldinger SM, Acquadro MA. Concepts in pain management. *Clin Podiatr Med Surg*. 2007;24(2):333–351.
5. Gkotsoulias EN, Simonson DC, Roukis TS. Outcomes and safety of endoscopic tarsal tunnel decompression: a systematic review. *Foot Ankle Spec*. 2014;7(1):57–60.

ADDITIONAL READING

- Reichert P, Zimmer K, Wnukiewicz W, et al. Results of surgical treatment of tarsal tunnel syndrome. *Foot Ankle Surg*. 2015;21(1):26–29.
- Tu P. Heel pain: diagnosis and management. *Am Fam Physician*. 2018;97(2):86–93.

CLINICAL PEARLS

- TTS is often underdiagnosed due to low clinician suspicion.
- Many cases of TTS can be managed conservatively with relative rest from exercise, biomechanical control, and anti-inflammatory drugs.
- Identification of surgically treatable causes is necessary to avoid permanent nerve compression, sensory deficits, and motor weakness.
- Early surgical intervention of intrinsic causes and persistent syndromes despite conservative management improves outcomes.

TEMPOROMANDIBULAR JOINT INJURY

Daniel C. Herman, MD, PhD, FAAPMR, FACSM, CAQSM • Giorgio A. Negron, MD

BASICS

Temporomandibular joint (TMJ) injuries, although relatively uncommon, do occur in sport. Players in collision sports (e.g., football, field hockey, soccer, lacrosse) may be at particular risk, along with divers.

DESCRIPTION

- TMJ complex consist of the mandibular condyle inserting into the mandibular fossa of the temporal bone (1).
- Temporomandibular disorders (TMD) are a myriad of painful conditions involving the TMJ, muscles of mastication, and surrounding bony/soft tissue parts:
  - TMD are categorized as intra-articular or extra-articular.
  - Trauma, dentoskeletal malocclusion, and bruxism are important contributors.
- If pain persists >3 mo, it is considered chronic.
- Up to 70% of sufferers may have displacement of the articular disk (typically anteromedially), made up of fibrocartilage (2,3).
- Osteoarthrosis is another common cause of TMJ pain.
- May be related to whiplash injuries, hyperextension associated with cervical trauma, or related acceleration-deceleration injuries in sport (2)

EPIDEMIOLOGY

Incidence

- Clinical symptoms of TMD affect 10–15% of the adult population (~5% seeking treatment at some point in their lives) (1).
- Incidence depict by bimodal peaks between 20 and 40 yr of age (1).
- Predominant gender: female > male (2:1, although this ratio may be reversed in athletes)

RISK FACTORS

- ~1/3 of TMD sufferers report a previous history of macrotrauma.
- Psychosocial conditions such as fibromyalgia, depression, and anxiety are risk factors for the development of chronic temporomandibular dysfunction (1,4).

GENERAL PREVENTION

- Use of mouth guards in sport may provide protection against traumatic causes:
  - Omission of use carries 1.6 to 1.9 times risk of orofacial trauma (5).
- Proper technique in sports-specific activities
- Avoidance of repetitive or unilateral chewing

COMMONLY ASSOCIATED CONDITIONS

In cases of trauma, other facial injuries may be related:

- Mandibular or other orofacial fractures
- Cervical neck injury may occur in whiplash-type injuries.

DIAGNOSIS

- Primarily based on history and physical exam findings
- Exclude other causes of unilateral facial or head pain.

HISTORY

- History of pain with jaw movement (particularly repetitive chewing), headache, and/or ear discomfort (1)
- Related history of oromaxillofacial trauma

PHYSICAL EXAM

- On inspection, look out for facial asymmetry, swelling, mastication muscle hypertrophy, and uncorrected deviation on maximum mouth opening (2).
- Limited range of motion of the mandible
- Tenderness over the muscles of mastication is most consistent with TMD.
- Tenderness over TMJ capsule, surrounding neck and shoulder muscles
- A "popping," "clicking," or "locking" sensation may be noted with jaw movement (1):
  - First click upon jaw opening may be associated with anterior disk displacement; second click when closing indicates recapture of displaced disk.
  - Crepitus may indicate osteoarthritis.
- Pain when clenching jaw
- Assess for dentoskeletal malocclusion:
  - TMJ dislocation and mandibular jaw fracture both present with malocclusion.
  - To determine fracture from TMJ injury, index finger may be pressed outward along the interior border of mandible (pain and movement of bone segment indicates jaw fracture) (5)[C].

DIFFERENTIAL DIAGNOSIS

- Mandibular fracture
- Myocardial ischemia
- Carotid or vertebral artery dissection
- Intracranial hemorrhage (subarachnoid hemorrhage)
- Temporal arteritis
- Multiple sclerosis (MS) may present with pain similar to trigeminal neuralgia.
- Trigeminal or glossopharyngeal neuralgia
- Postherpetic neuralgia (1)
- Vascular headache
- Dental abnormalities
- Salivary gland disorder, otitis media, external otitis, and sinusitis
- Elongated styloid process pain often is precipitated by swallowing or turning the head.
- Autoimmune conditions (systemic lupus erythematosus [SLE], Sjögren, rheumatoid arthritis) (1)

DIAGNOSTIC TESTS & INTERPRETATION

- No specific laboratory tests are indicated.
- Imaging not necessary for diagnosis; may be helpful to rule out other disorders with similar symptoms
- Initial studies include transcranial and transmaxillary plain radiography and/or panoramic radiography.
- Magnetic resonance imaging (MRI) to further evaluate joint pathology and disk position (ultrasound if MRI not available) (1,2)

TREATMENT

- Typically treated as outpatients with pain medication, muscle relaxants, and warm compresses
- In general, symptoms from acute injury resolve within 7 to 10 days, although a significant percentage of patients may have long-term sequelae.
- Prehospital:
  - Evaluate patient to rule out other more serious injuries:
    - Cervical spine injuries
    - Orofacial fractures
    - Dental abscess (1)
  - In acute injuries, conservative measures are applied:
    - Protection from further injury
    - Icing
    - Nonsteroidal anti-inflammatory drugs (NSAIDs) for pain relief if indicated
    - Decreased stimulation (i.e., chewing) on affected side
- Emergency department (ED) treatment:
  - Pain control
  - Radiographs to rule out other injuries as clinically indicated (plain film, computed tomography [CT])
  - For TMJ dislocation, you may perform digital intraoral reduction (bimanual traction) (5)[C]:
    - May use local anesthesia for auriculotemporal nerve block
  - For severe bruxism, refer to dentist or oral and maxillofacial surgeon for occlusal splints (1)[C].

MEDICATION

- NSAIDs (preferably naproxen) as first line (1)[A]
- Muscle relaxants to improve muscle spasms
- Additional adjunct therapies:
  - Tricyclic antidepressants (mainstay management for chronic conditions) (1)[C]
  - Intra-articular and local injections of anesthetics or steroids for severe cases (1)[A]
  - Inconclusive evidence for hyaluronic acid injection (1)[A]

ISSUES FOR REFERRAL

- Pain or loss of function uncontrolled by the preceding may benefit from referral to maxillofacial or orofacial surgeons (1)[C].
- Surgery is rarely required but may consist of:
  - Arthrocentesis and arthroscopy.
  - Hemiarthroplasty.
  - Osteotomy.
  - Total joint replacement is considered a salvage procedure.

ADDITIONAL THERAPIES

- Warm/cold compresses
- Biofeedback (1)[C]
- Acupuncture to treat myofascial pain
- Physical therapy exercises to strengthen muscles of mastication, maintain range of motion (1)[C]
- Although not studied extensively, a mouthpiece or mouth guard may help to relieve some postinjury pain.

ONGOING CARE

DIET

- A soft diet may be effective in reducing pain severity during episodes.
- Chewing gum also may make symptoms worse.

PROGNOSIS

Typically self-limited but can progress to a chronic state of inflammation and pain

REFERENCES

1. Gauer RL, Semidey MJ. Diagnosis and treatment of temporomandibular disorders. *Am Fam Physician*. 2015;91(6):378–386.
2. De Rossi SS, Greenberg MS, Liu F, et al. Temporomandibular disorders: evaluation and management. *Med Clin North Am*. 2014;98(6):1353–1384.
3. Liddell A, Perez DE. Temporomandibular joint dislocation. *Oral Maxillofac Surg Clin North Am*. 2015;27(1):125–136.
4. Young EJ, Macias CR, Stephens L. Common dental injury management in athletes. *Sports Health*. 2015;7(3):250–255.
5. Fillingim RB, Ohrbach R, Greenspan JD, et al. Potential psychosocial risk factors for chronic TMD: descriptive data and empirically identified domains from the OPPERA case-control study. *J Pain*. 2011;12(Suppl 11):T46–T60.

ADDITIONAL READING

- Marbach JJ. Tempomandibular pain dysfunction syndrome. History, physical examination, and treatment. *Rheum Dis Clin North Am*. 1996;22(3):477–498.
- Tanaka E, Detamore MS, Mercuri LG. Degenerative disorders of the temporomandibular joint: etiology, diagnosis, and treatment. *J Dent Res*. 2008;87(4):296–307.

CLINICAL PEARLS

- Consideration of possible underlying psychosocial factors may significantly aid in the treatment of TMD.
- The practitioner should take care at the time of presentation to evaluate for more serious masquerading conditions.
- Although acute cases typically resolve within 1 to 2 wk, close follow-up should be scheduled for consideration of additional treatment options in order to prevent progression to chronic pain states.

TFCC (TRIANGULAR FIBROCARTILAGE COMPLEX) TEARS

Stephen R. Paul, MD, CAQSM

BASICS

- TFCC tears are part of the spectrum of ulnar-sided wrist pain. Often with clicking, they can be disabling to the athlete.
- The TFCC acts as a primary stabilizer to the distal radioulnar joint (DRUJ) and a cushion to the ulnar-sided carpal bones, transmitting up to 18% of the load on the wrist (1)[C].
- TFCC tears are either traumatic or degenerative or combination of both.
- Traumatic tears may be acute or acute on chronic, repetitive events.
- Traumatic tears are either from acute collision (axial load with rotation, hyperpronation-supination, or traction) or repetitive injury (chronic loading of ulnar wrist).

DESCRIPTION

- The TFCC has five major components as described by Palmer (1)[C]:
  - TFC proper, the articular disc distal to the ulna
  - Meniscus homologue (ulnocarpal meniscus)
  - Radioulnar ligaments (dorsal and volar)
  - Sheath of the extensor carpi ulnaris (ECU)
  - Ulnar collateral ligament
- Fibers of the TFCC originate on the distal radius, inserting on the distal ulna, base of the ulnar stylus, and extending to lunate (ulnolunate ligament), triquetrum (lunotriquetral ligament), and base of the 5th metacarpal.
- TFCC acts as a stabilizer of the DRUJ (pronation, supination, volar and dorsal movement) and a cushion for the ulnocarpal forces.
- The periphery of the TFCC is vascular, and the central aspect is avascular, therefore, peripheral lesions often do well with repair.

EPIDEMIOLOGY

- Degenerative tears are seen with advancing age. Chan noted in a systematic review that the prevalence of TFCC abnormalities ranged from 27% in the youngest group (<30 yr) to 49% in patients >70 yr regardless of symptoms (2)[C].
- Iordache noted that magnetic resonance imaging (MRI) scans revealed TFCC abnormalities with a similar prevalence in asymptomatic participants: 34% in <30-yr-olds and 100% in those >60 yr (3)[C].
- Degenerative tears often are seen in an older population.
- Traumatic tears are seen frequently in the athletic population.

ETIOLOGY AND PATHOPHYSIOLOGY

- The thickness of the TFCC is inversely related to the ulnar variance (the more ulnar plus, the thinner the TFCC).
- In neutral mechanics, with axial load on, the load on the forearm is 82% at the distal radius and 18% at the TFCC; with removal of the TFCC, the radius takes 95% of the load (1)[C].
- Palmer classified TFCC tears in to two types: traumatic and degenerative (1)[C]:
  - Traumatic:
    - 1A: central perforation
    - 1B: ulnar avulsion ± distal ulnar fracture
    - 1C: avulsion from lunate or triquetrum
    - 1D: avulsion from sigmoid notch of radius
  - Degenerative:
    - 2A: TFCC wear
    - 2B: TFCC wear + lunate and/or ulnar chondromalacia
    - 2C: TFCC perforation + lunate and/or ulnar chondromalacia
    - 2D: TFCC perforation + lunate and/or ulnar chondromalacia + ligament tear
    - 2E: TFCC perforation + lunate and/or ulnar chondromalacia + ligament tear + ulnocarpal arthritis
- Several mechanisms have been described to cause TFCC tears.
- Axial loading the ulnar side of the wrist with a rotational force (often a fall on an outstretched hand)
- Hyperrotation with hyperpronation or hypersupination
- Traction to the ulnar side of the wrist
- Chronic repetitive loading the ulnar carpus

RISK FACTORS

- Type of sport can lead to tears from collision, falling on outstretched hand, and hyperrotation or traction.
- Racquet sports (tennis, racquetball), pole vault, gymnastics, golf, weight training (bench press), hockey (collision and hyperrotation with a slapshot), and water skiing (traction)
- Positive ulnar variance is associated with TFCC tears.
- Distal radius fractures are associated with tears of the TFCC. Symptomatic nonunion of the ulnar styloid is also associated with tear of the TFCC (often with distal radius fractures).

COMMONLY ASSOCIATED CONDITIONS

- Positive ulnar variance (result of distal radius fracture or congenital) can cause increased load of ulnar carpus on TFCC.
- Distal radius fractures can result in disruption of radial-ulnar aspect of TFCC (DRUJ instability) or increased ulnar variance.
- Nonunion of base of the ulnar styloid fracture may result in symptomatic TFCC tears.
- Instability (subluxation or dislocation) of the DRUJ, midcarpus, or triquetrum-lunate
- Ulnar impaction syndrome (abutment syndrome, impingement syndrome) with positive ulnar variance and risk factors (sport, repetitive trauma): There is central tear to TFCC, and chondromalacia develops in the lunate, triquetrum, and ulnar head.

DIAGNOSIS

HISTORY

- In athletes, there is a history of:
  - Acute trauma such as a fall on an outstretched hand, especially with ulnar load or ulnar deviation.
  - Traction or hyperrotation.
  - Previous Colles fracture.
  - Previous dislocated/subluxed DRUJ.
  - "Insignificant" wrist injury.
- Overuse and repetitive trauma to the ulnar side of the wrist as seen in club and racquet sports
- Patients often report ulnar-sided pain ± clicking.
- Weak hand grip
- Subjective sense of wrist instability
- Pain with pronation, supination, or extension with axial load

PHYSICAL EXAM

- TFCC impaction/load/compression test: Axially load the wrist and ulnar deviate; a positive test reproduces pain ± click.
- May have pain/weakness with isometric resisted wrist flexion (patient tries to lift table in supination); this is seen with dorsal-sided peripheral tears.
- Pain/weakness pushing out of a chair (wrist extension with axial load)
- The fovea sign describes point tenderness at the recess of the TFCC with a sensitivity of 95.2% and specificity of 86.5% correctly identifying TFCC injury. The fovea lies between the ulnar styloid process and the flexor carpi ulnaris (FCU) tendon. Distally, it is bounded by the pisiform bone and proximally by the volar surface of the ulnar head.
- Tests to rule out associated instability:
  - Shuck test (excessive anteroposterior [AP] glide with either fixed ulna in relation to radius or vice-versa in pronation, supination, and neutral)
  - AP translation of triquetrum to fixed lunate
  - AP translation of lunate to fixed triquetrum
  - Ulnar compression test: Squeeze ulnar head against sigmoid notch of distal radius.
- Diagnostic injection with lidocaine to either the ECU, FCU tendons, the TFCC interval, or the DRUJ—sigmoid notch may be useful to differentiate the source of pain

DIFFERENTIAL DIAGNOSIS

- Tendinopathy (ECU, FCU)
- DRUJ instability (dislocation, subluxation) and arthritis
- Carpal instability (lunotriquetral, midcarpal)
- Fracture (distal radius, ulnar styloid nonunion, triquetrum, hamate, pisiform)
- Ulnar carpal impingement (ulnar abutment syndrome)
- Kienböck disease

DIAGNOSTIC TESTS & INTERPRETATION

Initial Tests (lab, imaging)

- Radiographs: Lateral and posteroanterior [PA] in neutral, zero rotation to rule out associated fractures and determine ulnar variance. Presurgical assessment could include PA in full pronation with hand grip view to accentuate the ulnar variance.
- MRI, especially high-resolution scanners with experienced radiologists, is useful to detect TFCC pathology, with sensitivity and specificity reported as high as 92% and 89%, respectively (4)[C].
- MR arthrography with traction reduces vacuum effect and improves visualization of the TFC and ligament tears and is a good option for elite athletes, presurgical study or if there are unexplained clinical symptoms in lieu of a prior nonarthrographic MRI. Note: MRI arthrography can better delineate intrinsic ligament tears and the articular surface cartilage (4)[C].
- Peripheral lesions of the TFCC are difficult to image with MRI, and arthroscopy remains the gold standard for diagnosing TFCC pathology in addition to being therapeutic. The trampoline sign is when a surgical probe fails to spring back when peripheral tears exist (4)[C].
- MR arthrogram and high-resolution dedicated MRI are improving in accuracy to diagnose TFCC tears.
- Peripheral lesions are difficult to diagnose with imaging.

Diagnostic Procedures/Other

Diagnostic injection with lidocaine in to ECU, FCU, TFCC space, DRUJ, midcarpus, or lunotriquetral may help to differentiate pain.

TREATMENT

- Initial treatment for traumatic and symptomatic degenerative tears is conservative, for up to 8 to 12 wk and includes:
  - Nonsteroidal anti-inflammatory drugs (NSAIDs), relative rest (avoid painful activities):
    - Immobilization (ulnar deviation, slight volar flexion) in a short arm cast for 4 to 6 wk, if traumatic
    - Followed by physical therapy and use of a removable splint (5)[C]
- McAdams (5)[C] and Rettig (6)[C] recommend more aggressive approach for high-level athletes:
  - A trial of immobilization of the wrist for 2 to 3 wk if distal DRUJ is stable
  - Arthroscopic surgery if that fails or there is any associated instability
- Care to not load the ulnar wrist or load in pronosupination is important.
- Peripheral lesions often will heal owing to the improved vascularity.
- Injections with corticosteroids are often tried, but there is no evidence for efficacy to support this approach.
- If there is instability of the DRUJ (distal ulna is dorsal), immobilization in 30 degrees of supination for 4 wk followed by gradual return to neutral for the next 2 wk (5)[C]
- Surgery is indicated if symptoms persist or there is failure to improve after a short course of immobilization, any instability of the DRUJ or lunotriquetral, and positive ulnar variance (5)[C].

MEDICATION

Trial of NSAIDs for pain

ISSUES FOR REFERRAL

- If any instability to the DRUJ or lunotriquetral is noted, refer for arthroscopy (6)[C].
- If the wrist is stable and not responding to initial immobilization, refer for arthroscopy (6)[C].

ADDITIONAL THERAPIES

For competitive, elite athletes, a more aggressive approach has been recommended (6)[C].

SURGERY/OTHER PROCEDURES

- Anderson found no significant clinical outcomes for TFCC repair with either open or arthroscopic technique in 75 patients over 10 yr. But, although not significant, there were more complaints of superficial ulnar nerve pain in the open repair group. Also, female gender was associated with a higher rate of reoperation (7)[C].
- For Palmer type 1A lesions, arthroscopic débridement/repair is recommended (7)[C].
- For Palmer type 1B/C/D, arthroscopy with mini open repairs is performed (5)[C].
- Palmer 2A/B arthroscopic débridement (Consider osteotomy if + ulnar variance.) (5)[C]
- Palmer 2C/D with neutral ulna variance, no lunotriquetral instability—arthroscopic débridement (5)[C]
- Palmer 2C/D if ulna variance $<$2 mm, arthroscopy and:
  - Without lunotriquetral instability—wafer procedure indicated
  - With lunotriquetral instability—osteotomy indicated
- Palmer 2C/D with ulna variance $>$2 mm arthroscopy and osteotomy (5)[C]
- Palmer 2E arthroscopy has mixed results, often a salvage surgery is performed (5)[C].
- For degenerative Palmer type 2 lesions, ulnar variance is assessed as well as midcarpal stability and wear:
  - If ulnar variance is 3 mm or less, wafer procedure is recommended.
  - If ulnar variance is $>$3 mm, wafer + ulnar shortening is recommended (6)[C].
  - Wafer procedure is arthroscopic decompression of the ulnocarpal joint with débridement of the TFCC.

ONGOING CARE

FOLLOW-UP RECOMMENDATIONS

After initial injury, follow-up should be at 2 to 3 wk to gauge response to immobilization.

PROGNOSIS

- Return to play:
  - McAdams (5)[C] recommends a conservative approach postoperatively to avoid ulnar synovitis: 6 wk of immobilization in a short arm or Muenster cast followed by 6 wk of progressive range of motion and strength, with full return to sport at 3 mo postoperatively.
  - Rettig (6)[C] recommends return to restricted sport (golf and tennis) 4 to 6 wk after débridement of central TFCC tear (type 1A) and 3 to 4 mo after repair.
- Prognosis:
  - If no associated instability of DRUJ or lunotriquetral and no positive ulnar variance, long-term results are good.
  - McAdams (5)[C] reported excellent results for return to play with improvement in pain relief after arthroscopic surgery in 14 of 16 high-level athletes. The two who did not return to play at 3 mo had DRUJ instability and ulnar-carpal abutment; both returned to play after an additional period of time postoperatively, 5 to 7 mo (5)[C].

COMPLICATIONS

Previously undiagnosed carpal or DRUJ instability or ulnar-carpal abutment syndrome

REFERENCES

1. Palmer AK. Triangular fibrocartilage complex lesions: a classification. *J Hand Surg Am*. 1989;14(4):594–606.
2. Chan JJ, Teunis T, Ring D. Prevalence of triangular fibrocartilage complex abnormalities regardless of symptoms rise with age: systematic review and pooled analysis. *Clin Orthop Relat Res*. 2014;472(12):3987–3994.
3. Iordache SD, Rowan R, Garvin GJ, et al. Prevalence of triangular fibrocartilage complex abnormalities on MRI scans of asymptomatic wrists. *J Hand Surg Am*. 2012;37(1):98–103.
4. Ng AWH, Griffith JF, Fung CSY, et al. MR imaging of the traumatic fibrocartilaginous complex tear. *Quant Imaging Med Surg*. 2017;7(4):443–460.
5. McAdams TR, Swan J, Yao J. Arthroscopic treatment of triangular fibrocartilage wrist injuries in the athlete. *Am J Sports Med*. 2009;37(2):291–297.
6. Rettig AC. Athletic injuries of the wrist and hand: part II: overuse injuries of the wrist and traumatic injuries to the hand. *Am J Sports Med*. 2004;32(1):262–273.
7. Anderson ML, Larson AN, Moran SL, et al. Clinical comparison of arthroscopic versus open repair of triangular fibrocartilage complex tears. *J Hand Surg Am*. 2008;33(5):675–682.

ADDITIONAL READING

- Ahn AK, Chang D, Plate AM. Triangular fibrocartilage complex tears: a review. *Bull NYU Hosp Jt Dis*. 2006;64(3 4):114–118.
- Coggins CA. Imaging of ulnar-sided wrist pain. *Clin Sports Med*. 2006;25(3):505–526.
- Dumontier C. Physical examination of wrist instabilities. https://mo-journal.com/posts/physical-examination-of-wrist-instabilities-247. Accessed March 7, 2018.
- Nagle DJ. Triangular fibrocartilage complex tears in the athlete. *Clin Sports Med*. 2001;20(1):155–166.
- Palmer AK, Werner FW. Biomechanics of the distal radioulnar joint. *Clin Orthop Relat Res*. 1984;(187):26–35.
- Smith TO, Drew B, Toms A, et al. Diagnostic accuracy of magnetic resonance imaging and magnetic resonance arthrography for triangular fibrocartilaginous complex injury: a systematic review and meta-analysis. *J Bone Joint Surg Am*. 2012;94(9):824–832.
- Steinberg B. Acute wrist injuries in the athlete. *Orthop Clin North Am*. 2002;33(3):535–545.
- Tay SC, Tomita K, Berger RA. The "ulnar fovea sign" for defining ulnar wrist pain: an analysis of sensitivity and specificity. *J Hand Surg Am*. 2007;32(4):438–444.

CLINICAL PEARLS

- Ulnar-sided wrist pain has been described as the "low back pain" of the wrist due to the complexity of the functional anatomy, of which the TFCC contributes.
- A detailed history and careful examination can demystify this condition and lead to diagnosis of TFCC tears with or without resultant instability of the DRUJ, lunotriquetral intervals. This is also important rather than relying only on obtaining radiographs.
- Early referral for MRI imaging or arthroscopy is indicated when suspecting TFCC tears in the athlete, with any instability of the DRUJ or lunotriquetral intervals or when the TFCC fails to improve with conservative management after a short period of immobilization.
- The key to long-term treatment success in large part depends on positive ulnar variance—if present, consider referral to evaluate for ulnar shortening procedure.

THORACIC OUTLET SYNDROME

Brent Pickett, DO • Jeffrey R. Bytomski, DO, FAOASM

BASICS

DESCRIPTION

- Neurogenic or vascular symptoms in the upper extremity due to compression of the neurovascular bundle (brachial plexus and subclavian vessels) by skeletal and/or muscular structures above the 1st rib and behind the clavicle
- Symptoms are variable and based on the structure that is compressed or irritated.

ALERT
Three types:
- Neurogenic: >95% of cases
- Venous: 4% of cases
- Arterial: <1% of cases

RISK FACTORS

- Repetitive work

ALERT
Overhead athletes: swimmers, pitchers, weight lifters, volleyball and tennis players

- Poor posture
- Middle-aged female
- Congenital abnormalities:
  - Cervical rib
  - Abnormally long transverse process of C7
  - Anomalous fibromuscular band in the thoracic outlet
- Trauma
- Obesity

ETIOLOGY AND PATHOPHYSIOLOGY

- Brachial plexus nerve roots, subclavian artery, and subclavian vein pass through the scalene triangle formed by the 1st rib, anterior scalene muscles, and middle scalene muscles.
- Increased risk of positional compression of the neurovascular bundle at the thoracic outlet due to:
  - Congenital anatomic predisposition (cervical rib, abnormally long transverse process of C7, anomalous fibromuscular band)
  - Acquired extrinsic factors (anterior scalene hypertrophy, pectoralis minor tightness, poor posture causing decreased diameter of the costoaxillary canal, trauma, shortening of the scalene muscles due to active trigger points)
- Upper extremity venous thrombosis or Paget-Schroetter syndrome:
  - Overhead athletes may develop "effort thrombosis" due to repetitive shoulder hyperabduction and external rotation, which can compress the axillary-subclavian veins, damage the intimal lining, and transiently restrict venous flow. Over time, this creates a favorable environment for thrombus formation.

DIAGNOSIS

Thoracic outlet syndrome is largely a clinical diagnosis.

HISTORY

- Neurogenic and vascular symptoms related to certain positions
- Worse with lifting heavy objects, overhead activities, shoulder abduction, and external rotation
- Neurogenic:
  - Arm, shoulder, and neck pain
  - Paresthesias and numbness:
    - Frequently seen in the ulnar distribution
  - Headaches
  - Cramping of forearm muscles
  - Difficulty with fine motor skills of the hand
  - Sensory loss, motor weakness, atrophy (late findings)
  - Gilliatt-Sumner hand: severe wasting of the abductor pollicis brevis and, to a lesser extent, the interossei and hypothenar muscles
- Venous:
  - Pain
  - Edema
  - Cyanosis
  - Feeling of heaviness in the arm or hand
  - Venous distension of the arm and hand
- Arterial (often asymptomatic until embolization occurs):
  - Ischemic pain
  - Paresthesias and numbness
  - Claudication
  - Cool extremity
  - Pallor
  - Decreased distal pulse
  - Pulsating lump above the clavicle

PHYSICAL EXAM

- Swelling or discoloration of the affected extremity
- Muscle atrophy
- Decreased or absent distal pulse with activity or position changes
- Bruit auscultated in the supraclavicular space
- Provocative testing (low overall sensitivity and specificity):
  - Elevated arm stress test:
    - Arms abducted above the head in a "stick-em-up" position
    - Patient opens and closes fists at moderate speed for 3 min.
    - Positive test if position reproduces pain or paresthesias
  - Upper limb tension tests:
    - Position 1: Abduct arms to 90 degrees.
    - Position 2: Extend wrists.
    - Position 3: Tilt head to one side—ear to shoulder—then, tilt head to other side.
    - Positions 1 and 2 should cause ipsilateral pain, and position 3 should cause contralateral pain.
    - Strongest response is an onset of symptoms with position 1 and an increase in severity with positions 2 and 3.
  - Adson maneuver (original diagnostic test described in the 1920s):
    - Neck extended and turned to the affected side while the shoulder is slightly abducted and extended
    - Feel for radial pulse while patient takes a deep breath.
    - Positive test if pulse lost and symptoms reproduced
    - False positives are common.
  - Wright test:
    - Affected arm is progressively hyperabducted and externally rotated.
    - Positive test if radial pulse lost
  - Allen test:
    - Flex elbow to 90 degrees; abduct and externally rotate the shoulder.
    - Patient rotates head away from the test arm.
    - Positive test if radial pulse lost

DIFFERENTIAL DIAGNOSIS

- Cervical disc disorders
- Rotator cuff tear/impingement syndrome
- Brachial plexus neuritis
- Carpal tunnel syndrome
- Ulnar nerve entrapment
- Complex regional pain syndrome
- Polymyalgia rheumatica
- Fibromyalgia
- Subclavian steal
- Vasculitis
- Raynaud disease
- Multiple sclerosis
- Tumors of the spinal cord
- Pancoast tumor
- Neurofibroma
- Adhesive capsulitis
- Glenohumeral/acromioclavicular osteoarthritis

DIAGNOSTIC TESTS & INTERPRETATION

Initial Tests (lab, imaging)

- Consider hypercoagulable workup in venous thoracic outlet syndrome and patients with arterial thrombosis (1,2)[C].
- X-rays of the cervical spine and chest: useful to evaluate for a cervical rib or other thoracic pathology (2,3,4,5,6)[C]
- X-rays of the shoulder (2,4)[C]
- Magnetic resonance imaging (MRI): helpful to determine the location and cause of compression or to identify an anomalous fibrous band (4)[C]
- Duplex ultrasound (US): to document degree of stenosis, presence of an aneurysm, or confirm thrombosis (2,4)[C]

Diagnostic Procedures/Other

- Electromyogram (4,5,6)[C]
- Nerve conduction studies (4,5,6)[C]
- Arteriography/venography: reserved for cases of suspected arterial or venous thoracic outlet syndrome and for surgical planning (2,4,5)[C]

TREATMENT

- Conservative therapy is the initial approach, except in cases of thromboembolic phenomena with acute vascular occlusion, stenosis, arterial dilatation, or progressive neurologic deficits.
- Medications (2)[C]:
  - Nonsteroidal anti-inflammatory drugs (NSAIDs)
  - Muscle relaxants
  - Tricyclic antidepressants or selective serotonin reuptake inhibitors (SSRIs)
- Activity modification (2)[C]
- Weight loss (4)[C]
- Physical therapy (2,4)[C]:
  - Postural retraining
  - Strengthening of muscles that elevate the shoulder girdle
  - Pectoral and scalene stretching/strengthening
  - Scapulothoracic mobility
  - Trigger point treatment
  - Soft tissue mobilization
- Botox injections (4)[C]:
  - Computed tomography (CT)-guided injections into the scalene muscles
  - Consider as a short term adjunct to nonoperative therapy with physical therapy or as a bridge to surgery.
- Venous thoracic outlet syndrome with thrombus present (4)[C]:
  - Thrombolytics and anticoagulation

SURGERY/OTHER PROCEDURES

- Surgery is an option for neurogenic thoracic outlet syndrome that has not responded to aggressive nonoperative treatments or for patients with vascular compromise/thrombus formation (2,4)[C].
- CT-guided scalene block with local anesthetic to relax the anterior scalene muscle and lower the 1st rib to relieve the tension on the brachial plexus. If the injection provides symptomatic relief, it indicates likely benefit of a 1st rib resection/anterior scalenectomy (2,4)[C].

ONGOING CARE

FOLLOW-UP RECOMMENDATIONS

- Surgical referral if signs of vascular compromise or severe neurogenic symptoms are present
- Surgical referral when a cervical rib or extra-long transverse process of C7 is associated with loss of sensation, muscle atrophy, or weakness
- Surgical referral if symptoms persist despite an adequate course of aggressive therapy

COMPLICATIONS

- Poststenotic dilatation of the subclavian artery resulting in aneurysm formation and the potential for thromboembolism to the affected upper extremity (arterial thoracic outlet syndrome)
- Pulmonary embolism, residual symptoms, and high recurrence rate (venous thoracic outlet syndrome)
- Progressive motor deficits (neurogenic thoracic outlet syndrome)

REFERENCES

1. Farrar T, Rankin G, Chatfield M. Venous thoracic outlet syndrome: approach to diagnosis and treatment with focus on affected athletes. *Curr Sports Med Rep*. 2014;13(2):81–85.
2. Fugate MW, Rotellini-Coltvet L, Freischlag JA. Current management of thoracic outlet syndrome. *Curr Treat Options Cardiovasc Med*. 2009;11(2):176–183.
3. Daniels B, Michaud L, Sease F Jr, et al. Arterial thoracic outlet syndrome. *Curr Sports Med Rep*. 2014;13(2):75–80.
4. Nichols AW. Diagnosis and management of thoracic outlet syndrome. *Curr Sports Med Rep*. 2009;8(5):240–249.
5. Sanders RJ, Hammond SL, Rao NM. Diagnosis of thoracic outlet syndrome. *J Vasc Surg*. 2007;46(3):601–604.
6. Stewman C, Vitanzo PC Jr, Harwood MI. Neurologic thoracic outlet syndrome: summarizing a complex history and evolution. *Curr Sports Med Rep*. 2014;13(2):100–106.

CLINICAL PEARLS

- Thoracic outlet syndrome is a largely clinical diagnosis, although radiographic studies can be helpful if diagnosis is unclear.
- Treatment is often conservative, consisting of activity modification, physical therapy, and medication for pain.
- Surgical referral is reserved for patients with severe neurologic/vascular compromise or refractory symptoms despite adequate treatment.

THORACIC SPINE INJURY

Kenneth Vitale, MD, FAAPMR

BASICS

DESCRIPTION

- Thoracic spine fracture:
  - Rarely seen in sports but potentially catastrophic injury: higher risk in collision sports (e.g., hockey, football, wrestling)
  - The spinal column is divided into three distinct columns (Denis three-column theory) (1)[C]; if two of three are disrupted, the spinal column traditionally is considered unstable and should refer urgently.
  - **Anterior column**: anterior longitudinal ligament (ALL), anterior annulus, and anterior 2/3 of vertebral body
  - **Middle column**: posterior 1/3 of vertebral body, posterior annulus, and posterior longitudinal ligament (PLL)
  - **Posterior column**: posterior bony arch and posterior ligamentous complex (PLC) (supraspinous and interspinous ligaments, ligamentum flavum, facet capsule)
  - PLC now considered most critical predictor of stability (three-column theory only moderately reliable in determining stability)
  - Typically, **stable** fractures:
    - Transverse process, spinous process, or isolated articular fracture
    - Pars interarticularis fracture (more common in lumbar spine)
    - Compression fracture (axial, flexion, or lateral compression force); if anterior compression >40–50%, likely PLC disrupted and unstable
    - Extension injury: facet, lamina, spinous process fracture, disruption of ALL

ALERT

Typically, **unstable** fractures:

- Burst fracture (higher energy axial compression with centripedal displacement)
- Flexion-rotation injury (slice fracture): PLC typically fails and unstable.
- Fracture-dislocation injury: Bilateral facet dislocation (jumped facets) occurs, typically unstable as all three columns disrupted.
- Flexion-distraction (Chance fracture, seatbelt injury): most common at thoracolumbar junction, posterior and middle column fractures

- Thoracic discogenic pain and disk herniation:
  - Often challenging diagnosis, relatively rare
  - The three basic structures of normal vertebral disks:
    - Nucleus pulposus: gelatinous core, composed mostly of water and proteoglycans
    - Annulus fibrosus: concentric collagen lamellae surrounding nucleus; outer third innervated and may be clinically painful if tear present
    - Vertebral endplates: aid in the diffusion of nutrients into the disks, absorb hydrostatic pressure of axial loading, prevent nucleus from herniating into vertebral body

ALERT

Thoracic disk herniations rare (~1% of all herniated nucleus pulposus [HNP]):

- **Central**: higher potential for spinal cord injury; monitor for weakness, spasticity, hyperreflexia, abnormal gait, bowel/bladder incontinence
- **Centrolateral**: Often in younger patients with history of trauma may have contralateral pain and sensory changes resembling Brown-Séquard syndrome.
- **Lateral**: may cause radicular pain to rib area and visceral sites

- Muscular contusions: caused by a direct blow with intramuscular bleeding, often contact sports or falls. Check for potential rib fracture, pneumothorax/hemothorax, and pulmonary contusion.
- Musculoligamentous strain/sprain:
  - Stretch tear of thoracic muscles/and or ligaments
  - Seen most frequently in twisting/turning sports
- Facet syndrome:
  - Facet dysfunction/irritation and capsule microtears can lead to mild subluxation, synovitis, and fibrosis.
  - May have localized pain and rib asymmetry
  - Diagnosis of exclusion if no other injury
- Scheuermann (juvenile) kyphosis:
  - Osteochondrosis of thoracic vertebral ossification centers with at least 5% anterior wedging of at least three consecutive thoracic vertebrae
  - Often asymptomatic (~20% adolescents report pain)

ALERT

Spinal tumors:

- Pediatric Considerations: Maintain high index of suspicion in younger patients with night pain, fevers, systemic symptoms; persistent back pain in adolescents is never considered "normal."
- Vertebral tumors: primary (rare, usually younger adults, grow slowly; osteosarcoma most common malignant tumor) and metastatic (more common; painful with constitutional symptoms)
- Extramedullary tumors: usually benign, grow slowly and therefore are found in middle age and older individuals. (meningioma, schwannoma, neurofibroma)
- Intramedullary tumors: also, usually benign and found later in life but surgical excision difficult (intramedullary lipoma most common thoracic; astrocytoma, ependymoma common in cervical)
- Vertebral column most common site for bone metastases (30–70% cancer patients develop spine metastases: breast, lung, thyroid, kidney, prostate, colon, lymphoma, melanoma, sarcoma, myeloma.)

EPIDEMIOLOGY

- Thoracic spine fractures:
  - 19–50% thoracolumbar fractures result in neurologic damage and spinal cord compression.
  - 15% of spinal fractures occur in sports; third most common etiology after Motor vehicle accident (45%) and falls (20%):
    - In sports-related injuries, the most common cause of fracture is water sports (65%).
    - Of water sports, diving is most common (60%).
  - Male-to-female ratio of spinal fractures 4:1
  - Mean age: 24 ± 12 yr
- Scheuermann kyphosis: 5% of general population; typically seen at 10 to 15 yr, slight male predominance
- Facet syndrome: 15% (up 40%) of back pain (including lumbar) thought to be facet-mediated pain
- Disc disease: There is evidence of degenerative disc disease and disc herniation in up to 58% of athletes (vs. 38% control population); type and intensity of sport may accelerate degeneration.

ETIOLOGY AND PATHOPHYSIOLOGY

- The thoracic spine is very rigid owing to the rib cage and the costovertebral articulations.
- T2–T10 better protected from ribs and facet orientation in coronal plane (limits motion, allows rotation)
- T11–L2 injuries more common due to fulcrum effect (>50% of thoracolumbar injuries); cervicothoracic and thoracolumbar junction susceptible to shear and flexion-extension forces
- Extreme flexion-extension plus axial load are not well tolerated and may lead to injury.
- Thoracic spine fracture:
  - Most thoracic spine fractures occur at thoracolumbar junction region (T11–L2).
  - Rotational or extension forces may fracture the pars interarticularis and damage facets.
- Thoracic discogenic pain:
  - Up to 90% of herniated disks are due to degenerative processes. With aging, disc water content decreases, leading to decreased disc height and loss of axial absorption capacity.
  - Trauma may be implicated in up to 10–20%, typically a twisting/torsional movement.
- Facet syndrome:
  - Acute excessive motion that traumatizes joint versus chronic overuse

Genetics

Scheuermann kyphosis:

- True incidence probably higher because diagnosis often missed or misattributed to poor posture
- 74% heritability pattern (autosomal dominant)
- Histology shows disorganized endochondral ossification, collagen reduction, increased end plate mucopolysaccharides

RISK FACTORS

- Scheuermann kyphosis:
  - Possible additional risk factor from repetitive flexion sports at young age (e.g., water skiing has a higher prevalence)
  - Scheuermann may predispose to subsequent thoracic HNP.
- Facet syndrome:
  - Often in sports with powerful hyperextension or extremes of spinal range of motion (ROM) (e.g., gymnasts and figure skaters)
  - Facet syndrome can lead to facet osteoarthritis.
- Sport-specific risk factors:
  - Football players have increased risk of degenerative disc disease, facet degeneration, and chronic back pain proportional to their years of involvement in sport.
  - Weight lifting is also associated with degenerative disc disease and musculoligamentous sprains/strains.
  - Endurance athletes also may be at risk (e.g., butterfly swimmers and rowers are at risk for rib subluxation from the transverse processes) (often 6th or 7th rib).
  - Disk herniation is seen in any athletes participating in axial rotation sports, such as golf.

DIAGNOSIS

- Rapid evaluation of airway, breathing, and circulation (ABCs)
- Primary and secondary trauma survey
- Detailed spine and neurologic exam, with specific attention to bony deformity or tenderness and lower extremity neurologic deficits
- Any midline tenderness, distracting injury, or intoxication mandates plain-film spine radiography.

HISTORY

- Thoracic spine fracture:
  - Significant force is required for thoracic vertebral fractures, so associated injuries may obscure symptoms directly related to thoracic fractures.
  - Common symptoms:
    - Pain or tenderness:
      - Localized—usually midline
      - Referred—paraspinals, ribs, anterior chest wall, and/or visceral pain
    - Paresthesia or dysesthesia

ALERT

Bowel or bladder incontinence, saddle anesthesia, leg weakness, and gait instability indicates possible spinal cord injury.

- Thoracic discogenic pain and disc herniation:
  - Most commonly insidious onset without history of trauma
  - Pain is the most common symptom (60% of patients), may be band-like, dull, localized to the thoracic spine or referred to visceral, sternal, or inguinal regions.
  - Paresthesias and dysesthesias present in 25% of patients, typically dermatomal
  - Abdominal and intercostal weakness present in 17% of patients; suspect myelopathy if lower extremities affected.
  - Bladder symptoms present in only 2% of patients, suspect cord compression (and bowel incontinence) (2,3)[B].
- Muscular strains: typically, mild pain following a sporting activity
- Scheuermann kyphosis:
  - Symptoms are typically insidious onset with no history of major trauma.
  - Often seen with history of repetitive microtrauma, osteoporosis, osteochondrosis, necrosis of the ring apophysis, and/or tight hamstrings

PHYSICAL EXAM

- Thoracic spine fracture:
  - Localized soft tissue deformity

ALERT
Paraspinal muscle spasm:

- Assess for leg or saddle paresthesia, weakness or paraplegia, spasticity and hyperreflexia, all signs of spinal cord injury.
  - Reflexes: Hyperactive reflexes signify upper motor neuron lesions; hypoactive reflexes signify lower motor neuron lesions (spinal cord ends ~L1–L2).

ALERT
For initial spinal shock phase—hypotension, bradycardia, hyporeflexia

- Thoracic discogenic pain and disc herniation:
  - Musculoskeletal findings often nonspecific but may reveal local myofascial pain and stiffness
  - Sensory deficits to light touch or pinprick along a thoracic dermatomal pattern
  - Motor examination should include testing muscle strength, flexibility, and tone:
    - Include abdominal muscles; T9 and T10 lesions can affect lower abdominal muscles but spare upper abdominal muscles.
    - Lower extremity weakness and spasticity or hyperreflexia is serious, indicating myelopathy.
  - In isolated thoracic discogenic pain, upper extremity reflexes are normal (otherwise cervical injury) and lower extremity reflexes are normal (otherwise, suspect lumbosacral pathology or spinal cord injury) (2,3)[B].
- Scheuermann kyphosis:
  - Thoracic hyperkyphosis deformity that does not correct with passive extension
  - Compensatory lumbar hyperlordosis common
  - Tight hip flexors, hamstrings, lumbar fascia

DIFFERENTIAL DIAGNOSIS

- Arthritis (degenerative and rheumatoid)
- Spondyloarthropathy (e.g., ankylosing spondylitis)
- Congenital malformation (e.g., spina bifida)
- Pathologic fracture
- Spinal infection
- Paget disease

DIAGNOSTIC TESTS & INTERPRETATION

- Spinal tumors: Must rule out tumor when a patient has nocturnal back pain or significant constitutional symptoms.
- Complete blood count (CBC) with differential, erythrocyte sedimentation rate (ESR), C-reactive protein
- Otherwise, labs generally not indicated
- Pain or tenderness, MVA, or falls from height are indications for anteroposterior (AP) and lateral plain-film views of the spine.
- Thin-cut computed tomography (CT) scan is indicated in any patient with evidence of spinal fracture or ligamentous injury on plain films, or in patients with normal or inadequate plain films and significant pain or tenderness with mechanism for severe injury (4)[B].
- Thoracic spine fracture:
  - CT scan is more sensitive and specific than plain radiographs for the detection of thoracic spine fractures and should be used in any patient with a traumatic injury suspicious for fracture based on history, exam, or initial plain films.
  - Magnetic resonance imaging (MRI) ideal for spinal cord and ligamentous injury
- Thoracic discogenic pain and disc herniation:
  - Plain radiographs can be used but primarily to rule out fracture, cancer, or infection.
  - X-ray signs, however, can suggest disk herniation:
    - Disk calcification is present in up to 70% of patients with thoracic disk herniation versus only 4–6% of patients without herniation.
    - Other signs of disc degeneration: osteophyte formation, disc space narrowing, kyphosis
  - MRI: best visualization of the disc; should be urgently ordered if symptoms suggest spinal cord injury
  - CT myelography: less used now because MRI widely available and has contrast risk; visualizes lateral herniations and disc calcification well (2,3,5)[A]
- Scheuermann kyphosis: Plain radiographs are usually diagnostic:
  - Irregular appearing vertebral endplates
  - Anterior disc space narrowing
  - Wedging of >5 degrees of three adjacent vertebrae
  - Kyphosis of >40 degrees with apex typically T7–T9 (5)[B]
- Spinal tumors:
  - Start with plain x-ray, however, may not show abnormality until there is 30–50% loss of cancellous bone.
  - Technetium-99m bone scan is sensitive but not specific; can find smaller metastases than x-rays
  - 18F positron emission tomography shows improved specificity; good for metastatic spread
  - MRI, especially with gadolinium, demonstrates soft tissue and osseous changes well (5)[B].

TREATMENT

- Thoracic spine fracture:
  - Stable fractures are often treated with brace immobilization (e.g., a thoracolumbosacral orthosis [TLSO] can immobilize a stable [<50% height loss] thoracic compression fracture).
  - Orthosis often needed 6 to 12 wk
  - Unstable fractures or any neurologic deficit likely require surgical intervention.
- Thoracic discogenic pain:
  - Conservative; largely involves activity modification and gradual reintroduction of exercise as tolerated (6)[C]
  - Typically avoid epidural injection or surgery, unless refractory symptoms (2)[B]
  - Early surgical consult indicated for lower extremity symptoms
- Muscular contusions:
  - Conservative treatment: ice to reduce pain, limit bleeding and swelling
  - Moist heating pad after 72 hr
  - Gentle massage after initial pain has resolved
  - Analgesics as needed for pain
  - Restrict activity until pain-free ROM, full strength.
  - Physical therapy (PT) for ROM, strengthening, core stabilization exercises, teach biomechanics (5)[A]
- Muscular strains:
  - Conservative treatment with PT, including gradual mobilization and core stabilization (6)[C]
  - Nonsteroidal anti-inflammatory drugs (NSAIDs) as needed
- Facet syndrome:
  - Conservative; rest, avoid triggering activity.
  - PT with manual therapy techniques (6,7)[C]
  - Teach postural correction to prevent recurrence.
  - If no response, consider an intra-articular facet injection of corticosteroid and local anesthetic for diagnostic and therapeutic value.

- Scheuermann kyphosis:
  - PT to stretch tight hamstring muscles, hip flexors, and lumbar fascia; core strengthening; maximize posture and sagittal balance (8)[C].
  - Consider a brace in skeletally immature patients with fixed thoracic kyphosis >50 degrees (8)[C].
  - Milwaukee brace for high thoracic curves; Boston brace for lower thoracic curves (apex below T7) (8)[C]
  - Surgery is rarely indicated despite deformity, and indications are unclear; decision for surgery needs to be individualized based on symptoms and patient self-perception (8)[C].

MEDICATION

- Thoracic spine fracture with neurologic deficit:
  - High-dose steroid protocol: Solu-Medrol (methylprednisolone) 30 mg/kg intravenous (IV) bolus within 8 hr of injury, followed by 5.4 mg/kg/hr for the next 23 hr (4)
- Other causes of back pain: analgesics/NSAIDs PRN

ADDITIONAL THERAPIES

- Soft tissue mobilization, massage, trigger point therapy, and other manual therapy services can be helpful ancillary treatments for chronic thoracic pain (6,7)[C].
- Posture classes and methods (e.g., yoga, Pilates, Feldenkrais, many others) also can be considered for chronic symptoms.
- Emergency department (ED) treatment:
  - Perform all needed resuscitation and diagnostic tests with the patient in full spinal immobilization.
  - If spinal cord injury is suspected, administer high-dose steroids and consult a neurosurgeon or orthopedic spine surgeon urgently.
  - If spinal fracture or instability is suspected without neurologic impairment, order stat CT scan/MRI and consult neurosurgery or orthopedic spine surgery.
  - Pain control should be administered as soon as possible. NSAIDs, opiates, and benzodiazepines are the mainstays of treatment.

ADMISSION, INPATIENT, AND NURSING CONSIDERATIONS

- Follow the ABCs of trauma resuscitation.
- Airway intervention should be done with inline cervical immobilization.
- Preserve residual spinal cord function and prevent further injury by stabilizing the spine.
- Admission criteria:
  - Unstable spinal column injury
  - Spinal cord injury
  - Ileus
  - Severe intractable pain
  - Concomitant other injury/polytrauma
  - Patients with significant fracture or spinal cord injury should be treated in a regional trauma center.
- Discharge criteria:
  - Stable minor fractures after orthopedic or neurosurgical evaluation

ONGOING CARE

PATIENT EDUCATION

Keys to prevent recurrence include postural correction, core strengthening, and teaching proper biomechanics.

PROGNOSIS

Most thoracic injuries respond well to relative rest, activity modification, PT, and gradual reintroduction of activities.

REFERENCES

1. Denis F. The three column spine and its significance in the classification of acute thoracolumbar spinal injuries. *Spine (Phila Pa 1976)*. 1983;8(8):817–831.
2. Cornips EM. Crippling upper back pain after whiplash and other motor vehicle collisions caused by thoracic disc herniations: report of 10 cases. *Spine (Phila Pa 1976)*. 2014;39(12):988–995.
3. Brown CW, Deffer PA, Akmakjian J, et al. The natural history of thoracic disc herniation. *Spine (Phila Pa 1976)*. 1992;17(Suppl 6):S97–S102.
4. Chiles BW III, Cooper PR. Acute spinal injury. *N Engl J Med*. 1996;334(8):514–520.
5. Curtis C, d'Hemecourt P. Diagnosis and management of back pain in adolescents. *Adolesc Med State Art Rev*. 2007;18(1):140–164.
6. Masaracchio M, Kirker K, Collins CK, et al. An intervention-based clinical reasoning framework to guide the management of thoracic pain in a dancer: a case report. *Int J Sports Phys Ther*. 2016;11(7): 1135–1149.
7. Aiken DL, Vaughn D. The use of functional and traditional mobilization interventions in a patient with chronic thoracic pain: a case report. *J Man Manip Ther*. 2013;21(3):134–141.
8. de Mauroy J, Weiss H, Aulisa A, et al. 7th SOSORT consensus paper: conservative treatment of idiopathic & Scheuermann's kyphosis. *Scoliosis*. 2010;5:9.

ADDITIONAL READING

- Diaz J Jr, Cullinane D, Altman D, et al. Practice management guidelines for the screening of thoracolumbar spine fracture. *J Trauma*. 2007;63(3): 709–718.
- Nannapaneni R, Marks SM. Posterolateral thoracic disc disease: clinical presentation and surgical experience with a modified approach. *Br J Neurosurg*. 2004;18(5):467–470.
- Papagelopoulos P, Mavrogenis A, Savvidou O, et al. Current concepts in Scheuermann's kyphosis. *Orthopedics*. 2008;31(1):52–60.
- Ye C, Sun T, Li J, et al. Patterns of sports- and recreation-related spinal cord injuries in Beijing. *Spinal Cord*. 2009;47(12):857–860.

CLINICAL PEARLS

- 73% of thoracic herniations are asymptomatic; therefore, consider avoiding thoracic MRI during workup unless there is a concern for spinal cord injury.
- Return to play only when the athlete is pain free, neurologically intact, with normal ROM, and normal strength.
- If suspicious for a spine fracture or spinal cord injury, immobilize the patient on a spine board immediately.
- Patients with neurologic deficit, weakness, bowel/bladder symptoms, or significant gait instability should be transported directly to a trauma center.

TIBIAL STRESS FRACTURE

Andrew J.M. Gregory, MD, FAAP, FACSM

BASICS

Stress fracture of the tibia refers to an overuse injury of the bone as a result of repetitive loading that overwhelms its capacity to heal and must be differentiated from medial tibial stress syndrome, which is not a stress fracture. In general, stress fractures of the tibia can be classified into low-risk or high-risk stress fractures. The more common low-risk stress fracture of the tibia occurs on the posterior medial aspect of the bone (compression side) and heals well if treated appropriately. The less common high-risk stress fracture of the tibia occurs on the anterior aspect of the bone (tension side) and often does not heal well even when treated appropriately.

EPIDEMIOLOGY

- Incidence unknown, but fairly common
- Prevalence unknown, but fairly common
- 19–64% of all stress fractures
- Predominantly younger athletes (<20 yr old)
- Predominantly female athletes
- No difference in race

Incidence

Incidence of tibial stress fractures is not known and varies greatly among sports and studies.

Prevalence

Prevalence of tibial stress fractures is not known and varies between sports and studies.

ETIOLOGY AND PATHOPHYSIOLOGY

Insoles may reduce femoral and tibial stress fractures (1)[B].

Genetics

Little is known about the genetic predisposition for stress fracture other than osteopenia.

RISK FACTORS

- Previous history of stress fractures
- Track and field athletes
- Female gender
- Younger age
- Increase in training volume or intensity
- Multisport athletes
- Osteopenia/osteoporosis
- Disordered eating
- Oligomenorrhea/amenorrhea
- Chronic steroid use

GENERAL PREVENTION

Most stress fractures can be prevented by:

- Gradual increases in activity (the 10% rule: no more than a 10% increase in load—intensity, duration, or frequency per week).
- Appropriate footwear (properly fitted running shoes, orthotics if indicated).
- Appropriate nutrition (matching energy intake with expenditure; nutrition consult may be appropriate).

COMMONLY ASSOCIATED CONDITIONS

Female athlete triad or any of the signs:

- Osteopenia/osteoporosis: chronic steroid use
- Amenorrhea/oligomenorrhea: either primary or secondary
- Energy imbalance: disordered eating, excess exercise

DIAGNOSIS

- Primarily based on history and physical examination and a high index of suspicion based on risk factors
- X-rays can be helpful if positive but are often unremarkable.
- Hallmark is point tenderness on physical examination.
- It is important to distinguish anterior stress fractures (the dreaded black line) from posteromedial ones because the prognosis is much worse.

HISTORY

- Pain in the shin area:
  - Severe enough to limit activity
  - Worse with activity and better with rest
  - Night pain
  - Worsens over time if the activity is continued
  - Often associated with an increase in training duration, frequency, or intensity
  - Usually no associated injury
- Assess for risk factors:
  - Training history should include days per week, hours per day and intensity, and footwear (how often changed and what type).
  - Dietary history (calories, foods avoided, and vitamin D and calcium intake; weight changes)
  - Menstrual history (frequency, birth control pills, prior to birth control)
  - Family or personal history of stress fractures or osteoporosis/osteopenia
  - Medications known to decrease bone density (contraceptives, glucocorticoids, antiseizure medications)
  - Supplements (sex hormones or precursors, vitamin D, calcium)

PHYSICAL EXAM

- Focal tenderness to palpation on examination is the primary method for diagnosis of a stress fracture.
- Palpate for fracture callus, step-off, or crepitus.
- Hop test: pain at the site with hopping on one leg → be cautious with this because high index of suspicion can worsen fracture.
- Fulcrum test: pain at the site with bending the long bone over a fulcrum (table edge or examiner's leg)
- Tuning fork test: pain at the site when applying the tuning fork to a bony prominence of the same bone not the site of injury
- Examine foot type and function for biomechanical factors that predispose to stress fracture (pes planus, pes cavus, heavy heel strike).
- X-rays can be helpful in diagnosing stress fractures but is often negative initially.
- History and clinical examination are often all that is necessary.
- Magnetic resonance imaging (MRI) is the gold standard for diagnosis.
- Bone scan or computed tomography (CT) scan can be useful adjuncts.

DIFFERENTIAL DIAGNOSIS

- Medial tibial stress syndrome (shin splints)
- Osteoarthritis of the knee
- Chronic exertional compartment syndrome
- Popliteal artery entrapment syndrome
- Pes anserine bursitis
- Osgood-Schlatter disease
- Posterior/anterior tibialis tendonitis
- Superficial nerve entrapment
- Other bony processes: bone cysts, osteoid osteoma, tumor, infection

DIAGNOSTIC TESTS & INTERPRETATION

Initial Tests (lab, imaging)

Initial approach:

ALERT

- X-rays:
  - May be negative through course; often negative for 3+ wk; shows a lucency or fracture callus
  - For anterior cortical fractures, shows the "dreaded black line"
  - Sensitivity ranged from 12% (0–29%) to 56% (39–72%) (2).
  - Specificity ranged from 88% (55–100%) to 96% (87–100%) (2).
- Bone scan:
  - Sensitivity ranged from 50% (23–77%) to 97% (90–100%) (2).
  - Specificity ranged from 33% (12–53%) to 98% (93–100%) (2).
  - Poor accuracy (52%)
  - Helpful in multiple areas of concern, such as bilateral tibia or if MRI is not possible
- MRI:
  - Gold standard (2)[B]
  - Sensitivity ranged from 68% (45–90%) to 99% (95–100%) (2).
  - Specificity from 4% (0–11%) to 97% (88–100%) (2)
  - Best at demonstrating the exact location and extent of injury; accuracy (90%) (3)[B]
  - Shows fracture line on T1 and edema on T2
- CT scan:
  - Not useful in the acute setting
  - Sensitivity ranged from 32% (8–57%) to 38% (16–59%) (2).
  - Specificity from 88% (55–100%) to 98% (91–100%) (2)
  - Useful in assessing healing of fractures

- Musculoskeletal ultrasound (MSK US):
  - Sensitivity ranged from 43% (26–61%) to 99% (95–100%) (2).
  - Specificity ranged from 13% (0–45%) to 79% (61–96%) (2).
- Follow-up and special considerations:
  - X-rays will show the fracture healing in most cases; look for callus formation.
  - Bone scan can remain positive for over a year; therefore, not useful to determine healing
  - MRI may continue to show edema after the fracture is asymptomatic.
  - CT is useful for assessing fracture healing for fractures that are difficult to see on plain film.

Diagnostic Procedures/Other

Occasionally, stress fractures can be confused with tumor on imaging. A biopsy of the anterior tibia should be avoided if possible because it may increase the risk of nonunion.

TREATMENT

- Treatment of most stress fractures of the tibia is the same as other stress fractures, which is to remove the offending activity (usually impact activity).
- However, the treatment of anterior tibial stress fractures is quite different:
  - Posterior medial tibial stress fractures can be allowed to continue to participate in limited activity as pain allows. Decrease practice to allow more participation in games.
  - Anterior tibial stress fractures (the dreaded black line) should not continue to participate because of the risk of fracture completion and/or nonunion; requires prolonged non–weight-bearing or often surgery for internal fixation and/or bone grafting to heal
- Prehospital:
  - PRICE:
    - Protection: bracing
    - Rest
    - Ice
    - Compression
    - Elevation
  - Acetaminophen
  - Walking boot or long Aircast, crutches if necessary based on the amount of pain with weight-bearing
- Emergency department (ED) treatment:
  - Continued PRICE
  - Acetaminophen
  - Avoidance of scheduled nonsteroidal anti-inflammatory drugs (NSAIDs)
  - Walking boot
  - Crutches as needed
  - Consider non–weight-bearing or surgery for anterior tibial stress fractures or nonunion of tibial stress fractures.
  - Addressing other risk factors: nutritional, menstrual, osteopenia

MEDICATION

- No medications currently available to help stress fracture healing but can treat with pain medications.
- Pain medications with anti-inflammatory drugs may be contraindicated because they may delay the healing of fractures.

ISSUES FOR REFERRAL

- Most athletes with anterior tibial stress fractures should be referred for surgical treatment (4).
- Conservative treatment with casting and strict non–weight-bearing for 2 to 3 mo can be considered but still may result in nonunion.

ADDITIONAL THERAPIES

- Measures to alleviate the pain associated with stress fractures include ice, acetaminophen, a controlled ankle movement (CAM) walker boot, and crutches.
- Some evidence that use of a pneumatic or stirrup brace may shorten the time to return to activity (5)[B].
- Physical therapists can check and possibly correct poor biomechanics. Foot orthoses were not found to be effective for prevention of tibial stress fractures (6).

SURGERY/OTHER PROCEDURES

Surgical treatment of anterior tibial stress fractures consists of intermedullary nailing, with or without bone graft (3).

COMPLEMENTARY & ALTERNATIVE MEDICINE

Bone stimulators: Current evidence is insufficient to conclude a benefit in improving the rate of union in patients with a fresh fracture, osteotomy, delayed union, or nonunion or on time to healing in tibial stress fractures or a reduction in pain (1)[A].

ADMISSION, INPATIENT, AND NURSING CONSIDERATIONS

Not applicable in most cases

ONGOING CARE

- Low-risk stress fractures of the tibia: Ongoing activity modification and pain management is usually sufficient.
- High-risk stress fractures of the tibia require intermedullary nailing and grafting or non–weight-bearing and casting for 8 to 12 wk, after which intermedullary nailing and grafting still may be necessary (approximately 70% require surgery) (4).

DIET

- Nutritional evaluation is important, not only for healing of the current fracture but also for prevention of recurrence.
- Current recommendations from the National Osteoporosis Foundation are 1,000 mg of calcium and 400 to 800 IU of vitamin D daily for adults age <50 yr.

PATIENT EDUCATION

- Athletes should understand that training, nutrition, biomechanical, and footwear errors must be remedied.
- Athletes with a prior stress fracture are at increased risk for a future stress fracture.

PROGNOSIS

- Good for low-risk stress fractures of the tibia
- Poor for high-risk stress fractures of the tibia

COMPLICATIONS

- Posteromedial stress fractures of the tibia: potential for slower healing if continued participation is allowed
- Anterior stress fractures of the tibia: Risk of nonunion and delayed or partial union is high, requiring surgery (3).

REFERENCES

1. Mollon B, da Silva V, Busse JW, et al. Electrical stimulation for long-bone fracture-healing: a meta-analysis of randomized controlled trials. *J Bone Joint Surg Am*. 2008;90(11):2322–2330.
2. Wright AA, Hegedus EJ, Lenchik L, et al. Diagnostic accuracy of various imaging modalities for suspected lower extremity stress fractures: a systematic review with evidence-based recommendations for clinical practice. *Am J Sports Med*. 2016;44(1):255–263.
3. Mallee WH, Weel H, van Dijk CN, et al. Surgical versus conservative treatment for high-risk stress fractures of the lower leg (anterior tibial cortex, navicular and fifth metatarsal base): a systematic review. *Br J Sports Med*. 2015;49(6):370–376.
4. Robertson GA, Wood AM. Return to sports after stress fractures of the tibial diaphysis: a systematic review. *Br Med Bull*. 2015;114(1):95–111.
5. Whitelaw GP, Wetzler MJ, Levy AS, et al. A pneumatic leg brace for the treatment of tibial stress fractures. *Clin Orthop Relat Res*. 1991;(270):301–305.
6. Bonanno DR, Landorf KB, Munteanu SE, et al. Effectiveness of foot orthoses and shock-absorbing insoles for the prevention of injury: a systematic review and meta-analysis. *Br J Sports Med*. 2017;51(2):86–96.

ADDITIONAL READING

- Busse JW, Kaur J, Mollon B, et al. Low intensity pulsed ultrasonography for fractures: systematic review of randomised controlled trials. *BMJ*. 2009;338:b351.
- Kaeding CC, Yu JR, Wright R, et al. Management and return to play of stress fractures. *Clin J Sport Med*. 2005;15(6):442–447.
- Snyder RA, Koester MC, Dunn WR. Epidemiology of stress fractures. *Clin Sports Med*. 2006;25(1):37–52.

SEE ALSO

Other stress fracture chapters

CLINICAL PEARLS

- Distinguish low-risk from high-risk stress fracture based on imaging and exam.
- Tenderness to palpation is the main physical examination finding.
- MRI is the imaging study of choice.
- Evaluate for training errors.
- Evaluate for additional risk factors.

TIBIALIS POSTERIOR TENDINOPATHY

Alicia Chitanand, DO • Kenneth P. Barnes, MD, MSc, CAQSM, FACSM

BASICS

DESCRIPTION

- Overuse injury resulting in tendon degeneration with pain typically located posterior to the medial malleolus
- Various presentations of condition divided into three stages:
  - Stage 1: mild swelling, medial ankle pain, normal but painful heel rise, and no foot or ankle deformity
  - Stage 2: progressive flattening of the arch, flexible hindfoot, abducted midfoot, incompetent or ruptured tendon, and inability to perform a heel rise
  - Stage 3: all signs of stage 2 except the hindfoot deformity is fixed
- Synonym(s): posterior tibial tendon dysfunction; posterior tibial tendinopathy

EPIDEMIOLOGY

- Incidence of 2.3–3.6% in runners presenting to sports medicine clinics in earlier studies (1)
- Posterior tibial tendon dysfunction is the major cause of acquired flatfoot deformity in adults.

RISK FACTORS

- Recent increase or change in training or type of activity
- Surgical or accidental trauma to the foot
- 60% of cases in patients >50 yr of age associated with hypertension (HTN), diabetes, and obesity; no association of these factors with younger patients
- Severe pronation of the foot with planovalgus foot deformity
- Association with rheumatoid arthritis and seronegative inflammatory disease
- Prior exposure to steroids; local injection reported as a possible cause of rupture

DIAGNOSIS

HISTORY

- Pain along the length of the posterior tibialis tendon, particularly near the medial malleolus
- May relate to a recent change in activity frequency, type, and intensity
- Medial arch pain
- Occasional radiation of pain into the medial calf area
- Symptoms usually worsen with prolonged or strenuous activity, especially activities with a strong push-off motion.
- Initially painful but normal heel raise progressing to gait changes and inability to toe-raise

PHYSICAL EXAM

- Tender posterior tibialis tendon, especially posterior to the medial malleolus
- Medial ankle and possible foot swelling
- Flattened longitudinal arch compared with unaffected foot
- Increased hindfoot valgus and "too many toes sign," where more toes are seen laterally when viewing the patient from behind (late finding)
- Single-limb heel-rise test: Patient stands on affected foot and attempts to rise up on the ball of the foot while the other foot is off the ground. With tendinopathy, patients will be able to raise the affected heel, although with pain. Repetitive heel raises may show some weakness and pain in the tendon with persistent valgus hindfoot position through the toe raise.
- Tendon strength testing: foot plantarflexed and everted, then resist patients attempt to invert the foot (Avoid dorsiflexion because anterior tibialis may help to invert the foot.)

DIFFERENTIAL DIAGNOSIS

- Flexor hallucis or flexor digitorum longus tendinopathy
- Subluxation or dislocation of the posterior tibialis tendon
- Tarsal tunnel syndrome or other entrapment neuropathy
- Stress fracture to the navicular or accessory navicular (will present as point tenderness over the navicular)
- Fracture of sustentaculum, medial talar process, or talar dome (with acute trauma)

DIAGNOSTIC TESTS & INTERPRETATION

- Often clinical diagnosis and imaging not required
- Radiographs are often normal but may show minimal angular changes in earlier stages. Weight-bearing anteroposterior and lateral plain radiographs of the foot, plus anteroposterior, lateral, and mortise views of the ankle, should be obtained.
- A recent study showed that high-resolution ultrasound (HRUS) in an experienced ultrasonographer can be more accurate than 3T magnetic resonance imaging (MRI) in diagnosing posterior tibialis tendon dysfunction after reviewed intraoperatively (1)[B].

TREATMENT

- Early treatment is essential to prevent progression of stage 1 to 2 or 3.
- Use the Education, Unloading, Reloading, and Prevention (EdUReP) model for nonsurgical management of tendinopathy (2)[A]:
  - Education: 5 A's construct for behavioral counseling: assess, advise, agree, assist, and arrange
  - Unloading: over-the-counter (OTC) or custom orthotics for medial arch support; relative rest (cross-training—pool running or swimming as tolerated). It is preferred to use an orthosis with ankle stirrup support and medial longitudinal arch support (3)[B].

- Reloading: controlled reloading with focused concentric or eccentric exercises, transition to weight-support training (treadmill in pool) and weaning from unloading braces or orthotics. One study of 36 patients randomly assigned to: custom orthoses and calf stretching; custom orthoses, calf stretching, and a concentric exercise program; or custom orthoses, calf stretching, and an eccentric exercise program; all three groups improved pain after 3 mo, most effective in eccentric exercise group (4)[B]
- Prevention: prevention of disease progression and disease recurrence through gradual resumption of activity

- Studies have found that treatment with an orthosis and gastroc soleus stretches with or without structured exercises can be effective for patients with stage 1 or 2 posterior tibial tendon dysfunction (3)[B].

MEDICATION

Focus on pain control because inflammation is likely only during the initial phase of symptoms.

ALERT

Local steroid injections into the synovial sheath are not recommended and have been associated with tendon rupture.

SURGERY/OTHER PROCEDURES

- Stage 1 or 2 should be treated conservatively for ~3 to 4 mo before surgery is considered:
  - Tendon sheath release, scar tissue excision, and partial synovectomy are the typical surgical management approach.
  - Posterior tibial tendon sheath endoscopy has been shown to be effective at reducing pain and decreased need for more invasive surgeries (4,5)[C].
- Stage 3 disease has a fixed deformity, and tendon reconstruction will not correct the problem. Subtalar or triple arthrodesis is usually needed to block hindfoot motion.

COMPLEMENTARY & ALTERNATIVE MEDICINE

Glyceryl trinitrate patches, extracorporeal shock wave therapy, and sclerotherapy have not been evaluated specifically with posterior tibialis tendinopathy, and a recommendation cannot be made for their use.

REFERENCES

1. Arnoldner MA, Gruber M, Syrè S, et al. Imaging of posterior tibial tendon dysfunction—comparison of high-resolution ultrasound and 3T MRI. *Eur J Radiol*. 2015;84(9):1777–1781.
2. Davenport TE, Kulig K, Matharu Y, et al. The EdUReP model for nonsurgical management of tendinopathy. *Phys Ther*. 2005;85(10):1093–1103.
3. Houck J, Neville C, Tome J, et al. Randomized controlled trial comparing orthosis augmented by either stretching or stretching and strengthening for stage II tibialis posterior tendon dysfunction. *Foot Ankle Int*. 2015;36(9):1006–1016.
4. Wadehra A, Fallat LM, Jarski RJ. Surgical management of stage 2 adult and pediatric acquired flatfoot without tendon transfer or arthrodesis: a retrospective study. *J Foot Ankle Surg*. 2018;57(4):658–663.
5. Bernasconi A, Sadile F, Welck M, et al. Role of tendoscopy in treating stage II posterior tibial tendon dysfunction. *Foot Ankle Int*. 2018;39(4):433–442.

ADDITIONAL READING

- Alvarez RG, Marini A, Schmitt C, et al. Stage I and II posterior tibial tendon dysfunction treated by a structured nonoperative management protocol: an orthosis and exercise program. *Foot Ankle Int*. 2006;27(1):2–8.
- Andres BM, Murrell GA. Treatment of tendinopathy: what works, what does not, and what is on the horizon. *Clin Orthop Relat Res*. 2008;466(7): 1539–1554.
- Augustin JF, Lin SS, Berberian WS, et al. Nonoperative treatment of adult acquired flat foot with the Arizona brace. *Foot Ankle Clin*. 2003;8(3): 491–502.
- Chao W, Wapner KL, Lee TH, et al. Nonoperative management of posterior tibial tendon dysfunction. *Foot Ankle Int*. 1996;17(12):736–741.
- Geideman WM, Johnson JE. Posterior tibial tendon dysfunction. *J Orthop Sports Phys Ther*. 2000;30(2):68–77.
- Krause F, Bosshard A, Lehmann O, et al. Shell brace for stage II posterior tibial tendon insufficiency. *Foot Ankle Int*. 2008;29(11):1095–1100.
- Premkumar A, Perry MB, Dwyer AJ, et al. Sonography and MR imaging of posterior tibial tendinopathy. *AJR Am J Roentgenol*. 2002;178(1):223–232.
- Richie DH Jr. Biomechanics and clinical analysis of the adult acquired flatfoot. *Clin Podiatr Med Surg*. 2007;24(4):617–644.

CLINICAL PEARLS

- Posterior tibialis tendinitis is caused by overuse and needs relative rest. This can be done by orthotic use, bracing, or cam walker. A home exercise program and cross-training with pool activities can be beneficial in the long term for posterior tibialis tendinitis.
- Stage 1 and 2 can be treated conservatively.
- Most patients will need ~3 to 4 mo of therapy and treatment before they are able to return to previous activities.
- Even patients with a flattened arch and functionally incompetent tendon can be treated nonoperatively. The need for surgery hinges on the progression of symptoms and adherence to treatment and therapy. Definitive treatment for patients with a fixed hindfoot deformity is surgery, however.

TILLAUX FRACTURES: ANTERIOR TIBIA-FIBULA LIGAMENT AVULSION

David Johnson, MD • Michael Y. Yang, MD

BASICS

DESCRIPTION

- Salter-Harris (SH) type III avulsion fracture of the lateral distal tibial epiphysis
- Occurs with traumatic external rotatory force pulling on the anterior inferior talofibular ligament
- Transitional fracture, classically seen in adolescent girls ages 13 to 15 yr and boys ages 15 to 17 yr with a partially closed physis
- Synonyms: Tillaux-Chaput fracture; juvenile Tillaux fracture; transitional fracture of distal tibia
- Described by Paul Jules Tillaux in 1892 (1)

EPIDEMIOLOGY

- Relatively uncommon—15% of all juvenile injuries of the long bones involve the epiphyseal growth plate, and 2.9% of these injuries are juvenile Tillaux fractures (2)
- Adolescent ankle injuries typically within 1 yr from physeal closure. The anterior-lateral portion of the plate closes last.
- Tensile stress applied to the anterior tibiofibular ligament, which inserts on the anterolateral aspect of the distal tibial epiphysis

RISK FACTORS

- Peak incidence: girls 13 to 15 yr of age and boys 15 to 17 yr of age during the 12- to 18-mo mo period when the distal tibial physis is fusing centrally but not yet laterally
- Traumatic, forceful external rotation of the foot

DIAGNOSIS

HISTORY

- Forceful supination and external rotation with compression stress
- Also seen with internal rotation of the lower leg on a firmly planted foot
- Acute anterolateral ankle pain
- Reported pain with bearing weight

PHYSICAL EXAM

- Mild swelling and/or ecchymosis
- Tenderness over the anterolateral ankle and syndesmosis region
- Limited active ankle range of motion (ROM)
- Pain with passive ankle motion
- Weight-bearing—limited
- Examine for concurrent fibular injury.
- Extremity neurovascular examination

DIFFERENTIAL DIAGNOSIS

- Ankle or syndesmosis injury/sprain
- Triplanar fracture: more severe transitional fracture (SH IV) that fractures through the posterior distal tibial metaphysis
- Talar dome injury/osteochondritis dissecans
- Distal fibular physeal injury

DIAGNOSTIC TESTS & INTERPRETATION

- Radiography: ankle anteroposterior (AP), lateral, and mortise views
- Consider comparison of uninjured ankle to assess physeal closure.
- Computed tomography (CT): Patients with transitional distal tibial fractures as well as patients with displaced SH III and SH IV fractures may benefit from CT to better determine fracture pattern, amount of displacement, and need for surgery (3)[C].

TREATMENT

Nonsurgical:

- Initial: immobilization, non–weight-bearing, ice, elevation, acetaminophen and nonsteroidal anti-inflammatory drugs (NSAIDs)
- Nondisplaced or minimally displaced fractures (<2 mm) can be treated nonoperatively (4)[B].
- Closed reduction by positioning foot in internal rotation and slight inversion sufficient if postreduction interfragment gap is <2 mm (5)[B]
- *Postreduction evaluation*: neurovascular exam and repeat radiographs: ankle AP, lateral, and mortise views

- *Immobilization*:
  - Initial—compressive bulky dressing or fracture boot
  - 4-wk non–weight-bearing in a long leg cast with knee partially flexed stabilizes intra-articular rotational component (4)[B].
  - After initial 4 wk, may bear weight as tolerated for 2 to 4 wk in a short leg cast, cam walker, or rigid shell boot

SURGERY/OTHER PROCEDURES

- Indicated if ≥2 mm of displacement
- Open reduction with internal fixation of fracture (5)[C]
- Successful treatment also described using percutaneous fixation assisted arthroscopically (4)[C]
- Overall good reported surgical outcomes (5,6)
- Prognosis uniformly good after closed reduction and percutaneous fixation techniques if residual displacement is <2.5 mm (6)[C]

ADDITIONAL THERAPIES

Rehabilitation:

- Sport-specific drills
- Strengthening of dynamic stabilizers
- Proprioception training
- Proper shoe wear

ONGOING CARE

FOLLOW-UP RECOMMENDATIONS

For nonsurgically treated:

- Follow-up with x-rays, typically every 2 wk
- Evaluate for varus or valgus deformity.
- After 4 wk of immobilization, progress to walking cast or cam walker for 2 to 4 wk.

PROGNOSIS

- Generally good outcomes if treated
- Early arthritis: risk based on displacement
- Physeal arrest rare and typically of low concern given patients are near physeal closure
- Many patients are able to return to full activity after 3 mo postinjury.

REFERENCES

1. Cassas KJ, Jamison JP. Juvenile Tillaux fracture in an adolescent basketball player. *Phys Sportsmed*. 2005;33(2):30–33.
2. Spiegel PG, Cooperman DR, Laros GS. Epiphyseal fractures of the distal ends of the tibia and fibula. A retrospective study of two hundred and thirty-seven cases in children. *J Bone Joint Surg Am*. 1978;60(8):1046–1050.
3. Nenopoulos A, Beslikas T, Gigis I, et al. The role of CT in diagnosis and treatment of distal tibial fractures with intra-articular involvement in children. *Injury*. 2015;46(11):2177–2180.
4. Tiefenboeck TM, Binder H, Joestl J, et al. Displaced juvenile Tillaux fractures: surgical treatment and outcome. *Wien Klin Wochenschr*. 2017;129(5–6):169–175.
5. Choudhry IK, Wall EJ, Eismann EA, et al. Functional outcome analysis of triplane and Tillaux fractures after closed reduction and percutaneous fixation. *J Pediatr Orthop*. 2014;34(2):139–143.
6. Feng SM, Sun QQ, Wang AG, et al. "All-Inside" arthroscopic treatment of Tillaux-Chaput fractures: clinical experience and outcomes analysis. *J Foot Ankle Surg*. 2018;57(1):56–59.

ADDITIONAL READING

Habusta SF, Griffin EE. *Fractures, Tillaux*. Treasure Island, FL: StatPearls Publishing; 2018.

CLINICAL PEARLS

- Possible complications include posttraumatic arthritis and asymmetric physeal growth.
- If treated nonoperatively, 4 wk non–weight-bearing followed by 2 to 4 wk in a walking cast or cam walker. If stabilized with internal fixation, consensus is >4 wk non–weight-bearing and cast immobilization 4 to 12 wk (4)[C].
- Return to sports after >12 wk if well-healed on x-ray, pain-free with activity, and have full ROM and strength.
- Peroneal strengthening and proprioception training are essential rehab components.
- Proper mechanics and proper shoe wear

TINEA GLADIATORUM (CAPITIS, CORPORIS, CRURIS, PEDIS)

Philipp J. Underwood, MD, FAAEM, FACEP, FAAFP, CAQSM, RDMS

BASICS

DESCRIPTION

- This group of topical fungal infections commonly affects athletes, particularly wrestlers. They are classified by site of infection: Tinea capitis involves the scalp and hairline; tinea corporis involves the trunk, face, or extremities; tinea cruris involves inguinal folds; tinea pedis involves the feet. Infection is caused by a dermatophyte, most commonly from the *Trichophyton*, *Epidermophyton*, and *Microsporum* species. This is typically an infection of the stratum corneum that results in thickening of the epidermis and scale formation. Majocchi granuloma is an infection of the dermis, usually as a result of fungal entry through hair follicles.
- Synonym(s): ring worm (tinea corporis); jock itch (tinea cruris); athlete's foot (tinea pedis); tinea gladiatorum (most commonly *Trichophyton tonsurans* and *Trichophyton rubrum*)

EPIDEMIOLOGY

ALERT

Varies from 25–35% of all wrestlers during any given season

- 10–20% lifetime risk for nonathletes
- More common in African Americans and Asians
- 2 to 20 days from inoculation to subsequent development of identifiable skin lesions

RISK FACTORS

- Spread by direct contact with a pet or human carrier
- Fomite transmission may occur from wrestling mats, pieces of athletic equipment, shower floor, and so forth.

GENERAL PREVENTION

- Good personal hygiene
- Do not share towels or clothing.
- Wipe down surfaces before and after use.
- Wash clothing in hot water (60°C) (1).

DIAGNOSIS

Scraping of the leading edge of the skin plaque and preparation with potassium hydroxide (KOH) 5–20% can be examined under the microscope. This will reveal hyphae and pseudohyphae, which are diagnostic of tinea infection. For *tinea capitis*, spores are visualized by KOH preparation of the hair shaft. *Microsporum canis* may fluoresce bright green under a Wood lamp. Fungal culture using Sabouraud dextrose agar also can be used, but in athletes, use is limited by time and expense involved. Most tinea infections do not fluoresce under Wood light examination.

HISTORY

- Determine when and where lesions appeared and exposure history.
- Are other wrestlers and wrestling partners on the team are infected?

PHYSICAL EXAM

- Lesions present with erythema, pruritus, and scaling.
- Tinea capitis: two distinct types:
  - Black dot: most common form seen in United States and most commonly caused by *T. tonsurans*. Usually children and elderly. Erythematous, scaling patch that enlarges slowly. Hairs break off flush with scalp causing alopecia, which may be permanent.
  - Gray patch: uncommon in United States and caused by *M. canis* contracted usually from dogs and cats. Erythematous, scaling patch that enlarges slowly. Hairs break off 1 to 2 mm above the scalp.
- Tinea corporis: circular, erythematous, scaling plaques with central clearing on trunk, face, and extremities
- Tinea cruris: pruritic, scaling, erythematous patches in inguinal folds and/or medial thighs. If lesions present on penis or scrotum, consider candidal infection rather than tinea.
- Tinea pedis: pruritic, erythematous scaly skin along the sole of foot. Cracking and maceration of the web spaces also may be present. Bullous form will have bullae or vesicles filled with clear fluid.

DIFFERENTIAL DIAGNOSIS

- Tinea capitis: alopecia areata, impetigo, psoriasis, seborrhea, trichotillomania
- Tinea corporis: impetigo, eczema, psoriasis, contact or atopic dermatitis, drug eruption, cutaneous herpes, lupus, pityriasis rosea
- Tinea cruris: contact dermatitis, candidal intertrigo, erythrasma, psoriasis, seborrhea
- Tinea pedis: eczema, contact or atopic dermatitis, dyshidrosis, pitted keratolysis, psoriasis

TREATMENT

MEDICATION

- Primary treatment for tinea corporis, cruris, and pedis is with topical antifungal agents. Primary treatment for tinea capitis is oral antifungal agents.
- Initial treatment also may include a topical corticosteroid. This may help reduce the associated pruritus and erythema; however, this may exacerbate tinea infections and can lead to treatment failure.
- Azoles were slightly less effective in clinical cure compared to azoles + steroid combination (2).
- Tinea capitis and diffuse, multiple lesions in other areas should be treated with oral antifungal agents.
- When using oral agents, give consideration to drug interactions, potential for toxicity, and cost of medication.
- Prevention is key: Emphasize proper personal hygiene; use dry, cotton clothing; and keep athletic equipment disinfected properly.
- Tolnaftate and clotrimazole only suppress the fungus and are not cidal.
- Naftifine is both fungicidal and fungistatic.
- Shampooing hair and body with selenium (Selsun Blue) may be useful prophylaxis.
- Failure to treat all areas simultaneously may result in treatment failure.

- *Tinea capitis* requires oral treatment:
  - Griseofulvin: Treat for 6 wk. Monitor complete blood count (CBC), liver function tests (LFTs). Side effects: photosensitivity, headache, neutropenia, elevated LFTs, paresthesia, rash; pregnancy Category C:
    - Adults: 500 mg microsize or 330 to 375 mg ultramicrosize daily for 6 wk
    - Children: 11 mg microsize/kg/day or 7.3 mg ultramicrosize/kg/day for 6 wk
  - Terbinafine: Treat for 4 wk. Monitor CBC, LFTs; pregnancy Category B:
    - 10 to 20 kg: 62.5 mg daily
    - 20 to 40 kg: 125 mg daily
    - >40 kg: 250 mg daily
  - Itraconazole: Treat for 2 to 6 wk. Monitor LFTs. Caution: hypoglycemia with sulfonylureas, rhabdomyolysis with HMG-CoA reductase inhibitors; pregnancy Category C:
    - Adults: 100 mg daily up to 200 mg BID
    - Children: 3 to 5 mg/kg daily
  - Fluconazole: Treat for 2 to 4 wk. Increased international normalized ratio (INR) on warfarin; pregnancy Category C:
    - Adults: 200 mg daily
    - Children: 6 mg/kg/day
- *Tinea corporis, cruris, and pedis*: Topical antifungals are first-line treatment. Topical nystatin is ineffective; oral therapy for failed topical, extensive lesions or immunocompromised:
  - *Topical therapy*: Treat for 2 to 6 wk (continue treatment additional week after resolution of rash):
    - Naftifine: Gel, apply twice daily; cream, apply once daily.
    - Terbinafine: Apply once to twice daily.
    - Ciclopirox: Apply twice daily.
    - Clotrimazole: Apply twice daily.
    - Econazole: Apply once daily.
    - Ketoconazole: Apply once daily.
    - Miconazole: Apply twice daily.
    - Oxiconazole: Apply once to twice daily.
    - Sertaconazole: Apply twice daily.
    - Sulconazole: Apply once to twice daily.
    - Tolnaftate: Apply twice daily.
  - Oral therapy: Treat for 2 to 6 wk:
    - Griseofulvin: 500 mg daily OR 500 mg BID OR 250 mg TID
    - Fluconazole: 150 to 200 mg once weekly for 2 to 4 wk or 400 mg one-time dose
    - Itraconazole: 100 to 200 mg daily
    - Terbinafine: 250 mg daily

ADDITIONAL THERAPIES

Prophylaxis for tinea gladiatorum:

- Recommended for recurrent episodes (exclude immunocompromised state)
- Use by some prior to wrestling tournaments or during season:
  - Fluconazole: 200 mg once weekly
  - Itraconazole: 400 mg once every 2 mo

ONGOING CARE

ALERT

Wrestling return to play:

- National Collegiate Athletic Association (NCAA): A minimum of 2 wk of systemic antifungal therapy is required for scalp lesions. A minimum of 72 hr of topical therapy is required for skin lesions. Wrestlers with extensive and active lesions will be disqualified. Activity of treated lesions can be judged either by use of KOH preparation or a review of therapeutic regimen. Wrestlers with solitary or closely clustered, localized lesions will be disqualified if lesions are in a body location that cannot be "properly covered" (a gas-permeable dressing, e.g., Opsite, Tegaderm, Bioclusive, Duoderm, and then covered by elastic/stretch tape). The disposition of tinea cases will be decided on an individual basis as determined by the examining physician and/or athletic trainer (NCAA Sports Medicine Handbook 2009 to 2010).
- National Federation of State High School Associations (NFHS): tinea lesions (ringworm scalp, skin): oral or topical treatment for 72 hr on skin and 14 days on scalp (NFHS revised/approved April 2008)

FOLLOW-UP RECOMMENDATIONS

Most infections are easily treated with topical or oral antifungal agents; therefore, referral is rare. However, for cases that do not respond as expected, further evaluation to rule out an immunocompromised state or other systemic illness should be considered.

REFERENCES

1. Amichai B, Grunwald MH, Davidovici B, et al. The effect of domestic laundry processes on fungal contamination of socks. *Int J Dermatol*. 2013;52(11):1392–1394.
2. El-Gohary M, van Zuuren EJ, Fedorowicz Z, et al. Topical antifungal treatments for tinea cruris and tinea corporis. *Cochrane Database Syst Rev*. 2014;(8):CD009992.

CLINICAL PEARLS

- All areas of tinea infection need to be treated simultaneously to reduce risk of reinfection.
- Prevention strategies can reduce the risk to the participant and others.
- Consider oral fluconazole for extensive and resistant lesions as well as prophylaxis.

TRACHEAL AND LARYNGEAL INJURIES

Jeffrey P. Feden, MD, FACEP, CAQSM • Razib Khaund, MD

BASICS

DESCRIPTION

- Injuries to the larynx and trachea may result from either blunt or penetrating trauma involving the head, neck, or upper chest.
- Although they are relatively uncommon and sometimes subtle, these potentially life-threatening injuries must not be overlooked.

EPIDEMIOLOGY

- Laryngotracheal (LT) trauma occurs at an estimated frequency from 1/5,000 to 1/30,000 emergency department (ED) visits.
- Laryngeal injuries comprise <1% of blunt and 7% of penetrating trauma cases; only 10% result from athletic trauma (1).
- Mortality is as high as 20% and 40% for penetrating and blunt injuries, respectively (2).

ETIOLOGY AND PATHOPHYSIOLOGY

- LT trauma may cause obstructive edema, submucosal hematomas, cartilage fractures, mucosal tears, or complete LT separation.
- Low-velocity trauma may cause soft tissue swelling, lacerations, contusions, and abrasions.
- High-velocity trauma may injure laryngeal muscles and nerves.
- Forceful compression to the chest against a closed glottis may cause laryngeal fractures and mucosal disruption.

RISK FACTORS

- Contact and collision sports
- Sports with high-velocity projectiles (i.e., baseball, hockey, lacrosse)
- Motor sports

COMMONLY ASSOCIATED CONDITIONS

- Penetrating trauma is associated with additional injury to the chest, esophagus, vasculature, or nerves in 86% of cases; esophageal injury occurs 50% of the time.
- Blunt trauma is associated with intracranial injury (17%), cervical spine injury (13%), chest injury (13%), and esophageal injury (13%) (2).
- Pneumothorax may accompany distal tracheal injuries.

DIAGNOSIS

HISTORY

Signs or symptoms may be absent initially in up to 1/3 of those with LT trauma.

PHYSICAL EXAM

- Dysphonia (e.g., hoarseness) and neck/throat pain are most common (3)[C].
- Cough, hemoptysis, odynophagia, respiratory distress, stridor
- Loss of anatomic landmarks, anterior cervical tenderness, sternoclavicular (SC) crepitus, cervical ecchymosis, or hematoma

DIAGNOSTIC TESTS & INTERPRETATION

Initial Tests (lab, imaging)

- Chest radiograph to evaluate for associated trauma
- Cervical spine radiographs to evaluate for cervical spine injury
- Plain radiographs may show hyoid bone elevation or prevertebral air.
- Computed tomography (CT) imaging of the cervical region is recommended if the airway is stable because it provides additional anatomic detail useful for management decisions.

Diagnostic Procedures/Other

- Flexible bronchoscopy is the preferred initial method for evaluating the stable airway.
- Fiberoptic laryngoscopy may provide more detail about laryngeal anatomy and vocal cord function.

TREATMENT

- Prehospital:
  - Initial treatment focuses on the primary survey and airway, breathing, and circulation (ABCs) in accordance with Advanced Trauma Life Support guidelines.
  - Control the airway and immobilize the cervical spine.
  - Rapidly transport to the nearest ED while continuing to manage the airway.
  - Oral airways, combitubes, and laryngeal mask airways fail to provide a definitive airway by virtue of their supraglottic position.
  - Orotracheal intubation and cricothyroidotomy may be contraindicated in cases of significant trauma or complete LT separation; either must be undertaken with extreme caution to avoid losing the airway or causing greater injury.
- ED treatment:
  - Airway management is the priority (3)[C].
  - Prompt assessment of the stable airway includes fiberoptic laryngoscopy in consultation with ear, nose, throat (ENT) specialist, followed by close observation, further imaging with CT scan, or surgical management in the operating room (3)[C].
  - Preferred management of an unstable airway includes awake tracheotomy under local anesthesia in the operating room (2)[C].

ADDITIONAL THERAPIES

- Observation in an intensive care unit (ICU) for at least 24 hr is indicated for significant LT trauma that does not require emergent surgical intervention.
- Some patients may develop signs or symptoms up to 48 hr after injury.
- Monitor for signs of progressive airway compromise, and prepare for the possibility of urgent tracheotomy.
- Humidified air and head of the bed elevation
- Serial endoscopic examinations
- Vocal rest
- Minimize laryngeal irritation from gastric acid with H_2 blockers or proton pump inhibitors.
- Antibiotics and systemic corticosteroids are controversial.
- Use narcotic pain medications and sedatives with caution to avoid their effects of respiratory depression.
- Following initial treatment, prompt phoniatric evaluation is mandatory for all patients.
- Speech therapy may be required to restore vocal quality or to avoid permanent restrictions of phonation.

SURGERY/OTHER PROCEDURES

- Indications for surgery include initial airway instability, progressive airway decline despite conservative treatment, and complex LT injuries.
- Operative interventions range from tracheotomy to open reduction and internal fixation (ORIF) of the injured cartilaginous structures.
- 25–80% of patients with LT trauma will require surgery.

ONGOING CARE

- Long-term treatment goals involve restoring the anatomy, airway patency, and vocal quality.
- All athletes should be sent for phonic and speech therapy evaluations; speech therapy may be necessary to restore vocal quality.

PATIENT EDUCATION

- Dysphonia is the most common and problematic complication after LT trauma.
- Phoniatric evaluation is essential, and speech therapy may be important even after minor injuries.

PROGNOSIS

- Prognosis depends on injury severity, but complications may be avoided by early diagnosis and proper initial management.
- Voice disorders typically are associated with the most severe injuries, but even minor injuries can cause permanent problems with phonation.
- Most patients can expect excellent airway patency and good voice quality following LT trauma that has been recognized and treated appropriately.
- Prognosis is worse for those with late presentations (who already may have laryngeal stenosis).

COMPLICATIONS

- Dysphonia, hoarseness, voice fatigue, and poor vocal control are most common.
- Vocal cord paralysis owing to recurrent laryngeal nerve injury
- Permanent phonic disorders owing to laryngeal scarring or infection

REFERENCES

1. Paluska SA, Lansford CD. Laryngeal trauma in sport. *Curr Sports Med Rep*. 2008;7(1):16–21.
2. Atkins BZ, Abbate S, Fisher SR, et al. Current management of laryngotracheal trauma: case report and literature review. *J Trauma*. 2004;56(1): 185–190.
3. Mendis D, Anderson JA. Blunt laryngeal trauma secondary to sporting injuries. *J Laryngol Otol*. 2017;131(8):728–735.

ADDITIONAL READING

- Becker M, Duboé PO, Platon A, et al. MDCT in the assessment of laryngeal trauma: value of 2D multiplanar and 3D reconstructions. *AJR Am J Roentgenol*. 2013;201(4):W639–W647.
- Bhojani RA, Rosenbaum DH, Dikmen E, et al. Contemporary assessment of laryngotracheal trauma. *J Thorac Cardiovasc Surg*. 2005;130(2):426–432.
- Kim JD, Shuler FD, Mo B, et al. Traumatic laryngeal fracture in a collegiate basketball player. *Sports Health*. 2013;5(3):273–275.

CLINICAL PEARLS

- LT trauma may be immediately life threatening.
- Diagnosis often requires a high index of suspicion.
- Prompt recognition and airway management are essential.
- Complications and airway compromise may not develop until 24 to 48 hr following injury.
- Consideration of associated traumatic injuries is also important.

TRANSIENT OSTEOPOROSIS OF THE HIP

Uziel Sauceda, MD, ABFM certified • Eric Yuan, MD

BASICS

DESCRIPTION

- Transient osteoporosis of the hip (TOH) is a clinical presentation of acute hip pain, characterized by bone marrow edema of the femoral head, bone resorption, and subsequent resolution.
- Also known as primary bone marrow edema of proximal femur
- Similar bone marrow edema syndromes happen in the knee, ankle, and foot.

EPIDEMIOLOGY

- Condition is rare and of unknown incidence or prevalence; most information derived from case series
- Common in middle age men, average age of 40 yr with wide age of distribution
- Also common in females in 3rd trimester of pregnancy
- Rare in children

ETIOLOGY AND PATHOPHYSIOLOGY

- Etiology largely unknown, still debated whether it is part of early avascular necrosis (AVN)
- Other authors propose it is a subset of complex regional pain syndrome type 1 (1).
- Proposed pathophysiology involves an initial insult, followed by edema leading to separation of bone trabeculae, and then increased bone resorption. Resorption is self-limited, and last stage involves resolution of edema, pain, and return of bone formation.
- Inferred from histologic findings
- Initial insult: trauma, microfracture, infection, ischemic injury, venous hypertension, surgery, drugs, alcohol, or neurovascular dysfunction

RISK FACTORS

- Pregnancy, alcohol, abnormal vascularity, inflammatory state, mechanical injury, osteogenesis imperfecta, hypothyroid, neurologic and metabolic derangements
- Drugs: thiazolidinediones, serotonin reuptake inhibitors, nonsteroidal anti-inflammatory drugs (NSAIDs), steroids, and HIV protease inhibitors (2)
- Many risk factors are same as initial insult proposed in pathophysiology.

COMMONLY ASSOCIATED CONDITIONS

- Pregnancy
- Osteogenesis imperfecta
- Migratory osteoporosis
- Generalized low bone mass

DIAGNOSIS

Note that TOH is diagnosis of exclusion; therefore, a thorough evaluation for more common etiologies is warranted.

HISTORY

- Often spontaneous onset of acute unilateral or bilateral hip pain without obvious causal factor or trauma
- 3rd trimester of pregnancy
- Often unable to bear weight
- Ask about recent new medicine, illicit substances, alcohol, smoking, or new activity. Presentation can vary from vague pain to severe pain and immobility.

PHYSICAL EXAM

- Pain may be out of proportion to exam findings.
- Antalgic gait
- Decrease in full range of motion (ROM), along with pain, specifically on internal/external rotation
- Percussion of hip bone causes pain at affected side.
- Various exam maneuvers may cause pain of hip and are unlikely to be specific.

DIFFERENTIAL DIAGNOSIS

- Osteoarthritis
- Infection: septic hip joint, osteomyelitis
- Tumor: metastasis versus primary versus benign (osteoid osteoma)
- Fracture: acute, compression, or stress type
- Femoro-acetabular impingement
- Chondral defect: labral tear, osteochondritis dissecans
- AVN
- Inflammatory joint disease
- Radicular pain

DIAGNOSTIC TESTS & INTERPRETATION

- There are no lab tests specific for TOH.
- To evaluate for systemic disease: complete blood count with differential, blood urea nitrogen (BUN)/creatinine and electrolytes, liver enzymes, and coagulation panel. Erythrocyte sedimentation rate (ESR) and C-reactive protein (CRP) help in determining if there is underlying inflammatory component.
- *X-ray*: may be normal, but evaluate for osteopenia (compared to contralateral) and obvious tumors or fractures
- *Bone scan*: increased uptake at femoral head; seen in all phases of condition and persists for weeks after clinical improvement
- *Dual energy x-ray absorptiometry (DEXA)*: may show osteoporosis
- *Magnetic resonance imaging (MRI) with or without contrast*: best confirmation test (3)[C]
- Differentiate AVN versus TOH.
- High signal intensity on T2 sequences, homogenous, without distinct border or focal defect, located on femoral head. Edema may extend to neck or intertrochanteric region.
- Joint effusion is often seen.
- Subchondral changes indicates more AVN diagnosis (subchondral radiolucency crescent sign).

TREATMENT

GENERAL MEASURES

- The majority have self-limited course and complete resolution with conservative management within 6 mo (ranges from 4 to 12 mo).
- Analgesia should be tailored to individual; may include short course of opioids if severe
- Minimize weight-bearing/rest, analgesics, and ultrasound therapy (2,3)[C].
- Suppression of bone resorption or induction of bone formation may shorten recovery time (2,3)[C].
- Surgical treatment usually not required, unless symptoms refractory or femoral head fracture present

MEDICATION

- *Bisphosphonate therapy*:
  - Alendronate PO: 70 mg/wk:
    - Average recovery of 6 mo in 8 cases (3)[C]
  - Pamidronate intravenous (IV): Dosing varies in separate case reports: 45 mg q3d for 3 doses or 60 mg q7d for 4 doses (3)[C]:
    - Clinical recovery of 2 mo in 15 cases
- *Other bone remodeling agents*:
  - Calcitonin nasal: 200 IU daily for 4 to 6 wk (3)[C]:
    - Recovery in 4.7 mo in 6 cases
  - Teriparatide: 20 μg daily:
    - Recovery in 4 wk in 1 case (3)[C]
  - Iloprost: a prostacyclin analogue. Thought to increase vessel dilation and reduce permeability; can improve symptom of pain (3)[C]

Pregnancy Considerations

- Exposure to bisphosphonates before conception or during pregnancy may affect fetal skeletal mineralization, shorten gestational age, or cause birth defects/abortion.
- Calcitonin preferred because it doesn't cross placenta and safe to use during pregnancy (3)[C]

ISSUES FOR REFERRAL

- Refer to orthopedics if any suspicion of AVN or underlying femoral fracture.
- If considering medical therapy, consult endocrinology for recommendation on dosage and duration because there are no formal guidelines.

ADDITIONAL THERAPIES

- *Hyperbaric oxygen therapy* (4)[C]
- In 41 total patients, half underwent combination analgesics and hyperbaric oxygen (O_2), whereas the control was treated with only analgesics.
- It showed improvement in Western Ontario and McMaster Universities Osteoarthritis Index (WOMAC) scores as well as MRI findings at 3 mo.

SURGERY/OTHER PROCEDURES

- Core decompression therapy (2)[C]: usually used for AVN treatment of femoral head
- Has not been shown to improve outcomes more than medical therapy; data is limited to case reports.
- Best left for patients that pain is unable to be controlled with conservative treatment

ONGOING CARE

FOLLOW-UP RECOMMENDATIONS

- Follow-up MRI usually done; timing of repeat study uncertain; not unreasonable to repeat at 6 mo
- Weight-bearing activity as tolerated; unclear when high impact activity can resume but likely when minimal imaging findings and patient clinically improved

PATIENT EDUCATION

- Emphasize importance of limited weight-bearing while symptomatic.
- Smoking cessation, alcohol moderation, and optimization of diet rich in calcium/vitamin D may help (2)[C].
- Medication to alter bone resorption is off-label and needs full informed consent.
- Diagnosis is self-limited and will resolve with time.

PROGNOSIS

- Limited data to suggest long-term abnormalities after TOH resolves
- Recurrence months to years afterward at a separate skeletal site (contralateral hip) is known to happen and suggests a diagnosis of regional migratory osteoporosis (2).

COMPLICATIONS

- Fracture is rare: subchondral, femoral neck, or subcapital; more frequently seen in females.
- Progression to AVN or osteonecrosis is rare.

REFERENCES

1. Vaishya R, Agarwal AK, Kumar V, et al. Transient osteoporosis of the hip: a mysterious cause of hip pain in adults. *Indian J Orthop*. 2017;51(4):455–460.
2. Patel S. Primary bone marrow oedema syndromes. *Rheumatology (Oxford)*. 2014;53(5):785–792.
3. Asadipooya K, Graves L, Greene LW. Transient osteoporosis of the hip: review of the literature. *Osteoporos Int*. 2017;28(6):1805–1816.
4. Capone A, Podda D, Ennas F, et al. Hyperbaric oxygen therapy for transient bone marrow oedema syndrome of the hip. *Hip Int*. 2011;21(2):211–216.

ADDITIONAL READING

- Diwanji SR, Cho YJ, Xin ZF, et al. Conservative treatment for transient osteoporosis of the hip in middle-aged women. *Singapore Med J*. 2008;49(1):e17–e21.
- Fessel J. There are many potential medical therapies for atraumatic osteonecrosis. *Rheumatology (Oxford)*. 2013;52(2):235–241.
- Mirza R, Ishaq S, Amjad H. Transient osteoporosis of the hip. *J Pak Med Assoc*. 2012;62(2):196–198.
- Thiryayi WA, Thiryayi SA, Freemont AJ. Histopathological perspective on bone marrow oedema, reactive bone change and haemorrhage. *Eur J Radiol*. 2008;67(1):62–67.

CLINICAL PEARLS

- TOH is a diagnosis of exclusion; evaluate for common causes of hip pain before diagnosing.
- MRI is imaging modality of choice and is able to distinguish between AVN and TOH.
- Most patients will recover with conservative treatment of rest, analgesia, and maintenance of ROM within 6 mo.
- Follow-up at least every 3 mo recommended after proper pain control
- Use endocrine consult if considering using medications to alter bone resorption.
- Surgical management is last resort.

TRICEPS TENDINITIS

Adam Culver, MD • Anthony Martin, MD, CAQSM • David E. Price, MD, FAAFP, CAQSM

BASICS

DESCRIPTION

- Inflammation of the triceps tendon at or proximal to the insertion onto the olecranon
- Classically an overuse injury due to repetitive extension of the elbow or extreme force placed on the tendon
- May result from direct trauma

EPIDEMIOLOGY

- Uncommon, but higher prevalence observed in certain groups (see "Risk Factors")
- Male predominance (1)
- Has been described through a wide range of ages (1)

ETIOLOGY AND PATHOPHYSIOLOGY

Inflammation or swelling of the triceps tendon due to excessive force or repetitive use

RISK FACTORS

- Certain sports such as professional weight lifting, professional football (American), softball players (1)
- Use of anabolic steroids and history of local corticosteroid injections may also predispose to injury (2).
- Systemic disorders, including renal osteodystrophy, hyperparathyroidism, and diabetes mellitus (2)
- Commonly associated with posterior impingement, presence of loose bodies, classic tennis elbow, history of elbow arthroplasty, high-intensity interval training (2)

GENERAL PREVENTION

- Proper form when lifting weights
- Avoid excessive weight or force when utilizing triceps.
- Dynamic warm-up prior to repetitive use of triceps or weight lifting

COMMONLY ASSOCIATED CONDITIONS

- Olecranon bursitis
- Triceps tendon rupture (1)
- Lateral epicondylitis (1)

DIAGNOSIS

HISTORY

- Increasing pain in the posterior elbow over several weeks that worsens over course of the day and associated with occasional morning stiffness
- Improvement can be seen with periods of inactivity.

PHYSICAL EXAM

- Pain in the posterior elbow
- Pain on full extension/flexion of the elbow
- Tenderness/swelling at or above the triceps insertion onto the olecranon
- Increased pain with resisted extension of the elbow
- Possible weakness with elbow extension (may be indicative of tendon rupture)

DIFFERENTIAL DIAGNOSIS

- Olecranon fracture/stress fracture
- Olecranon bursitis
- Triceps rupture
- Subtendinous bursitis
- Cervical radiculopathy
- Posterior interosseous neuropathy

DIAGNOSTIC TESTS & INTERPRETATION

- Anterior/posterior and lateral plain films may be helpful if concerned for tendon avulsion (3)[B].
- Ultrasound may be useful in distinguishing between triceps tendonitis and olecranon bursitis if the physical exam is unclear (4)[B].
- Ultrasound may distinguish acute versus chronic pathology with increased tendon thickness, hypoechogenicity of tendon fibers, and calcific deposits within the tendon being found in chronic pathology (often called tendinopathy) (3)[B].
- Magnetic resonance imaging (MRI) is rarely needed.

TREATMENT

- Long-term treatment:
  - Prevention is vital in high-risk populations such as weight lifters, carpenters/construction workers, or guitar players; the key to prevention is dynamic warm-up, avoiding excessive force, and taking frequent breaks within activity.
  - Injection of platelet-rich plasma (PRP) is likely effective for improving function and decreasing pain intensity in the long term (5)[A].

- Acute treatment:
  - RICE: rest, ice, compression, elevation:
    - Rest: Avoid any that which may exacerbate symptoms.
    - Ice: Use ice packs in the painful area for 5 to 10 min 3 to 4 times/day; may also perform ice massage
    - Compression: wrapping the affected area with an elastic bandage, strap, or brace
    - Elevation: If swelling is present, elevation will help alleviate the swelling.
  - Nonsteroidal anti-inflammatory drugs (NSAIDs) are also a mainstay of therapy.

MEDICATION

- Anti-inflammatories: NSAIDs (e.g., ibuprofen, etodolac)
- Acetaminophen

ISSUES FOR REFERRAL

- If history, physical exam, or other imaging studies suggest signs of tendon rupture, including profound weakness with elbow extension, referral to orthopedic surgery is necessary for potential surgical intervention.
- For high-risk patients, physical therapy may be beneficial to ensure proper form and stretching.

ADDITIONAL THERAPIES

- Special considerations:
  - Limit ice to 10 min 3 or 4 times daily to avoid cubital tunnel damage of the ulnar nerve.
- Rehabilitation:
  - Graduated eccentric strengthening following period of rest
  - French stretch: (i) Clasp fingers together with hands above head; (ii) keep elbows close to head; (iii) reach down behind head attempting to touch back; (iv) hold, and then repeat.
  - French press: as with stretch, except holding a dumbbell
  - Towel stretch: (i) injured arm overhead with uninjured reaching behind back; (ii) one end of towel in each hand; (iii) pull, hold, and repeat.

SURGERY/OTHER PROCEDURES

- Surgical intervention should be considered after a minimum of 1 yr of conservative management (3,6)[C].
- Rare, but operative treatment described with elliptical resection of diseased tissue

ONGOING CARE

FOLLOW-UP RECOMMENDATIONS

Return to sport/activity when no longer tender at or above tendon insertion, strength regained, and full range of motion

REFERENCES

1. Taylor S, Hannafin J. Evaluation and management of elbow tendinopathy. *Sports Health*. 2012;4(5):384–393.
2. Keener JD, Sethi PM. Distal triceps tendon injuries. *Hand Clin*. 2015;31(4):641–650.
3. Donaldson O, Vannet N, Gosens T, et al. Tendinopathies around the elbow part 2: medial elbow, distal biceps and triceps tendinopathies. *Shoulder Elbow*. 2014;6(1):47–56.
4. Blankstein A, Ganel A, Givon U, et al. Ultrasonographic findings in patients with olecranon bursitis. *Ultraschall Med*. 2006;27(6):568–571.
5. Fitzpatrick J, Bulsara M, Zheng MH. The effectiveness of platelet-rich plasma in the treatment of tendinopathy: a meta-analysis of randomized controlled clinical trials. *Am J Sports Med*. 2017; 45(1):226–233.
6. Sibley PA, Harman TW, Bamberger HB. Triceps tendinopathy. *J Hand Surg Am*. 2015;40(7): 1446–1448.

CLINICAL PEARLS

- Evidence suggests that the increased risk of rupture with injection serves as a contraindication to direct tendon injection with corticosteroid.
- Emerging evidence for PRP and its ability to promote faster healing and decrease pain may be beneficial in these types of injuries.

TRICEPS TENDON RUPTURE

Christopher Miles, MD, CAQSM • Matthew Horn, MD

BASICS

DESCRIPTION

Triceps rupture occurs when the triceps tendon becomes detached from its insertion on the olecranon after an elbow injury (1).

EPIDEMIOLOGY

Incidence

- Least common of all tendon injuries (0.78%) (1,2)
- Average age: 45.6 yr old (2)
- Predominant sex: male (2)
- Most common sports: soccer, weight lifters/bodybuilders (especially with concomitant anabolic steroid use) (1,2)

Pediatric Considerations

- Insertion of triceps tendon ossifies at age of 9 yr, so it is not visible on radiographs before this age (3).
- In children with open growth plates, triceps tendon rupture injury typically causes avulsion of epiphysis with subsequent Salter-Harris type I or II injury (3).

ETIOLOGY AND PATHOPHYSIOLOGY

- Triceps muscle composed of long, lateral, and medial heads (4):
  - Long head originates from the infraglenoid tuberosity on the scapula.
  - Lateral head originates from the posterior-lateral portion of the humerus and the lateral intermuscular septum.
  - Medial head extends from distal to spiral groove to trochlea.
  - All three heads insert on the olecranon.
- Overloading an extended elbow (1)
- Abrupt eccentric contraction of triceps muscles (1)
- Direct posterior elbow trauma (4)

RISK FACTORS

- Extrinsic factors (1,2):
  - Local steroid injection
  - Degenerative arthritic changes
  - Olecranon bursitis
  - Recent elbow arthroplasty
  - Anabolic steroid use
  - Fluoroquinolone use
- Intrinsic factors (1,2):
  - Chronic renal failure
  - Secondary hyperparathyroidism
  - Hypocalcemic tetany
  - Rheumatoid arthritis
  - Marfan syndrome
  - Osteogenesis imperfecta
  - Systemic lupus erythematosus
  - Insulin-dependent diabetes

GENERAL PREVENTION

- Properly warm up and stretch prior to physical activity.
- Ensure accurate weight-lifting techniques.
- Avoid local steroid injections and anabolic steroid use.
- Ensure proper rehabilitation from elbow arthroplasty (1,5).

COMMONLY ASSOCIATED CONDITIONS

- Olecranon fracture (intra-articular)
- Triceps tendinosis
- Triceps contusion
- Avulsion fracture of the olecranon
- Radial head fracture
- Olecranon bursitis (1,2)

DIAGNOSIS

HISTORY

- Fall on outstretched hand (4)[C]
- Direct elbow trauma (4)[C]
- Patients may feel a pop with resisted elbow extension such as with weight lifting or daily activities (1)[C].

PHYSICAL EXAM

- Swelling and ecchymosis at posterior elbow near triceps insertion site (5)[C]
- Elbow tender to palpation (4)[C]
- Palpable gap at, or proximal, to olecranon tip (1)[C]
- Decreased range of motion (ROM) with elbow extension (4)[C]
- Pain with active elbow extension (4)[C]
- Positive Viegas test (modified Thompson test). With this technique, lack of elbow extension after proximal compression of muscle mass can suggest a diagnosis of complete rupture (1)[C].

DIFFERENTIAL DIAGNOSIS

- Elbow strain
- Olecranon bursitis
- Radial head fracture
- Distal humerus fracture (1)[C]

DIAGNOSTIC TESTS & INTERPRETATION

- Anteroposterior (AP) and lateral elbow radiographs: "flake sign" (Dunn-Kusnezov sign) seen on lateral radiograph (1)[C],(2)[A],(4)[C]
- Ultrasound: triceps tendon rupture (1)[C]
- Magnetic resonance imaging (MRI) elbow: gold standard if above inconclusive despite clinical suspicion (1)[C]; also necessary for guiding management and preoperative planning (6)[C]
- Partial versus complete triceps tendon tears (4)[A],(5)[C]:
  - Partial rupture affecting $<50\%$ of tendon:
    - Diagnosed on exam or MRI:
      - Exam findings: Patient can perform active elbow extension against gravity with strength $>3/5$ (6)[C].
  - Partial rupture affecting $>50\%$ of tendon or complete ruptures:
    - Diagnosed on exam or MRI:
      - Exam findings: patient with significant loss of triceps extension with strength $<3/5$ (6)[C]

ALERT

It is important to note that active elbow extension may be preserved with a 10% tear or even a 95% tear because of lateral triceps expansion to the forearm fascia (6)[C]. MRI is most useful for determining the percentage of tears and hence is of paramount help in preoperative management (6)[C].

TREATMENT

GENERAL MEASURES

- Ice and acetaminophen or nonsteroidal anti-inflammatory drugs (NSAIDs) initially are appropriate.
- Arm should be placed in sling with 90 degrees or less of flexion initially after the injury. A posterior splint may be applied if necessary but should be in 90 degrees or less of flexion.

ISSUES FOR REFERRAL

Refer all patients with complete or partial triceps rupture $>50\%$ to orthopedics for surgical consultation.

ADDITIONAL THERAPIES

- Conservative (1)[C]:
  - Weeks 1 to 6: immobilization:
    - Immediate immobilization with 30 degrees elbow flexion by splint or brace
  - Weeks 6 to 12: ROM:
    - Gradually increase ROM with adjustable angle elbow brace after 6 wk.
    - Full ROM targeted by 12 wk postinjury
  - Weeks 12 and on: strengthening:
    - Goal of full extension strength by 6 to 9 mo posttreatment
  - Shoulder, wrist, and hand ROM exercises may be started immediately.
  - After immobilization, physical therapy is important.
- Physical therapy
- Current studies are investigating the use of platelet-rich plasma (PRP) for partial ruptures.

SURGERY/OTHER PROCEDURES

Complete triceps rupture or partial triceps tendon rupture >50% (1)[C]:

- Primary repair of tendon within 3 wk of initial rupture
- Transosseous cruciate technique most common (4)[C]
- ~90% return rate to reinjury activity level after surgery (2)[A]
- Postoperative physical therapy:
  - Weeks 0 to 6: postoperative adjustable elbow splint at 20 degrees flexion, increasing flexion by 10 degrees every week with passive elbow extension
  - Weeks 6 to 12: active elbow extension
  - Weeks 12 and on: active elbow extension against resistance
- Complete triceps rupture untreated within the first 6 wk following rupture (4)[C]:
  - Triceps reconstruction
  - Achilles tendon allograft with a calcaneal bony attachment considered in some cases (4)[C]

ONGOING CARE

FOLLOW-UP RECOMMENDATIONS

Routine follow-up at 4 to 6 wk (transition from immobilization to ROM), 12 wk (transition from ROM to strengthening), and 6 mo (medical clearance) (1,6)

PATIENT EDUCATION

Triceps extension ROM and strengthening exercises to begin after immobilization

PROGNOSIS

- Nonoperative treatment of partial tears generally resulted in full ROM and subjective strength within 3 to 9 mo (4).
- Primary repair of partial tears typically resulted in full ROM and subjective strength by 3 to 6 mo (4).
- Primary repair of complete tears generally resulted in full ROM by 3 mo and baseline subjective strength by 6 mo (4).
- Total triceps reconstruction typically resulted in some loss of ROM and full subjective strength by 2 to 3 yr (4).

COMPLICATIONS

- Complete rupture untreated within the first 6 wk; will likely require triceps reconstruction
- Partial rupture that progresses into complete rupture during conservative therapy
- Postoperative rerupture
- Postoperative wounds given thin subcutaneous tissue at posterior elbow
- Complex regional pain syndrome
- Compartment syndrome
- Heterotopic ossification
- Residual flexion contractures between 5 and 20 degrees (1)

REFERENCES

1. Demirhan M, Ersen A. Distal triceps ruptures. *EFORT Open Rev*. 2016;1(6):255–259.
2. Dunn JC, Kusnezov N, Fares A, et al. Triceps tendon ruptures: a systematic review. *Hand (N Y)*. 2017;12(5):431–438.
3. Paramanathan V, Brookfield S, Menon D. Paediatric triceps avulsion fracture identified with ultrasound. *Int J Surg Case Rep*. 2013;4(10):923–925.
4. Tom JA, Kumar NS, Cerynik DL, et al. Diagnosis and treatment of triceps tendon injuries: a review of the literature. *Clin J Sport Med*. 2014;24(3):197–204.
5. Bunshah JJ, Raghuwanshi S, Sharma D, et al. Triceps tendon rupture: an uncommon orthopaedic condition. *BMJ Case Rep*. 2015;2015:bcr2014206446. doi:10.1136/bcr-2014-206446.
6. Sharma SC, Singh R, Goel T, et al. Missed diagnosis of triceps tendon rupture: a case report and review of literature. *J Orthop Surg (Hong Kong)*. 2005;13(3):307–309.

ADDITIONAL READING

- Aunon-Martin I, Prada-Canizares A, Jimenez-Diaz V, et al. Treatment of a complex distal triceps tendon rupture with a new technique: a case report. *Arch Trauma Res*. 2016;5(1):e32221.
- Foulk DM, Galloway MT. Partial triceps disruption: a case report. *Sports Health*. 2011;3(2):175–178.
- Mair SD, Isbell WM, Gill TJ, et al. Triceps tendon ruptures in professional football players. *Am J Sports Med*. 2004;32(2):431–434.
- Mancini F, Bernardi G, De Luna V, et al. Surgical repair of isolated triceps tendon rupture using a suture anchor technique: a case report. *Joints*. 2017;4(4):250–252.

CLINICAL PEARLS

- Triceps rupture should be included in differential diagnosis of every patient with an acute elbow injury (6).
- Significant swelling increases risk of missing diagnosis initially because it hinders ability to localized pain and gap at insertion site of triceps tendon on the olecranon (5).
- It is important to categorize triceps ruptures as partial or complete because this guides treatment (1,6).
- It is important to note that active elbow extension may be preserved with a 10% tear or even a 95% tear because of lateral triceps expansion to the forearm fascia (6).
- Consider point of care (POC) ultrasound if rupture not visualized on radiographs, especially in children (3).
- MRI is most useful for determining the percentage of tears and hence is of paramount help in preoperative management (6).
- Delay in surgical repair past 3 wk from injury increases risk of requiring triceps reconstruction and worse functional outcomes postoperatively (1).

TRIGGER FINGER

Miranda Gordon-Zigel, MD • Rahul Kapur, MD, CAQSM

BASICS

DESCRIPTION
- Also called flexor tenosynovitis
- Type of stenosing tenosynovitis
- Nodule on flexor tendon catching on first annular (A1) pulley
- Can affect any digit; occasionally, multiple digits
- Ring and middle digit involvement most common in adults
- Almost exclusively thumb in children
- Diffuse versus nodular versus "congenital" (pediatric trigger thumb)

EPIDEMIOLOGY
- Predominant gender: female > male (3 to 6 times more common in females)
- Predominant age: bimodal: age <8 yr and 55 to 60 yr
- Seen more commonly in dominant hand
- Lifetime risk 2.6% in general population but 10% in diabetics
- In children, 25% will have bilateral involvement.

Incidence
28 cases/100,000 population

ETIOLOGY AND PATHOPHYSIOLOGY
- Inflammation of flexor digitorum superficialis (FDS) tendon leading to nodule formation
- A1 pulley spans from volar plate of distal metacarpal to base of proximal phalanx.
- Nodule catches on A1 pulley during finger flexion, leading to pain.
- Pain often greatest at metacarpophalangeal (MCP) joint
- Generally idiopathic
- Activity or occupation that involves repetitive use of the fingers
- Results from repetitive trauma but also occasionally sepsis from secondary infection (e.g., tuberculosis)

RISK FACTORS
- Diabetes, rheumatoid arthritis (RA), connective tissue disorders
- Repetitive trauma with compressive force against MCP area (e.g., arc welding)

GENERAL PREVENTION
Activity modification

COMMONLY ASSOCIATED CONDITIONS
- Diabetes
- RA
- Hypothyroidism
- Amyloidosis
- Mucopolysaccharidosis
- Connective tissue disorders

DIAGNOSIS

HISTORY
- Painful catching/clicking with finger flexion or extension
- Pain over MCP; may refer to palm or proximal interphalangeal (PIP) joint
- Digit may be locked, usually in flexion.
- Stiffness develops with prolonged symptoms.

PHYSICAL EXAM
- Tender, palpable nodule on flexor tendon, just proximal to MCP
- Active fist closing reproduces lock/snap.

DIFFERENTIAL DIAGNOSIS
- Dupuytren contracture
- Carpal tunnel syndrome
- Gamekeeper's thumb
- RA
- Tendon sheath ganglion
- Suppurative tenosynovitis

DIAGNOSTIC TESTS & INTERPRETATION

Initial Tests (lab, imaging)
- Lab not indicated, except to evaluate associated systemic disease
- Imaging not indicated; x-rays may be considered to rule out differentials.

Diagnostic Procedures/Other
None; steroid injection is both therapeutic and diagnostic.

TREATMENT

GENERAL MEASURES
- Activity modification
- Splinting of MCP joint at 10 to 15 degrees of flexion × 6 to 10 wk:
  - Reduces tendon motion in sheath
  - Allows resolution of surrounding synovitis
  - 93% with partial or full symptom resolution after 10 wk (1)[A]
  - Distal interphalangeal (DIP) immobilization showed a negative effect (1)[A].

MEDICATION

First Line

Injected corticosteroids (see "Surgery/Other Procedures" below)

Second Line

Nonsteroidal anti-inflammatory drugs (NSAIDs) may help with pain relief; no specific evidence but commonly recommended

SURGERY/OTHER PROCEDURES

- Corticosteroid injection into tendon sheath:
  - Palmar or dorsolateral approach to avoid neurovascular bundle
  - Subcutaneous (SC) infiltration equal or superior to intrasheath injection (2)[B]
  - May require repeat injection in 1 mo
  - Up to 93% complete or partial reduction of symptoms in nodular type (3)[A]
  - Only 50% response in diffuse type or diabetes
- Surgical release of A1 pulley:
  - Open or percutaneous procedure
  - First-line treatment for locked digit or pediatric trigger thumb, although there is increasing argument toward conservative management for the latter
  - Indicated if repeat injections ineffective
  - 97% complete resolution of symptoms (3)[A]

ONGOING CARE

FOLLOW-UP RECOMMENDATIONS

Patient Monitoring

May see increased glucose level following steroid injection in diabetes

PROGNOSIS

- Excellent; over 90% symptom resolution with steroid or surgical therapy
- 23–63% of pediatric trigger digits may resolve spontaneously.

COMPLICATIONS

- If untreated:
  - PIP joint flexion contracture
  - Distal triggering from FDS tendon degeneration
- Of injection:
  - Fat atrophy and necrosis
  - Local skin depigmentation
  - Theoretical risk of tendon rupture
- Of surgical release:
  - Bowstringing of flexor tendon
  - Second annular (A2) pulley injury
  - Digital nerve injury
  - Infection
  - Long-term scar tenderness

REFERENCES

1. Lunsford D, Valdes K, Hengy S. Conservative management of trigger finger: a systematic review [published online ahead of print December 28, 2017]. *J Hand Ther*. doi:10.1016/j.jht.2017.10.016.
2. Kazuki K, Egi T, Okada M, et al. Clinical outcome of extrasynovial steroid injection for trigger finger. *Hand Surg*. 2006;11(1–2):1–4.
3. Nimigan AS, Ross DC, Gan BS. Steroid injections in the management of trigger fingers. *Am J Phys Med Rehabil*. 2006;85(1):36–43.

ADDITIONAL READING

- Akhtar S, Bradley MJ, Quinton DN, et al. Management and referral for trigger finger/thumb. *BMJ*. 2005;331(7507):30–33.
- Giugale J, Fowler J. Trigger finger: adult and pediatric treatment strategies. *Orthop Clin North Am*. 2015;46(4):561–569.
- Ryzewicz M, Wolf JM. Trigger digits: principles, management, and complications. *J Hand Surg Am*. 2006;31(1):135–146.

CLINICAL PEARLS

- Clinical diagnosis by painful catching at MCP joint
- Corticosteroid injection is safe and highly effective first-line treatment.
- Surgical release provides excellent results when conservative measures fail.
- Trigger finger in diabetics is less likely to respond to steroid therapy.

TROCHANTERIC BURSITIS

Stephen Carek, MD • Daniel C. Herman, MD, PhD, FAAPMR, FACSM, CAQSM

BASICS

DESCRIPTION

Historically, the condition of pain and tenderness in the area of the greater trochanter had been referred to as *trochanteric bursitis*. Recent literature has referred to this condition as *greater trochanteric pain syndrome*. This change has come about owing to the recognition that the etiology of this pain can be from multiple sources, including the bursa and gluteal tendons or the iliotibial band. This includes tendinosis and tendon tears of the gluteus medius and gluteus minimus that insert on the greater trochanter (1).

EPIDEMIOLOGY

- Incidence peaks between the 4th and 6th decades of life.
- Predominant gender: female > male (4:1)
- Common in runners

ETIOLOGY AND PATHOPHYSIOLOGY

- Etiology of bursitis:
  - Inflammation of the bursae can come from repetitive friction between the bony structures of the trochanter and the muscle, tendon, or fascial tissue that overlies the bursae.
  - Inflammation of the bursae also can come about owing to direct trauma to the lateral hip.
- Etiology of tendinopathy:
  - Tendon changes can come about from acute or chronic overuse of a muscle tendon unit.
  - Weakness or tightness of the muscle tendon unit contributes to this condition.

RISK FACTORS

- Ipsilateral or contralateral hip arthritis
- Degenerative changes of the lumbar spine
- Degenerative changes of the knees
- Leg-length discrepancy
- Total hip arthroplasty
- Obesity
- Fibromyalgia
- Iliotibial band syndrome
- Weakness of hip abductors and/or external rotators of the hip
- Pes planus
- Excessive or rapidly increased activity
- Training on hard or banked surfaces
- Poorly cushioned shoes
- Limitation of internal rotation of the hip
- Local trauma

Genetics

No genetic predisposition is known.

GENERAL PREVENTION

- Strengthening of hip external rotators and hip abductors
- Stretching of muscles around the hip
- Avoid sudden increase in activity (including intensity, duration, or pace).
- Avoid exercise on banked surfaces.
- Proper shoe wear
- Avoid direct trauma (use protection when appropriate).
- Weight loss (if appropriate)

COMMONLY ASSOCIATED CONDITIONS

See "Risk Factors."

DIAGNOSIS

HISTORY

- Pain localized to the area of the lateral hip is the key historical finding. This pain may radiate down the lateral thigh or into the groin.
- Pain is often aggravated by:
  - Prolonged walking.
  - Rising after sitting.
  - Lying on affected side.
  - Squatting.
  - Climbing.
- Patient also may report other related conditions as seen in "Risk Factors."

PHYSICAL EXAM

- Tenderness over the greater trochanter is the key diagnostic finding.
- Pain reported within 30 sec of standing on the affected limb (LR = 12) (2)
- Other exam tests may be positive but are less specific and lack sensitivity:
  - Pain with extremes of passive rotation, abduction, or adduction
  - Pain with resisted hip abduction and external or internal rotation
  - Positive Trendelenburg sign
- Other testing to evaluate for associated conditions:
  - Positive Patrick-FABERE (flexion, abduction, external rotation, extension) testing for sacroiliac joint dysfunction or hip joint pathology
  - Ober test for iliotibial band flexibility
  - Flexion and extension of hip for hip joint pathology
  - Leg-length measurement for leg-length discrepancy
  - Foot inspection for pes planus or overpronation
  - Lower extremity neurologic assessment for lumbar radiculopathy or neuromuscular disorders

DIFFERENTIAL DIAGNOSIS

A wide variety of conditions should be considered:

- Lumbosacral disc disease
- Spinal stenosis
- Radiculopathy
- Degenerative disease of the hip
- Osteonecrosis of the hip
- Stress fracture of the hip
- Slipped capital femoral epiphysis
- Fracture
- Contusion
- Soft tissue infection

DIAGNOSTIC TESTS & INTERPRETATION

Initial Tests (lab, imaging)

- Blood tests are not altered by this condition.
- Imaging is not essential for the diagnosis.
- If radiography is done, it should include anteroposterior view and frog-leg lateral view of the affected hip.
- Radiographs typically are normal but can show irregular bone formation or bony spurring at the greater trochanter owing to chronic bursitis or chronic tendinopathy.
- Radiographs also may show associated degenerative disease of the hip joint or the lumbar spine.

Diagnostic Procedures/Other

- Advanced imaging is rarely necessary.
- Detection of abnormalities on magnetic resonance imaging (MRI) is a poor predictor of clinical syndrome.
- Ultrasound can be used to aid in diagnosis and management of gluteal tendon tears and may be more accurate than MRI (3)[A].

TREATMENT

GENERAL MEASURES

- Multimodal conservative approach including (4)[A]:
  - Ice
  - Analgesics
  - Nonsteroidal anti-inflammatory drugs (NSAIDs)
  - Minimize aggravating activities such as running or prolonged standing or walking.
  - Avoid lying on affected side and consider placing a pillow between knees while sleeping.
- Physical therapy or home exercises program focusing on (5)[A]:
  - Strengthening (including hip abductors and external rotators of the hip)
  - Stretching (including the piriformis and iliotibial band)
  - Address flexibility of hip and low back.
- Corticosteroid injection (5)[A]:
  - Ultrasound-guided injection may be helpful for patient with large body habitus.
- Extracorporeal shock wave therapy
- Platelet-rich plasma (PRP) injections for refractory cases (4,6)[C]
- Deep friction massage of greater trochanteric, gluteal, and iliotibial band areas
- Weight loss (if applicable)
- Address leg-length discrepancy (if applicable).
- Address pes planus or overpronation (if applicable).

MEDICATION

- Analgesics:
  - Acetaminophen 1,000 mg PO TID
- NSAIDs:
  - Ibuprofen 800 mg PO TID
  - Naproxen 500 mg PO TID
  - Others
- Injectable corticosteroids:
  - 1 mL of dexamethasone 4 mg/mL
  - 1 mL of triamcinolone 40 mg/mL
- Anesthetics:
  - Injection of anesthetic alone can be diagnostic.
  - Should be used along with corticosteroids during injection
  - 5 mL of 1% lidocaine, 5 mL of 0.5% bupivacaine, or a combination of both can be used.

ISSUES FOR REFERRAL

- Recalcitrant pain and failure of conservative treatments
- Septic bursitis

SURGERY/OTHER PROCEDURES

- Surgery is rarely needed and should be reserved for recalcitrant cases that have failed conservative measures.
- Various surgical procedures have been described. They include:
  - Open surgery with fenestration or release of the iliotibial band and excision of the subgluteal bursae.
  - Arthroscopic bursectomy.
  - Gluteal tendon repair.

ONGOING CARE

COMPLICATIONS

- Bursal thickening and fibrosis
- Tendon thickening, fibrosis, or tearing

REFERENCES

1. Redmond JM, Chen AW, Domb BG. Greater trochanteric pain syndrome. *J Am Acad Orthop Surg*. 2016;24(4):231–240.
2. Grimaldi A, Mellor R, Nicolson P, et al. Utility of clinical tests to diagnose MRI-confirmed gluteal tendinopathy in patients presenting with lateral hip pain. *Br J Sports Med*. 2017;51(6):519–524.
3. Grimaldi A, Mellor R, Hodges P, et al. Gluteal tendinopathy: a review of mechanisms, assessment and management. *Sports Med*. 2015;45(8):1107–1119.
4. Mautner K, Colberg RE, Malanga G, et al. Outcomes after ultrasound-guided platelet-rich plasma injections for chronic tendinopathy: a multicenter, retrospective review. *PM R*. 2013;5(3):169–175.
5. Lustenberger DP, Ng VY, Best TM, et al. Efficacy of treatment of trochanteric bursitis: a systematic review. *Clin J Sport Med*. 2011;21(5):447–453.
6. Fitzpatrick J, Bulsara MK, O'Donnell J, et al. The effectiveness of platelet-rich plasma injections in gluteal tendinopathy: a randomized, double-blind controlled trial comparing a single platelet-rich plasma injection with a single corticosteroid injection. *Am J Sports Med*. 2018;46(4):933–939.

ADDITIONAL READING

- Korakakis V, Whiteley R, Tzavara A, et al. The effectiveness of extracorporeal shockwave therapy in common lower limb conditions: a systematic review including quantification of patient-rated pain reduction. *Br J Sports Med*. 2018;52(6):387–407.
- Paluska SA. An overview of hip injuries in running. *Sports Med*. 2005;35(11):991–1014.
- Williams BS, Cohen SP. Greater trochanteric pain syndrome: a review of anatomy, diagnosis and treatment. *Anesth Analg*. 2009;108(5):1662–1670.

CLINICAL PEARLS

- Trochanteric bursitis, also referred to as greater trochanteric pain syndrome, is best diagnosed with tenderness of the lateral hip and reproduced pain with single leg stance.
- Treatment modalities including ice, analgesics, anti-inflammatories, physical therapy, and steroid injections are reasonable first-line interventions for pain and improved function.
- Ultrasound is an emerging diagnostic tool and can be used to assist in guidance for injections.

TURF TOE

Holly J. Benjamin, MD, FAAP, FACSM • Abdullah Hasan-Pratt, MD

BASICS

1st metatarsophalangeal (MTP) joint sprain

DESCRIPTION

- Forced hyperextension of the 1st MTP, resulting in sprain of the plantar capsuloligamentous complex (PLC) as well as chondral and osseous injuries
- The common factors resulting in turf toe injury are hard playing surfaces, light flexible footwear, and axial loading.

EPIDEMIOLOGY

- The overall incidence and prevalence remains unknown, with the majority of available data emanating from smaller studies.
- The incidence of this injury has increased over the years secondary to athletic fields being covered by artificial turf as well as increased flexibility of the toe box in athletic shoes.
- Within college football, the overall incidence of turf toe injuries obtained over 5 yr via the NCAA's Injury Surveillance System (ISS) was 0.062 per 1,000 athlete exposures (1).

ALERT

In NCAA football players, there was an 85% higher risk of turf toe injury on third-generation "artificial fill turf"(0.087 per 1,000) as compared to natural grass (0.047 per 1,000), where artificial nonfill surfaces (Astroturf) had a rate of 0.057 per 1,000 (not significantly different than grass 0.017, 0.36) (1).

- The proposed theory for this discrepancy in injuries seen on different playing surfaces is that MTP hyperextension is increased with increased traction (i.e., less give as compared to grass and Astroturf).
- Although turf toe is seen more often in football, it also occurs in basketball, dancing, soccer, tennis, volleyball, and wrestling.
- There seem to be no differentiating ethno-cultural, sex-related, or age-related determinants connected to turf toe (1).

ETIOLOGY AND PATHOPHYSIOLOGY

- The MTP joint bears the majority of a person's body weight (40–60%) during walking, increasing up to 2- to 3-fold during running, and up to an 8-fold increase during jumping.
- In the acute setting, 80% of turf toe typically occur during an applied downward force, where the great toe is dorsiflexed beyond its biomechanical limits, resulting in tear of the capsule about the neck of the 1st MTP (2).
- In a minority of cases, forced plantarflexion ("sand toe") and valgus/varus mechanisms can also lead to symptoms consistent with turf toe.

RISK FACTORS

- Artificial turf and playing surfaces
- Athlete's experience and years of sports participation
- Athlete's position while playing sport
- Athlete's weight, where higher forces are transmitted with increased weight
- Flattening of the 1st MTP
- Football players (defensive and offensive running backs, wide receivers, linemen)
- Foot pronation
- Hallux degenerative joint disease
- Increased ankle dorsiflexion
- Increased friction between athletic shoe and turf
- Increased toe box flexibility and decreased number of cleats in the shoe
- Prior 1st MTP joint injury
- Pes planus (2)

GENERAL PREVENTION

- Early identification of athletes with prior MTP injuries or existing ankle injuries requiring range of motion (ROM)-limiting support or braces is key toward preventative measures.
- Limited ROM at the MTP, specifically limited dorsiflexion <60 degrees, can also predispose athletes to injuries secondary to hyperextension.
- Through vigilant screening during preparticipation physicals, as well as at early signs of MTP injury, the use of orthotic and rigid insoles can reduce the progression of injury and minimize inactive time secondary to injury.

COMMONLY ASSOCIATED CONDITIONS

In addition to plantar plate rupture, excessive forefoot hyperextension may also injure the articular cartilage, sesamoids, and subchondral bone resulting in fracture.

DIAGNOSIS

HISTORY

- Acute forced hyperextension of MTP joint resulting in painful weight-bearing, pain with ROM, and especially pain with applied pressure to MTP during running or jumping (toeing off)
- Swelling, tenderness, and possibly ecchymosis/bruising will also be reported.

PHYSICAL EXAM

- Swelling of 1st MTP, with or without ecchymosis
- Tenderness to palpation of MTP joint
- Decreased active ROM
- Pain with dorsiflexion and passive ROM
- Laxity within the ligamentous capsule and instability of MTP joint may be seen in severe injury, resulting in a positive Lachman test.
- Grading system:
  - Grade 1 injuries are a capsular strain without loss of its functional integrity. Clinically, there is mild edema and pain but no bruising, and ROM is preserved.
  - Grade 2 injuries represent partial thickness tearing of the plantar plate and capsular structures. Clinically, there is both edema and ecchymosis of the 1st MTP, loss of ROM, moderate pain, and often have an antalgic gait.
  - Grade 3 injuries are acute injuries with complete disruption of the PLC or occasionally chronic dysfunction is considered a grade 3 injury. The plantar plate may be completely avulsed from the metatarsal neck, and impaction of the metatarsal head may occur during full extension of the joint. Clinically, there is marked edema and ecchymosis, severe pain to palpation, and they rarely can bear weight or ambulate during the immediate postinjury period (3).

DIFFERENTIAL DIAGNOSIS

- Gout
- Plantar plate rupture
- 1st distal metatarsal or proximal phalangeal fracture
- Osteoarthritis of 1st MTP (hallux rigidus)
- Sesamoiditis
- Sesamoid stress fracture
- Flexor or extensor hallucis tendonitis

DIAGNOSTIC TESTS & INTERPRETATION

- Initial imaging should include anteroposterior, lateral, and oblique radiographs.
- If plantar tenderness, sesamoid views should also be obtained.
- Magnetic resonance imaging (MRI) can be obtained to evaluate soft tissue edema or the true extent of the plantar plate injury but is often not required (4).
- The resulting earlier, more accurate diagnosis has changed the course of conservative treatment, provided a road map for potential surgery when indicated, and decreased overall morbidity (4).
- Grade 1 sprain:
  - X-ray: normal appearance
  - MRI: edema of any portion of the PLC, no tear
- Grade 2 sprain:
  - X-ray: normal appearance
  - MRI: partial tear of any portion of the PLC, edema if acute
- Grade 3 sprain:
  - X-ray: possible fracture, sesamoid retraction, or diastasis of bipartite sesamoid
  - MRI: Full-thickness tear of any portion of the PLC, bony edema, sesamoid retraction, or diastasis of bipartite sesamoid

TREATMENT

GENERAL MEASURES

- Grade 1 sprain:
  - Ice, elevation, and nonsteroidal anti-inflammatory drugs (NSAIDs)
  - Toe spica taping with activity, which restricts excessive dorsiflexion
  - Gentle ROM exercises can be initiated typically 3 to 5 days postinjury. Initial exercise consists of passive plantar flexion to prevent sesamoid adhesions while protecting the healing soft tissues.
- Grade 2 sprain:
  - Ice, elevation, and NSAIDs
  - Toe spica taping with activity as well as orthotics such as stiff sole/turf toe plate
  - Gentle passive ROM exercises as tolerated, but explosive, push off activities should be restricted until low impact exercise is tolerated without pain or limitation; usually up to 2 wk
- Grade 3 sprain:
  - Treatment similar to grade 2 sprains
  - Weight-bearing as tolerated, with use of crutches if pain with ambulation
  - Prolonged progression typical due to severity of symptoms; clearance optimal when has progressed with weight-bearing and has returned to preinjury performance level; often up to 8 wk

MEDICATION

- NSAIDS are used primarily to reduce pain.
- Steroid injections are not recommended.

ADDITIONAL THERAPIES

- Treatment of turf toe depends largely on the grade of injury. Once identified, some grade 1 and many grade 2 and grade 3 injuries should be referred to a foot and ankle specialist for definitive treatment (5).
- Physical therapy can aid greatly in both acute management with gentle ROM techniques as well as in chronic cases where repeated injuries have resulted in restricted ROM at 1st MTP (5).

SURGERY/OTHER PROCEDURES

- In the acute setting, surgery is only indicated in plantar plate rupture, sesamoid fracture, severe chondral injury, or significant fracture dislocation at MTP (6).
- In chronic turf toe, surgery may become a viable option if ROM is significantly limited affecting return to preinjury performance level, osteonecrosis of sesamoid, or persistent pain/instability despite conservative therapy (6).

ONGOING CARE

More severe or recurrent cases may require a rigid-soled shoe or rigid forefoot orthotic when participating in sports.

PROGNOSIS

The prognosis for full return to preinjury performance level is usually good unless repeated injury without fully healing or chronic injuries resulting in instability or limited ROM.

COMPLICATIONS

Chronic or severe cases can lead to significantly limited ROM, which can predispose to recurrent injury, so early controlled ROM is recommended after injury to minimize the risk of this complication.

REFERENCES

1. George E, Harris AH, Dragoo J, et al. Incidence and risk factors for turf toe injuries in intercollegiate football: data from the National Collegiate Athletic Association Injury Surveillance System. *Foot Ankle Int*. 2014;35(2):108–115.
2. Childs SG. The pathogenesis and biomechanics of turf toe. *Orthop Nurs*. 2006;25(4):276–282.
3. McCormick JJ, Anderson RB. Rehabilitation following turf toe injury and plantar plate repair. *Clin Sports Med*. 2010;29(2):313–323.
4. Crain JM, Phancao JP. Imaging of turf toe. *Radiol Clin North Am*. 2016;54(5):969–978.
5. Allen LR, Flemming D, Sanders TG. Turf toe: ligamentous injury of the first metatarsophalangeal joint. *Mil Med*. 2004;169(11):xix–xxiv.
6. Doty J, Coughlin M. Turf toe repair: a technical note. *Foot Ankle Spec*. 2013;6(6):452–456.

ADDITIONAL READING

- Clanton TO, Ford JJ. Turf toe injury. *Clin Sports Med*. 1994;13(4):731–741.
- Crain JM, Phancao JP, Stidham K. MR imaging of turf toe. *Magn Reson Imaging Clin N Am*. 2008; 16(1):93–103.
- Kubitz ER. Athletic injuries of the first metatarsophalangeal joint. *J Am Podiatr Med Assoc*. 2003;93(4):325–332.
- Mullen JE, O'Malley MJ. Sprains—residual instability of subtalar, Lisfranc joints, and turf toe. *Clin Sports Med*. 2004;23(1):97–121.
- Rodeo SA, O'Brien S, Warren RF, et al. Turf-toe: an analysis of metatarsophalangeal joint sprains in professional football players. *Am J Sports Med*. 1990; 18(3):280–285.
- Watson TS, Anderson RB, Davis WH. Periarticular injuries to the hallux metatarsophalangeal joint in athletes. *Foot Ankle Clin*. 2000;5(3):687–713.

CLINICAL PEARLS

- Common injury; clinical diagnosis with adjunctive radiographs typical; MRI is not often needed.
- Return to play and progression of all three grades of sprains depending on severity of symptoms and all must complete a gradual, functional progression over a period of 1 to 8 wk typically.
- Early return to play is associated with chronic pain and a higher complication rate, particularly for grade III injuries.
- Corticosteroid injections have no role in the acute treatment of this condition.

ULNAR COLLATERAL LIGAMENT INJURIES OF THE ELBOW

Jason L. Zaremski, MD, CAQSM, FAAPMR, FACSM • Daniel C. Herman, MD, PhD, FAAPMR, FACSM, CAQSM

BASICS

DESCRIPTION

- Sprain or tearing of the ulnar collateral ligament (UCL) of the elbow secondary to acute or chronic valgus stress leading to pain, instability, and dysfunction
- Two main mechanisms: chronic deterioration of the UCL owing to repetitive valgus overload or, less commonly, an acute traumatic rupture

EPIDEMIOLOGY

- Most UCL injuries are seen in baseball players, but they also can be seen in wrestlers, javelin throwers, tennis players, football players, volleyball players, and in acute trauma victims.
- UCL injuries are more common in skeletally mature athletes, but the incidence in skeletally immature athletes is rising.
- Predominant gender: male > female
- Although the exact prevalence of UCL injury is unknown, there has been a definite increase in the number of surgical reconstructions performed in professional, collegiate, and high school athletes in recent years (1).

ETIOLOGY AND PATHOPHYSIOLOGY

- The UCL is the primary restraint to valgus stress of the elbow in flexion.
- The UCL is composed of three ligaments: the anterior bundle, posterior bundle, and transverse ligament.
- The anterior bundle, which is composed of an anterior and posterior band with reciprocal functions, is the most important medial stabilizer of the elbow. Rupture of the anterior bundle is considered a complete tear of the UCL.
- The posterior bundle provides secondary restraint beyond 90 degrees of flexion.
- The transverse ligament is an extension of the joint capsule and does not contribute to valgus stability.
- Repetitive valgus load to the elbow is absorbed primarily by the UCL and the forearm flexor muscles.
- Over time, the UCL becomes overloaded, and microtraumatic tears occur, potentially leading to altered throwing kinematics.
- Cumulative microtrauma can lead to rupture of the UCL.
- Altered mechanics lead to decreased throwing accuracy and velocity.
- Acute rupture can occur in a previously attenuated ligament or in a normal ligament subjected to extreme valgus stress, such as an elbow dislocation.

RISK FACTORS

- Participation in sport that demands repetitive excessive valgus stress to the elbow, such as high-velocity throwing or overhead activity, is a risk factor for chronic injury.
- Contact sports or sports with significant fall risk are a factor in acute injury.
- Sport specialization, excessive throwing, poor pitching mechanics, and weak links in the kinetic chain

GENERAL PREVENTION

- Athletes who participate in throwing or overhead sports should be on a conditioning program that includes core stabilization, rotator cuff and forearm muscle strengthening, and posterior capsule stretching.
- Athletic technique should be reviewed to minimize valgus stress to the elbow.
- Throwing athletes should have a 3- to 4-mo rest from throwing per 12 mo (2).

COMMONLY ASSOCIATED CONDITIONS

- Valgus extension overload syndrome: radiocapitellar and posteromedial olecranon impingement
- Ulnar neuritis or subluxation
- Osteochondral loose bodies

DIAGNOSIS

HISTORY

- In acute rupture, the athlete may experience sudden pain, sometimes with an audible pop, and cannot resume play.
- Chronic injuries present as persistent, insidious medial elbow pain, often accompanied by decreased command and velocity of throwing.

PHYSICAL EXAM

- Tenderness along the sublime tubercle
- Joint effusion and ulnar nerve tenderness may be present.
- Flexion contracture with pain at terminal extension is common.
- Valgus stress test: The examiner stabilizes the arm and flexes the elbow to 30 degrees; valgus stress is applied. The test is positive if the athlete has pain, apprehension, or instability.
- Milking maneuver: The forearm is supinated and the elbow flexed to 90 degrees; the examiner applies a valgus stress by pulling on the thumb while palpating along the UCL. Pain, apprehension, or instability indicates MCL injury, but this test can give a high number of false-positive results.
- Moving valgus stress test: This test is highly sensitive and specific for UCL injury. A constant valgus stress is placed on the elbow as the joint is moved through the arc of flexion and extension. The test is positive if the athlete's pain is reproduced between 70 and 120 degrees of flexion.

DIFFERENTIAL DIAGNOSIS

- Flexor/pronator tendonitis or rupture
- Ulnar neuritis or subluxation
- Medial triceps subluxation
- Loose bodies
- Olecranon osteophytosis
- Medial epicondyle avulsion
- Pronator syndrome

DIAGNOSTIC TESTS & INTERPRETATION

- X-rays: Three-view series of the elbow should be performed to evaluate for osteophytes, calcifications within the ligament or soft tissues, osteochondral damage, and loose bodies.
- Stress x-rays may show joint widening compared with the contralateral elbow; a difference in joint opening of >1 mm suggests UCL injury (3)[B].
- Ultrasound (US) also can reveal disruption of the UCL in the hands of an experienced user (stress US compared to the uninjured side may be particularly helpful).

- Magnetic resonance imaging (MRI) arthrography is superior to MRI alone to diagnose UCL tears (3).
- MRI can visualize attenuation, partial tearing, or complete tearing of the UCL as well as evaluate the articular surface and surrounding soft tissue structures. Image enhancement is possible with saline or gadolinium.
- Arthroscopy can evaluate and treat associated articular injuries but cannot visualize the UCL well. Stress testing under arthroscopy, however, can be diagnostic of UCL tear (4)[C].

TREATMENT

GENERAL MEASURES

- Acute treatment: Acute injuries should be treated with rest from sport, ice, nonsteroidal anti-inflammatory drugs (NSAIDs), and sling immobilization if pain is substantial with movement. Caution should be used to avoid direct ice application over the ulnar nerve.
- Long-term treatment:
  - Sprain but not partial tear, consisting of edema seen on imaging but no definitive tear, should be treated with rehabilitation, including sports-specific training.
  - Low-grade partial tear injuries are treated with removal from sport followed by prolonged rehabilitation and sports-specific training.
  - High-grade partial tears, particularly distally, as well as complete ruptures are treated with surgical reconstruction in the high-demand throwing athlete.
- Orthobiologic treatment (5)[B]:
  - There is some evidence that platelet-rich plasma can successfully improve outcomes versus rest and rehabilitation alone in low-grade partial tears.
- Rehabilitation (6):
  - Range of motion (ROM) exercises begin after pain decreases.
  - Once pain free, strengthening begins with wrist flexor and extensor groups followed by scapular stabilizers.
  - Throwing and valgus stresses are restricted for at least 6 wk.
  - A structured sports-specific program, such an interval throwing program, is begun when the athlete has full strength and painless valgus testing.
  - Athletes are rested at any period when they experience pain.

SURGERY/OTHER PROCEDURES

- Surgery is indicated for complete rupture or failure of 3 to 6 mo of conservative management in a high-demand competitive athlete.
- In some cases with proximal or distal insertional UCL partial thickness tears, UCL repair and augmentation rather than reconstruction may be a viable option. However, the research and surgical outcomes is minimal at the time of publication of this text.
- Surgical reconstruction of the UCL is performed using the palmaris longus, toe extensor, or other tendon graft through a muscle-splitting approach in the flexor-pronator bundle.
- Surgery is followed by lengthy postoperative rehabilitation:
  - After 10 to 14 days of immobilization, ROM exercises are initiated.
  - Hinged bracing is usually recommended until 6 wk.
  - At that time, strengthening exercises begin.
  - Valgus stress is avoided until 4 mo postoperatively.
  - An interval throwing program is initiated at approximately 4 mo with soft tosses.
  - This is advanced in intervals, with return to competitive throwing allowed at 9 to 12 mo if the athlete is pain free with full strength and ROM.
  - Athletes are rested at any step if pain recurs.
- Return to play after reconstruction ranges is typically at least 12 mo, longer if the athlete is an overhead throwing athlete and pitches or is a javelin thrower.
- Most modern techniques allow >90% of athletes to return to sport, although there is a slight decrease of returning to sport at previous level of competition (67–92%) (4)[A].

REFERENCES

1. Erickson BJ, Nwachukwu BU, Rosas S, et al. Trends in medial ulnar collateral ligament reconstruction in the united states: a retrospective review of a large private-payer database from 2007 to 2011. *Am J Sports Med*. 2015;43(7):1770–1774.
2. MLB.com. Pitch smart. https://m.mlb.com/pitchsmart/pitching-guidelines/. Accessed March 28, 2018.
3. Roedl JB, Gonzalez FM, Zoga AC, et al. Potential utility of a combined approach with US and MR arthrography to image medial elbow pain in baseball players. *Radiology*. 2016;279(3):827–837.
4. Peters SD, Bullock GS, Goode AP, et al. The success of return to sport after ulnar collateral ligament injury in baseball: a systematic review and meta-analysis. *J Shoulder Elbow Surg*. 2018;27(3):561–571.
5. Dines JS, Williams PN, ElAttrache N, et al. Platelet-rich plasma can be used to successfully treat elbow ulnar collateral ligament insufficiency in high-level throwers. *Am J Orthop (Belle Mead NJ)*. 2016;45(5):296–300.
6. Ellenbecker TS, Wilk KE, Altchek DW, et al. Current concepts in rehabilitation following ulnar collateral ligament reconstruction. *Sports Health*. 2009;1(4):301–313.

CLINICAL PEARLS

- UCL injuries are predominantly seen in high-velocity throwing or overhead athletes.
- Pain, apprehension, or laxity appreciated on valgus testing of the elbow should lead to MRI arthrography and/or US imaging to evaluate the integrity of the UCL.
- Most UCL sprains and low-grade tears injuries respond to rehabilitation and sports-specific training, but surgical reconstruction should be considered in high-level athletes that have high-grade partial tears and rupture.

ULNAR COLLATERAL LIGAMENT INJURY OF THUMB (SKIER'S THUMB)

Corey Carson, MD, CAQSM

BASICS

DESCRIPTION

- Synonym(s): skier's thumb; gamekeeper's thumb
- Sprain of the ulnar collateral ligament (UCL) of the 1st metacarpophalangeal (MCP) joint with or without a bony avulsion from the insertion on the phalanx
- Stener lesion:
  - Displacement of the ruptured ligament proximal to the adductor pollicis aponeurosis, effectively preventing healing without surgical intervention
  - Incidence with a complete tear is reported between 64% and 87% (1).

EPIDEMIOLOGY

- As high as 50 per 100,000 and 10 times more likely than radial collateral ligament injuries
- Represents 5–7% of all skiing injuries and second in frequency only to knee injuries in skiers

RISK FACTORS

Ski poles likely increase the risk of UCL injury:

- Wrist straps on the ski poles do not likely increase the risk of UCL injury further.

DIAGNOSIS

Avulsion of bony fragment at the insertion of UCL on the phalanx may be associated with this condition.

HISTORY

- Stress to the thumb in extended and/or abducted position
- Usually in skiing but often occurs in other sports, such as football and mixed martial arts
- Historically called gamekeeper's thumb as a reference to chronic UCL injuries suffered by gamekeepers while twisting the necks of small game like rabbits while hunting

PHYSICAL EXAM

- Diagnosis may be made based on physical examination if the examination is done within a couple of hours.
- Pain, swelling, and muscle spasm may make clinical diagnosis of a complete tear difficult if the examination is performed later:
  - Local anesthetic may be helpful for the diagnosis in these cases (2)[C].
- Pain at the origin and insertion of the UCL
- Swelling and tenderness over the ulnar aspect of the 1st MCP joint
- Mild-to-complete instability on stress testing of UCL with MCP joint in flexion, depending on whether it is a 1st-, 2nd-, or 3rd-degree sprain:
  - Tested at 0 and 30 degrees of metacarpal phalangeal joint flexion
  - There is significant side-to-side variability in UCL testing in noninjured individuals (3)[B]:
    - Most important physical finding is lack of an end point because this indicates complete ligament disruption.

DIFFERENTIAL DIAGNOSIS

- Radial collateral ligament sprain
- Metacarpal fracture
- Proximal phalanx fracture
- MCP sprain

DIAGNOSTIC TESTS & INTERPRETATION

- X-rays (posteroanterior [PA]/lateral) (2):
  - Rule out bony avulsion or other fractures.
  - Stress x-rays to determine if the tear is partial (usually treated conservatively) or complete (often treated surgically)
  - Because of associated muscle spasm, many clinicians advise local anesthetic infiltration before x-rays.
  - "Sag sign": Volar subluxation of the proximal phalanx in relation to the metacarpal at the MCP joint may indicate UCL injury (2).
- Ultrasound (US):
  - Excellent accuracy when performed by an experienced ultrasonographer (4)[C]:
    - Full thickness tears are characterized by nonvisualization of the UCL and visualization of a heterogeneous mass proximal to the MCP joint representing the retracted ligament known as a "stump sign."
- Magnetic resonance imaging (MRI) (5):
  - Ordered to diagnose whether there is a complete tear or to evaluate for a Stener lesion: 96% sensitivity and 95% specificity

TREATMENT

- Ice, elevation, and immobilization should be used immediately after the injury for protection and pain control.
- Partial tears:
  - Nonsurgical treatment is generally successful for these injuries (1,2)[C].
- Protection with thumb spica splint or cast:
  - 2 to 4 wk of immobilization followed by 2 to 4 wk of protection during activity
  - Start range of motion after period of immobilization.
  - Progress to strengthening exercises as symptoms allow.
- Complete tears:
  - If a Stener lesion can be ruled out with MRI or MR arthrogram, good results can be expected with conservative treatment (i.e., brace or cast) (1,2)[C].
  - If a Stener lesion is present, treatment should be surgical (1,2)[C].

- If the presence of a Stener lesion cannot be determined, management is controversial. Because surgical repair generally yields excellent results, surgery is preferred by many clinicians. However, even after failure of nonoperative treatment at anywhere from 1 mo to >6 yr, nearly all patients achieve complete pain relief and normal strength, stability, and range of motion after surgical reconstruction (6)[A]. Therefore, some clinicians will treat patients with a trial of conservative treatment and reserve surgery for patients who continue to have symptoms.
- Avulsion fractures:
  - If avulsion-type fracture is present, treatment is a thumb spica cast for 4 to 6 wk (1,2)[C]:
    - Casting may be modified to a hand-based thumb spica (wrist out) as symptoms allow.

MEDICATION

Acetaminophen or nonsteroidal anti-inflammatory drugs (NSAIDs) are generally adequate for pain control.

ADDITIONAL THERAPIES

- Rehabilitation may be helpful in regaining full range of motion and strength postoperatively or in those with difficulty regaining motion and strength after conservative treatment.
- Early range of motion may be acceptable postoperatively (2)[C].

SURGERY/OTHER PROCEDURES

- Acute operative treatment (1,2):
  - Several different surgical techniques for repair are used and will depend on the exact nature of the injury and surgeon experience.
  - Cast or splint is used for 4 to 6 wk at which time range of motion and strengthening exercises are initiated.
  - Full unrestricted activity is generally allowed at 12 wk.
  - Protected activity may be allowed sooner depending on the surgical technique and surgeon preference.
- Chronic operative treatment (6)[A]:
  - Generally requires surgical reconstruction of the UCL.
- Patients generally experience excellent clinical outcomes after surgical treatment of both acute and chronic UCL injury without any significant difference between repair and reconstruction for acute and chronic injury, respectively.

ONGOING CARE

- Surgery is the preferred treatment for chronic instability (6)[A].
- Conservative treatment is limited to bracing and strengthening exercises.

PROGNOSIS

- Prognosis is excellent for partial UCL injuries (1,3)[C].
- Prognosis is excellent for complete tears treated surgically (6)[A].

COMPLICATIONS

- Most common complication is instability, resulting in decreased pinch strength:
  - Long-term instability increases the risk of osteoarthritis.
- Other complications are related to surgical interventions (local numbness and infection).

REFERENCES

1. Baskies MA, Lee SK. Evaluation and treatment of injuries of the ulnar collateral ligament of the thumb metacarpophalangeal joint. *Bull NYU Hosp Jt Dis*. 2009;67(1):68–74.
2. Johnson JW, Culp RW. Acute ulnar collateral ligament injury in the athlete. *Hand Clin*. 2009;25(3):437–442.
3. Malik AK, Morris T, Chou D, et al. Clinical testing of ulnar collateral ligament injuries of the thumb. *J Hand Surg Eur Vol*. 2009;34(3):363–366.
4. Melville D, Jacobson JA, Haase S, et al. Ultrasound of displaced ulnar collateral ligament tears of the thumb: the Stener lesion revisited. *Skeletal Radiol*. 2013;42(5):667–673.
5. Plancher KD, Ho CP, Cofield SS, et al. Role of MR imaging in the management of "skier's thumb" injuries. *Magn Reson Imaging Clin N Am*. 1999;7(1):73–84.
6. Samora JB, Harris JD, Griesser MJ, et al. Outcomes after injury to the thumb ulnar collateral ligament—a systematic review. *Clin J Sport Med*. 2013;23(4):247–254.

ADDITIONAL READING

- Avery DM III, Caggiano NM, Matullo KS. Ulnar collateral ligament injuries of the thumb: a comprehensive review. *Orthop Clin North Am*. 2015;46(2):281–292.
- Avery DM III, Inkellis ER, Carlson MG. Thumb collateral ligament injuries in the athlete. *Curr Rev Musculoskelet Med*. 2017;10(1):28–37.

CLINICAL PEARLS

Timing for return to play depends on severity and whether surgery is performed. Incomplete tears usually are treated with splinting for 4 to 8 wk, with range of motion exercises and strengthening beginning after 3 wk. A protective splint should be worn for sports until range of motion and strength have returned to normal, usually within 6 to 8 wk of injury. If surgery is performed, range of motion and strengthening exercises usually begin 6 wk after surgery. A protective splint usually is prescribed until range of motion and strength have returned to normal.

ULNAR IMPACTION SYNDROME

Emily Levy, MD, CAQSM

BASICS

DESCRIPTION

- Ulnar impaction syndrome (also referred to as ulnocarpal abutment or ulnocarpal impaction syndrome) is a degenerative condition of the ulnar-sided wrist due to excessive load across the ulnocarpal joint.
- It occurs most often with positive ulnar variance. In the normal wrist, 20% of the load goes through the ulna and 80% through the radius. With greater ulnar variance, loads approaching 40% can go through the distal ulnar joint (1).
- It can result in a myriad of pathology, including triangular fibrocartilage complex (TFCC) deterioration, degeneration of the ulnar head, lunate, triquetrum, and/or lunotriquetral interosseous ligament (LTIL).
- Ulnar impaction syndrome is also seen in neutral or negative variance due to dynamic impaction during high-impact activities.

EPIDEMIOLOGY

Little is known about the demographics of ulnar impaction syndrome.

ETIOLOGY AND PATHOPHYSIOLOGY

- Biomechanical changes causing excessive loading across the ulnocarpal joint are responsible for degeneration of the TFCC and articular surfaces of the ulnar head, lunate, and triquetrum.
- Positive variance of just 2 mm will increase the load through the ulna from 20% to 40%.
- Ulnar impaction syndrome can also occur in neutral or negative variance due to activities that increase axial loading and rotation leading to a dynamic variance.
- Patients with distal radial fracture malunion often acquire this condition when the balance of the distal radial ulnar joint (DRUJ) is altered and the ulna develops a positive variance in relation to the radius.

Genetics

Positive ulnar variance is more prevalent in Asians, and therefore incidence may be higher, but further studies need to be done (1).

RISK FACTORS

- Not well studied
- Any condition leading to ulnar positive variance traumatic injury
- Repetitive forceful loading of the wrist in pronation and ulnar deviation, such as gymnasts, boxers, and athletes of racquet sports (2)

GENERAL PREVENTION

Prevention in the repetitive loading population includes activity modification and functional bracing when needed. In patients with acquired ulnar impaction syndrome, most commonly secondary to traumatic shortening of the distal radius, open reduction and internal fixation of the radius is done to recreate a balanced wrist joint.

COMMONLY ASSOCIATED CONDITIONS

- Scapholunate dissociation
- TFCC tears
- Lunotriquetral ligament tears
- Radial shortening from Colles fracture

DIAGNOSIS

The diagnosis of ulnar impaction syndrome is a clinical one assisted by radiographic findings.

HISTORY

- Pain on the dorsal-ulnar side of DRUJ
- Pain with pronation and ulnar deviation of wrist
- Pain with axial loading

PHYSICAL EXAM

- Painful range of motion (ROM) especially with rotation and ulnar deviation
- Positive ballottement test
- Positive ulnocarpal stress test
- Positive fovea test

DIFFERENTIAL DIAGNOSIS

- Pisotriquetral arthritis
- DRUJ arthrosis
- Neuritis of the dorsal cutaneous branch of the ulnar nerve
- Extensor carpi ulnaris (ECU) subluxation or tendinopathy
- Isolated TFCC tear

DIAGNOSTIC TESTS & INTERPRETATION

- Complete wrist radiograph series, including posteroanterior (PA) wrist to evaluate ulnar variance
- A pronated grip PA radiograph to evaluate for dynamic ulnar variance
- Radiographic identification of subchondral sclerosis and cystic changes, particularly around the distal ulna and ulnar carpal bones, the lunate and the triquetrum

- Magnetic resonance imaging (MRI) of the wrist without contrast may aid in identifying bony edema and chondral lesions but is not required for diagnosis.

TREATMENT

GENERAL MEASURES

Nonoperative treatment is first line and includes rest and/or immobilization for 6 to 12 wk, nonsteroidal anti-inflammatory drugs (NSAIDs), and local corticosteroids (2).

SURGERY/OTHER PROCEDURES

- If nonoperative treatment fails, surgical intervention is indicated.
- Surgical intervention is done to decrease load across the ulnocarpal joint or sometimes just to decompress the TFCC when there is a central lesion (3).
- Gold standard surgical option is ulnar shortening osteotomy (USO) often with wrist arthroscopy to evaluate TFCC, LTIL, and articular surfaces (4).
- May consider wafer procedure, which is a partial distal ulnar resection of the dome of the ulnar head
- These two surgical techniques have been found to have similar outcomes of pain relief and wrist function, but USO group required more revisions and delayed union (5,6).
- Wafer shortens by 2 to 3 mm, does not fix stylocarpal impaction if present, and does not improve dorsal subluxation, if present.
- If acquired positive ulnar variance due to radius, may correct radius as opposed to ulna

COMPLEMENTARY & ALTERNATIVE MEDICINE

There are several other surgical methods, including the Sauvé-Kapandji procedure and Darrach procedure, which have not yet shown superiority to the USO (7).

ONGOING CARE

PROGNOSIS

- More studies are needed for prognosis of nonoperative treatment.
- A systematic review of operative treatment showed a 100% satisfaction rate for arthroscopic wafer procedure, 89% for open wafer procedure, and 84% for USO (5)[A].
- 88% of patients report being satisfied to very satisfied following USO at average of 10-yr follow-up (4)[B] despite 30% of patients requiring hardware removal.

COMPLICATIONS

Surgical complications include need for hardware removal in USO, nonunion, and need for revision procedures.

REFERENCES

1. Sammer DM, Rizzo D. Ulnar impaction. *Hand Clin*. 2010;26(4):549–557.
2. Biswas S. Ulnolunate impaction syndrome. *Eplasty*. 2015;15:ic2.
3. Löw S, Herold A, Unglaub F, et al. Treatment of ulnar impaction syndrome with and without central TFC lesion. *J Wrist Surg*. 2018;7(2):133–140.
4. Fufa DT, Carlson MG, Calfee RP, et al. Mid-term results following ulna shortening osteotomy. *HSS J*. 2014;10(1):13–17.
5. Stockton DJ, Pelletier ME, Pike JM. Operative treatment of ulnar impaction syndrome: a systematic review. *J Hand Surg Eur Vol*. 2015;40(5): 470–476.
6. Katz DI, Seiler JG III, Bond TC. The treatment of ulnar impaction syndrome: a systematic review of the literature. *J Surg Orthop Adv*. 2010;19(4): 218–222.
7. Yu YD, Wu T, Tian FT, et al. Ulnar impaction syndrome with different operative methods: a comparative biomechanical study. *Int J Clin Exp Med*. 2015;8(4):5715–5722.

ADDITIONAL READING

Möldner M, Unglaub F, Hahn P, et al. Functionality after arthroscopic debridement of central triangular fibrocartilage tears with central perforations. *J Hand Surg Am*. 2015;40(2):252–258.e2.

CLINICAL PEARLS

- Ulnar impaction syndrome is a degenerative condition involving the abutment of the ulna onto the carpal bones.
- Diagnosis is clinical, aided by radiographic findings.
- If patients do not improve with a course of nonoperative treatment, ulnar-sided osteotomy or wafer procedure is typically performed depending on which structures are affected.

ULNAR TUNNEL SYNDROME

Richard Okragly, MD • Amanda Chaney, DO, FAAFP, CAQSM

BASICS

DESCRIPTION

- Compression of the ulnar nerve in Guyon canal at the level of the wrist
- Guyon canal is bordered by the volar carpal ligament, transverse retinacular ligament, and laterally by the hook of the hamate.
- The superficial sensory branch and/or the deep motor branch of the ulnar nerve can be involved.
- Synonyms: handlebar palsy; Guyon canal syndrome
- Types (based on the Shea and McClain classification):
  - I—combined sensory and motor deficit
  - II—motor deficit only
  - III—sensory deficit only

ETIOLOGY AND PATHOPHYSIOLOGY

- Guyon canal is located in the base of the hand on the ulnar side:
  - The borders of Guyon canal are:
    - Pisiform (medially).
    - Hook of the hamate (laterally).
    - Volar carpal ligament/pisohamate ligament (volar, roof).
    - Transverse retinacular ligament (floor).
- Injury to the nerve is caused by trauma to wrist and pressure over the hypothenar eminence.
- A true motor, true sensory, or mixed injury pattern can be seen, depending on the location of compression.
- The mixed (motor and sensory) type is due to compression in the proximal aspect of Guyon canal before the division of the ulnar nerve into superficial and deep branches (type I).
- True motor type is due to compression of the ulnar nerve at the level of the lower wrist (type II).
- True sensory type is due to compression of the superficial branch of the ulnar nerve at the distal aspect of Guyon canal (type III).

RISK FACTORS

- Environmental trigger factors:
  - Repetitive occupational wrist trauma (occupational neuritis)
  - Baseball catchers
  - Cyclists (1)
  - Hockey goalies
  - Golf and racquet sports
  - Martial arts
  - Wheelchair athletes
  - Cross-country skiing
  - Weight lifters
- Anatomical
- Ganglion cyst
- Hook of hamate/pisiform fracture
- Deviant hypothenar muscles
- Ulnar artery aneurysm

GENERAL PREVENTION

- Avoid excessive pressure to ulnovolar aspect of palm.
- Avoid repetitive wrist trauma.
- Ergonomic bicycle grips and/or gloves

COMMONLY ASSOCIATED CONDITIONS

- Cubital tunnel syndrome
- Carpal tunnel syndrome
- Radial nerve compression
- Hook of hamate fractures
- Martin-Gruber ulnar-median anastomosis (15% of population)
- Riche-Cannieu deep ulnar-median anastomosis
- Hypothenar hammer syndrome

DIAGNOSIS

HISTORY

- Ring (4th) and small (5th) finger paresthesias with variable weakness of grip
- Localized pain and tenderness over Guyon canal
- Paresthesias or vascular compromise (coldness and pallor of the 4th and 5th digits, cyanosis, and pain) if the ulnar artery is involved
- Coincidental involvement of the median nerve is common (tingling or numbness or weakness or pain in the 2nd and 3rd digits and the lateral aspect of the 4th digit) (2,3,4)[C].

PHYSICAL EXAM

- Depending on the location of the lesion, motor, sensory, or mixed signs may be elicited.
- Sensory (2,3,4)[C]:
  - Positive Tinel sign at the pisiform, affecting the medial aspect of the 4th digit and all of the 5th digit
  - Sensory loss at tip of little finger
  - Hypoesthesia on volar sensory branch without involvement of dorsal sensory branch
- Motor (2,3,4)[C]:
  - Weakness with resistance of adductor pollicis and all interossei muscles
  - Late atrophy of the first dorsal interosseous muscle
  - Positive Wartenberg sign: abduction of the small finger due to interosseous and lumbrical compromise
  - Positive Froment sign: activation of flexor pollicis longus to substitute for adductor pollicis
  - Decreased grip strength (40% due to ulnar-innervated muscles)
  - Ulnar claw hand with paralysis of the deep motor branch

DIFFERENTIAL DIAGNOSIS

- Proximal ulnar entrapment (elbow, cervicothoracic spine)
- Calcific tendonitis of flexor carpi ulnaris tendon
- Carpal instability
- Arthropathy of pisotriquetral joint
- Ligamentous wrist injury
- Ulnar artery thrombosis
- Hypoesthesia on dorsal sensory branch does *not* involve compression in Guyon canal.

DIAGNOSTIC TESTS & INTERPRETATION

Initial Tests (lab, imaging)

Generally, imaging is not needed to make the diagnosis but can be used to establish the etiology or rule out other diagnoses (2,3,4,5,6)[C]:

- Radiographs to exclude carpal instability and fracture at hook of hamate or pisiform: carpal tunnel view
- Computed tomography (CT) scan to exclude hook of the hamate fractures
- Doppler ultrasound (US) to exclude thrombosis
- Magnetic resonance imaging (MRI) to exclude ganglion cyst or lipoma as space-occupying lesions and evaluate areas of muscle denervation
- US imaging to assess ulnar nerve within the ulnar tunnel

Diagnostic Procedures/Other

Electromyogram (EMG) studies to document ulnar nerve pathology (2,3,4,5,6)[C] and localize area of compression

TREATMENT

Prehospital:

- Avoid aggravating activities, including but not limited to (3,4)[C]:
  - Repetitive hand motions and activities.
  - Heavy grasping and gripping.
  - Resting the palm against hard surfaces.

MEDICATION

First Line

Nonsteroidal anti-inflammatory drugs (NSAIDs) (3,4)[C]

Second Line

Local injection of corticosteroids (3,4)[C]

ADDITIONAL THERAPIES

- Conservative treatment to include (2,3,5)[C]:
  - Splinting
  - Padding of gloves and handlebars
  - Physical therapy
  - Rest
- Adjust activity to avoid repetitive wrist trauma (2,3,5)[C].
- Adjusting bicycle fit to reduce hand/wrist pressure

SURGERY/OTHER PROCEDURES

- Fascial release to free the aponeurosis around Guyon canal (2,3,5,6,7)[C]
- Surgery to remove compressive ganglion (2,3,6)[C]
- Hook of hamate excision in setting of fracture

ONGOING CARE

FOLLOW-UP RECOMMENDATIONS

- Following surgery, proper wound care and pain control are essential.
- Return to full activity 4 to 8 wk following surgical decompression (3)[C].

REFERENCES

1. Brubacher JW, Leversedge FJ. Ulnar neuropathy in cyclists. *Hand Clin*. 2017;33(1):199–205.
2. Anto C, Aradhya P. Clinical diagnosis of peripheral nerve compression in the upper extremity. *Orthop Clin North Am*. 1996;27(2):227–236.
3. Plancher KD. The athletic elbow and wrist, part II: common overuse injuries. *Clin Sports Med*. 1996; 15:347–353.
4. Baker CL Jr. Overuse injuries in the upper extremity. *Clin Sports Med*. 2001;20:603–605.
5. Cass S. Upper extremity nerve entrapment syndromes in sports: an update. *Curr Sports Med Rep*. 2014; 13(1):16–21.
6. Beltran J, Rosenberg ZS. Diagnosis of compressive and entrapment neuropathies of the upper extremity: value of MR imaging. *AJR Am J Roentgenol*. 1994; 163(3):525–531.
7. Chen SH, Tsai TM. Ulnar tunnel syndrome. *J Hand Surg Am*. 2014;39(3):571–579.

ADDITIONAL READING

Green DP. *Green's Operative Hand Surgery*. Vol 2. 2nd ed. London, United Kingdom: Churchill Livingstone Publishing; 1988:1452–1454.

CLINICAL PEARLS

- Numbness and tingling in the hand are not always signs of carpal tunnel syndrome.
- A good history and physical examination are necessary to accurately diagnose this condition.
- Nerve conduction velocity (NCV)/EMG can be normal if tested during first few weeks of symptoms.
- Serial EMGs can be used to determine if conservative treatment is effective or if further management is warranted.

ULTRAVIOLET KERATITIS

Carrie Zaslow, MD • Tracy Zaslow, MD, FAAP, CAQSM

BASICS

- Also known as photokeratitis or solar keratitis
- Acute syndrome occurs after exposure of the eyes to ultraviolet (UV) radiation.
- Painful but usually self-limited

DESCRIPTION

Exposure to various forms of UV radiation leads to redness, pain, tearing, and photophobia in association with epithelial defects of the cornea and conjunctival injection.

ETIOLOGY AND PATHOPHYSIOLOGY

- Cornea transmits light in visible spectrum.
- Cornea absorbs light in UV spectrum:
  - 10–20% of light in UVA spectrum is absorbed.
  - Nearly 100% of UVC light is absorbed and a substantial amount of UVB (1).
- Damage to the cornea in UV keratitis:
  - Results from absorption of light at the transition point between UVB and UVC (290 nm)
  - Occurs from absorption in the corneal epithelium, the most anterior part of the cornea
  - Causes surface epithelial cells to die and desquamate
  - Damaged cells contain epithelial nociceptor terminal axons that are destroyed, leading to corneal pain secondary to stimulation of the subepithelial nerve plexus.
  - Tear film also primarily disrupted by UV exposure.

Genetics

No genetic association

RISK FACTORS

- UV exposure to unprotected eyes associated with various recreational and occupational activities (2,3)
- Sources of exposure:
  - Welder's arc burns
  - Snow blindness
  - High-voltage-line short circuits
  - Other solar exposure
  - Sunlamps
  - Damaged metal halide lamps
  - Aquaria disinfection lamps
  - Laboratory or germicidal UV lamps

GENERAL PREVENTION

The mode of prevention depends on the type of exposure:

- Recreational sun exposure: well-fitting sunglasses that meet the American National Standards Institute (ANSI) standards with protection against most UV-A and UV-B radiation
- Occupational exposure to solar and artificial-solar UV sources: UV-blocking safety goggles in accordance with ANSI
- Occupational exposure to metal halide or mercury vapor lamps: Adherence to the U.S. Food and Drug Administration (FDA) Radiological Health Program is recommended.

COMMONLY ASSOCIATED CONDITIONS

Facial/eyelid edema and erythema, resulting from the same UV exposure injury

DIAGNOSIS

- Accurate history, including:
  - Type of exposure
  - Timing and duration of exposure
  - Use of protective eyewear
- Visual acuity
- Complete bilateral ocular exam, including:
  - Extraocular movements
  - Slit-lamp exam with and without fluorescein stain of conjunctiva/sclera/cornea
  - Slit-lamp exam of anterior chambers (checking for cell and flare)
  - Intraocular pressure
  - Lenses
  - Eversion of the lids to check for foreign bodies
  - pH exam (to rule out chemical keratitis)

HISTORY

- Exposure without protective eyewear 6 to 12 hr prior to onset of symptoms (4)
- To assess amount of UV radiation with exposure, need to know time of day, season, hemisphere, clouds and haze, atmospheric scattering, and ground reflection
- Symptoms (usually bilateral):
  - Intense pain
  - Photophobia
  - Foreign body sensation
  - Mild to moderate decrease in visual acuity
  - Increased lacrimation

PHYSICAL EXAM

- Topical anesthetic generally is needed to obtain a good physical exam.
- Penlight exam:
  - Tearing, injection, chemosis of the bulbar conjunctiva, and corneal haziness
  - No discharge present in the tarsal conjunctiva; lack of discharge distinguishes photokeratitis from infectious conjunctivitis.
  - Pupils are usually relatively miotic and react sluggishly.
- Fluorescein exam: confluent superficial punctuate staining between the lids
- Slit-lamp exam:
  - Eversion of the eyelids should not reveal a foreign body.
  - Superficial punctate staining of the cornea
  - Corneal edema and anterior chamber reaction (cell and flare) may be seen.
- A thorough eye exam including fluorescein staining and slit-lamp exam generally is sufficient for diagnosis.

DIFFERENTIAL DIAGNOSIS

- Foreign body of the cornea or eyelids
- Intraocular foreign body
- Corneal abrasion
- Thermal burns
- Toxic epithelial keratopathy (from exposure to chemicals or drugs)
- Exposure keratopathy
- Nocturnal lagophthalmos
- Conjunctivitis
- Stevens-Johnson syndrome
- Infectious keratitis
- Neurotrophic keratopathy
- Contact lens–related problems
- Trauma
- Dry eye syndrome
- Scleritis

DIAGNOSTIC TESTS & INTERPRETATION

Initial Tests (lab, imaging)

- Is typically a clinical diagnosis
- If intraocular foreign body suspected as comorbid condition: Orbit x-ray, computed tomography (CT), ultrasound, ultrasound biomicroscopy, or magnetic resonance imaging (MRI) can aid in diagnosis and localization; MRI and CT best if globe injury suspected (4)[B]

Diagnostic Procedures/Other

pH of tear lake: To distinguish from a chemical burn, check pH of tear lake in lower conjunctival fornix; pH should be normal in UV keratitis.

TREATMENT

GENERAL MEASURES

- Treatment is supportive.
- Severe pain from the syndrome should be treated with oral analgesics.
- Although they do have a role in the physical exam, topical anesthetics should *never* be prescribed.
- Emergency department (ED) treatment:
  - Oral analgesics:
    - Mild oral narcotics may be necessary.
    - Pain control is important to allow patient to sleep, thus creating an anatomic patch.
  - Cycloplegic drops:
    - Will help to relieve photophobia
    - Will induce pupil dilation and inhibit accommodation (causing blurring of near vision)
    - Short-acting agents (i.e., cyclopentolate) preferable to avoid long-lasting pupil dilation that can be uncomfortable for patient
  - Antibiotic ointment:
    - To provide prophylaxis against superinfection
    - Has secondary effect of providing lubrication and increasing comfort
  - Pressure patch (optional):
    - Only to be used in very reliable patients who have scheduled follow-ups
    - On the worse eye for 24 hr
    - May provide some relief
    - Has not been proven to aid in expeditious healing

MEDICATION

- Antibiotic ointment (prescribed 3 to 4 times per day for 2 to 3 days):
  - Erythromycin
  - Bacitracin
  - Polymyxin-bacitracin
- Cycloplegics:
  - Cyclopentolate 1%
  - Homatropine 2–5%
  - Scopolamine 0.25%

ADMISSION, INPATIENT, AND NURSING CONSIDERATIONS

- Initial stabilization:
  - Topical anesthesia helps to obtain:
    - More accurate documentation of visual acuity.
    - More thorough eye exam and fluorescein staining.
    - Do not prescribe on outpatient basis: interferes with healing and worsens keratitis.
- Admission criteria:
  - Patients requiring bilateral patching with severely decreased visual acuity and whose social circumstances make it impossible for the patient to take care of his or her own needs
- Discharge criteria:
  - Nearly all patients may be discharged from the ED following treatment.
  - Lesions usually heal completely within 24 to 48 hr.
  - Ophthalmologist referral for patients who have other eye disorders or for those who fail to improve significantly after 24 hr

ONGOING CARE

- Corneal surface regenerates in 24 to 72 hr.
- Surface regeneration leads to symptom resolution.

FOLLOW-UP RECOMMENDATIONS

- Reexamination in 24 to 48 hr
- If symptoms improved: Patient can continue with topical antibiotics QID and discontinue cycloplegic.
- If symptoms not improved and superficial punctate staining is still present: Continue treatment with cycloplegics and antibiotics, and refer to ophthalmologist.

Patient Monitoring

Long-term monitoring is generally unnecessary.

Patients should be counseled on using protective eyewear.

PATIENT EDUCATION

Depending on their daily activities, patients should be referred to the appropriate resource to learn about protective eyewear:

- ANSI (www.ANSI.org)
- FDA Radiological Health Program (www.FDA.gov)

PROGNOSIS

Generally, acute, single episodes heal without long-term sequelae.

COMPLICATIONS

Chronic UV exposure can lead to other sequelae:

- Cutaneous melanoma
- Ocular melanoma
- Erythema
- Cataract
- Pinguecula/pterygium
- Nonmelanocytic skin cancer

REFERENCES

1. Young A. Acute effects of UVR on human eyes and skin. *Prog Biophys Mol Biol*. 2006;92(1):80–85.
2. Izadi M, Jonaidi-Jafari N, Pourazizi M, et al. Photokeratitis induced by ultraviolet radiation in travelers: a major health problem. *J Postgrad Med*. 2018;64(1):40–46.
3. Kwon DH, Moon JD, Park WJ, et al. Case series of keratitis in poultry abattoir workers induced by exposure to the ultraviolet disinfection lamp. *Ann Occup Environ Med*. 2016;28:3.
4. Loporchio D, Mukkamala L, Gorukanti K, et al. Intraocular foreign bodies: a review. *Surv Ophthalmol*. 2016;61(5):582–596.

ADDITIONAL READING

- American National Standards Institute: www.ANSI.org
- Bagheri N, Wajda B, eds. *The Wills Eye Manual: Office and Emergency Room Diagnosis and Treatment of Eye Disease*. 7th ed. Philadelphia, PA: Wolters Kluwer; 2016.
- U.S. Food and Drug Administration: www.FDA.gov
- Verma AS, Dwarika D, Bhola RM, et al. Photokeratitis following the manipulation of aquaria disinfection lamps. *Emerg Med J*. 2007;24(3):232.

CLINICAL PEARLS

- A patient with eye pain should not be prescribed topical anesthetic eye drops.
- Abuse of these drops can lead to neurotrophic keratopathy, a loss of corneal sensation leading to epithelial defects.
- Patients must be counseled about use of protective eyewear.

URETERAL, BLADDER, AND URETHRAL TRAUMA

Robert J. Baker, MD, PhD, FAAFP, FACSM

BASICS

DESCRIPTION

- Sports-related trauma to the trunk and/or perineum can result in contusion, laceration, or complete transection of the ureter, bladder, or urethra.
- Injury to the genitourinary (GU) tract is overall uncommon. Lower GU tract injuries from blunt or penetrating mechanisms can involve the bladder, urethra, or the external genitalia.
- Ureteral, bladder, and urethral injuries may be associated with pelvic fractures.

EPIDEMIOLOGY

Injury to the GU tract is overall uncommon.

ALERT
Fractures of the pelvis can result in injuries to the urethra, bladder, and ureters.

- Ureteral injury is very rare compared with other GU organs, and traumatic ureteral injury rarely occurs in isolation from blunt trauma, but if present, is highly associated with concomitant injuries.
- Ureteral injuries account for 1% of all GU injuries.
- Bladder injuries (contusion or rupture) occur in approximately 1.6% of blunt abdominal trauma:
  - Extraperitoneal in 60% and intraperitoneal in 30%
- With posterior urethral injuries, there is a concomitant bladder injury 15% of the time.
- Although males are susceptible to blunt injury of the urethra, this type of injury is uncommon in females.
- Impingement of the bulbous urethra against the pubic symphysis results in urethral injuries from the straddle mechanism.
- Straddle injuries in females may result in labial hematoma and urinary retention. These injuries have been reported in in-line skating.
- Most posterior urethral injuries occur by a shearing mechanism.

ETIOLOGY AND PATHOPHYSIOLOGY

Bladder injuries are broadly classified as extraperitoneal (i.e., injury confined to extraperitoneal space) or intraperitoneal (i.e., injury communicating with the peritoneum).

Genetics

- No specific genetic predisposition for GU injuries
- However, genetic malformations and solitary kidney are often diagnosed in young children after workup for GU trauma.

RISK FACTORS

- In children with multiple injuries, GU injuries are common (1)[C].
- Although rare, avulsion of the ureter secondary to blunt trauma is known to occur in children (2)[B].
- Rupture of the bladder may occur following blunt or penetrating trauma. The bladder is especially at risk for injury when full (1,3,4)[C].
- The abdominal position of the bladder, in childhood, places it at greater risk for traumatic injury (1,3,5)[C].
- Bladder injuries often occur in association with pelvic fractures (3,5)[A].

GENERAL PREVENTION

Appropriate protective equipment for contact sports is recommended.

COMMONLY ASSOCIATED CONDITIONS

- Urethral injuries in children may result from a straddle mechanism (i.e., direct trauma to the perineum commonly due to contact with the crossbar of a bicycle) (3,5)[A].
- Patients admitted with multiple trauma injuries will have associated GU injuries 10% of the time (1)[A].

DIAGNOSIS

HISTORY

- Ureter: trauma to the back or flank, hematuria, expanding flank mass (2)[C]:
  - Suspect traumatic ureteral injury if: (i) an appropriate mechanism of injury; (ii) new symptoms of fever, flank pain, sepsis, and/or ileus occur following initial trauma stabilization; or (iii) following pelvic surgery (2)[C].
- Bladder: hematuria, urethrorrhagia, or inability to void following a traumatic injury to the abdomen (3)[C]
- Urethra: trauma to the pelvis possibly resulting in fracture, urethrorrhagia, hematuria, inability to void, and lower abdominal or perineum pain (4)[C]

PHYSICAL EXAM

- Clinical features that should increase suspicion for lower GU tract injury include suprapubic tenderness, hematuria, blood at the urethral meatus, and difficulty voiding, although these are nonspecific (2)[C].
- Ureter: flank pain, flank mass (urine or hematoma), lower abdominal pain, urinary urgency, hematuria, fever, chills, rarely shock (1,2)[C]
- Bladder: hematuria, urethrorrhagia, or inability to void (2)[C]
- Urethra: urethrorrhagia and inability to void, especially if pelvic fracture is present or suspected, rectal exam reveals a floating or absent prostate; ecchymosis and swelling of the external genitalia (2)[C]
- Localized tenderness: ureter, flank pain; bladder, abdominal pain; urethra, perineum pain
- Peritoneal signs can occur with extravasation, especially of the bladder (2)[C].
- Look for ecchymosis in the pubic area or perineum (2)[C].
- Findings consistent with pelvic fracture (1,5)[C]

DIFFERENTIAL DIAGNOSIS

- Hematuria: kidney contusion, kidney laceration, sports-induced hematuria, kidney failure, renal calculi, cystitis
- Inability to void: kidney failure, renal calculi, kidney laceration, prostatic hypertrophy, cauda equina

DIAGNOSTIC TESTS & INTERPRETATION

Initial Tests (lab, imaging)

ALERT
Hematuria on urinalysis, although nonspecific, can be an indication of lower collecting system injury (urethra, bladder, ureter) (1,2)[C].

- The degree of hematuria is not necessarily correlated with the degree of injury. Small urethral injuries may present with significant gross blood. Large ureteral injuries may present with microscopic hematuria (4)[C].
- Hematuria is present in <1/2 of patients with a ureteral injury (2)[C].
- Plain x-rays can identify associated injuries (e.g., pelvic fractures, lower rib fractures, and spinal vertebrae fractures), which may raise suspicion of a GU injury (5)[C].
- Ureter: in hemodynamically stable patients, contrast-enhanced computed tomography (CT) scan of the abdomen/pelvis recommended to diagnosis of ureteral injury:
  - Identification of ureteral injuries requires a delay of 5 to 10 min after the administration of intravenous (IV) contrast to allow contrast to reach the ureters.
- Bladder: Retrograde cystography can establish presence of bladder rupture (2)[B].
- Urethra: Retrograde urethrography is diagnostic (6)[C].
- Children: Some recommend all children should be imaged if they have gross hematuria or >50 red blood cells (RBCs) per high-power field (5)[C].
- Ultrasound (US) is not reliable at differentiating urine and blood. Thus, US is not the imaging technique to use in patients with high risk of bladder injury (6)[B].

Follow-Up Tests & Special Considerations

- Direct inspection of the ureters in the operating room is the most sensitive method to assess for ureteral injury (2)[B].
- IV dyes (e.g., methylene blue, indigo carmine) can be used to aid the assessment looking for dye leakage along the course of the ureter (2,3,4)[B].

Diagnostic Procedures/Other

When CT of the abdomen/pelvis and CT cystogram are both needed for the evaluation of pelvic trauma, the CT cystogram should be performed after the corticomedullary phase of the CT scan (to assess possible kidney injury) or the arterial phase (to assess other injuries).

- Waiting will prevent extravasated bladder contrast from obscuring vascular injuries that may benefit from urgent angioembolization (2,6)[A].

Test Interpretation

- Pelvic fracture patterns associated with high risk of GU injury are pubic rami fractures of all four rami, ipsilateral rami fracture with massive posterior disruption of the sacrum, sacroiliac joint, or ilium (2)[B].
- Pelvic fracture patterns associated with low risk are single rami fractures, ipsilateral rami fractures without ring disruption (2)[B].
- Very little risk of ureteral injury with isolated fractures of acetabulum, ilium, and sacrum (6)[C]

TREATMENT

GENERAL MEASURES

ALERT

Because these injuries are often associated with trauma and multiple injuries, stabilization of the patient is the most important (2)[C].

- Signs of shock may be present and should be addressed immediately (2)[C].
- Other more life-threatening organ trauma, renal injuries, for example, likely will need to be addressed first (2)[C].
- Analgesia: Oral analgesia may be adequate; however, pain from associated trauma may require intramuscular (IM) or IV administration of strong narcotics (6)[C].
- Prognosis is good for full recovery if the injury is diagnosed early and treated appropriately (2)[A].
- Most patients will require urologic consultation and possible surgical intervention (6)[C].

ALERT

- Urinary drainage is an essential aspect of the acute management of a suspected lower GU tract injury. Blind catheter passage prior to lower GU tract imaging is discouraged (2,6)[B].
- Co-management should address concerns regarding the placement of any suprapubic catheters in patients who are likely to need surgery to repair pelvic fractures (2)[C].
- Bladder injuries are broadly classified anatomically as extraperitoneal (i.e., injury confined to extraperitoneal space) simple or complex or intraperitoneal (i.e., injury communicating with the peritoneum) (3)[C].
  - Complex extraperitoneal bladder injuries include bladder neck injury, open pelvic fracture with impinging bone into the bladder, concomitant rectal and/or vaginal injury (2,3,6)[A].
- The management of bladder injuries is according to anatomic classification (3)[A]:
  - Simple extraperitoneal bladder injuries, begin with conservative management with urethral catheter drainage alone, are safe with a high rate of spontaneous bladder healing (3)[C].
  - Complex extraperitoneal bladder injuries are managed with early surgical repair rather than bladder catheter drainage alone. These injuries are not likely to heal with urethral catheter drainage alone (3)[C].
  - Early repair is also reasonable for patients with pelvic fracture who require open reduction/fixation or who have other indications for laparotomy (3)[C].
- Traumatic intraperitoneal bladder injuries should be repaired because they are typically large and will not heal with catheter drainage (3)[C].

ISSUES FOR REFERRAL

Referral to trauma and general surgery is emergent if a lower collecting system injury is suspected.

ADDITIONAL THERAPIES

- Special considerations:
  - Ureteral fistulas and strictures can occur as a result of missed injuries or from entrapment associated with fibrosis from healed dislocation of sacroiliac joints (2)[C].
  - IV pyelogram should be performed prior to the cystogram (2)[C].
  - Retrograde urethrography should be performed prior to catheterization in the male athlete who has sustained a pelvic fracture and is unable to void following the trauma (3)[C].
- Rehabilitation:
  - No specific rehabilitation, but general reconditioning is usually required following the period of convalescence
  - Following surgical procedures, rehabilitation exercises directed at the back or pelvic musculature may be necessary.

SURGERY/OTHER PROCEDURES

- Ureteral injuries generally require some form of treatment:
  - Minimal blunt ureteral injuries and partial penetrating injuries may be amenable to ureteral stenting.
  - Ureteral repair should be performed when injury is identified at the time of laparotomy, if possible.
  - For severe injuries, ligation of the ureter with urinary drainage and delayed reconstruction may be necessary.
  - Transection of the ureter requires prompt repair, ureteropyelostomy (1,2)[C].
- Any bladder rupture associated with pelvic fracture where penetration of the bladder by a bony spicule is possible is best managed with surgical dèbridement (1,2)[C].
- Intraperitoneal rupture of the bladder is appropriately treated with transperitoneal exploration, dèbridement, and repair (6)[C].
- Initial management of urethral injuries remains controversial. Although early exploration and realignment have been successful, lower complication rates have been found with conservative treatment and delayed realignment (6)[C].

ONGOING CARE

FOLLOW-UP RECOMMENDATIONS

- Delayed diagnosis of ureteral injury can result in nephrectomy (6)[C].
- Small, uncomplicated extraperitoneal rupture of the bladder may be managed nonoperatively with a urethral catheter for 7 to 14 days (2)[C].

Patient Monitoring

- Repeat imaging is recommended prior to catheter removal to ensure that bladder or urethral healing has occurred, regardless of whether the injury was managed conservatively or required surgery (2)[C].
- Bladder injuries requiring surgery are repaired with a two-layer closure with urethral catheter drainage for 2 to 3 wk (2)[C].
- Dual catheter drainage (suprapubic tube, urethral catheter drainage) may be warranted in select circumstances (2)[C].
- Cystography is recommended prior to catheter removal to ensure complete healing has occurred regardless of whether the injury was managed conservatively or required surgery (2)[C].
- Avoidance of imaging for simple intraperitoneal repairs has also been advocated (2)[C].

PROGNOSIS

Full recovery and return to sports is expected but will be influenced by surgical procedure.

REFERENCES

1. McGeady JB, Breyer BN. Current epidemiology of genitourinary trauma. *Urol Clin North Am*. 2013;40(3):323–334.
2. Phillips B, Holzmer S, Turco L, et al. Trauma to the bladder and ureter: a review of diagnosis, management, and prognosis. *Eur J Trauma Emerg Surg*. 2017;43(6):763–773.
3. Gomez RG, Ceballos L, Coburn M, et al. Consensus statement on bladder injuries. *BJU Int*. 2004;94(1):27–32.
4. Chapple C, Barbagli G, Jordan G, et al. Consensus statement on urethral trauma. *BJU Int*. 2004;93(9):1195–1202.
5. Styn NR, Wan J. Urologic sports injuries in children. *Curr Urol Rep*. 2010;11(2):114–121.
6. Morey AF, Brandes S, Dugi DD III, et al. Urotrauma: AUA guideline. *J Urol*. 2014;192(2):327–335.

ADDITIONAL READING

- Asplund C, Barkdull T, Weiss BD. Genitourinary problems in bicyclists. *Curr Sports Med Rep*. 2007;6(5):333–339.
- Bryan ST, Coleman NJ, Blueitt D, et al. Bladder problems in athletes. *Curr Sports Med Rep*. 2008;7(2):108–112.
- Gross JA, Lehnert BE, Linnau KF, et al. Imaging of urinary system trauma. *Radiol Clin North Am*. 2015;53(4):773–788.
- Johnsen NV, Dmochowski RR, Young JB, et al. Epidemiology of blunt lower urinary tract trauma with and without pelvic fracture. *Urology*. 2017;102:234–239.
- Kong JP, Bultitude MF, Royce P, et al. Lower urinary tract injuries following blunt trauma: a review of contemporary management. *Rev Urol*. 2011;13(3):119–130.
- Lumen N, Kuehhas FE, Djakovic N, et al. Review of the current management of lower urinary tract injuries by the EAU Trauma Guidelines Panel. *Eur Urol*. 2015;67(5):925–929.
- Pariser JJ, Pearce SM, Patel SG, et al. National patterns of urethral evaluation and risk factors for urethral injury in patients with penile fracture. *Urology*. 2015;86(1):181–185.

CLINICAL PEARLS

- Suspect traumatic ureteral injury if (i) an appropriate mechanism of injury; (ii) new symptoms of fever, flank pain, sepsis, and/or ileus occur following initial trauma stabilization; or (iii) following pelvic surgery.
- Clinical features that should increase suspicion for lower GU tract injury include suprapubic tenderness, hematuria, blood at the urethral meatus, and difficulty voiding, although these are nonspecific.
- Repeat imaging is recommended prior to catheter removal to ensure that bladder or urethral healing has occurred, regardless of whether the injury was managed conservatively or required surgery.
- Retrograde cystography (fluoroscopic or CT imaging) is the only imaging study to establish a diagnosis of bladder injury.

VENOUS THROMBOEMBOLISM IN ATHLETES

William M. Collins, DO • Alejandro Centurion, MD

BASICS

DESCRIPTION

- Venous thromboembolism (VTE) is a condition in which a blood clot (thrombus) forms in a vein.
- When a thrombus occurs in the "deep veins" of the extremities or pelvis, it is called a deep vein thrombosis (DVT).
- A thrombus in the lung is called a pulmonary embolism (PE).
- A thrombus can limit blood flow through the vein, causing swelling and pain.
- Most commonly, venous thrombosis occurs in the "deep veins" in the legs, thighs, or pelvis (DVT).
- DVT can also occur in upper extremity veins (effort thrombosis).
- In most cases, PE is caused by a DVT when part of a blood clot breaks off and lodges in the lung.

EPIDEMIOLOGY

Incidence

- Estimated 900,000 affected in the United States yearly (1 to 2 per 1,000)
- 60,000 to 100,000 die per year due to VTE.
- Affects ~1 to 2 in 1,000 people every year
- Rates increase with age and are higher in males compared to females.
- There are no data on incidence of VTE in athletes.

ETIOLOGY AND PATHOPHYSIOLOGY

Virchow triad of venous stasis, vessel wall injury, and coagulation abnormality are considered the primary mechanisms for the development of venous thrombosis.

Genetics

Genetic defects such as factor V Leiden mutation or protein C or S deficiencies are associated with DVTs.

RISK FACTORS

- Older age
- Active cancer
- Antiphospholipid syndrome
- Estrogen therapy
- Pregnancy or peripartum
- Personal or family history of VTE
- Obesity
- Autoimmune and chronic inflammatory diseases
- Heparin-induced thrombocytopenia
- Surgery
- Trauma or fracture
- Central venous catheter or pacemaker
- Hospitalization
- Nursing-home residence
- Immobilization during travel (>4 hr)
- Paresis or paralysis
- Factor V Leiden
- Prothrombin mutation
- Antithrombin deficiency
- Protein C deficiency
- Protein S deficiency
- Non-O blood group
- It is postulated that athletes may be at increased risk of VTE due to long travel distances and direct trauma to tissues, although the claim is mostly supported by case studies and expert opinion (1).

GENERAL PREVENTION

- Avoid prolonged immobility.
- Hydrate adequately.
- Consider compression stockings when immobilized.
- Caution when using birth control; use low-estrogen pills when possible.
- Prophylaxis for hospitalized patients

COMMONLY ASSOCIATED CONDITIONS

- Malignancy accounts for 1/5 of all cases.
- The list of risk factors is inclusive of associated conditions.

DIAGNOSIS

Wells criteria for DVT (1)[A]:

Active cancer within 6 mo	+1
Paralysis or immobilization of lower extremity	+1
Immobilization at least 3 days OR surgery in the previous 4 weeks	<4 wk +1
Tenderness/cord along vein	+1
Entire leg swollen	+1
Calf circumference >3 cm vs. other leg	+1
Alternative diagnosis likely	−2
Interpretation	
High probability	+3
Moderate probability	+1–2
Low probability	0

Wells criteria for PE (1)[A]

Clinical signs and symptoms of DVT	+3
PE no. 1 diagnosis *or* equally likely	+3
Heart rate >100	+1.5
Immobilization at least 3 days *or* surgery in the previous 4 wk	+1.5
Previous, objectively diagnosed PE or DVT	+1.5
Hemoptysis	+1
Malignancy with treatment within 6 mo or palliative	+1
Interpretation	
High probability	>6
Moderate probability	+2–6
Low probability	<2

- A low or intermediate pretest probability of PE/DVT (Wells) with a negative D-dimer effectively rules out PE/DVT.
- A high pretest probability with a negative D-dimer still warrants further evaluation with imaging.
- A positive D-dimer warrants further imaging with computed tomography (CT) angiography or V/Q scan if CT not available.

HISTORY

- Many patients are asymptomatic; however, the classic symptoms of DVT are swelling, pain, and discoloration in the involved extremity.
- Clinical signs and symptoms of PE as the primary manifestations occur in 10% of patients with confirmed DVT.
- Signs of PE are dyspnea, chest pain, cough, hemoptysis, and symptoms of DVT.

PHYSICAL EXAM

- Signs of DVT: Inspection of the extremity may reveal ipsilateral edema and erythema: >1- to 2-cm circumferential difference in leg.
- Palpation of the extremity may reveal a palpable cord, increased warmth, and superficial venous dilation.
- Homans sign: Passive dorsiflexion of the ankle elicits pain in the calf.
- Phlegmasia cerulea dolens: reddish purple lower extremity from venous engorgement and obstruction
- Signs of pulmonary embolus: tachycardia; tachypnea; low-grade fever; and abnormal electrocardiogram (ECG) S wave in lead I, Q wave in lead III, inverted T wave in lead III (S1Q3T3)

DIFFERENTIAL DIAGNOSIS

- Superficial thrombophlebitis
- Cellulitis
- Torn muscles and ligaments
- Ruptured Baker cyst
- Bilateral edema (seen with heart, kidney, or liver disease) is rarely caused by DVT.
- Prior DVT and postphlebitic syndrome
- Arterial insufficiency
- Arthritis
- Lymphangitis
- Extrinsic compression of iliac vein secondary to tumor, hematoma, or abscess
- Hematoma
- Lymphedema
- Neurogenic pain
- Prolonged immobilization or limb paralysis
- Stress fractures or other bony lesions
- Varicose veins

DIAGNOSTIC TESTS & INTERPRETATION

- No blood test diagnoses or excludes DVT with complete certainty.
- D-dimer (enzyme-linked immunosorbent assay [ELISA] technique) has sensitivities around 95% (2)[A].
- Complete blood count (CBC) and prothrombin time (PT)/partial thromboplastin time (PTT) as baseline measurements

- Labs for idiopathic DVT include factor V Leiden, prothrombin, serum homocysteine, factor VIII level, lupus anticoagulant, protein C and S levels, antithrombin activity, and anticardiolipin antibodies.
- DVT: ultrasound (US) (gold standard) (2)[A]:
  - Sensitivities and specificities vary by vein with more accuracy in the proximal veins.
  - Sensitivities of 89–96%
  - Specificities of 94–99%
  - US is recommended for patients with high pretest probability (Wells criteria) in the lower extremities.
  - Duplex scanning (combination of color Doppler and B-mode US)
- Venography is the historic gold standard:
  - Accurate but invasive
  - Associated with dye reactions
  - Can precipitate phlebitis
- PE: CT angiography (gold standard) (1,3)[A]:
  - With intermediate to high risk, the positive predictive value is 92–96% (3)[A].
  - In high clinical risk, negative predictive value is 60% (3)[A].
- Contraindication in those with kidney failure
- V/Q scan if CT angiography not available

TREATMENT

Outpatient treatment:

- Anticoagulation (1,4,5)[A]
- Factor Xa inhibitors or direct thrombin inhibitors (DTI) are considered treatment of choice (4)[A]:
  - Oral agents
  - Do not require laboratory monitoring
  - Excellent safety profile
- Low-molecular-weight heparin (LMWH) is considered if DTI/factor Xa inhibitors are unavailable or cost prohibitive.
- Warfarin is considered as last option given need for continuous monitoring of international normalized ratio (INR).
- Contraindications:
  - Active internal bleeding
  - Uncontrolled hypertension (HTN)
  - Significant recent trauma or surgery
  - Central nervous system (CNS) tumor
- Treatment duration (5)[A]:
  - Provoked DVT/PE: Recommend 3 mo of anticoagulation.
  - Unprovoked first time DVT/PE: Recommend 3 mo of anticoagulation and discussion of risk–benefit of indefinite anticoagulation at completion of 3 mo:
    - Low-or moderate-risk bleeding, recommend indefinite anticoagulation
    - High risk, recommend 3 mo of anticoagulation

MEDICATION

- Rivaroxaban 15 mg PO BID with food for 21 days, then 20 mg PO daily with food afterward (4,5)[A]
- Apixaban 10 mg PO BID for 7 days, then 5 mg PO BID afterward
- Dabigatran 150 mg PO BID
- Enoxaparin: 1 mg/kg subcutaneous (SC) BID
- Return to play (6)[C]:
  - Although anticoagulation remains the mainstay for DVT/VTE treatment, in recent decades there has been a shift from initial bed rest to early mobilization.
  - Athletes are encouraged to begin light ambulation within 24 hr of starting medical anticoagulation therapy (e.g., walking).
  - Weeks 1 to 3: reintroduction to activities of daily living
  - Week 4: begins engaging in non–weight-bearing activities (e.g., swimming)
  - Week 5: progresses to nonimpact-loading exercises (e.g., cycling)
  - Week 6: begins impact-loading exercises (e.g., running)
  - Week 6+: A gradual transition to sport-specific protocols as well as an increase in the duration and intensity of training may be initiated.
  - Progression through return-to-play protocol should be based on the athletes' achievement and symptomatic improvement rather than based on a fixed timeline.
  - Athletes are not advised to participate in contact sports while on anticoagulation (6)[C].

ISSUES FOR REFERRAL

Cardiology, pulmonary, hematology, or anticoagulation clinic is appropriate if the physician is uncomfortable with managing patients with DVT.

ONGOING CARE

FOLLOW-UP RECOMMENDATIONS

Patient Monitoring

No monitoring required for DTI or factor Xa inhibitors. INR levels should be evaluated frequently until stable with a target range between two and three (if using warfarin).

PATIENT EDUCATION

When patients are traveling, they should sit in seats that allow leg extension, take hourly walking breaks, wear loose clothing, and avoid crossing their legs.

PROGNOSIS

PE will occur in 50% of untreated patients with DVT within days or weeks. If the DVT was caused by a thrombophilic disorder, the risk of repeat episode may be high.

COMPLICATIONS

Review all secondary disease or negative reactions that may occur during the course of an illness, that usually aggravate the illness, and any possible preventive measures. In addition, differentiate between acute/chronic, likelihood of complication, and common/rare.

REFERENCES

1. Di Nisio M, Van Es N, Büller HR. Deep vein thrombosis and pulmonary embolism. *Lancet*. 2016;388(10063):3060–3073.
2. Segal JB, Eng J, Tamariz LJ, et al. Review of the evidence on diagnosis of deep venous thrombosis and pulmonary embolism. *Ann Fam Med*. 2007;5(1):63–73.
3. Wilbur J, Shian B. Diagnosis of deep venous thrombosis and pulmonary embolism. *Am Fam Physician*. 2012;86(10):913–919.
4. Robertson L, Kesteven P, McCaslin JE. Oral direct thrombin inhibitors or oral factor Xa inhibitors for the treatment of deep vein thrombosis. *Cochrane Database Syst Rev*. 2015;(6):CD010956.
5. Kearon C, Akl EA, Ornelas J, et al. Antithrombotic therapy for VTE disease: CHEST guideline and expert panel report. *Chest*. 2016;149(2):315–352.
6. Depenbrock PJ. Thromboembolic disorders: guidance for return-to-play. *Curr Sports Med Rep*. 2011;10(2):78–83.

ADDITIONAL READING

- Berkowitz JN, Moll S. Athletes and blood clots: individualized, intermittent anticoagulation management. *J Thromb Haemost*. 2017;15(6):1051–1054.
- Bishop M, Astolfi M, Padegimas E, et al. Venous thromboembolism within professional American sport leagues. *Orthop J Sports Med*. 2017;5(12):2325967117745530. doi:10.1177/2325967117745530.
- Centers for Disease Control and Prevention. Venous thromboembolism (blood clots). https://www.cdc.gov/ncbddd/dvt/data.html. Accessed September 24, 2018.
- Eichner ER. Clots and consequences in athletes. *Curr Sports Med Rep*. 2014;13(5):287–288.
- Heit JA, Spencer FA, White RH. The epidemiology of venous thromboembolism. *J Thromb Thrombolysis*. 2016;41(1):3–14.
- Hirsh J, Hoak J. Management of deep vein thrombosis and pulmonary embolism. A statement for healthcare professionals. Council on Thrombosis (in consultation with the Council on Cardiovascular Radiology), American Heart Association. *Circulation*. 1996;93(12):2212–2245.
- Hull CM, Harris JA. Cardiology patient page. Venous thromboembolism and marathon athletes. *Circulation*. 2013;128(25):e469–e471.
- Mall NA, Van Thiel GS, Heard WM, et al. Paget-Schroetter syndrome: a review of effort thrombosis of the upper extremity from a sports medicine perspective. *Sports Health*. 2013;5(4):353–356.

CLINICAL PEARLS

- A DVT is associated with risk factors noted in Virchow triad of:
  - Venous stasis of an alteration in normal blood flow.
  - Vascular endothelial injury.
  - Hypercoagulability.
- Essential workup includes a Doppler US (duplex scanning) of the affected extremity and CT angiography of chest if concerned for PE.
- DTI or factor Xa inhibitors considered treatment of choice for outpatient management
- Factor Xa inhibitors or DTI are considered treatment of choice for PE and DVT.
- Athletes are not advised to participate in contact sports while on anticoagulation.

VOCAL CORD DYSFUNCTION

Sarah Merrill, MD, CAQSM

BASICS

DESCRIPTION

Vocal cord dysfunction (VCD) is not uncommon but often missed diagnosis in both athletes and nonathletes (1,2). VCD—also known as paradoxical vocal fold motion—is caused by inappropriate adduction of the vocal cords that results in temporary partial airway obstruction (1,3). VCD can cause significant appearing symptoms of stridor, wheezing, and apparent upper airway obstruction during exercise (1,2,3,4). Due to these distinctive symptoms, patients or athletes with VCD are frequently misdiagnosed and subjected to unnecessary testing and invasive procedures, such as intubation or tracheostomy (3). VCD is typically a diagnosis of exclusion after most serious etiologies are excluded (5).

EPIDEMIOLOGY

Incidence

- Due to widespread underdiagnosis, it is difficult to accurately assess incidence and prevalence (3).
- VCD has a noted female adolescent predominance but is also seen in males and in patients from pediatrics to geriatrics (1,2).

Prevalence

Prevalence estimates vary widely from 4% to 30% of adults (2).

ETIOLOGY AND PATHOPHYSIOLOGY

- Normally, the true vocal cords open (abduct) on inspiration and close (adduct) on expiration (1,4).
- Paradoxical vocal cord motion occurs when the true vocal cords inappropriately adduct on inspiration, causing a temporary and reversible partial airway obstruction and transient airway narrowing (1,3,5). The degree of the obstruction varies (1,3).
- Exercise, underlying asthma, inhaled irritants or allergens, rhinosinusitis, or gastroesophageal reflux disease (GERD) can precipitate or exacerbate VCD (2,3).
- Although precipitants have been identified, no reliable causative factor has been identified (1,2).

Genetics

There is no established genetic component to VCD (4).

RISK FACTORS

There is a higher rate of VCD in patients with asthma and previous intubation (1,3).

GENERAL PREVENTION

Avoidance of known triggers (1,3,4)

COMMONLY ASSOCIATED CONDITIONS

- Asthma
- Exercise-induced bronchoconstriction (EIB)
- Exercise-induced asthma (EIA) (2,3,5)

DIAGNOSIS

HISTORY

- Patients will typically report episodes of dyspnea on exertion, wheezing sometimes progressing to stridor, and cough (1,2,3). These episodes are typically brought on by increased activity, often leading to false or incompletely accurate diagnosis of EIA (1,2). However, stress, environmental allergens, GERD, or chemical irritants can also trigger episodes (1,2,3).
- Patients may complain of dyspnea, choking sensation, dysphonia, wheezing, and cough during these episodes (1,2). However, symptoms are typically mild and intermittent (1,2).
- VCD symptoms tend to occur *during* peak exercise or immediately following exercise and can last for hours to days (2,5). Symptoms typically stop and start precipitously (5). EIA/EIB symptoms tend to occur 15 to 20 min *after* exercise and athletes have *expiratory* wheezing (2,5). Laryngospasms tend to last a few seconds to minutes (2).
- Symptoms are not typically relieved with albuterol (2,3).

PHYSICAL EXAM

- Physical exam outside of the acute episode may be normal (3,4).
- During an acute episode, adventitious breath sounds and/or stridor can be heard on *both* inspiration and expirations, most prominently over the anterior neck (1,2,3).
- Unlike asthma, symptoms are more prominent with inspiration than expiration (1,3).
- Although patients exhibit apparent air hunger, they often have a normal PaO_2 (>97% O_2 saturation). When there is a decrease in PaO_2, it is usually due to hypoventilation (2,3).

DIFFERENTIAL DIAGNOSIS

- Asthma
- EIA
- EIB
- Presence of foreign body
- Vocal cord tumor
- Laryngospasm
- Laryngeal angioedema
- Vocal fold paresis
- GERD
- Nerve injury after cervical or thyroid surgery
- Irritant exposure
- Rhinosinusitis
- Prolapse of supraglottic tissue
- Tracheomalacia
- Laryngomalacia
- Psychogenic stridor

DIAGNOSTIC TESTS & INTERPRETATION

Initial Tests (lab, imaging)

- Spirometry is often used initially for patients with exertional dyspnea. A flattened inspiratory limb and forced expiratory flow (FEF) 50/forced inspiratory flow (FIF) 50 >1 suggests extrathoracic obstruction consistent with VCD but is not sensitive. Up to 70% of patients can also have a positive methacholine challenge (1,2,3).
- Asthma typically shows limited expiratory flow-volume curve (1,2).
- Flexible laryngoscopy is considered the gold standard for diagnosis (5). Laryngoscopy performed during or immediately following exercise (continuous laryngoscopy exercise [CLE] test) reveals inspiratory and early expiratory adduction of the anterior 2/3 of the true vocal cords (1,2,3).

Follow-Up Tests & Special Considerations

- Impulse oscillometry can be used in patients who cannot cooperate with spirometry, such as children (2,3).
- 4D computed tomography (CT) has been used experimentally in a small number of patients (2).

TREATMENT

- **Acute management:**
  - Because episodes are often self-limiting, reassurance and supportive measures can be effective (1).
  - Encourage patient to pant, which forces abduction of the vocal cords. Breathing through a straw or diaphragmatic breathing can produce similar results (1,5).
  - Inhalation of a combination of helium and oxygen (heliox) to reduce airway resistance (1)
  - Continuous positive airway pressure (CPAP) (4)
- **Long-term management:**
  - Education of patient and family members regarding diagnosis (1,4)
  - Avoidance of known triggers (1,3,4)
  - Referral to speech language pathologist for behavioral speech and voice therapy (1,3,5)
  - Speech therapy generally focuses on respiratory retraining and abortive techniques for acute episodes, laryngeal and whole body relaxation techniques, vocal hygiene, and phonation retraining if appropriate (1,5).

MEDICATION

First Line

- Case studies have shown some benefit with use of inhaled anticholinergics such as ipratropium prior to exercise (1,4).
- Generally, inhaled β_2-agonists (albuterol) do not ease symptoms of VCD unless there is a concomitant asthma component to symptoms (2,3).

SURGERY/OTHER PROCEDURES

In severe, recalcitrant cases, long-term tracheostomy has been performed (1).

ONGOING CARE

Education of athletes, parents, and coaches regarding symptoms and treatments are essential for avoiding unnecessary hospitalizations and procedures.

REFERENCES

1. Deckert J, Deckert L. Vocal cord dysfunction. *Am Fam Physician*. 2010;81(2):156–159.
2. Fretzayas A, Moustaki M, Loukou I, et al. Differentiating vocal cord dysfunction from asthma. *J Asthma Allergy*. 2017;10:277–283.
3. Morris MJ, Christopher KL. Diagnostic criteria for the classification of vocal cord dysfunction. *Chest*. 2010;138(5):1213–1223.
4. Hoyte FC. Vocal cord dysfunction. *Immunol Allergy Clin North Am*. 2013;33(1):1–22.
5. Barnes, KP. Exercise-induced bronchoconstriction and vocal cord dysfunction in athletes: a brief overview. *Athl Train Sports Health Care*. 2010;2(2):52–56.

CLINICAL PEARLS

- VCD results from the true vocal cords inappropriately adducting on inspiration.
- VCD resulting in exertional dyspnea typically peaks during maximal exertion. EIA/EIB, however, typically causes dyspnea 15 to 20 min after activity.
- VCD can be accurately diagnosed by CLE test done during or immediately following exercise.
- Exercise-induced VCD is most common in adolescent females.

WARTS

Kathleen Weber, MD, MS • Shannon Powers, DO

BASICS

DESCRIPTION

Warts (verrucas) are caused by a human papillomavirus (HPV) infection, resulting in a variety of lesions on the skin and mucous membranes. Several different HPV genotypes are associated with warts, as is noted below.

EPIDEMIOLOGY

- >150 different genotypes of HPV have been identified (1,2).
- Cutaneous HPV infections, three types:
  - Common warts (verruca vulgaris): 70%:
    - HPV types 1 to 5, 7, 27, 29 (3)
  - Plantar warts (verruca plantaris): 25–30%:
    - HPV types 1 to 4, 27, 29, 57 (3)
  - Flat warts (verruca plana): 3–4%:
    - HPV types 3, 10, 28, 29 (3)
- 10–20% of children will develop cutaneous warts, with the peak incidence occurring between 12 and 16 yr.
- Mucosal HPV infections:
  - Most common are genital warts (condyloma acuminatum).
  - Estimated prevalence rate of HPV genital infection in the U.S. adult population is 10–20% (4).

ETIOLOGY AND PATHOPHYSIOLOGY

- HPV infects epithelial tissues and mucous membranes.
- The virus infects the mucosa or the basal layer of the skin, causing cellular proliferation and vascular growth, resulting in a mucosal or skin lesion (4).
- Incubation period, once exposed, varies from weeks to more than a year.

RISK FACTORS

- Cutaneous HPV infections:
  - Transmission: direct or indirect contact; minor superficial abrasions of the skin promote infection.
  - Autoinoculation occurs especially in younger children.
  - Risk factors: immunocompromised
- Mucosal HPV infections:
  - Transmission: sexual contact; contact with contaminated objects; autoinoculation; vertical transmission during vaginal delivery (4)
  - Risk factors: unprotected sexual relations, multiple sex partners, immunocompromised

GENERAL PREVENTION

- Cutaneous lesions: no restrictions for participation; coverage recommended
- Mucosal lesions: condoms recommended but not completely effective
- Anogenital warts: The importance of Pap smears should be stressed; screen for other sexually transmitted diseases (1).
- Quadrivalent HPV vaccination is indicated for use in patients who are between 9 and 26 yr of age, which targets HPV types 6, 11, 16, and 18; not recommended for pregnant women (1,5)
- Ideally, young women should be vaccinated before they have sexual intercourse for the first time (1).
- Male circumcision may decrease male transmission rates (5).

COMMONLY ASSOCIATED CONDITIONS

- Cutaneous HPV infection: Warts may regress spontaneously; immunocompromised individuals may be refractory to all treatment.
- Condylomata recur commonly despite therapy.
- Condylomata are associated with cervical dysplasia and cervical squamous cell carcinoma, invasive carcinoma of genitalia, and anal squamous cell carcinoma.

DIAGNOSIS

Warts are usually diagnosed based on their appearance (2,5).

HISTORY

- Cutaneous and anogenital warts are usually asymptomatic, but plantar warts can cause discomfort during activities.
- Without treatment, the wart can remain for months to years.
- Diagnosis is usually made by characteristic appearance of lesions (2,5).

PHYSICAL EXAM

- Verruca vulgaris (common warts):
  - Skin-colored papule, hyperkeratotic with horny surface
  - Normal skin markings are disrupted.
  - Pathognomonic for warts are red-black dots seen on the surface.
  - Can be one or multiple lesions
  - Typically, asymptomatic but may be painful, especially if located over areas of pressure
  - Distribution: fingers, hands (most common), knees; may occur anywhere
- Verruca plantaris (plantar warts):
  - Skin-colored papule with coarse, keratotic surface; has characteristic red-black dots
  - Normal skin markings are disrupted.
  - Painful, especially if located over areas of pressure
  - Distribution: plantar surface of foot
- Verruca plana (flat warts):
  - Skin colored or lightly pigmented; well-defined, smooth, flat, or slightly elevated papules
  - Variety of shapes: round, oval, linear
  - Sizes vary from pinhead to a few millimeters.
  - Numbers range from a few to hundreds.
  - Distribution: face; dorsum of the hands; extremities, especially shins
  - Most commonly seen in children and less common in adolescents and adults
- Condylomata acuminata (anogenital warts):
  - Skin colored, slightly pigmented, or pink
  - Range from soft, tiny isolated papules, filiform, and often pedunculated sessile papules to cauliflower masses (4)
  - Distribution: glans penis, prepuce, shaft, labia, vagina, cervix, perianal area, urethra, bladder, rectum, and oral cavity (4)
  - Most asymptomatic or subclinical; may go unrecognized

DIFFERENTIAL DIAGNOSIS

- Verruca vulgaris: callus, guttate psoriasis, molluscum contagiosum, seborrheic keratosis
- Verruca plantaris: callus, corn
- Verruca plana: lichen planus, molluscum contagiosum, seborrheic keratosis, moles, skin tags
- Condylomata acuminata: lichen planus, pearly penile papules, skin tags, squamous cell carcinoma, condyloma lata due to secondary syphilis, seborrheic keratosis, vulvar intraepithelial neoplasia (5)

DIAGNOSTIC TESTS & INTERPRETATION

Diagnostic Procedures/Other

- Subclinical lesions on the genital skin can be visualized as white patches by applying 5% acetic acid to the suspected area.
- Confirmed by biopsy if diagnosis unclear by exam

TREATMENT

MEDICATION

First Line

- Self-administered:
  - For cutaneous infections: salicylic acid preparations (10–40%) (2,3)[A]. Apply once or twice daily for 6 to 12 wk pending preparation.
  - For mucosal lesions: imiquimod 5% cream (5)[A]. Apply 3 times per week (alternating every other day) for up to 16 wk.
- Clinician administered:
  - For cutaneous infections: cryosurgery (liquid nitrogen): Apply to wart and surrounding normal tissue (1 to 2 mm) for ~10 sec; repeat every 2 wk as needed for up to four treatments (may be painful) (3,5)[B].
  - For mucosal lesions: trichloroacetic acid 80% (4)[B]. Apply 1 to 3 times per week and repeat as needed.

ISSUES FOR REFERRAL

Referral to a dermatologist or gynecologist should be considered in recalcitrant warts or immunocompromised patients.

ADDITIONAL THERAPIES

- There is some evidence supporting use of 5-fluorouracil for treatment of both cutaneous infections and mucosal lesions (2,5)[B].
- For mucosal lesions: Podofilox and sinecatechins can be used as self-administered therapies. Podophyllin can be used as a clinician-administered therapy (5)[B].
- Podofilox and podophyllin are contraindicated during pregnancy (5)[C].
- Although used for cutaneous infections, there is limited evidence of effectiveness for use of duct tape; duct tape is sometimes used in conjunction to treatment with salicylic acid (3)[B].
- There is limited evidence of effectiveness for use of pulsed dye laser (PDL) for treatment of cutaneous infections and mucosal lesions (3)[B].

SURGERY/OTHER PROCEDURES

- For cutaneous infections: excision, electrocautery, CO_2 laser surgery (2)[C], and intralesional injections (bleomycin, *Candida*, or mumps skin antigen) (2,3,6)[B]
- For mucosal lesions: cryosurgery as described earlier (5)[B], electrocautery or excision (4)[A], CO_2 laser (5)[C]

ONGOING CARE

FOLLOW-UP RECOMMENDATIONS

Patient Monitoring

- Papanicolaou tests screening for cervical cancer at age 21 yr (exception: can consider screening earlier if HIV positive or immunocompromised)
- In cases of extensive or recalcitrant anogenital warts, consider diagnostic evaluation for immunodeficiency, especially HIV (2).

PATIENT EDUCATION

- Advise to observe for recurrence of infection.
- Counsel on associated risk of sexually transmitted infection (STI) transmission.
- Ensure eligible patients are up to date on HPV vaccine series (5).

COMPLICATIONS

- Skin irritation
- Infection
- Pain from procedure
- Damage to tendon or nerve

REFERENCES

1. Kahn JA. HPV vaccination for the prevention of cervical intraepithelial neoplasia. *N Engl J Med*. 2009;361(3):271–278.
2. Sterling JC, Gibbs S, Haque Hussain SS, et al. British Association of Dermatologists' guidelines for the management of cutaneous warts 2014. *Br J Dermatol*. 2014;171(4):696–712.
3. Mulhem E, Pinelis S. Treatment of nongenital cutaneous warts. *Am Fam Physician*. 2011;84(3): 288–293.
4. Scheinfeld N, Lehman DS. An evidence-based review of medical and surgical treatments of genital warts. *Dermatol Online J*. 2006;12(3):5.
5. Karnes JB, Usatine RP. Management of external genital warts. *Am Fam Physician*. 2014;90(5): 312–318.
6. Kruter L, Saggar V, Akhavan A, et al. Intralesional bleomycin for warts: patient satisfaction and treatment outcomes. *J Cutan Med Surg*. 2015;19(5):470–476.

ADDITIONAL READING

- Committee on Practice Bulletins—Gynecology. Practice Bulletin No. 168: cervical cancer screening and prevention. *Obstet Gynecol*. 2016;128(4):e111–e130.
- Cordoro KM, Ganz JE. Training room management of medical conditions: sports dermatology. *Clin Sports Med*. 2005;24(3):565–598.
- Herman BE, Corneli HM. A practical approach to warts in the emergency department. *Pediatr Emerg Care*. 2008;24(4):246–254.
- Yan J, Chen SL, Wang HN, et al. Meta-analysis of 5% imiquimod and 0.5% podophyllotoxin in the treatment of condylomata acuminata. *Dermatology*. 2006;213(3):218–223.

CLINICAL PEARLS

- Warts are a result of HPV infection, which can result in common warts, plantar warts, flat warts, and anogenital warts.
- Warts are usually diagnosed based on history and clinical appearance.
- First-line therapy for cutaneous warts is salicylic acid or cryotherapy.
- First-line therapy for mucosal warts is imiquimod or trichloroacetic acid.
- Consider immune deficiency in cases of extensive or recalcitrant warts.

WOLFF-PARKINSON-WHITE (WPW) SYNDROME

Giselle Aerni, MD • Aaron L. Baggish, MD, FACC, FACSM

BASICS

DESCRIPTION

A disorder of cardiac conduction caused by accessory pathways between the atria and ventricles leading to ventricular preexcitation

EPIDEMIOLOGY

Incidence

New cases are diagnosed in the general population at a rate of 0.004% per year.

Prevalence

- 0.1–0.3% of general population affected:
  - No difference in the athletic population
- Predominant gender: male > female
- 10–48% of pediatric cases present with sudden cardiac death (SCD) as the initial event.
- Patients with Wolff-Parkinson-White (WPW) have 0.1–0.45% risk of SCD per year:
  - Accounts for 1% of SCD in athletes

ETIOLOGY AND PATHOPHYSIOLOGY

- Presence of at least one accessory electrical pathway that bypasses the atrioventricular (AV) node allowing for premature electrical impulse delivery and ventricular preexcitation and reentrant tachyarrhythmias utilizing the bypass track and AV node
- Associated arrhythmias:
  - Reentrant type A (orthodromic):
    - Most common form of WPW associated arrhythmia, not typically associated with SCD risk but common cause of symptoms
    - Antegrade limb is the AV nodal conduction system, and the retrograde limb is the accessory pathway.
    - A circuit is created that potentiates reentrant narrow complex supraventricular tachycardia (SVT).
  - Reentrant type B (antidromic):
    - Less common than type A
    - The circuit operates in the opposite direction manifesting as a wide complex tachycardia.
  - Atrial fibrillation:
    - Not caused by WPW but if conducted down the accessory pathway can degenerate into ventricular fibrillation, triggering SCD

Genetics

- 3–4% of the cases are familial.
- Genetic abnormality (*PRKAG2* gene), which also causes marked left ventricular hypertrophy:
  - Inheritance pattern is autosomal dominant.

COMMONLY ASSOCIATED CONDITIONS

- Ebstein anomaly
- Hypertrophic cardiomyopathy
- Ventricular septal defect
- Atrial septal defect
- Corrected transposition of the great arteries

DIAGNOSIS

HISTORY

- Patients may present as incidental finding on electrocardiogram (ECG) and otherwise asymptomatic (WPW pattern).
- Symptoms of WPW syndrome may include:
  - Palpitations.
  - Chest pain.
  - Dyspnea.
  - Dizziness.
  - Weakness.
  - Fatigue.
  - Nausea.
  - Light-headedness.
  - Syncope.
- Initial presenting symptom may be SCD.

PHYSICAL EXAM

- Tachycardia:
  - Regular (reentrant SVT)
  - Irregular (atrial fibrillation)
- Signs of instability:
  - Hypotension
  - Chest pain
  - Change in mental status
  - Rales

DIFFERENTIAL DIAGNOSIS

- AV nodal reentry SVT
- Atrial fibrillation
- Ventricular fibrillation
- Ventricular tachycardia
- ECG:
  - PR interval <120 ms during sinus rhythm in adults and <90 ms in children
  - Delta wave: slurring of initial portion of the QRS complex
  - QRS duration >120 ms in adults and >90 ms in children
  - Secondary ST- and T-wave changes
- ECG findings in symptomatic or unstable patients:
  - SVT
  - Atrial fibrillation
  - Ventricular tachycardia
  - Ventricular fibrillation

DIAGNOSTIC TESTS & INTERPRETATION

Diagnostic Procedures/Other

- Echocardiogram: structural heart disease
- Holter monitor or external event monitor: useful in documenting paroxysmal tachyarrhythmias
- Exercise stress test: useful in risk assessment
- Electrophysiology (EP) study:
  - Elucidates the accessory pathway(s)
  - Determines inducibility of AV reciprocating tachycardia (AVRT)
  - Indications:
    - Risk stratification for asymptomatic athletes (1)[C]
- Risk stratification is one of the most important goals of diagnostic workup in WPW:
  - Low-risk findings:
    - Asymptomatic athletes demonstrating abrupt loss of preexcitation with exercise or increased heart rates
    - Intermittent WPW on ECG traditionally considered low risk but does not rule out presence of high-risk pathways found on EP
  - High-risk findings:
    - Persistence of delta wave during maximal effort limited exercise testing
    - Multiple different morphologies of delta waves suggest multiple accessory pathways.
    - Shortest preexcited R-R interval (SPERRI) of <250 ms in adults and <220 ms in children on EP study during induced atrial fibrillation

TREATMENT

MEDICATION

- Antiarrhythmic medications are less effective than transcatheter ablation for treatment of WPW.
- Additionally, antiarrhythmic medications can hinder athletic performance.

ISSUES FOR REFERRAL

- All athletes with identified WPW on ECG should be referred to cardiology.
- Risk stratification is initial goal to guide management.
- Athletes who are symptomatic or have high-risk pathways deserve full discussion of risks and benefits of noninvasive and invasive treatment strategies and activity participation.

SURGERY/OTHER PROCEDURES

- Transcatheter ablation (radiofrequency ablation [RFA] and cryoablation) is first-line treatment with potential for definitive cure and should be considered in those who are symptomatic or who have high-risk pathways.
- RFA is gold standard due to higher success rate with lower recurrence (2)[C]:
  - Efficacy is 95% (3)[B].
  - Recurrent accessory pathway conduction up to 10% at 1 yr depending on location of pathway (3)[B]
  - Complications (total 4%) include right bundle branch block (RBBB) (0.5%), left bundle branch block (LBBB) (0.1%), valve regurgitation (0.3%), hematoma at catheter site (1.4%), and AV block (0.9%) (4)[B].
- Recurrent accessory pathway can usually be successfully treated with repeated RFA:
  - 25% of repeat RFA were done in patients with Ebstein anomaly (5)[B].

ADMISSION, INPATIENT, AND NURSING CONSIDERATIONS

- Patients with stable sustained tachycardia or any signs of instability require acute treatment.
- Stable patients with narrow complex, regular tachycardia:
  - Vagal maneuvers such as Valsalva
  - Right carotid artery massage:
    - Auscultate the artery first for bruit, which would be contraindication to massage.
  - Fluid replacement and Trendelenburg position if the patient has mild hypotension
  - Pharmacologic conversion if carotid massage fails:
    - Adenosine 6-mg rapid intravenous (IV) push; if ineffective, repeat with 12 mg; children: 0.1 mg/kg rapid IV push
- Stable patients with irregular wide-complex tachycardia:
  - Procainamide is the drug of choice: 6 to 13 mg/kg IV at 0.2 to 0.5 mg/kg/min until arrhythmia controlled, up to a total dose of 1,000 mg and then 2 to 6 mg/min.

ALERT

Never use calcium channel blockers, β-blockers, or digoxin. These medications block the AV node and lead to conduction occurring exclusively down the faster accessory pathway, resulting in fatal ventricular dysrhythmias.

- Unstable patients:
  - Synchronized cardioversion

ONGOING CARE

FOLLOW-UP RECOMMENDATIONS

- Return to sport 2 to 4 wk after catheter ablation
- No guidelines on frequency of surveillance on asymptomatic athletes with initially identified low-risk pathways

PROGNOSIS

- Successfully ablated WPW patients not known to have persistently elevated SCD risk
- Nonablated WPW patients had a higher long-term death risk than ablated patients (6)[B].
- Atrial fibrillation rates are high, long term, and not affected by ablation (6)[B].

REFERENCES

1. Zipes DP, Link MS, Ackerman MJ, et al. Eligibility and disqualification recommendations for competitive athletes with cardiovascular abnormalities: Task Force 9: arrhythmias and conduction defects: a scientific statement from the American Heart Association and American College of Cardiology. *Circulation*. 2015;132(22):e315–e325.
2. Cohen MI, Triedman JK, Cannon BC, et al. PACES/HRS expert consensus statement on the management of the asymptomatic young patient with a Wolff-Parkinson-White (WPW, ventricular preexcitation) electrocardiographic pattern: developed in partnership between the Pediatric and Congenital Electrophysiology Society (PACES) and the Heart Rhythm Society (HRS). Endorsed by the governing bodies of PACES, HRS, the American College of Cardiology Foundation (ACCF), the American Heart Association (AHA), the American Academy of Pediatrics (AAP), and the Canadian Heart Rhythm Society (CHRS). *Heart Rhythm*. 2012;9(6):1006–1024.
3. Van Hare GF, Javitz H, Carmelli D, et al; and Participating Members of the Pediatric Electrophysiology Society. Prospective assessment after pediatric cardiac ablation: recurrence at 1 year after initially successful ablation of supraventricular tachycardia. *Heart Rhythm*. 2004;1(2):188–196.
4. Van Hare GF, Javitz H, Carmelli D, et al. Prospective assessment after pediatric cardiac ablation: demographics, medical profiles, and initial outcomes. *J Cardiovasc Electrophysiol*. 2004;15(7):759–770.
5. Lu C, Wu M, Chen H, et al. Epidemiological profile of Wolff-Parkinson-White syndrome in a general population younger than 50 years of age in an era of radiofrequency catheter ablation. *Int J Cardiol*. 2014;174(3):530–534.
6. Bunch TJ, May HT, Bair TL, et al. Long-term natural history of adult Wolff-Parkinson-White syndrome patients treated with and without catheter ablation. *Circ Arrhythm Electrophysiol*. 2015;8(6):1465–1471.

ADDITIONAL READING

- Baggish AL, Shah AB. MY APPROACH to the athlete with Wolff-Parkinson-White Syndrome (WPW). *Trends Cardiovasc Med*. 2018;28(2):154–155.
- Ceresnak SR, Dubin AM. Wolff-Parkinson-White syndrome (WPW) and athletes: Darwin at play? *J Electrocardiol*. 2015;48(3):356–361.
- Di Mambro C, Drago F, Milioni M, et al. Sports eligibility after risk assessment and treatment in children with asymptomatic ventricular pre-excitation. *Sports Med*. 2016;46(8):1183–1190.
- Di Mambro C, Russo MS, Righi D, et al. Ventricular pre-excitation: symptomatic and asymptomatic children have the same potential risk of sudden cardiac death. *Europace*. 2015;17(4):617–621.
- Mah DY, Sherwin ED, Alexander ME, et al. The electrophysiological characteristics of accessory pathways in pediatric patients with intermittent preexcitation. *Pacing Clin Electrophysiol*. 2013;36(9):1117–1122.
- Rao AL, Salerno JC, Asif IM, et al. Evaluation and management of Wolff-Parkinson-White in athletes. *Sports Health*. 2014;6(4):326–332.
- Sethi KK, Dhall A, Chadha DS, et al. WPW and preexcitation syndromes. *J Assoc Physicians India*. 2007;55(Suppl):10–15.

CLINICAL PEARLS

- Classic ECG findings are shortened PR interval and presence of delta wave.
- Asymptomatic athletes should be evaluated for the purpose of risk stratification for primary determination of the role of RFA.
- Symptomatic athletes presenting with symptoms clearly attributable to WPW-associated tachyarrhythmias should be considered for RFA prior to return to athlete participation.
- RFA is first-line treatment for patients who are symptomatic or asymptomatic with high-risk pathways.
- AV nodal blocking agents should not be used in the management of acute tachyarrhythmias among patients with known or suspect WPW physiology.

Appendix A
MUSCULOSKELETAL RADIOGRAPHY

Tudor Hughes, FRCR

When ordering radiographic studies, it is important to know the most appropriate study to answer the questions at hand. To this end, it is necessary to know which images are obtained when a certain series is requested and the advantages of each series and projection. Although all centers will have slightly different series, what follows is a general guideline.

As a general rule, computed tomography (CT) is a useful adjunct for intra-articular fracture preoperative planning in larger joints, where the fractured bone is to be repaired rather than replaced, or complex areas, such as the carpal or tarsal regions. Although CT does involve a significant dose of ionizing radiation, this is of most concern centrally rather than peripherally. A full x-ray series of the pelvis or lumbar spine can give a higher radiation dose and less useful information than coned-down CT of the area of interest.

Ultrasound (US) is an ideal inexpensive way of assessing superficial soft tissues for both trauma and masses. It has the distinct advantage of being dynamic, imaging the patient in real time as they move, and also being interactive with the patient, assessing their points of pain.

Magnetic resonance imaging (MRI) is a useful method for assessing the soft tissues for injury or mass, the bones for occult injuries, and bone marrow changes.

UPPER EXTREMITIES

FINGERS

For 2nd to 5th digits. Specifically to look at one finger for trauma, foreign body, or localized mass. A marker should be applied, particularly on the lateral projection. Consider US for radiolucent foreign body. Consider MRI or US for mass or tendon lesion/injury.

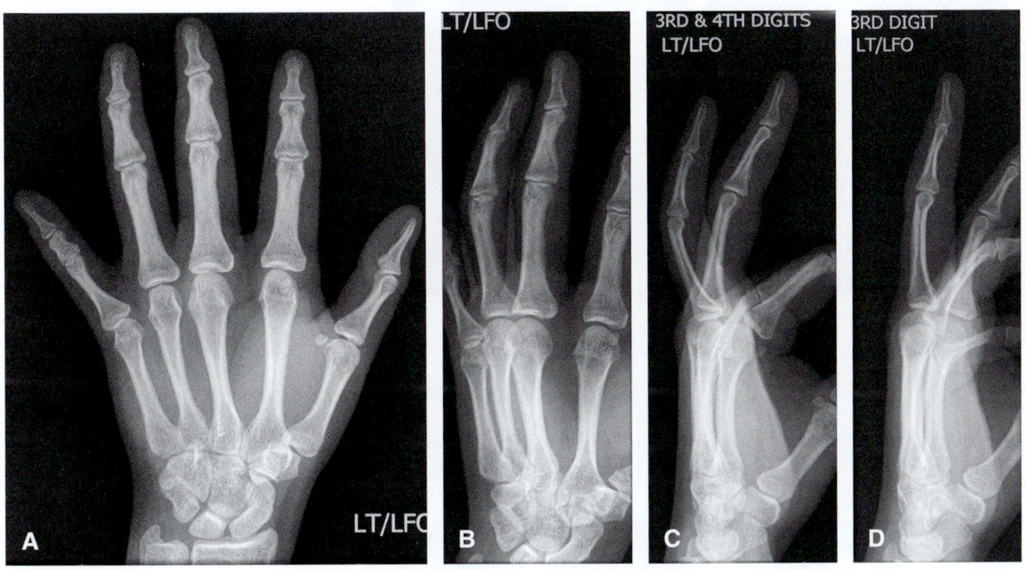

FIGURE 1. A: PA hand. B: Oblique of fingers. C, D: Lateral of fingers.

THUMB

Specifically to look at the thumb for trauma, foreign body, or localized mass. Good for ulnar collateral ligament (UCL) avulsion. A marker should be applied. Consider US for radiolucent foreign body. Consider MRI or US for mass, UCL injury (without or with Stener lesion) or tendon lesion/injury. Stress views are no longer encouraged for acute UCL injury for fear of converting to a Stener lesion but may be useful later on to assess stability.

Musculoskeletal Radiography

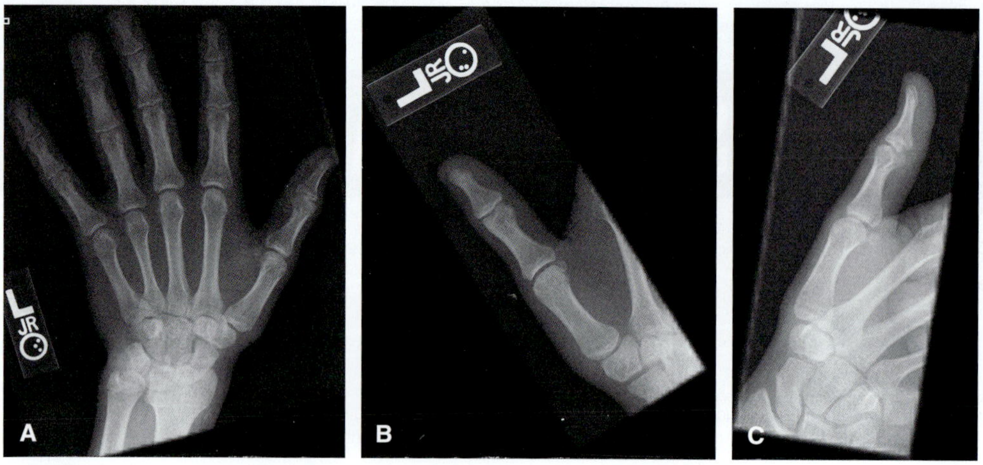

FIGURE 2. A: PA hand. B: PA thumb. C: Lateral thumb.

HAND
Routine

This includes an off-axis view of the wrist but should not be used to assess wrist alignment. Good overview for hand pain. May need additional wrist views if pain is proximal or difficult to localize. Important to have fingers spread on lateral view so that all volar plates are well visualized. MRI or US may be useful adjuncts to look at adjacent soft tissues.

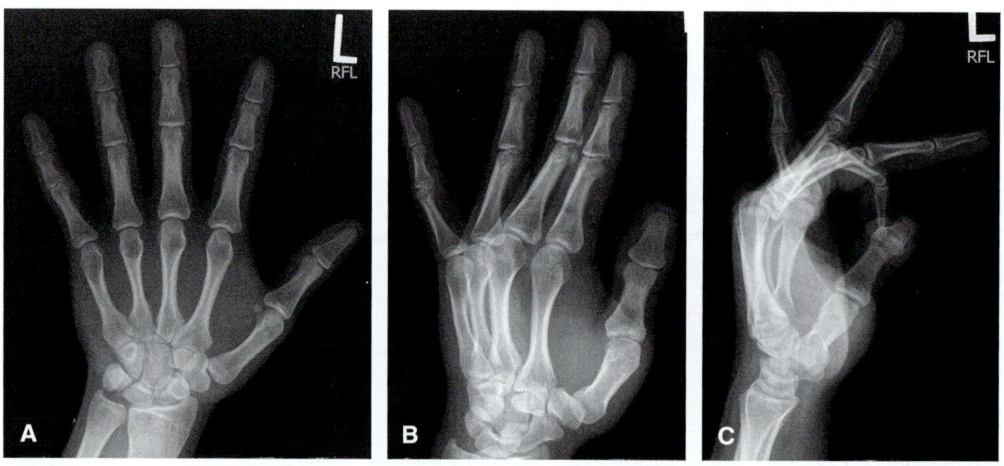

FIGURE 3. A: PA of hand. B: Oblique of hand. C: Lateral of hand.

HAND
Arthritis Survey

Some centers prefer pronated obliques over supinated ball catcher (Norgaard) obliques. Both of these are good for overall assessment of arthritis, individual erosions, soft tissue swelling, and distribution. MRI and US are useful adjuncts to assess the soft tissues, for synovitis joint fluid, and are said to be more sensitive for erosions.

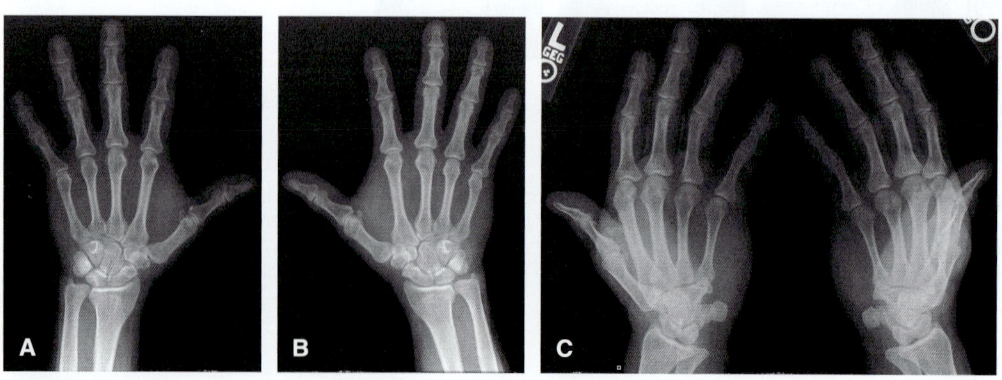

FIGURE 4. A, B: PA of each hand. C: AP Norgaard projection (ball-catcher's position).

WRIST

Nontrauma, Infection

For typical wrist pain evaluations, including arthritis or mass. Good for carpal alignment. US: good for soft tissue masses, tendon pathology. CT scan may be a useful adjunct to assess for occult scaphoid fractures and for healing as well as other occult injuries, such as hook of hamate fracture. CT is often used in the preoperative workup of intra-articular distal radial fractures. MRI is good for occult fractures, Kienböck disease, avascular necrosis (AVN) of lunate or scaphoid, triangular fibrocartilage tears, or intercarpal ligament injuries.

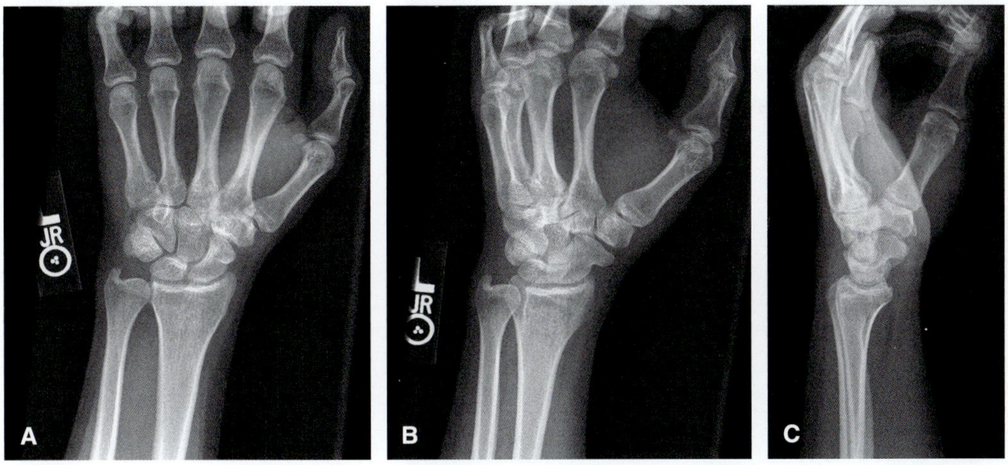

FIGURE 5. A: PA wrist. B: Ulnar oblique wrist. C: Lateral wrist.

Trauma

Additional scaphoid views include oblique and ulnar deviation with cranial angulation. These are good to assess for most aspects of trauma, including fracture, subluxation, or dislocation. Of note, the lateral view can only be used to assess alignment when the volar aspect of the pisiform projects between the scaphoid and capitate. MRI is a useful adjunct to assess for occult injury, intercarpal ligament injury, triangular fibrocartilage complex injury, mass, or synovitis.

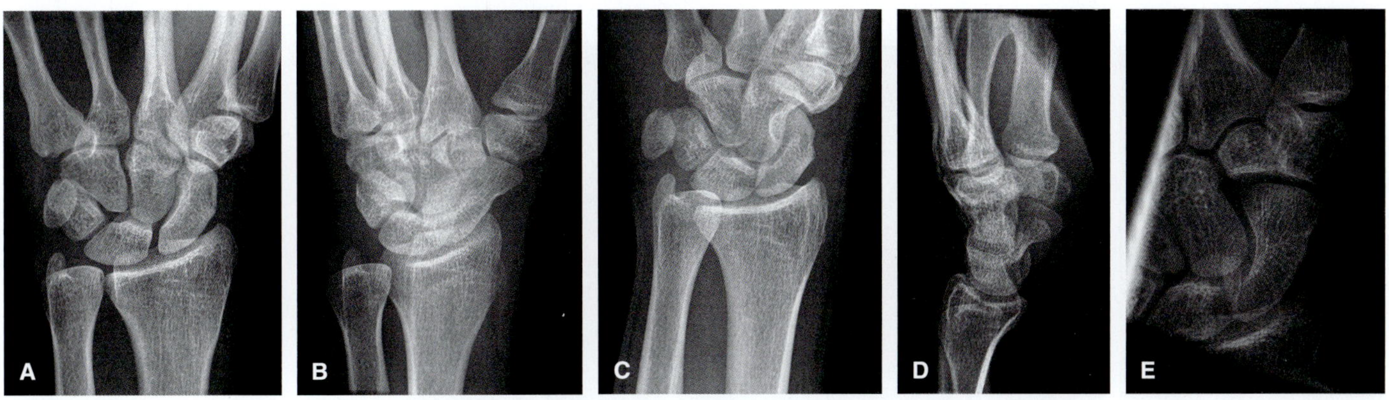

FIGURE 6. A: PA wrist. B: Ulnar oblique wrist. C: Radial oblique wrist. D: Lateral wrist. E: Navicular view.

Additional Views

Clenched fist views taken anteroposterior (AP) are useful for occult cases of scapholunate ligament disruption. Clenching the fist pushes the carpal bones apart. Carpal tunnel view is good for looking for hook of hamate, trapezial ridge fractures, or carpal tunnel syndrome posttrauma/wrist fracture. CT is another good way to assess for occult carpal fractures. MRI without or with intra-articular dilute gadolinium is good to assess for internal derangement.

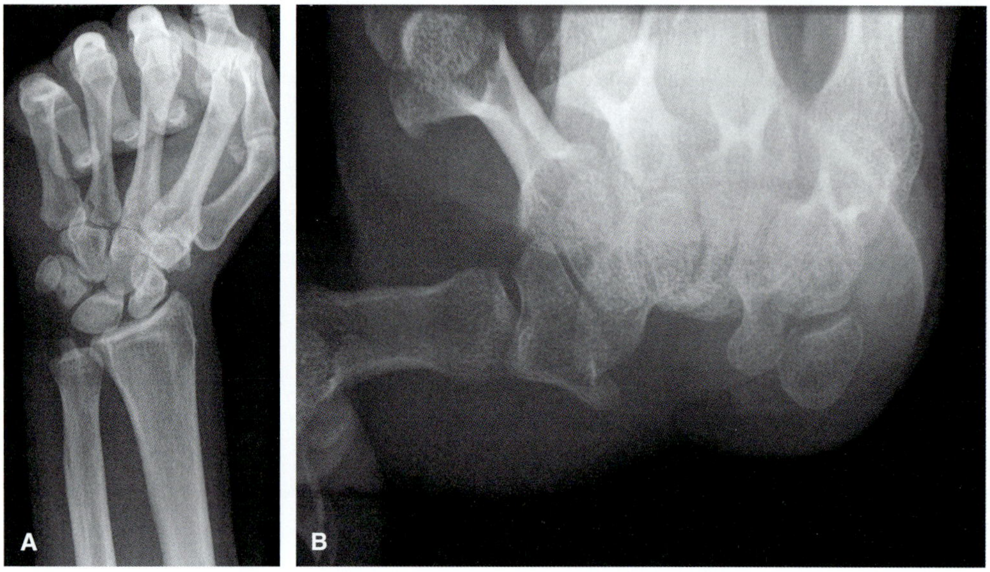

FIGURE 7. A: Clenched fist. B: Carpal tunnel views.

FOREARM

Good for trauma, mass, foreign body, cellulitis/osteomyelitis, or abscess. It is important that the elbow rotates through 90 degrees between the AP and lateral so that two identical views of the ulna are not obtained. Consider US or MRI to assess for mass or soft tissue injury.

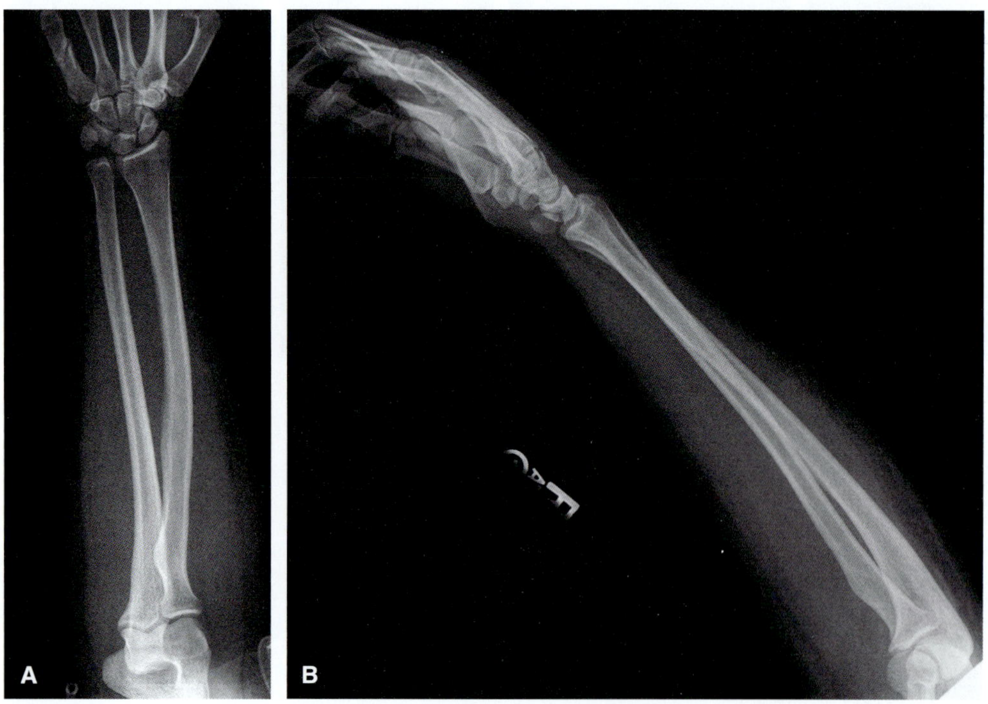

FIGURE 8. A: AP forearm. B: Lateral forearm.

ELBOW

Nontrauma

Chronic injuries, arthritis, foreign bodies, and infection. Lateral is good for effusion and olecranon bursitis. AP is good for epicondylar enthesopathy and osteophytes. Consider US or MRI for soft tissue mass.

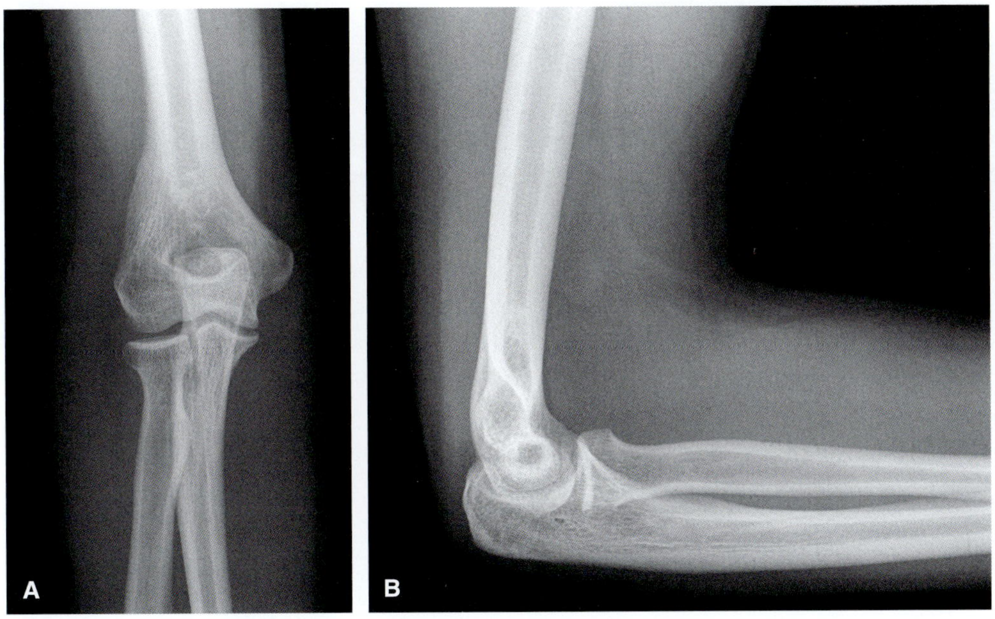

FIGURE 9. A: AP elbow. B: Lateral elbow.

Trauma

Good to assess for otherwise occult radial head fractures. Often, AP, lateral, and radial head are enough for trauma. US or MRI can assess for ligamentous or tendon injuries.

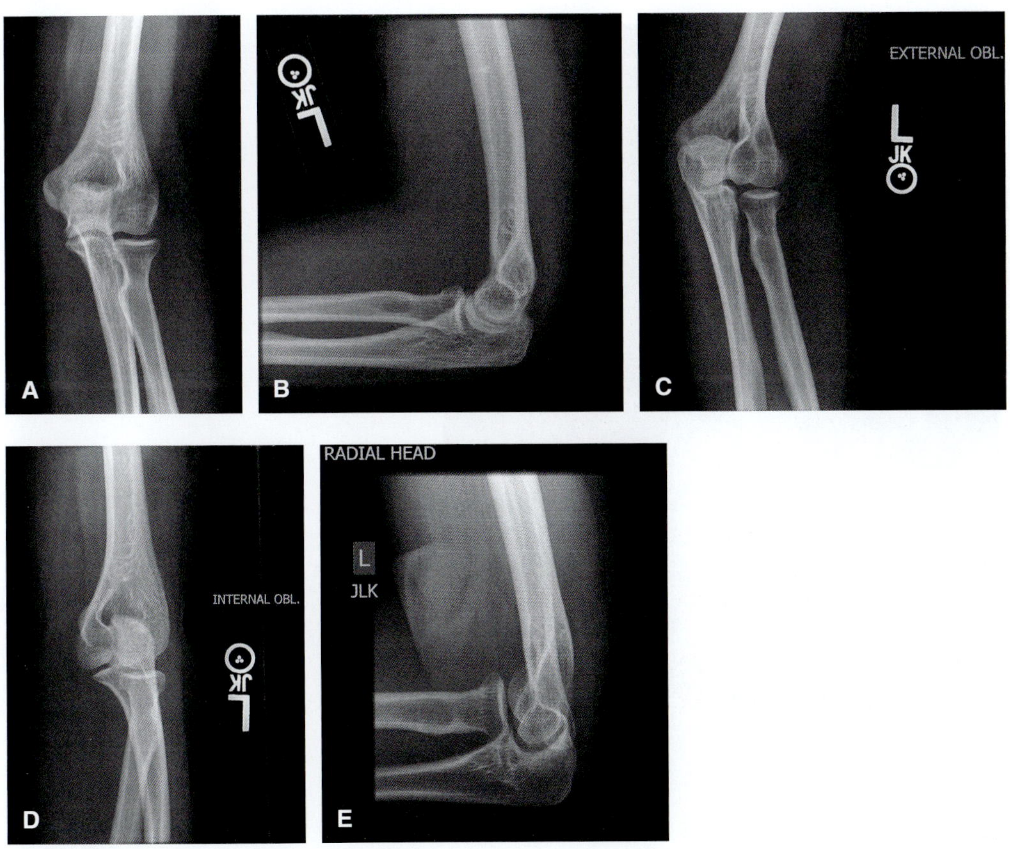

FIGURE 10. A: AP. B: Lateral. C: Lateral (external or radial) oblique. D: Medial (internal or ulnar) oblique. E: Radial head view.

Additional Views

Good to assess for radio opaque causes of cubital tunnel syndrome, such as osteophytes. Consider US or MRI for further assessment of cubital tunnel.

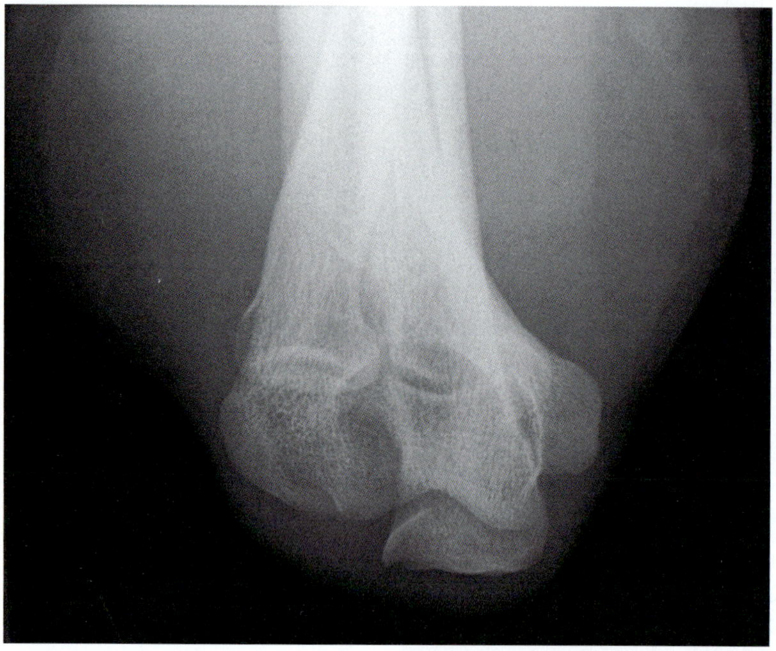

FIGURE 11. Cubital tunnel view.

HUMERUS

To assess for trauma, infection, mass, or foreign body. Both the shoulder and elbow should be included on the study in both projections, but they should not be overinterpreted on such limited views.

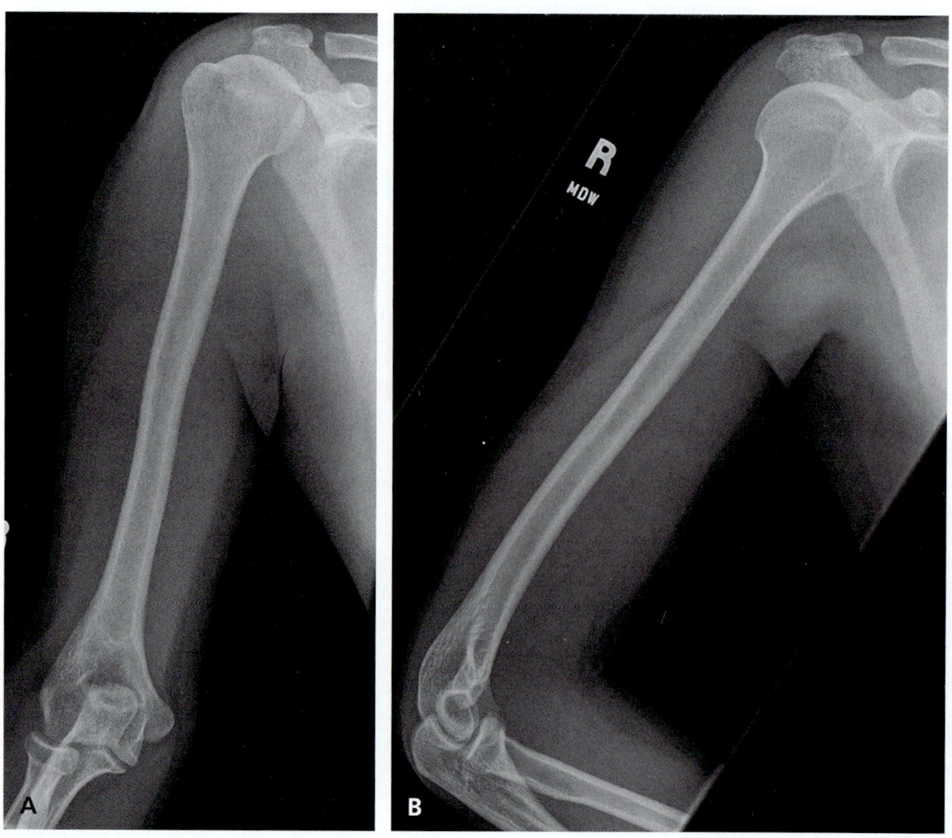

FIGURE 12. A: AP/external rotation. B: Lateral/internal rotation.

SHOULDER

Nontrauma, Chronic Pain

Shoulder series vary widely between institutions. Good to assess for location of hydroxyapatite, osteoarthrosis, and other degenerative changes. US or MRI is best to assess for rotator cuff tears. If a rotator cuff tear is seen on plain films by reduced acromiohumeral distance, then MRI is better than US to show the degree of retraction and atrophy, if the patient is a candidate for repair. MRI is best for glenoid labral pathology for which an MRI arthrogram will give additional information. CT is useful in the preoperative planning of shoulder arthroplasty to assess for bone stock and any intra-articular glenoid fracture.

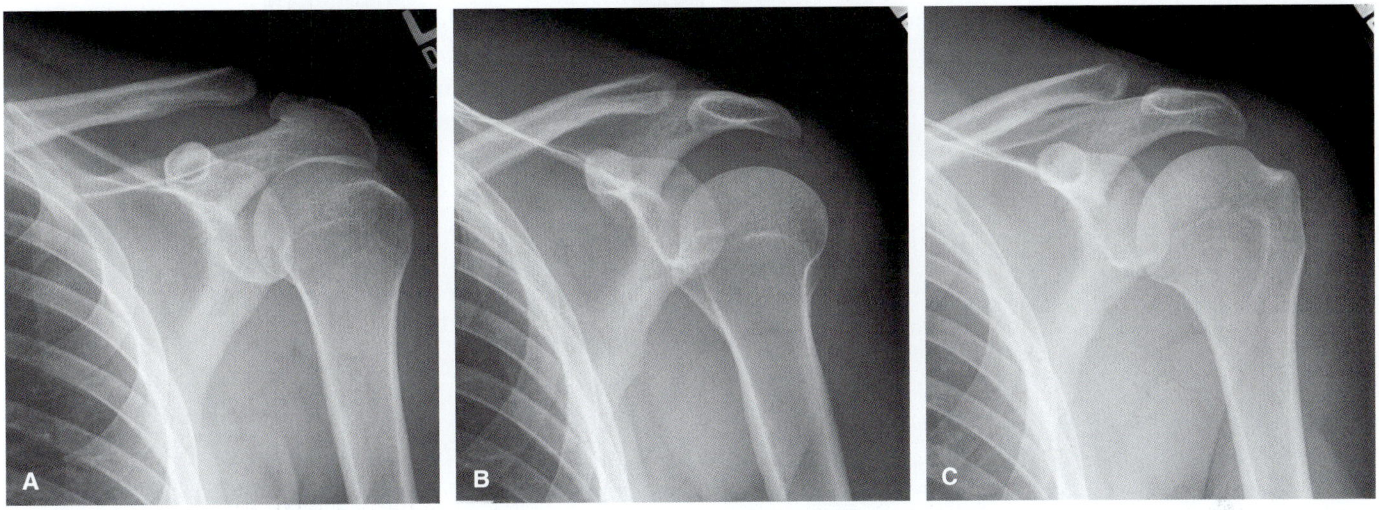

FIGURE 13. A: AP neutral. B: AP internal rotation. C: AP external rotation.

Trauma, Acute Injuries

To evaluate for humeral neck/tuberosity fractures and shoulder dislocations. CT is useful to assess for Hill-Sachs lesions and bony Bankart. MRI can be difficult to interpret acutely due to blood tracking into the rotator cuff from tuberosity fractures. Subacutely, MRI may be useful to assess for accompanying internal derangement.

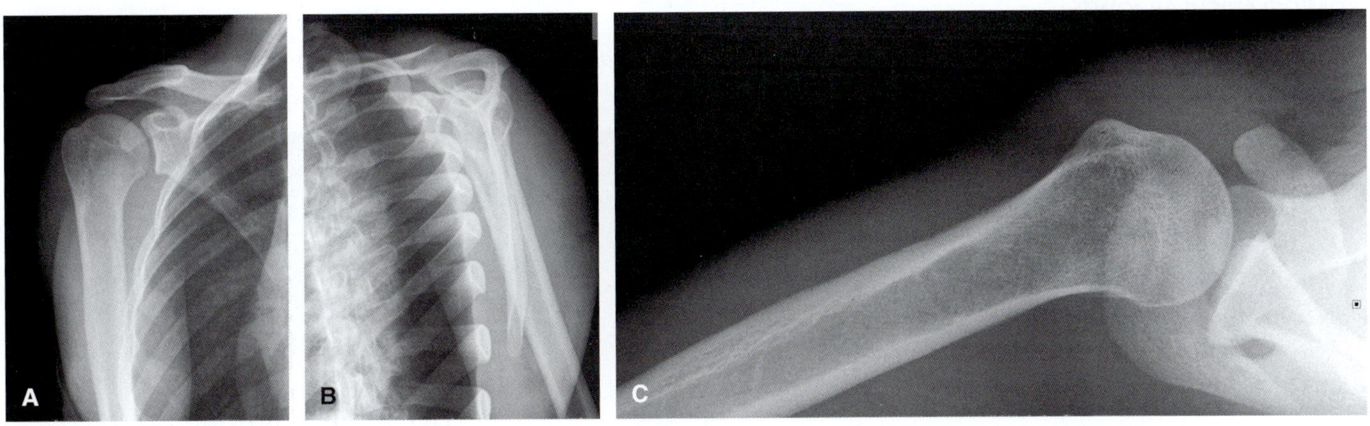

FIGURE 14. A: AP scapula, neutral rotation. B: Lateral "Y" view. C: Axillary view, as tolerated by patient.

Additional Views

Outlet view is good to look at subacromial space to assess for causes of external shoulder subacromial impingement. It can also be used to localize calcium in the rotator cuff. Stryker notch view is good for Hill-Sachs lesions, but most are seen on neutral rotation AP shoulder. Westpoint view is good for detecting bony Bankart lesions, but consider CT. Velpeau view can be a useful adjunct to assess for dislocation in a patient who cannot raise their arm.

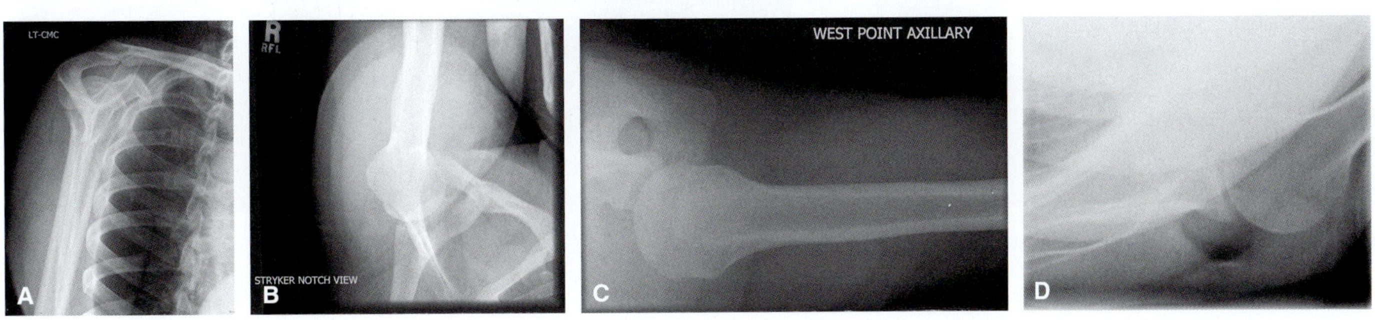

FIGURE 15. A: Supraspinatus view (outlet, Bigliani method). B: Westpoint. C: Stryker. D: Velpeau.

SCAPULA

Good for trauma, scapulothoracic syndrome. Consider CT for trauma workup to assess for glenoid involvement. MRI can assess for scapulothoracic friction syndromes.

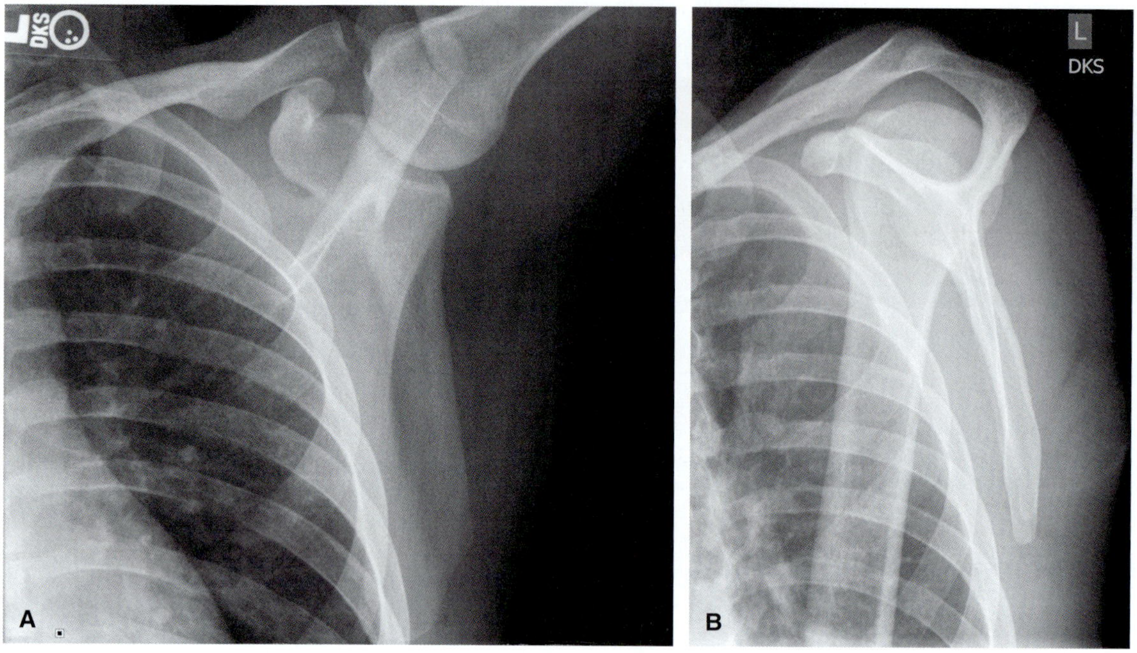

FIGURE 16. A: AP scapula. B: Lateral scapula.

ACROMIOCLAVICULAR JOINTS

These are routinely assessed on AP shoulder views. Views without and with weights to look for occult type 1 separations usually do not alter management but can make the diagnosis. May be useful in legal cases. Consider MRI to assess for deltotrapezial disruption in type 3 or higher injuries.

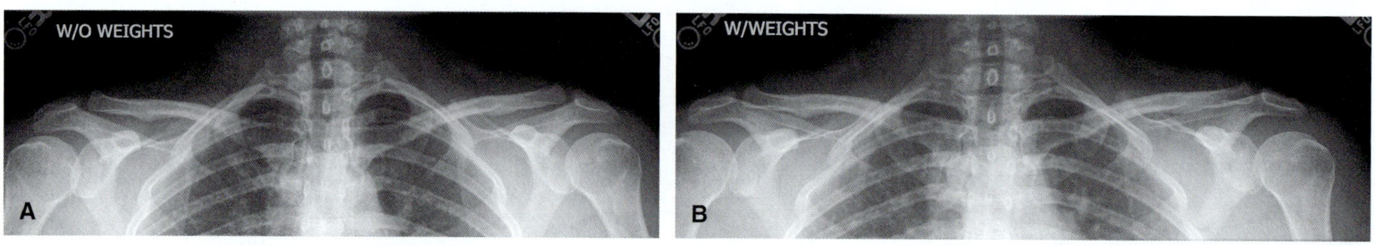

FIGURE 17. A: AP without weights. B: AP with weights.

CLAVICLES

Good for clavicle fractures. Medial clavicle fractures can be difficult to see. Consider CT for possible medial clavicle fractures.

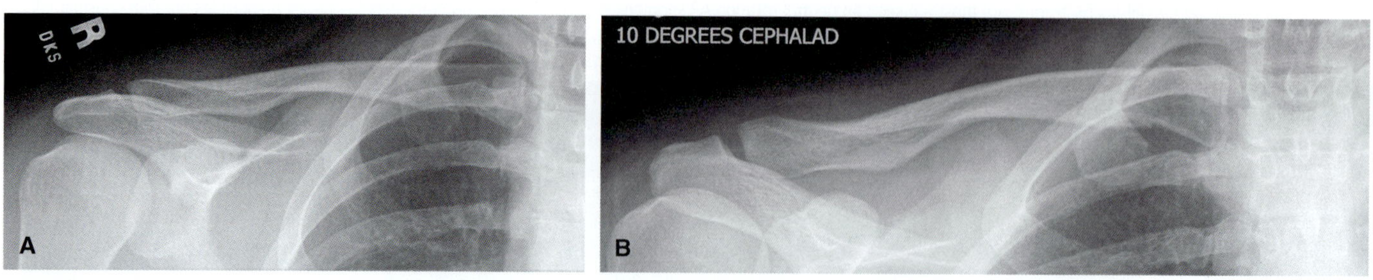

FIGURE 18. A: AP, 0-degree tube angle. B: AP, 10-degree cephalad angle.

LOWER EXTREMITIES

TOES

For 1st to 5th digits. Specifically to look at one toe for trauma, foreign body, or localized mass. Socks off. A marker should be applied. The lateral view should have the affected toe lifted or depressed clear of the others. Consider US for radiolucent foreign body. Consider MRI or US for mass or tendon lesion/injury.

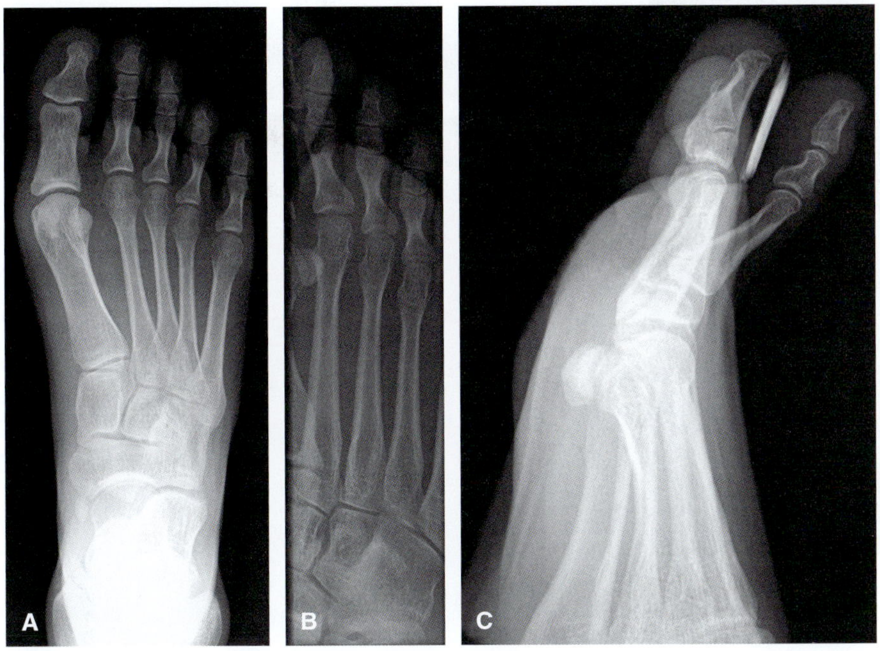

FIGURE 19. A: AP foot. B: Medial oblique of affected toe(s). C: Lateral of toe(s).

FOOT

Perform all three views for trauma and nontrauma cases. A limited two-view foot is discouraged. Weight-bearing to assess foot alignment. Non–weight-bearing if painful to stand or looking for a foreign body or mass. Non–weight-bearing if ulcer and looking for osteomyelitis. Always remove socks.

Consider US for Morton neuroma, plantar fasciitis, or superficial mass. CT is good for full assessment of Lisfranc injuries; MRI good for occult fracture or mass.

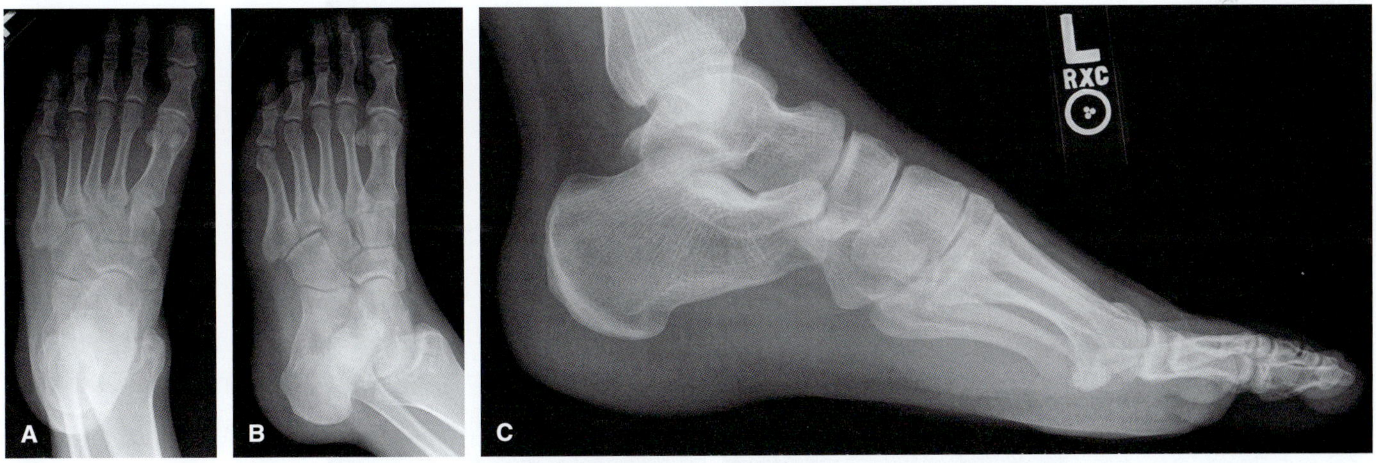

FIGURE 20. A: AP (dorsoplantar). B: Medial oblique. C: Lateral (mediolateral projection).

Sesamoid View

Good to look at sesamoid alignment with metatarsal head in hallux valgus, to assess metatarsal sesamoid osteoarthrosis, or to look for fracture of sesamoid.

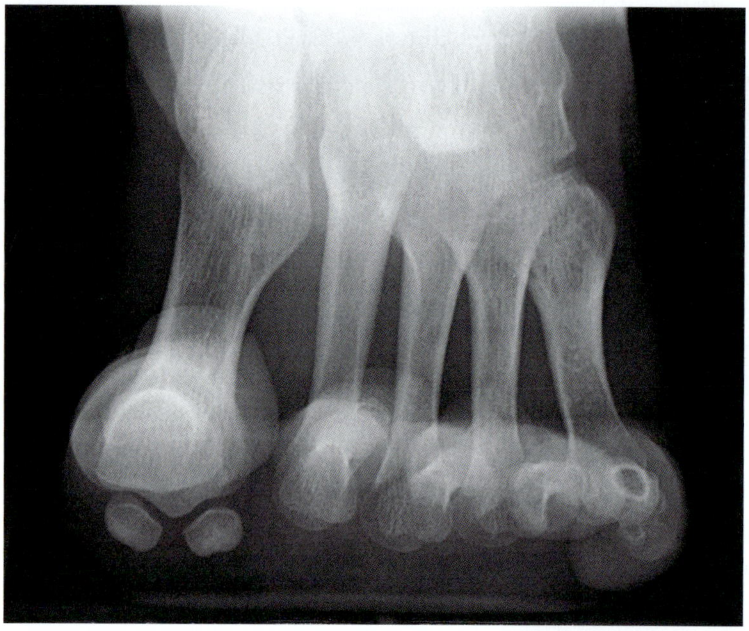

FIGURE 21. Sesamoid projection.

Os Calcis

Weight-bearing for alignment or non–weight-bearing for mass or if too painful to stand. Good for trauma and heel alignment. This should be the preferred study for heal pain rather than a foot series. The posterior subtalar joint and middle subtalar facet are often well visualized on the axial or Harris Beath view. Consider CT for full preoperative assessment of calcaneal fractures.

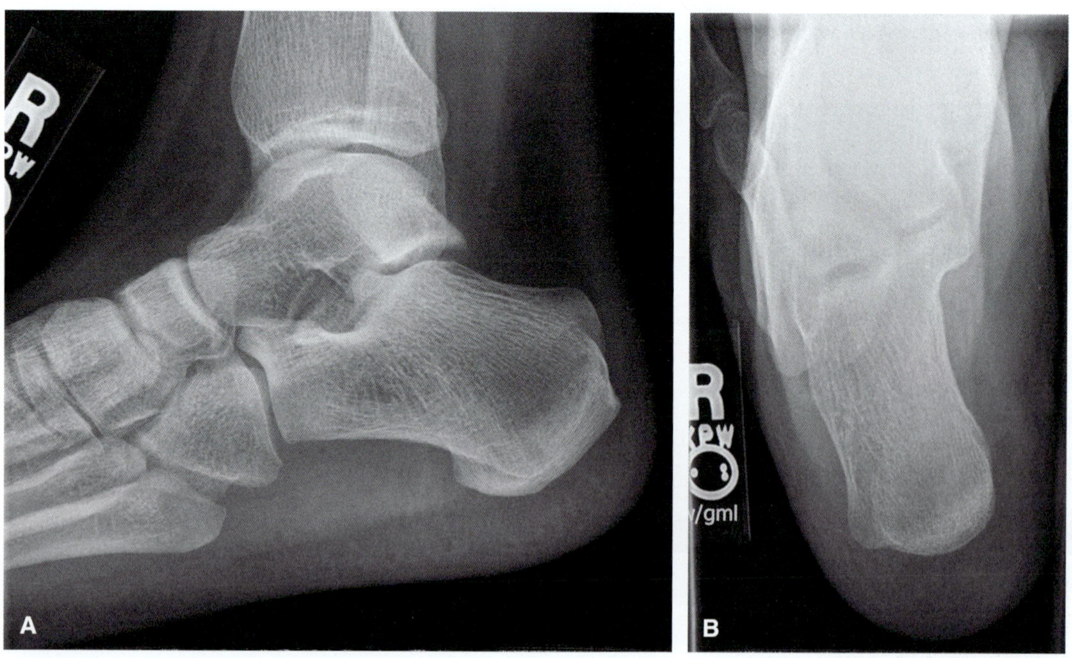

FIGURE 22. A: Lateral calcaneus mediolateral projection. B: PA axial plantodorsal.

ANKLE

Weight-bearing if alignment being assessed or non–weight-bearing if trauma or looking for mass.

Ideal for all acute ankle injuries. The base of 5th metatarsal should be included in case the ankle pain originates from there. For heel pain, use heel or calcaneal projections. US is useful to assess tendon injuries. CT is good for complex hindfoot fractures. MRI is good to assess the tendons and ligaments for masses and occult fractures.

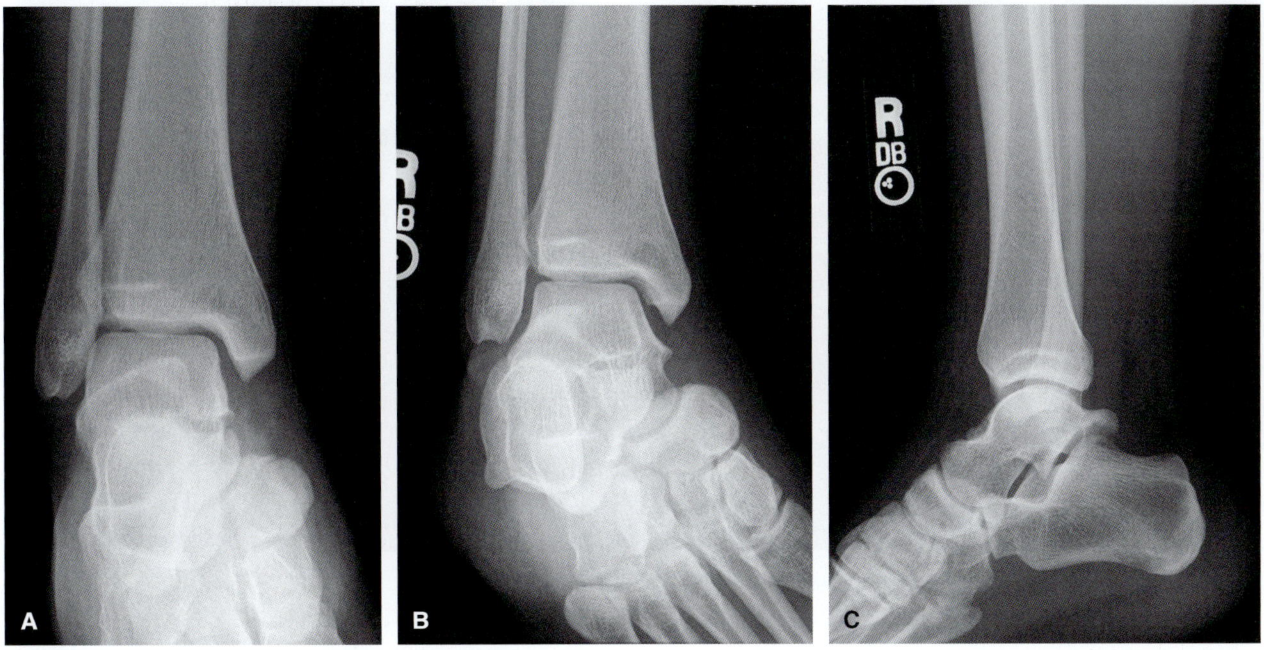

FIGURE 23. A: AP ankle. B: Mortise ankle. C: Mediolateral lateral.

Posterior Subtalar Joint

The Broden view is a useful adjunct view to look at the posterior subtalar joint to assess for intra-articular fractures and arthritis.

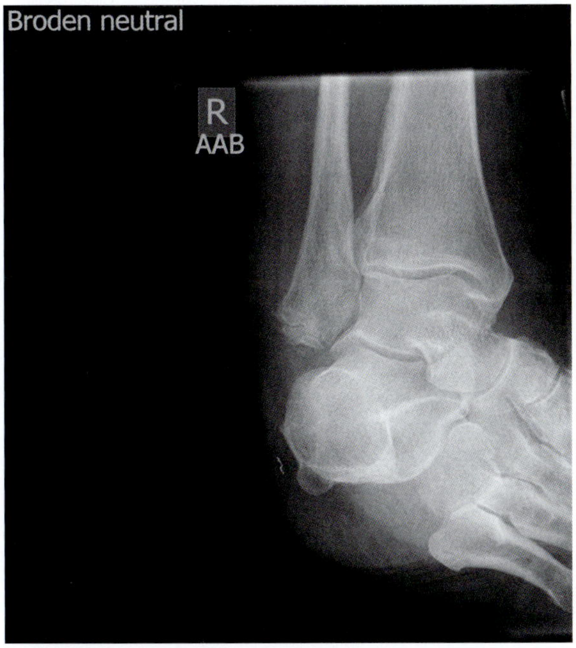

FIGURE 24. Broden view of posterior subtalar joint.

Weight-Bearing Views of the Ankle

Weight-bearing views are useful to eliminate the effects of a large joint effusion from widening or straightening the ankle mortise.

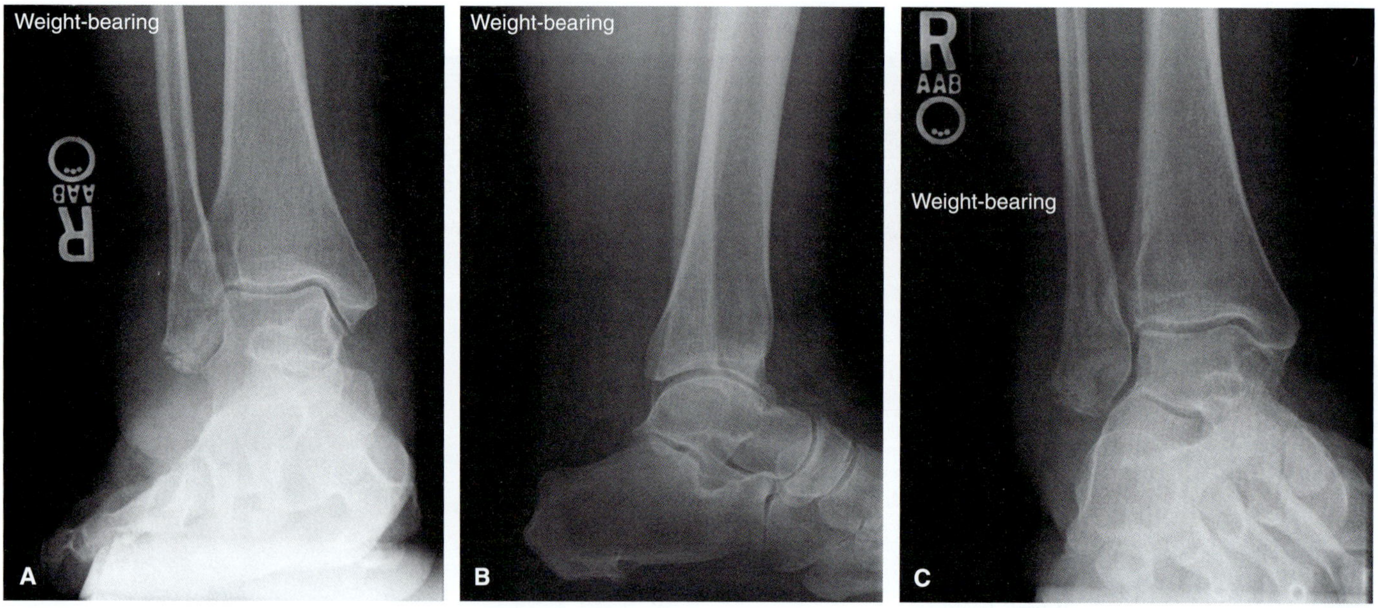

FIGURE 25. A: AP weight-bearing ankle. B: Mortise weight-bearing ankle. C: Mediolateral lateral weight-bearing ankle.

Stress Views of the Ankle

These give more functional information than MRI about ligamentous laxity and are useful in planning treatment for unstable ankles. It is important to have the other side for comparison.

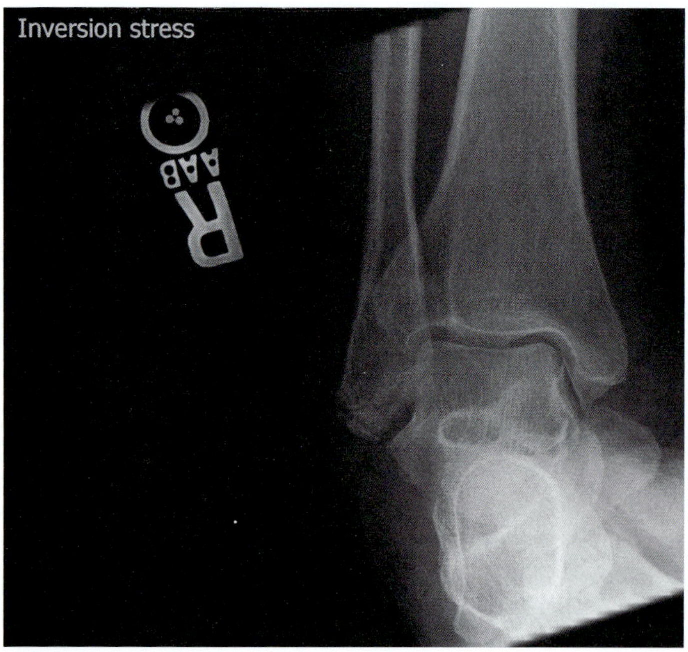

FIGURE 26. AP ankle with varus stress.

TIBIA/FIBULA

This should include both the ankle and knee joints. The ankle and knee should not be overinterpreted on these off-axis views. Good for trauma, foreign body, mass, cellulitis. For stress fractures, consider MRI or bone scan.

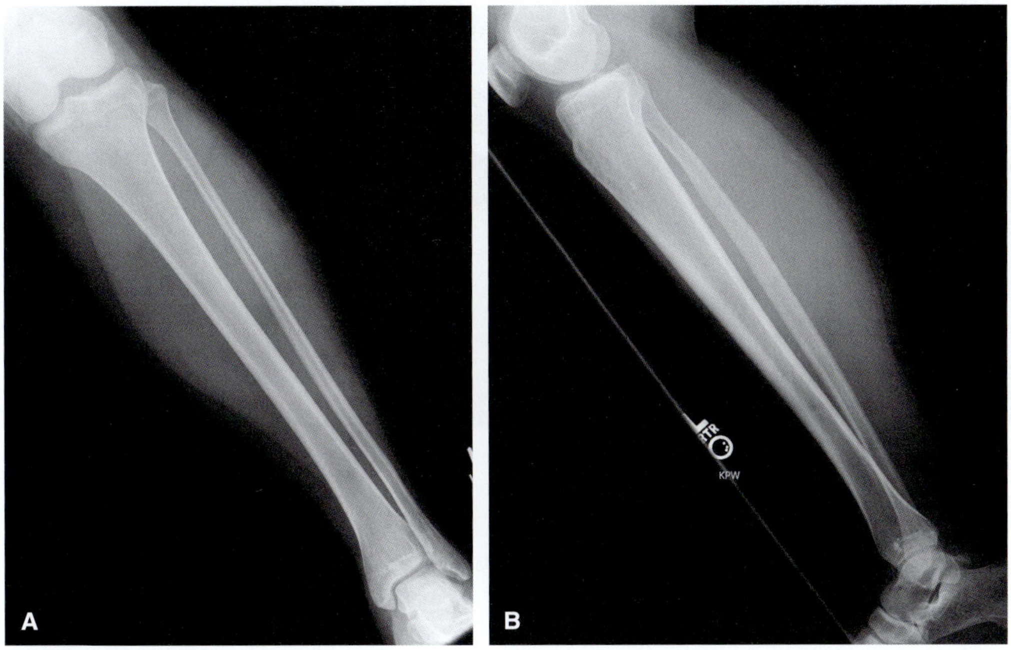

FIGURE 27. A: AP. B: Mediolateral lateral.

KNEE

Nontrauma, Chronic Injury

Good for initial arthritis assessment. MRI is useful to assess for internal derangement but is of less value when there is obvious osteoarthrosis on radiographs.

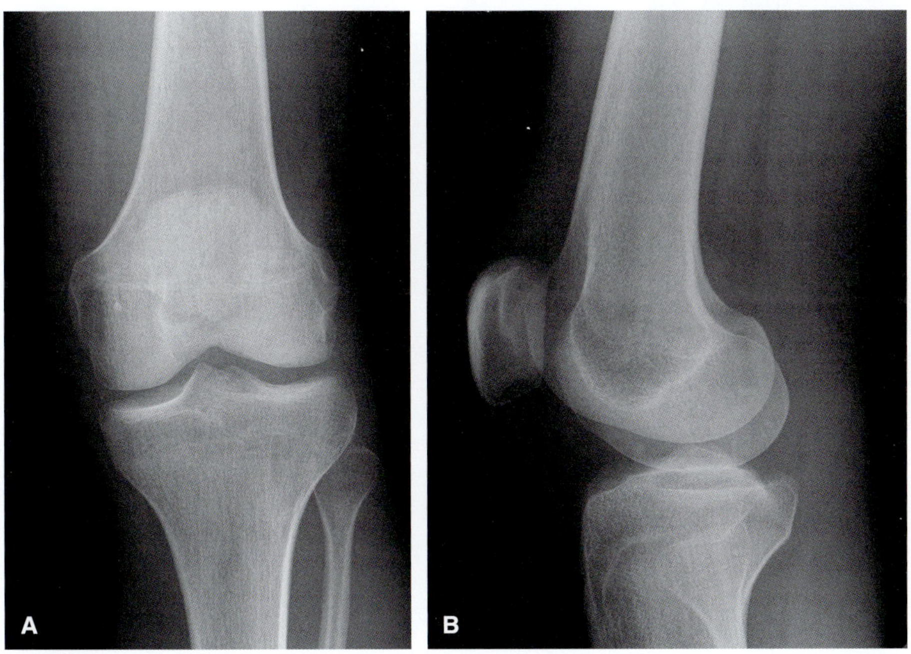

FIGURE 28. A: AP. B: Mediolateral lateral.

Trauma, Acute Injury

Shoot through lateral added to assess for a lipohemarthrosis; if present, a fracture must be sought. CT is a useful adjunct to assess for occult tibial plateau fractures and to plan surgery with fractures seen on radiographs. MRI being used increasingly to assess accompanying soft tissue injuries in cases of tibial plateau fractures.

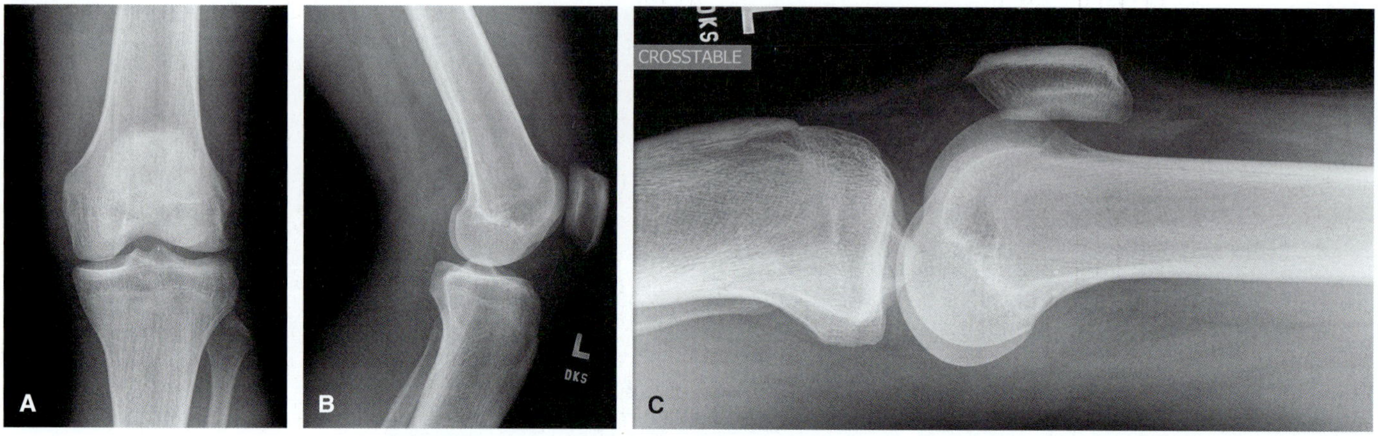

FIGURE 29. A: AP. B: Mediolateral lateral. C: Lateromedial crosstable lateral.

Additional Views

Rosenberg view: This weight-bearing posteroanterior (PA) view with flexion is useful to show both the intercondylar notch and the joint space formed by the more posterior femoral condyle.

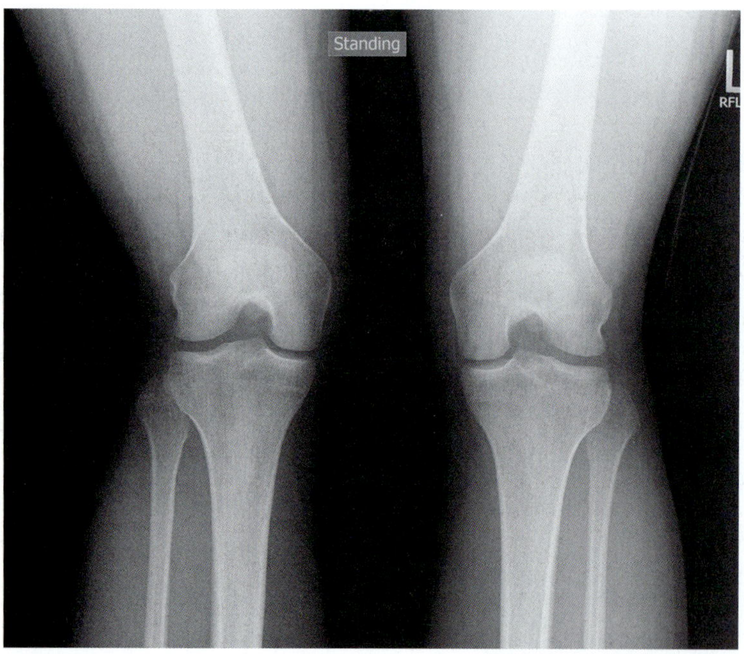

FIGURE 30. Rosenberg view.

Oblique views: Traditionally used to assess for occult tibial plateau fractures; still useful but now often replaced by CT or MRI.

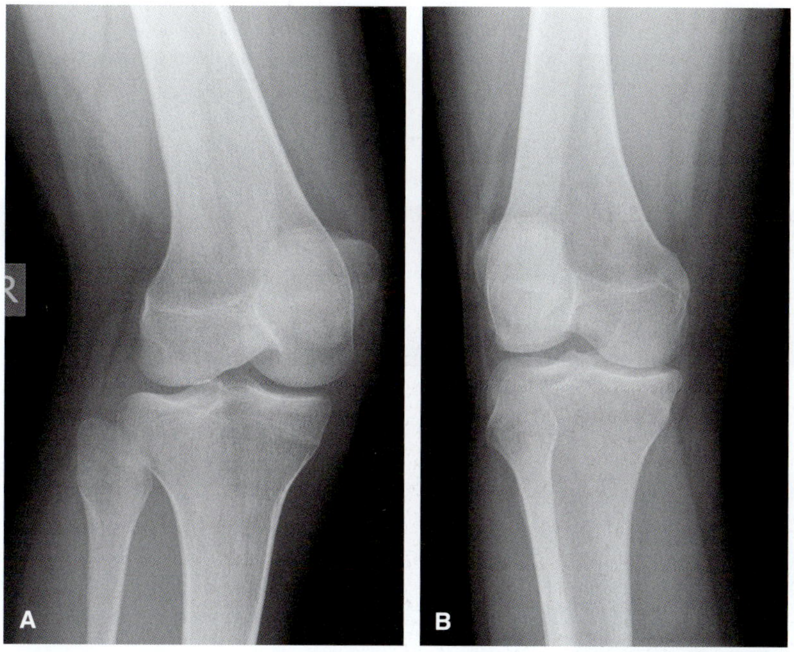

FIGURE 31. A: Medial oblique. B: Lateral oblique.

Patella: Initially, a routine knee is performed in cases of trauma.

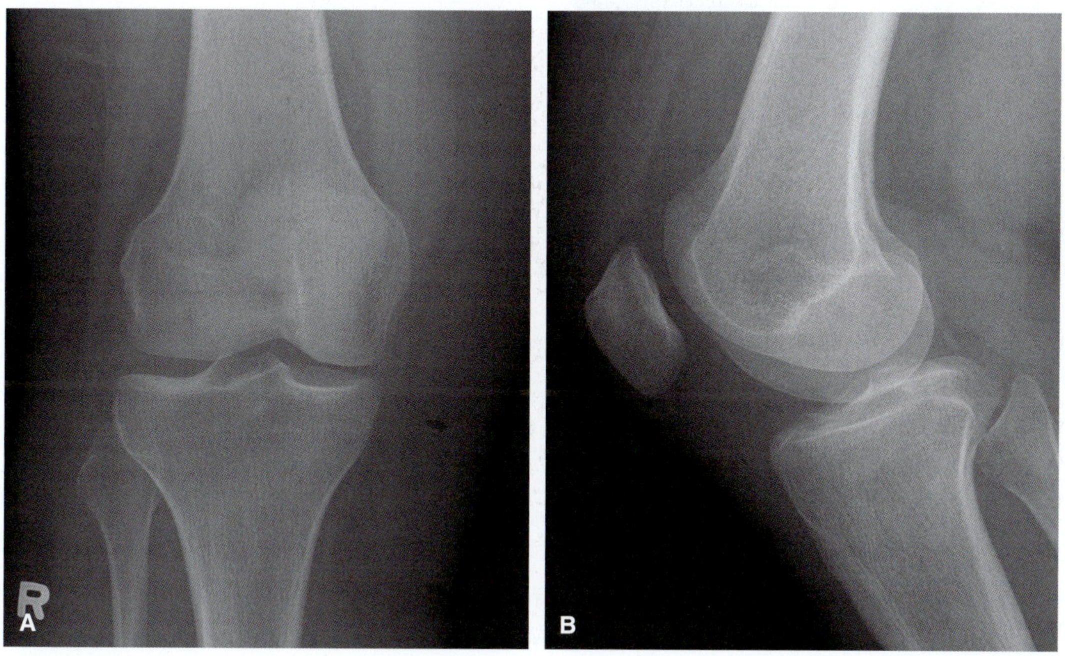

FIGURE 32. A: PA knee. B: Mediolateral lateral.

Additional Views

Merchants view is good to assess patella alignment in cases of subluxation, dislocation, or tracking problems. These are taken at 30 degrees of flexion, the angle at which the patella is most unstable. It is taken caudal cranial and includes both knees. The sunrise axial projection is taken kneeling of just the affected the knee.

FIGURE 33. Merchants (bilateral patellar view).

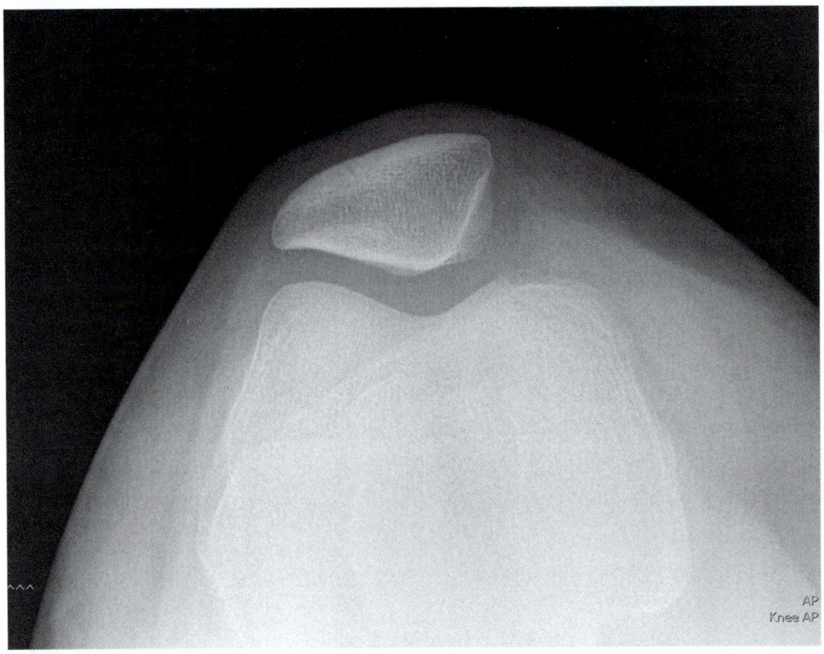

FIGURE 34. Axial projection (unilateral sunrise method).

FEMUR

Acute Injury, Trauma

Views of the femur should include both the hip and knee. The trauma series has a crosstable lateral of both the hip and knee so that the patient does not have to move.

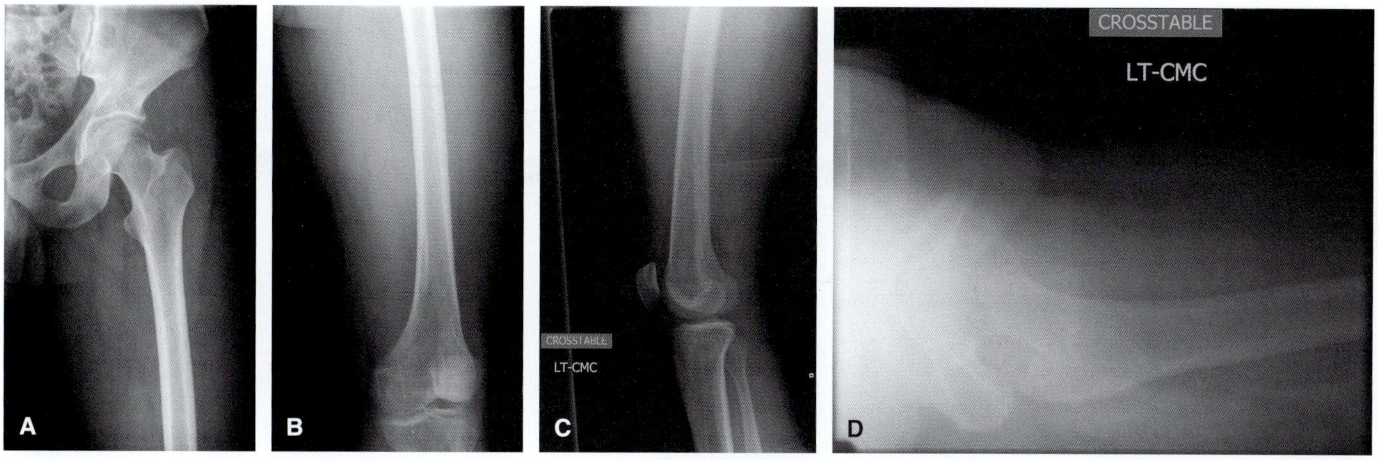

FIGURE 35. A: AP proximal. B: AP distal. C: X-table lateral femur to include knee joint. D: Inferosuperior lateral to include proximal femur and hip joint for unilateral injury.

Nonacute Injury

The views include both the hip and the knee, but the hip is a frog lateral and the knee is a rolled mediolateral. For soft tissue mass, consider MRI.

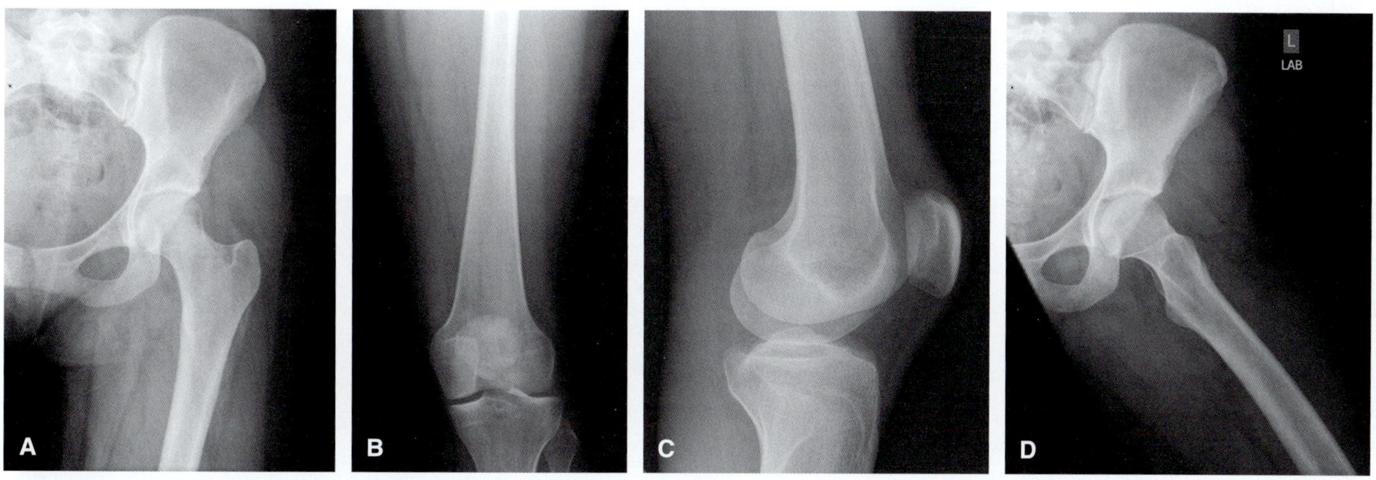

FIGURE 36. A: AP to include hip and proximal femur. B: AP to include knee and distal femur. C: Mediolateral lateral to include knee. D: Lateral frog-leg hip.

PELVIS

Include Both Hips on Image

Good initial screening test for acute trauma. Good for ill-defined pain or metastatic search. Consider CT for full assessment of pelvic trauma.

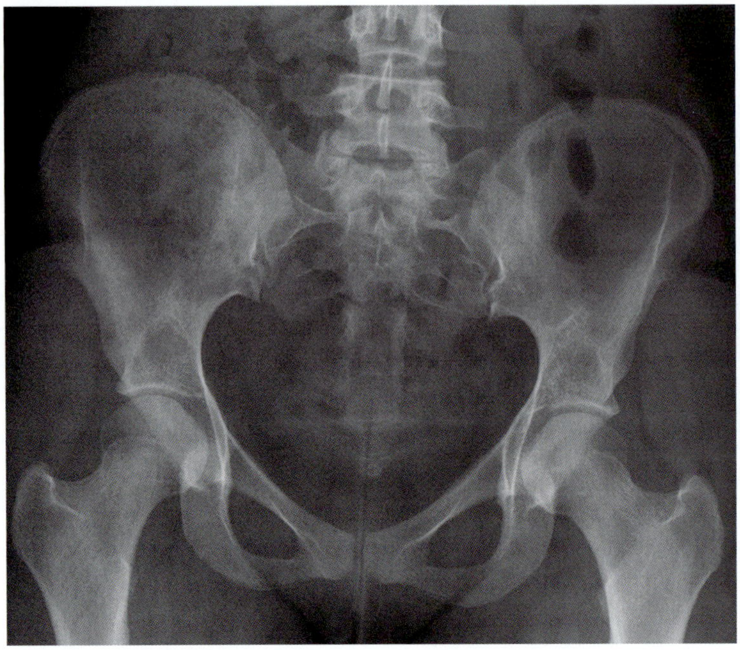

FIGURE 37. AP pelvis.

Hips

Trauma, Acute Injury: AP pelvis and a crosstable lateral to assess for hip pain localized to one side of the pelvis/hip.

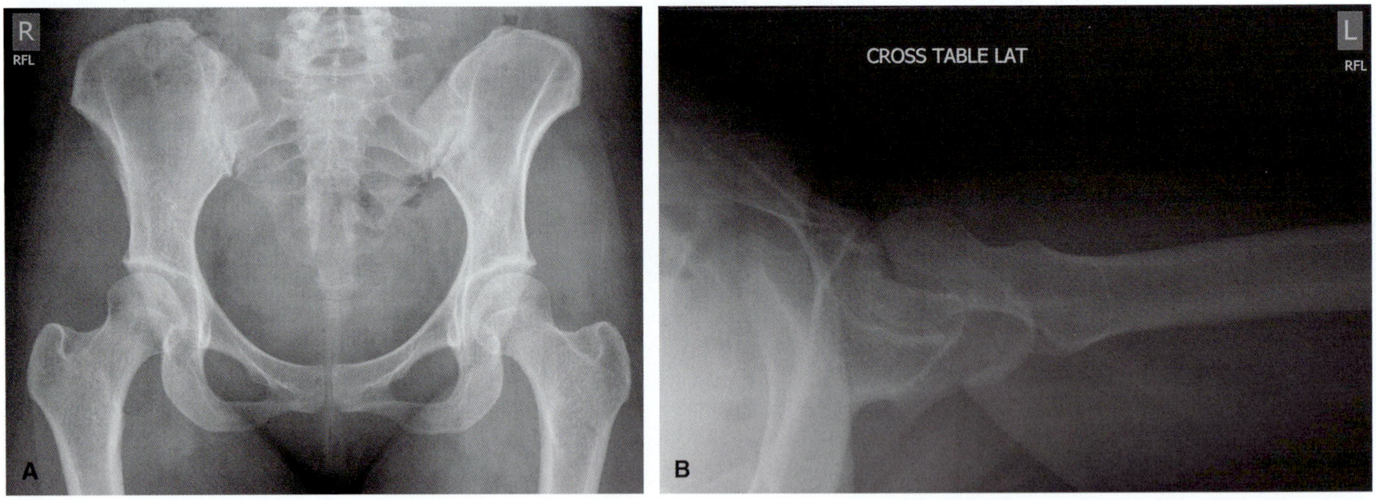

FIGURE 38. A: AP pelvis. B: Inferosuperior lateral to include proximal femur and hip joint for unilateral injury.

Nontrauma, Chronic Injury: The crosstable lateral is replaced by a frog lateral. The frog leg can be bilateral or unilateral depending on the pain. MRI is an excellent way to assess hip pain if the radiographs show only minimal abnormality. MRI arthrogram can give useful additional information about the labrum.

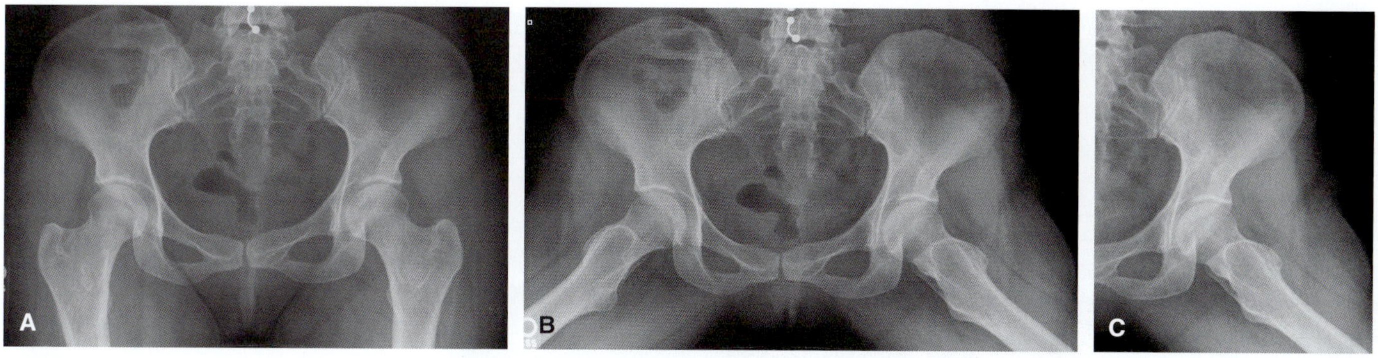

FIGURE 39. A: AP pelvis. B: Bilateral frog leg. C: or Frog-leg lateral of affected hip.

Sacroiliac Joints
Good initial screening test for sacroiliitis. MRI is more sensitive and saves radiation to the gonads.

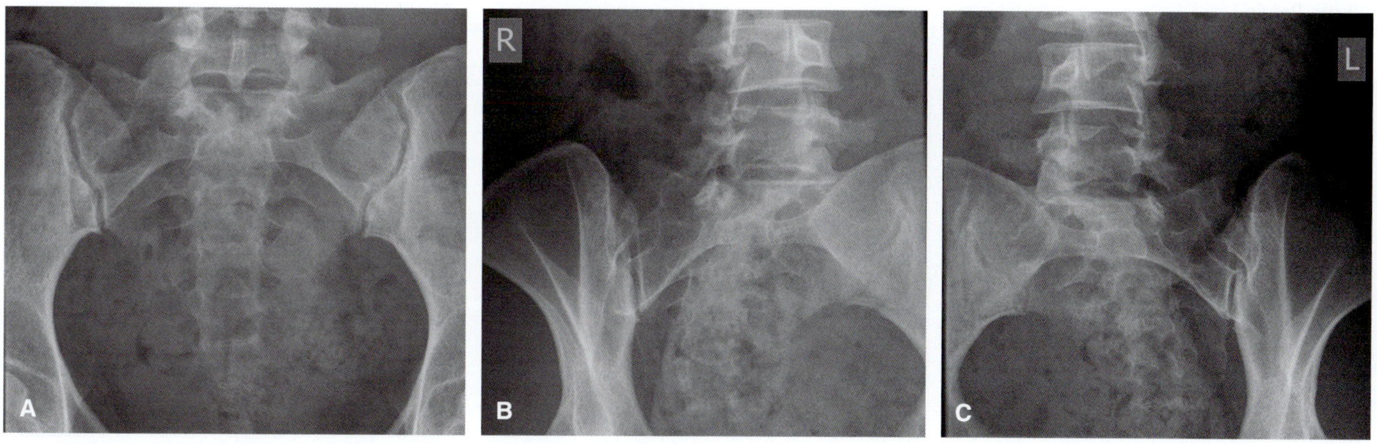

FIGURE 40. A: AP pelvis. B: AP oblique of right sacroiliac joint. C: AP oblique of left sacroiliac joint.

Acetabulum (Judet Views)
Good for assessing acetabular fractures but now usually replaced by oblique images of whole pelvis; requires four images: two right posterior oblique (RPO) and two left posterior oblique (LPO) images, collimated to affected side only.

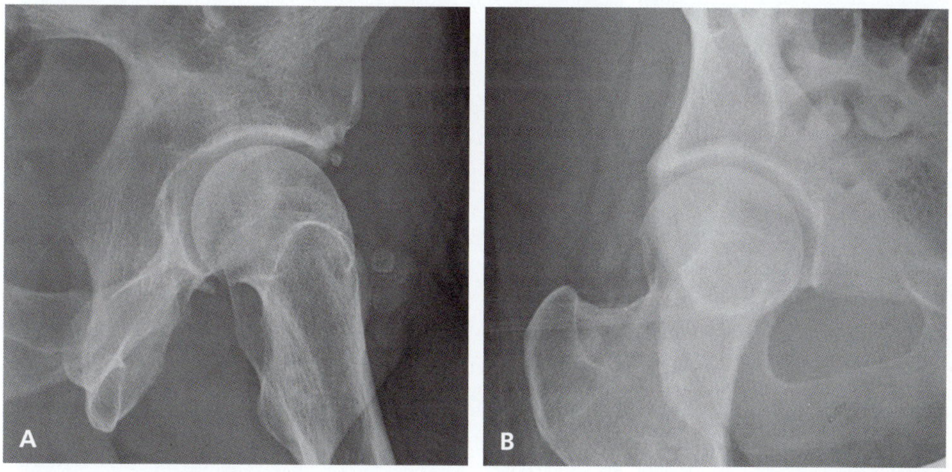

FIGURE 41. A: Left iliac LPO. B: Right obturator LPO. *(continued)*

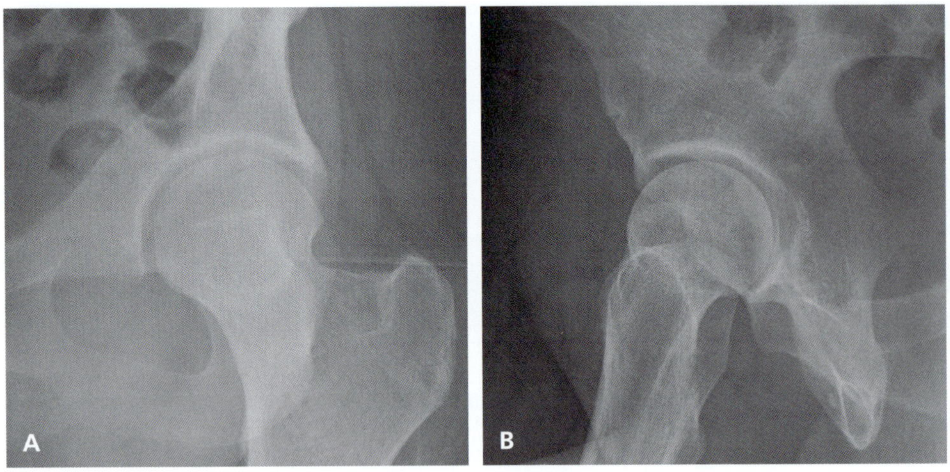

FIGURE 41. (*Continued*) C: Left obturator RPO. D: Right iliac RPO.

Oblique Pelvis

Also good for assessing fractures about the acetabular. CT is good for the initial assessment, but when there is a need to follow up fractures, oblique views are usually used.

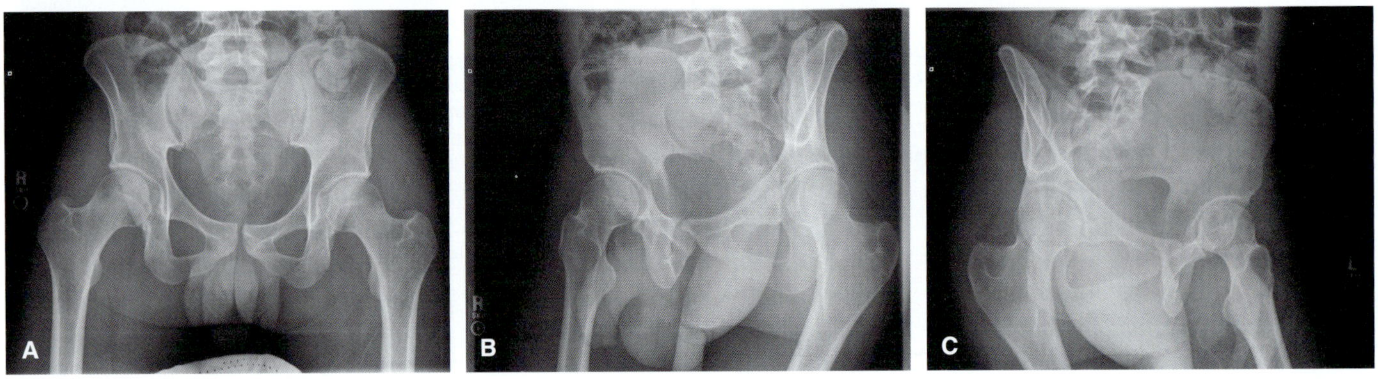

FIGURE 42. A: AP pelvis. B: RPO. C: LPO.

Inlet/Outlet

Good to assess for pelvic fractures involving the pubic rami and sacrum. CT is good for the initial assessment, but when there is a need to follow up fractures at these locations, inlet and outlet views are usually used.

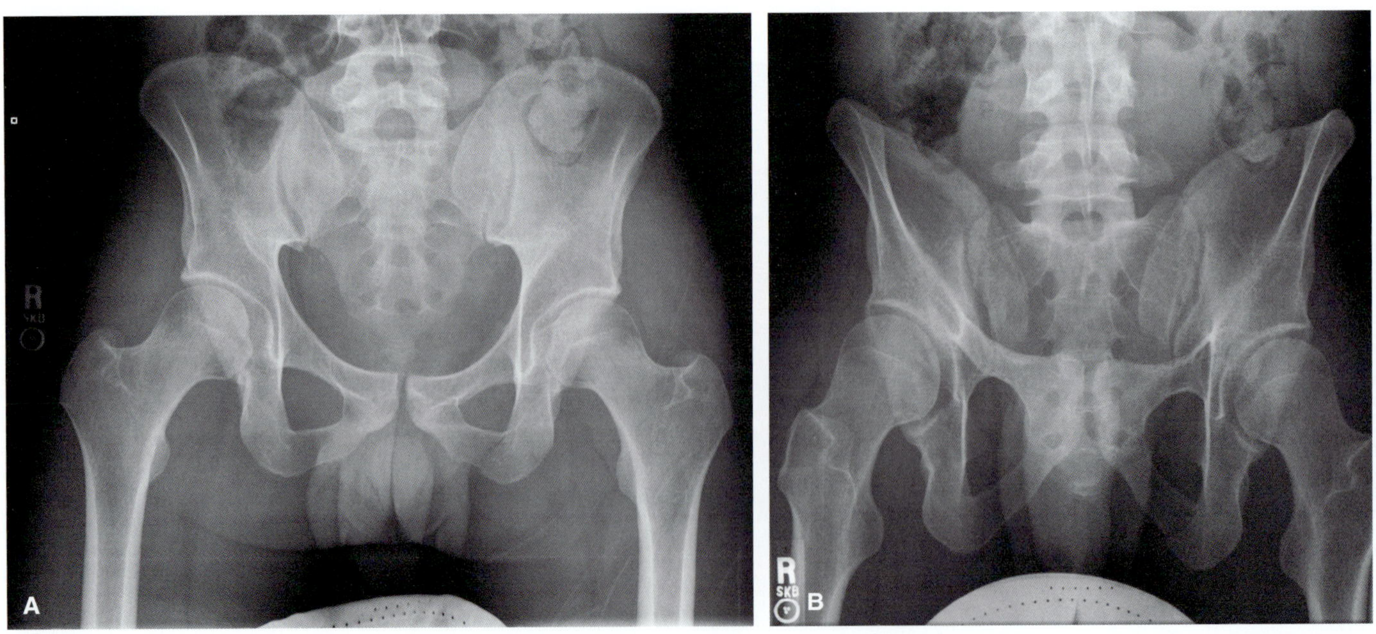

FIGURE 43. A: AP pelvis. B: AP axial outlet view. (*continued*)

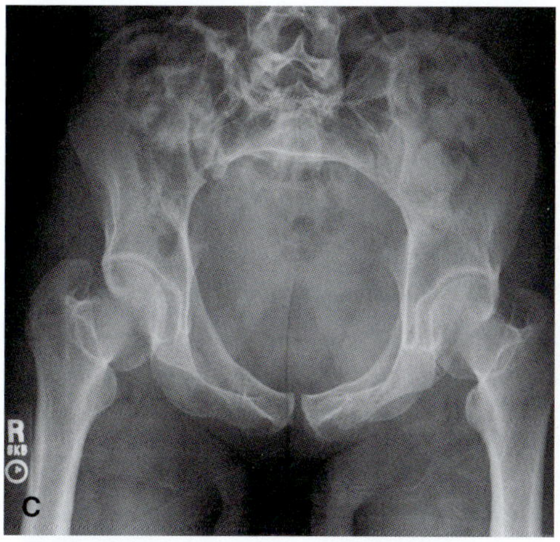

FIGURE 43. (*Continued*) C: AP axial inlet view.

VERTEBRAL COLUMN

SKULL

Not used very often because most indications for a skull radiograph are better served by a CT; can still be used to assess shunt continuity.

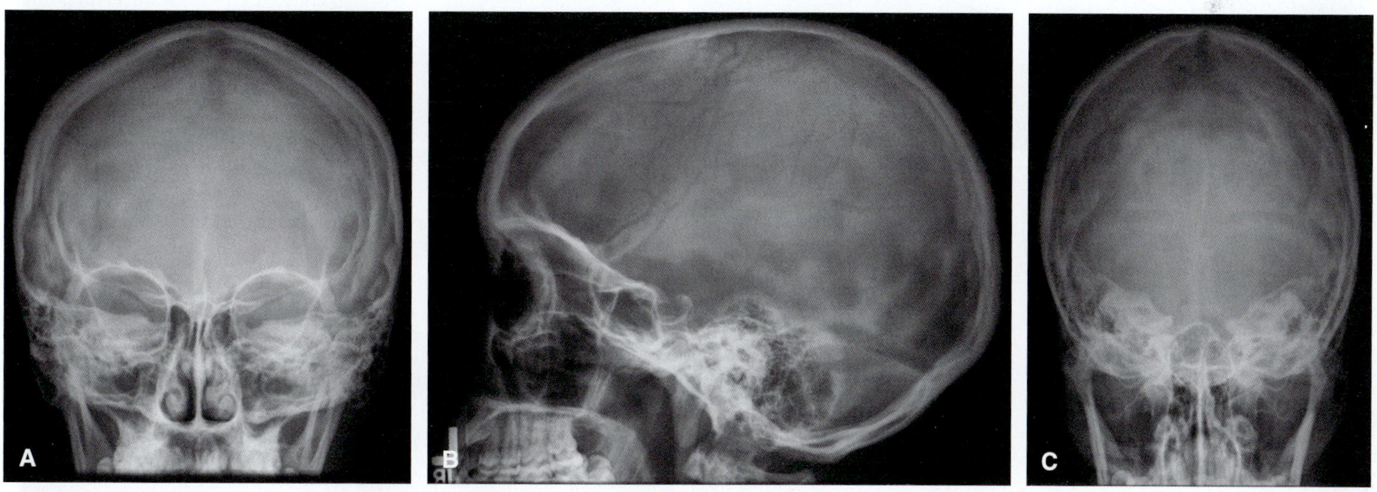

FIGURE 44. A: PA skull. B: Lateral skull. C: Townes view.

FACE

Good initial screening test for facial trauma. If found, these will usually be followed up with CT to show the full extent.

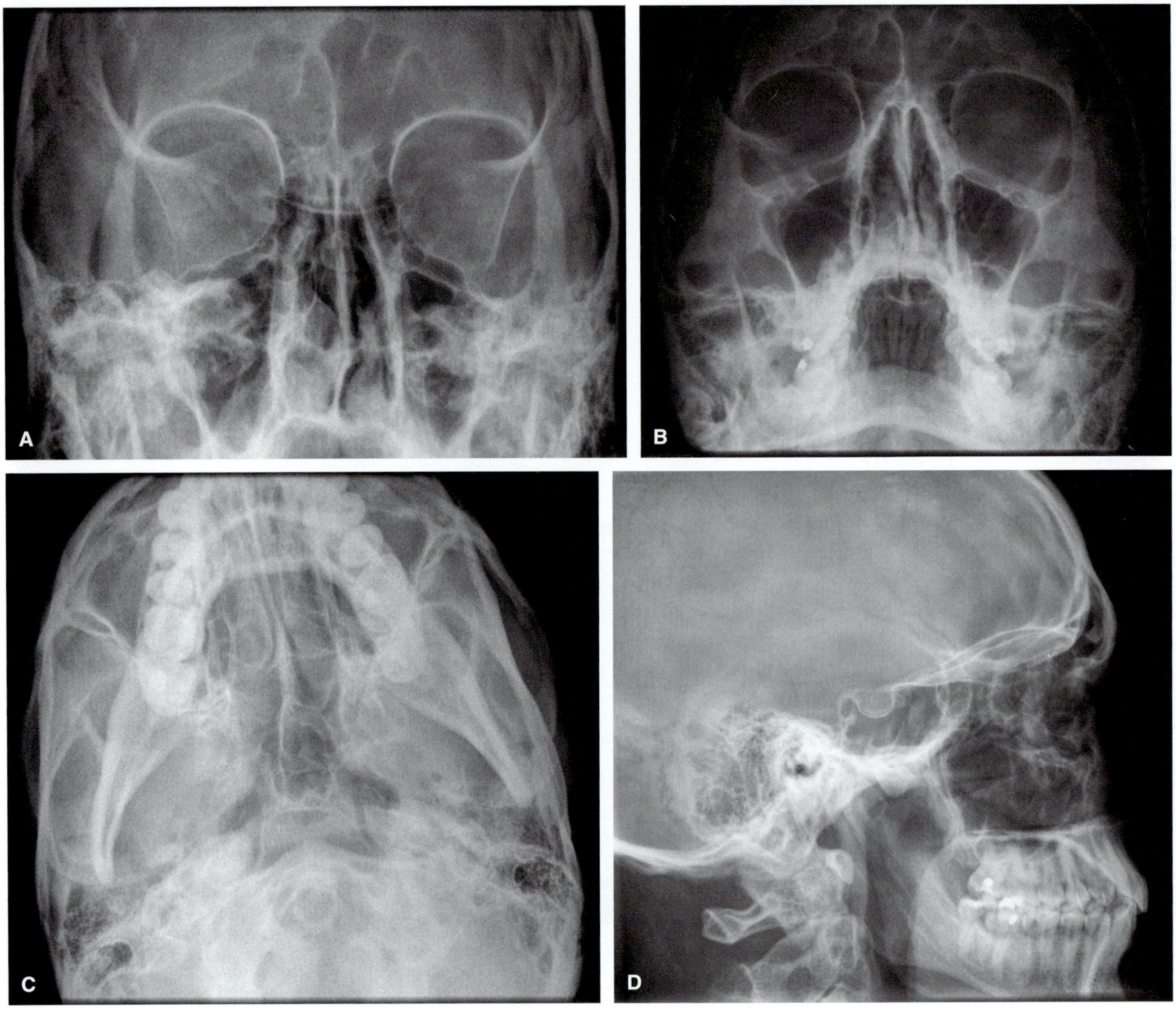

FIGURE 45. A: Occipitofrontal. B: Occipitomental. C: Occipitomental with 30-degree cranial angulation. D: Lateral face.

ORBITS

Useful to look for any destructive bony lesion about the orbit; replaced by CT when available

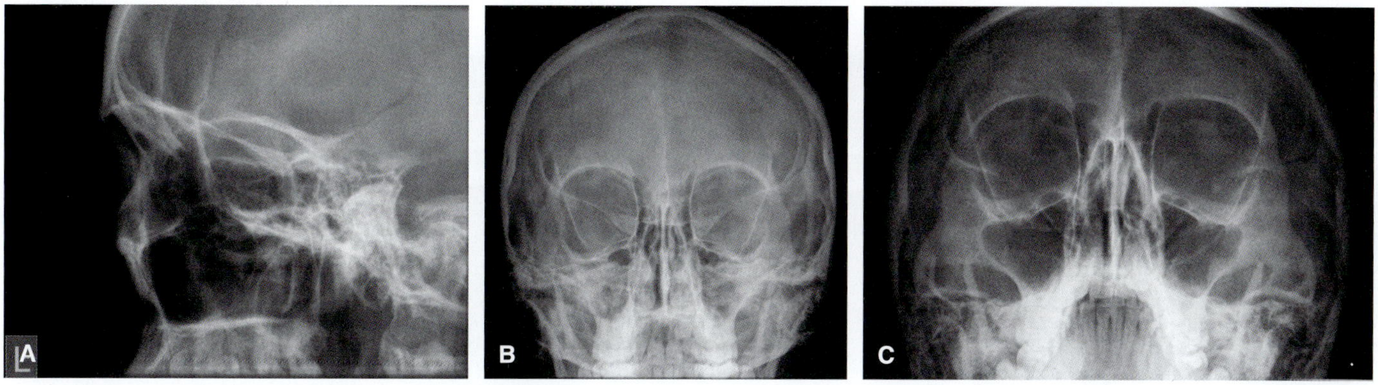

FIGURE 46. A: Lateral face. B: Occipitofacial. C: Occipitomental.

EYES

Only indication would be to look for a radiopaque metal foreign body within the globe of the eye, usually prior to MRI. By just the eyes looking up and down, it is possible to see if the body moves with the globe or is elsewhere.

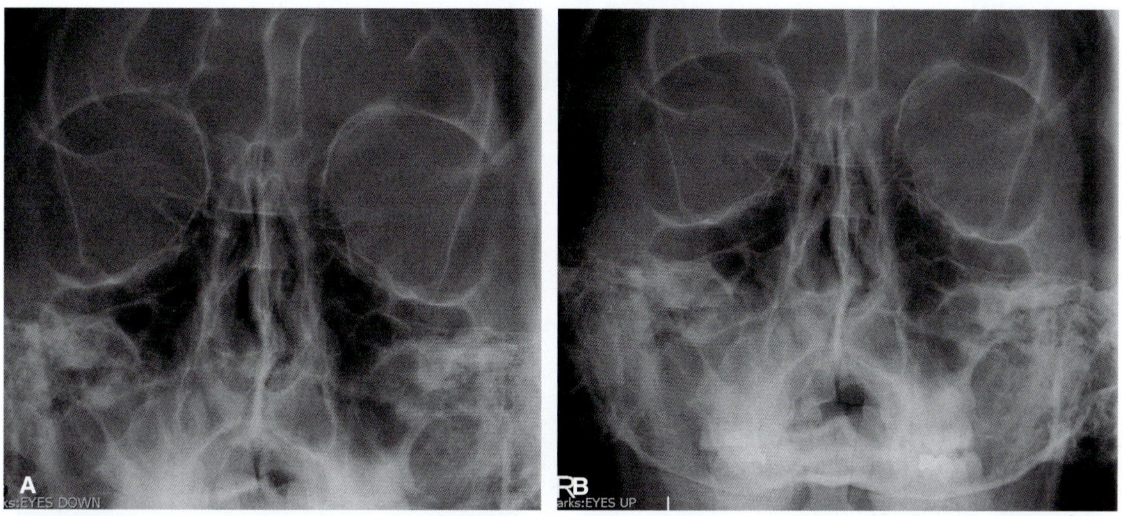

FIGURE 47. A: Occipitofacial looking up. B: Occipitofacial looking down.

MANDIBLE

The first investigation to look for mandible trauma but also used to look for disease related to the teeth and their sockets. CT is a useful adjunct for mandibular trauma. The oblique views are labeled, such that the side marker represents the inferiorly projecting side of the mandible.

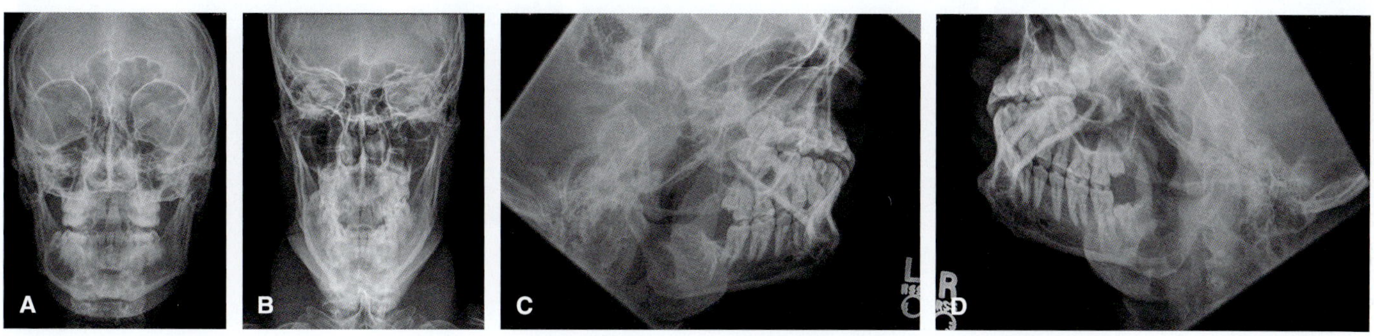

FIGURE 48. A: Occipitofacial. B: AP axial. C: Left inferosuperior oblique. D: Right inferosuperior oblique.

NASAL BONE

Used to assess for nasal trauma. Can also be used to show the septum in cases of nasal septal destruction but would usually be replaced by CT for the latter. Many advocate not radiographing the nose for 7 to 10 days until the swelling has subsided and then only if the patient is unhappy with the appearance. Bilateral lateral views are probably overdoing things.

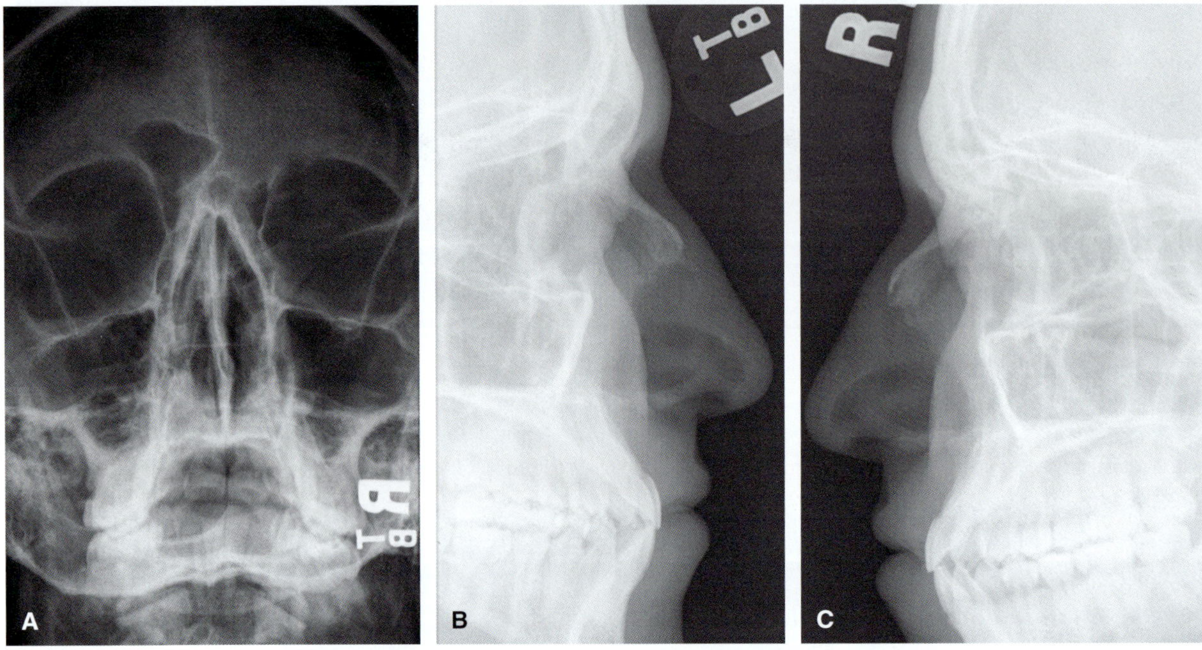

FIGURE 49. A: Coned-down occipitofacial. B: Left lateral soft tissue exposure. C: Right lateral soft tissue exposure.

CERVICAL SPINE

Complete

Include a swimmer's view if C7–T1 junction is not well visualized on the lateral view, and a Fuchs' view if the odontoid is suboptimal on the open mouth odontoid view. Such a full series is rarely used and would be replaced by CT for acute trauma and CT or MRI for chronic pain/radiculopathy. Oblique views, such as these, would be difficult in the trauma setting and would be done as trauma obliques with the patient supine and the beam angled obliquely.

They can be useful to show the posterior elements, particularly at the cervicothoracic junction where it may otherwise be difficult.

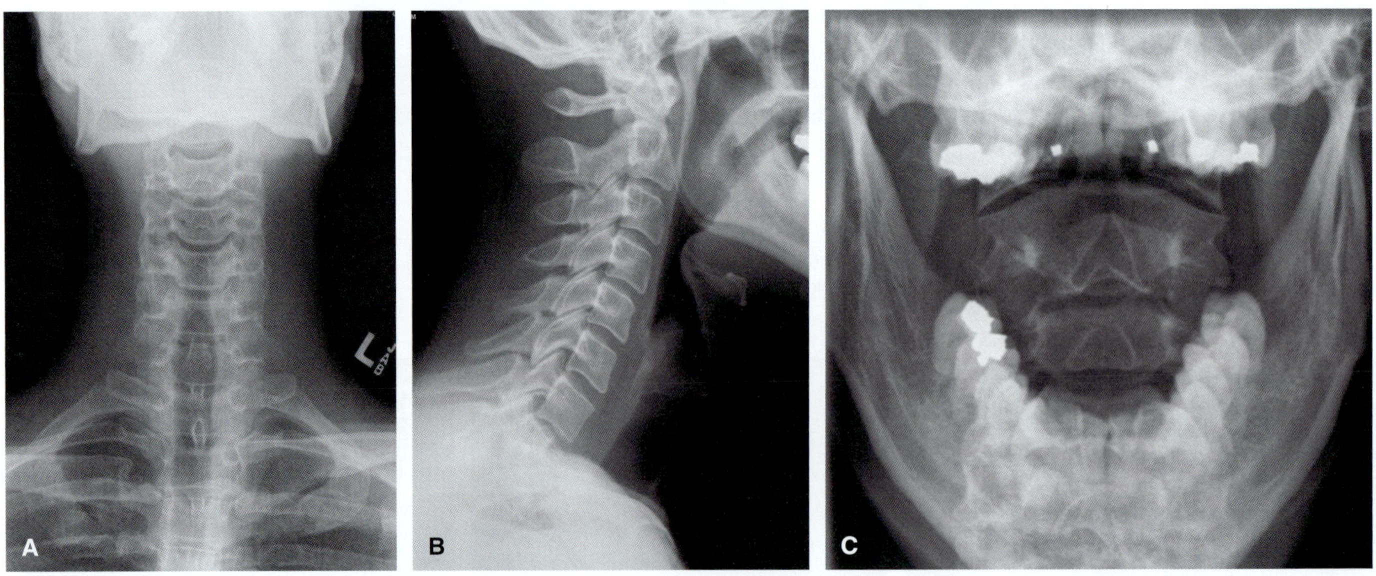

FIGURE 50. A: AP. B: Lateral. C: AP odontoid (open mouth). (*continued*)

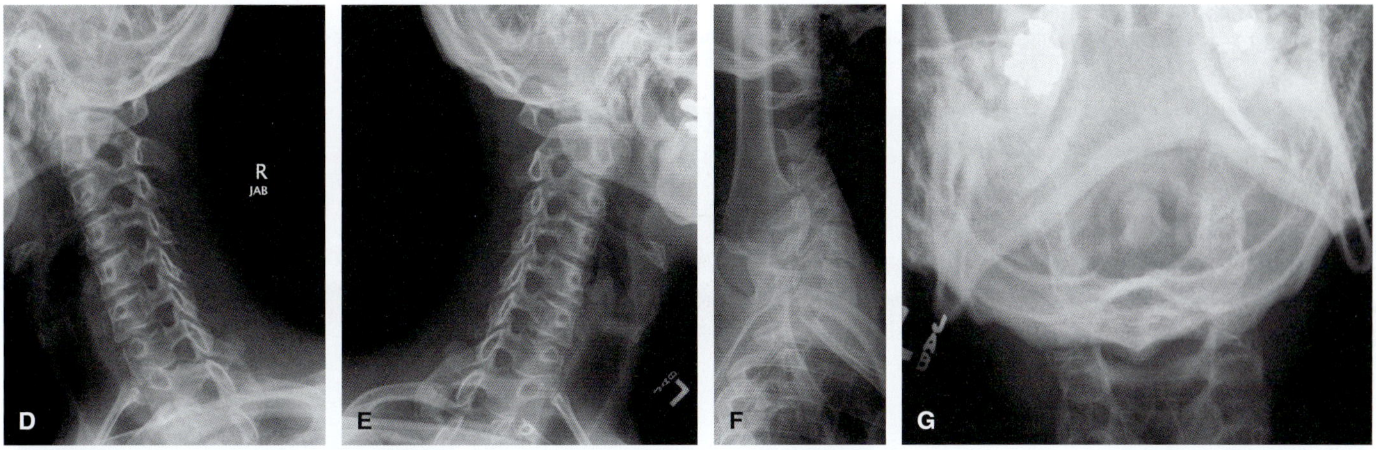

FIGURE 50. (*Continued*) D: Right anterior oblique (wrongly labeled). E: Left anterior oblique. F: Swimmer's view to visualize C7–T1. G: Fuchs' view.

Limited

A more reasonable series for acute trauma. Follow-up or chronic pain would usually emphasize the area of interest.

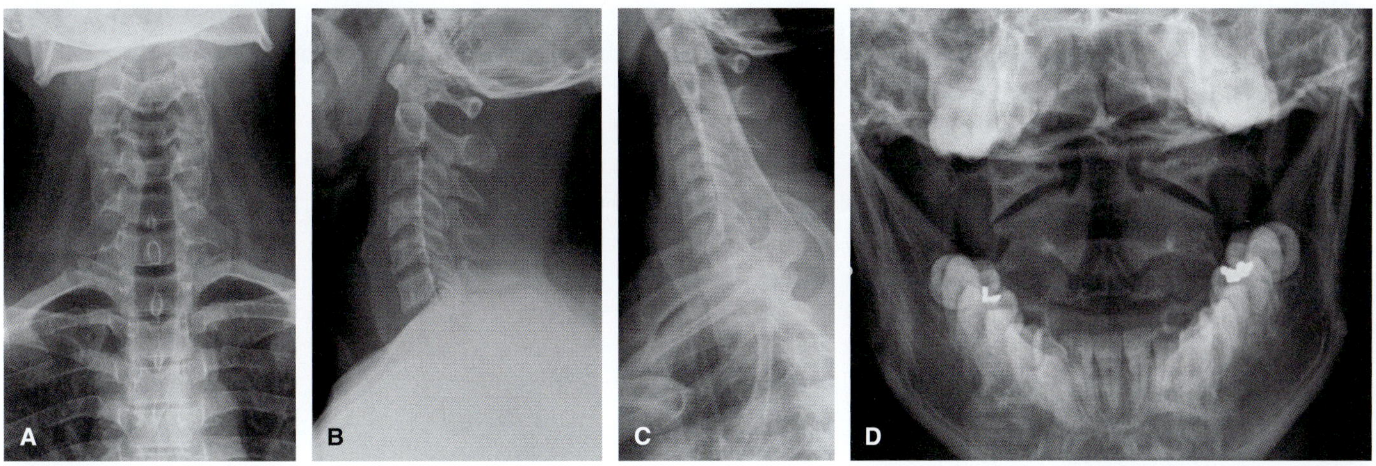

FIGURE 51. A: AP. B: Lateral. C: AP odontoid (open mouth). D: Swimmer's view.

Flexion–Extension Series
The best way to assess for cervical stability. They cannot be obtained acutely after trauma when there will likely be spasm but should be delayed for 10 days.

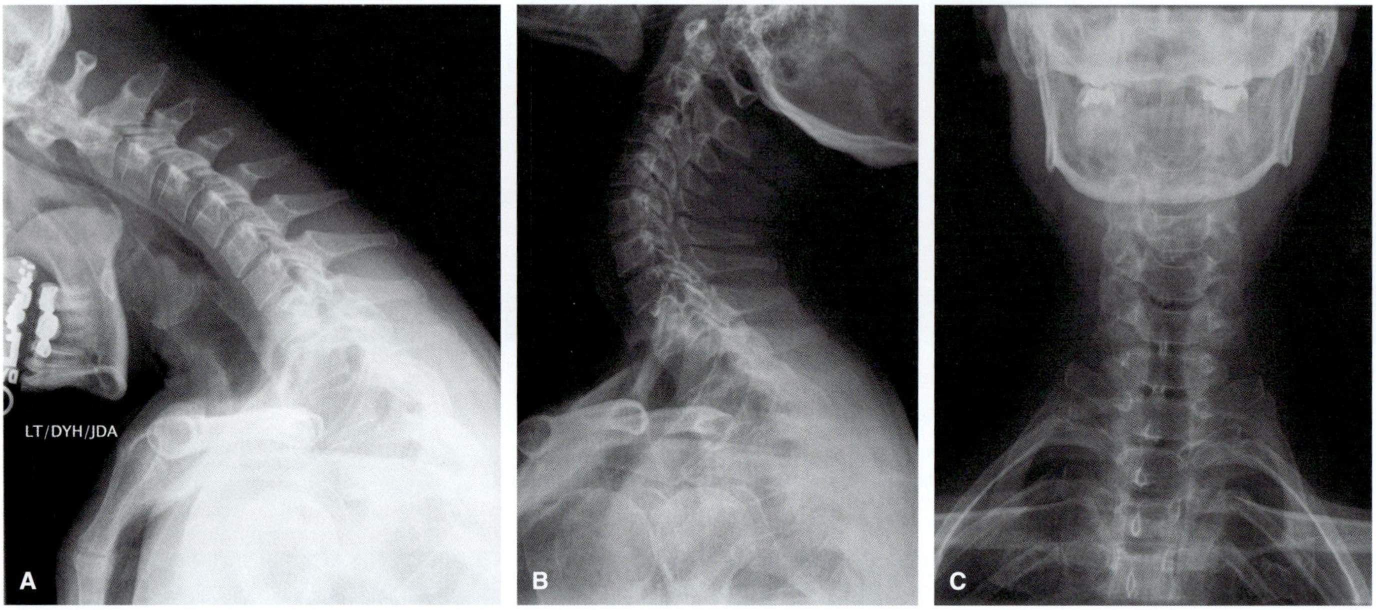

FIGURE 52. A: Flexion lateral. B: Extension lateral. C: AP.

THORACIC SPINE

Good initial assessment of pain and trauma. The lateral view may need to be augmented by a swimmer's view to show the cervicothoracic junction.

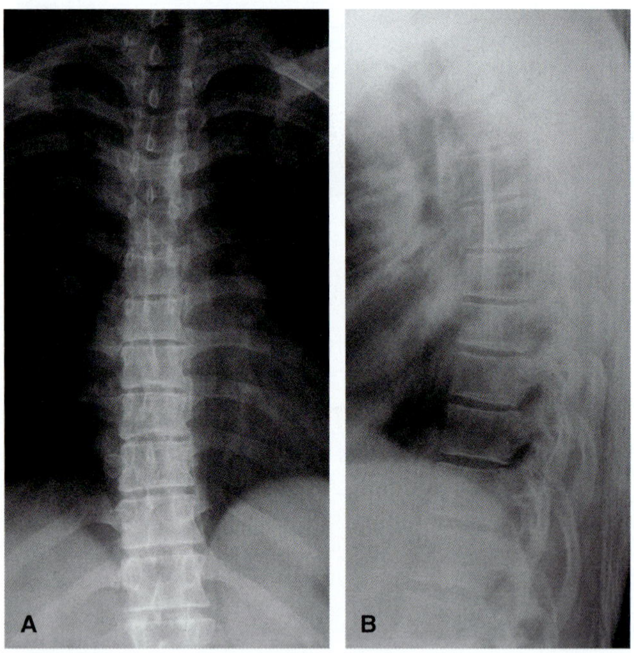

Figure 53. A: AP thoracic spine. B: Lateral thoracic spine.

Additional Views

The lateral view may need to be augmented by a swimmer's view to show the cervicothoracic junction. CT is used to characterize any fractures seen and MRI in cases of long tract signs.

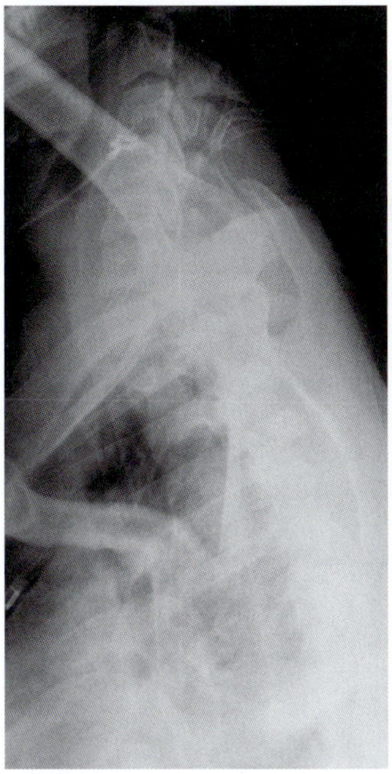

FIGURE 54. Swimmer's view of cervicothoracic junction.

LUMBAR SPINE

Routine Imaging

The images vary from center to center. Some will include an AP pelvis, others just AP and lateral lumbar spine. Good to assess for acute trauma, alignment, spondylolysis, and spondylolisthesis. CT is usually performed if trauma is seen on the radiographs. MRI is useful in cases of radiculopathy.

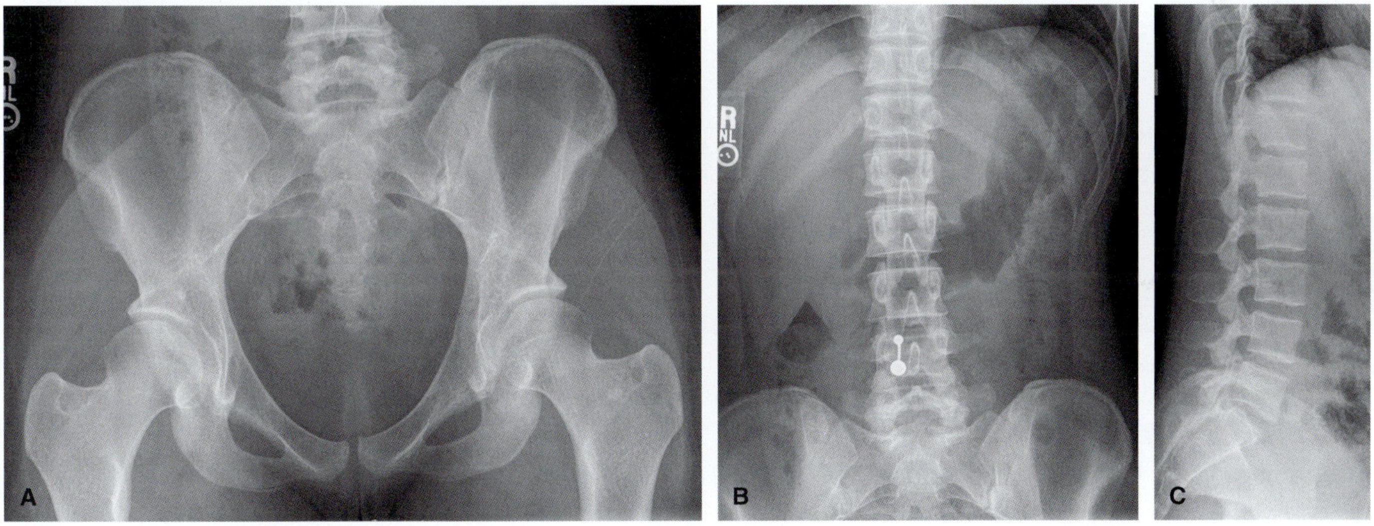

FIGURE 55. A: AP pelvis. B: AP lumbar spine. C: Lateral lumbar spine.

Additional Views

For follow-up flexion–extension exams, a neutral lateral is not needed. These extra images start to incur a large radiation dose for little extra information and are not encouraged. Oblique views allow visualization of the facet joints and can show pars defects, although these are often better seen on the lateral view. The flexion–extension views are to look for instability in the preoperative planning of possible spinal fusion or the postoperative assessment of fusion. The coned-down lateral view of the lumbosacral junction is useful because often this region is oblique on the lateral lumbar spine.

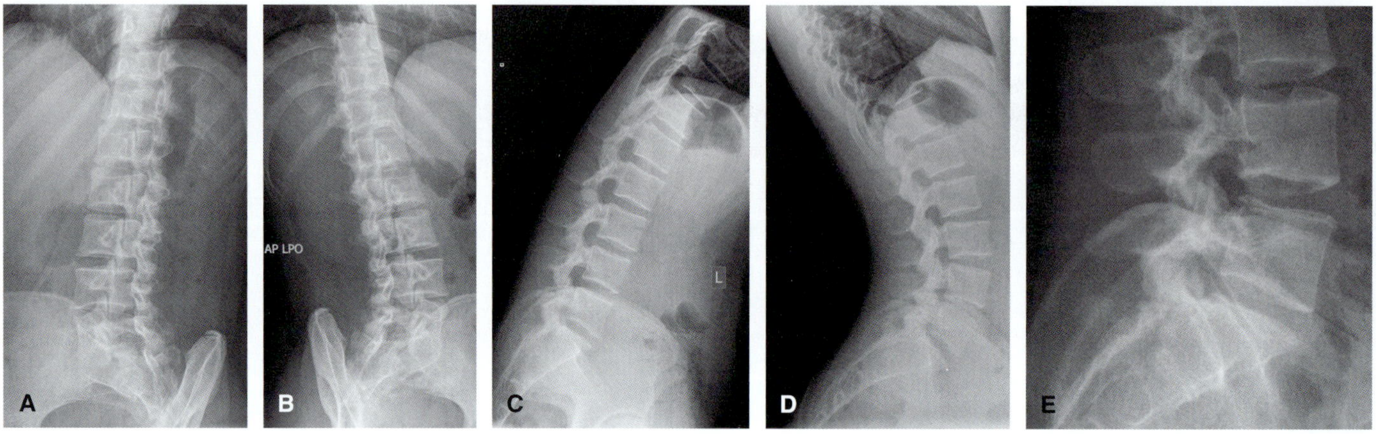

FIGURE 56. A: Right posterior oblique lumbar spine. B: Left posterior oblique lumbar spine. C: Flexion lateral lumbar spine. D: Extension lateral lumbar spine. E: L5–S1 lateral.

SACRUM

Often difficult to see even with good radiographs due to bowel gas and feces. Not usually imaged separately from the pelvis in trauma; can be used to look for lesions affecting the sacral plexus.

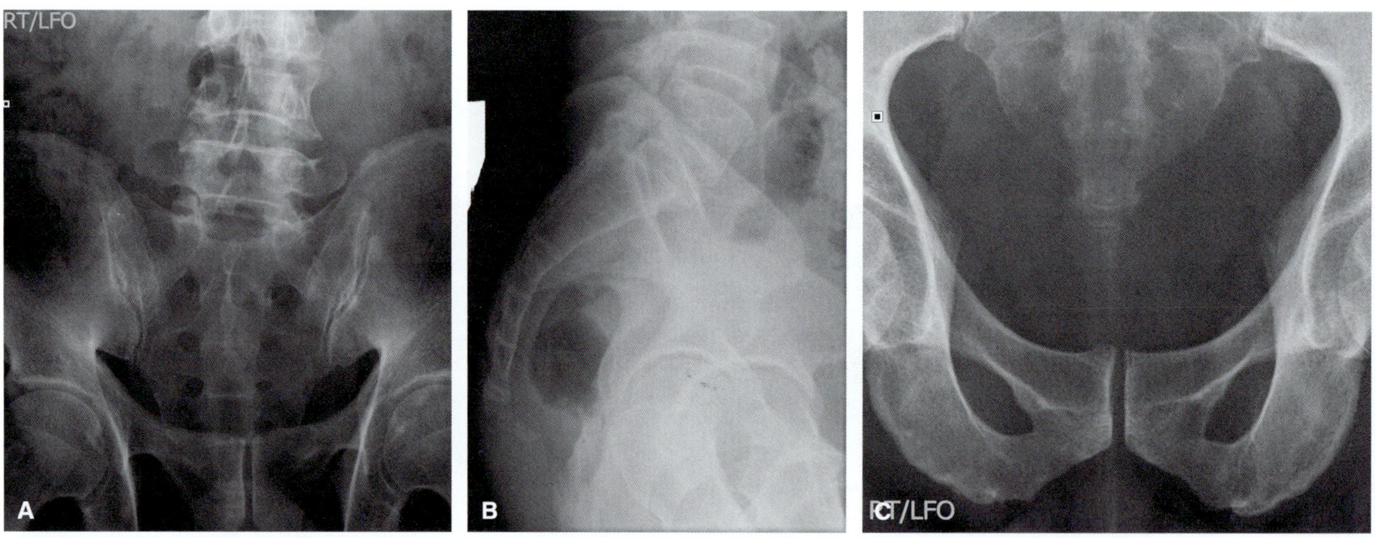

FIGURE 57. A: AP cranial. B: Lateral. C: AP caudal.

COCCYX

Used in cases of coccydynia. The coccyx has a wide variety of shapes and angles and is often inconclusive for the radiation dose used.

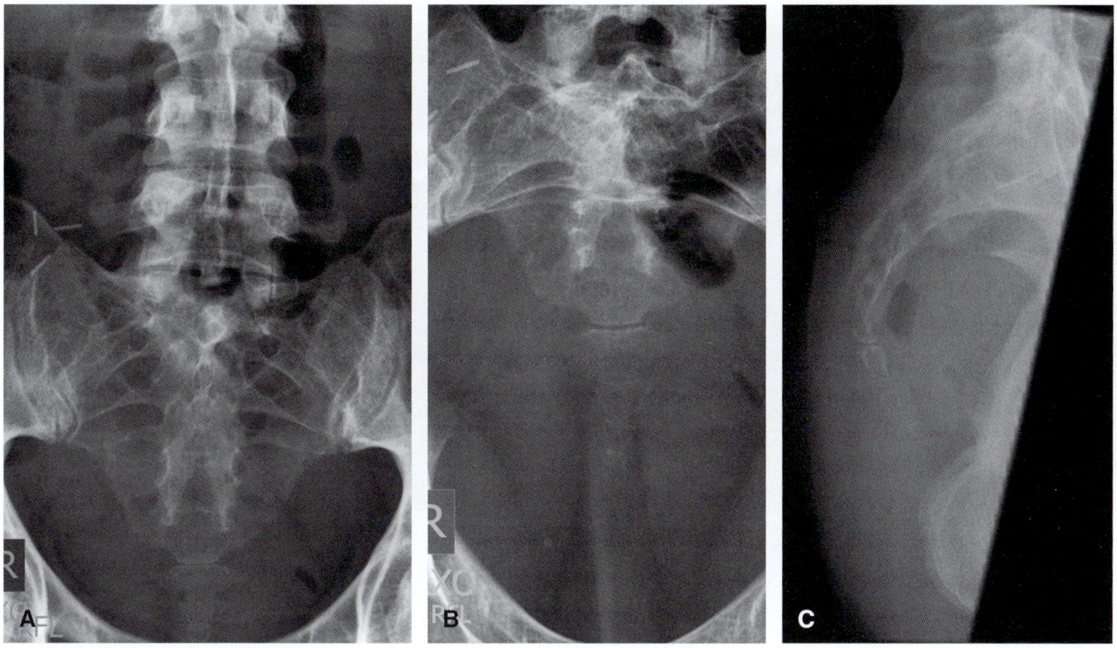

FIGURE 58. A: AP. B: AP caudal. C: Lateral.

SCOLIOSIS SERIES

Used to measure the Cobb angle and look for progression; also used to look for underlying congenital vertebral anomaly.

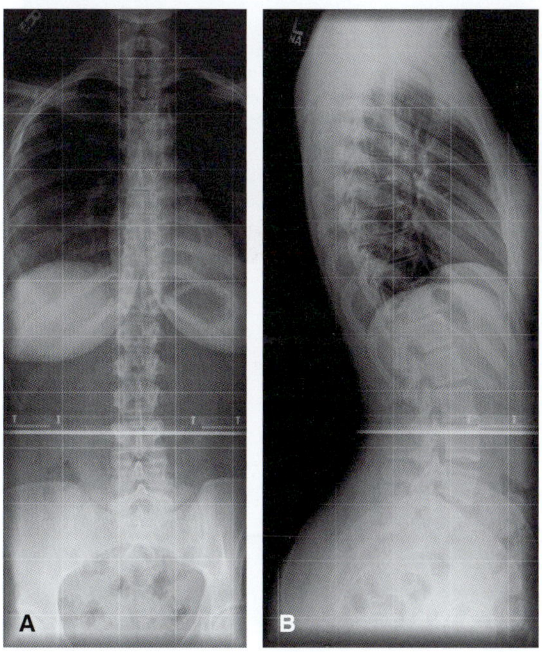

FIGURE 59. A: PA taken weight-bearing. B: Lateral taken weight-bearing.

Additional Views

Views taken erect, leaning to the left and to the right are useful to look for mobile and fixed segments of scoliosis in planning surgery.

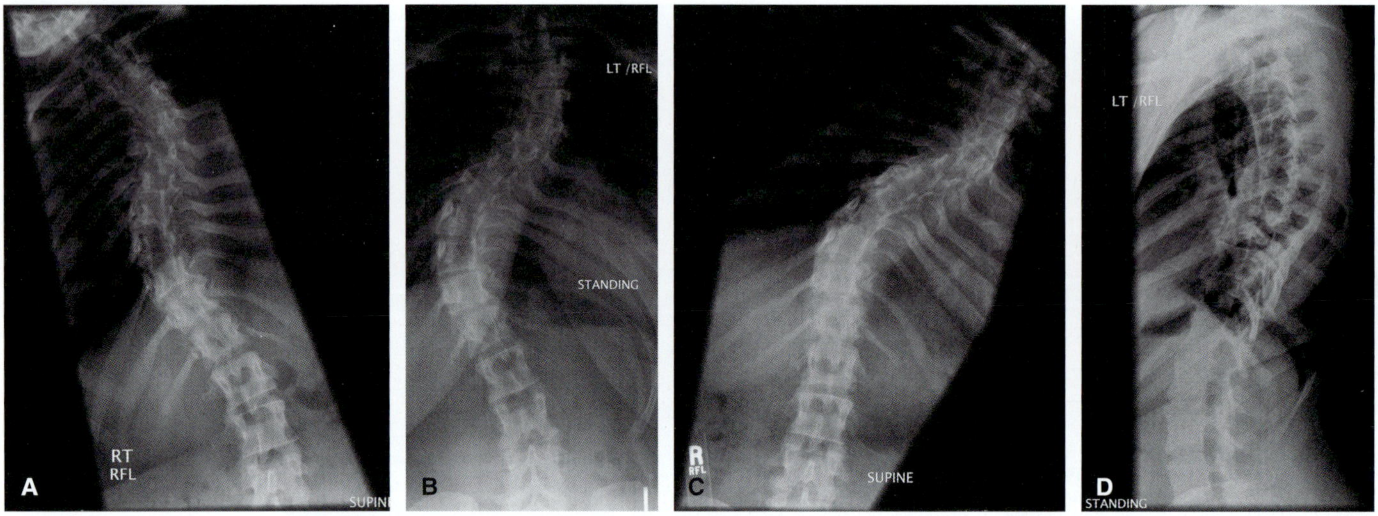

FIGURE 60. A: AP best bend right. B: AP erect. C: AP best bend left. D: Standing Lateral.

MISCELLANEOUS BONE STUDIES

SCAN-O-GRAM

Used to measure leg length. Coned-down views are taken of the iliac crests, hips, knees, and ankles with a ruler behind the patient. The beam being centered on each area of interest will reduce artifact due to parallax.

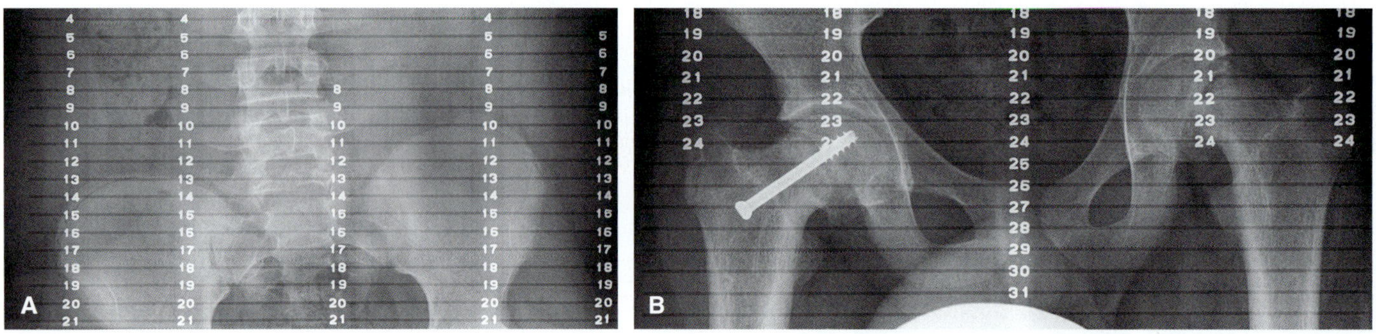

FIGURE 61. A: AP wing of pelvis. B: AP hip joint.

LEG ALIGNMENT—INCLUDES JOINTS FROM HIP TO ANKLE

Patient upright, equal weight in each foot. Both leg alignment and leg length can be assessed on this study if weight-bearing. The weight-bearing line passes from the middle of the femoral head to the middle to the tibial plafond and should pass between the tibial eminences. This determines varus or valgus deformity at the knees. Used for pre- and postoperative assessment of total knee arthroplasty.

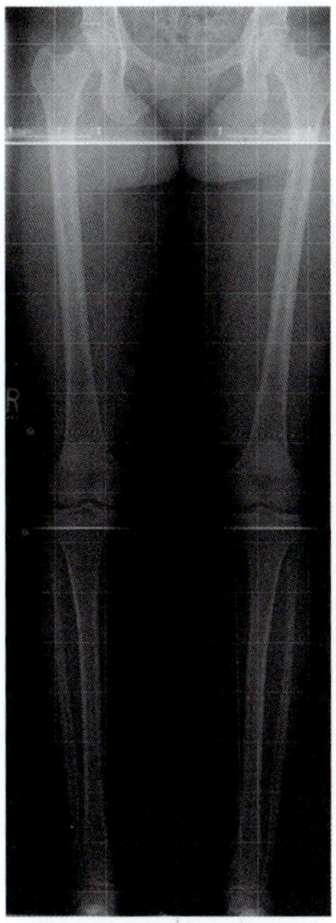

FIGURE 62. AP both legs.

ARTHRITIS JOINT SURVEY

This could include up to; AP/lateral C-spine, AP/lateral T-spine, AP/lateral L-spine, AP bilateral shoulders, AP/lateral bilateral knees, AP pelvis, AP, oblique and lateral bilateral hands (to include wrists), AP/lateral bilateral ankles (include heel on lateral views), AP/oblique bilateral feet. Because this would be a large radiation dose, it is often better to tailor this to the regions of pain.

METASTATIC BONE SURVEY

This varies from one center to another and could include from 5 to 30 images. The most important areas to image are the axial skeleton and the proximal appendicular skeleton. A full survey would include left lateral skull, AP/lateral C-spine, AP/lateral L-spine, AP/lateral bilateral humerus (to include shoulders), AP/lateral bilateral forearms, AP ribs bilaterally, AP/lateral T-spine, AP pelvis, AP/lateral bilateral femurs, AP/lateral bilateral tibia/fibulas. This is likely to be replaced by whole body MRI in the near future.

BONY THORAX

RIBS

For most acute rib injuries, the protocol is a PA erect chest exam to evaluate for pneumothorax. Only patients with pathologic fractures or patients who have undergone a bone scan should be imaged for rib fractures. Legal cases may also require documentation of fracture. It is important to have a "bb" at the site of pain and for the technologist to annotate if the bb is anterior or posterior.

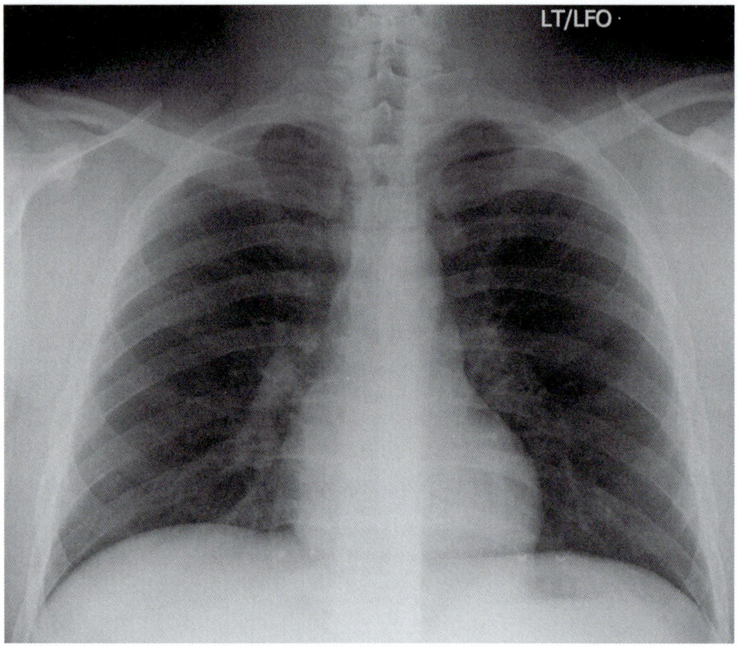

FIGURE 63. PA chest only. If history is acute rib injury.

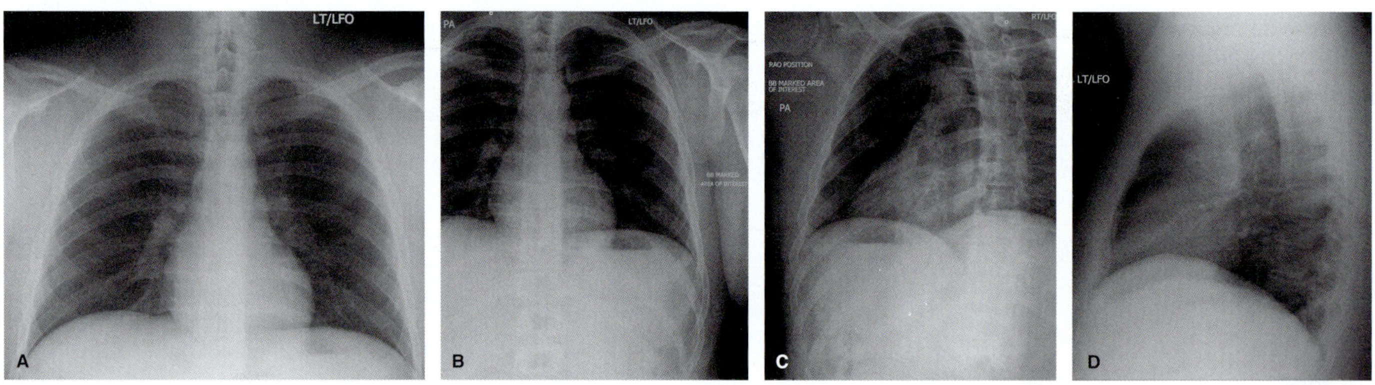

FIGURE 64. Post bone scan or pathologic fractures. A: AP or PA ribs—dependent on site of injury. B, C: Affected side closest to Bucky oblique ribs. D: Lateral Ribs.

STERNUM

Even on good radiographs, visualization of the sternum is limited. The study of choice is CT.

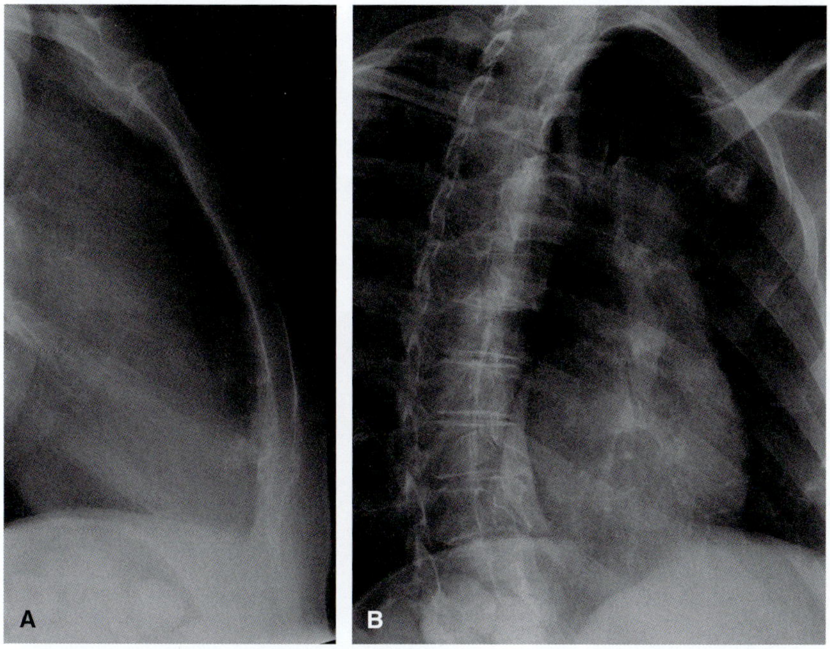

FIGURE 65. A: Lateral. B: Right anterior oblique.

STERNOCLAVICULAR JOINTS

Study of choice is CT. These are very poorly visualized radiographically. A useful sign is a difference in height of the anterior ends of the ribs.

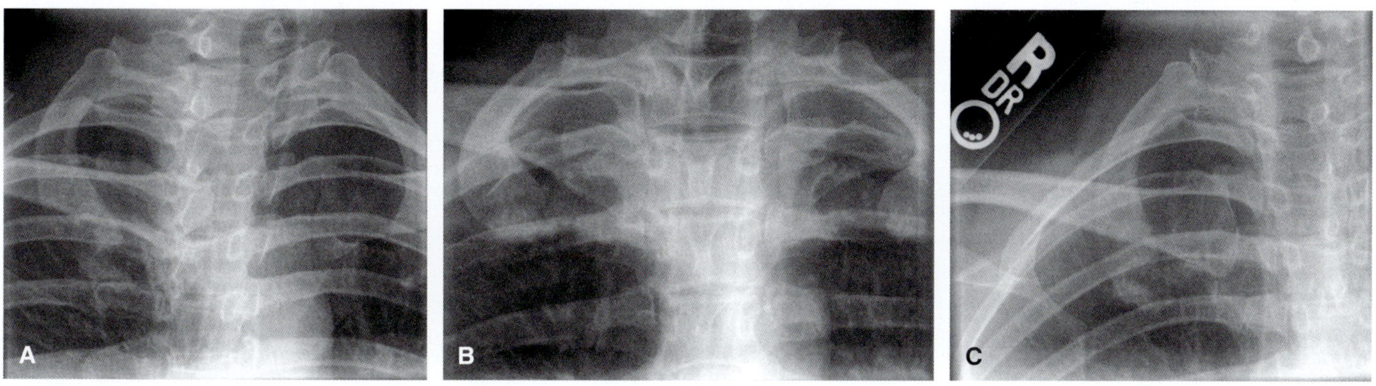

FIGURE 66. A: PA. B: AP axial. C: Coned-down PA.

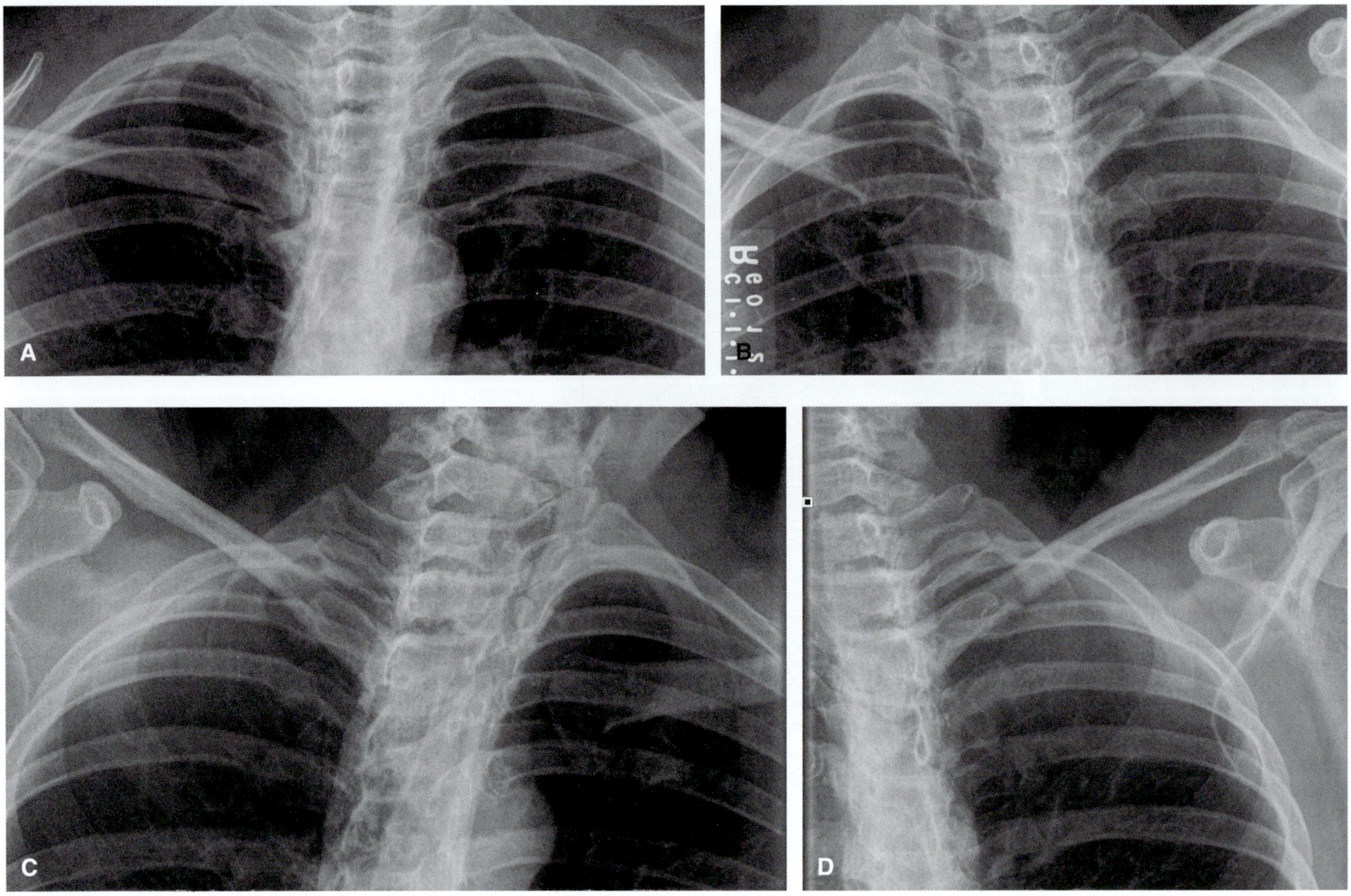

FIGURE 67. A–D: PA and obliques.

Appendix B

JOINT AND SOFT TISSUE INJECTION

Michal Kalli Hose, MD • Anna P. Quan, MD

INTRODUCTION

Joint and soft tissue injections are valuable tools in the treatment of common musculoskeletal conditions. When musculoskeletal pain persists despite use of noninvasive conservative modalities including oral and topical nonsteroidal anti-inflammatory drugs (NSAIDs), activity modification, splinting, ice, heat, and physical therapy, joint injections may provide temporary pain relief and improve function.

INDICATIONS FOR JOINT INJECTIONS

Diagnostic

- Injection of local anesthetic can provide temporary pain relief to allow a more accurate musculoskeletal physical exam (e.g., evaluate for rotator cuff tear vs. weakness secondary to pain).
- Analysis of joint fluid aspirates can assist in the diagnosis of multiple conditions including:
  - Gout/pseudogout (crystal analysis).
  - Septic arthritis (elevated white blood cell [WBC] and/or positive Gram stain and culture).
  - Trauma (hemarthrosis).

Therapeutic

- Decrease pain.
- Increase range of motion (ROM) and function.
- Improve quality of life.

Conditions

- Crystalline arthropathies
- Osteoarthritis
- Inflammatory arthritis
- Bursitis
- Tendonosis
- Ganglion cysts
- Nerve entrapments
- Fasciitis
- Trigger points

CONTRAINDICATIONS

Absolute

- Infection (overlying cellulitis)
- Lack of informed consent
- Allergy to injection medications
- Injection into weight-bearing tendons such as Achilles and patella due to high risk of rupture

Relative

- Brittle or uncontrolled diabetes
- Coagulopathy (safe in patients with international normalized ratio [INR] <3.5)
- Previous joint replacement/hardware
- History of avascular necrosis
- History of steroid or hyaluronic acid (HA) flare

SUPPLIES

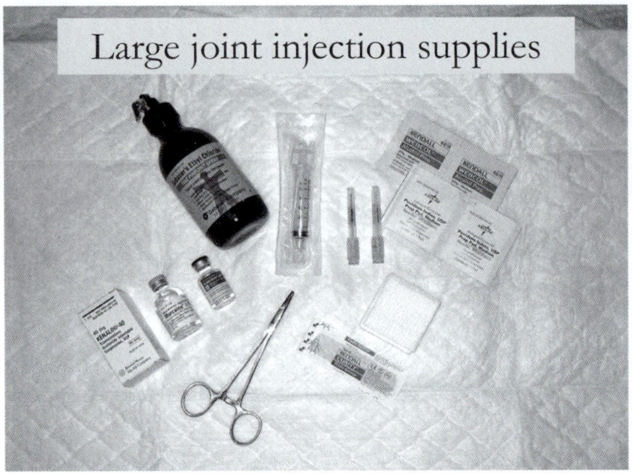

- Nonsterile gloves
- Syringes: 3 to 5 ml, or larger volumes if aspiration is planned (10, 20, 60 ml)
- Needles:
  - 18 gauge for drawing up fluid or anti–stick needle/connector
  - 16 to 18 gauge for large aspirations or HA injections
  - 21 to 22 gauge 1.5 inches standard size for medium to large joints or HA injections
  - 25 gauge 1.5 inches or 25 gauge 5/8 inches standard size for small joints
  - 21- to 22-gauge 3.5-inch spinal needles often needed for ultrasound-guided hip injections and trochanteric bursa injections in large patients
- Betadine × 3 or chlorhexidine swabs × 45 sec
- Alcohol swabs
- Gauze
- Band-Aids
- Topical vapocoolant spray, such as ethyl chloride
- Hemostat clamp

LOCAL ANESTHETIC

- Topical anesthetic can be useful for temporary pain relief or to aid in diagnosis.
- The choice of anesthetic depends on formulary availability and desired duration of action.
- In general, lidocaine has a quick onset of 3 to 5 min with 1- to 2-hr duration, and bupivacaine has a 5-min onset with 3- to 4-hr duration.
- Bupivacaine or lidocaine with epinephrine can be used in certain areas for possible prolonged benefit of the injection but should not be used when injecting digits or smaller joints.

CORTICOSTEROID

- Corticosteroids can reduce inflammation which may decrease local pain and swelling.
- Lower solubility steroids have longer duration of action.
- To avoid suppression of hypothalamic-pituitary-adrenal axis, limit to 3 to 4 injections per year and be especially cautious for those with HIV on protease inhibitors.
- Based on in vitro, animal, and radiologic studies, intra-articular (IA) use of local anesthetics and cortisone may have detrimental effects on human articular cartilage and chondrocytes. Although the clinical significance of these studies is unclear, the clinical relationship between local anesthetic exposure and chondrolysis requires further study.

Table 1. Properties of Injectable Corticosteroids

Corticosteroid	Relative Anti-inflammatory Potency	Solubility	Biological Half-life
Hydrocortisone	1	High	8–12 hr
Triamcinolone (Kenalog)	5	Intermediate	12–36 hr
Methylprednisolone (Depo–Medrol)	5	Intermediate	12–36 hr
Betamethasone (Celestone Soluspan)	25	Low/high	26–54 hr
Dexamethasone (Decadron LA)	25	High	26–54 hr

From McNabb JW. *A Practical Guide to Joint & Soft Tissue Injections*. 3rd ed. Philadelphia, PA: Wolters Kluwer; 2015.

Table 2. Equivalent Dosages of Injectable Corticosteroids

Corticosteroid Preparation	Equivalent Dose/Volume
Kenalog	40 mg/mL
Depo-Medrol	40 mg/mL
Celestone Soluspan	6 mg/mL
Decadron LA	8 mg/mL

From McNabb JW. *A Practical Guide to Joint & Soft Tissue Injections*. 3rd ed. Philadelphia, PA: Wolters Kluwer; 2015.

VISCOSUPPLEMENTATION

- Sodium hyaluronate is a glycosaminoglycan found in normal joint fluid.
- In osteoarthritis, the concentration of sodium hyaluronate is lower.
- Synthetic formulations of sodium hyaluronate are derived from rooster combs.
- Available products:
  - Synvisc and Synvisc-One (Genzyme)
  - Gel-One (Zimmer)
  - Hyalgan (Fidia)
  - Supartz FX (Bioventus)
  - Orthovisc (Anika Therapeutics)
  - Euflexxa, previously named Nuflexxa (Savient)
  - Monovisc (Anika Therapeutics)
  - Gel-Syn (Institut Biochimique SA)
  - HYMOVIS (Fidia)
- Lack of high-powered evidence showing therapeutic efficacy
- Consider for patients failing conservative therapy or when corticosteroids are contraindicated.
- Contraindicated in patients with allergies to avian proteins or eggs (those agents with avian proteins).

TECHNIQUE

- The specific techniques for each joint are discussed in each joint section.
- In general, the following techniques should be followed:
  - Identify the anatomic landmarks and mark the entry site with the cap of the needle.
  - Cleanse the area with Betadine/chlorhexidine and alcohol.
  - Spray topical ethyl chloride vapocoolant (if available) to decrease needle entry pain.
  - Insert the needle to the proper depth for the specific injection site.
  - Inject the steroid/analgesic mixture. There should be free flow (without resistance) of the medication.
  - Remove the needle and apply pressure with gauze.
  - Apply a Band-Aid.

COMPLICATIONS

- Major risks of corticosteroid injections include bleeding, infection, tendon rupture, steroid flare, fat pad or soft tissue atrophy, and skin depigmentation.
- Steroid flare (crystal synovitis) is treated with rest, ice, NSAIDs and usually resolves spontaneously after 24 to 36 hr.
- HA flare can also be treated with rest, ice, NSAIDs and usually resolves spontaneously after several days. HA flare can be more drastic than steroid flare, and severe flares may require synovial aspiration and cultures to distinguish between pseudosepsis and true infection.
- The estimated risk of causing septic arthritis from arthrocentesis is low, on the order of 0.01%.

AFTERCARE

- While the local anesthetic is in effect, the patient will have less proprioceptive feedback from the joint, so patients are recommended to rest the injected joint for several hours.
- Educate the patient to monitor for signs or symptoms of infection including fever, erythema, warmth, or increasing pain.
- Ice is an effective modality for pain control following an injection.
- Activities can generally be resumed after 3 to 5 days as tolerated after a cortisone injection. Patients may notice that HA has a longer lag time (1 to 2 wk) before pain relief is noted.
- Encourage the patient to keep a pain and activity journal to record duration of pain relief and improved function. This information helps the patients make a personalized informed decision of whether to repeat injection therapy in the future.

INFORMED CONSENT

- Every invasive procedure (including joint aspirations or injections) should include a detailed informed consent.
- Lawsuits have occurred over complications to joint injections, and, in these situations, having an informed consent signed and kept with the patient's medical record is of utmost importance. Alternatives include careful informed consent discussed with the patient or guardians and documented in the record.
- The informed consent includes documentation that the patient is competent to make decisions and that a discussion of the risks and benefits of an injection have been reviewed.

BILLING/CODING

- Current Procedural Terminology (CPT) codes should be used to accurately assign the proper codes for the procedures performed.
- ICD10 codes and CPT codes will be listed with each joint or soft tissue injection discussed.

BIBLIOGRAPHY

- Agur AM, Dalley AF. *Grant's Atlast of Anatomy*. 12th ed. Philadelphia, PA: Lippincott Williams & Wilkins; 2009.
- Bannuru RR, Schmid CH, Kent DM, et al. Comparative effectiveness of pharmacologic interventions for knee osteoarthritis: a systematic review and network meta-analysis. *Ann Intern Med*. 2015;162(1):46–54.
- Blair B, Rokito AS, Cuomo F, et al. Efficacy of injections of corticosteroids for subacromial impingement syndrome. *J Bone Joint Surg Am*. 1996;78(11):1685–1689.
- Bowman S, Awad ME, Hamrick MW, et al. Recent advances in hyaluronic acid based therapy for osteoarthritis. *Clin Transi Med*. 2018;7(1):6.
- Brown GA. AAOS clinical practice guideline: treatment of osteoarthritis of the knee: evidence-based guideline, 2nd edition. *J Am Acad Orthop Surg*. 2013;21(9):577–579.
- Buchbinder R, Green S, Youd JM. Corticosteroid injections for shoulder pain. *Cochrane Database Syst Rev*. 2003;(1):CD004016.
- Cardone DA, Tallia AF. Diagnostic and therapeutic injection of the elbow region. *Am Fam Physician*. 2002;66(11):2097–2100.
- Cardone DA, Tallia A. Diagnostic and therapeutic injection of the hip and knee. *Am Fam Physician*. 2003;67(10):2147–2152.
- Cardone DA, Tallia A. Joint and soft tissue injection. *Am Fam Physician*. 2002;66(2):283–288.
- Carolina Orthopaedic & Sports Medicine Center: http://www.orthogastonia.com
- Esenyel C, Demirhan M, Esenyel M, et al. Comparison of four different intra-articular injection sites in the knee: a cadaver study. *Knee Surg Sports Traumatol Arthrosc*. 2007;15(5):573–577.
- Griffin LY, ed. *Essentials of Musculoskeletal Care*. 3rd ed. Rosemont, IL: American Academy of Orthopaedic Surgeons; 2005.
- Hochberg MC, Altman RD, April KT, et al. American College of Rheumatology 2012 recommendations for the use of nonpharmacologic and pharmacologic therapies in osteoarthritis of the hand, hip, and knee. *Arthritis Care Res (Hoboken)*. 2012;64(4):465–474.
- Jackson DW, Evans N, Thomas B. Accuracy of needle placement into the intra-articular space of the knee. *J Bone Joint Surgery Am*. 2002;84-A(9):1522–1527.
- Kang MN, Rizio L, Prybicien M, et al. The accuracy of subacromial corticosteroid injections: a comparison of multiple methods. *J Shoulder Elbow Surg*. 2008;17(Suppl 1):61S–66S.
- Lievense A, Bierma-Zeinstra S, Schouten B, et al. Prognosis of trochanteric pain in primary care. *Br J Gen Pract*. 2005;55(512):199–204.
- Luc M, Pham T, Chagnaud C, et al. Placement of intra-articular injection verified by the backflow technique. *Osteoarthritis Cartilage*. 2006;14(7):714–716.
- McNabb JW. *A Practical Guide to Joint & Soft Tissue Injection & Aspiration*. Philadelphia, PA: Lippincott Williams & Wilkins; 2005.
- Piper SL, Kramer JD, Kim HT, et al. Effects of local anesthetics on articular cartilage. *Am J Sports Med*. 2011;39(10):2245–2253.
- Safran MR, McKeag DB, Van Camp SP. *Manual of Sports Medicine*. Philadelphia, PA: Lippincott-Raven Publishers; 1998.
- Saunders S. *Injection Techniques in Orthopaedic and Sports Medicine*. 2nd ed. Philadelphia, PA: WB Saunders; 2002.
- Shbeeb MI, O'Duffy JD, Michet CJ Jr, et al. Evaluation of glucocorticosteroid injection for the treatment of trochanteric bursitis. *J Rheumatol*. 1996;23(12):2104–2106.
- Smidt N, vad der Windt DA, Assendelft WJ, et al. Corticosteroid injections, physiotherapy, or a wait-and-see policy for lateral epicondylitis: a randomised controlled trial. *Lancet*. 2002;359(9307):657–662.
- Stephens MB, Beutler AI, O'Connor FG. Musculoskeletal injections: a review of the evidence. *Am Fam Physician*. 2008;78(8):971–976.
- Tallia AF, Cardone DA. Diagnostic and therapeutic injection of the ankle and foot. *Am Fam Physician*. 2003;68(7):1356–1362.
- Tallia AF, Cardone DA. Diagnostic and therapeutic injection of the shoulder region. *Am Fam Physician*. 2003;67(6):1271–1278.
- Tallia AF, Cardone DA. Diagnostic and therapeutic injection of the wrist and hand region. *Am Fam Physician*. 2003;67(4):745–750.
- Zuber T. Knee joint aspiration and injection. *Am Fam Physician*. 2002;66(8):1497–1500, 1503–1504, 1507.

CREDITS LIST

Figures 2, 13, 14, 28, 32, and 33 from McNabb JW. *A Practical Guide to Joint & Soft Tissue Injection & Aspiration: An Illustrated Text for Primary Care Providers*. 2nd ed. Philadelphia, PA: Lippincott Williams & Wilkins; 2010.
Figures 3, 7, 17, 18, 29, 36, 41, 42, and 49 from McNabb JW. *A Practical Guide to Joint & Soft Tissue Injection & Aspiration*. Philadelphia, PA: Lippincott Williams & Wilkins; 2005.
Figures 6, 21, 27, and 34 from Agur AMR, Dalley AF. *Grant's Atlas of Anatomy*. 14th ed. Philadelphia, PA: Wolters Kluwer; 2017.
Figures 8, 30, 31, 35, and 37 from McNabb JW. *A Practical Guide to Joint & Soft Tissue Injections*. 3rd ed. Philadelphia, PA: Wolters Kluwer; 2015.
Figure 9 from Wiesel SW, Williams GR Jr, Ramsey ML, et al. *Operative Techniques in Shoulder and Elbow Surgery*. 2nd ed. Philadelphia, PA: Wolters Kluwer; 2016.
Figure 11 from Moore KL, Dalley AF II, Agur AMR. *Clinically Oriented Anatomy*. 8th ed. Philadelphia, PA: Wolters Kluwer; 2017.
Figure 19 from Penny SM. *Introduction to Sonography and Patient Care*. Philadelphia, PA: Wolters Kluwer; 2016.
Figure 23 from Detton AJ. *Grant's Dissector*. 16th ed. Philadelphia, PA: Wolters Kluwer; 2017.
Figures 25 and 47 from Anderson MK. *Foundations of Athletic Training: Prevention, Assessment, and Management*. 6th ed. Philadelphia, PA: Wolters Kluwer; 2017.
Figure 38 from McConnell T, Hull K. *Human Form, Human Function: Essentials of Anatomy & Physiology*. Philadelphia, PA: Lippincott Williams & Wilkins; 2011.
Figure 45 from Bucci C. *Condition-Specific Massage Therapy*. Baltimore, MD: Wolters Kluwer Health/Lippincott Williams & Wilkins; 2012.

TRIGGER POINT INJECTION

INDICATIONS

- Trigger points occur due to focal areas of muscular pain and spasm and often involve the back muscles.
- There is no clear evidence of benefit for trigger point injections, but anecdotally, some patients report reduced pain after trigger point injections.
- There are real risks of pneumothorax with legal actions taken against providers involved.
- ICD10:
  - G44.229 Chronic tension-type headache, not intractable
  - M54.2 Cervicalgia
  - M79.0 Rheumatism, unspecified
  - M79.7 Fibromyalgia

ANATOMY

- The anatomy depends on the location of the trigger point injection.
- The injection is performed over the tender nodule, which is usually in the muscles surrounding the scapula.

SUPPLIES
- Gloves
- Betadine or chlorhexidine and alcohol swabs
- 3-mL syringe with 25-gauge 5/8- to 1-inch needle
- 1 mL 1% lidocaine
- ½ mL (20 mg) Kenalog or equivalent (optional)
- Ethyl chloride
- Gauze
- Band-Aid

TECHNIQUE
- Palpate the tender nodule and mark with needle cap.
- Cleanse the skin with alcohol swab and then Betadine × 3 or chlorhexidine × 45 sec.
- Apply ethyl chloride until skin turns white.
- Injection site is directly into the nodule.
- A fanning technique can be used to disperse the fluid in various directions, which can be helpful in large nodules.

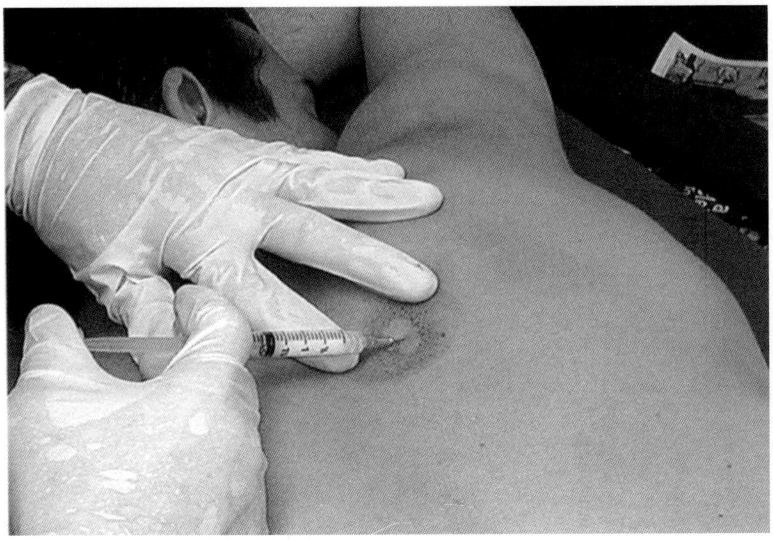

- Remove needle and apply pressure with gauze, gently massaging material.
- Apply Band-Aid.

AFTERCARE
- Instruct patient that the area may be numb for several hours after the procedure and that pain may be present for several days.
- Instruct patient that the cortisone usually takes effect within 72 hr.
- Instruct patient to return to your office if they develop redness, swelling, or increased pain at the injection site.

CPT CODE
- 20552 Injection(s); single or Multiple trigger point(s), 1 or 2 muscles
- 20553 Injection(s); single or Multiple Trigger Point(s), 3 or more muscles

SUBACROMIAL INJECTION

INDICATIONS
- Subacromial injections are useful for diagnostic and therapeutic purposes.
- Any condition along the spectrum of rotator cuff diseases that cause subacromial pain syndrome may respond to corticosteroid injection.
- Injections are indicated once conservative therapy (activity modification, NSAIDS, physical therapy) has failed; however, in some cases, an injection given prior to physical therapy can allow patients to perform their therapy better and with less pain.
- Subacromial corticosteroid injection provides short-term pain relief that is greater than placebo and at least equal to NSAID therapy – evidence rating B.
- ICD10:
  - S43.42 Sprain of rotator cuff capsule
  - S46.0 Injury of muscle(s) and tendon(s) of the rotator cuff of shoulder
  - M75.10 Unspecified rotator cuff tear or rupture, not specified as traumatic
  - M75.40 Impingement syndrome of unspecified shoulder

ANATOMY
- The subacromial space is bordered superiorly by the coracoacromial ligament stretching between the coracoid process and acromion.
- The contents of the subacromial space include the subacromial bursa, supraspinatus tendon, and tendon of the long head of the biceps.

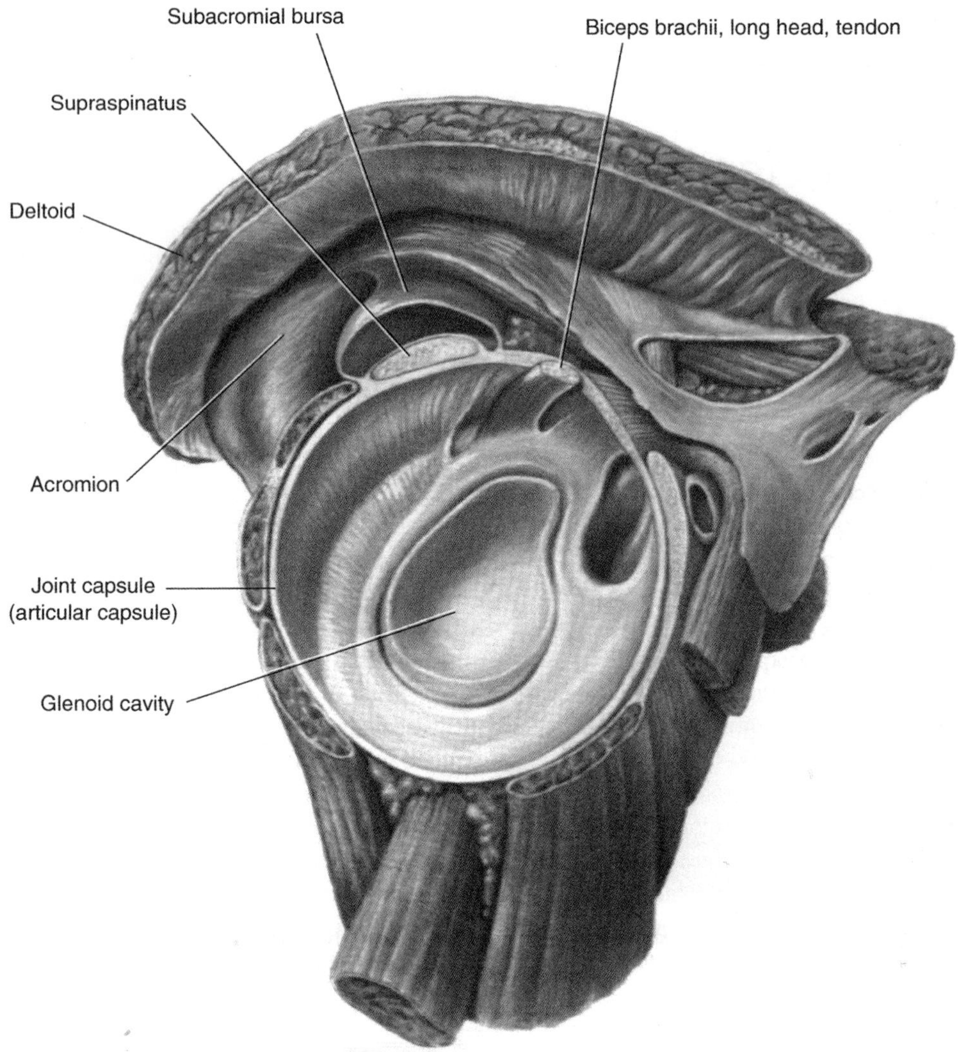

SUPPLIES
- Gloves
- Betadine/chlorhexidine and alcohol swabs
- 5-mL syringe with 22-gauge or 25-gauge 1½-inch needle
- 4-mL anesthetic (can combine 2 mL 1% lidocaine and 2 mL 0.25% bupivacaine [Marcaine])
- 1 mL (40 mg) Kenalog or equivalent
- Ethyl chloride
- Gauze
- Band-Aid

TECHNIQUE
- There are three approaches to the subacromial injection: anterior, lateral, and posterolateral.
- Given the increased risk of pneumothorax with the anterior approach, we do not recommend this approach.
- Determine which approach you will use and mark the area with the needle cap.
- Lateral approach: The lateral edge of the acromion is palpated:
  - Cleanse the skin with alcohol swab and then Betadine × 3 or chlorhexidine × 45 sec.
  - Apply ethyl chloride until the skin turns white.
  - The needle is inserted at the midpoint of the acromion and angled slightly upward under the acromion to full length (up to hub of needle).

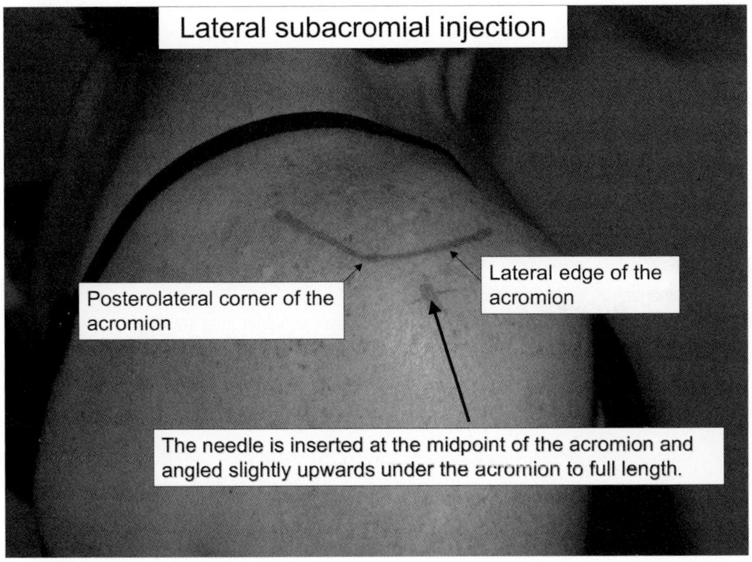

- Posterolateral approach: The distal, lateral, and posterior edges of the acromion are palpated, and the soft spot 1 cm below the posterolateral corner is marked:
  - Cleanse the skin with alcohol swab and then Betadine × 3 or chlorhexidine × 45 sec.
  - Apply ethyl chloride until the skin turns white.
  - The needle is inserted 1 cm inferior to the posterolateral edge of the acromion. The needle is directed toward the opposite nipple (coracoid).

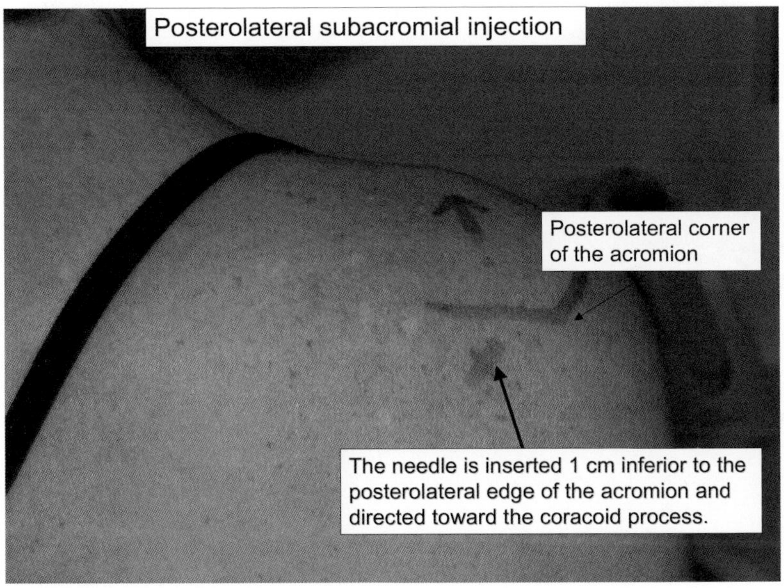

- Never inject under pressure—steroid injected directly into a tendon may cause tendon rupture.
- Remove needle and apply pressure with gauze.
- Apply Band-Aid.
- Have patient perform Codman exercises or arm swings to disperse the fluid through the bursa.

AFTERCARE
- Instruct patient that the shoulder may be numb for several hours after the procedure and that pain may be present for several days.
- Instruct patient that the cortisone usually takes effect within 72 hr.
- After 5 to 7 days, the patient can resume his or her regular activity, and you should recommend starting ROM and rotator cuff strengthening exercises.
- Instruct patient to return to your office if they develop redness, swelling, or increased pain at the injection site.

CPT CODE
- 20610 Arthrocentesis, aspiration and/or injection; major joint or bursa (e.g., shoulder, hip, knee, subacromial bursa); without ultrasound guidance
- 20611 Arthrocentesis, aspiration and/or injection; major joint or bursa (e.g., shoulder, hip, knee, subacromial bursa); with ultrasound guidance, with permanent recording and reporting

GLENOHUMERAL JOINT INJECTION

INDICATIONS

- Glenohumeral injections are useful for patients with shoulder pain secondary to osteoarthritis or rheumatoid arthritis.
- Glenohumeral injections can aid in improving ROM with physical therapy for patients with adhesive capsulitis or frozen shoulder.
- Injections are indicated once conservative therapy (activity modification, NSAIDS, physical therapy) has failed.
- ICD10:
  - M19.019 Primary osteoarthritis, shoulder
  - M19.219 Secondary osteoarthritis, shoulder (rotator cuff arthropathy)
  - M75.00 Adhesive capsulitis of unspecified shoulder

ANATOMY

- The glenohumeral joint is a ball and socket joint composed of the clavicle, scapula, and humerus.
- The glenoid cavity is very shallow but contains a lip of fibrous tissue called the glenoid labrum, which deepens the glenoid and increases shoulder joint stability.

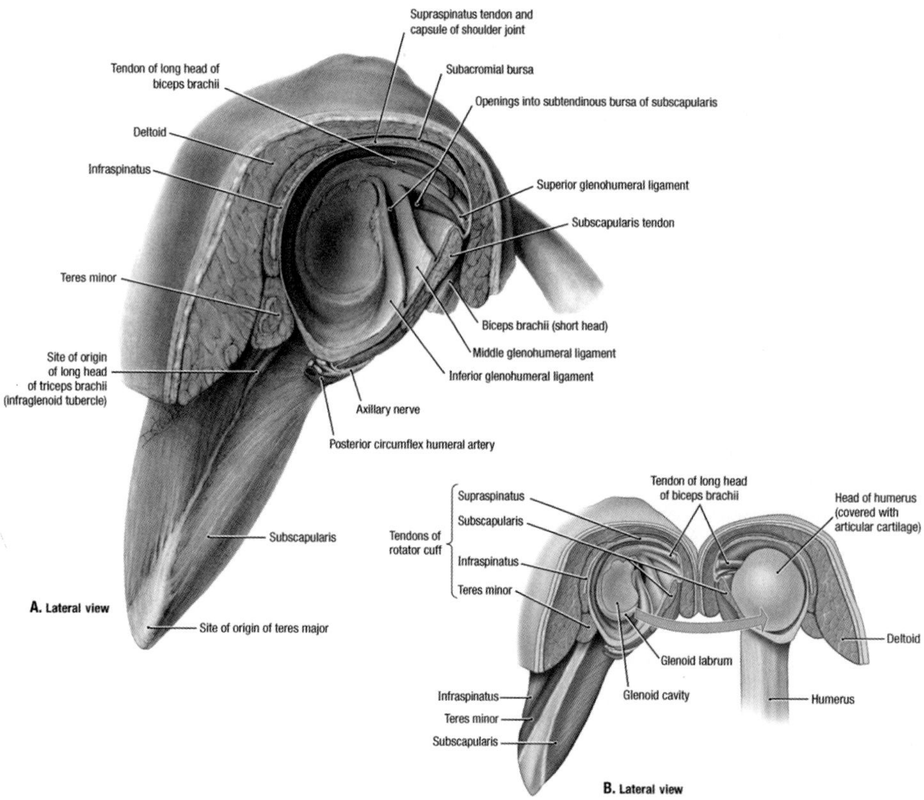

A. Lateral view

B. Lateral view

SUPPLIES

- Gloves
- Betadine/chlorhexidine and alcohol swabs
- 3-mL syringe with 22-gauge or 25-gauge 1½-inch needle
- 1 to 2 mL anesthetic
- 1 mL (40 mg) Kenalog or equivalent
- Ethyl chloride
- Gauze
- Band-Aid

TECHNIQUE

- The glenohumeral joint can be approached from the anterior or posterior direction.
- The posterior approach is preferable because both subacromial and glenohumeral injections can be done through one needle stick.
- Posterior approach: The distal, lateral, and posterior edges of the acromion are palpated, and the soft spot 1 cm below the posterolateral corner is marked with the needle cap:
  - Cleanse the skin with alcohol swab and then Betadine × 3 or chlorhexidine × 45 sec.
  - If available, have an assistant distract (pull down) and externally rotate the arm.
  - Apply ethyl chloride until the skin turns white.
  - The needle is inserted just inferior to the posterolateral edge of the acromion. The needle is directed anteriorly and may need to be walked into the joint.
  - Accuracy can be significantly improved with ultrasound guidance.

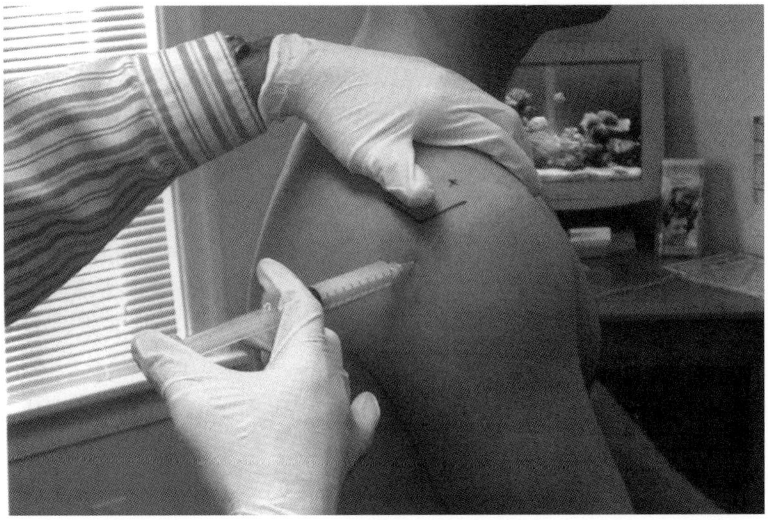

- Anterior approach: The head of the humerus is palpated and the joint space determined and marked with the needle cap:
  - The needle should be placed just medial to the head of the humerus and 1 cm lateral to the coracoid process. The needle is directed posteriorly and slightly superiorly and laterally. If the needle hits against bone, it should be pulled back and redirected at a slightly different angle.

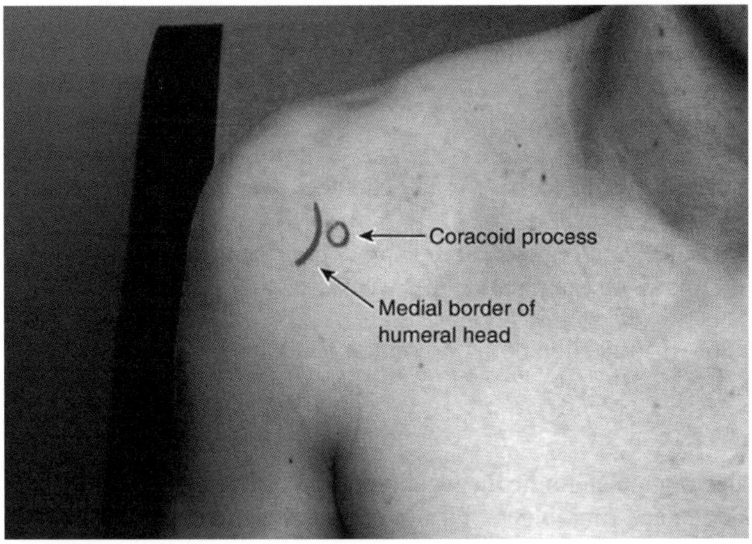

- Never inject under pressure—steroid injected directly into a tendon may cause tendon rupture.
- Remove needle and apply pressure with gauze.
- Apply Band-Aid.
- Have patient perform Codman exercises or arm swings to disperse the fluid through the glenohumeral joint.

AFTERCARE
- Instruct patient that the shoulder may be numb for several hours after the procedure and that pain may be present for several days.
- Instruct patient that the cortisone usually takes effect within 72 hr.
- After 5 to 7 days, the patient can resume his or her regular activity.
- Instruct patient to return to your office if they develop redness, swelling, or increased pain at the injection site.

CPT CODE
- 20610 Arthrocentesis, aspiration and/or injection; major joint or bursa (e.g., shoulder, hip, knee, subacromial bursa); without ultrasound guidance
- 20611 Arthrocentesis, aspiration and/or injection; major joint or bursa (e.g., shoulder, hip, knee, subacromial bursa); with ultrasound guidance, with permanent recording and reporting

ACROMIOCLAVICULAR JOINT INJECTION

INDICATIONS
- Acromioclavicular (AC) joint injections are indicated for patients with shoulder pain due to pathology of the AC joint.
- Injections are indicated once conservative therapy (activity modification, NSAIDS) has failed.
- ICD10:
  - M25.519 Pain in unspecified shoulder
  - M19.019 Primary osteoarthritis, unspecified shoulder

ANATOMY

- The AC joint can be palpated as a narrow indentation at the distal end of the clavicle, about one thumb's width medial to the lateral edge of the acromion.
- The joint line runs obliquely medially at approximately a 20-degree angle.

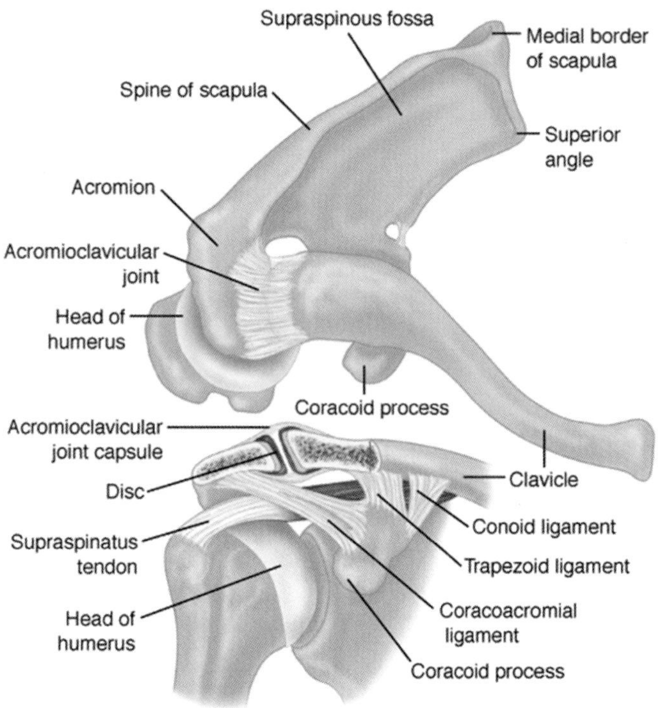

SUPPLIES

- Gloves
- Betadine/chlorhexidine and alcohol swabs
- 3-mL syringe with 25-gauge 5/8- to 1-inch needle
- ½ mL 1% lidocaine
- ½ mL (20 mg) Kenalog or equivalent
- Ethyl chloride
- Gauze
- Band-Aid

TECHNIQUE

- Palpate the depression of the AC joint at the distal clavicle and mark it with the needle cap.
- Cleanse the skin with alcohol swab and then Betadine × 3 or chlorhexidine × 45 sec.
- Apply ethyl chloride until skin turns white.
- Insert the needle at a 15- to 20-degree angle (needle pointed more medially).

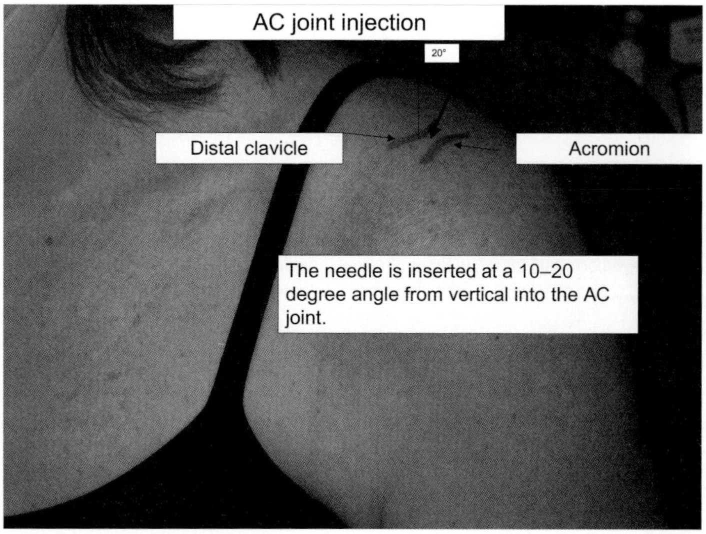

- Viewing the x-rays prior to injection can help determine the exact angle of the AC joint. Ultrasound guidance will dramatically help with accuracy and reduce pain of the injection.
- Inject the fluid into the joint.
- Remove needle and apply pressure with gauze.
- Apply Band-Aid.

AFTERCARE
- Instruct patient that the shoulder may be numb for several hours after the procedure and that pain may be present for several days.
- Instruct patient that the cortisone usually takes effect within 72 hr.
- Instruct patient to return to your office if he or she develops redness, swelling, or increased pain at the injection site.
- Avoid repetitive or heavy overhead lifting.

CPT CODE
- 20600 Arthrocentesis, aspiration and/or injection; small joint or bursa (e.g., fingers, toes); without ultrasound guidance
- 20604 Arthrocentesis, aspiration and/or injection; small joint or bursa (e.g., fingers, toes); with ultrasound guidance, with permanent recording and reporting

ELBOW JOINT INJECTION

INDICATIONS
- Elbow injections are useful for the treatment of elbow pain due to arthritis from either trauma, osteoarthritis, or rheumatoid arthritis.
- Injections are indicated once conservative therapy (activity modification, NSAIDS, physical therapy) has failed.
- ICD10:
  - M25.529 Pain in unspecified elbow
  - M19.029 Primary osteoarthritis, unspecified elbow
  - M19.229 Secondary osteoarthritis, unspecified elbow

ANATOMY
- The elbow joint is composed of the ulnohumeral, radiocapitellar, and proximal radioulnar joints.
- The elbow joint can be approached via the triangle formed by the lateral olecranon, head of the radius, and lateral epicondyle.

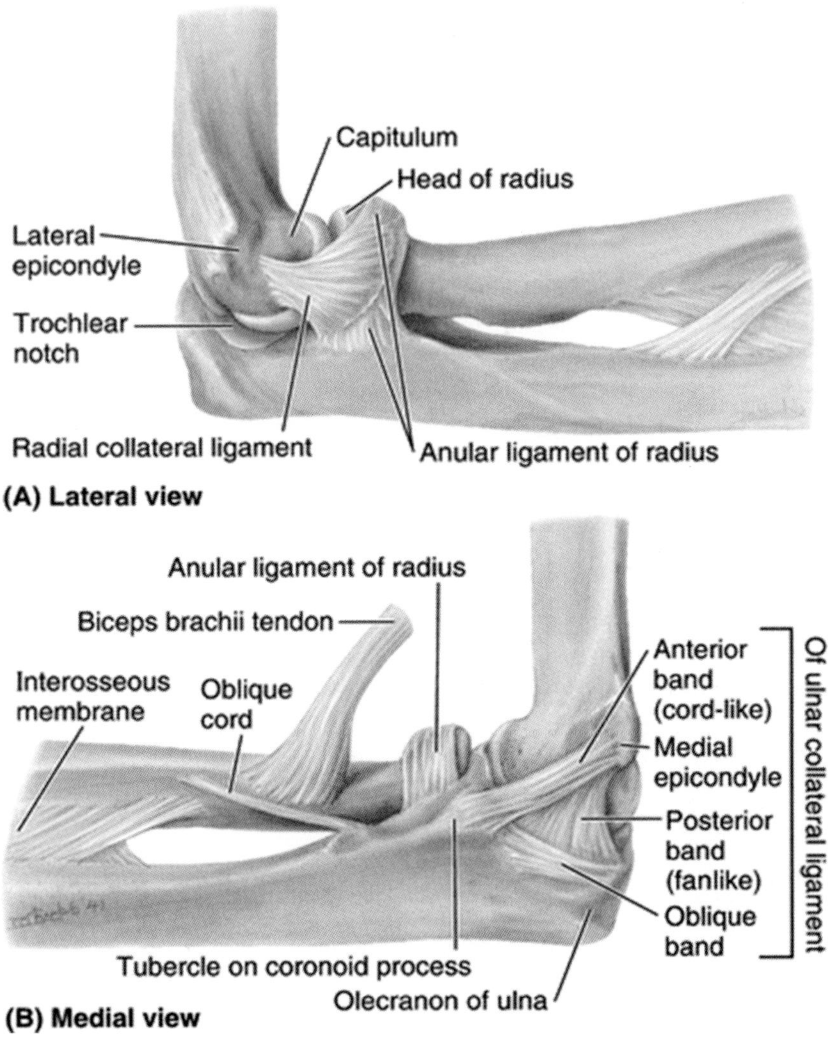

(A) Lateral view

(B) Medial view

SUPPLIES
- Gloves
- Betadine/chlorhexidine and alcohol swabs
- 3-mL syringe with 25-gauge 1-inch needle
- 5- to 10-mL syringe with 20-gauge or 22-gauge needle if aspirating
- 1 mL 1% lidocaine without epinephrine
- ½ mL (20 mg) Kenalog or equivalent
- Ethyl chloride
- Gauze
- Band-Aid

TECHNIQUE
- Place the patient's arm on the table at a 45-degree angle.
- Mark the soft depression in the center of the triangle formed by the lateral olecranon, head of the radius, and lateral epicondyle with the needle cap.
- Cleanse the skin with alcohol swab and then Betadine × 3 or chlorhexidine × 45 sec.
- Apply ethyl chloride until the skin turns white.
- The needle is inserted into the elbow joint between the lateral epicondyle and the radial head.

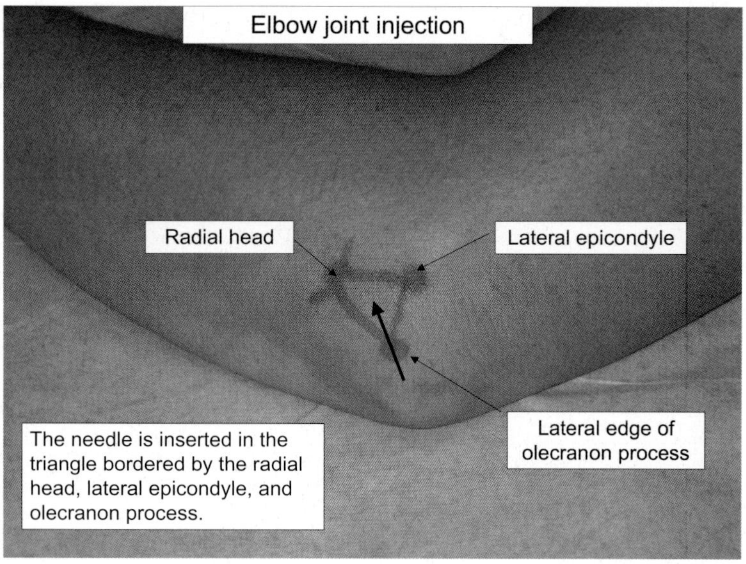

- If aspirating, remove as much fluid as possible and then stabilize the needle in the joint, twist off the syringe, and place the 3-mL syringe containing cortisone mixture on the needle.
- Inject the fluid into the joint.
- Remove needle and apply pressure with gauze.
- Apply Band-Aid.
- Instruct the patient to perform flexion/extension ROM exercises to disperse the fluid within the joint.

AFTERCARE
- Instruct patient that the elbow may be numb for several hours after the procedure and that pain may be present for several days.
- Instruct patient that the cortisone usually takes effect within 72 hr.
- After 3 to 5 days, the patient can resume his or her regular activity.
- Instruct patient to return to your office if they develop redness, swelling, or increased pain at the injection site.

CPT CODE
- 20605 Arthrocentesis, aspiration and/or injection; intermediate joint or bursa or ganglion cyst (e.g., temporomandibular, acromioclavicular, wrist, elbow or ankle, olecranon bursa); without ultrasound guidance
- 20606 Arthrocentesis, aspiration and/or injection; intermediate joint or bursa or ganglion cyst (e.g., temporomandibular, acromioclavicular, wrist, elbow or ankle, olecranon bursa); with ultrasound guidance, with permanent recording and reporting

EPICONDYLITIS INJECTION

INDICATIONS
- Epicondylitis injections are indicated for the treatment of lateral (tennis elbow) or medial (golfer's elbow) epicondylitis.
- Lateral epicondylitis injections are very common in primary care.
- Injections are indicated once conservative therapy (activity modification, NSAIDS, splinting, physical therapy) has failed.
- Corticosteroid injection reduces short-term (<6 wk) symptoms from lateral epicondylitis, but physical therapy is superior to steroid injection after 6 wk:
  - Evidence rating A
- ICD10:
  - M77.10 Lateral epicondylitis, unspecified elbow
  - M77.00 Medial epicondylitis, unspecified elbow

ANATOMY

- The origin of the common extensor tendon is at the lateral epicondyle.

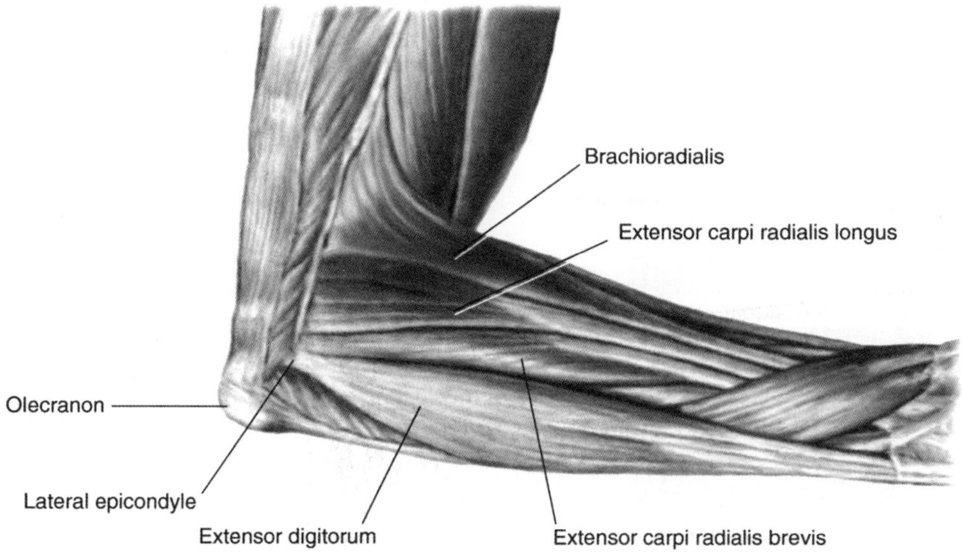

- The origin of the common flexor tendon is at the medial epicondyle.
- The epicondyles are very superficial, which increases the risk of skin depigmentation and atrophy with cortisone injections.

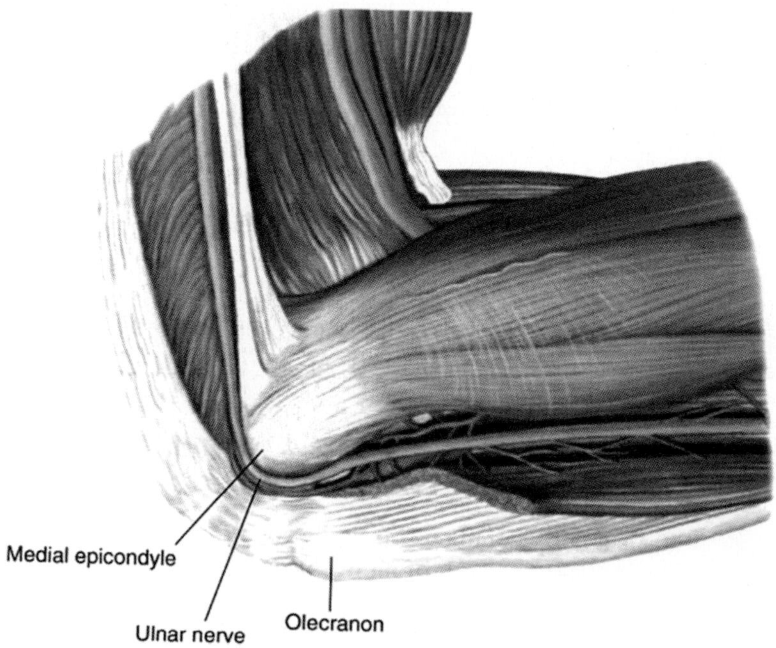

SUPPLIES

- Gloves
- Betadine/chlorhexidine and alcohol swabs
- 3-mL syringe with 25-gauge 5/8- or 1-inch needle
- ½ mL 1% lidocaine without epinephrine
- ½ mL (20 mg) Kenalog or equivalent
- Ethyl chloride
- Gauze
- Band-Aid

TECHNIQUE

- Lateral epicondyle: Place the patient's arm on the table at a 45-degree angle with the lateral elbow facing up:
  - Palpate the area of most tenderness over the epicondyle and mark this with the cap of the needle.
  - Cleanse the skin with alcohol swab and then Betadine × 3 or chlorhexidine × 45 sec.
  - Apply ethyl chloride until the skin turns white.

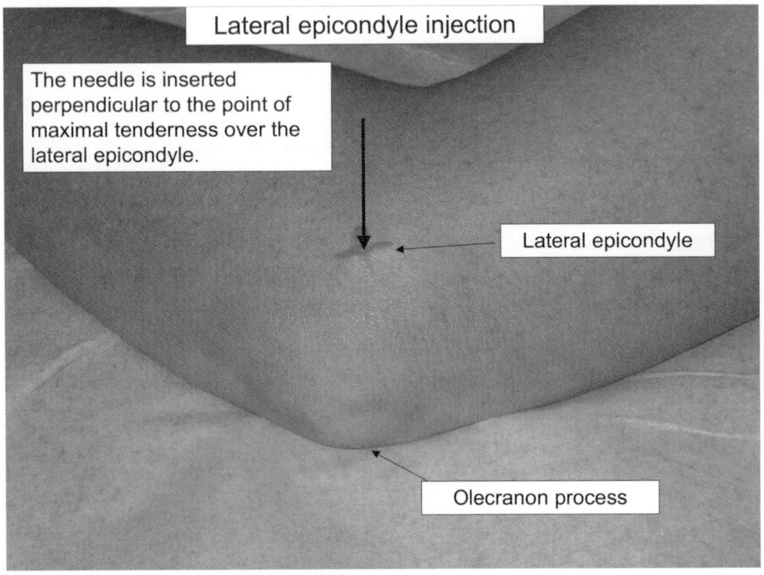

  - The needle is inserted down to the bone of the lateral epicondyle.
  - Inject the fluid into the area. If there is resistance of flow, then back the needle slightly out so the hub of the needle is not against bone and then inject.
  - Take care not to inject cortisone while withdrawing the needle because this superficial tracking of cortisone can increase the risk of skin atrophy and depigmentation.
  - Remove needle and apply pressure with gauze.
  - Apply Band-Aid.
- Medial epicondyle: Place the patient's arm on the table at a 45-degree angle with the medial elbow facing up:
  - Palpate the area of most tenderness over the epicondyle and mark this with the cap of the needle.
  - Cleanse the skin with alcohol swab and then Betadine × 3 or chlorhexidine × 45 sec.
  - Apply ethyl chloride until the skin turns white.
  - The needle is inserted down to the bone of the medial epicondyle.

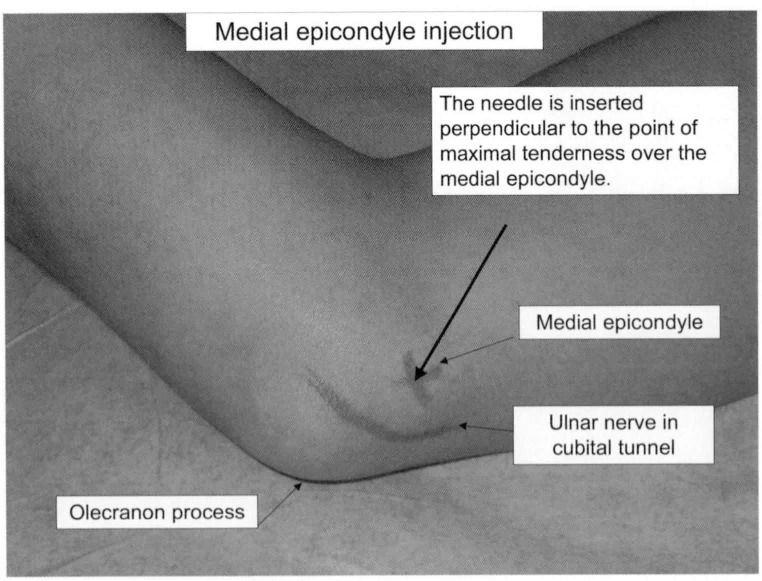

– Take care not to inject the ulnar nerve because it traverses posterior to the medial epicondyle in the cubital tunnel. If the patient experiences pain or numbness in the ulnar nerve distribution while the needle is inserted, then back out and reposition the needle more anteriorly before injecting cortisone. At this time, doing this injection without ultrasound guidance increases the risks of injury to the ulnar nerve.
– Inject the fluid into the area. If there is resistance of flow, then back the needle slightly out so the hub of the needle is not against bone and then inject.
– Take care not to inject cortisone while withdrawing the needle because this superficial tracking of cortisone can increase the risk of skin atrophy and depigmentation.
– Remove needle and apply pressure with gauze.
– Apply Band-Aid.

AFTERCARE

- Instruct patient that the elbow may be numb for several hours after the procedure and that pain may be present for several days.
- In addition, anesthetic spreading from the injection posteriorly may affect the ulnar nerve, and transient ring and pinky finger numbness may occur.
- Instruct patient that the cortisone usually takes effect within 72 hr.
- NSAIDS and ice can be used to control postprocedure pain.
- Consider an elbow extension splint to rest the elbow and/or wrist splint to avoid wrist flexion/extension for 1 to 2 wk to allow the injection to take effect.
- The patient should avoid repetitive wrist extension or flexion.
- Instruct patient to return to your office if they develop redness, swelling, or increased pain at the injection site.

CPT CODE

- 20551 Injection(s) of single tendon origin or insertion

WRIST INJECTION

INDICATIONS

- Wrist injections are useful for the treatment of wrist pain due to arthritis from either trauma, osteoarthritis, or rheumatoid arthritis.
- Injections are indicated once conservative therapy (activity modification, NSAIDS, splinting, physical therapy) has failed.
- ICD10:
  - M25.539 Pain in unspecified wrist
  - M19.039 Primary osteoarthritis, unspecified wrist
  - M06.839 Other specified rheumatoid arthritis, unspecified wrist

ANATOMY

- The wrist joint capsule is not continuous but has septa, which makes the wrist injection sometimes difficult.
- The radiocarpal joint can be palpated just distal to the distal radius in a depression near the scapholunate articulation.

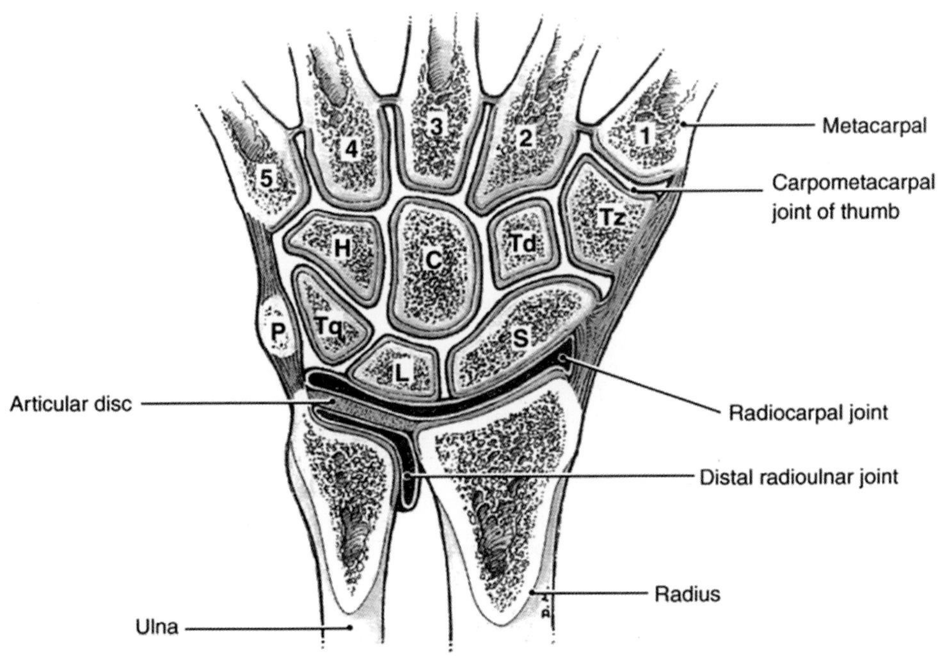

SUPPLIES

- Gloves
- Betadine/chlorhexidine and alcohol swabs
- 3-mL syringe with 25-gauge 5/8- or 1-inch needle
- 5- to 10-mL syringe with 20-gauge or 22-gauge 5/8- or 1-inch needle for aspiration
- ½ mL 1% lidocaine without epinephrine
- ½ mL (20 mg) Kenalog or equivalent
- Ethyl chloride
- Gauze
- Band-Aid

TECHNIQUE

- Palpate the depression distal to the distal radius near the scapholunate articulation.
- Mark this area with the cap of the needle.
- Cleanse the skin with alcohol swab and then Betadine × 3 or chlorhexidine × 45 sec.
- Apply ethyl chloride until the skin turns white.
- The needle is inserted into the wrist joint.

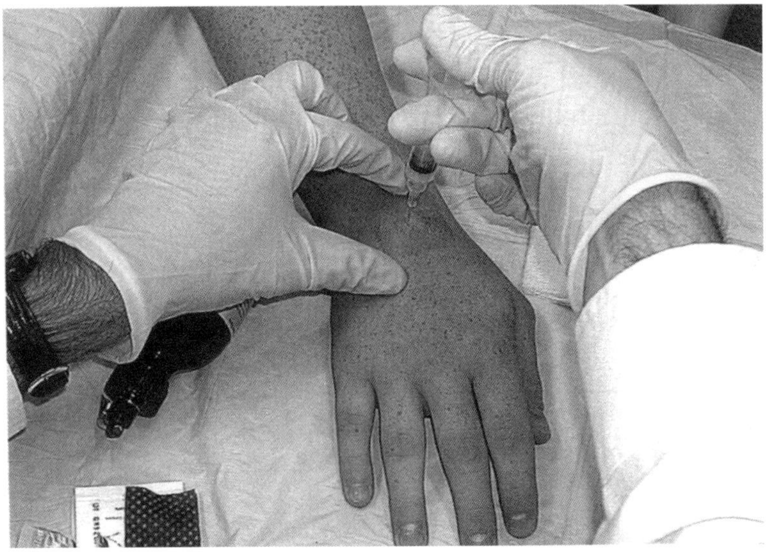

- If aspirating, withdraw fluid with 5- to 10-mL syringe, then stabilize needle and exchange 3-mL syringe containing steroid mixture and inject.
- If injecting, use 3-mL syringe with 25-gauge 1-inch needle and inject fluid into joint.
- The fluid should flow easily without resistance. If there is resistance, reposition the needle by either advancing or withdrawing the needle until the flow of fluid is smooth.
- Remove needle and apply pressure with gauze.
- Apply Band-Aid.
- Have patient perform wrist flexion and extension exercises to disperse the fluid through the wrist joint.

AFTERCARE

- Instruct patient that the wrist may be numb for several hours after the procedure and that pain may be present for several days.
- Instruct patient that the cortisone usually takes effect within 72 hr.
- After 3 days, the patient can resume his or her regular activity.
- Consider use of wrist splint for 1 to 2 wk after injection.
- Instruct patient to return to your office if they develop redness, swelling, or increased pain at the injection site.

CPT CODE

- 20605 Arthrocentesis, aspiration and/or injection; intermediate joint or bursa (e.g., temporomandibular, acromioclavicular, wrist, elbow or ankle, olecranon bursa); without ultrasound guidance
- 20606 Arthrocentesis, aspiration and/or injection; intermediate joint or bursa (e.g., temporomandibular, acromioclavicular, wrist, elbow or ankle, olecranon bursa); with ultrasound guidance, with permanent recording and reporting

DE QUERVAIN TENOSYNOVITIS INJECTION

INDICATIONS

- de Quervain tenosynovitis injections are indicated for the treatment of tenosynovitis over the radial aspect of the wrist.
- These injections are very common in primary care.
- Injections are indicated once conservative therapy (activity modification, NSAIDS, occupational therapy, splinting) has failed.
- ICD10:
  - M65.4 Radial styloid tenosynovitis [de Quervain]

ANATOMY

- The dorsal wrist has six compartments containing tendons.
- The 1st dorsal compartment contains the abductor pollicis longus and the extensor pollicis brevis tendons.
- de Quervain tenosynovitis occurs when the tendon sheath becomes inflamed and thickened causing pain, swelling, and occasional triggering.

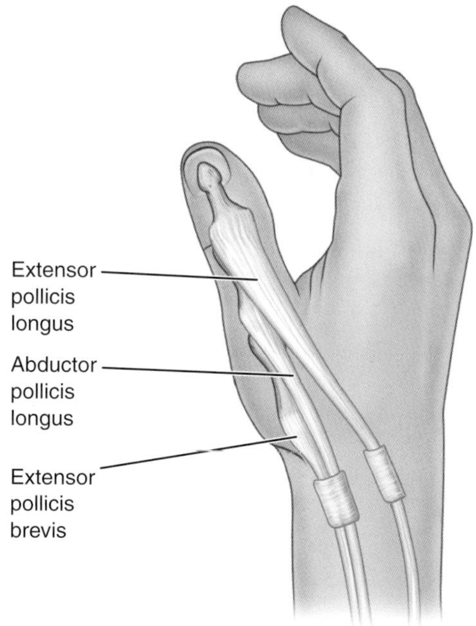

SUPPLIES
- Gloves
- Betadine/chlorhexidine and alcohol swabs
- 3-mL syringe with 25-gauge 5/8- or 1-inch needle
- ½ mL 1% lidocaine without epinephrine
- ½ mL (20 mg) Kenalog or equivalent
- Ethyl chloride
- Gauze
- Band-Aid

TECHNIQUE
- Palpate the area of most tenderness over the 1st dorsal compartment and mark this with the needle cap.
- Cleanse the skin with alcohol swab and then Betadine × 3 or chlorhexidine × 45 sec.
- Apply ethyl chloride until the skin turns white.
- The needle is inserted into the tendon sheath between the abductor pollicis longus and extensor pollicis brevis tendons at ~30-degree angle.
- Ultrasound dramatically increases accuracy of this injection and improves outcomes.

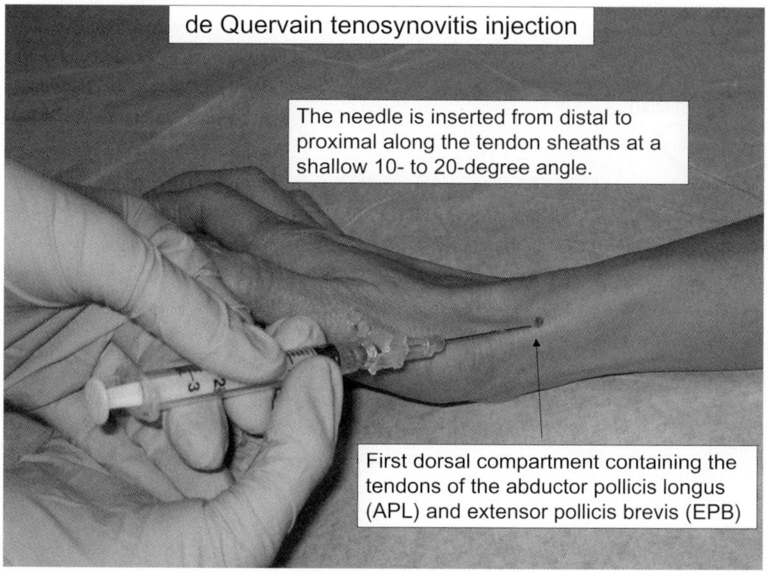

- Inject the fluid into the sheath. If there is resistance to flow, then the needle is likely in a tendon and should be backed slightly out until free flow is obtained.
- An elliptical shaped bulge occurs with the injection of the bolus of fluid into the sheath.
- Take care not to inject cortisone while withdrawing the needle because this superficial tracking of cortisone can increase the risk of skin atrophy and depigmentation.
- Remove needle and apply pressure with gauze.
- Gently massage the fluid up and down along the tendon sheath.
- Apply Band-Aid.

AFTERCARE

- Instruct patient that the wrist may be numb for several hours after the procedure and that pain may be present for several days.
- Instruct patient that the cortisone usually takes effect within 72 hr.
- NSAIDS and ice can be used to control postprocedure pain.
- Consider a thumb spica wrist splint to rest the tendons for 1 to 2 wk to allow the injection to take effect.
- The patient should avoid repetitive thumb abduction and/or extension.
- Instruct patient to return to your office if they develop redness, swelling, or increased pain at the injection site.

CPT CODE

- 20500 Injection(s); single tendon sheath, or ligament, aponeurosis

1ST CARPOMETACARPAL JOINT INJECTION

INDICATIONS

- 1st carpometacarpal (CMC) (thumb) injections are useful for the treatment of thumb pain due to arthritis.
- Injections are indicated once conservative therapy (activity modification, NSAIDS, thumb spica splinting) has failed.
- ICD10:
  - M18.0 Bilateral primary osteoarthritis of first carpometacarpal joints
  - M18.1 Unilateral primary osteoarthritis of first carpometacarpal joint
  - M18.2 Bilateral post-traumatic osteoarthritis of first carpometacarpal joints
  - M18.3 Unilateral post-traumatic osteoarthritis of first carpometacarpal joint
  - M18.11 Unilateral primary osteoarthritis of first carpometacarpal joint, right hand
  - M18.12 Unilateral primary osteoarthritis of first carpometacarpal joint, left hand

ANATOMY

- The thumb CMC joint is composed of the saddle-shaped base of the 1st metacarpal as it articulates with the trapezium.
- The thumb CMC joint can be approached on the extensor surface proximal to the 1st metacarpal, taking care to avoid the radial artery and extensor pollicis tendons.

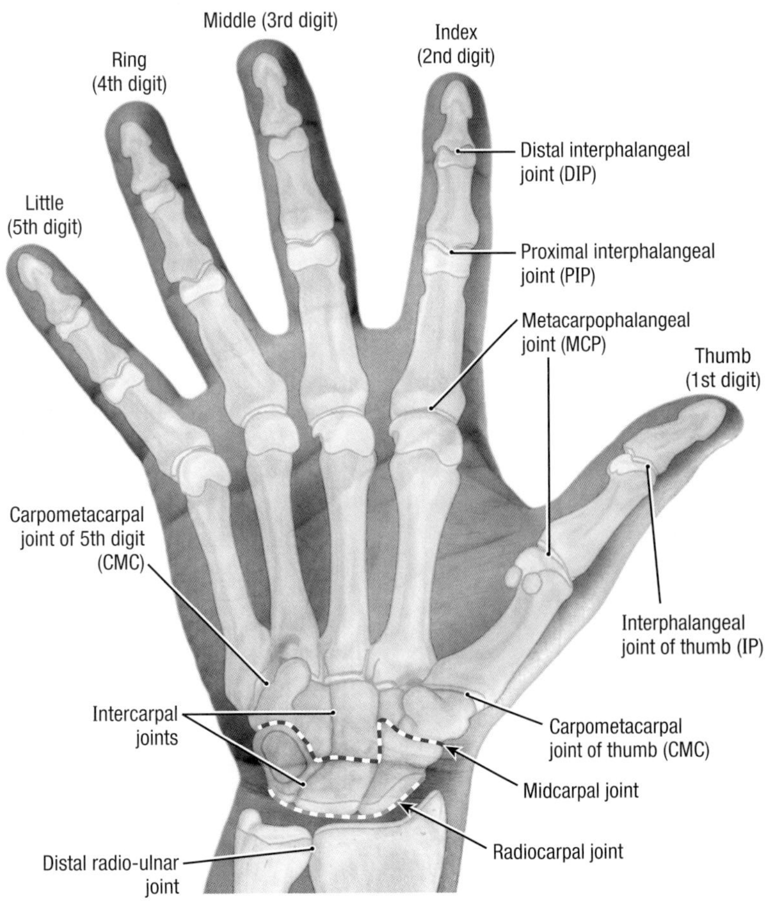

SUPPLIES

- Gloves
- Alcohol swabs
- Betadine or chlorhexidine swabs
- 18-gauge needle for drawing up medications or Medic anti-stick needle
- 3-mL syringe with 25-gauge 1-inch needle for injection
- ½ mL 1% lidocaine without epinephrine (if using)
- ½ mL (20 mg) triamcinolone suspension (Kenalog) or equivalent
- Ethyl chloride
- Gauze
- Band-Aid

TECHNIQUE

- Place the patient's hand and forearm on the table palm down.
- Palpate the CMC joint between the base of the 1st metacarpal and the wrist trapezium between the extensor pollicis longus and extensor pollicis brevis tendons.
- Mark the depression at the base of the 1st metacarpal with needle cap.
- Cleanse the skin with alcohol swab and then Betadine × 3 or chlorhexidine × 45 sec.
- Apply ethyl chloride for topical cooling.
- To avoid the radial artery, the needle should enter on the ulnar side of the extensor pollicis brevis tendon. Distraction of the thumb can increase the space to get the needle into the joint.
- Corticosteroid alone can be injected without anesthetic, given the small size of the CMC joint. Usually, not more than ½ mL volume will fit into the joint space.

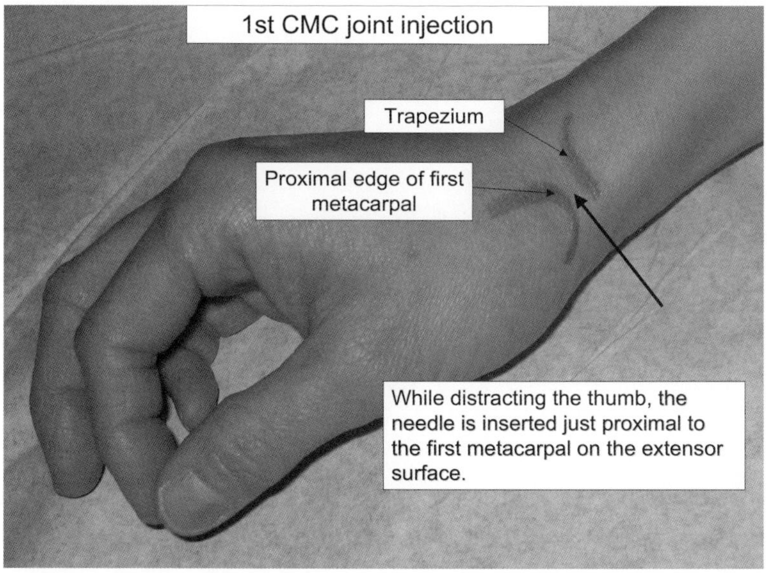

- Inject the corticosteroid into the CMC joint.
- Remove needle and apply pressure with gauze.
- Apply Band-Aid.

AFTERCARE

- Instruct patient that the thumb may be numb for several hours after the procedure and that pain may be present for several days.
- Instruct patient that the cortisone usually takes effect within 48 to 72 hr.
- Suggest the patient wear the thumb spica splint for the next 1 to 2 wk with daily thumb extension stretches.
- After 3 to 5 days, the patient can resume his or her regular activity.
- Instruct patient to return to your office if they develop redness, swelling, or increased pain at the injection site.

CPT CODE

- 20600 Arthrocentesis, aspiration and/or injection; small joint or bursa (e.g., fingers, toes); without ultrasound guidance
- 20604 Arthrocentesis, aspiration and/or injection; small joint or bursa (e.g., fingers, toes); with ultrasound guidance, with permanent recording and reporting

CARPAL TUNNEL INJECTION

INDICATIONS

- Carpal tunnel injections are useful for the treatment of wrist pain due to median nerve compression at the carpal tunnel from either trauma, overuse, or rheumatoid arthritis.
- Injections are indicated once conservative therapy (activity modification, NSAIDs, splinting, physical therapy) has failed.
- Local corticosteroid injections for carpal tunnel syndrome provide greater symptom relief for 1 mo after injection compared with placebo (number needed to treat [NNT] = 2) and oral corticosteroids. However, significant symptom relief after 1 mo has not been demonstrated following injection.
- ICD10:
  - G56.00 Carpal tunnel syndrome, unspecified upper limb

ANATOMY

- The carpal tunnel is bounded by the carpal bones dorsally and the transverse carpal ligament (flexor retinaculum) ventrally.
- The contents of the tunnel include the median nerve and flexor tendons of the hand.

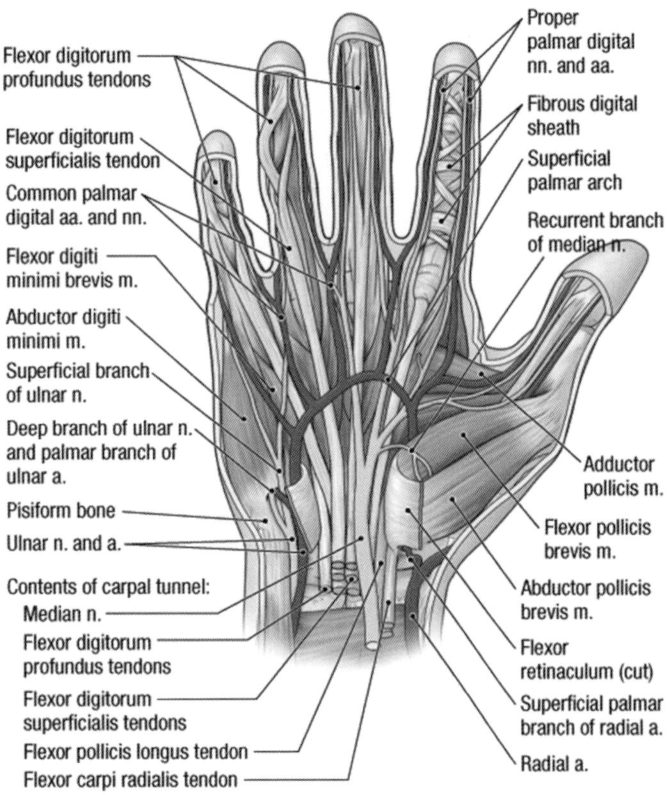

SUPPLIES

- Gloves
- Betadine/chlorhexidine and alcohol swabs
- 3-mL syringe with 25-gauge 1½-inch needle
- 1½ mL 1% lidocaine without epinephrine
- ½ mL (20 mg) Kenalog or equivalent
- Ethyl chloride
- Gauze
- Band-Aid

TECHNIQUE

- Have the patient lay the hand palm up on the table and make a fist with slight wrist flexion.
- Observe the tendons of the palmaris longus (10% of the population will not have one) and the flexor carpi radialis.
- Mark a spot with the needle cap 4 cm proximal to the distal palmar crease between the two tendons mentioned above.
- Cleanse the skin with alcohol swab and then Betadine × 3 or chlorhexidine × 45 sec.
- With the fist clenched and the wrist slightly flexed, the needle is inserted at a shallow angle (~20 degrees) along the tendon sheath, aiming toward the ring finger. Have the patient slowly extend the wrist and fingers noticing the needle advance toward the carpal tunnel. This indicates proper needle placement.

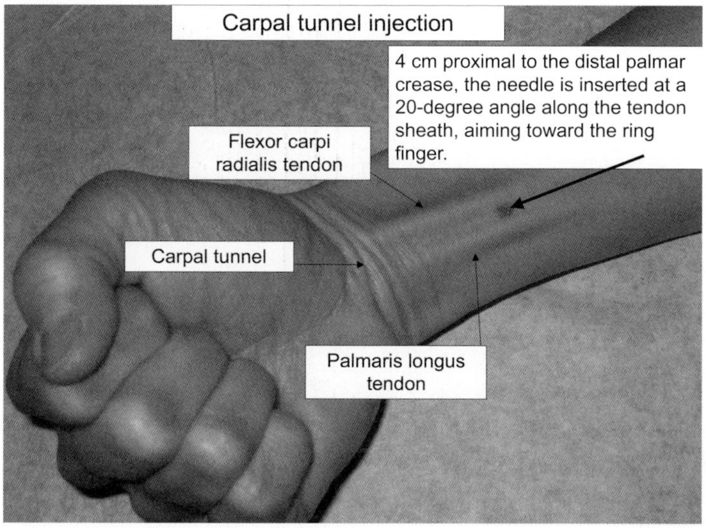

- Ask the patient if they feel any increased pain or numbness. If they do, remove the needle because it may be in the median nerve.
- DO NOT INJECT INTO THE MEDIAN NERVE.
- The fluid should flow easily without resistance. If there is resistance, reposition the needle by repeating the technique from the beginning.
- Remove needle and apply pressure with gauze.
- Massage the fluid distally toward the carpal tunnel.
- Apply Band-Aid.

AFTERCARE

- Instruct patient that the wrist may be numb for several hours after the procedure and that pain may be present for several days.
- Instruct patient that the cortisone usually takes effect within 72 hr.
- After 3 days, the patient can resume his or her regular activity.
- Recommend continued use of wrist splint for 1 to 2 wk after injection.
- Instruct patient to return to your office if they develop redness, swelling, or increased pain at the injection site.

CPT CODE

- 20526 Injection, therapeutic, carpal tunnel

TRIGGER FINGER INJECTION

INDICATIONS

- Trigger fingers occur when a flexor tendon nodule repetitively gets stuck under the annular pulley on the palmar aspect of the finger.
- Injections are indicated once conservative therapy (activity modification, splinting, NSAIDs) has failed.
- ICD10:
  - M65.30 Trigger finger, unspecified finger

ANATOMY

- Nodule or thickening occurs in the flexor tendon, which catches on the A-1 proximal pulley making finger extension difficult.

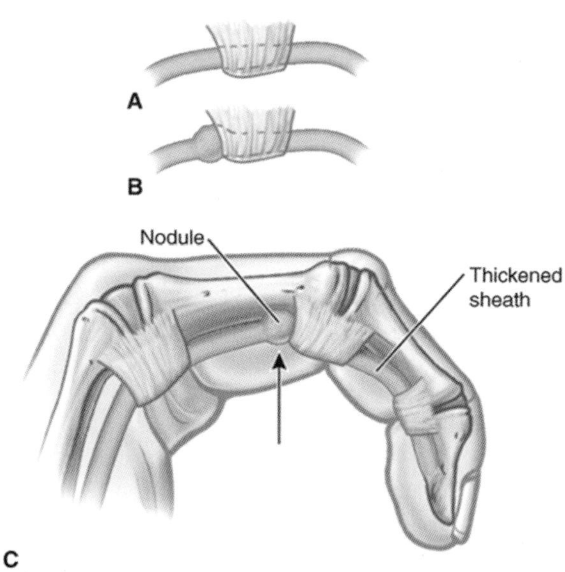

SUPPLIES
- Gloves
- Betadine/chlorhexidine and alcohol swabs
- 3-mL syringe with 25-gauge 5/8- to 1-inch needle
- ½ mL 1% lidocaine
- ½ mL (20 mg) Kenalog or equivalent
- Ethyl chloride
- Gauze
- Band-Aid

TECHNIQUE
- Palpate the tender nodule on the palm of the hand and mark with needle cap.
- Cleanse the skin with alcohol swab and then Betadine × 3 or chlorhexidine × 45 sec.
- Apply ethyl chloride until skin turns white.
- Injection site is either directly into the nodule or at the proximal interphalangeal digital crease.

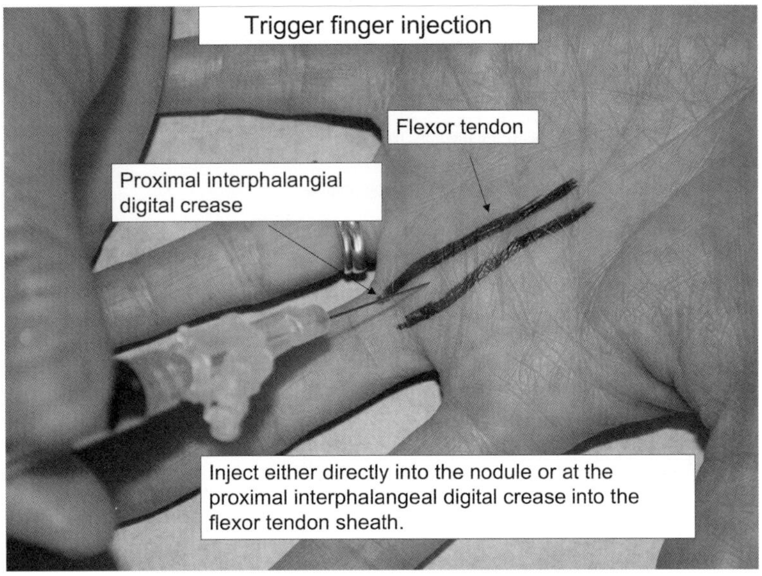

- Insert needle at a 45-degree angle—when you feel rubbery resistance, you are at the level of the tendon. Back needle out slowly until it is no longer in tendon and the fluid flows easily within the tendon sheath.
- Never inject under pressure—steroid injected directly into a tendon may cause tendon rupture.
- Remove needle and apply pressure with gauze, gently massaging material along tendon.
- Apply Band-Aid.

AFTERCARE
- Instruct patient that the finger may be numb for several hours after the procedure and that pain may be present for several days.
- Instruct patient that the cortisone usually takes effect within 72 hr.
- The use of a finger splint after an injection for 1 to 2 wk can increase the efficacy of the injection.
- After 3 days, start extension exercises—hold finger in extension 10 sec × 10 times for one set. Complete three sets per day.
- Instruct patient to return to your office if they develop redness, swelling, or increased pain at the injection site.
- Avoid repetitive gripping or use padded gloves for any vibrating tools (i.e., jackhammers).

CPT CODE
- 20550 Injection(s); single tendon sheath, or ligament, aponeurosis (e.g., plantar "fascia")

GANGLION CYST INJECTION

INDICATIONS
- Most ganglion cysts resolve spontaneously, with conservative treatment including splinting. Home efforts to rupture the cyst by hitting it with a heavy book are not recommended.
- Aspiration and corticosteroid injection can be considered for ganglion cysts if patients complain of symptoms such as pain, limited ROM, paresthesias, or aesthetic considerations.

- Aspiration and steroid injection is effective without recurrence in 27–67% of cases.
- ICD10:
  - M67.40 Ganglion, unspecified site
  - M67.44 Ganglion, hand
  - M67.479 Ganglion, unspecified ankle and foot

ANATOMY

- Ganglion cysts are the most common soft tissue tumors of the hand and wrist, more commonly in women (3:1).
- These thick mucin-filled cysts may out pouch from synovial or tendon sheaths from trauma or repetitive irritation.
- Ganglion cysts are often connected to an underlying ligament or joint, most commonly at the scapholunate joint (60–70%), and next most frequently at the volar wrist (20–25%), and thirdly at the palmar flexor tendon sheath (10–12%).

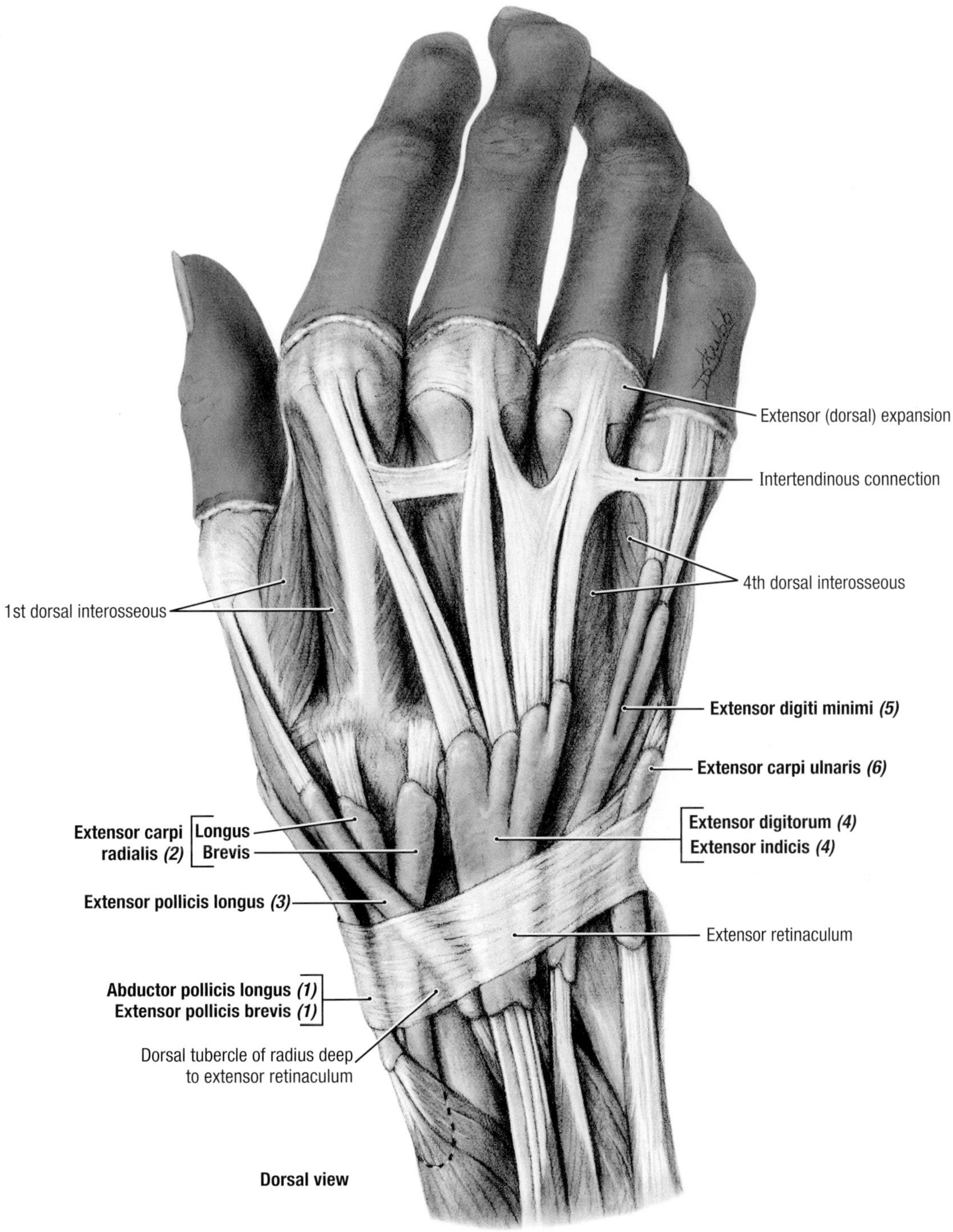

SUPPLIES

- Gloves
- Alcohol swabs
- Betadine or chlorhexidine swabs
- 18-gauge needle for drawing up medications or Medic anti-stick needle
- 5- to 10-mL syringe with 18- to 22-gauge 1-inch needle if aspirating viscous cyst contents
- 3-mL syringe with 22-gauge 1-inch needle if injecting
- ½ to 1 mL 1% lidocaine without epinephrine (if using)
- ½ mL 40 mg/mL (20 mg) triamcinolone suspension (Kenalog) or equivalent
- Ethyl chloride
- Gauze
- Band-Aid

TECHNIQUE

- Position the patient in sitting position with his or her arm on the table with the ganglion cyst facing upward.
- Cleanse the skin with alcohol swab and then Betadine × 3 or chlorhexidine × 45 sec.
- Apply ethyl chloride for topical cooling.
- Aspirate using the 18-gauge needle—the thick mucoid cyst contents may be difficult to aspirate and may actually be more effectively milked out of the puncture site after the needle is removed.

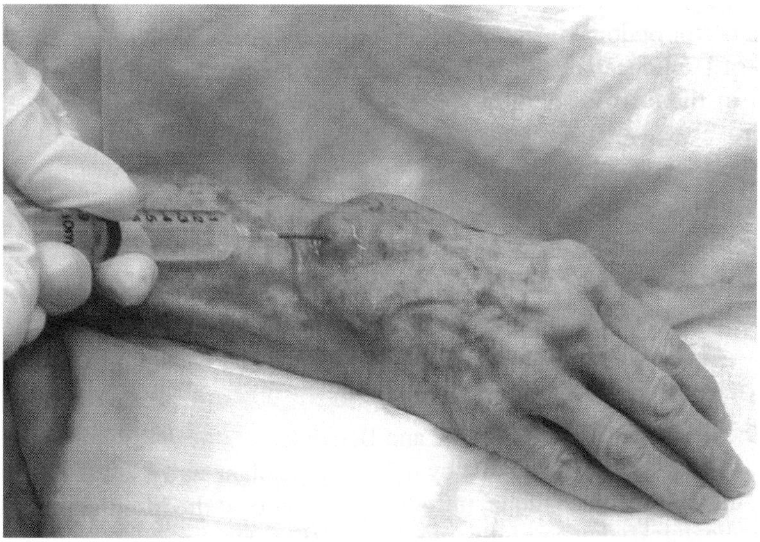

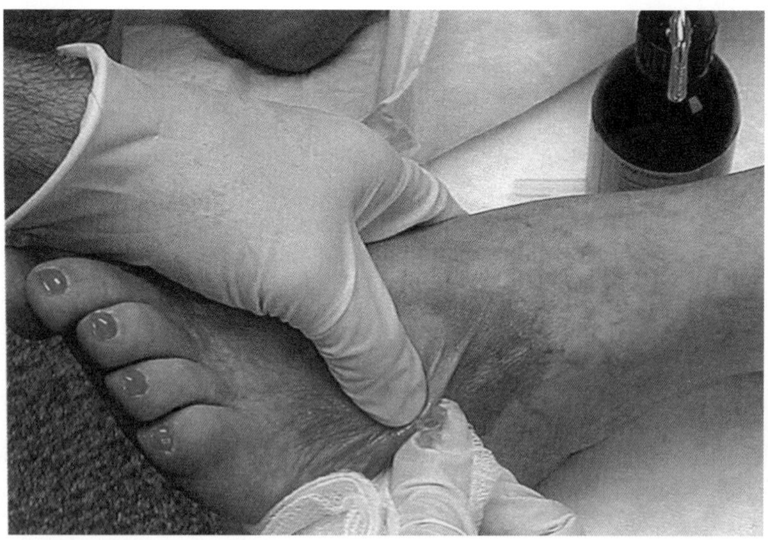

- First, aspirate the cyst contents if possible and then stabilize the needle position with a hemostat, remove the aspiration syringe, secure the syringe with the steroid mixture, and inject.
- Remove needle and apply pressure with gauze.
- Band-Aid

AFTERCARE

- Apply pressure dressing.
- Instruct patient to return to your office if they develop redness, swelling, or increased pain at the injection site.
- Ganglion cyst recurrence is common—consider referral to hand orthopedics for surgical ganglionectomy if patients continue to experience pain and discomfort from the ganglion cyst.

CPT CODE

- 20612 Aspiration and/or injection of ganglion cyst(s) any location
- 20605 Arthrocentesis, aspiration and/or injection; intermediate joint, bursa, or ganglion cyst (e.g., temporomandibular, acromioclavicular, wrist, elbow or ankle, olecranon bursa); without ultrasound guidance
- 20606 Arthrocentesis, aspiration and/or injection; intermediate joint, bursa, or ganglion cyst (e.g., temporomandibular, acromioclavicular, wrist, elbow or ankle, olecranon bursa); with ultrasound guidance, with permanent recording and reporting

TROCHANTERIC BURSA INJECTION

INDICATIONS

- Corticosteroid injection is an accepted treatment for trochanteric bursitis or greater trochanteric pain syndrome caused by chronic hip pressure, limping, leg length discrepancies, acute trauma, hip surgery, or repetitive trauma, such as from iliotibial band friction.
- Trochanteric bursa injections are indicated if pain persists despite conservative therapy, including avoiding direct pressure and repetitive trauma, ice, NSAIDs, and stretching of the iliotibial band, tensor fascia lata, external hip rotators, hip flexors, and quadriceps.
- A randomized controlled trial showed prolonged benefit from early corticosteroid injection for trochanteric bursitis.
- Another randomized controlled study of patients who received trochanteric bursa corticosteroid injections demonstrated a 2.7 relative risk of recovery at 5 yr, with the conclusion that early steroid injection may help prevent chronic bursitis pain.
- ICD10:
  - M70.60 Trochanteric bursitis, unspecified hip
  - M70.61 Trochanteric bursitis, right hip
  - M70.62 Trochanteric bursitis, left hip

ANATOMY

- The trochanteric bursa lies superficial to the greater trochanter of the femur, between the trochanteric process and the gluteus medius/iliotibial tract.
- Tenderness to palpation over the trochanteric process is the classic finding for trochanteric bursitis.

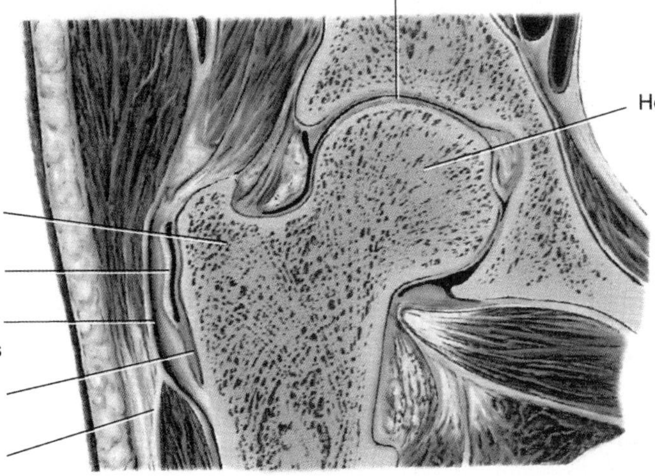

SUPPLIES

- Alcohol swabs
- Betadine or chlorhexidine swabs
- 18-gauge needle for drawing up medications or Medic anti-stick needle
- 6-mL syringe with 21- to 22-gauge 1½- to 2-inch needle for thin patients
- 21- to 22-gauge 3.5-inch spinal needle may be needed for heavier patients.
- 5 mL 1% lidocaine without epinephrine and/or 0.25% bupivacaine
- 1 mL 40 mg/mL (40 mg) triamcinolone suspension (Kenalog) or equivalent
- Ethyl chloride
- Gauze
- Band-Aid

TECHNIQUE

- Lay the patient in lateral recumbent position, with the affected side up.
- Flex the patient's hip at 50 degrees, and flex the knees 60 to 90 degrees.
- Palpate the greater trochanteric process and identify the point of maximal tenderness, which usually corresponds well to the most superficial point of bony prominence. Mark this area with the needle cap.
- Cleanse the skin with alcohol swab and then Betadine × 3 or chlorhexidine × 45 sec.
- Apply ethyl chloride for topical cooling.
- Position the needle perpendicular to the skin and advance toward the site of maximal trochanteric tenderness.
- Advance the needle until the tip reaches bone level to ensure delivery of the steroid below the tendon. Never inject under pressure, which may indicate placement within the tendon.
- Withdraw the needle 2 to 3 mm to remain within the trochanteric bursa.

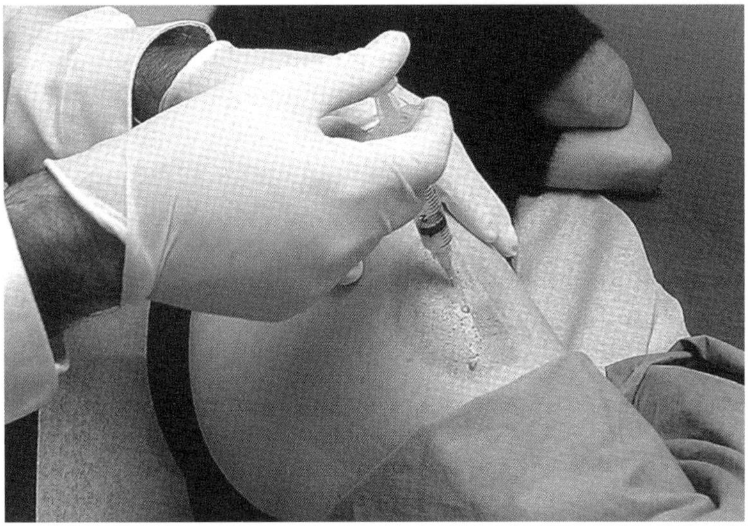

- For acute bursitis, the 5 to 6 ml of corticosteroid and lidocaine can be directly injected into the bursa.
- For chronic bursitis, a clockwise peppering motion may help break up scar tissue—each time, the needle should reach the level of bone and then inject.
- Crepitus can often be felt at the needle tip if chronic scarring/bursitis/tendonitis is present.
- Remove needle and apply pressure with gauze.
- Band-Aid

AFTERCARE

- Warn patients that pain relief from the cortisone anti-inflammatory effect may not start until 2 to 3 days postinjection.
- Avoid direct pressure or trauma to the trochanteric bursa.
- Rest 3 days and then restart stretches of the iliotibial band, hip flexors, and extensors.
- Instruct patient to return to your office if they develop redness, swelling, or increased pain at the injection site.
- Injection can be repeated in 6 to 12 wk if pain relief was <50%.

CPT CODE

- 20610 Arthrocentesis, aspiration and/or injection; major joint or bursa (e.g., shoulder, hip, knee, subacromial bursa); without ultrasound guidance
- 20611 Arthrocentesis, aspiration and/or injection; major joint or bursa (e.g., shoulder, hip, knee, subacromial bursa); with ultrasound guidance, with permanent recording and reporting

OLECRANON BURSA INJECTION

INDICATIONS

- Olecranon bursa aspiration is useful to relieve swelling in acute bursitis or to diagnose gouty bursitis or infectious bursitis (most often *Staphylococcus aureus*). Olecranon bursa steroid injections are useful for the treatment of chronic bursitis.
- Most acute traumatic olecranon bursitis episodes are self-limited.
- Injections are indicated once conservative therapies (rest, ice, compression with elbow sleeve, elevation, avoidance of direct pressure, NSAIDs) have failed.
- ICD10:
  - M70.20 Olecranon bursitis, unspecified elbow
  - M70.21 Olecranon bursitis, right elbow
  - M70.22 Olecranon bursitis, left elbow

ANATOMY

- The olecranon bursa overlies the olecranon process at the proximal ulna.
- Olecranon bursitis is visible as posterior elbow swelling, often described as a golf ball or goose egg over the elbow tip.

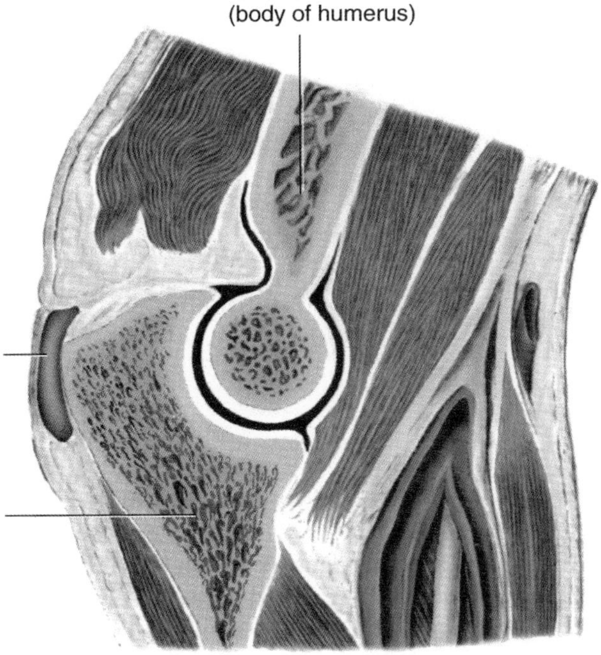

SUPPLIES

- Gloves
- Alcohol swabs
- Betadine or chlorhexidine swabs
- 18-gauge needle for drawing up medications or Medic anti-stick needle
- 3-mL syringe with 25-gauge 1-inch needle if injecting
- 5- to 10-mL syringe with 18- to 22-gauge needle if aspirating
- 1 mL 1% lidocaine without epinephrine
- ½ mL 40 mg/mL (20 mg) triamcinolone suspension (Kenalog) or equivalent
- Ethyl chloride
- Gauze
- Band-Aid

TECHNIQUE

- Place the patient's arm on the table at maximal elbow flexion to accentuate the swelling.
- Palpate over the olecranon bursa for fluctuance.
- Cleanse the skin with alcohol swab and then Betadine × 3 or chlorhexidine × 45 sec.
- Apply ethyl chloride for topical cooling.
- Aim the needle perpendicular to the olecranon bursa.
- Aspirate bursa fluid until the bursa is flat.

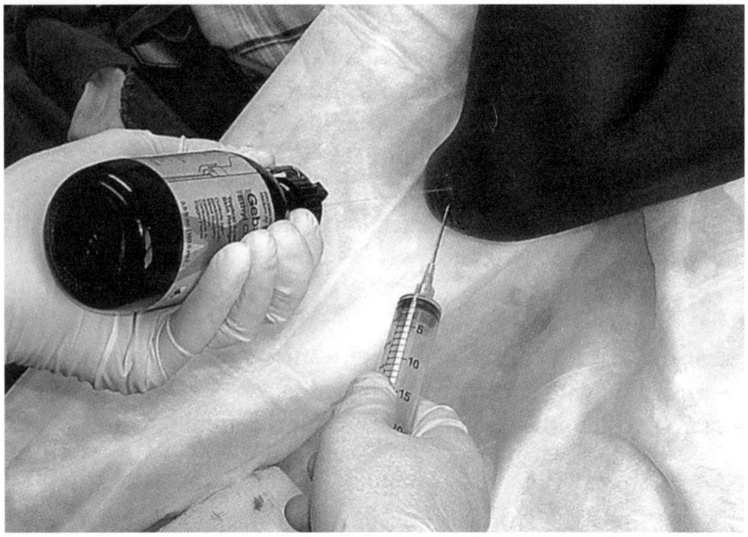

- If infection has been ruled out, inject steroid/lidocaine into bursa.
- Remove needle and apply pressure with gauze.
- Band-Aid

AFTERCARE

- A compressive elbow sleeve may help prevent fluid reaccumulation.
- Avoid direct pressure or trauma to the elbow.
- For recalcitrant olecranon bursitis, consider a posterior splint or elbow pads for 1 to 2 wk after the steroid injection.
- Instruct patient to return to your office if they develop redness, swelling, or increased pain at the injection site.

CPT CODE

- 20605 Arthrocentesis, aspiration and/or injection; intermediate joint or bursa (e.g., temporomandibular, acromioclavicular, wrist, elbow or ankle, olecranon bursa); without ultrasound guidance
- 20606 Arthrocentesis, aspiration and/or injection; intermediate joint or bursa (e.g., temporomandibular, acromioclavicular, wrist, elbow or ankle, olecranon bursa); with ultrasound guidance, with permanent recording and reporting

PREPATELLAR BURSA INJECTION

INDICATIONS

- Acute trauma, repetitive pressure, or rarely infection can cause inflammation and swelling in the prepatellar bursa.
- Prepatellar aspiration may be performed to relieve acute pressure and swelling.
- Corticosteroid injection is a second-line therapy for chronic prepatellar bursitis after the failure of conservative therapy, including avoidance of direct pressure, rest, ice, and NSAIDs.
- ICD10:
  - M70.40 Prepatellar bursitis, unspecified knee
  - M70.41 Prepatellar bursitis, right knee
  - M70.42 Prepatellar bursitis, left knee

ANATOMY

- The prepatellar bursa lies between the patella and the overlying skin.
- Prepatellar bursitis is visible as a well-circumscribed region of swelling over the patella.
- Prepatellar bursitis should be differentiated from patellar fracture or IA knee effusion.

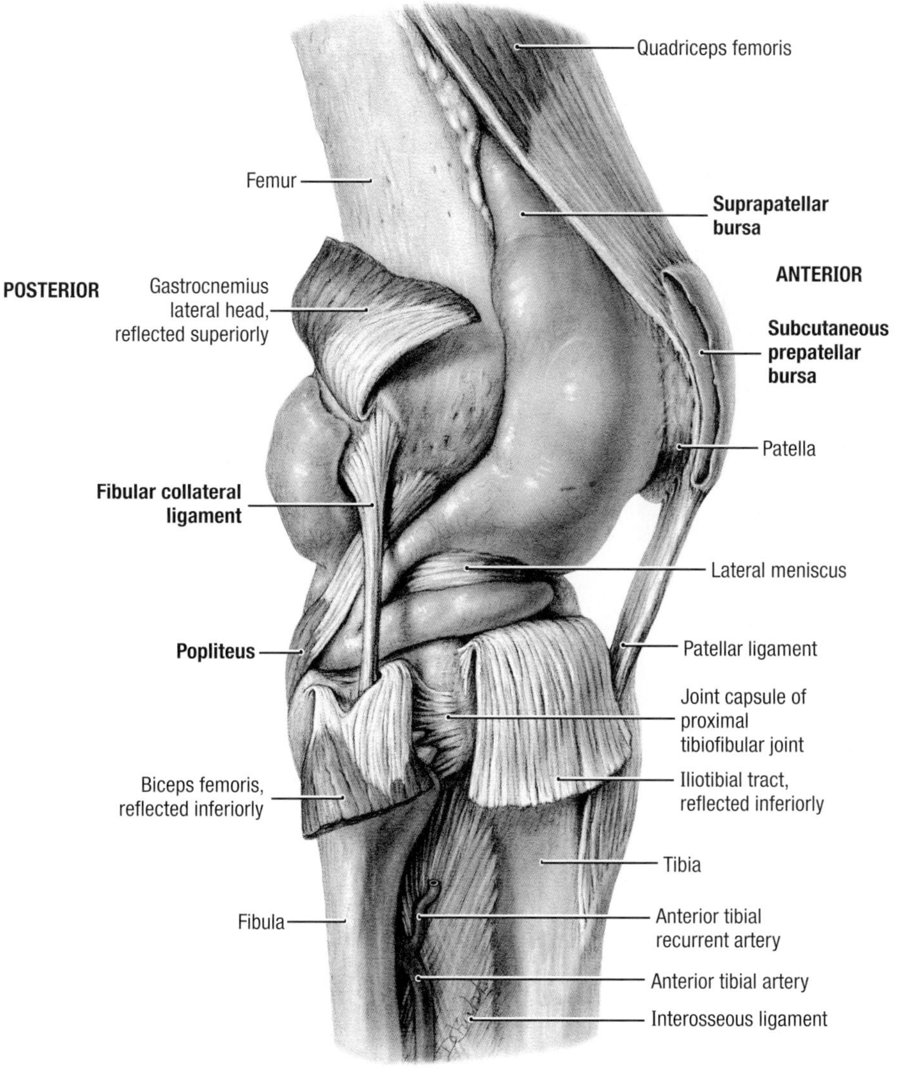

Lateral view

SUPPLIES

- Gloves
- Alcohol swabs
- Betadine or chlorhexidine swabs
- 18-gauge needle for drawing up medications or Medic anti-stick needle
- 5- to 10-mL syringe with 18- to 22-gauge 1-inch needle if aspirating
- 1 mL 1% lidocaine without epinephrine (optional)
- ½ mL 40 mg/mL (20 mg) triamcinolone suspension (Kenalog) or equivalent (optional)
- Ethyl chloride
- Gauze
- Band-Aid

TECHNIQUE

- Position the patient in supine position with the knee flexed at 30 degrees on a pillow.
- Position the affected leg with patella facing upward.
- Cleanse the skin with alcohol swab and then Betadine × 3 or chlorhexidine × 45 sec.
- Apply ethyl chloride for topical cooling.
- The prepatellar bursa swelling should be clearly visible.
- Aspirate by approaching from the side of the visible prepatellar swelling.

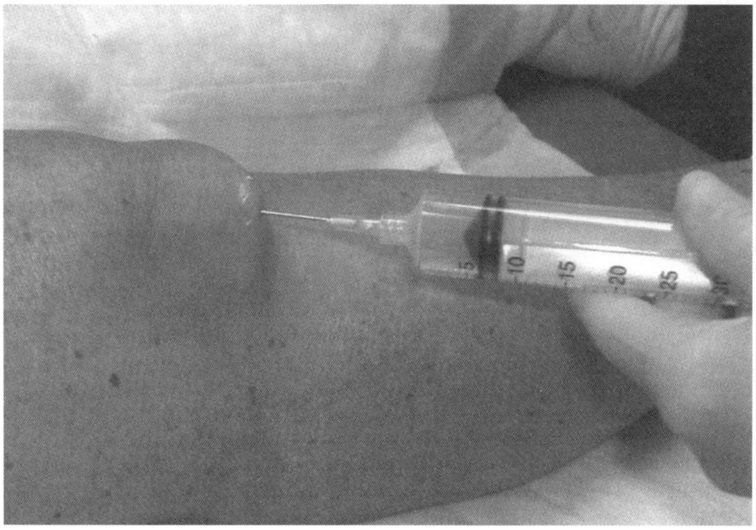

- Aspirate first, then stabilize the needle position with a hemostat while changing to the syringe with the steroid/lidocaine mixture, and then inject.
- Remove needle and apply pressure with gauze.
- Band-Aid

AFTERCARE

- Apply pressure dressing.
- Rest for 3 days.
- Continue the rest, ice, compression, and elevation (RICE) conservative therapy.
- Remind patients to avoid direct pressure on their patellas or to use knee pads if kneeling is required for work.
- Instruct patients to return to your office or urgent care if they develop redness, swelling, or increased pain at the injection site.

CPT CODE

- 20605 Arthrocentesis, aspiration and/or injection; intermediate joint or bursa (e.g., temporomandibular, acromioclavicular, wrist, elbow or ankle, olecranon bursa); without ultrasound guidance
- 20606 Arthrocentesis, aspiration and/or injection; intermediate joint or bursa (e.g., temporomandibular, acromioclavicular, wrist, elbow or ankle, olecranon bursa); with ultrasound guidance, with permanent recording and reporting

PES ANSERINE BURSA INJECTION

INDICATIONS

- Trauma or repetitive friction over the anserine bursa can cause inflammation that worsens with knee flexion or rotation.
- Corticosteroid injections may be considered early in the course of treatment for anserine bursitis, along with the conservative therapy of NSAIDs, rest, ice, and stretching.
- ICD10:
  - M70.51 Other bursitis of knee, right knee
  - M70.52 Other bursitis of knee, left knee

ANATOMY

- The pes anserine bursa lies between the conjoined tendon of the sartorius, gracilis, and semitendinosus muscles and the tibial insertion of the medial collateral ligament.
- Diagnosis is made by tenderness to palpation over the anserine bursa, ~2 cm below the medial joint line at the proximal medial tibia.
- Swelling is not usually visible with anserine bursitis.

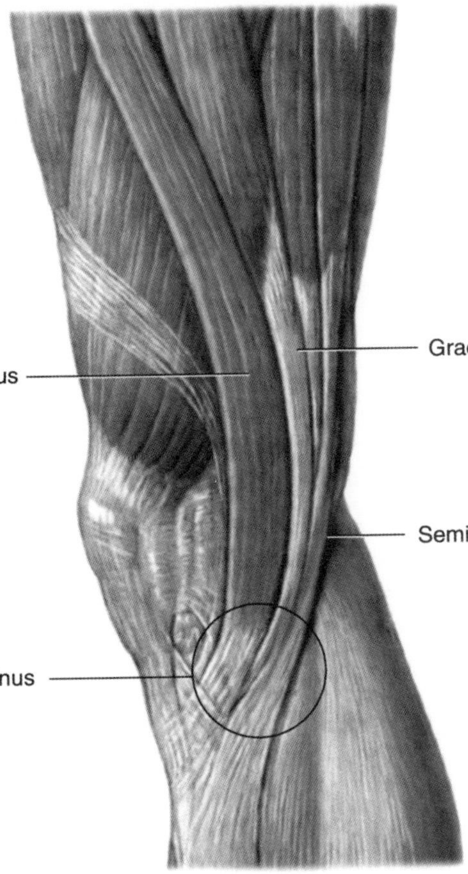

SUPPLIES
- Gloves
- Alcohol swabs
- Betadine or chlorhexidine swabs
- 18-gauge needle for drawing up medications or Medic anti-stick needle
- 3-mL syringe with 25-gauge 1-inch needle
- 1 mL 1% lidocaine without epinephrine
- ½ mL 40 mg/mL (20 mg) triamcinolone suspension (Kenalog) or equivalent
- Ethyl chloride
- Gauze
- Band-Aid

TECHNIQUE
- Lay the patient in supine position.
- Position the affected leg with the medial joint line accessible.
- Identify the anserine bursa 1 to 2 cm below the middle of the medial joint line.
- The point of maximal tenderness along the medial tibial plateau often serves to identify the ideal injection site—mark this site with the needle cap.
- Cleanse the skin with alcohol swab and then Betadine × 3 or chlorhexidine × 45 sec.
- Apply ethyl chloride for topical cooling.
- Insert the needle perpendicular to the skin.
- Advance the needle to the level of bone to find the bursa space between the conjoined tendons and the tibia.
- Inject the steroid/lidocaine mixture into the bursa—resistance to flow should be minimal.

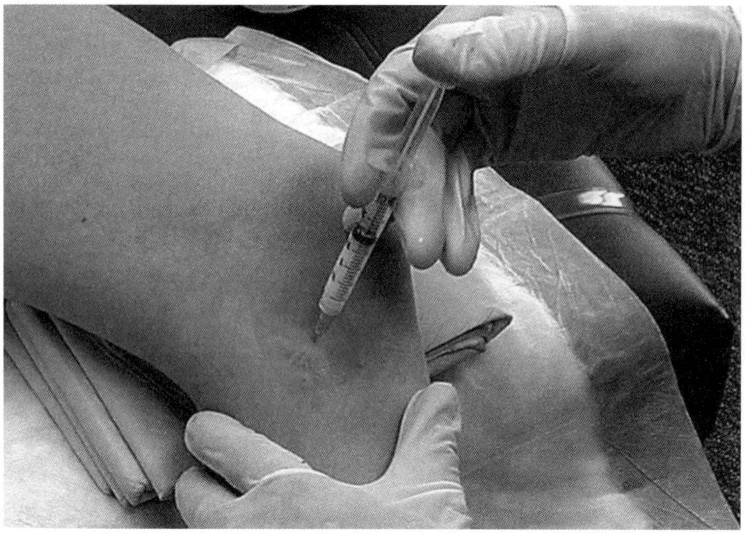

- Remove needle and apply pressure with gauze.
- Band-Aid

AFTERCARE
- Rest 3 days and then resume stretching exercises.
- A physical therapy referral to develop a stretching plan for the knee adductors and quadriceps, especially the vastus medialis, may help prevent recurrence.
- Sleeping with a cushion between the knees may help decrease direct pressure on the anserine bursa.
- Instruct patient to return to your office if they develop redness, swelling, or increased pain at the injection site.

CPT CODE
- 20605 Arthrocentesis, aspiration and/or injection; intermediate joint or bursa (e.g., temporomandibular, acromioclavicular, wrist, elbow or ankle, olecranon bursa); without ultrasound guidance
- 20606 Arthrocentesis, aspiration and/or injection; intermediate joint or bursa (e.g., temporomandibular, acromioclavicular, wrist, elbow or ankle, olecranon bursa); with ultrasound guidance, with permanent recording and reporting

KNEE JOINT INJECTION

INDICATIONS
- Knee joint aspiration is useful in the diagnosis of knee effusions (i.e., to diagnose crystalline disease, hemarthrosis, or rule out infection) and for the reduction of pain and pressure from effusions.
- Corticosteroid injection of the knee is indicated for the treatment of osteoarthritis, crystalline disease, or synovitis in rheumatoid arthritis.
- HA viscosupplementation injections are U.S. Food and Drug Administration (FDA)-approved for knee osteoarthritis.
- Knee injection therapy may be appropriate if knee pain continues despite evidence-based conservative therapy (activity modification, weight loss, acetaminophen, oral or topical NSAIDs, physical therapy, ice, heat).
- Strength of evidence for IA knee injection therapies is strongest for corticosteroid (Category 1A). In a recent large meta-analysis assessing pain relief at 3 mo posttreatment, IA corticosteroid had a larger effect size than IA placebo, oral placebo, oral acetaminophen, and all other oral treatments.
- Strength of evidence for HA injections is more controversial because many of the HA studies were funded by pharmaceutical companies. 2012 guidelines by ACR list HA use as no recommendation, and current American Academy of Orthopedic Surgeons recommends against HA use, due to an effect size no better than NSAIDS, with higher risk of side effects. However, anecdotally, many patients report longer relief with HA injections than corticosteroid.
- No guidelines currently recommend use of newer injectable agents including platelet-rich plasma, immunologics, or botulinum toxin because evidence is still developing.
- Concerns regarding chondrotoxic effects from lidocaine, bupivacaine, or other IA anesthetics are mainly based on cell culture, animal studies, and high-dose exposure in operating room procedures. Evidence for harm in small doses in a single IA exposure is lacking. However, if patients are concerned, the knee injections can be done without IA anesthetic agents.
- ICD10:
  - M17.0 Bilateral primary osteoarthritis of knee
  - M17.10 Unilateral primary osteoarthritis, unspecified knee
  - M17.2 Bilateral post-traumatic osteoarthritis of knee
  - M17.3 Unilateral post-traumatic osteoarthritis of knee

ANATOMY
- The knee joint consists of the femoral–tibial and femoral–patellar joints, with stabilization from the anterior and posterior cruciate ligaments and the medial and lateral collateral ligaments.

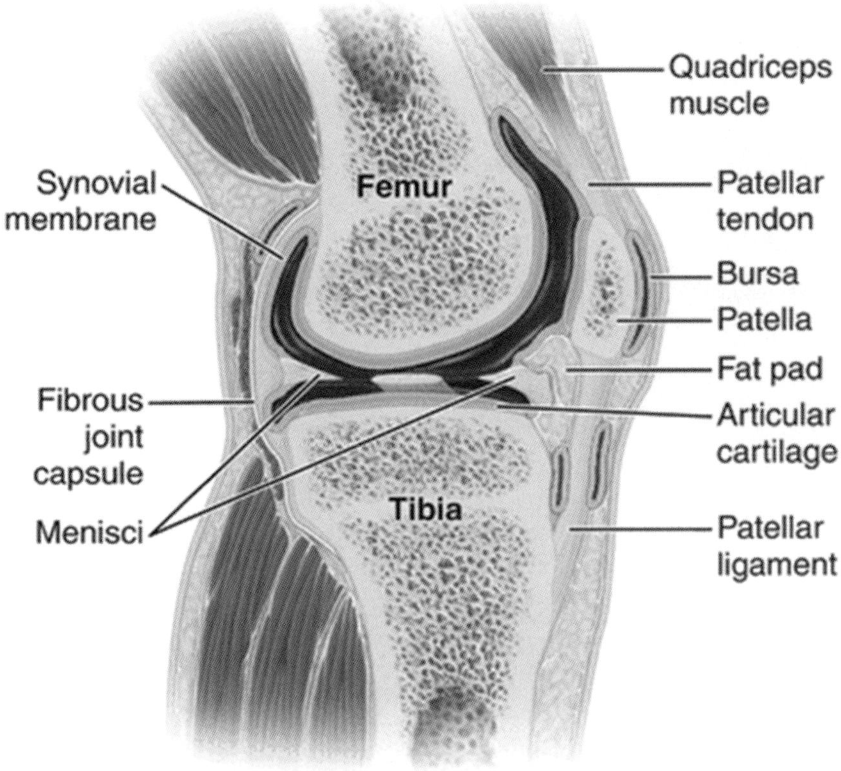

Sagittal section

SUPPLIES

- Gloves
- Alcohol swabs
- Betadine or chlorhexidine swabs
- 18-gauge needle for drawing up medications or Medic anti-stick needle
- 3-mL syringe with 25-gauge 1-inch needle for injection
- 20- to 60-mL syringe with 18- to 22-gauge 1½-inch needle if aspirating
- 5- to 10-mL syringe with 21- to 22-gauge 1½-inch needle for injecting
- 5 to 7 mL 1% lidocaine without epinephrine and or 0.25% bupivacaine (if using)
- 1 mL 40 mg/mL (40 mg) triamcinolone suspension (Kenalog) or equivalent
- Ethyl chloride
- Gauze
- Band-Aid

TECHNIQUE

- The knee joint can be aspirated or injected from multiple approaches, including the anterior medial or lateral approach with the knee flexed to 90 degrees, or a superior or midpatellar approach with the knee in extension.
- For the anterior approach, the patient is seated with the knee flexed at 90 degrees. The needle is inserted in the "soft spot" demarcated by the patella, patellar tendon, tibial plateau, and distal femoral condyle. The needle angle is parallel to the floor and aimed slightly posterior.

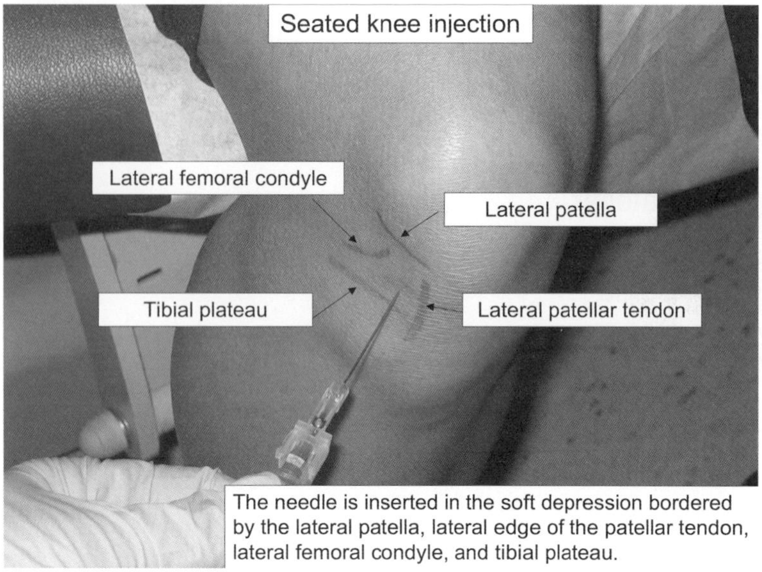

The needle is inserted in the soft depression bordered by the lateral patella, lateral edge of the patellar tendon, lateral femoral condyle, and tibial plateau.

- The anterior seated approach has the advantage of less bony discomfort but had a success rate of 70–75% in a trial comparing knee injection techniques. The supine lateral midpatellar approach had a higher success rate of 93% in the same study and may be a more reliable access to the knee joint in larger patients.
- For the supine medial or lateral midpatellar approach, position the patient's knee either in full extension, which gives the most patellar mobility, or slightly flexed at 5 degrees with a rolled towel supporting underneath. The needle is advanced parallel to the floor directed straight toward the patellar midpole.

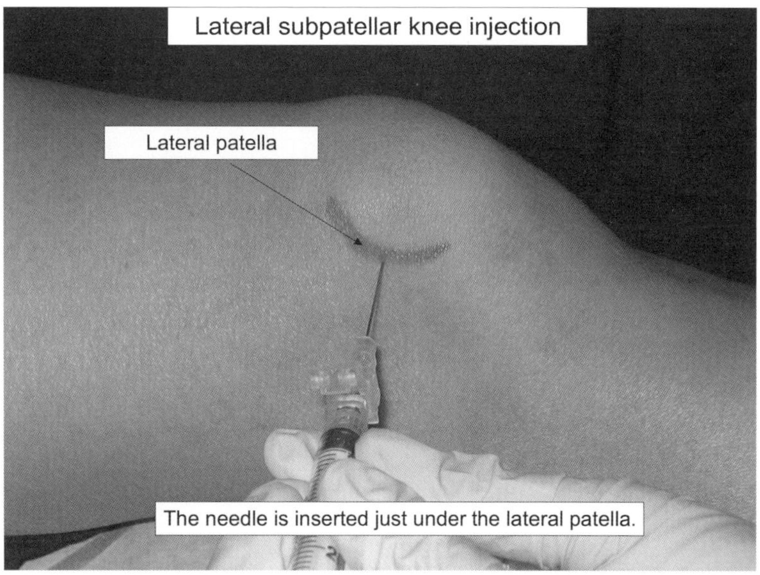

The needle is inserted just under the lateral patella.

- For the superior approach, draw lines from the superior and lateral borders of the patella—at the intersection of these lines, insert the needle at a 45-degree angle directed toward the middle of the patella.

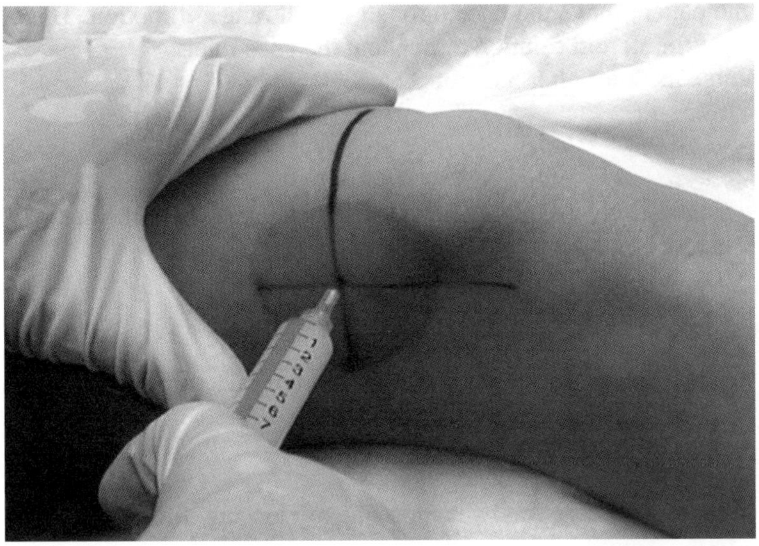

- After selecting an injection approach, mark the entry point with a pen or needle cap.
- Cleanse the skin with alcohol swab and then Betadine × 3 or chlorhexidine × 45 sec.
- Apply ethyl chloride for topical cooling.
- If draining an effusion, be careful not to move the needle during negative pressure aspiration.
- Keep the needle hub and syringe tip sterile during syringe transfers.
- Gentle pressure on the suprapatellar bursa may facilitate more complete drainage of the effusion.
- After aspiration, remove the aspiration syringe and connect the therapeutic syringe securely.
- Inject the therapeutic medication into the joint—there should be minimal resistance to flow.
- Remove needle and apply pressure with gauze.
- Apply Band-Aid.

AFTERCARE

- Lidocaine lasts 4 to 6 hr; bupivacaine can last up to 12 hr—avoid heavy exercise while the IA anesthetics are in effect because the decreased proprioceptive feedback may increase risk of falls.
- Patients may have mild discomfort at the injection site and can use ice or NSAIDs to mitigate pain until the injection takes effect.
- Inform your patient that steroids may take 2 to 3 days, and HA may take up to several weeks to take effect.
- After 3 to 5 days, the patient can resume his or her regular activity and advance as tolerated.
- Instruct patient to return to your office if they develop redness, swelling, or increased pain at the injection site.
- Recommend continued isometric quadriceps strengthening, low-impact exercise, and weight loss.
- Repeat injection can be done after 3 mo if the steroid injection afforded adequate pain relief—average duration of effect for joint steroid injections is 4 wk.

CPT CODE

- 20610 Arthrocentesis, aspiration and/or injection; major joint or bursa (e.g., shoulder, hip, knee, subacromial bursa); without ultrasound guidance
- 20611 Arthrocentesis, aspiration and/or injection; major joint or bursa (e.g., shoulder, hip, knee, subacromial bursa); with ultrasound guidance, with permanent recording and reporting

ANKLE JOINT INJECTION

INDICATIONS

- Ankle aspiration is useful for the diagnosis of ankle effusions (i.e., to diagnose crystalline disease or rule out infection).
- Corticosteroid injection to the ankle is indicated for the treatment of ankle arthritis, crystalline disease, or synovitis in rheumatoid arthritis.
- Injections are indicated once conservative therapy (activity modification, NSAIDs, physical therapy) has failed.
- ICD10:
  - M19.071 Primary osteoarthritis, right ankle and foot
  - M19.072 Primary osteoarthritis, left ankle and foot
  - M19.079 Primary osteoarthritis, unspecified ankle and foot
  - M19.279 Secondary osteoarthritis, unspecified ankle and foot

ANATOMY

- The ankle joint consists of the articulation of the tibiotalar and talofibular joints.
- The ankle joint space can be approached either medially or laterally.

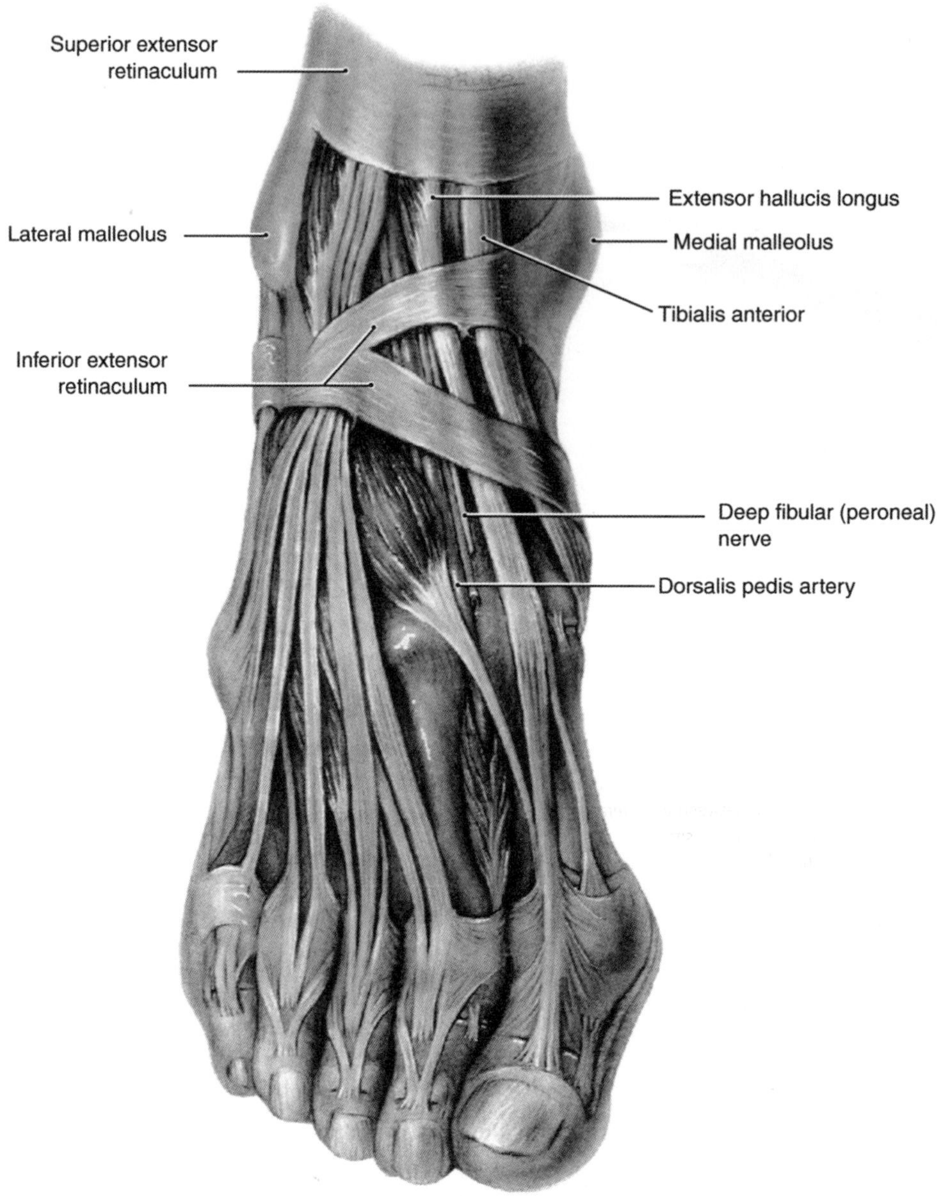

SUPPLIES

- Gloves
- Alcohol swabs
- Betadine or chlorhexidine swabs
- 18-gauge needle for drawing up medications or Medic anti-stick needle
- 3-mL syringe with 25-gauge 1-inch needle for injection
- Extra 3- to 5-mL syringes if needed for aspiration of effusion
- ½ to 1 mL 1% lidocaine without epinephrine (if using)
- ½ mL 40 mg/mL (20 mg) triamcinolone suspension (Kenalog) or equivalent
- Ethyl chloride
- Gauze
- Band-Aid

TECHNIQUE

- The patient can be in a sitting or supine position.
- Medial approach: Identify the soft spot between the anterior tip of the medial malleolus and the medial edge of the tibialis anterior tendon:
  - Palpate down to feel the tibiotalar joint line—mark this site with the needle cap.
  - Cleanse the skin with alcohol swab and then Betadine × 3 or chlorhexidine × 45 sec.
  - Apply ethyl chloride for topical cooling.

– Advance the needle in a posterolateral direction and inject.
– Having an assistant apply mild eversion/plantarflexion pressure may help to open the joint.
– Remove needle and apply pressure with gauze.
– Apply Band-Aid.

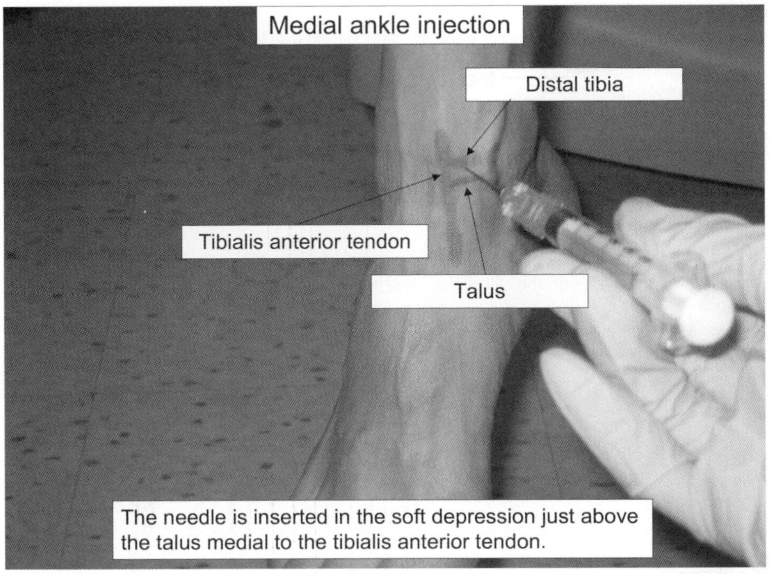

- Lateral approach: Identify the triangular depression between the lateral tibia, fibula, and the talus:
  – Palpate down to feel the tibiotalar joint line—mark this site with the needle cap.
  – Cleanse the skin with alcohol swab and then Betadine × 3 or chlorhexidine × 45 sec.
  – Apply ethyl chloride for topical cooling.
  – Advance the needle in a posteromedial direction.
  – If aspirating, remove as much fluid as possible and then stabilize the needle in the joint with a hemostat and switch between the aspiration and therapeutic syringes. Keep the needle hub and syringe tips sterile.
  – After securing the therapeutic syringe, inject the steroid/lidocaine mixture.
  – Remove needle and apply pressure with gauze.
  – Apply Band-Aid.

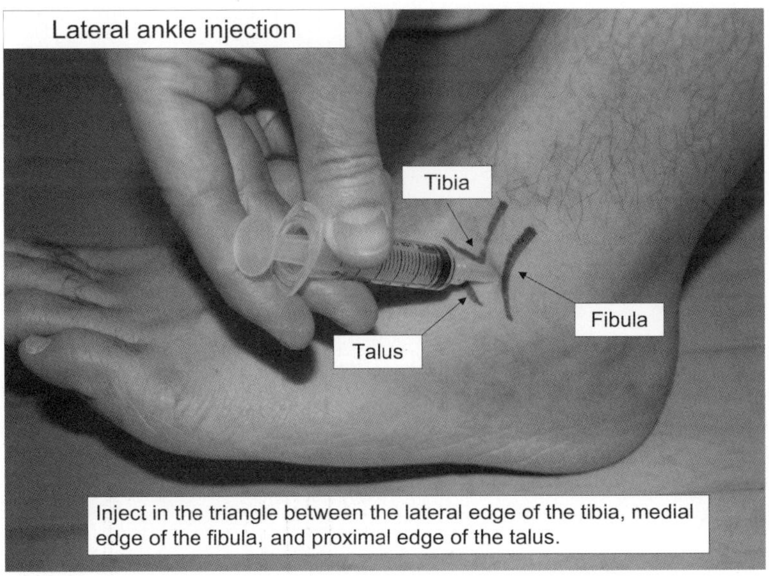

AFTERCARE

- Lidocaine lasts 4 to 6 hr; bupivacaine can last up to 12 hr—avoid heavy exercise while the IA anesthetics are in effect because the decreased proprioceptive feedback may increase risk of falls.
- Patients may have mild discomfort at the injection site and can use ice or NSAIDs to mitigate pain until the injection takes effect.
- Inform your patient that steroids may take 3 days to take effect.
- If pain is improved, start ankle rehabilitation with ROM exercises, strengthening band flexion/extension exercises.
- Instruct patient to return to your office if they develop redness, swelling, or increased pain at the injection site.
- Repeat injection can be done after 3 mo if the steroid injection afforded adequate pain relief—average duration of effect for joint steroid injections is 4 wk.

CPT CODE

- 20605 Arthrocentesis, aspiration and/or injection; intermediate joint or bursa (e.g., temporomandibular, acromioclavicular, wrist, elbow or ankle, olecranon bursa); without ultrasound guidance
- 20606 Arthrocentesis, aspiration and/or injection; intermediate joint or bursa (e.g., temporomandibular, acromioclavicular, wrist, elbow or ankle, olecranon bursa); with ultrasound guidance, with permanent recording and reporting

PLANTAR FASCIA INJECTION

INDICATIONS

- Excessive stretching and repetitive trauma can lead to microtears of the plantar fascia from its insertion on the calcaneus. These microtears can lead to chronic inflammation and pain at the calcaneal insertion or along the entire plantar fascia.
- Conservative treatment includes stretching, arch-supporting orthotics, heel pads, NSAIDs, and nighttime plantar fascia splints. Patients can roll pressure along their arch/heel with a tennis ball or frozen water bottle.
- Corticosteroid injection is a second-line therapy after the failure of conservative therapy, given the higher risk of complications, including fat pad atrophy and rupture of the plantar fascia.
- ICD10:
  - M72.2 Plantar fascial fibromatosis

ANATOMY

- The plantar fascia supports the medial longitudinal arch of the foot and stretches between the base of the phalanges and the medial tuberosity of the calcaneus.
- The plantar fascia lies deep to the fat layer of the heel.
- On physical exam, the plantar fascia insertion point on the calcaneus is usually markedly tender to palpation.

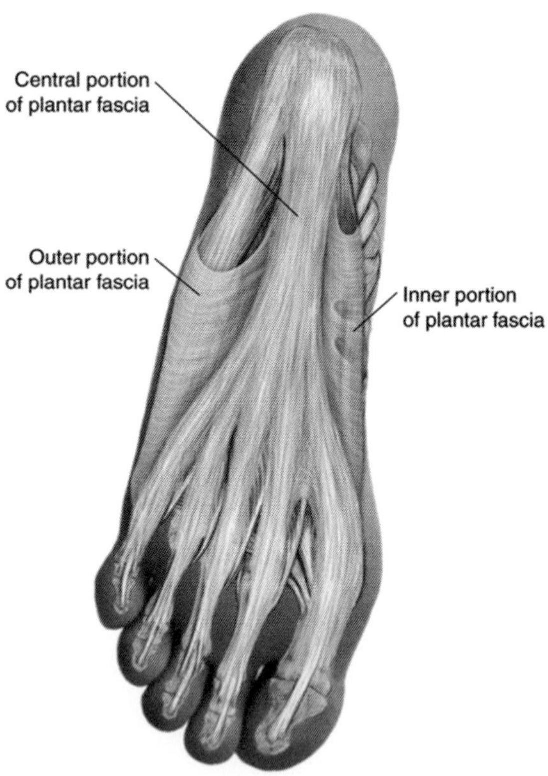

SUPPLIES

- Gloves
- Alcohol swabs
- Betadine or chlorhexidine swabs
- 18-gauge needle for drawing up medications or Medic anti-stick needle
- 3-mL syringe with 25-gauge 1.5-inch needle for injection

- ½ mL 1% lidocaine without epinephrine (if using)
- ½ mL 40 mg/mL (20 mg) triamcinolone suspension (Kenalog) or equivalent
- Ethyl chloride
- Gauze
- Band-Aid

TECHNIQUE

- Position the patient in the lateral recumbent position with the painful side down.
- Position the affected foot medial side up.
- Palpate the maximal point of tenderness at the plantar fascia insertion on the calcaneus, usually in the middle of the heel—this gives the injection target depth along the width of the heel.
- Find the medial edge of the calcaneus and mark with needle cap—this marks the injection point along the length of the foot.
- Cleanse the skin with alcohol swab and then Betadine × 3 or chlorhexidine × 45 sec.
- Apply ethyl chloride for topical cooling.
- Inject perpendicular to the medial foot, aiming just distal to the calcaneal edge in order to avoid the heel fat pad.
- If the calcaneus is reached with the needle tip, walk the needle off the bony edge and then down to the depth of the point of maximal tenderness.
- Inject the steroid/lidocaine mixture.
- Remove needle and apply pressure with gauze.
- Apply Band-Aid.

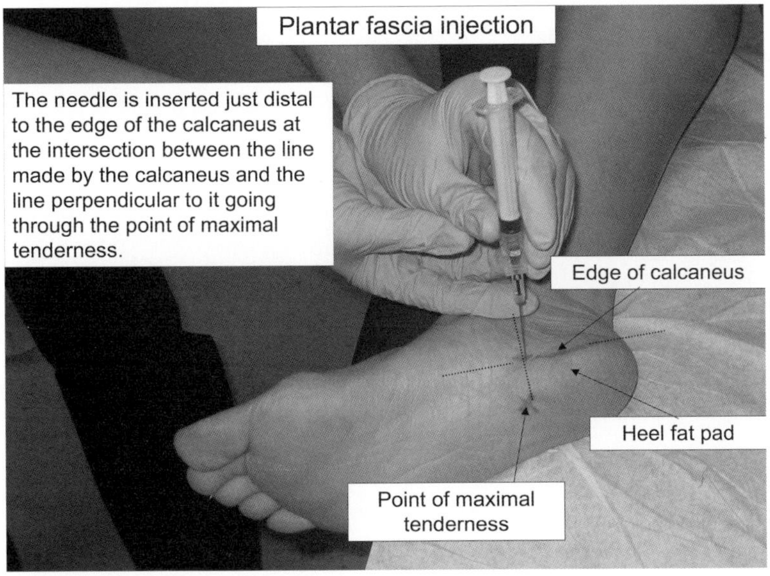

AFTERCARE

- Apply pressure dressing.
- Rest 3 days.
- Continue the RICE conservative therapy and consistent plantar fascia stretching.
- Instruct patient to return to your office if they develop redness, swelling, or increased pain at the injection site.

CPT CODE

- 20550 Injection(s); single tendon sheath, or ligament, aponeurosis (e.g., plantar "fascia")

MORTON NEUROMA INJECTION

INDICATIONS

- Morton neuroma results from irritation of the interdigital nerve in the foot from repetitive compressive trauma, such as compression from tight or high-heeled shoes.
- Injections are indicated once conservative therapies (shoes with a wider metatarsal box, metatarsal pads, orthotic arch supports, NSAIDs) have failed.
- ICD10:
  - G57.6 Lesion of plantar nerve: Morton's metatarsalgia

ANATOMY

- Morton neuroma usually develops between the 2nd and 3rd or between the 3rd and 4th metatarsal heads.
- Tenderness to palpation between the metatarsal heads usually confirms the diagnosis.

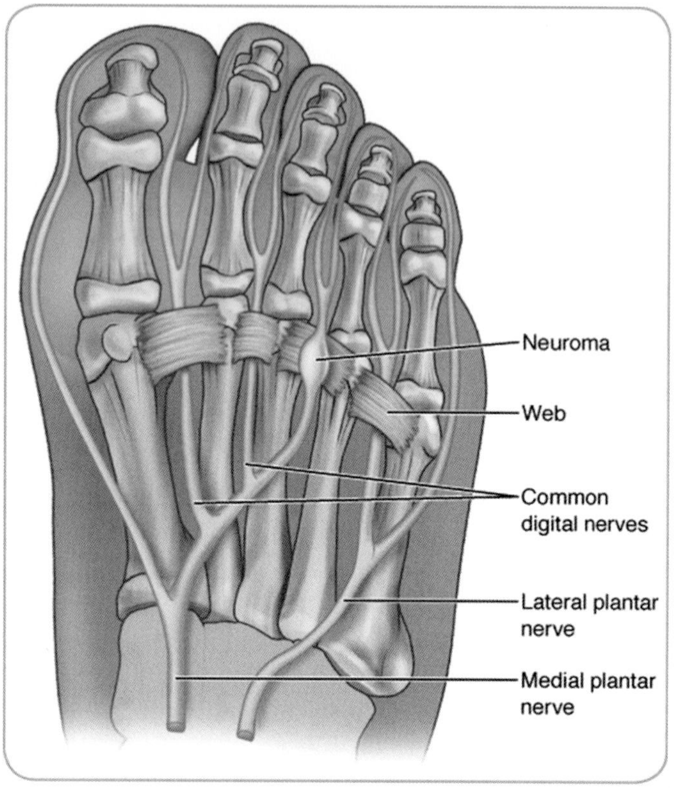

SUPPLIES
- Gloves
- Alcohol swabs
- Betadine or chlorhexidine swabs
- 18-gauge needle for drawing up medications or Medic anti-stick needle
- 3-mL syringe with 25-gauge 1-inch needle for injection
- ½ mL 1% lidocaine without epinephrine (if using)
- ½ mL 40 mg/mL (20 mg) triamcinolone suspension (Kenalog) or equivalent
- Ethyl chloride
- Gauze
- Band-Aid

TECHNIQUE
- Lay the patient in a supine position with a bent knee and the foot flat on the table.
- Identify the point of maximal tenderness between the metatarsal heads on the dorsal foot—mark entry site with needle cap.
- Cleanse the skin with alcohol swab and then Betadine × 3 or chlorhexidine × 45 sec.
- Apply ethyl chloride for topical cooling.
- Advance the needle at a 45-degree angle proximally toward the point of maximal tenderness or nodule—aim toward the heel and stop at the level of the interdigital fullness.
- Do not inject at the level of the plantar fat pad to avoid fat pad atrophy.
- Remove needle and apply pressure with gauze.
- Apply Band-Aid.

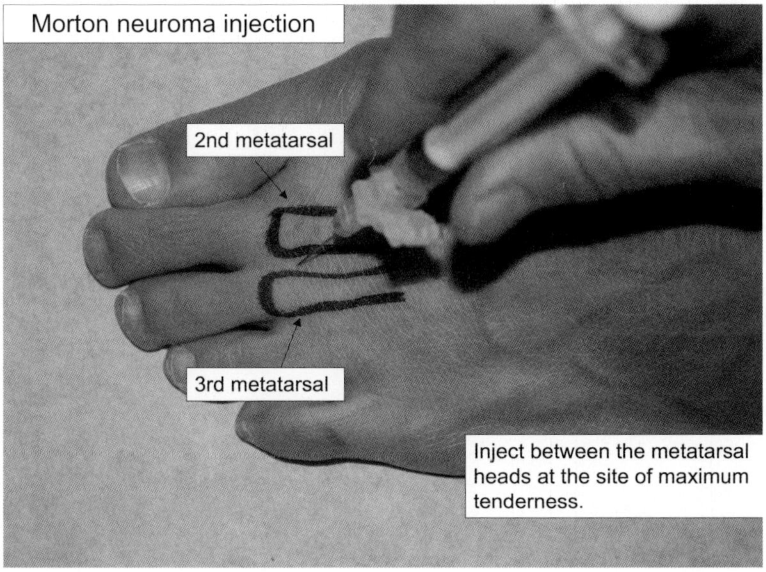

AFTERCARE

- Lidocaine lasts 4 to 6 hr; bupivacaine [Marcaine] can last up to 12 hr.
- However, steroid effect may take 2 to 3 days to decrease inflammation.
- Advise continued proper footwear, metatarsal pads, and orthotics. Gel toe spacers may relieve nerve pressure.
- Instruct patient to return to your office if they develop redness, swelling, or increased pain at the injection site.
- Repeat injection can be done after 3 mo if the steroid injection afforded adequate pain relief—average duration of effect for joint steroid injections is 4 wk.

CPT CODE

- 64450 Injection, nerve block, therapeutic, other peripheral nerve or branch

1ST METATARSOPHALANGEAL INJECTION

INDICATIONS

- Aspiration of the 1st metatarsal phalangeal joint is useful in the diagnosis of gout and pseudogout.
- Therapeutic steroid injection can be a useful adjunct therapy for 1st metatarsophalangeal (MTP) osteoarthritis, rheumatoid arthritis, or crystal arthropathies.
- ICD10:
  - M79.673 Pain in unspecified foot
  - S93.523 Sprain of metatarsophalangeal joint of unspecified great toe
  - M19.079 Primary osteoarthritis, unspecified ankle and foot
  - M19.179 Post-traumatic osteoarthritis, unspecified ankle and foot
  - M10.00 Gout

ANATOMY

- The MTP joint line is palpable on the dorsal surface of the foot.

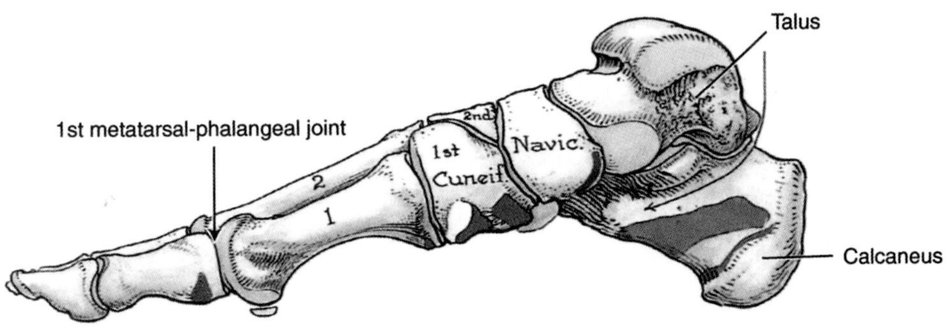

SUPPLIES

- Gloves
- Betadine/chlorhexidine and alcohol swabs
- 3-mL syringe with 25-gauge 5/8- to 1-inch needle
- 1 mL 1% lidocaine without epinephrine
- ½ mL (20 mg) Kenalog or equivalent
- Ethyl chloride
- Gauze
- Band-Aid

TECHNIQUE

- Lay the patient in a supine position with a bent knee and the foot flat on the table.
- Flex and extend the 1st MTP joint to identify the joint line and mark with needle cap.
- Cleanse the skin with alcohol swab and then Betadine × 3 or chlorhexidine × 45 sec.
- Apply ethyl chloride for superficial numbing.
- Distal traction may help open the joint space.
- Aim the needle distally toward the toe and enter at a 60-degree angle to match the joint slope.
- The joint lies fairly superficially, and the injection solution should flow freely within the joint.
- Remove needle and apply pressure with gauze.
- Apply Band-Aid.

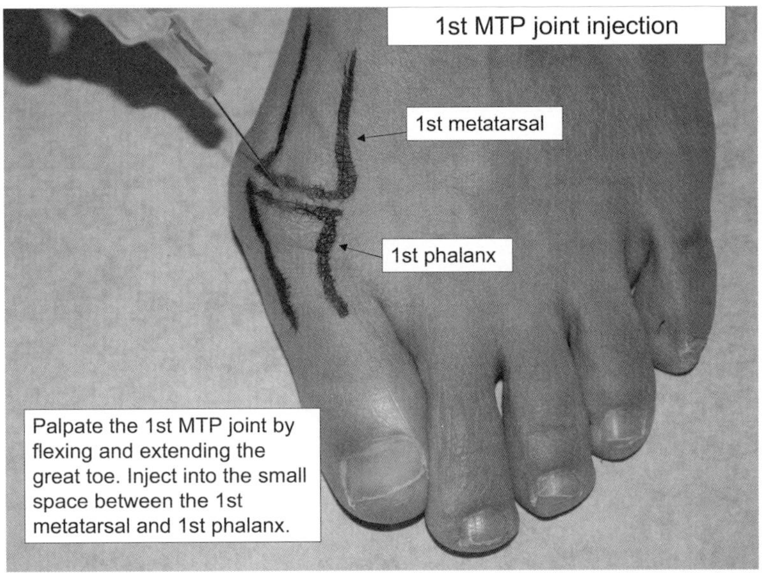

AFTERCARE

- Instruct patient that the toe may be numb for several hours after the procedure and that pain may be present for several days.
- Instruct patient that the cortisone usually takes effect within 72 hr.
- Advise continued proper footwear and arch supports for proper walking mechanics.
- Instruct patient to return to your office if they develop redness, swelling, or increased pain at the injection site.
- If helpful, repeat injection can be done after 3 mo—average duration of effect for steroid injections is 4 wk.

CPT CODE

- 20600 Arthrocentesis, aspiration and/or injection; small joint or bursa (e.g., fingers, toes); without ultrasound guidance
- 20604 Arthrocentesis, aspiration and/or injection; small joint or bursa (e.g., fingers, toes); with ultrasound guidance, with permanent recording and reporting

INDEX

E

F

M

Q

R

S

T

U

V

W

Y

Z